GUIDE TO
CLINICAL
NEUROLOGY

GUIDE TO CLINICAL NEUROLOGY

Edited by

J. P. MOHR, M.S., M.D.

Sciarra Professor of Clinical Neurology
Department of Neurology
College of Physicians and Surgeons of Columbia University
Attending Neurologist
Neurological Institute
Columbia-Presbyterian Medical Center
New York, New York

J. C. GAUTIER, M.D.

Membre de l'Académie Nationale de Médecine
Professor of Neurology and Consultant Physician
Hôpital de la Salpêtrière
Paris

With illustrations by R. J. Demarest

Churchill Livingstone
New York, Edinburgh, London, Melbourne, Tokyo

Library of Congress Cataloging-in-Publication Data

Guide to clinical neurology / edited by J.P. Mohr, J.C. Gautier ; with
   illustrations by R. Demarest.
      p. cm.
   Includes bibliographical references and index.
   ISBN 0-443-08927-2
   1. Neurology. I. Mohr, J. P. II. Gautier, J. C.
   [DNLM: 1. Nervous System Diseases. WL 140 G946 1995]
RC346.G85 1995
616.8—dc20
DNLM/DLC
for Library of Congress   95-8195
                                             CIP

Distributed in the United Kingdom by Churchill Livingstone, Robert Stevenson House, 1–3 Baxter's
Place, Leith Walk, Edinburgh EH1 3AF, and by associated companies, branches, and representatives
throughout the world.

Accurate indications, adverse reactions, and dosage schedules for drugs are provided in this book,
but it is possible that they may change. The reader is urged to review the package
information data of the manufacturers of the medications mentioned.

The Publishers have made every effort to trace the copyright holders for borrowed material.
If they have inadvertently overlooked any, they will be pleased to make the necessary
arrangements at the first opportunity.

Acquisitions Editor: *Kerry Willis*
Assistant Editor: *Ann Ruzycka*
Production Editor: *David Terry*
Production Supervisor: *Sharon Tuder*
Cover Design: *Paul Moran*

Printed in the United States of America

First published in 1995   7 6 5 4 3 2 1

To our wives,
Joan S. Mohr and Madeleine Gautier,
who have valiantly shared the peaks and troughs of the effort

Contributors

Allen J. Aksamit, Jr., M.D.

Associate Professor, Department of Neurology, Mayo Medical School; Consultant, Department of Neurology, Mayo Clinic, Rochester, Minnesota

M. Zuheir Al-Kawi, M.D.

Associate Professor, Department of Medicine, King Faisal University, Alkhobar, Saudi Arabia; Head, Section of Neurology, and Chairman, Department of Medicine, King Faisal Specialist Hospital and Research Centre, Riyadh, Saudi Arabia

O. Appenzeller, M.D.

Professor Emeritus, Departments of Neurology and Medicine; President, New Mexico Health Enhancement and Marathon Clinics Research Foundation, Albuquerque, New Mexico

David R. Borchelt, M.D.

Instructor, Department of Pathology, Johns Hopkins University School of Medicine, Baltimore, Maryland

John C. M. Brust, M.D.

Professor of Clinical Neurology, Department of Neurology, College of Physicians and Surgeons of Columbia University; Director, Department of Neurology, Harlem Hospital Center, New York, New York

Didier Cros, M.D.

Director, Electromyography Unit, Clinical Neurophysiology Laboratory, Department of Neurology, Massachusetts General Hospital, Boston, Massachusetts

Larry E. Davis, M.D., F.A.C.P.

Professor, Departments of Neurology and Microbiology, University of New Mexico School of Medicine; Chief, Neurology Service, Albuquerque Veterans Affairs Medical Center, Albuquerque, New Mexico

Stephen M. Davis, M.D., F.R.A.C.P.

Associate Professor, Department of Medicine, University of Melbourne Faculty of Medicine, Melbourne, Victoria, Australia; Director, Department of Neurology, Royal Melbourne Hospital, Parkville, Victoria, Australia

Lisa M. DeAngelis, M.D.

Associate Professor, Department of Neurology, Cornell University Medical College; Chief, Neurology Service, Department of Neurology, Memorial Sloan-Kettering Cancer Center, New York, New York

Salvatore DiMauro, M.D.

Lucy G. Moses Professor, Department of Neurology, College of Physicians and Surgeons of Columbia University, New York, New York

B. Eymard, M.D.

Consultant, Department of Neurology, Hôpital de la Salpêtriére, Paris, France

R. S. J. Frackowiak, M.D., F.R.C.P.

Professor, Wellcome Department of Cognitive Neurology, Institute of Neurology, London, England

J. C. Gautier, M.D.

Professor, Department of Neurology, and Consultant Physician, Hôpital de la Salpêtriére, Paris, France

Steven Gulevich, M.D.

Associate Medical Director, Center for Occupational Neurology and Neurotoxicology, Colorado Neurological Institute, Englewood, Colorado

John J. Halperin, M.D.

Professor, Department of Neurology, Cornell University Medical College, New York, New York; Chairman, Department of Neurology, North Shore University Hospital, Manhasset, New York

Stephen L. Hauser, M.D.

Betty Anker File Professor and Chair, Department of Neurology, University of California, San Francisco, School of Medicine, San Francisco, California

J. J. Hauw, M.D.

Professor, Department of Pathology, Paris University Faculty of Medicine; Head, Department of Neuropathology, Hôpital de la Salpêtriére, Paris, France

M. G. Hennerici, M.D.

Professor and Chairman, Department of Neurology, University of Heidelberg Faculty of Medicine, Klinikum Mannheim, Germany

J. A. Hicks, B.Sc.(Hon), M.B.Ch.B., Dip.Obs., M.R.C.G.P.

Research Fellow, Department of Psychiatry, University of Toronto Faculty of Medicine, Toronto, Ontario, Canada

Michael Hoffmann, M.D., F.C.P.(SA)

Consultant in Neurology, Departments of Medicine and Vascular Surgery, University of Natal Faculty of Medicine, Natal, South Africa; Director, Stroke Unit, Entabeni Hospital, Durban, South Africa

Jeffery D. Kocsis, M.D.

Professor, Departments of Neurology and Neurobiology, Yale University School of Medicine, New Haven, Connecticut; Associate Director, PVA/EPVA Neuroscience Research Center, Veterans Administration Hospital, West Haven, Connecticut

Vassilis E. Koliatsos, M.D.

Assistant Professor, Departments of Pathology, Neurology, and Neuroscience, Johns Hopkins University School of Medicine, Baltimore, Maryland

Dale J. Lange, M.D.

Associate Professor, Department of Neurology, College of Physicians and Surgeons of Columbia University; Director, Neuromuscular Laboratory, Neurological Institute; Director, Eleanor and Lou Gehrig MDA/ALS Center, Columbia-Presbyterian Medical Center; Associate Attending Neurologist, Department of Neurology, Presbyterian Hospital, New York, New York

H. Lassman, M.D.

Professor, Research Unit for Experimental Neuropathology, Austrian Academy of the Sciences, and Professor of Neuropathology, Institute of Neurology, Vienna, Austria

A. Lieberman, M.D.

Chief, Section of Movement Disorders, Barrows Neurological Institute, Phoenix, Arizona

P. Loiseau, M.D.

Consultant Professor, Department of Neurology, Bordeaux University Faculty of Medicine, Bordeaux, France

Lee J. Martin, M.D.

Assistant Professor, Department of Pathology, Johns Hopkins University School of Medicine, Baltimore, Maryland

Ayrton S. Massaro, M.D.

Attending Neurologist, Escola Paulista de Medicina-Universidade Federal de São Paulo, São Paulo, Brazil

F. Mauguière, M.D., Ph.D.

Professor, Department of Neurology, Claude Bernard University Faculty of Medicine; Head, Department of Functional Neurology and Epileptology, Neurological Hospital, Lyon, France

J. P. Mohr, M.S., M.D.

Sciarra Professor of Clinical Neurology, Department of Neurology, College of Physicians and Surgeons of Columbia University; Attending Neurologist, Neurological Institute, Columbia-Presbyterian Medical Center, New York, New York

E. Oribe, M.D., F.A.C.P.

Clinical Assistant Professor, Department of Neurology, Cornell University Medical College, New York, New York; Chief, Division of Neurology, Department of Medicine, Catholic Medical Center of Brooklyn and Queens, Jamaica, New York

Donald L. Price, M.D.

Professor, Departments of Pathology, Neurology, and Neuroscience, Johns Hopkins University School of Medicine; Director, Division of Neuropathology, Johns Hopkins Hospital, Baltimore, Maryland

W. Rautenberg, M.D.

Associate Professor, Department of Neurology, University of Heidelberg Faculty of Medicine, Klinikum Mannheim, Germany

Edward P. Richardson, Jr., M.D.

Bullard Professor of Neuropathology Emeritus, Harvard Medical School; Neuropathologist, Charles S. Kubik Laboratory for Neuropathology, Department of Pathology, and Senior Neurologist, Neurology Service, Massachusetts General Hospital, Boston, Massachusetts

Gustavo C. Román, M.D.

Clinical Professor, Department of Neurology, University of Texas Medical School at San Antonio, San Antonio, Texas; Clinical Professor, Department of Neurology, Georgetown University School of Medicine, Washington, D.C.; Formerly Chief, Neuroepidemiology Branch, National Institute of Neurological Diseases and Stroke, National Institutes of Health, Bethesda, Maryland

Neil L. Rosenberg, M.D.

Associate Clinical Professor, Division of Clinical Pharmacology and Toxicology, Department of Medicine, University of Colorado School of Medicine; Medical Director, Center for Occupational Neurology and Neurotoxicology, Colorado Neurological Institute, Denver, Colorado

Lewis P. Rowland, M.D.

Henry and Lucy Moses Professor and Chairman, Department of Neurology, College of Physicians and Surgeons of Columbia University; Director, Neurology Service, Neurological Institute, Columbia-Presbyterian Medical Center, New York, New York

C. M. Shapiro, D.Sc.(Hon), M.B.B.C.A.B., Ph.D., M.R.C.(Psych), F.R.C.P.(C)

Professor, Department of Psychiatry, and Director, Neuropsychiatry Program, University of Toronto Faculty of Medicine, Toronto, Ontario, Canada

Sangram S. Sisodia, M.D.

Assistant Professor, Department of Pathology, Johns Hopkins University School of Medicine, Baltimore, Maryland

Ruth D. Snow, M.D.

Assistant Professor, Department of Radiology, University of South Alabama College of Medicine; Director, Division of Magnetic Resonance Imaging, Department of Radiology, University of South Alabama Medical Center, Mobile, Alabama

A. Spina-Franca, M.D.

Professor Emeritus, Department of Neurology, São Paulo University Medical School; Researcher, Department of Neurology, Hospital das Clinicas, Centro de Investigacoes em Neurologia, São Paulo, Brazil

P. H. St. George-Hyslop, M.D.

Assistant Professor, Division of Neurology, Department of Medicine, Centre for Research in Neurodegenerative Diseases, University of Toronto Faculty of Medicine; Consultant, Department of Medicine, The Toronto Hospital, Toronto, Ontario, Canada

W. Steinke, M.D.

Associate Professor, Department of Neurology, University of Heidelberg Faculty of Medicine, Klinikum Mannheim, Germany

Antonio Uccelli, M.D.

Professor, Department of Neurology, University of Genoa School of Medicine, Genoa, Italy

K. Vass, M.D.

Associate Professor of Neurology, Institute of Neurology, Austrian Academy of the Sciences, Vienna, Austria

Stephen G. Waxman, M.D.

Professor and Chairman, Department of Neurology, Yale University School of Medicine; Neurologist-in-Chief, Yale-New Haven Hospital, New Haven, Connecticut; Director, PVA/EPVA Neuroscience Research Center, Veterans Administration Hospital, West Haven, Connecticut

J. P. Williams, M.D.

Professor, Department of Radiology, University of South Alabama College of Medicine; Director, Division of Neuroradiology, University of South Alabama Medical Center, Mobile, Alabama

Preface

Some thirty years ago, at about 6:30 A.M. on the neurology wards of the Massachusetts General Hospital in Boston, two young neurologists, one American, the other French, found that they shared many interests in clinical neurology. This stemmed in part from a common admiration for the senior neurologists at the institution, leading among them C. Miller Fisher, Raymond D. Adams, and E. Pierson Richardson, Jr. In addition, the American party was keenly interested in the French way of life (including neurology), and the French party had a particular interest in the American-English language and the American way of thinking (including neurology).

During the following years, agreeing or disagreeing on neurologic issues, they met several times a year, either in the United States or in France, in town or in the country, the latter being, in their opinion, where neurologists' minds are best able to think about the art of the neurologic clinical examination.

After exchanging experiences and views over a period of threescore years, one night during dinner they and their spouses felt that it could be useful to put on paper some salient output of this informal and unusual partnership.

Here is the *Guide to Clinical Neurology*, the product of this collaboration, bearing a title that as best as possible reflects the American-French bridge represented in this book. It is intended for those just beginning, as well as those already experienced, in the subject of neurology. And, as most seasoned neurologists enjoy reading good writing on clinical neurology, we hope that some colleagues will take pleasure in some of the chapters.

While attempting to take into account the most modern investigations into neurologic diseases, we have striven never to forget that such facilities are not yet available in many parts of the world. Therefore, the prime value of clinical data has been stressed and some techniques described that, although in more fortunate places are no longer performed, still must be resorted to elsewhere.

A good illustration tells more than a long paragraph. We have been fortunate to have the eminent Robert J. Demarest as our illustrator. Those few readers newly exposed to his work will, no doubt, be convinced of his unsurpassed talents.

Along the way, the snags, difficulties, and doubts experienced during the writing have been greatly eased by our many collaborators, who enthusiastically subscribed to the idea of a new book on clinical neurology. Many thanks are due to our coauthors and also to the young clinicians and researchers who generously devoted much time in reviewing and criticizing early manuscripts: Drs. J. J. Aron, C. Duyckaerts, A. Dürr, N. Isenberg, J. J. Hauw, S. H. Lee, G. Lascault, R. M. Lazar, J. M. Léger, R. S. Marshall, H. Mast, R. B. Libman, J. Philippon, C. Pierrot-Deseilligny, N. V. Ramani, and R. L. Sacco.

We also wish to thank those colleagues who have let us reproduce materials from their archives, among them many of the unacknowledged computed tomography and magnetic resonance scans from Dr. A. Khandji, and fundus photographs from Drs. D. Aron-Rosa, M. Behrens, and P. Le Hoang.

Having bet on us, Churchill Livingstone has given constant and full support. Special thanks are due to William Schmitt and Robert Hurley, who undertook the original acquisition; Kerry Willis, Senior Editor; Ann Ruzycka, Assistant Editor, David Terry, Senior Production Editor, and Charlie Lebeda, Design Manager. Each of them tried unfailingly to accommodate the sometimes divergent needs of the contributors and editors during manuscript and figure preparation and during the production process. We wish to express our gratitude for their forbearance, kindness, and close collaboration.

J. P. Mohr, M.D., J. C. Gautier, M.D.

Contents

Color plates follow page 176.

Section I
Basic Pathophysiology

1

Neuronal Death: Studies of Amyotrophic Lateral Sclerosis, Alzheimer's Disease, and Their Animal Models

Donald L. Price, Sangram S. Sisodia,
Vassilis E. Koliatsos, David R. Borchelt,
and Lee J. Martin

The death of neurons can result from a variety of processes (e.g., anoxia, ischemia, trauma, and toxins, to name the more obvious). Currently, however, the term *neuronal death* is reserved for the poorly understood decline in the number of neurons in the so-called "degenerative diseases," an appellation that reflects our ignorance of the basic processes at work.

Two of the major neurologic diseases that typify degenerative disease, amyotrophic lateral sclerosis (ALS) (see Ch. 63) and Alzheimer's disease (see Ch. 60), have provided the impetus for detailed study and recent, rapid advances in the understanding of the biologic processes that may account for them. These fields of achievement warrant description in a book of this kind and serve as a point of departure for what follows in the text. The hopes these advances carry show that neurology, far from the contemplative field it is considered to be by some is a paradigm of the most active research and progress.

Many human neurologic disorders, including ALS and Alzheimer's disease, are characterized by selective degeneration of different subsets of neurons, resulting in distinct clinical syndromes. In this review, we discuss some of the key issues in investigations of neuronal disorders, and we use ALS and Alzheimer's disease to illustrate important principles.

Beginning in middle or late life, ALS or motor neuron disease usually manifests as muscle weakness and atrophy frequently accompanied by spasticity and hyperreflexia. Electrodiagnostic studies disclose fibrillations, fasciculations, and giant polyphasic potentials; muscle biopsies demonstrate denervation atrophy (see Ch. 63). Alzheimer's disease, the most common cause of dementia in late life, manifests as a gradual loss of memory, followed by progressive deterioration of thought, judgment, language skills, praxis, visual-spatial perceptions, mood, behavior, and the ability to manage personal affairs (see Ch. 60). Both disorders are usually inexorably progressive; patients become increasingly incapacitated and die of aspiration pneumonia, pulmonary emboli, or other intercurrent medical illnesses.

ALS and Alzheimer's disease share many features (Table 1-1). In both diseases, age is a major risk factor. Moreover, specific genes influence the expression of these diseases. For example, approximately 10 percent of cases of both Alzheimer's disease and ALS are familial. In early-onset familial cases, mutations have been identified in genes located on chromosome 21 (i.e., superoxide dismutase 1 [SOD1] in ALS and the amyloid precursor protein [APP] in Alzheimer's disease). ALS and Alzheimer's disease selectively affect subsets of nerve cells, and vulnerable neurons develop cytoskeletal pathologic features and eventually die. Autopsies of individuals with neurodegenerative disease almost invariably show end-stage disease, making it difficult to reconstruct the evolution and mechanisms of cellular degeneration.

Table 1-1. Comparison of Motor Neuron Disease and Alzheimer's Disease

	Motor Neuron Disease	Alzheimer's Disease
Familial	~10%	~10%
Sporadic	Majority	Majority
Putative onset	FALS, midlife Sporadic, late life	FAD, midlife Sporadic, late life
Duration	3–5 years	8–12 years
Signs	Paralysis, spasticity	Dementia
Chromosomal loci	21 (FALS) 5 (spinal muscular atrophy 1–3) X (Kennedy's disease)	21 + 14 (early-onset FAD) 19 (late-onset FAD and sporadic AD)
Gene (chromosome)	SOD1 (21) in some FALS families	APP (21) in some FAD families apoE (late-onset FAD and sporadic AD)
Vulnerable cells	Upper and lower motor neurons	Brainstem monoaminergic neurons Basal forebrain cholinergic neurons Nerve cells in amygdala, hippocampus, and neocortex
Cytoskeletal pathologic finding	Neurofilamentous axonal swellings	Neurofibrillary tangles Neurites Neuropil threads
Amyloid	—	$A\beta$ deposits (parenchyma/vessels)
Death of neurons	Severe	Severe
Animal models	Axotomy-induced retrograde degeneration Certain toxic axonopathies HCSMA Spontaneously occurring murine models Neurofilament gene transgenic mice SOD1 mutation transgenic mice	Aged nonhuman primates, bears, dogs APP transgenic mice In vivo injection of $A\beta$

Abbreviations: $A\beta$, β-amyloid protein; AD, Alzheimer's disease; apoE, apolipoprotein E; APP, amyloid precursor protein; FAD, familial Alzheimer's disease; FALS, familial amyotrophic lateral sclerosis; HCSMA, hereditary canine spinal muscular atrophy; SOD1, superoxide dismutase 1.

Therefore, the mechanisms of selective vulnerability, cytoskeletal dysfunction, and cell death that involve at-risk populations of neurons are not yet well understood. The character, dynamics, and evolution of the cellular pathology and the mechanisms of this cell dysfunction/death are difficult to study in humans. Investigators have thus turned increasingly to studies of animal models that recapitulate some of the features of the human disease. Animal models can be particularly useful for defining the causes of disease, characterizing the evolution of the pathologic findings, analyzing pathogenic mechanisms, and testing novel therapeutic approaches. Such models of ALS and Alzheimer's disease have begun to be developed.

MOTOR NEURON DISEASE

Human Disorder

Clinical Features

Classical ALS (see Ch. 63), with a worldwide prevalence of more than 4 to 6 per 100,000, usually begins in late life, whereas spinal muscular atrophies are more common in infancy and childhood.

Genetics

Approximately 10 percent of cases of adult-onset ALS are familial and show autosomal dominant inheritance associated with age-dependent penetrance. In 13 different pedigrees with familial ALS, 11 different missense mutations (see Ch. 4) in Cu/Zn SOD1 have been discovered. SOD1, a member of a family of metalloenzymes characterized by their ability to dismutate O_2^-, is encoded by an aproximately 15-kilobase-pair gene that consists of five exons on chromosome 21. SOD1 catalyzes the conversion of O_2^-, the product of spontaneous and enzyme-catalyzed oxidation, into H_2O_2 and O_2. Behaving as a reductant or oxidant, O_2^- gives rise to reactive molecules that can injure cells by a variety of mechanisms, including direct DNA damage, increase in intracellular free calcium, protein oxidation, and lipid peroxidation.

Other forms of motor neuron disease show different patterns of inheritance. Juvenile spinal muscular atrophy has an autosomal recessive inheritance; most cases show linkage to DNA markers on chromosome 5q. Kennedy's disease, an adult-onset X-linked recessive bulbospinal muscular atrophy, is caused by triplet-repeat mutations in exon one of the androgen receptor gene (X q11–12).

Selective Vulnerability of Specific Neural Systems

Weakness and muscle atrophy are attributable to selective dysfunction and degeneration of large motor neurons of the brainstem and spinal cord, whereas the spasticity, hyperreflexia, and extensor plantar signs result from lesions of upper motor neurons.

Neuropathologic Findings

Affected motor neurons show phosphorylated neurofilaments and ubiquitin immunoreactivities in perikarya, intracytoplasmic inclusions, neurofilamentous swellings of proximal axons, reductions in the caliber of distal axons, wallerian degeneration, and eventually, cell degeneration. End-stage disease is characterized by reduced numbers of motor neurons in brainstem nuclei and spinal cord and loss of large pyramidal neurons in the motor cortex. These lesions are accompanied by the degeneration of axons in peripheral motor nerves (denervation atrophy of muscle) and of corticospinal tracts (denervation of target fields).

Etioiogic Factors and Mechanisms

The factors involved in the dysfunction and death of neurons in motor neuron disease include genetic factors (i.e., mutations of SOD1 and androgen receptor); oxidative injury; excitotoxicity, possibly mediated by glutamate receptors; and perturbations in the neuronal cytoskeleton.

Animal Models

In animal models, studies of alterations in the biology of neurofilaments have provided evidence that neurofibrillary axonal pathology, similar to those that occur in ALS, is related to alterations in the axonal transport of neurofilament proteins. However, it is clear that the mechanisms that cause the pathology of motor neurons in ALS will only be fully understood when we have animal models that are faithful to the human disease and that can be examined in detail with a variety of neurobiologic strategies.

Several models of motor neuron disease exist, for example, axotomy-induced retrograde degeneration, toxic axonopathies (i.e., intoxication with β,β'-iminodipropionitrile [IDPN]), Brittany spaniels with hereditary canine spinal muscular atrophy (HCSMA), several spontaneously occurring murine models, transgenic mice that overexpress deleted or mutated neurofilament genes, and transgenic mice that express mutated SOD1. Below, we briefly review, with emphasis on investigations from our laboratories, current studies of several of these animal models.

Axotomy-Induced Retrograde Responses of Neurons

Axonal transsection is the simplest model of motor neuron disease. Known classically as wallerian degeneration, it involves several distinctive effects. At the lesion site, fast anterograde and retrograde transport are interrupted, and the proximal and distal stumps of axons accumulate membranous elements and transport endogenous and exogenous proteins. Axotomized neurons show chromatolysis; reduced levels of choline acetyltransferase (ChAT); alterations in levels of specific messenger RNA (mRNA) and proteins, such as neurofilament proteins, peripherin, and tubulin; aberrant distributions of cytoskeletal proteins (i.e., phosphorylated neurofilaments in perikarya); and changes in the transport of some of these proteins. For example, after axotomy, levels of neurofilament gene expression are reduced, whereas levels of β-tubulin and peripherin mRNA increase. Axonal transport studies have shown that the amounts of neurofilament proteins that enter axons are decreased and that a wave of reduced axonal caliber moves down the axon at the rate of transport of neurofilament proteins. Eventually, the synthesis of neurofilament proteins returns to normal, and axonal caliber is restored. These observations are consistent with the concept that neurofilaments are one determinant of axonal caliber. After axotomy, markers for neurotransmitter-related components decrease; in adult motor neurons, nerve growth factor receptor (p75^{NGFR}) expression increases. The p75^{NGFR} immunoreactivity is present exclusively in axotomized neurons, as verified by the colocalization of p75^{NGFR} immunoreactivity with a fluorescent retrograde tracer injected at the crush site. When motor neurons reach targets, p75^{NGFR} immunoreactivity disappears, indicating that p75^{NGFR} expression is closely linked with disconnection of the cells from the target.

Axotomy models have been used to study processes that lead to cell death and to test therapies that preserve cell phenotype and promote cell survival. For example, when the facial nerves of neonatal rats or the L4-5 ventral roots of adult rats are transsected close to the cell bodies, motor neurons undergo a series of retrograde changes that include chromatolysis, loss of transmitter phenotype (ChAT immunoreactivity), and accumulation of phosphorylated neurofilaments in perikarya. Subsequently, 70 to 80 percent of motor neurons die. Recently, four lines of evidence have been presented to show that brain-derived neurotrophic factor (BDNF) is a trophic factor for motor neurons. This neurotrophin is expressed in the local environment and in muscle targets of motor neurons, and muscle expression is upregulated by denervation. Motor neurons express the gene that encodes p145^{trkB}, a receptor involved in BDNF signal transduction. BDNF is transported selectively to α-motor neurons from skeletal muscles. In the facial nerve axotomy model, gelfoam that contains human recombinant BDNF apposed to the proximal stump reduces cell death to 20 percent in the vehicle-treated group. This study, and other work, suggest that BDNF has a trophic effect on motor neurons. Neurotrophin-4/5 has similar effects on motor neurons in this paradigm, whereas nerve growth factor and neurotrophin-3 have no effect. The effects of BDNF and neurotrophin-4/5 on motor neurons raise the possibility that administration of the neurotrophin may be useful in treating animals, including transgenic mice with familial ALS-related SOD1 mutations, that develop the motor neuron disease phenotype.

Intoxication With IDPN

The administration of IDPN causes accumulation of maloriented arrays of neurofilaments in proximal motor axons that leads to proximal swelling and distal atrophy of axons. This pathologic finding, similar to that identified in cases of HCSMA and ALS and in some aged individuals, is likely to be caused by selective impairment in the slow transport of neurofilament proteins, subsequent to the dissociation of neurofilaments from microtubules.

Hereditary Canine Spinal Muscular Atrophy

At present, HCSMA is the best-characterized spontaneously occurring model of motor neuron disease. This autosomal dominant disease in Brittany spaniels is characterized by weakness and atrophy of the skeletal muscles with sparing of eye movements and sphincters.

Mating affected dogs to affected dogs produces an accelerated disease associated with tetraplegia by 3 to 4 months of age. Heterozygous animals become weak at approximately 6 months and are severely paralyzed at 2 to 3 years. Chronically affected dogs show mild weakness. All HCSMA phenotypes develop neurofilamentous swellings in the proximal axons of motor neurons, a pathologic finding virtually identical to that occurring in cases of ALS.

Transport of the neurofilament triplet proteins is impaired, and reductions occur in perikaryal size and axonal diameters, abnormalities that are interpreted to reflect growth arrest and axonal atrophy. In some motor neurons, ChAT immunoreactivity is reduced.

Progressive Motor Neuronopathy

This autosomal recessive murine disease presents as hindlimb paralysis and progresses to quadriparesis and death 6 to 7 weeks after birth. Histologic examination shows neurogenic muscular atrophy, degeneration of motor axons, and slight chromatolysis of spinal motor neurons.

Murine Motor Neuron Degeneration

Originally recognized as a spontaneous adult-onset neurologic disease that occurs in C57BL/6 mice of both sexes, murine motor neuron degeneration is an autosomal dominant disease that maps to the proximal arm of chromosome 8. Motor abnormalities begin in the hindlimbs. Eventually, the animals show little spontaneous movement and die before 1 year of age. The disease was considered to be a motor neuron disease because reduced mobility is a major clinical sign and the original studies that focused on motor neurons were interpreted to show selective pathologic findings in these nerve cells. However, recent investigations have shown that these mice develop widespread abnormalities of neurons, including accumulation of lipofuscin and adenosine triphosphate synthase, subunit 9(c). These abnormalities are characteristic of neuronal ceroid lipofuscinosis, and murine motor neuron degeneration is now considered a murine form of neuronal ceroid lipofuscinosis.

Transgenic Mice That Express Constructs of Neurofilament Genes

Recently, transgenic lines with neurofilament gene constructs have been produced. Transgenic mice that express the mouse neurofilament-L (68-kD polypeptide neurofilament subunit) gene under the transcription control of a strong MSV long-terminal repeat promoter showed transgene expression in a number of tissues, including skeletal muscle, lens, and kidney. These mice did not initially exhibit neurologic disorders but, when two independent high-expressing neurofilament-L lines were mated, transgenic mice accumulated neurofilament-L to approximately fourfold the normal level in sciatic nerve, and spinal motor neurons developed accumulations of neurofilaments in perikarya, swelling of proximal axons, evidence of mild axonal degeneration, and skeletal muscle atrophy. When human neurofilament-H (200-kD polypeptide neurofilament subunit) was expressed in transgenic mice, animals developed neurologic signs and neurofilamentous pathology (i.e., accumulations of filaments in cell bodies, axonal swellings, axonal degeneration, death of motor neurons, and denervation atrophy).

More recently, transgenic mice that express neurofilament-M (150- to 160-kD polypeptide neurofilament subunit) transgenes deleted of the carboxy-terminal 50 amino acids have been shown to develop more severe abnormalities of motor neurons. Finally, transgenic mice with a point mutation in the conserved region of the carboxy-terminal portion of the rod domain of neurofilament-M develop severe hindlimb weakness associated with extensive accumulation of neurofilaments in motor neuron cell bodies and dendrites, swollen proximal axons, severe wallerian degeneration of motor axons, and death of motor neurons.

SOD1 Transgenic Mice

The recent discovery that mutations in the Cu/Zn SOD1 gene are linked to familial ALS suggests that transgenic strategies that introduce SOD1 mutations into mice may be able to produce models of familial ALS. As noted above, the SODs, a family of metalloenzymes, are characterized by their ability to convert O_2^- into O_2 and H_2O_2 and include SOD1, a soluble homodimer distributed in the cytoplasm and nucleus of many mammalian cells; Mn SOD2, a homotetrameric mitochondrial matrix enzyme localized to chromosome 6; and EC-SOD3, a homotetrameric, glycosylated Cu/Zn enzyme localized to the extracellular space and coded for by a gene on chromosome 4. SOD1, made up of five exons, is coded for by an approximately 15-kilobase gene on chromosome 21.

Transgenic mice that harbor a human SOD1 gene and approximately 800 base pairs of the SOD regulatory sequences are reported to show abnormal nerve terminals in distal muscles and tongue. Neuromuscular junctions are characterized by withdrawal and destruction of terminals, multiple small terminals, decreased ratios of terminal area to postsynaptic membranes, and complex and hyperplastic secondary folds. These observations have been interpreted to indicate that overexpression of the SOD1 gene is associated with abnormalities of motor neurons, possibly similar to those described in aged rodents and in individuals with Down syndrome.

Recent transgenic approaches have taken advantage of the demonstration of the finding that some cases of familial ALS are linked to mutations in SOD. It has recently been shown that mice that overexpress SOD1 and harbor a glycine-to-alanine substitution of amino acid 93 (i.e., G93A variant) develop weakness of the limbs and die by 5 to 6 months of age. A similar phenotype occurs in mice that express the SOD mutant (e.g., the G37R variant). These animals develop hindlimb weakness at 3.5 to 4 months of age and usually die 4 weeks after the onset of neurologic disease. The animals show loss of motor neurons, wallerian degeneration in the ventral roots, and denervation atrophy. G37R mice develop cytoskeletal abnormalities and axonal swellings. The findings of these studies are consistent with the concept that the disease results from dominant gain-of-function mutations in the SOD1 gene. The availabilities of these models, generated by the creation of mice with human SOD1 mutations, provide an extraordinary opportunity to study issues of causality, disease mechanisms, and therapies.

ALZHEIMER'S DISEASE

Human Disease

Clinical Disease

The clinical features of Alzheimer's disease are considered in Chapter 60. Cases of senile dementia are usually classified on the basis of criteria formulated by the NINCDS-ADRDA joint task force, as possible, probable, or definite Alzheimer's disease. The clinical course of Alzheimer's disease may vary considerably, but most patients show declines in mental status, usually at a rate of three to four points per year on the Blessed Information-Memory-Concentration test and two to three points per year on the Mini-Mental State Examination.

Clinical histories, physical examinations, neuropsychological testing, and a variety of diagnostic assessments are used to exclude other causes of dementia and to determine the possibility or probability of a diagnosis of Alzheimer's disease. Neuroimaging studies, positron emission tomography, and singlephoton emission computed tomography can show decreased regional glucose metabolism and blood flow in the parietal and temporal lobes, with involvement of other cortical areas at later stages (see Ch. 60). However, at present, short of the examination of brain biopsy, there are no tests to establish the diagnosis of Alzheimer's disease in living subjects.

Genetics

The principal identified risk factors for Alzheimer's disease are age and genetic influences. Several genetic loci have been linked to disease in early-onset familial Alzheimer's disease. Mutations in APP at position 717 in APP-770 have been identified in 11 early-onset families. In these cases, mutations replace the normally occurring valine residue with either isoleucine, glycine, or phenylalanine. Two related Swedish families with early-onset familial Alzheimer's disease harbor a double mutation in the APP gene, which results in a substitution of Lys-Met to Asn-Leu at residues 670 and 671 (of APP-770). In addition, mutations at residues 693 or 692 of APP-770, in which a Glu is substituted by Gln or Ala is substituted by Gly, respectively, have been linked to disease in two unrelated Dutch families with hereditary cerebral hemorrhage with amyloidosis-Dutch. In more than 80 percent of cases of early-onset familial Alzheimer's disease, a compelling linkage has been demonstrated to markers on chromosome 14.

More recently, investigators have identified a genetic locus, positioned on the proximal long arm of chromosome 19 and thought to be apolipoprotein E (apoE), which shows linkage to late-onset and sporadic Alzheimer's disease. ApoE, a 34-kD glycoprotein, is one of 10 apolipoproteins that mediate the metabolism of plasma lipoprotein particles. It is a principal component of very low-, intermediate-, and high-density lipoproteins and chylomicrons, which transport cholesterol and other lipids. The three major isoforms of apoE (i.e., E2, E3, and E4) are products of three alleles expressed at a single gene locus. Individuals with one or two copies of the apoE4 allele exhibit an increased risk for late-onset familial and sporadic Alzheimer's disease. In patients with late-onset familial Alzheimer's disease, the apoE4 allelic frequency is 0.50 compared with 0.16 in age-matched controls, whereas, in sporadic Alzheimer's disease, apoE4 shows an allelic frequency of 0.40. In an autopsy series of cases of late-onset Alzheimer's disease, there was a significant association between the presence of the apoE4 allele and increased parenchymal and vascular deposits of the β-amyloid protein (Aβ).

Neuronal Systems Vulnerable in Alzheimer's Disease

Correlative neuropathologic-neurochemical studies have shown that clinical symptoms and signs in cases of Alzheimer's disease are associated with abnormalities that involve neuronal populations in the basal forebrain cholinergic system and monoaminergic brainstem systems (i.e., locus ceruleus and raphe complex) and the anterior thalamus, hippocampus, neocortex, and amygdala.

A consistent lesion in Alzheimer's disease is the degeneration of cholinergic neurons in the medial septum, diagonal band, and nucleus basalis, which provide the principal cholinergic innervation of amygdala, hippocampus, and neocortex of primates. These cells develop neurofibrillary tangles and neurites (abnormalities that usually are part of senile plaques) and, eventually, undergo atrophy and cell death. Reductions occur in levels of acetylcholine and the activities of ChAT and acetylcholinesterase. With age, the hippocampus exhibits some decline in ChAT activity; however, in Alzheimer's disease, the decrements are very severe. Levels of cortical ChAT activity appear to correlate with the degree of dementia. Neurons of the locus ceruleus and raphe also exhibit perikaryal pathologic findings (i.e., neurofibrillary tangles). The axons and terminals of these cells may form neurites, and noradrenergic and serotoninergic markers may be decreased in target fields. In some cases of Alzheimer's disease, neurons of the anterior nucleus of the thalamus also show evidence of degeneration, and neurites are present in target fields of these

cells (e.g., retrosplenial cortex). The amygdala is also damaged by disease.

Characteristic pathologic findings also occur in the hippocampus and medial temporal lobe. Pyramidal neurons, particularly those in entorhinal cortex, CA1, and CA2, are severely affected in AD (see Ch. 25). These lesions involve, for the most part, glutamatergic systems that disconnect hippocampus and neocortex. Glutamatergic pyramidal neurons in layers III and V of neocortex are selectively destroyed by the disease process. Also affected are interneurons, some of which use corticotropin-releasing factor or somatostatin as transmitters. Levels of somatostatin, somatostatinergic binding sites, and corticotropin-releasing hormone are reduced in the neocortex, whereas binding sites for corticotropin-releasing hormone are increased. Other cortical peptidergic systems do not appear to be altered significantly, but some peptidergic neurons develop neurites associated with senile plaques.

The mechanisms that lead to dysfunction and death of these neurons are not well understood but may involve excitotoxicity, Aβ toxicity, and the activation of proteases. The principal consequence of these lesions is a diminution of synaptic inputs in a variety of brain regions.

Cytoskeletal Pathology in Neurons

Many affected neurons exhibit neurofibrillary tangles, neuropil threads, and neurites. Neurofibrillary tangles are filamentous inclusions in perikarya and dendrites, whereas neurites and neuropil threads are altered neuronal processes. These lesions are enriched 15-nm straight filaments and, more importantly, insoluble paired helical filaments, which consist principally of phosphorylated isoforms of tau. The phosphorylation of tau appears to be linked to the formation of the straight filaments that become increasingly modified and cross-linked to form insoluble paired helical filaments. Tau phosphorylation alters the stability of microtubules, with subsequent effects on intracellular transport, cellular geometry, and neuronal viability. Other neurofibrillary tangle-associated epitopes include ubiquitin, microtubule-associated protein-2, neurofilament proteins (particularly phosphorylated epitopes of the 200-kD protein), and possibly Aβ. Neurites show epitopes related to paired helical filaments, APP, ubiquitin, neurofilaments, and neurotransmitter markers. Because neurofibrillary tangles, neurites, and neuropil threads contain similar cytoskeletal constituents, these fibrillar inclusions are believed to be generated by common mechanisms.

Amyloid

A principal hallmark of Alzheimer's disease is the presence of deposits of Aβ in parenchyma, particularly in the hippocampus and neocortex. Extracellular

Aβ deposits are generally associated with neurites in senile plaques, but Aβ is also present in preamyloid deposits and within the walls of leptomeningeal and cerebral vessels. A 39 to 43 amino acid peptide, Aβ is composed of 11 to 15 amino acids of the transmembrane domain and 28 amino acids of the extracellular domain of larger APP. The APP gene, which encompasses approximately 400 kb of DNA, gives rise to alternatively spliced APP mRNA that encode Aβ-containing proteins of 695, 714, 751, and 770 amino acids.

APPs are type I integral membrane glycoproteins that mature through the constitutive secretory pathway and acquire N- and O-linked oligosaccharides, sialic acid, tyrosine sulfate, and phosphate. Depending on the cell type and level of transient expression, a fraction (10 to 30 percent) of newly synthesized APP appears on the cell surface, and some of these molecules are cleaved between positions 16 and 17 of amyloid, which results in the release of soluble APP into the conditioned medium. The presence of soluble APP in human cerebrospinal fluid that contains amyloid epitopes suggests that similar processing events occur in vivo. This important processing pathway precludes Aβ amyloidogenesis by directing cleavage within the amyloid peptide region.

The protease responsible for endoproteolytic cleavage of APP at the cell surface has not been identified and, for convenience, has been termed α-secretase. To examine the specificity of α-secretase, detailed substitution, deletion, and insertion mutagenesis of the residues that surround the APP cleavage site were examined in transfection assays. These studies revealed that α-secretase is highly unusual in that it has relaxed primary sequence specificity at the cleavage site but appears to cleave APP substrates at a defined distance from the plasma membrane. Interestingly, the production of soluble APP is severely compromised by amino acid replacements proximal to the α-secretase cleavage site that destabilizes the α-helical structure of the β-peptide sequence. Proteases with similar chemical properties are likely to be responsible for "shedding" of ectodomains from a wide variety of transmembrane molecules, including the transforming growth factor-α precursor and c-kit ligand.

Secreted APP isoforms that contain Aβ epitopes are present in the cerebrospinal fluid. A fraction of cell-surface APP is also internalized and degraded by endosomal-lysosomal pathways. Processing through the endosomal-lysosomal pathway results in the production of fragments that contain the entire Aβ region and the APP carboxy-terminus and are, hence, potentially amyloidogenic. Recent reports indicate that peptides similar to Aβ (β1-40) and truncated forms of Aβ (approximately β 17–40) are secreted constitutively by culture cells and are present in the cerebrospinal fluid.

The cellular and molecular mechanisms of Aβ generation are not entirely understood, but several recent studies have clarified these processes. For example, despite excitement created by the discovery of potential amyloidogenic fragments generated in endosomal-lysosomal pathways, several lines of evidence now suggest that the lysosomal degradation of APP is unlikely to contribute to the production of Aβ. Kinetic studies show that Aβ is released in parallel to soluble APP and that Aβ is not detected in purified lysosomes. In addition, Aβ production is not inhibited by leupeptin, an inhibitor of lysosomal protease function. Finally, Aβ is released by cultured fibroblasts from patients with I-cell disease, in which proteases do not target to lysosomes. However, agents that interfere with pH gradients (i.e., ammonium chloride and chloroquine) inhibit the production of Aβ, which suggests that Aβ may be generated in acidic compartments (i.e., endosomes or late Golgi). Furthermore, diminished levels of soluble Aβ are released from cells that express APP deleted of the entire cytoplasmic tail. These results suggest indirectly that the reinternalization of APP from the cell surface may favor the generation of Aβ. Preliminary studies showing Aβ generation from surface-labeled APP support this model. Although these studies suggest that Aβ may be produced and released in vitro and in vivo, the relationship of these Aβ-related fragments to deposits of Aβ isolated from patients with Alzheimer's disease (which is principally 42 to 43 amino acids) is not clear.

Until recently, many believed that Aβ is generated by aberrant metabolism of the precursor. One model predicted that membrane damage incurred in the brains of individuals with Alzheimer's disease and allowed protease to act on APP with subsequent liberation of the partially hydrophobic Aβ peptide from the bilayer. This concept had to be reevaluated when it was discovered that Aβ was detectable in the conditioned medium of a wide variety of cultured cells and in human cerebrospinal fluid. Most Aβ peptides secreted in these settings are Aβ1-40. Significantly, Aβ1-42/Aβ1-43, admixed with Aβ1-40, appears to be the predominant Aβ species in senile plaque amyloid. Most importantly, Aβ1-42/43, which nucleates rapidly and is not soluble, may serve as a seed for aggregates of Aβ deposits. Moreover, the Aβ deposits may interact with other moieties, (e.g., apoE and apoJ) to enhance the formation of Aβ fibrils.

As described earlier, several mutations in the APP gene are linked to diseases characterized by deposition of amyloid in the brain. In these cases, the mutations either flank or reside within the Aβ peptide region. In recent studies, a combination of biochemical and enzyme-linked immunosorbent assays were used to demonstrate that cells transfected with APP complementary DNA that encodes the "717" substitutions secrete a higher percentage of long Aβ peptides (i.e., Aβ1-42) relative to cells that express wild-type APP. These studies are particularly notable because physicochemical studies have indicated that amyloid formation is a nucleation-dependent phenomenon and that the carboxy-terminus of Aβ may be a critical determinant of the rate of amyloid formation. As hypothesized earlier, these studies argue that β1-42 and/or β1-43, rather than Aβ1-40, may be the pathogenic proteins in Alzheimer's disease. However, it is possible that β1-40 could aggregate as a result of prior "seeding" by trace amounts of Aβ1-42 fibrils. Support for the idea that Aβ1-42/43 are critical for amyloid formation emerged recently from studies in which end-specific antibodies (i.e., reagents that uniquely recognize Aβ1-40 or Aβ1-42) were used in immunocytochemical studies of brains with Alzheimer's disease. These studies convincingly demonstrated that the bulk (more than 95 percent) of senile plaques consist of Aβ1-42. In addition, a mutation in APP that leads to a Glu-Gln substitution at position 693, corresponding to amino acid 22 of Aβ, is associated with hereditary cerebral hemorrhage with amyloidosis-Dutch, a disease in which Aβ is deposited around blood vessels. In vitro studies indicate that Aβ peptides that contain this mutation are more prone to aggregate into fibrils. More recently, a double mutation at codons 670 and 671 has been demonstrated in two large, related Swedish families with early-onset Alzheimer's disease. This double mutation results in substitution of the normal Lys-Met dipeptide to Asn-Leu. Tissue culture cells transfected with complementary DNA that encoded this mutant polypeptide secrete six- to eightfold higher levels of Aβ-containing peptides compared with cells transfected with wild-type constructs.

Finally, in one newly described family with a mutation at codon 692 of APP (substitution of Gly for Ala), affected individuals show both presenile dementia and cerebral hemorrhages. Recent studies indicate that this Gly-Ala substitution alters the amino-terminal microheterogeneity of secreted Aβ, including the appearance of several hydrophobic species that might contribute to the potential for fibrillogenesis.

Animal Models

Aged Nonhuman Primates

These animals develop age-associated impairments in performance on cognitive and memory tasks early in the third decade of life. Our laboratory has behaviorally characterized a colony of rhesus monkeys that range from 3 to 34 years of age. These behavioral investigations indicate that cognitive and memory deficits in rhesus monkeys appear late in the second dec-

ade and become more evident in the mid-to-late 20s. Impairments in performance of certain spatial abilities occur in some animals in their late teens. However, in other test categories, behavior is not altered until the third decade of life. Behavioral deficits that occur in aged nonhuman primates closely resemble those that occur in aged humans.

These impairments in performance on specific behavioral tasks are thought to be associated, in individual animals, with the deposition of amyloid and the formation of neurites. In many old animals, Aβ appears as diffuse deposits, in the cores of senile plaques, and around blood vessels. The earliest lesions in the parenchyma include the presence of slightly enlarged neurites (i.e., distal axons, nerve terminals, and dendrites) and preamyloid deposits. Neurites often contain membranous elements, mitochondria (some degenerating), lysosomes, APP, phosphorylated neurofilaments, synaptophysin, and transmitter markers. In individual plaques, APP- and synaptophysin-immunoreactive neurites are often surrounded by a halo of distorted neuropil and Aβ immunoreactivity. The presence of APP-like immunoreactivity in neuronal perikarya, axons, and neurites within Aβ-containing plaques suggests that neurons can serve as one source for some Aβ deposits. In addition, the proximity of Aβ to reactive astrocytes and microglia and to vascular cells suggests that these populations of nonneuronal cells may participate in the formation of Aβ. Neurites appear to represent disconnected axons and swollen dendrites. Research that focuses on Aβ amyloidogenesis investigates the interactions of cells (i.e., neurons, astroglia, astrocytes, and vascular cells), colocalized proteins (i.e., α_1-antichymotrypsin, apoE, SP40, 40 [apolipoprotein J]), and constituents of the complement cascade.

Transgenic Mice

Transgenic approaches can directly test whether the expression of exogenous wild-type or mutant APP or the expression of Aβ-containing fragments is involved in the pathogenesis of Alzheimer's disease-type abnormalities. Over the past few years, several groups have attempted to produce mice with Aβ deposits using complementary DNA and yeast artificial chromosome-based transgenic technologies. Some of these efforts are reviewed below. Unfortunately, although a variety of transgenic lines have been developed, with one possible exception, these animals have not developed the brain abnormalities characteristic of Alzheimer's disease.

On the basis of in situ hybridization studies, which indicate an increase in levels of transcripts that encode APP-751 in hippocampal neurons in Alzheimer's disease, several investigators attempted to produce transgenic mice that overexpress human APP-751 in brain. The initial report describing transgenic mice that expressed APP-751 showed poorly resolved extracellular Aβ deposits and A68-immunoreactive processes in the cortex. More recent studies from this group report that the murine deposits closely resemble the preamyloid deposits in the brains of young adults with Down syndrome or patients with early-stage Alzheimer's disease. The authors used a human Aβ-specific antibody and several other Aβ antibodies to visualize diffuse deposits. Such observations, however, await confirmation.

The finding that several missense mutations in APP are genetically linked to pedigrees with early-onset Alzheimer's disease has led investigators to assess the phenotype of transgenic mice that overexpress mutant APP. In one such study, transgenes that encode *myc* epitope-tagged human APP-695 (HuAPP-695myc) or HuAPP-695myc that harbor the APP-717 mutation were placed under the transcriptional control of the hamster prion gene promoter, and several lines of transgenic mice were generated with these constructs. No developmental or pathologic abnormalities were evident in "wild-type" animals despite abundant HuAPP-695myc expression in all neurons of the central nervous system. The level of total APP was elevated approximately 2.5-fold in wild-type lines. Remarkably, mice that expressed mutant APP at levels similar to or slightly higher than wild-type expressors showed markedly reduced life spans (50 to 100 days). Death was not preceded by wasting, could not be attributed to a specific injury, and was not accompanied by amyloid plaques or neurofibrillary tangles. The biochemical or physiologic bases for the premature death phenotype are presently uncertain.

The overexpression of APP, as occurs in individuals with Down syndrome, is thought to lead to the premature deposition of Aβ in the brain. To mimic the trisomic APP dosage imbalance observed in individuals with Down syndrome, a yeast artificial chromosome that contained approximately 650 kilobases of human genomic DNA, including the APP gene, was transfected into embryonic stem cells. Embryonic stem cells that contained stably integrated yeast artificial chromosome DNA were microinjected into mouse blastocysts, and chimeric mice were generated. After breeding, it was established that human APP sequences were transmitted to the mouse germline. Furthermore, human APP mRNA is actively transcribed in mouse tissue, and the splicing pattern of human APP transcripts in transgenic mouse tissue mirrored the endogenous pattern of alternatively spliced mRNA. With antibodies specific for human APP, Western blot analysis of transgenic mouse brain extracts revealed that human APP contributed approximately 40 percent of total APP levels. No Alzheimer's disease-type pathology was demonstrable in young (<2 months) animals. Furthermore, no pathologic findings were observed in animals as old as 14 months. Ongoing additional breeding approaches are intended to increase human APP gene copy number and, hence, APP levels. The yeast artificial chromosome-embryonic stem cell strategy can be used to introduce modified human APP yeast artificial chromosome that encode familial Alzheimer's disease mutations into the mouse germline and to determine whether the presence of these mutations predisposes to Aβ deposition and, possibly, other brain abnormalities that occur in individuals with Alzheimer's disease. Moreover, these mice produced by transgenic strategies will allow analyses of the sequential biochemical, cellular, and molecular pathologic results characteristic of early-onset familial Alzheimer's disease.

CONCLUSIONS

The identification of specific genetic mutations in familial Alzheimer's disease and familial ALS has ushered in a new and exciting era of research aimed at clarifying the relationship between genetic lesions and the cause and/or pathogenesis of these devastating human neurodegenerative diseases. At present, neither the mechanisms of selective vulnerability, cytoskeletal abnormalities, and cell death nor the character, dynamics, and evolution of cellular pathology of vulnerable populations of neurons are well understood. Nevertheless, recent studies have provided compelling evidence that simple animal models can be generated (e.g., transgenic mice that express familial ALS-linked mutant SOD1 genes) to recapitulate some of the features of the human disease. These animal models will be particularly useful for defining the causes of disease, characterizing the evolution of pathologic findings, analyzing the pathogenetic mechanisms, and most importantly, offering in vivo paradigms in which rational therapeutic strategies can be developed.

ACKNOWLEDGMENTS

The authors thank their many colleagues at The Johns Hopkins Medical Institutions and other institutions for stimulating discussions and for contributions to the work reviewed, especially Drs. John W. Griffin, Don W. Cleveland, Michael K. Lee, Philip C. Wong, Z.-S. Xu, Linda C. Cork, John D. Gearhart, Paul N. Hoffman, Lary C. Walker, Bruce Lamb, and Cheryl A. Kitt.

These investigations were supported by grants from the U.S. Public Health Service (NS 20471 and AG 05146), The Robert L. and Clara G. Patterson Trust,

The Metropolitan Life Foundation, the American Health Assistance Foundation, and funds from the Claster family. Drs. Price and Koliatsos are recipients of a Leadership and Excellence in Alzheimer's Disease (LEAD) award and a Javits Neuroscience Investigator Award (NIH NS 10580).

ANNOTATED BIBLIOGRAPHY

Avraham KB, Sugarman H, Rotshenker S, Groner Y. Down's syndrome: morphological remodelling and increased complexity in the neuromuscular junction of transgenic CuZn-superoxide dismutase mice. J Neurocytol 1991;20:208–15.

In mice, hindlimb muscles, nerve terminal length, number of nerve terminal branching points, and incidence of sprouting that results in synapse formation increased with advanced age and in CuZn-SOD1 transgenic mice.

Borchelt DR, Shen J, Johannsdottir R et al. Premature death in transgenic mice expressing the Alzheimer's amyloid precursor protein, abstracted. Soc Neurosci Abstr 1994; 20:636.

Unexplained short life span.

Corder EH, Saunders AM, Strittmatter WJ et al. Gene dose of apolipoprotein E type 4 allele and the risk of Alzheimer's disease in late onset families. Science 1993;261: 921–3.

Risk for Alzheimer's disease increased from 20 to 90 percent, and mean age at onset decreased from 84 to 68 years.

Cork LC, Griffin JW, Munnell JF et al. Hereditary canine spinal muscular atrophy. J. Neuropathol Exp Neurol 1979;38:209–21.

Descriptions of this then newly recognized disorder.

Cork LC, Masters C, Beyreuther K, Price DL. Development of senile plaques. Relationships of neuronal abnormalities and amyloid deposits. Am J Pathol 1990;137: 1383–92.

The initial stages of neurite formation and parenchymal amyloid deposits may be independent of the appearance of vascular amyloid.

Doyu M, Sobue G, Mukai E et al. Severity of X-linked recessive bulbospinal neuronopathy correlates with size of the tandem CAG repeat in androgen receptor gene. Ann Neurol 1992;32:707–10.

Studies in 26 Japanese patients from 21 families with X-linked recessive bulbospinal neuronopathy showed the number of CAG repeats significantly correlated with the age at onset.

Griffin JW, Clark AC, Parhad I et al. The neuronal cytoskeleton in disorders of the motor neuron. Adv Neurol 1991; 56:103–13.

Review article.

Griffin JW, Hoffman PN, Clark AW et al. Slow axonal transport of neurofilament proteins: impairment by β,β'-iminodipropionitrile administration. Science 1978;202: 633–5.

Selectively impairs slow axonal transport.

Griffin JW, Price DL, Engel WK, Drachman DB. The pathogenesis of reactive axonal swellings: role of axonal transport. J Neuropathol Exp Neurol 1977;36:214–27.

Anterograde and retrograde transport carries membranous organelles.

Gurney ME, Pu H, Chiu AY et al. Motor neuron degeneration in mice that express a human Cu,Zn superoxide dismutase mutation. Science 1994;264:1772–5.

Haass C, Koo EH, Mellon A et al. Targeting of cell-surface beta-amyloid precursor protein to lysosomes: alternative processing into amyloid-bearing fragments. Nature 1992;357:500–3.

Description of a second processing pathway for Aβ and a suggestion that it may be responsible for generating amyloid-bearing fragments in Alzheimer's disease.

Haass C, Schlossmacher MG, Hung AY et al. Amyloid beta-peptide is produced by cultured cells during normal metabolism [see comments]. Nature 1992;359:322–5.

The production of Aβ in soluble form in vitro and in vivo during normal cellular metabolism raises issues whether it is a true disease effect.

Harding AE. Inherited neuronal atrophy and degeneration predominantly of lower motor neurons. In Dyck PJ, Thomas PK, Griffin JW et al. (eds). Peripheral Neuropathy. 3rd Ed. WB Saunders, Philadelphia, 1993, p. 1051.

Text article.

Hoffman PN, Thompson GW, Griffin JW, Price DL. Changes in neurofilament transport coincide temporally with alterations in the caliber of axons in regenerating motor fibers. J Cell Biol 1985;101:1332–40.

Most neurofilaments in motor fibers move continuously in an anterograde direction. The transport of neurofilaments plays an important role in regulating axonal caliber.

Iwatsubo T, Odaka A, Suzuki N et al. Visualization of Aβ42(43)-positive and Aβ40-positive senile plaques with end-specific Aβ-monoclonal antibodies: evidence that an initially deposited Aβ species is Aβ1-42(43). Neuron, in press

Jarrett JT, Lansbury PT Jr. Seeding "one-dimensional crystallization" of amyloid: a pathogenic mechanism in Alzheimer's disease and scrapie? Cell 1993;73:1055–8.

Review article.

Koliatsos VE, Clatterbuck RE, Winslow JW et al. Evidence that brain-derived neurotrophic factor is a trophic factor for motor neurons in vivo. Neuron 1993;10:359–67.

BDNF rescues motor neurons from degeneration and may also play a role in the normal physiology of these cells.

Koliatsos VE, Crawford TO, Price DL. Axotomy induces nerve growth factor receptor immunoreactivity in spinal motor neurons. Brain Res 1991;549:297–304.

Immunocytochemical study of the onset, course, and specificity of nerve growth factor-receptor upregulation after distal or proximal crush of the sciatic nerve. Findings suggest target-derived factors participate in the regulation of nerve growth factor-receptor gene expression in adult motor neurons.

Martin LJ, Sisodia SS, Koo EH et al. Amyloid precursor protein in aged nonhuman primates. Proc Natl Acad Sci U S A 1991;88:1461–5.

APP immunoreactivity in neuronal perikarya, dendrites, axons, and neurites in Aβ-containing plaques is consistent with a hypothesis that neurons can serve as one source of brain amyloid.

Pardo CA, Rabin BA, Palmer DN, Price DL. Accumulation of the adenosine triphosphate synthase subunit C in the mnd mutant mouse. A model for neuronal ceroid lipofuscinosis. Am J Pathol 1994;144:829–35.

Descriptions of the utility of this mouse model.

Price DL, Borchelt DR, Walker LC, Sisodia SS. Toxicity of synthetic Aβ peptides and modeling of Alzheimer's disease. Neurobiol Aging 1992;13:623–5.

Review article.

Price DL, Martin LJ, Clatterbuck RE et al. Neuronal degeneration in human diseases and animal models. J Neurobiol 1992;23:1277–94.

Review article.

Price DL, Sisodia SS. Cellular and molecular biology of Alzheimer's disease and animal models. Annu Rev Med 1994;45:435–42.

Review article.

Rosen DR, Siddique T, Patterson D et al. Mutations in Cu/Zn superoxide dismutase gene are associated with familial amyotrophic lateral sclerosis. Nature 1993;362:59–62.

Genetic linkage shown between familial ALS and a gene that encodes a cytosolic, Cu/Zn-binding SOD1.

Sisodia SS, Koo EH, Beyreuther K et al. Evidence that β-amyloid protein in Alzheimer's disease is not derived by normal processing. Science 1990;248:492–5.

Altered APP processing may results in the release and subsequent deposition of intact Aβ.

Stadtman ER. Protein oxidation and aging. Science 1992; 257:1220–4.

Review article discussing systems that generate oxygen free radicals that catalyze the oxidative modification of proteins.

Strittmatter WJ, Saunders AM, Schmechel D et al. Apolipoprotein E: high-avidity binding to β-amyloid and increased frequency of type 4 allele in late-onset familial Alzheimer disease. Proc Natl Acad Sci USA 1993;90: 1977–81.

Significant association found between apoE4 allele and late-onset familial Alzheimer's disease.

Suzuki N, Cheung TT, Cai X-D et al. An increased percentage of long amyloid β protein secreted by familial amyloid β protein precursor (βAPP^{717}) mutants. Science 1994;264:1336.

Williams DB, Windebank AJ. Motor neuron disease, in Dyck PJ, Thomas PK, Griffin JW et al. (eds). Peripheral Neuropathy. 3rd Ed. WB Saunders, Philadelphia, 1993, pp. 1028–50.

Text article.

Wisniewski HM, Terry RD. Morphology of the aging brain, human and animal. Prog. Brain Res 1973;40:167–86.

Review article.

2

Molecular and Cellular Pathophysiology of Demyelinating Disorders

Stephen G. Waxman and Jeffery D. Kocsis

Damage to the myelin sheath without transsection of the axon (demyelination) is one of the cardinal pathologic changes in inflammatory demyelinating diseases of the central nervous system (CNS), including multiple sclerosis. Demyelination also occurs in spinal cord compression (e.g., caused by the expansion of epidural tumors that grow within the spinal canal adjacent to the spinal cord) and in nonpenetrating spinal cord injury. In fact, as early as 1906, Gordon Holmes described demyelination in association with spinal cord compression in a patient with tuberculous paraplegia. Within the peripheral nervous system (PNS), demyelination occurs in the Guillain-Barré syndrome and as a component of the pathologic characteristics in many other neuropathies.

Although the axon is preserved in demyelinating disorders, damage to the myelin sheath, irrespective of whether it occurs secondary to traumatic injury, inflammation, or other causes, can produce profound abnormalities in the conduction of action potentials that are associated with severe functional impairment. Because the axon maintains its integrity and the axon membrane is intact in demyelinating disorders, attention in the laboratory has focused on the question, "How does demyelination produce clinical deficits?" Moreover, because many patients with multiple sclerosis experience remissions, in which there is clinical recovery despite the apparent persistence of demyelination in the brain and spinal cord, much attention has been focused on the corollary issue, "How does clinical recovery occur in patients with demyelination of central axons?"

In attempting to answer these questions, neuroscientists have had to examine biophysical mechanisms of action potential propagation in normal myelinated axons, which depend on the distribution of specialized protein molecules (including voltage-sensitive ion channels) along the axon, and have studied the changes in the axon that occur subsequent to demyelination. Over the past decade, there have been significant advances in our understanding of the molecular architecture of the myelinated axon membrane and its implications for the pathophysiology of demyelinating disorders. This chapter first describes the molecular organization and biophysics of normal myelinated axons and then reviews the pathophysiology of demyelination and the basis for recovery of function following damage to the myelin sheath.

CONDUCTION IN MYELINATED AXONS

In nonmyelinated axons (e.g., the giant axon in the squid and C-fibers in human peripheral nerves), the action potential creeps along the fiber micron by micron, in a continuous manner. In contrast, in myelinated axons, the action potential propagates in a *saltatory* (from the Latin for *jump*) manner, "jumping" in a discontinuous fashion from one node of Ranvier to the next. Saltatory conduction is facilitated by the myelin sheath, which has a high electrical resistance and a low capacitance; these properties permit the myelin to function as an insulator. In normal myelinated axons, the internodal conduction time (the time required for propagation from one node of Ranvier to the next) is about 20 μs.

The different modes of conduction in myelinated and nonmyelinated fibers are reflected in different

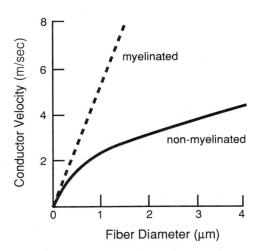

Figure 2-1. Graph showing the relationship between conduction velocity and axon diameter for nonmyelinated and myelinated axons. Myelination results in an increase in conduction velocity.

conduction velocities. In nonmyelinated fibers, conduction speed is proportional to the square root of diameter and ranges up to 2 m/s. In myelinated fibers, on the other hand, conduction velocity increases linearly with diameter and can be greater than 50 m/s. As a result of their different conduction velocity-diameter relationships, conduction velocity is higher in myelinated axons than in nonmyelinated fibers of the same size (Fig. 2-1). Thus, one consequence of myelination is an increased conduction velocity. Another consequence of myelination is greater efficiency of conduction. Myelinated axons can conduct action potentials at higher frequencies and require less energy per action potential than nonmyelinated axons.

As noted below, the consequences of demyelination can be predicted from these factors. As might be expected, demyelination is associated with a reduction in the speed of propagation (i.e., decreased conduction velocity). As described below, however, demyelination is also associated with other abnormalities of conduction, including conduction failure. This is due, at least in part, to the manner in which the myelinated axon membrane is constructed.

Ion Channel Organization of Myelinated Axons

Na$^+$ and K$^+$ Channel Distribution

The electrical properties of axons depend on the presence of specialized molecules in the axon membrane: voltage-sensitive Na$^+$ channels, which depolarize the axon, and K$^+$ channels, which tend to repolarize it. Although these channels seem to be distributed at random along nonmyelinated axons (where they support continuous conduction), the distribution of channels

within the axolemma of myelinated mammalian axons is nonuniform.

Na$^+$ channels in myelinated axons are clustered in high density at the nodes of Ranvier, where action potentials are generated. The density of Na$^+$ channels at the node is higher than in almost any other membrane. Voltage-clamp and saxitoxin binding studies demonstrate that about 1,000 Na$^+$ channels per square micron are present at the node. In contrast, there seem to be less than 25 Na$^+$ channels per square micron in the internodal axon membrane (i.e., the axon membrane between the nodes of Ranvier), which is normally covered by the myelin.

Voltage-clamp studies show that, after acute demyelination, a K$^+$ current is unmasked together with a capacitative current as the internodal axon membrane is exposed, reflecting the presence of K$^+$ channels in the internodal axon membrane, as described below. The internodal K$^+$ current and capacity are not matched, however, by a corresponding increase in Na$^+$ current. This shows that the acutely demyelinated axon membrane (which was formerly internodal) contains few Na$^+$ channels. The paucity of Na$^+$ channels in the internodal axon membrane provides another reason, in addition to the loss of the insulating sheath per se, for impaired conduction after demyelination. The small number of internodal sodium channels is insufficient in most axons to support conduction.

The heterogeneous distribution of Na$^+$ channels in myelinated axons is paralleled by a complementary distribution of at least one type of K$^+$ channel. Although Na$^+$ channels in myelinated axons are aggregated at the node of Ranvier, early voltage-clamp studies of the nodes of Ranvier in mammalian PNS in the late 1970s suggested that K$^+$ channels were sparsely represented at the node. In agreement with these observations in mammalian peripheral myelinated axons, application of K$^+$ channel blocking drugs (such as 4-aminopyridine [4-AP]) had minimal effects on the duration of the action potentials recorded from intact myelinated axons of the central nervous system (which could not be voltage clamped). These results suggested that, in the PNS and CNS, there are few, if any, 4-AP-sensitive K$^+$ channels at the nodes of Ranvier. Although K$^+$ currents are not prominent at the node in normal myelinated axons, large K$^+$ currents sensitive to 4-AP become apparent after demyelination. These observations suggested that 4-AP-sensitive K$^+$ channels (which have been termed *fast* K$^+$ channels, as described below) are present in the internodal or paranodal part of the axon membrane where they are covered by the myelin. Observations during early stages of development (prior to the maturation of myelin sheaths) and after demyelination showed that 4-

AP can significantly affect the action potential waveform of premyelinated and demyelinated axons. This finding confirmed that 4-AP-sensitive K^+ channels are indeed present in the axon membrane under the myelin (Fig. 2-2).

This picture of a mirror-image distribution of Na^+ and K^+ channels at the node and internode dominated early thinking about axonal organization and continues to provide a basis for understanding axonal pathophysiology. However, this picture is, in fact, a simplification of axonal channel distribution. Several

additional channels and ion-exchange proteins have been found in the mammalian axon membrane over the past few years, and a complex distribution of K^+ channels along myelinated axons, as described below, has emerged. Nevertheless, the segregation of Na^+ channels at the node and fast K^+ channels in the internodal axon membrane under the myelin has important implications for the pathophysiology of demyelination.

Two Types of K⁺ Channels in Myelinated Axons

The idea that there are two types of K^+ channels in myelinated axons arose from experiments that used electrotonus measurements and intra-axonal recordings from intact peripheral nerves and CNS axon tracts and was subsequently confirmed with voltage-clamp methods to study isolated peripheral nerve fibers. These distinct K^+ channel types are best recognized in immature or demyelinated axons where the paranodal axon-myelin junctions (which normally seal the myelin to the axon on either side of the node, thereby isolating the internodal part of the axon membrane from the extracellular space) are either immature or disrupted. The first type of K^+ channel (which we termed *fast*) is blocked by 4-AP and the second (which we termed *slow*) is blocked by tetraethylammonium (TEA). The fast 4-AP-sensitive K^+ channel has more rapid kinetics than the TEA-sensitive channel, and it can contribute to repolarization of the action potential and to an early and brief afterhyperpolarization that follows the action potential. The slow TEA-sensitive channel activates more slowly and produces a longer lasting afterhyperpolarization that follows repetitive firing of the axon and modulates burst activity so as to participate in spike-frequency adaptation. These distinct K^+ channels are localized in different parts of the axon membrane. The 4-AP-sensitive fast K^+ channels are located in the axon membrane under the myelin at the paranode or internode. In contrast, the TEA-sensitive slow K^+ channels are present in the axon membrane at the node of Ranvier.

In addition to these two types of channels, which are highly selective for K^+, both PNS and CNS myelinated axons have other channels, termed *inwardly rectifying channels*, that use both K^+ and Na^+ as charge carriers. These inward rectifier channels are activated by hyperpolarization. When open, they mediate a depolarization. The inward rectifier appears to maintain the excitability of the axon at an appropriate level during hyperpolarizations that are evoked by other K^+ channels and Na^+, K^+ adenosine triphosphatase (ATPase). Figure 2-3 summarizes our current understanding of the distribution of Na^+ and K^+ channels on myelinated axons. The distribution of these chan-

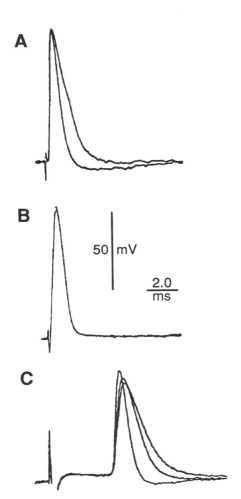

Figure 2-2. Masking of 4-AP-sensitive K^+ channels by the myelin sheath. Recordings from **(A)** premyelinated axon (at an early stage of development, before myelin is formed), **(B)** myelinated axon, and **(C)** experimentally demyelinated axon. In each case, two action potentials are juxtaposed, one recorded under control conditions and a second after the axon is exposed to the K^+ channel blocking drug 4-AP. Action potential repolarization is delayed by 4-AP in premyelinated (Fig. A) and demyelinated (Fig. C) axons, but there is no effect in the myelinated (Fig. B) axon, which indicates that the 4-AP-sensitive K^+ channels are covered by the myelin sheath.

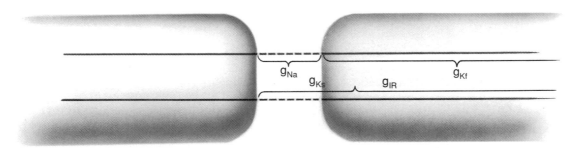

Figure 2-3. Diagram showing ion channel organization of the myelinated axon. Na$^+$ channels (g$_{Na}$) are clustered in the axon membrane at the node; 4-AP-sensitive (fast) K$^+$ channels (g$_{Kf}$) have a complementary distribution.

nels along the axon has important implications for pathophysiology.

Na$^+$, K$^+$ Adenosine Triphosphatases and Na$^+$-Ca^{++} Exchangers

Ionic homeostasis in axons is maintained by specialized protein molecules, including Na$^+$, K$^+$-ATPase. This ATP-consuming molecule, embedded within neural membranes, extrudes three Na$^+$ ions for every two K$^+$ ions it imports into the axon and is thus termed the *electrogenic ion pump*. It has long been known that, during periods of high-frequency impulse activity in peripheral nerves, activation of a ouabain-sensitive Na$^+$, K$^+$ ATPase can produce membrane hyperpolarization. Recently, electrophysiologic studies have demonstrated that the activation of Na$^+$, K$^+$-ATPase in myelinated axons within the CNS can produce a hyperpolarization, which is accompanied by decreased excitability of the axon. The localization of Na$^+$, K$^+$-ATPases (i.e., nodal versus internodal) remains controversial. However, membrane hyperpolarization caused by enhanced electrogenic pump activity has been demonstrated on demyelinated axons, which suggests that Na$^+$, K$^+$-ATPase activity may oppose depolarization (and thus interfere with the generation of action potentials) in the demyelinated (formerly internodal) axonal membrane. It appears likely that the Na$^+$, K$^+$-ATPase-mediated hyperpolarization can contribute to conduction block at sites of demyelination.

There is also another specialized molecule, termed the *Na$^+$-Ca$^+$ exchange* protein, which is located in the axon membrane. Under normal conditions, this molecule uses the electrochemical gradient of sodium (which is present in much higher concentrations outside the axon) to extrude calcium ions from the cytoplasm in exchange for sodium in a manner that does not require ATP. Recent studies have shown that, following anoxic injury to CNS white matter (as can occur as a result of strokes), axons depolarize and there is a massive influx of sodium. This collapses the sodium gradient. As a result, the Na$^+$-Ca$^+$ exchange molecule operates in a different mode, carrying Ca$^+$ ions backward into the axoplasm. This provides a pathway, even in the absence of synapses or excitatory transmitters and their receptors, for an influx of calcium, which injures the axon; it also accounts for the sensitivity of myelinated CNS axons to anoxia. This mode of axonal injury may also be important following trauma to the spinal cord, which, like anoxia, leads to depolarization and sodium influx into CNS myelinated axons and triggers a damaging increase in intracellular calcium.

ABNORMAL CONDUCTION IN DEMYELINATED AXONS

As noted above, the myelin serves as a high-resistance, low-capacitance insulator that shunts the action current from one node to the next. In addition, the axon itself exhibits a complex organization, and the molecular machinery responsible for generation of action potentials (i.e., high densities of Na$^+$ channels) is confined to the nodes of Ranvier. In view of these specializations, one might expect that the axon would conduct action potentials in an abnormal manner following damage to the myelin sheath.

Indeed, it is now recognized that demyelinated axons exhibit a variety of abnormal modes of conduction. These are illustrated schematically in Figure 2-4 and are discussed below.

Decreased Conduction Velocity and Conduction Block

In moderately demyelinated fibers, there is a reduction in conduction velocity. The internodal conduction time can be prolonged from its normal value (20 μs) to nearly 500 μs. Thus, the time required for the action potential to propagate along the axon is increased. When looked at from the point of view of the entire population of axons in a nerve or tract, there is also a corollary abnormality of conduction, termed

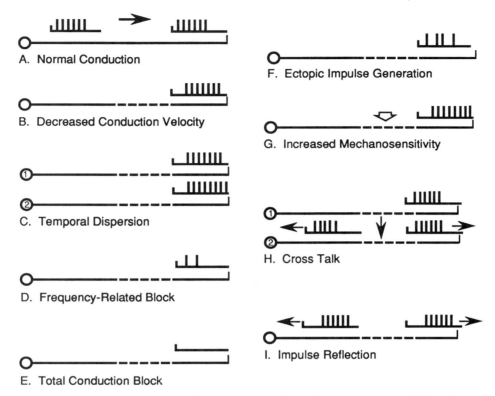

Figure 2-4. (A–I) Abnormal modes of action potential conduction at sites of demyelination (dotted lines).

temporal dispersion (i.e., loss of synchrony of the action potentials carried by different axons that are demyelinated to different degrees). As a result of temporal dispersion, a front of action potentials in different axons within the nerve or tract, which should converge *synchronously* on a postsynaptic target, impinges on the postsynaptic cell in a staggered manner, thus interfering with temporal summation.

More severely demyelinated fibers exhibit *conduction block* (see Ch. 12). When conduction block occurs, action potentials do not propagate through the injured part of the axon. Conduction block may be frequency related so that low-frequency impulse trains, or the first few action potentials within a train, are propagated relatively reliably through the lesion, with loss only of high-frequency impulse trains or the action potentials traveling late within a series. Alternatively, the most severe conduction abnormality is *total conduction block,* in which none of the action potentials can propagate through the lesion.

Positive Conduction Abnormalities

Still other abnormal modes of impulse conduction in demyelinated axons are "positive" in the Jacksonian sense because they involve *hyperexcitability* or genera-

tion of *extra* impulses. These modes of conduction include abnormal (ectopic) impulse generation and increased mechanosensitivity. Abnormal cross-talk between axons and reflection of impulses back from sites of pathologic involvement can also interfere with information trafficking.

Correlation Between Abnormal Conduction and Clinical Deficits

The human CNS appears to be somewhat resilient to changes in conduction time. This is manifested, for example, by the observation of prolonged latencies in the visual-evoked potential (VEP), in patients who have recovered from optic neuritis. Many of these patients have recovered full visual acuity, normal visual fields, and so forth. Nevertheless, the VEP (which provides an estimate of the conduction time from the retina to the visual cortex) can show a prolonged latency, which represents a "footprint" of residual demyelination that has still not been repaired by the formation of new myelin in these patients. Patients with multiple sclerosis can exhibit excellent vision despite increases in latency of the VEP of tens of milliseconds. This is a good example of the *functional plasticity* of the human CNS.

Although slowed conduction velocity per se does not necessarily cause neurologic deficits, temporal dispersion can have important clinical sequelae. It is well known, for example, that early in the course of demyelinating neuropathies (e.g., early in Landry-Guillain-Barré syndrome and diabetic neuropathy) distal tendon reflexes (e.g., ankle jerks) are reduced or abolished. This is probably explained by a loss of synchrony in afferent action potentials (produced by small degrees of slowing, which result in temporal dispersion) so that temporal summation is lost at the central synapse, where it normally mediates the monosynaptic stretch reflex.

In contrast to slowed conduction velocity, which can remain asymptomatic, conduction block results in a loss of neural information. Thus, it is a major cause of clinical deficits. As noted below, a variety of strategies are being examined by neuroscientists working in laboratories throughout the world in an effort to reverse conduction block in demyelinated axons.

Positive conduction abnormalities also have important clinical sequelae. Increased mechanosensitivity, for example, probably accounts for Tinel's sign (paresthesias elicited by percussion over a diseased peripheral nerve) and Lhermitte's sign (pins-and-needles paresthesia that radiates down the spine and into the limbs and is elicited by flexion of the neck, which stretches the cervical spinal cord and elicits abnormal mechanosensitivity if there is damage to dorsal column axons).

Mechanisms of Conduction Failure in Demyelinated Axons

Several factors contribute significantly to conduction block and decreased conduction velocity at sites of demyelination: the reduced current density in the demyelinated region as a result of the loss of myelin, the paucity of Na^+ channels in the demyelinated axon region, the unmasking of internodal K^+ channels (which had previously been covered by the myelin), and hyperpolarization induced by Na^+, K^+-ATPase activity at sites of demyelination.

Figure 2-5 shows the idealized paths of current flow in normal and demyelinated axon regions. Current generated by the influx of Na^+ ions during the action potential in a normal region of a myelinated fiber (Fig. 2-5A) is shunted without attenuation toward the next node because of the high resistance and low capacitance of the overlying myelin sheath. As a result of its high resistance and low capacitance, the myelin that covers the internode allows for the rapid transfer of charge and reliable activation of the next node. Thus, conduction occurs in myelinated axons with a rapid velocity and a high "safety factor." In contrast, when the myelin is damaged (Fig. 2-5B), the current generated by Na^+ channel activation at a given node is no longer focused on the next node by the insulating sheath but is rather distributed throughout the demyelinated region. The result is a decreased current density and increased charging time of the axon membrane, which can result in either conduction slowing or block.

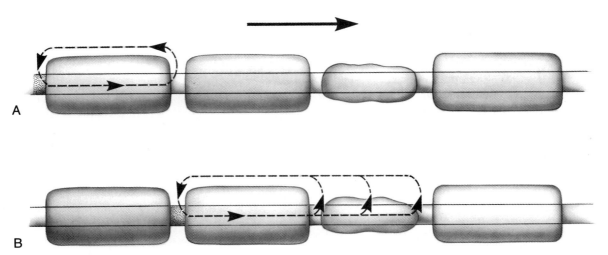

Figure 2-5. Current flow during conduction of the action potential (dotted area) in **(A)** normal region of a myelinated axon and **(B)** in a demyelinated zone. Current flow is shown by dashed arrows. The high-resistance, low-capacitance myelin normally acts as insulation, shunting the current to the next node of Ranvier to ensure rapid, reliable conduction (Fig. A). In demyelinated regions, there is loss of current because of damage to the insulator, so that current is dissipated (Fig. B). As a result, conduction is slowed or blocked.

As discussed above, the density of Na$^+$ channels in the axon membrane is much lower in the internodal part of the axon than at the node of Ranvier. Following acute demyelination, the newly exposed internodal membrane contains an insufficient number of Na$^+$ channels to sustain action potential conduction. Therefore, the nonuniform distribution of Na$^+$ channels along the axon is an important determinant of action potential failure following acute demyelination. In addition, the distribution of K$^+$ channels and pumps, such as Na$^+$, K$^+$-ATPase, appear to contribute to conduction block after demyelination. The unmasking of K$^+$ channels that are normally located under the myelin results in their activation so that they will "clamp" the axon membrane close to the K$^+$ equilibrium potential, E_K, and thus tend to hyperpolarize the axon after demyelination. Moreover, demyelinated axon regions are hyperpolarized by Na$^+$, K$^+$-ATPase activity. Therefore, conduction block in demyelinated axons appears to result from a combination of changes in passive current flow (because of the loss of the myelin per se), inadequate excitability (as a result of the low Na$^+$ channel density in the internodal axon membrane), and hyperpolarization from activation of internodal conductances K$^+$ and electrogenic pumps.

Molecular Plasticity in Demyelinated Axons

Although the density of Na$^+$ channels in the internodal axon membrane is too low to support conduction after acute demyelination, human demyelinating diseases, such as multiple sclerosis, and some experimental models are characterized by remissions characterized by at least partial recovery of the functions lost with demyelination. For example, following a bout of optic neuritis, in which vision is lost as a result of demyelination of the optic nerve or tract, most patients with multiple sclerosis experience an improvement in vision. These remissions occur despite a paucity of remyelination within the CNS. These observations indi-

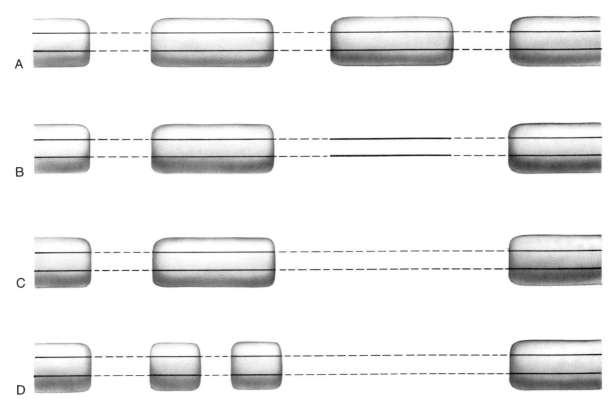

Figure 2-6. Diagram showing postulated events involved in recovery of conduction in demyelinated axon. **(A)** In normally myelinated axon, Na$^+$ channels (dashed lines) are clustered at the nodes of Ranvier. **(B)** After damage to the myelin, the internodal axon membrane is exposed but contains an insufficient density of Na$^+$ channels to support conduction. **(C)** In chronically demyelinated axons, the internodal axon membrane acquires a higher-than-normal density of Na$^+$ channels, so that it can support action potentials. **(D)** Formation of short myelin sheaths at the edge of the demyelinated zone also promotes conduction because the action potential now has to propagate a shorter distance before it invades the demyelinated zone.

cate that recovery of conduction in chronically demyelinated axons can mediate clinical recovery in demyelinating diseases. For conduction to occur through demyelinated axon regions, the axon membrane must acquire enough Na$^+$ channels to support action potential generation. It is now clear that the demyelinated axon membrane can reorganize so that it has a Na$^+$ channel density that is higher than that in a normal internodal axon membrane (Fig. 2-6). For example, immunocytochemical studies have shown the deposition of new Na$^+$ channels in the chronically demyelinated axon membrane. Electrophysiologic studies show changes in conduction that are consistent with increased Na$^+$ channel distribution in demyelinated axolemma. Hot spots of Na$^+$ channels can develop at zones that are destined to become new, remyelinated nodes and can support discontinuous conduction, even before remyelination in peripheral nerve. In other demyelinated axons, conduction can become continuous (similar to the mode of conduction in nonmyelinated axons), as a result of the acquisition of a density of Na$^+$ channels sufficient to support conduction along extended domains within the demyelinated (former internodal) region. The molecular mechanisms responsible for this Na$^+$ channel plasticity are not fully understood and are under study in several laboratories. This reorganization of Na$^+$ channels in demyelinated axons may be dependent on interactions with glial cells.

PHARMACOLOGIC RESTORATION OF CONDUCTION

The distribution of ion channels and pumps on demyelinated axons suggests the possibility of developing pharmacologic agents that might reverse conduction block at sites of demyelination. Drugs that prolong the action potential would be expected to overcome conduction block in demyelinated axons because the increased inward current associated with a prolonged action potential would produce greater depolarization of the axon membrane at the site of demyelination. It is well established that lowering the temperature of demyelinated axons, which prolongs the action potential by altering Na$^+$ channel kinetics, can lead to restoration of conduction. As might be expected, clinical deficits in multiple sclerosis can be improved transiently by lowering the patient's body temperature (conversely, those with multiple sclerosis experience transient worsening of clinical status when the temperature is elevated, e.g., by a fever or in a hot shower).

Pharmacologic studies on the restoration of conduction at sites of experimental demyelination have been carried out with agents that prolong Na$^+$ channel conductance by blocking inactivation and that block the

activation of K$^+$ channels. Prolongation of the action potential and improved conduction are seen in demyelinated spinal roots, sciatic nerve, and dorsal column axons after application of the K$^+$ channel blocking agent 4-AP, which shows preferential blocking effects on fast K$^+$ channels.

Reversal of conduction block in an experimental model of focal demyelination is illustrated in Figure 2-7. A focally demyelinated axon was stimulated on both sides of the lesion, and recordings were obtained with microelectrodes to determine whether action potentials could propagate through the demyelinated zone (Fig. 2-7A). Before treatment with K$^+$ channel blocking drugs, action potentials did not conduct through the lesion (Fig. 2-7B). Thus, there was conduction block at the site of demyelination. To examine whether conduction failure could be reversed by the blockade of fast K$^+$ channels, the nerve was then exposed to 4-AP. As seen in Figure 2-7C, conduction failure in this demyelinated axon was reversed by 4-

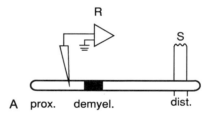

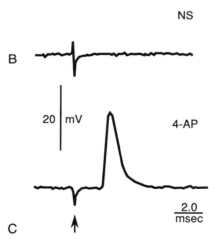

Figure 2-7. Reversal of conduction block in a demyelinated axon with the experimental drug 4-AP. **(A)** An axon, demyelinated in the area marked in black, is stimulated at S, and electrical signals are recorded on the other side of the lesion (R) to determine whether action potentials propagate through the lesion. **(B)** In the absence of potassium channel blockade, there is conduction failure. **(C)** After exposure to the K$^+$ channel blocking drug 4-AP, conduction proceeds through the lesion.

AP. These in vitro results indicate that conduction block in demyelinated axons can be overcome with 4-AP. As discussed above, 4-AP may have a specific action on demyelinated axons because, in normal myelinated axons, the 4-AP-sensitive K^+ channels in the internode are covered by myelin. Phase I trials of 4-AP after traumatic spinal cord injury in dogs have suggested increased sensibility to painful stimuli and increased ability to place the hindlimb after treatment with this drug.

Clinical studies have been carried out to examine the effectiveness of 4-AP and the related drug 3,4-diaminopyridine as a symptomatic therapy in multiple sclerosis and Lambert-Eaton syndrome (on the basis of the rationale that prolongation of the action potential by blockade of fast K^+ channels in the preterminal axon will result in increased neurotransmitter release). These studies report improved motor function in patients with Lambert-Eaton syndrome and some improvement in motor performance, reduction in scotoma size, and improved critical flicker fusion in patients with multiple sclerosis. Further studies will be required to assess the therapeutic potential of 4-AP and related compounds. Nevertheless, it has now been demonstrated, at a minimum, that it is possible to devise rational pharmacologic strategies that reverse conduction failure in demyelinated axons.

Inhibitors of Na^+, K^+-ATPase are also being studied as possible approaches to overcome conduction failure in demyelinated axons. For example, ouabain reduces the hyperpolarization that is seen in demyelinated axons and can lead to restoration of conduction. Systemic application of digitalis improves the latency increase and frequency-following, as measured with somatosensory-evoked potentials in rats with focal demyelinating lesions of the spinal cord. Preliminary studies suggest that some patients with multiple sclerosis may show small clinical improvement concurrent with significant changes in evoked potentials after administration of intravenous digoxin (0.02 mg/kg of body weight). Further work in this area is underway and may be important in the development of symptomatic therapies for multiple sclerosis and related disorders.

INDUCTION OF REMYELINATION IN DEMYELINATED AXON REGIONS

Induction of remyelination is also being examined in some laboratories as an experimental approach that might promote functional recovery in demyelinated axons. To restore conduction, it may not be necessary to remyelinate the denuded axons fully. Remyelination with even abnormally thin myelin sheaths or short internodes can facilitate conduction, assuming that there is an adequate density of Na^+ channels at the nodes formed along the remyelinated axons. Partial remyelination, at the edge of a demyelinated lesion, may also facilitate conduction. Formation of short myelin segments, at the junction between normally myelinated and demyelinated axon regions, would be expected to overcome impedance mismatch and thus encourage impulse invasion into the demyelinated zone (Fig. 2-6D).

Several approaches have been taken to the induction of remyelination within the CNS. One approach focuses on inducing remyelination by existing glial cells. It appears likely that oligodendrocytes and Schwann cells form myelin sheaths after they are instructed to do so by contact with "recognition molecules" or "myelination-inducing molecules" produced by the axon. Molecular neuroscientists are examining the signals that control the initiation of myelination, with the goal of developing interventions that would promote myelin formation via residual oligodendrocytes. Alternative approaches that are being considered might utilize Schwann cells or other myelin-forming cells transplanted to the nervous system. Experimental studies have demonstrated that myelin can be formed by transplanted glial cells; such studies show this new myelin can result in improved conduction. These experimental approaches are relatively new, and it remains to be determined whether they will have therapeutic value.

The occurrence of remissions in multiple sclerosis (see Ch. 73) provides a striking example of the functional plasticity of the human CNS. As outlined above, neuroscientists are beginning to understand the ways in which the CNS can adaptively respond to injury so as to mediate functional recovery. Although this area is in its infancy, it seems not unduly optimistic to expect that, in the future, new therapeutic approaches may facilitate significant functional recovery after the CNS has been damaged by various pathologic insults, including demyelination.

ANNOTATED BIBLIOGRAPHY

Black JA, Kocsis JD, Waxman SG. Ion channel organization of the myelinated fiber. Trends Neurosci 1990;13:48–54.

A review of current understanding of ion channel localization in mammalian axons together with pathophysiologic implications.

Bostock H, Sears TA. The internodal axon membrane: electrical excitability and continuous conduction in segmental demyelination. J Physiol [Lond] 1978;280:273–301.

The first physiologic demonstration of Na^+ channel plasticity in chronically demyelinated axons.

Halliday AM, McDonald WI. Pathophysiology of demyelinating disease. BMJ 1977;33:21–7.

Superb review correlating clinical abnormalities, clinical electrophysiology, and basic mechanisms of symptom production.

Kocsis JD, Waxman SG. Absence of potassium conductance in central myelinated axons. Nature 1980;287:348–9.

Early demonstration of the absence of 4-AP-sensitive potassium channels at the node of Ranvier.

Rasminsky M. Hyperexcitability of pathologically myelinated axons and positive symptoms in multiple sclerosis, in Waxman SG, Ritchie JM (eds). Demyelinating Disease: Basic and Clinical Electrophysiology. Raven Press, New York, 1981, pp.289–98.

Excellent discussion of positive signs and symptoms in multiple sclerosis and their physiologic basis.

Ritchie JM, Rogart RB. The density of sodium channels in mammalian myelinated nerve fibers and the nature of the axonal membrane under the myelin sheath. Proc Natl Acad Sci USA 1977;72:211–5.

First study to use saxitoxin to study sodium channel distribution in myelinated fibers.

Sears TA, Bostock H. Conduction failure in demyelination: is it inevitable?, in Waxman SG, Ritchie JM (eds). Demyelinating Disease: Basic and Clinical Electrophysiology. Raven Press, New York, 1981, pp. 353–75.

Excellent discussion of conduction failure in demyelination and physiologic mechanisms that underlie recovery from conduction block.

Targ EG, Kocsis JD. 4-Aminopyridine leads to restoration of conduction in demyelinated rat sciatic nerve. Brain Res 1985;328:358–61.

Early demonstration of reversal of conduction block with 4-AP.

Waxman SG. Conduction in myelinated, unmyelinated, and demyelinated fibers. Arch Neurol 1977;34:585–90.

Early morphologic demonstration of the differential structure of the axon membrane at the node of Ranvier compared with the internode, together with a discussion of pathophysiologic implications.

Waxman SG, Ransom BR, Stys PK. Non-synaptic mechanisms of calcium-mediated injury in CNS white matter. Trends Neurosci 1991;14:461–8.

A review of the molecular mechanisms that underlie anoxic injury in white matter axons. This articles provides a basis for understanding the pathophysiology of lacunar stroke.

3

Inflammation in the Nervous System

H. Lassmann and K. Vass

The nervous system may be affected by the immune system in two different situations: immune surveillance and immune defense against potentially pathogenic agents. Both require the entry of immunocompetent cells into the nervous system, but once they have reached their destination, the task of the cells is fundamentally different. During immune surveillance, immune cells screen for possible pathogens but leave the elements of the nervous system untouched. During immune defense, by contrast, the pathogens that have already entered the nervous system have to be eliminated, and effective removal and destruction of the targets is required in the course of the inflammatory process. Such destruction and removal cannot be completely selective and also results in "bystander damage" to the surrounding tissue, although this has to be minimized as far as possible.

When basic pathogenetic aspects of inflammation in the nervous system are discussed, the following questions have to be addressed: (1) How do immunocompetent cells enter the nervous system under the conditions of immune surveillance or established inflammation? (2) Where and how in the nervous system is the specific antigen recognized by the immune system? (3) Are there special regulatory circuits that locally tune the sensitivity and degree of the immune reaction in the nervous system? (4) What immunologic mechanisms lead to the destruction and elimination of pathogens from the nervous system and what is their role in the induction of "bystander damage"? (5) How is the inflammatory reaction terminated and, in particular, how do inflammatory cells leave the nervous system during clearance of inflammatory lesions?

PRINCIPAL ASPECTS OF BRAIN INFLAMMATION
Entry of Inflammatory Cells Into the Nervous System

For a long time, the nervous system was considered to be an immunoprivileged organ. This concept was based on the existence of a blood-brain barrier, which impeded the entry of immunocompetent cells, antibodies, and immunologic mediators. As a consequence, the normal nervous system was thought to be not only devoid of hematogenous cells but also lacking in the expression of molecules such as class I or class II major histocompatibility complex (MHC) antigens, which are important for antigen recognition and presentation and are regulated by immune system-derived cytokines.

The concept of immune privilege, however, can no longer be maintained. For a long time, neurologists knew that the cerebrospinal fluid (CSF) of normal individuals contains a small number of hematogenous cells, in particular T lymphocytes, a sign that some entry occurred routinely. In addition, more recent neuropathologic studies revealed that, within the normal brain of laboratory animals and humans few lymphocytes and monocytes are present in meninges, perivascular spaces, and parenchyma. Class I and class II MHC molecules are present on meningeal and perivascular monocytic cell populations and may sometimes be found on parenchymal microglia and ependyma under normal conditions. All these data indicate that there is a continuous exchange of hematogenous cells between the circulation and the brain. A similar situation also holds true for serum proteins. As an example, immunoglobulins enter the central nervous system (CNS) through the normal blood-brain barrier only to a very limited degree. However, the barrier is not complete. Thus, the prolonged presence of high titers of autoantibodies in the blood may be involved in disease induction, as in paraneoplastic syndromes. Furthermore, certain cytokines may even pass the normal blood-brain barrier by an active transport mechanism.

Despite these insights, little is known on the turnover of hematogenous cells in the normal brain. Peri-

vascular and meningeal monocytes are largely replaced by newly ingrowing hematogenous cells within
1 to 3 months. On the contrary, the resident microglia
constitutes a stable pool with little replacement, even
under pathologic conditions.

T lymphocytes are present in the normal brain only

for short periods. After intravenous injection, T lymphocytes reach the brain within 3 hours and leave the
nervous system after 1 day. Only activated T lymphocytes are allowed to enter the brain through the intact
blood-brain barrier, whereas resting T cells are locked
out. These observations mean that, in the course of

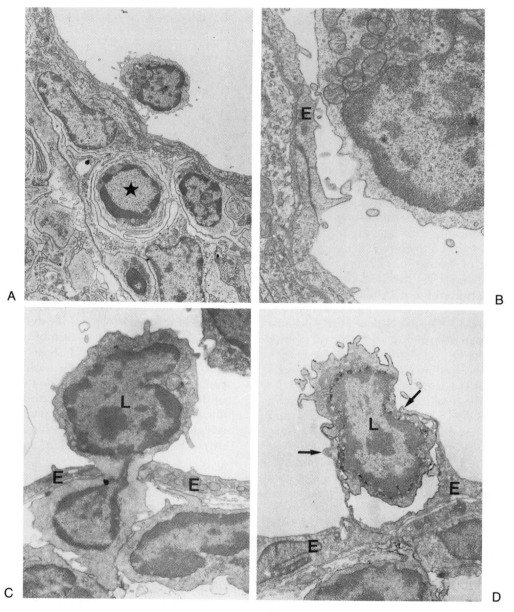

Figure 3-1. Migration of inflammatory cells through the blood-brain barrier. **(A)** Binding of inflammatory cell to the luminal surface of the endothelial cell as a first step in the transmigration process. In the
perivascular infiltrate, one lymphocyte (*star*) shows early nuclear changes of programmed cell death.
(× 4,000.) **(B)** Detail from Fig. A. Cell processes of endothelial cell (*E*) and leukocyte contact each other.
(× 20,000.) **(C)** Migration of a (probably activated) lymphocyte (*L*) through the endothelium of a meningeal vessel. The endothelial cell (*E*) has a smooth (nonactivated) surface. (× 13,000.) **(D)** T lymphocytes
(*L*), identified by immune electron microscopy for the α/β-T-cell receptor, is caught by cell processes of
"activated" cerebral endothelium (*E*). (× 9,000.)

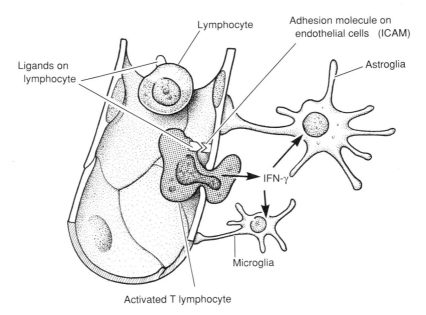

Figure 3-2. Immune surveillance in the normal brain. Only activated T lymphocytes can pass the blood-brain barrier. The normal, resting endothelium has only a very low expression of adhesion molecules. After specific antigen are encountered, T lymphocytes activate cells of the nervous system and endothelial cells by local production of cytokines (mainly interferon-γ).

peripheral immune activation, such as an acute infection, some activated T lymphocytes will pass the blood-brain barrier, enter the nervous system, and search for the respective antigen (Figs. 3-1 and 3-2). If the antigen is not present in the nervous system, the cells will disappear rapidly and without consequences. On the other hand, when the antigen is found by the activated T lymphocytes in the course of immune surveillance, an inflammatory reaction will be initiated.

The passage of inflammatory cells through the blood-brain barrier at the site of active inflammation is fundamentally different from that in the normal brain. Within a given inflammatory focus in the nervous system, only a small percentage (1 to 4 percent) of the inflammatory cells in fact are antigen specific. All other cells are secondarily recruited into the inflammatory focus and include T lymphocytes, B lymphocytes, monocytes/macrophages, and polymorphonuclear leukocytes. At this stage of inflammation, not only activated but also resting cells are recruited into the lesions, and it is the blood-brain barrier endothelium that actively catches and guides circulating immune cells into the established inflammatory focus (Figs. 3-1 and 3-3).

Another mechanism by which inflammatory cells can be attracted into the nervous system operates in bacterial meningitis and encephalitis. In this case, bacterial products and toxins, both directly or through other chemotactic factors such as interleukin-8, recruit effector cells, mainly granulocytes and macrophages, into the nervous system. This happens before a specific immune response against bacterial antigens can occur. Also, in this situation, the dynamics of the reaction in the nervous system differ from those in other organs. For instance, if lipopolysaccharide, one of the major immune stimulatory molecules of bacterial walls, is directly injected into the nervous system, recruitment of granulocytes requires much longer time and higher lipopolysaccharide concentrations compared with the situation after injection at other sites of the body.

Adhesion Molecules Mediate the Binding of Inflammatory Cells to the Blood-Brain Barrier Endothelium and Their Migration Through the Vessel Wall

Studies on immune surveillance of the nervous system reveal that T lymphocytes migrate through the blood-brain barrier in an antigen-independent manner. In addition, the recruitment of effector cells, such as monocytes, natural killer cells, or granulocytes, must involve antigen-independent adhesion mechanisms.

Recent in vitro and in vivo studies indicate that leukocyte adhesion molecules play a key role in the interaction between inflammatory cells and the vascular endothelium. Adhesion molecules are cell surface receptors that interact with specific partners on the surface of other cells or with extracellular matrix mole-

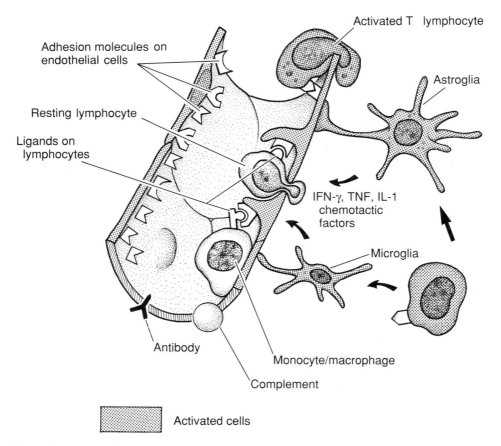

Figure 3-3. Inflammatory focus. Activated endothelial cells express higher levels of adhesion molecules and actively catch inflammatory cells. Only a small number are antigen-specific cells; the others are resting lymphocytes (T and B cells), monocytes, and polymorphonuclear leukocytes. Local production of cytokines and chemotactic factors by these cells and by autochthonous cells of the nervous system (astrocytes, microglial cells, and Schwann cells) helps to recruit more inflammatory cells of the blood-brain barrier.

cules. Biochemically, adhesion molecules can be classified into major groups:

The *selectins* are lectinlike proteins that specifically interact with carbohydrate moieties on cell surface proteins or lipids. Because selectins are glycoproteins, they also tend to interact in a homotypic way.

The *integrins* are heterodimeric proteins that are mainly involved in cell matrix interactions. They act as receptors for complement, fibronectin, vitronectin, fibrin, and other extracellular structures. They may, however, also mediate cell-to-cell interactions by binding to certain adhesion molecules of the immunoglobulin gene superfamily.

The *immunoglobulinlike adhesion molecules* are integral membrane proteins, which contain immunoglobulin loop domains in their extracellular portion. These molecules either interact with each other or with integrins. Other adhesion molecules may either be complex proteoglycans or may represent variable

proteins or lipids with conserved carbohydrate domains.

Migration of inflammatory cells through the vessel wall requires several consecutive steps. First, the cells mediate lose binding to the endothelial cells, reflected by a slow rolling along the endothelial surface. This initial binding step is mainly mediated by selectins. Then, the cells attach firmly to the endothelial cell surface. This second step is due to the interaction between integrins and immunoglobulinlike adhesion molecules. Finally, the cells penetrate the endothelial barrier and the subendothelial basement membrane. For this third step, hyaluronidase and, possibly, proteolytic enzymes together with active cell mobility are required. These steps of leukocyte emigration through the vascular wall are similar in all organs of the body, yet the nervous system differs in some aspects.

In comparison to vessels elsewhere in the body, blood-brain barrier endothelial cells mediate a lower basal level of adhesiveness toward leukocytes. This may explain why there is only a low exchange of inflammatory cells through the normal blood-brain barrier. There is, however, some expression of immunoglobulin adhesion molecules on endothelial cells (intercellular adhesion molecules [ICAM]) in normal brain endothelia, especially in venules. Activation of lymphocytes leads to conformational changes of leukocyte function-associated antigen 1 (LFA1), the binding partner of ICAMs. This is associated with a dramatic increase in the binding affinity between these two molecules. Only activated lymphocytes are able to bind to and pass through the normal blood-brain barrier endothelium (Fig. 3-4).

When an inflammatory focus is already established, a variety of other adhesion molecules are upregulated at the endothelial surface, which leads to recruitment of inflammatory cells into the lesions and is similar to that in other organs of the body (Fig. 3-4).

Apparently, selective patterns of cell recruitment exist because different types of inflammatory cells dominate different pathologic conditions. In a disease that is dominated by T lymphocytes, such as autoimmune encephalomyelitis, the interaction between vascular cell adhesion molecules and very late antigen 4 (Fig. 3-4) appears to be of critical importance for the maintenance of the inflammatory lesions. In contrast, in brain lesions that are predominantly mediated by macrophages, the interaction between ICAMs and LFA1 (Fig. 3-4) seems to be prominent. Although our understanding of the mechanisms is still fragmentary, interference with adhesion molecule function may lead to a promising area of anti-inflammatory therapy.

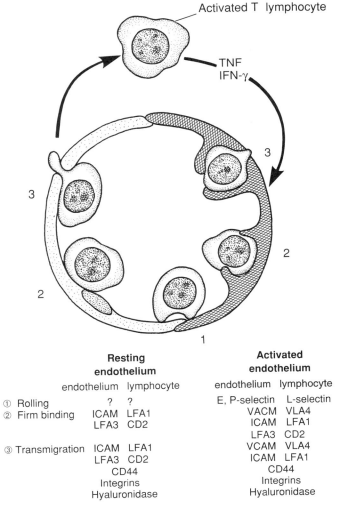

	Resting endothelium		Activated endothelium	
	endothelium	lymphocyte	endothelium	lymphocyte
① Rolling	?	?	E, P-selectin	L-selectin
② Firm binding	ICAM	LFA1	VACM	VLA4
	LFA3	CD2	ICAM	LFA1
			LFA3	CD2
③ Transmigration	ICAM	LFA1	VCAM	VLA4
	LFA3	CD2	ICAM	LFA1
		CD44		CD44
		Integrins		Integrins
		Hyaluronidase		Hyaluronidase

Figure 3-4. Transmigration of inflammatory cells through resting and activated endothelial cells of the blood-brain barrier.

The Role of Cytokines and Chemotactic Factors in Leukocyte Migration Through the Blood-Brain Barrier

Inflammatory mediators can be involved in the recruitment of leukocytes into the nervous system by two different means. First, they may directly attract inflammatory cells into the lesions. Such chemokines are locally produced, either by inflammatory cells or by local tissue components, and specifically attract neutrophils or monocytes. To perform their task, they have to reach and activate their target cells. When synthesized in the brain component, they have to pass the blood-brain barrier to reach leukocytes in the circulation or on the surface of cerebral endothelial cells. Therefore, they act only when the blood-brain barrier is predamaged in an inflammatory lesion. As an example, interleukin-8, although of critical importance in the inflammatory reaction of bacterial meningitis, does not induce inflammation when injected into the normal CSF. It is important to note that factors locally produced by the nervous system may have chemokine function. Recently, it was shown that neuropeptides, such as substance P, may have a chemotactic activity for macrophages. Thus, not only factors produced by the immune system are involved in leukocyte recruitment. Second, leukocyte recruitment to the brain also occurs by stimulating the expression of adhesion molecules on the endothelial surface. At present, the most important cytokines in this process are interleukin-1, tumor necrosis factor-α, and interferon-γ. However, in this setting, the blood-brain barrier also acts differently from other vascular systems in the body. As an example, atraumatic injection of tumor necrosis factor-α into the normal CNS has little or no effect on leukocyte recruitment. However, when the blood-brain barrier is predamaged, extensive inflammation is induced.

All the data on leukocyte migration through the blood-brain barrier suggest that traffic of inflammatory cells into the normal brain is kept minimal and selectively allows only those cells to enter that are absolutely required for immune surveillance. However, when inflammation is started, the secondary recruitment of leukocytes into the brain is accomplished in the same way and extent as everywhere else in the body.

Sites of Antigen Recognition for T-Cell-Mediated Inflammation

T lymphocytes can only be activated by specific antigens in the context of products of the MHC antigens. MHC antigens provide specialized binding sites for polypeptide chains and are predominantly expressed on bone marrow-derived cells. These cells must process putative antigenic proteins and polypeptide chains and combine them with either class I or class II MHC antigens by specific internal pathways.

Class I antigens predominantly combine with internal antigens, including viral proteins, whereas class II antigens generally combine with antigens taken up from the extracellular space into the endosomal/lysosomal pathway. Class I antigens activate CD8 antigen-expressing T lymphocytes; CD4 cells recognize antigen together with class II. The type of T cell that is activated, assisted by a locally produced cocktail of cytokines, then determines the further actions of the immune system, such as activation of effector pathways, stimulation of antibody production, or suppression of the immune reaction. Thus, MHC antigen-expressing cells, as the sites of antigen presentation, must have a prominent strategic position in the organization of an immune response.

Within the nervous system, a hierarchy of antigen-presenting, MHC-expressing cells with a peculiar spatial organization and a concentration along blood-brain interfaces is obvious. Under normal, resting conditions, MHC class I and II antigens can only be found on monocytic cells in meningeal and perivascular positions. Along with these constitutively MHC-expressing cells, some microglial cells with processes within the perivascular glia limitans and endoneurial macrophages in peripheral nerves are MHC positive. Class I antigens are also found on endothelial cells, whereas endothelial cells are mostly class II negative, at least under in vivo conditions. Meningeal and perivascular monocytic cells alone are sufficient as antigen-presenting cells in the induction of encephalitis, and there is good reason to regard these meningeal and perivascular cells as the first line of antigen presentation in immunologic defense of the brain.

During an inflammatory reaction, the intensity of MHC expression increases. In addition, almost all microglial cells become class I and II positive. Thus, for the CNS, the network of microglia can be regarded as the second line of defense.

The third line is the neuroectodermal cells, such as astrocytes, ependymal cells, and Schwann cells. Nerve cells, oligodendrocytes, and myelin are consistently negative for class II MHC antigens but, occasionally, can express class I. This is in line with the concept that there is no direct antigen presentation to CD4-positive lymphocytes on myelin or oligodendroglia in autoimmune demyelinating diseases and that the relevant antigens have to be liberated into the extracellular space to be processed and presented by specialized presenter cells. However, direct cytotoxic attack, mediated by class I-restricted, CD8-positive T cells or by γ/δ cells appears to be possible.

That MHC-expressing meningeal and perivascular monocytes are sufficient to mediate antigen presentation in autoimmune encephalomyelitis raises a question about the role of neuroectodermal cells in this process. In certain models of virus-induced demyelinating disorders, the genetic potential of antigen presentation by astrocytes was shown to correlate with disease susceptibility. In addition, the pathogenicity of autoimmune T-lymphocyte lines paralleled their ability to recognize antigen on astrocytes. Local upregulation of MHC expression within the CNS by various insults may precipitate inflammation in autoimmune encephalomyelitis.

However, a role for antigen-presenting astrocytes in the downregulation of CNS inflammation has to be considered. Under certain in vitro conditions, astrocytes, in the presence of a specific antigen, suppress rather than stimulate T-cell activation. This is in line with the poor proliferative response of T lymphocytes within brain lesions of autoimmune encephalomyelitis. Thus, astrocytes may be not as important as antigen presenters for the development of an inflammatory lesion, but rather they may be a central immunomodulatory cell within the CNS. This notion is further underlined by the great variety of cytokines

not only with stimulatory but also with suppressive action that can be produced by these cells.

Mechanisms of Tissue Damage in Inflammatory Lesions of the Nervous System

The presence of inflammatory cells within the nervous system may have deleterious consequences for local tissue. Damage can be induced either by antigen specific ways or in an antigen-independent manner (Fig. 3-5). T-cell-mediated antigen-specific damage in the CNS appears to be a rare phenomenon. This is mainly due to the poor expression of MHC antigens on neuroectodermal cells in the brain. However, in some models of virus encephalomyelitis, class I MHC-restricted T-cell-mediated cytotoxicity may contribute to the destruction of virus-infected neuroectodermal cells. In autoimmunity, in vitro studies show that antigen-presenting astrocytes or Schwann cells can be destroyed by class II-restricted T lymphocytes. This mechanism may play a role, especially in the mechanisms of demyelination in experimental and human inflammatory polyradiculoneuritis.

Recently, it was suggested that γ/δ- T lymphocytes

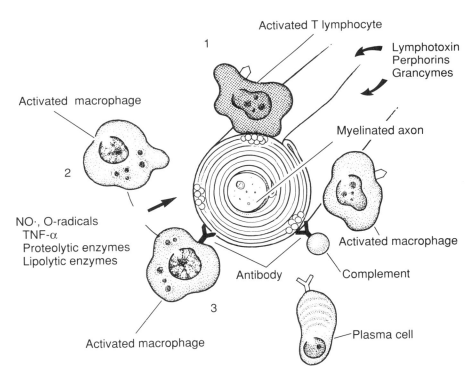

Figure 3-5. Tissue destruction by inflammatory cells. Within the nervous system, the most sensitive structures are oligodendrocytes and myelin sheaths. (*1*) Cytotoxic T lymphocytes can directly attack these structures. (*2*) Macrophages, activated by local T cells, can induce tissue damage by a variety of mechanisms ("bystander" damage). (*3*) The sensitivity of this macrophage-induced damage is dramatically increased if macrophages are opsonized by antibodies to surface eptiopes of the myelin sheath (antibody-dependent cellular cytotoxicity). (*4*) By binding of complement, antibodies themselves can induce demyelination.

may play an important role in demyelination in multiple sclerosis. Such γ-δ-T lymphocytes, which are directed against stress proteins, can selectively destroy oligodendrocytes in vitro. These cells are found in the inflammatory infiltrates of patients with multiple sclerosis and may therefore damage oligodendrocytes that are stressed in the course of the inflammatory reaction.

An effective and specific way to induce tissue damage in the nervous system is mediated by antibodies directed against antigens expressed on the surface of brain cells. These target antigens may either be foreign antigens in brain infections or may be autoantigens. In this situation, antibody-labeled structures are either recognized by activated macrophages or destroyed by activated complement. Because of the poor penetration through the normal blood-brain barrier, antibodies damage the nervous system, in general, only in the presence of a pre-existing inflammatory reaction induced by other immunologic means, such as a T-cell-mediated reaction.

Antibodies appear to play a major role in the pathogenesis of certain chronic virus-induced inflammatory diseases of the nervous system, such as subacute sclerosing panencephalitis. Furthermore, in inflammatory demyelinating disease, the presence of demyelinating antibodies may lead to widespread primary demyelination and, thus, may be especially important in the pathogenesis of multiple sclerosis.

A less specific way to induce tissue damage in the course of inflammation in the nervous system is by the activation of effector cells, especially of macrophages or granulocytes. In this case, the tissue can be damaged directly by the toxic products that are liberated from activated macrophages. These toxins include oxygen radicals, nitric oxide radicals, cytotoxic cytokines (such as tumor necrosis factor-α), and proteolytic and lipolytic enzymes. In addition, because of the increased blood-brain barrier permeability, cytotoxic serum proteins, such as complement components, enter the nervous system and also damage the tissue.

High local concentrations of these factors not only eliminate pathogens from the lesions but also induce a variable amount of "bystander damage" to nerve and glia cells. However, myelin and oligodendrocytes are by far the most sensitive in regard to the toxic action of complement and macrophage products. Thus, in chronic inflammatory conditions, myelin is damaged and lost to a greater extent than are other structures of the nervous system. This may explain in part why chronic autoimmune diseases of the CNS and peripheral nervous system reflect inflammatory demyelinating pathologic findings.

Especially in acute inflammatory brain diseases, a whole secondary cascade of events is triggered by the immunologic reaction. Inflammatory mediators act on the predamaged blood-brain barrier, increase its permeability, and induce vasogenic brain edema. In addition, the expression of endothelial adhesion molecules is upregulated; together with endothelial damage, this can lead to thrombosis and vascular occlusion. This further potentiates the tissue damage by ischemia. Toxic factors, liberated during tissue damage, such as excitotoxins or arachidonic acid metabolites, further potentiate the lesions and may induce cytotoxic brain edema. If this vicious circle is not stopped, life-threatening complications are inevitable. For all these reasons, the goal of therapy of inflammatory diseases of the nervous system is not only to eliminate responsible pathogens from the lesions. In all situations, therapeutic measures of immune suppression, antiedema therapy, and anticoagulation therapy have also to be considered.

Termination of Inflammation in the Central and Peripheral Nervous System

Surprisingly little is known on the mechanisms involved in the termination of an inflammatory response in the brain. Obviously, elimination of specific pathogens will eventually lead to clearance of inflammation from the nervous system in bacterial and viral encephalitis. However, even in autoimmune diseases such as acute disseminated encephalitis, inflammation subsides, although the target antigen cannot be eliminated from the nervous system.

Up to now, several different mechanisms have been identified that may be responsible for downregulation of the immune response in the nervous system. In autoimmune encephalomyelitis, recovery from the disease coincides with the peak of corticosteroid secretion in the adrenal glands. Furthermore, the susceptibility for autoimmune encephalomyelitis to some extent correlates with the steroid response evoked after immunization, and adrenalectomy massively potentiates the disease. Not surprisingly, high-dose corticosteroid therapy is effective in experimental and human inflammatory demyelinating diseases.

Another possible mechanism in the downregulation of brain inflammation is the local production of immunosuppressive cytokines. Transforming growth factor-β is one possible example. It is locally produced within inflammatory brain lesions of experimental animals and humans. Despite its having a variety of different effects on immune cells, this cytokine has been shown to suppress experimental autoimmune encephalomyelitis effectively.

Clearance of inflammation in the brain raises a question about the fate of inflammatory cells in the lesions. Recent evidence may explain the elimination

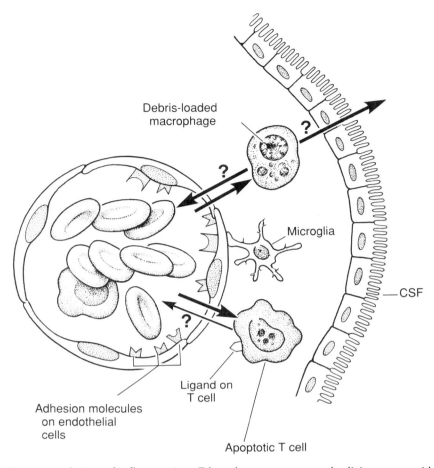

Debris-loaded
macrophage

?

?

Microglia

CSF

Ligand on
T cell

Adhesion molecules
on endothelial
cells

?

Apoptotic T cell

Figure 3-6. Downregulation of inflammation. T lymphocytes apparently disintegrate within the inflammatory focus. One possible mechanism is apoptosis. The clearing of loaded macrophages is so far not fully understood. They leave the nervous system either by the brain-blood barrier or by the ependyma into the CSF.

of inflammatory cells. Within the infiltrates in the CNS and peripheral nervous system, a large proportion of T lymphocytes show the typical morphologic alterations of apoptosis (programmed cell death). This indicates that most T lymphocytes do not leave the inflammatory focus in the brain but are locally destroyed when inflammation subsides. In contrast, programmed cell death in other inflammatory cells (monocytes, macrophages, or granulocytes) is exceptionally rare. These cells presumably leave the CNS, either through the CSF space or the brain-blood barrier, in an as yet undefined way (Fig. 3-6).

It is not resolved at present what mechanisms induce programmed cell death of T lymphocytes in inflammatory brain lesions. High doses of steroids can drive mature T cells into apoptosis. This may be an additional explanation for the beneficial action of steroid megadose therapy in multiple sclerosis. In addition, however, local factors, such as cytotoxic cytokines

or imbalanced signal transduction in the course of antigen presentation by neuroectodermal cells, may be even more important for the induction of T-lymphocyte apoptosis during spontaneous remissions of inflammatory brain diseases.

IMPLICATIONS FOR NEUROLOGIC DISEASE

Bacterial and Viral Infections of the Nervous System

The separation of the brain from the immune system by the blood-brain barrier and the particular mechanisms for cells of the immune system to pass the barrier has many consequences for the pathogenesis of bacterial or viral infections of the nervous system.

In bacterial meningitis, the concentration of bacteria within the CSF has to reach a critical concentration of 10^6 cells/ml before an inflammatory reaction starts. This apparently is due to the previously discussed fact that proinflammatory mechanisms induced by bacterial cell wall components are less effective in the nervous system compartments than elsewhere in the body. As a negative consequence, the bacterial load is already advanced when immunologic defense mechanisms are starting to work.

Another consequence of the mentioned peculiarities of the blood-brain barrier is that bacterial or viral antigens or whole organisms may become sequestered within the brain compartment. An example is human immunodeficiency virus (HIV) infection of the nervous system. HIV is carried into the brain by infected leukocytes in the course of immunosurveillance, and the infection of the brain occurs early after systemic infection. There it spreads into the stable pool of microglial cells, where it is protected from vigorous elimination by effector mechanisms that are effective in other tissues of the body. It remains in the CNS from the beginning of the incubation period of acquired immunodeficiency syndrome and will possibly also escape antiviral therapy.

Finally, infectious diseases of the nervous system may secondarily induce autoimmune reactions that by themselves may become pathogenic. Infection of laboratory animals with corona virus or measles virus, after a first episode of acute virus encephalitis, may lead to a more chronic demyelinating leukoencephalitis. In such animals, T lymphocytes that are specific for myelin basic protein can be recovered that can transfer the same disease to naive recipients. Such virus-induced autoimmunity may play a major role in the induction of human inflammatory demyelinating diseases, such as multiple sclerosis.

Autoimmunity and Nervous System Inflammation

Immunization of animals or humans with whole tissue or components of the CNS or peripheral nervous system leads, through autoimmunity, to acute or chronic inflammatory disease of the nervous system. The pathologic findings in these diseases are uniform. They mainly involve the white matter and are characterized by inflammation and demyelination. In humans, autoimmunity after sensitization against brain tissue may lead to acute disseminated leukoencephalitis, acute hemorrhagic leukoencephalitis, and multiple sclerosis-like syndromes.

The uniform induction of inflammatory demyelinating disease of the nervous system by autoimmunity led to the concept that only antigens in myelin sheaths are recognized during the autoimmune process. Indeed, for a long time, myelin basic protein, a major component of the myelin sheath, has been regarded as the sole target antigen for nervous system-specific autoimmunity.

However, antigens such as myelin basic protein are recognized by T cells not at the myelin sheath or in oligodendrocytes. In particular, the antigen has to be processed and presented in the context of MHC molecules by specialized presenter cells to be recognized by a T-cell-mediated immune response. As discussed earlier, constitutive MHC expression in the normal CNS is restricted to meningeal and perivascular monocytic cells, and antigen presentation by these cells alone is sufficient to induce a T-cell-mediated encephalitis. Thus, the major requirement for an antigen located within the CNS to become a target for T-cell-mediated autoimmune encephalitis is that it is liberated into the brain extracellular space in the course of physiologic turnover and, therefore, reaches the perivascular or meningeal pool of presenter cells. From these concepts, it can be predicted that not only myelin basic protein but also multiple CNS proteins may become targets in autoimmunologically mediated encephalomyelitis. After a more systematic search, it turned out that many more components of the CNS and peripheral nervous system may be recognized in the course of a pathogenic autoimmune response. They include myelin basic protein, proteolipid protein, myelin oligodendroglia glycoprotein, myelin-associated glycoprotein, and others. It can be predicted that this list of putative target antigens for cerebral autoimmune diseases will even grow longer in the coming years.

These recent discoveries have major implications for research in demyelinating diseases such as multiple sclerosis. The search for possible autoimmune responses has to be extended to many more antigens, and it is likely that the disease in different patients with multiple sclerosis is induced by autoimmune reactions against different antigens. This further implies that antigen-specific therapy may become difficult in patients with multiple sclerosis.

The multiplicity of possible target autoantigens for inflammatory demyelinating diseases raises another paradox: Why are the lesions concentrated in the white matter, and why is myelin primarily affected in these diseases? It now becomes clear that the distribution of the lesions has more to do with the density of draining veins and venules than with the presence of myelin. Furthermore, the dominance of demyelination may be explained in part by the higher susceptibility of myelin compared with that of other structures of the nervous system for macrophage-mediated cytotoxicity. Additional mechanisms, such as demyelinating autoantibodies, may also be important in the pathogenesis of multiple sclerosis.

Transplantation and Rejection of Brain Tissue

Contrary to other locations in the body, histoincompatible or even xenogenic nervous tissue may be tolerated for extended periods when transplanted directly into the brain. However, when a second peripheral transplantation is performed with incompatible tissue, the brain transplant is immediately rejected in parallel with the second peripheral transplant. A similar vigorous rejection of histoincompatible brain transplants can be provoked by generalized immune stimulation in the course of infections or cytokine treatment. Because T lymphocytes pass the blood-brain barrier only in an activated stage, this peripheral immune stimulation appears to be required to bring enough specific T cells into the CNS and to induce sufficient MHC antigen expression for effective rejection of a brain transplant. It is not clear yet whether brain transplant rejection is mediated mainly by class I or class II MHC-restricted T-cell responses.

It has been argued that MHC mapping is less crucial for transplantation of the brain compared with other tissues. Although this is true for a single transplant in individuals not exposed to infectious pathogens or other immune stimulation, this goal is neither easy to achieve nor desirable in transplanted patients. Thus, for brain tissue transplantation, the same rules of MHC mapping have to be followed as in the transplantation of other organs.

CONCLUSIONS

Because of its delicate function and its lack of regenerating capacity, the brain has to be surveyed by the immune system in a specially balanced way. This surveillance not only has to be sufficient to protect from infection and to eliminate pathogens, but it also has to keep secondary damage to the surrounding tissue as low as possible. This goal is achieved by several different means. First, the blood-brain barrier separates the brain from the immune system under normal conditions and allows only access of a small population of activated T lymphocytes for immune surveillance. Second, when inflammation is already established, local production of immune mediators can counteract the immunologic process. Third, T lymphocytes are efficiently eliminated from established inflammatory brain lesions by programmed cell death, a mechanism that also prevents overshooting inflammatory reactions. It is obvious that a failure of these mechanisms during infectious diseases or autoimmunity may lead to life-threatening conditions.

ANNOTATED BIBLIOGRAPHY

Gallagher RB (ed): Leucocyte-endothelial cell interaction. Immunol Today 1992;13:86–112.

A special issue, containing three extensive reviews on the interaction of granulocytes, lymphocytes, and platelets with endothelial cells.

Fontana A, Constam DB, Frei K et al. Modulation of the immune response by transforming growth factor beta. Int Arch Allergy Immunol 1992;99:1–7.

Review of the role of cytokines in brain inflammation with special reference to the inhibitory effects of transforming growth factor-beta.

Lassmann H (ed). Inflammation and the blood brain barrier. Brain Pathol 1991;1:88–123.

Special issue devoted to the interaction of inflammatory cells with the blood-brain barrier, containing four reviews on migration of inflammatory cells through the barrier, sites of antigen recognition in vivo, interaction of T cells and endothelial cells in vitro, and expression of adhesion molecules on cerebral vessels.

Lassmann H, Zimprich F, Rossler K, Vass K. Inflammation in the nervous system. Basic mechanisms and immunological concepts. Rev Neurol 1991;147:763–81.

Extensive review on basic aspects of brain inflammation, containing more than 230 references for further reading.

Mason D. Genetic variation in the stress response: susceptibility to experimental allergic encephalomyelitis and implications for human inflammatory disease. Immunol Today 1991;12:57–60.

Detailed summary of the role of the corticosteroid response in the regulation of autoimmune encephalomyelitis. Critical discussion of mechanisms that control and terminate inflammation.

Olsson T. Immunology of multiple sclerosis. Curr Opin Neurol Neurosurg 1992;5:195–202.

Summary and critical review of T- and B-cell responses against various target antigens in autoimmune encephalitis and multiple sclerosis.

Perry HV, Andersson PB, Gordon S. Macrophages and inflammation in the central nervous system. Trends Neurosci 1993;16:268–73.

Critical discussion on the mechanisms by which macrophages may damage brain tissue in the course of inflammation.

Quagliarello V, Scheld WM. Bacterial meningitis: pathogenesis, pathophysiology and progress. N Engl J Med 1992; 327:864–72.

Recent extensive review with complete survey of the current literature on the pathogenesis of bacterial meningitis.

Sloan DJ, Wood MJ, Charlton HM. The immune response to intracerebral neural grafts. Trends Neurosci 1991;14: 341–6.

Review on the immunologic reactions in brain tissue grafting, included in a special issue on general possibilities and problems of brain grafting.

4

Molecular Genetics of Neurologic Disease

P. H. St. George-Hyslop

BASIC MECHANISMS IN GENETIC DISEASES

Genetic diseases are the clinical result of an inherited aberration in a gene product (Table 4-1 provides a glossary of genetic terms used in this chapter) or in the expression of a gene that, on interacting with environmental and other genetic factors, leads to a physiologic defect as a disease phenotype. Because the mode of inheritance of a genetic disease trait can be easily identified by direct inspection of the segregation pattern within a family, genetic diseases tend to be classified according to the apparent mode of inheritance (autosomal recessive, autosomal dominant, sex-linked, and so forth). This mode of classification frequently reflects differences in the functional and clinically evident effect of the underlying mutation.

Recessive Traits

In recessive traits, the most common functional effect of disease mutations is either a gene product that has impaired function or the failure to generate a gene product in adequate quantities. At a molecular level, the mutations that underlie recessive traits are either single-base substitutions (also known as point mutations) or more extensive structural rearrangements of the genomic DNA sequence (e.g., duplications, deletions, or inversions). These mutations interfere with the genetic information encoded in genomic DNA or with its subsequent processing through transcription into RNA and translation into a peptide by at least five different molecular mechanisms (Figs. 4-1 and 4-2).

First, mutations can disrupt the normal function of the protein by the substitution of the wrong amino acid directly within catalytic or other functional sites of the protein. Such mutations are referred to as mis-sense mutations and are typically caused by single-base substitutions in coding sequences of genes. Missense mutations can also cause disease by either the substitution of amino acids in nonfunctional structural domains of the protein, which alter the tertiary structure of the protein with remote effects on the functional domains, or by the substitution of amino acids in domains important for the appropriate post-translational trafficking of the protein (Fig. 4-2B). Examples of the latter mechanism, which causes the protein to be targeted to the wrong cellular site, are certain mutations in acid maltase that cause adult forms of Pompe's disease (Table 4-2).

Second, mutations can cause disease by introducing nonsense or *stop codons* within the amino acid coding sequence of the gene. Stop codons, which prematurely terminate translation of the protein from the messenger RNA (mRNA), may be introduced by either a point mutation, which directly changes a *sense codon* to a *nonsense codon,* or by an insertion or deletion of bases in multiples other than three, which causes a shift in the three-base reading frame (Fig. 4-2C).

Third, mutations that involve an in-frame deletion or duplication remove part of the coding sequence but preserve the three-base codon reading frame. Such structural anomalies usually dramatically alter the tertiary structure and biochemical function of the resultant peptide (Fig. 4-2D).

Fourth, point mutations or deletions or duplications that involve the canonical splice-donor or splice-acceptor sequences 3' and 5' to each exon interfere with the correct splicing of RNA transcripts into mature mRNA (Fig. 4-2E). Mutations of this type result in mRNA sequences that cannot be translated appropriately and are usually also unstable.

Finally, the deletion of regulatory elements in the

Table 4-1. Glossary of Terms

Alleles	Alternative versions of genes (e.g., different DNA sequences at the same locus)
Autosome	One of the 22 nonsex-determining genes (i.e., not the X or Y chromosome)
Centromeric	Closer to the central portion of a chromosome
Codon	Sequence of three nucleotides in a DNA or RNA strand that provides the genetic information for the construction of a certain amino acid at a site in a protein chain
Exon	A portion of DNA that codes for a given section of a mRNA
Genome	Entire complement of genetic material in a cell
Genotype	Genetic constitution (e.g., nucleotide sequence) at a given locus
Heteroplasmy	Condition in which genetic brake-up of a tissue is highly variable
Homozygous	An individual with the same DNA sequence at the same site in the two parental chromosomes
Intron	A portion of DNA that lies between two exons and does not code for protein
Mb	Million base pairs
Meioses	The process of cell division during gametogenesis
Messenger RNA (mRNA)	An exact copy of a portion of a DNA sequence that is then transferred to the area in the cytoplasm where proteins are produced
Monomer	A single unit of a protein
Mutation	Abnormality in nucleotide sequence of a gene
Phenotype	A manifestation of a gentoype
RNA transcripts	The products of the copying of a DNA sequence to an RNA sequence
Sex-linked	Pertaining to the genes carried in the X or Y chromosome
Stochastic	A random distribution of a discrete variable
Telomeric	Closer to the terminal portion of a chromosome
Triplets	Triple sequences of nucleotides
Wild Type	Naturally occurring gene

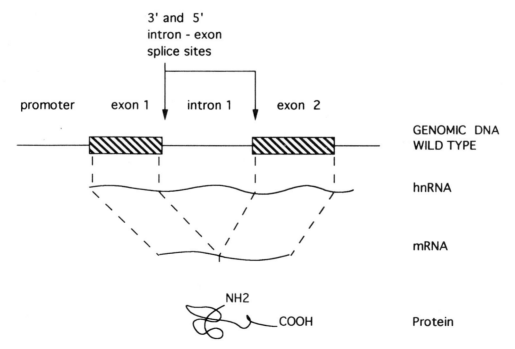

Figure 4-1. The structure of a typical gene encoded in genomic DNA includes regulatory elements at the 5′ and 3′ ends and protein coding sequences (exons) interspersed with noncoding sequences (introns). Heteronuclear RNA (hnRNA) is transcribed from the entire gene, including both exons and introns and some untranslated sequences at the 3′ and 5′ ends of the gene. Noncoding sequences are spliced out at specific canonical splicing sites at the beginning and ends of each exon, thereby creating the mature cytoplasmic mRNA. The mature mRNA is translated by the ribosomal apparatus in the cytoplasm to generate a peptide that may then undergo post-translational modifications (e.g., glycosylation or removal of signal peptides).

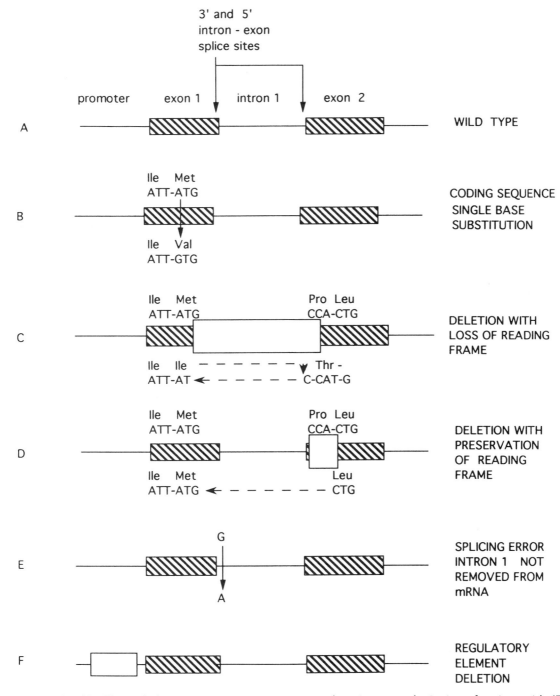

Figure 4-2. (A–F) Single base pair mutations may cause the missense substitution of amino acids (Fig. B) or the creation of a nonsense stop codon, which causes termination of protein translation from the mRNA template (not shown). Deletions and duplications simply remove or duplicate a section of the gene. If the deletion or duplication involves an exact multiple of three bases, the reading frame is preserved, and protein translation is preserved, leading to a truncated but often partially functional protein (Fig. D). Deletions or duplications that involve nucleotides in multiples other than three alter the reading frame and lead to either an aberrant sequence or more commonly to the creation of a stop codon because of the reading frame shift (Fig. C). Point mutations or deletions or duplications in the intron-exon splice sites lead to incomplete removal of the noncoding intronic sequences (Fig. E); mutations in regulatory sequences lead to defective transcription of the gene (Fig. F).

Table 4-2. Inherited Adult Neurologic Diseases in which the Disease Gene Has Been Identified[a]

Disease	Gene	Mutation
Duchenne's and Becker's muscular dystrophies	Dystrophin	Duchenne: point mutations or deletions with loss of reading frame; Becker: point mutations or deletions with preservation of reading frame
Hyperkalemic periodic paralysis; paramyotonia congenita; and acetolazamide-responsive myotonia congenita	Muscle sodium channel (SCN4A)	Point mutations
Malignant hyperthermia	Ryanodine receptor	Point mutation
Myotonic dystrophy	Myotonin protein kinase	Trinucleotide repeat 3′ untranslated region
Myotonia congenita (Thomsen's disease)	Muscle chloride channel (CLCN1)?	By linkage analysis and analogy to *adr* mouse phenotype; no mutations yet documented
Pompe's disease (glycogen storage disease II)	α-1,4-glucosidase (acid maltase)	Juvenile = point mutations in catalytic site; adult = point mutation that causes defective post-translational processing
McArdle's disease (glycogen storage disease V)	Muscle glycogen phosphorylase	Point mutation
Tarui disease (glycogen storage disease VII)	Phosphofructokinase Muscle isoenzyme	Point mutation
Carnitine palmitoyl transferase deficiency	Carnitine palmitoyl transferase	Point mutations
Congenital myasthenia	Acetylcholine receptor subunits or acetylcholinesterase?	By functional assays; no mutations yet documented
Familial amyloidotic polyneuropathy (Andrade)	Transthyretin	Point mutations
Familial amyloidotic polyneuropathy (Finnish)	Gelsolin	Point mutation
Charcot-Marie-Tooth (HMSN type 1b)	Myelin glycoprotein zero (MPZ)	Point mutation
Charcot-Marie-Tooth (HMSN type 1a)	Peripheral myelin protein-22 (PMP22)	Duplication or point mutation rarely
Hereditary pressure-sensitive neuropathy	Peripheral myelin protein-22 (PMP22)	Deletion
Hypertrophic dejerine-sottas disease (HMSN III)	Peripheral myelin protein-22 (PMP22) or myelin glycoprotein zero (MPZ)	Point mutations as for Charcot-Marie-Tooth types 1a and 1b
Refsum's disease	Phytannic acid oxidase	No mutations yet found
Acute intermittent porphyria	Porphobilinogen deaminase (uroporphyrinogen synthetase)	Point mutations or deletions, splice site mutations
Porphyria variegata	Protoporphyrinogen oxidase	No mutations yet found
X-linked spinobulbar muscular atrophy	Androgen receptor	Trinucleotide repeat
Familial amyotrophic lateral sclerosis (ALS1 subtype)	Cu/Zn superoxide dismutase	Point mutations
Icelandic hereditary cerebral hemorrhage with amyloidosis	Cystatin C	Point mutations
Dutch hereditary cerebral hemorrhage with amyloidosis	Amyloid precursor protein (APP)	Point mutation
Familial Alzheimer's disease (rare presenile-onset AD1 subtype)	Amyloid precursor protein (APP)	Point mutations
Familial Alzheimer's disease (late-onset AD2 subtype)	Apolipoprotein E	Dose-dependent allelic association with $Cys^{112}Arg$ (ε 4) variant; ε 2 allele may reduce risk of AD
Gerstmann-Strässler	Prion protein	Point mutations or insertions
Fatal familial insomnia	Prion protein	Point mutation

(continues)

Table 4-2 *(Continued)*.

Disease	Gene	Mutation
Huntington's disease	Huntingtin (IT15, unknown function)	Trinucleotide repeat (CAG) in 5′ coding
X-linked mental retardation (fragile X syndrome, FRAXA)	FMR1 (unknown function)	Trinucleotide repeat in 5′ untranslated region
Spinocerebellar ataxia type 1 (SCA1; Menzel-type OPCA)	Unnamed (unknown function)	Trinucleotide repeat
Dentatorubral-pallidoluysal Atrophy	B37 (unknown function)	Trinucleotide repeat
Wilson's disease	ATP7β (copper-transporting adenosine triphosphatase)	Point mutation or deletion
Hyperexplexia (jumping Frenchmen of Maine)	Glycine receptor subunit (GRA1)	Point mutation
Niemann-Pick (variants A-E)	Acid sphingomyelinase	Type A: nonsense/deletion; type B: missense point mutation
Metachromatic leukodystrophy	Arylsulfatase A	Point mutation or deletion, splice site mutations
Adrenoleukodystrophy	Adrenoleukodystrophy protein (?peroxisomal membrane protein)	Point mutation or deletion
Fabry's disease	α-Galactosidase	Point mutation or deletion
Tay-Sachs disease	Hexosaminidase A	Juvenile: deletion at exon 1, insertion at exon 11, splice site at intron 12; adult: point mutation exon
Pelizaeus-Merzbacher	Myelin proteolipid protein	Point mutation
von Recklinghausen's disease (neurofibromatosis I)	Neurofibromin (GAP-like protein)	Point mutations or deletions and other rearrangements
Bilateral acoustic neurofibromatosis (neurofibromatosis II)	Merlin (schwannomin) (membrane-anchoring structural protein)	Point mutations or deletions
Tuberous sclerosis type 2 (CHR 16 linked)	Tuberin (Gap like protein)	Deletions
Machado-Joseph disease	MJD1 (unknown function)	Trinucleotide repeat in 3′ coding sequence
Infantile and juvenile spinal muscular atrophy (SMAI–III)	Un-named (apoptosis inhibiting protein)	Point mutation/deletion
DOPA responsive dystonia	?GTP cyclohydrolase I	Point mutations; homozygous mutation is also associated with atypical hyperphenylaninemia
von Hippel-Lindau	VHLP (unknown function)	Point mutations or deletions
Chronic progressive external ophthalmoplegia (Kearns-Sayre)	Mitochondrial DNA	Deletions
Leber's optic atrophy	Mitochondrial ND4	Point mutations
Mitochondrial encephalomyopathy with ragged red fibers (MERRF) and myeloencephalopathy lactic acidosis and stroke (MELAS)	Mitochondrial transfer RNA genes	Point mutations

[a] The table lists each disease, the name or symbol for the wild-type gene, and the type of defects observed to date. Except where adult variants are known to exist, pediatric neurologic lipid storage diseases and disorders that affect amino acid metabolism are not included in this list. A comprehensive list of the latter disorders can be found in texts of classical biochemical genetics. Several disorders thought to be phenotypically distinct have been found to be genetically related by virtue of allelic mutations in the same gene (the phenotypic differences are sometimes explainable by different effects of the mutations observed in each phenotype). Conversely, some diseases with similar phenotypes are in fact caused by mutations in different genes. For each of the disorders listed in this table, an up-to-date inventory of known mutations can be accessed in the On-line Mendelian Inheritance in Man database at Johns Hopkins University.

gene, such as the promoter elements at the 5′ and 3′ ends of the gene, can result in inappropriate or inadequate gene expression (Fig. 4-2F).

Regardless of the molecular mechanisms involved, the defective protein derived from the mutant allele in recessive diseases does not affect the function of the protein derived from the normal wild-type allele. Thus, for autosomal genes, recessive mutations produce a phenotype only in subjects homozygous for the defect. Similarly, in X-linked recessive diseases, only hemizygous male and homozygous female recipients display the clinical phenotype. The archetype of recessive disorders are the enzymopathies, such as those involved in the glycogen storage pathways.

Dominant Traits

The types of genetic mutations encountered in dominantly inherited diseases are similar to those observed with recessive diseases. However, in contrast to recessive traits, the acquisition of a single defective allele of a dominant disease gene is sufficient to cause the disease phenotype. Thus, dominant diseases are characterized by disease in both heterozygous carriers, who carry one normal and one defective copy of the gene, and in homozygotes, who carry two defective copies of the gene.

In true dominant diseases (e.g., Huntington's disease, discussed below and in Ch. 77), the disease phenotype in subjects homozygous for the defective gene is indistinguishable from that in subjects with a single defective allele (heterozygotes). In co-dominant diseases (e.g., some types of late-onset Alzheimer's disease, discussed below and in Ch. 60), the heterozygote develops the disease, but the homozygote has a more severe phenotype.

The mechanisms by which the inheritance of a single defective allele causes a disease phenotype are diverse. Some dominant mutations probably cause a gain of function in which the added function is deleterious. Other dominant mutations exert a dominant negative effect whereby the defective allele functionally inactivates the wild-type allele as well. The best examples of dominant negative mutations are those that involve genes the proteins of which are subunits of polymeric proteins (e.g., superoxide dismutase 1 [SOD1] in familial amotrophic lateral sclerosis [ALS], discussed below). Still other dominant mutations may represent a loss of function in highly critical enzymes or structural proteins.

Complex Traits

Although the mode of inheritance of many genetic diseases of the nervous system is often obvious from simple inspection of clinical pedigrees as autosomal recessive, autosomal dominant, or sex-linked, it is clear that several common neurologic diseases display a more complex mode of transmission that does not seem to fit the simple rules of mendelian inheritance.

There are several potential explanations for these apparent anomalies. For instance, in some cases, the disease may not be a single-gene disorder but may in fact require the collusion of two or more different genetic loci with additive or multiplicative effects (polygenic traits). In other instances, the disease may have a single-gene defect as its genetic basis, but the penetrance and/or expression of that defect may be modified by other genes or by exogenous events. In

yet other familial diseases, the causative mutation itself may vary (e.g., unstable trinucleotide repeat diseases). This variation in the mutation itself is often correlated with the severity of symptoms and may obscure the simple mode of inheritance. Finally, some familial neurologic diseases do not show mendelian modes of inheritance because the DNA that carries the disease-causing mutation is not inherited according to mendelian rules for chromosomal inheritance (i.e., mitochondrial DNA). Examples of each of these mechanisms are discussed below.

VARIABLE DISEASE EXPRESSION CAUSED BY DEVIATIONS FROM CLASSICAL PATTERNS OF MENDELIAN INHERITANCE

Reduced Penetrance or Variable Phenotypic Expression

For some diseases, although the disease gene itself is inherited in a mendelian fashion, a proportion of the disease gene carriers may live a normal life without expressing the disease. Such diseases are referred to as having reduced or incomplete penetrance. Alternatively, the disease gene may be expressed in all gene carriers (complete penetrance), but the clinical phenotype may differ markedly between different family members (variable expressivity). Examples of the latter include Gilles de la Tourette's syndrome in which only a proportion of family members express the classical panoply of symptoms (see Ch. 77). If only those family members who express the classical features of Gilles de la Tourette's syndrome are considered, then the disease often appears to be nonfamilial. However, if other abnormal phenotypes, such as simple chronic motor tics and obsessive compulsive behavior are also included, the disease appears to be a fully penetrant autosomal dominant trait.

In diseases such as Gilles de la Tourette's syndrome, with reduced penetrance and/or variable expressivity, it is likely that the phenotypic variation arises mostly from the effects of other genetic or environmental factors that modify, block, or delay the expression of the defective alleles. An alternative but probably less common cause of phenotypic variation is the simple stochastic variation in expression of the disease gene itself. Importantly, in those diseases in which penetrance and expressivity are modified by other factors, it is possible that, if these other factors were identified, they might be exploited therapeutically.

Instability of the Mutation

Recently, at least five diseases of neurologic interest have been reported to result from a novel class of genetic mutations that involve the insertion/amplification of a variable number of trinucleotide repeat elements. These diseases include autosomal dominant myotonic dystrophy (see Ch. 82), X-linked recessive spinobulbar muscular atrophy (see Ch. 82), Huntington's disease (see Ch. 77), X-linked recessive fragile X syndrome (FRAXA), and spinocerebellar ataxia type 1 (see Ch. 64).

All of these diseases, but especially myotonic dystrophy, Huntington's disease, and FRAXA display the clinical phenomenon of anticipation with earlier onset and/or more severe symptoms in successive generations. In addition, in myotonic dystrophy and Huntington's disease, the parental origin of the defective chromosomes can have a significant effect on the phenotype in the affected offspring. In myotonic dystrophy, children born to mothers mildly affected with the disease (but not to affected fathers) may show severe congenital myotonic dystrophy and mental retardation. Similarly, children born to fathers with Huntington's disease may occasionally develop a more severe juvenile form that is characterized by the onset of a rapidly progressive dementia with rigidity in childhood or adolescence. Both of these phenomena were previously attributed to parental imprinting. However, it is now clear that they simply reflect sex differences in the degree of instability of the trinucleotide repeat (more unstable in female meioses in myotonic dystrophy and more unstable in male meioses in Huntington's disease).

Complex Modes of Transmission

Many diseases that display clear familial clustering of a disease trait do not show unequivocal mendelian inheritance (e.g., epilepsy and mental retardation). In such diseases, it is likely that some of the families that segregate the disease phenotype may have a single-gene disorder (e.g., juvenile myoclonic epilepsy on 6p, progressive myoclonus epilepsy on 21q, or FRAXA chromosome X). However, the majority probably represent a more complex situation in which alleles at more than one locus may contribute to the overall risk, either synergistically or additively. Such traits are frequently referred to as polygenic traits. (See the related discussion of variable penetrance above.)

To date, this type of disorder has been intractable to molecular dissection in human pedigrees. However, polygenic traits, such as epilepsy, diabetes, and hypertension, are being addressed in murine models by determining the genotype at multiple marker loci scattered uniformly across the genome and then searching for evidence of cosegregation of clusters of markers with an increased or decreased risk for the disease phenotype by statistical simultaneous search techniques. In mice, this strategy has recently led to the mapping of two probably cooperative loci that cause epilepsy in the EL strain of mice. The major

locus that accounts for much of the inherited risk maps to mouse chromosome 9 (d-se) (syntenic to human chromosome 3), with a lesser risk associated with a second locus on mouse chromosome 2 (Mpmv-28). Together these loci contribute approximately 50 percent of the variance in the quantitative trait (risk of seizures). Ultimately, a similar strategy should be applicable to human polygenic diseases, especially if candidate genes can first be identified using animal models.

Nonmendelian Modes of Transmission

Important sources of apparent nonmendelian inheritance of familially clustered disease with variable phenotypic expression are mutations in mitochondrial genes. Mitochondria contain a small amount of DNA that codes for some but not all mitochondrial proteins. However, two unique features of mitochondrial biology require that the inheritance of mitochondrial DNA does not follow classical mendelian models. First, mitochondria contain multiple copies of mitochondrial DNA and each cell contains multiple mitochondria. During cell division, these mitochondrial DNA molecules are randomly segregated into the daughter mitochondria by budding off, and the daughter mitochondria are randomly assorted into the daughter cells. This process, known as *cytoplasmic inheritance,* differs markedly from the predictable binary nature of mendelian nuclear or chromosomal inheritance. These processes of random allocation inherent in cytoplasmic transmission of mitochondrial DNA therefore provide ample opportunity for daughter cells to acquire widely differing loadings of mutant mitochondrial DNA. Some daughter cells acquire mitochondria without mutations; other daughter cells acquire mitochondria loaded with mutated mitochondrial DNA (heteroplasmy).

The second complication in the genetics of mitochondrial DNA arises from the fact that the mitochondria of the zygote (embryo) are contributed almost exclusively by the maternal gamete. These two observations therefore form the basis for the clinical observations of (1) maternal inheritance (because of the mode of transmission of mitochondria) and (2) often markedly variable expressivity (because of heteroplasmy) in mitochondrial diseases such as Leber's optic neuropathy, mitochondrial encephalomyopathy with ragged red fibers, and myeloencephalopathy lactic acidosis and stroke.

SPECIFIC DISEASE MECHANISMS

In this section, several diseases are used to illustrate specific examples of different genetic mechanisms that cause disease. Table 4-1 outlines additional inher-

Table 4-3. Inherited Adult Neurologic Diseases in which Only the Chromosomal Locations of the Disease Genes Are Known[a]

Disease	Locus	Status
Duchenne-like autosomal recessive muscular dystrophy	13q	Provisional
Fascioscapulohumeral dystrophy	4qter	Confirmed
Limb girdle dystrophy (proximal, type I)	5q	Provisional
Limb girdle dystrophy (Leyden-Möbius, type II)	15q + others	Confirmed
Riley-Day dysautonomia (HSAN III)	9q	Provisional
Familial spastic paraplegia	14q + others	Provisional
Friedreich's ataxia	9cen	Confirmed
Spinocerebellar atrophy	12q (SCA2, Holguin type) others (Holmes type)	Confirmed
Autosomal dominant dystonia	9q + others	Confirmed
X-linked dystonia parkinsonism (Lubag)	X	Provisional
Juvenile myoclonic epilepsy	6p + others	Confirmed
Progressive myoclonus epilepsy	21q	Confirmed
Benign familial neonatal seizures	20q (BFNC1)	Confirmed
	8q (BFNC2)	Provisional
Ceroid lipofuscinosis	16p (juvenile)	Confirmed
	1p (infantile)	Provisional
	Other (Late infantile)	
	Other (adult/Kuf)	
Tuberous sclerosis	9q (TSC1)	Confirmed
Familial alzheimer's disease	14q (AD3)	Confirmed
	19q (AD2)	Confirmed
	Others	

[a] Genetic linkage studies have established the approximate chromosomal locations of these genes. By convention, single reports of genetic linkage are considered provisional until replicated in a second independent dataset. Some disease phenotypes may be associated with genetic defects at more than one locus (i.e., display nonallelic or locus heterogeneity). Locus heterogeneity is suspected on the basis of the fact that some pedigrees do not cosegregate with the markers that show linkage in other pedigrees or is proved when a second locus is identified.

ited neurologic diseases that affect adults for which the disease gene has been characterized. Table 4-3 lists some diseases for which the actual gene defect has not yet been characterized but for which an approximate chromosomal location has been defined by genetic linkage studies. Further information on clinical and neuropathologic phenotypes of these diseases are found elsewhere in this text.

Conventional Autosomal Recessive Diseases

Phenylketonuria

The genetic mechanisms that underlie conventional autosomal recessive traits are best exemplified by the enzyme deficiency diseases that were discovered by classic biochemical approaches. Subsequent application of molecular genetic approaches have defined a broad range of mutations that give rise to these diseases. Because in-depth discussions of most of these diseases are provided in conventional textbooks of biochemical genetics, this chapter describes only one such disease, phenylketonuria, which has been well studied

at both the biochemical and molecular level and epitomizes these diseases.

Phenylketonuria is a recessive inherited trait characterized by mental retardation (treatable by dietary restriction of phenylalanine intake), epilepsy, abnormalities of gait and posture, a readily identifiable "mousy" body odor, and cutaneous stigmata, including light pigmentation and eczema. Conventional biochemical studies have determined that the underlying biochemical anomaly is defective function of phenylalanine hydroxylase (PAH). Recent molecular studies have shown that the gene encoding the PAH protein is 90 kilobases in size, maps to chromosome 12q22-q24.1, and produces a 2.4 kilobase mRNA transcript. Multiple mutations have now been detected in the PAH gene, including single-base substitutions, which result in nonsense mutations, missense mutations, and splicing mutations, as well as deletions. Many of the missense mutations are clustered in exon 7, which probably reflects the functional importance of this domain rather than the presence of a mutational hot spot within the gene. The frequencies of each of these mutations vary in different populations, which suggests that the mutations have not arisen from a single common founder but rather from multiple independent mutational events. Affected homozygotes can be either homozygous for the same mutation (especially in inbred pedigrees or in populations in which one mutation is especially predominant), or they may have inherited parental PAH genes with different mutations (i.e., they are, in fact, compound heterozygotes).

It has been suggested that heterozygous female carriers of phenylketonuria may have a reduced frequency of spontaneous abortions, possibly as a result of protection against the abortifacient Ochratoxin A in moldy foodstuffs. Similar competitive advantages for heterozygotes in selected envirnoments have been proposed to explain both regional and ethnic differences in the frequencies of certain diseases and to explain the persistence of diseases that are lethal in homozygotes.

Conventional X-Linked Diseases

Duchenne's and Becker's Muscular Dystrophies

Duchenne's muscular dystrophy (DMD) and Becker's muscular dystrophy (BMD) are two allelic disorders characterized by variable degrees of muscular dystrophy, cardiomyopathy, mental retardation, and other less common phenotypes that are inherited as X-linked recessive traits (see Ch. 82). BMD is clinically differentiated from DMD on the basis of a milder and less rapidly progressive phenotype. Recent positional cloning studies have identified a large gene, dystrophin, which spans 1 to 2 million billion pairs of DNA and contains at least 60 exons, and which generates a mature mRNA transcript of 16 kilobases that in turn encodes a 3,685 amino acid protein with a molecular weight of 427 kD. The dystrophin gene is predominantly expressed in brain and muscle cells (which explains the disease phenotype), but expression can be detected in many other tissues at low levels (illegitimate transcription). Transcripts in the brain and muscle differ in the site of the promoter used and the first exon.

Both DMD and BMD are associated with mutations in the dystrophin gene. Furthermore, in both DMD and BMD, the most common mutations are deletions within the gene, 70 percent of which occur in the distal half of the gene (most commonly one breakpoint is in intron 43). These deletions are often large (most greater than 137 kilobases), but the clinical phenotype correlates poorly with the size of the deletion. It appears that the differences in the severity of the phenotype between DMD and BMD are most closely associated with the presence or absence of dystrophin in muscle. In DMD, the mutations are most commonly deletions or duplications (65 percent of cases) that cause a shift in the reading frame and lead to failure to produce dystrophin (Fig. 4-2). As a result, subjects with DMD have virtually absent dystrophin immunoreactivity in muscle biopsies. In BMD, on the other hand, the mutations are also frequently large deletions (71 percent of cases), but they are "in-frame," so that an attenuated but partially functional protein is produced (which can be detected on immunoblots) (Fig. 4-2). However, about one-third of DMD and BMD cases do not have a gross structural abnormality of the dystrophin gene. In these cases, the mutations have usually turned out to be point mutations that cause a reading frame shift with absence of dystrophin production (the DMD phenotype) or missense mutations that lead to amino acid substitutions (the BMD phenotype). A few cases of BMD have been described with deletions of the muscle promoter of the dystrophin gene, leading to lower levels of full-sized dystrophin on immunoblots. A single case of DMD has been reported with a missense mutation in the actin-binding domain (Leu54Arg), which may indicate that this region is necessary for dystrophin stability and function.

Conventional Autosomal Dominant Disease

Familial Amyotrophic Lateral Sclerosis

Although familial ALS is transmitted as an autosomal dominant trait with age-dependent penetrance, the disease is known to be genetically heterogeneous (see Ch. 63). Some pedigrees show evidence for genetic linkage to chromosome 21, whereas other pedigrees with indistinguishable phenotypes can be excluded from chromosome 21. The gene on chromosome 21 that is associated with the chromosome 21 subtype of familial ALS (type 1) is the Cu, Zn SOD1, which exists functionally as a homopolymeric protein. Some, but not all, of the mutations discovered in the SOD1 gene in association with familial ALS type 1 have caused conformational changes in the mutant SOD1 monomer, which have resulted in both loss of function of the mutant monomer and inhibition of the wild-type monomer in heterodimers (i.e., a dominant negative effect). Consequently, because only the wild-type homopolymers remain functionally active, the overall cellular SOD1 activity is reduced by more than the 50 percent predicted for the inactivation of the mutant monomer alone. The explanation for the susceptibility of motor neurons to loss of SOD1 appears to be that these neurons normally require and express high levels of SOD1 to protect against superoxide radicals (O_2^-) and NO· species generated from a variety of sources but particularly by excitotoxic descending pathways.

Diseases With Unstable Trinucleotide Repeats

Huntington's Disease

Huntington's disease has long been the archetypal inherited neurodegenerative disease. In fact, it was one of the first genetic disorders to be tackled with the positional cloning strategies discussed below. Greater detail on the clinical, pathologic, and biochemical aspects of this disease is available in Chapter 77.

The genetic defect that causes Huntington's disease has been mapped to the distal short arm of chromosome 4 (4p). The genetic recombinational data and examination of the frequency of association between Huntington's disease and specific alleles of several 4p markers (allelic association or linkage disequilibrium studies) focused interest on a 2.5-megabase region of 4p near the marker D4S95, flanked proximally by the marker D4S125 and flanked distally by D4S168. Subsequently, the Huntington's disease gene itself was cloned from this region. The normal function of the gene (IT15, also known as Huntingtin) is currently unclear because the nucleotide and deduced amino acid sequence displays no known homology to other proteins within the usual databases. However, it appears that the molecular defect associated with Huntington's disease is the amplification of a trinucleotide $(CAG)_n$ repeat in the 5' translated region of the IT15 gene. In normal subjects, this trinucleotide repeat is less than 33 elements in size. In patients with Huntington's disease, the amplification is unstable and larger (more than 37). The size of the amplified element correlates inversely with the age of onset and severity of symptoms.

In addition to the fundamental goal of cloning the disease gene itself, molecular genetic studies of Huntington's disease have also provided solutions to problems that have tormented classical geneticists and clinicians alike. It is now clear that, despite the highly variable clinical phenotype, probably all cases of Huntington's disease arise from mutations at the same locus on chromosome 4p. The observation that juvenile cases arise more frequently when the father is the gene carrier is now adequately explained by the trinucleotide repeat being more unstable in male meioses, which allows the occurrence of larger amplifications with earlier and more severe clinical phenotypes in affected progeny from such meioses. However, in addition to the sex of the transmitting parent, the age of clinical onset is also affected by alleles at the Huntington's disease locus on the normal chromosome. For instance, the number of repeats on the normal paternal chromosome correlates with age of onset in maternally transmitted disease.

Another observation from molecular genetic studies that supports empirical clinical tenets is the observation that individuals who are very likely (more than 98 percent) to be homozygous for the Huntington's disease mutation are not phenotypically distinguishable from those with a single copy of the defect. This observation confirms the classical concept that Huntington's disease is a true autosomal dominant trait with complete but age-dependent penetrance.

Finally, despite the fact that disease-causing mutation in the IT15 gene is a highly variable amplification of a normally variable repeat element, the presence of strong linkage disequilibrium between Huntington's disease and specific alleles at markers near the IT15 gene suggests that only a limited number of ancestral chromosomes are actually susceptible to this pathologic amplification. The explanation for this is not yet known, although a similar phenomenon exists in myotonic dystrophy, in which strong evidence for linkage disequilibrium is also seen between myotonic dystrophy and markers near the myotonin-protein kinase gene.

Spinobulbar Muscular Atrophy

Spinobulbar muscular atrophy is a rare, X-linked recessive disorder characterized by mild testicular feminization, progressive lower motor neuron weakness in spinal and bulbar innervated musculature, and often mild sensory symptoms (see Ch. 82). The observation of mild feminization led to investigation of the androgen receptor gene on the X chromosome and to the observation that the disease-causing mutation is an amplification of a CAG triplet tract coding for a variable number polyglutamine tract in the androgen receptor protein. In normal individuals, this poly-CAG tract varies between 15 and 30 triplets; in affected subjects, the tract is between 40 and 50 triplets long with some variation in triplet tract length from generation to generation. The mechanism by which amplification of the polyglutamine tract in the androgen receptor gene leads to spinobulbar muscular atrophy is unknown.

Fragile X Mental Retardation Syndrome

FRAX is associated with the amplification of a CGG triplet repeat in noncoding sequences 5' to the AUG start codon of the FMR-1 gene. The FMR-1 gene itself is conserved in evolution, but even though its amino acid sequence has been deduced, its function is still unknown. In the normal population, the CGG triplet repeat in the FMR-1 gene varies from 6 to 54 triplets. In normal asymptomatic transmitting males (and females), the triplet is expanded to between 50 and 200 triplets. In symptomatic subjects, the triplet repeat is greater than 200 triplets in length. Triplet repeats greater than 50 are meiotically unstable because offspring of asymptomatic males and females who carry the premutation alleles (50 to 200 triplets) show larger variations in the number of alleles acquired than do offspring of subjects with less than 50 repeats. However, it appears that most meiotic events that give rise to the very large repeat amplifications (more than 200 triplets) necessary for symptomatic disease arise from female meioses.

Two explanations have been postulated to explain the mechanism by which a 5' triplet repeat might cause FRAX. The simplest is that the expanded triplet repeat simply perturbs the normal processing of the FMR-1 heteronuclear RNA into mRNA; a hypothesis that agrees with the observation of absent FMR-1 mRNA in symptomatic males. However, the observation that methylation of a CpG island near the 5' end of the FMR-1 gene correlates well with the absence of FMR-1 mRNA, and mental retardation suggests that methylation of promoter sequences near the amplified CGG triplet repeat may also be as important as a negative regulator of FMR-1 transcription. In fact, the necessity for both amplification of premutation alleles and methylation of the mutant gene provides an explanation for the following unusual type of anticipation observed in FRAX (Sherman paradox): mildly symptomatic males transmit the unstable premutation allele to their asymptomatic daughters, in whom the gene is both amplified and methylated (imprinted) during X inactivation. Although these daughters remain asymptomatic by virtue of the normal maternal X chromosome, they subsequently transmit the methylated and amplified FMR-1 allele to one-half of their own male offspring who do not erase the maternal methylation imprint and who become symptomatic.

Myotonic Dystrophy

The disease that causes the mutation in myotonic dystrophy (see Ch. 82) is the amplification of a CAG triplet repeat in the 3' untranslated mRNA of the myotonin-protein kinase gene on chromosome 19q. This gene is predicted to be a transmembrane protein with an amino-terminal adenosine triphosphate-binding domain, a protein kinase catalytic domain, and domains with homology to muscle structural proteins. The CAG triplet repeat in the normal population usually numbers less than 30. As in FRAX, subjects with 50 to 100 repeats are generally asymptomatic or only mildly affected, but these alleles are at high risk of further amplification in subsequent male or female meioses to produce symptomatic disease (more than 100 repeats). The mechanism by which amplification of the 3' triplet repeat leads to disease seems likely to be due to interference in myotonin-protein kinase gene expression.

Interestingly, like Huntington's disease, genetic linkage studies in myotonic dystrophy have shown

strong linkage disequilibrium between myotonic dystrophy and polymorphic DNA markers near the myotonin-protein kinase gene. This implies that there is a relatively small subset of founder chromosomes that are predisposed to the pathologic amplification of the GCT triplet.

Disorders With Complex Modes of Inheritance

Familial Alzheimer's Disease

Familial Alzheimer's disease is an archetypal complex genetic trait (see Ch. 60). Although familial aggregation of Alzheimer's disease has been recognized for some time, it has been difficult to discriminate whether such aggregation simply reflects random clustering as a result of the high frequency of Alzheimer's disease in the elderly population (at least 6 cases per 100 population in those older than the age of 65 years); nonrandom clustering caused by exposure of family members to shared environmental risks; or nonrandom clustering because of inherited factors. Several recent epidemiologic surveys, however, have now convincingly shown that a proportion of familially clustered Alzheimer's disease is inherited as a simple autosomal dominant trait with age-dependent penetrance, although the estimated proportion of cases of Alzheimer's disease with a monogenic basis is still disputed.

Genetic linkage studies in familial Alzheimer's disease pedigrees have revealed that a proportion of pedigrees predominantly with a presenile onset of this disease appear to cosegregate with several genetic markers clustered on the proximal long arm of chromosome 21 near the candidate gene that encodes the precursor of the β-peptide of senile plaques (the β-amyloid precursor protein gene [β-APP gene]). Subsequent studies confirmed that a small proportion of familial Alzheimer's disease cases (less than 0.03) are in fact due to a mutation in this gene. However, most such pedigrees are not associated with mutations in the β-APP gene.

The mechanism by which mutations in codon 717 lead to the familial Alzheimer's disease phenotype is unclear. It has been speculated that the mutations, which occur in a transmembrane domain of the β-APP protein, may disrupt the cell membrane; may lead to an unstable stem loop structure in the β-APP mRNA, causing differential processing and enhanced translation of the mutant mRNA; may disrupt the normal but as yet unknown function of β-APP; or may subtly alter the post-translational processing of β-APP. Currently, the last hypothesis has been experimentally examined and seems most likely.

A second familial Alzheimer's disease susceptibility locus has recently been discovered on chromosome

14q near the anonymous DNA markers D14S43 and D14S77. This locus is associated with a significant proportion of early-onset pedigrees that lack β-APP mutations. The identity of this gene is currently unknown, but it does not appear to be one of the obvious candidate genes already mapped to chromosome 14 (α_1-antichymotrypsin; c-fos, or cathepsin G).

Evidence of a third genetic locus associated with an inherited predisposition to Alzheimer's disease is provided by the observation that some cases of late-onset familial and late-onset sporadic Alzheimer's disease are associated with the inheritance of a specific, naturally occurring coding sequence polymorphism (Cys → Arg at codon 112, allele ε 4) of apolipoprotein E on chromosome 19. Inheritance of the ε 4 allele of apolipoprotein E is associated with increased risk for, and earlier age of onset, of Alzheimer's disease in a dose-dependent fashion. Thus, subjects homozygous for ε 4 have a higher risk and an earlier onset of symptoms than do subjects heterozygous for ε 4, who in turn have a higher risk and earlier onset than subjects without any ε 4 alleles. The mechanism of action of the ε 4 allele is unknown, but preliminary data have suggested that the apolipoprotein E ε 4 allele binds to β/A4 peptide more avidly than do the other alleles.

At least one other familial Alzheimer's disease susceptibility locus is thought to exist because several pedigrees have been described that show no evidence for linkage to chromosome 14, 19, or 21. However, further evidence for the complexity of genetic factors in Alzheimer's disease is provided by the recent observation of an interaction between the apolipoprotein E and the β-APP genotypes in determining the overall risk for Alzheimer's disease in members of pedigrees that segregate β-APP Val717Ile mutations.

Disorders That Are Both Infectious and Inheritable

Diseases of the Prion Gene

About 10 percent of cases with Creutzfeldt-Jakob Disease (CJD) and most cases of Gerstmann-Sträussler Syndrome (GSS) show strong familial aggregation and are thought to be transmitted as an autosomal dominant trait (see Ch. 50). To date, mutations in the human prion protein gene have been discovered at codon 53 (insertion of 48, 56, or 72 amino acids), codon 178 (missense point mutation leading to Asp → Asn substitution), and codon 200 (Glu → Lys substitution) in familial CJD and at codon 102 (Pro → Leu), codon 117 (Ala → Val), and 198 (Hp → Ser) in GSS. The inherited prion diseases appear to be transmitted as a true dominant trait, like Huntington's disease, because the clinical phenotype of a patient homozygous for the codon 200 mutation was indistinguishable from that of heterozygotes. Several benign polymorphisms have been detected at codon 53 (inserts of less than 48 amino acids), codon 117 (single base pair change that does not change the encoded amino acid), and at codon 129 (single base pair change that causes a Met → Val substitution). The homozygous state at codon 129 (Met/Met or Val/Val) has been associated with an increased risk for sporadic CJD, and individuals who are heterozygotes frequently have an atypical course whether the illness occurs in the context of familial CJD/GSS or in the context of sporadic CJD.

Similar observations have been made about the incubation period of natural and experimental scrapie, which shows genetic linkage to the prion protein gene. Recently, a mutation at codon 178 has been observed in a family that segregated a multisystem neurologic illness, a prominent symptom of which was fatal insomnia. The reason why mutations at this codon that would usually cause more typical features of CJD/GSS but instead cause this unusual symptom complex in some families is related to the 129 met/VAC polymorphism.

It has been suggested that the mutant prion protein (PrP^C) products in GSS and familial CJD may have an increased propensity to change conformation into the scrapie (PrP^{Sc}) isoform as a stochastic phenomenon, which once started is self-propagating. Whether the sporadic forms of CJD and GSS represent somatic mutations that cause the same cascade or are merely spontaneous conversion of the normal PrP^C isoform to PrP^{Sc} without a genetic alteration in somatic cells of the subject is unclear. Furthermore, the mechanism by which either mutated or normal PrP^{Sc} leads to fairly specific patterns of transmissible neurodegeneration remains to be elucidated. However, it is clear that the mutations in the prion protein gene are pathogenic because the disease phenotype can be inherited in, and transmitted from, transgenic mice that carry a mutation at codon 102, which suggests that the inherited forms of the prion diseases are functionally similar to the noninherited forms. The necessary role of an endogenous prion protein gene product for the development of these disease is amply demonstrated by the observation that transgenic mice that lack the prion protein gene appear developmentally and phenotypically normal but are resistant to scrapie.

Two-Hit Diseases: Disorders of Recessive Tumor-Suppressor Genes

Bilateral Acoustic Neurofibromatosis

The discovery that tumor cells frequently have deletions of selected chromosomal regions has led to the discovery of an unusual mode of transmission common to several types of inherited malignancies. In these disorders, a germline mutation confers a recessive predisposition to certain malignancies. Because these germline mutations are rare, most subjects are asymptomatic heterozygotes. The disorder is brought to clinical attention in heterozygotes by the occurrence of a second, somatic mutation that deletes the wild-type allele on the normal chromosome in selected somatic cells. Because these genes are presumably tumor-suppressor genes, homozygous loss arising from the action of these two mechanisms leads to multiple independent tumors.

The archetype of these disorders is neurofibromatosis type II. In this disorder, bilateral acoustic schwannomas, meningiomas, and schwannomas of the dorsal roots develop together with several other findings, such as presenile posterior cataracts. Analysis of tumors from subjects with neurofibromatosis type 2 and from some subjects with sporadic acoustic neuromas and meningiomas revealed somatic deletions of chromosome 22q. Subsequent positional cloning studies have led to the isolation of a gene encoding a 587-amino acid protein (named Merlin) with homology to proteins thought to link cytoskeletal and transmembrane proteins (moesin, ezrin, and radixin). Multiple germline mutations have now been found in this gene in subjects with neurofibromatosis type 2 (15 of 16 are nonsense mutations or deletions associated with a truncated protein). Tumors from these subjects had also lost the wild-type gene on the normal chromosome as a result of deletions in the tumor itself. Two subjects with sporadic acoustic neuromas were found to have had somatic nonsense mutations in one chromosome 22 and a somatic deletion in the other chromosome 22.

Similar mechanisms probably pertain in familial retinoblastoma and in the other phakomatoses, such as von Recklinghausen's disease (neurofibromatosis type 1) and von Hippel-Lindau disease. The inherited mutations of recessive tumor-suppressor genes that underlie these diseases are also thought to require a second somatic mutation to bring out the disease phenotype. In neurofibromatosis type 1, even the nontumor phenotypes, such as café au lait spots and Lisch nodules, are thought to arise from this two-hit mechanism. Indeed, it has been proposed that the extreme variability of the disease, both within and between families, can be adequately explained in this instance solely on the randomness by which the necessary second mutation occurs in different somatic cell types at different stages of development.

METHODS FOR GENETIC ANALYSIS OF INHERITED NEUROLOGIC DISEASE

The primary genetic defect that causes a disease phenotype can be identified by standard biochemical techniques if conventional biochemical or pathologic studies suggest a particular candidate gene (e.g., the identification of defective phenylalanine hydroxylase activity as a result of the discovery of abnormal phenylalanine metabolites in the urine of patients with phenylketonuria). However, in most diseases, conventional biochemical studies have not yet identified an immediately obvious candidate gene. Under these circumstances, it is still possible to identify the disease gene with a positional cloning strategy. This approach is based on the fact that genes located close together on the same chromosome (e.g., within 1 million nucleotides) tend to segregate together during gametogenesis; genes situated further apart on the same chromosome (e.g., within 10 million nucleotides) segregate nonrandomly but are occasionally separated by meiotic recombination events in proportion to the physical distance that separates them on the chromosome.

Genes situated on different chromosomes segregate at random. Thus, by comparing the segregation of the disease with that of a series of genetic markers specific for different chromosomal regions, it is possible eventually to find a subset of genetic markers that cosegregate with the disease trait and, thus, with the disease gene itself. Because the chromosomal location of the genetic markers is already known by virtue of the way in which they were isolated, the observation of genetic linkage allows the chromosomal location of the disease gene to be inferred.

Although the analysis of cosegregation of a polymorphic genetic marker with a disease locus can be assessed by simple inspection of pedigree data, it is usually necessary to establish that this pattern of coinheritance was not a chance event. This statistical analysis is accomplished by calculating the logarithm of the odds (or likelihoods) that the pattern of coinheritance had occurred because of genetic linkage relative to the likelihood that it was a chance event (lod score) allowing for occasional instances of meiotic recombination (usually 1, 5, 10, 20, 30, or 40 percent recombination frequencies). By convention, lod scores greater than +3.00 are taken to provide sufficient evidence to prove linkage; lod scores less than −2.00 are taken to exclude linkage at the stated recombination fraction. The recombination fraction that gives the highest lod score provides an estimate of the genetic distance (and thus physical distance) that separates the marker locus and the disease gene.

A critical reagent in this approach is the use of genetic markers that can be used to "tag" the paternal and maternal copies of each chromosome and differentiate them from each other and from all other copies of that chromosome that enter the pedigree by marriage in subsequent generations. By the tagging of chromosomes from the founder parents, it is possible to determine whether the disease segregates with a particular copy of the founder chromosomes (and is thus present in most or all of the currently living affected pedigree members and absent from the obligate escapee members of the pedigree(s) under analysis).

Classical studies used genetically variable (polymorphic) proteins, such as blood group antigens. However, more recent studies have used naturally occurring, usually innocent variations in the nucleotide sequence of genomic DNA. These DNA sequence variations are recognized as single-base substitutions that alter a restriction endonuclease cleavage site (restriction fragment length polymorphisms) or as the insertion or deletion of variable numbers of tandemly repeated sequences (microsatellite or simple sequence repeats and variable number tandem repeats). The latter classes of markers have greater variability and thus greater informativeness than the simple binary restriction fragment length polymorphisms and are now the standard type of marker used for initial linkage studies.

To facilitate efficient mapping of disease genes, the genetic markers have been isolated from most chromosomal regions and arranged into comprehensive genetic linkage maps that depict the relationship and distance between different markers. These maps, which are continuously updated and related to physical maps of the same chromosomal regions, can be obtained through computerized databases, such as the Genome Database at Johns Hopkins University.

The discovery of the approximate chromosomal location of a disease gene is usually the first of several steps that lead eventually to the cloning of the disease gene. Initially, the approximate location of the disease gene can be further refined with the same genetic linkage paradigm to discover additional markers that segregate more closely with the disease and can be used to define the centromeric and telomeric boundaries of a minimal cosegregating region. Once a narrow chromosomal location has been identified for the disease gene, the disease gene itself can be cloned from this minimal cosegregating region with a variety of techniques collectively termed positional cloning.

Briefly stated, these techniques involve cloning overlapping DNA fragments from the chromosomal region that carries the disease gene (chromosome walking) and screening each of these clones for transcribed or expressed sequences (i.e., genes). Expressed sequences from the chromosomal region of interest are then searched for mutations in subjects affected by the disease of interest.

PRACTICAL CONSIDERATIONS

From a practical point of view, a strong family history can frequently be elicited from relatives of patients afflicted with several disorders of neurologic interest (e.g., epilepsy, migraine, mental retardation, multiple sclerosis, bipolar illness, schizophrenia, or Alzheimer's disease). Inevitably, the question is raised as to the risk for recurrence in other family members. As an initial approach, it is necessary to document the extended family tree fully to ascertain whether this familial clustering unarguably reflects one of the rare instances of monogenic transmission of these disorders or whether it represents a more complex pattern of inheritance.

In the instances in which a monogenic pattern of inheritance is obvious, counseling is straightforward and, where possible, can take advantage of molecular genetic studies discussed in earlier sections.

These clinically applied molecular genetic studies can be either mutational analysis in diseases in which the disease gene(s) has (have) been identified or linkage analysis and haplotype comparison with known affected pedigree members when only the chromosomal location of the disease gene is known. The latter is feasible when the disease is known to be homogeneous or the pedigree is large enough to establish statistically significant evidence for linkage between the disease locus and the genetic markers in the particular pedigree that presents for genetic counseling. When the familial aggregation is less clear-cut, calculation of the risk is largely empirical, and is best handled by referral to a professional genetic counselor.

ANNOTATED BIBLIOGRAPHY

Beggs AH, Hoffman EP, Snyder J et al. Exploring the molecular basis for the variability among patients with Becker muscular dystrophy: dystrophin gene and protein studies. Am J Hum Genet 1991;49:54–67.

Becker muscular dystrophy.

Brice A, Mallet J. La génétique moléculaire: une nouvelle approche des neurosciences cliniques. Rev Neurol (Paris) 1991;147:1–16.

Thorough review including a detailed glossary of terms.

Collins FS. Positional cloning: let's not call it reverse anymore. Nature Genet 1992;1:3–6.

A review of positional cloning strategies.

Eisensmith RC, Woo SLC. Molecular basis of phenylketonuria and related hyperphenylalaninemias: mutations and polymorphisms in the human phenylalanine hydroxylase gene. Hum Mutat 1992;1:13–23.

A review of the molecular genetics of phenylketonuria that illustrates the types of molecular defects in recessive diseases.

Farrer LA, Myers RH, Connor L et al. Segregation analysis reveals evidence of a major gene for Alzheimer disease. Am J Hum Genet 1991;48:1026–33.

Gusella JF. DNA polymorphisms and human disease. Annu Rev Biochem 1986;55:831–4.

A review of the use of genetic linkage strategies to find disease genes.

Gusella JF, Huntington Disease Collaborative Group. A novel gene containing a trinucleotide repeat that is expanded and unstable on Huntington's disease chromosomes. Cell 1993;72:971–83.

Describes the isolation of the disease gene for Huntington's disease.

Hu X, Ray PN, Murphy EG et al. The frequency, distribution, and phenotype-genotype correlation. Am J Hum Genet 1990;46:682–95.

Duchenne muscular dystrophy.

Karlinsky H, Vaula G, Haines JL et al. Molecular and prospective phenotypic characterization of a pedigree with familial Alzheimer disease and a missense mutation in codon 717 of the β-amyloid precursor protein (APP) gene. Neurology 1992;42:1445–53.

Describes the phenotype and molecular genetics of Alzheimer's disease associated with mutations in the APP gene.

La Spada AR, Wilson EM, Lubahn DB et al. Androgen receptor gene mutation in X-linked spinal bulbar muscular atrophy. Nature 1991;352:77–9.

Characterization of the spinobulbar muscular atrophy gene defect as a pathologic expansion of a trinucleotide repeat element.

Myers RH, Leavitt J, Farrer LA et al. Homozygote for Huntington disease. Am J Hum Genet 1989;34:615–8.

Describes molecular evidence that Huntington's disease is a true dominant disorder.

Ott J. Human Genetic Linkage Analysis. Johns Hopkins University Press, Baltimore, 1984.

A text on methods of statistical genetic linkage analysis.

Palmer MS, Dryden AJ, Hughes JT, Collinge J. Homozygous prion protein genotype predisposes to sporadic Creutzfeldt-Jakob disease. Nature 1991;352:340–2.

Describes effect on susceptibility to CJD of polymorphisms within the prior protein gene.

Prusiner S. Molecular biology of prion diseases. Science 1991;252:1517–22.

Review biology of prion genes.

Rocca WA, Amaducci LA, Schoenberg BS. Epidemiology of clinically diagnosed Alzheimer's disease. Ann Neurol 1986;19:415–24.

Evidence for a genetic cause in many cases of Alzheimer's disease.

Rosen DR, Siddique T, Patterson D et al. Mutations in Cu/Zn superoxide dismutase gene are associated with familial amyotrophic lateral sclerosis. Nature 1993;362:59–62.

Describes mutations observed in familial ALS.

Saunders A, Strittmatter WJ, Schmechel S et al. Association of apoliprotein E allele e4 with the late-onset familial and sporadic Alzheimer disease. Neurology 1993;43:1467–72.

Association of late-onset familial and sporadic Alzheimer's disease with the apolipoprotein E gene.

Seizinger BR, Martuza RL, Rouleau G et al. Models for inherited susceptibility to cancer in the nervous system: a molecular-genetic approach to neurofibromatosis. Dev Neurosci 1987;9:144–53.

Reviews the recessive tumor-suppressor gene hypothesis.

St. George-Hyslop PH, Boulianne G. Molecular genetics of inherited neurodegenerative diseases, in Calne D (ed). Neurodegeneration. WB Saunders, New York, 1993.

A review of the application of molecular genetic techniques to neuroscience.

St. George-Hyslop P, Haines J, Rogaev E et al. Genetic evidence for a novel familial Alzheimer disease gene on chromosome 14. Nature Genet. 1992;2:330–4.

Describes a novel familial Alzheimer's disease gene locus on chromosome 14.

St. George-Hyslop PH, Tsuda T, Crapper DR, McLachlan et al. Alzheimer disease and possible gene interactions. Science 1994;263:537–8.

Describes evidence for interactions between different familial Alzheimer's disease loci.

Trofatter J, MacCollin M, Rutter JL et al. A novel moesin-ezrin-radixin-like gene is a candidate for the NF2 tumor suppressor gene. Cell 1993;72:791–800.

Describes the isolation of the neurofibromatosis type 2 gene.

Tsuda T, Munthasser S, Fraser P et al. Analysis of the functional effects of a mutation in SOD1 associated with familial amyotrophic lateral sclerosis. Neuron 1994;13:727–36.

Reviews the mechanisms of action of SOD1 mutations in ALS.

Upadhyaya M, Shen M, Cherryson A et al. Analysis of mutations at the neurofibromatosis 1 (NF1) locus. Hum Mol Genet 1992;1:735–40.

Describes mutations found in the neurofibromatosis type 1 gene.

5
Stroke

J. P. Mohr and J. C. Gautier

EPIDEMIOLOGY

As a cause of injury to the brain, stroke, taken as a single entity, is among the most important. All forms of stroke taken into account, the incidence averages approximately 180 per 100,000 per year (0.2 percent) worldwide with a prevalence of 500 to 600 per 100,000 (0.5 percent), a low of 250 per 100,000 being reported for the United Kingdom to as high as 900 per 100,000 in the Far East. Where data have been collected, the age-adjusted rates for initial stroke approach 109 per 100,000 for whites and 208 per 100,000 for blacks, in studies in the United States, with age-specific rates higher in blacks than in whites. Rates for subarachnoid hemorrhage are highest in young black women for reasons not explained. It remains uncertain whether the higher prevalence of risk factors for stroke in blacks accounts for this difference.

In 8 to 20 percent of patients the stroke is fatal within the first 30 days. For over 50 years the major cause of stroke has been ischemic infarction. Early recurrence of infarction adds to the neurologic deficit and functional disability and lengthens hospital stay. Stroke recurs after the first 30 days in 4 to 14 percent of patients per year, and 5-year survival averages only 60 percent.

Stroke Subtype

For generations it was widely taught that atherothrombosis was the leading cause of stroke. In the 1930s autopsy-based studies from a single hospital population, such as those at the Boston City Hospital reported by Aring and Merritt (1935), indicated that atherosclerosis accounted for over 70 percent of cases of stroke and embolism a mere 3 percent (Table 5-1). Considering the equally widespread view that little therapy existed for atherosclerosis, many students were easily persuaded that stroke was a disease with no treatment. Well into the 1960s and 1970s even prospective case series such as the Framingham Study diagnosed atherothrombotic brain infarction (grouping large-vessel atherothrombosis with lacunar infarction) as the most frequent cause of stroke, the frequency being somewhat lower than in the Boston City Hospital study but still accounting for 44 percent of the 693 cases of stroke and transient ischemic attack. Cerebral embolism was diagnosed more frequently, at 21 percent, while intracranial hemorrhage remained static at roughly 12 percent and other causes were diagnosed in 2 percent of cases (Table 5-1).

The Harvard Cooperative Stroke Registry, a prospective hospital-based study of 694 patients with stroke, also initially reported thrombotic infarction as the leading cause of stroke, using traditional acceptance of risk factors of hypertension and diabetes to infer the diagnosis of atherothrombosis when no other data were available. Yet only 36 percent of strokes were attributed to large-artery stenosis or thrombosis due to atherosclerosis. This cohort was the first to include lacunes as a diagnosis (see Ch. 35), the 17 percent ascribed to them being largely subtracted from the portion of stroke formerly attributed to atherosclerosis. By using more modern criteria, fully 31 percent were diagnosed as embolism, 10 percent were intracerebral hematoma, and 6 percent subarachnoid hemorrhage (Table 5-1). This study did not contain a separate category for infarcts whose cause remained undetermined. This effort was pioneered by the group at the Salpétrière in Paris, who as early at 1968 reported 28 percent of cases of infarction as being of undetermined cause. These studies, while having a negative effect on the diagnosis of large-artery atherosclerosis, helped encourage the view that embolism is a common form of stroke through the use of more liberal criteria for the diagnosis of embolism. The traditional requirements of atrial fibrillation and valvular

Table 5-1. Ischemic Stroke Subtype by Study and Year

Study	Year	Cases	Thrombosis			Embolism		Hemorrhage	
			Lac	Ath	TAP	Cryp	Emb	ICH	SAH
Boston City Hosp.	1935	407		81%ᵃ		3%ᵃ		15%ᵃ	
Rochester, MN	1954	548		75%		3%		10%	6%
Framingham, MA	1961	90		63%		15%		4%	18%
Salpêtrière, Paris	1968	122		43%		28%	16%		
Rochester, MN	1969	993		71%		3%		10%	5%
Harvard Registry	1976	802	17%	36%		20%		11%	7%
NINCDS Data Bank	1988	1802	19%	6%	4%	28%	14%	13%	13%

Abbreviations: Lac, lacune; Ath, large-artery severe stenosis or occlusion, attributed to atherosclerosis; TAP, tandem arterial pathology; Cryp, cryptogenic stroke (infarct of undetermined cause); Emb, cardiogenic embolism (atrial fibrillation, valvular disease, other cause); ICH, parenchymatous intracerebral hemorrhage; SAH, subarachnoid hemorrhage; NINCDS, National Institute of Neurological and Communicative Disorders and Stroke.

ᵃ Where no breakdown given, percentage includes all subtypes of thromboses, embolisms, or hemorrhages.

heart disease for a diagnosis of embolism were supplemented by angiographic data showing intracranial branch occlusion or a normal angiogram performed days after the stroke. More recent work, reflected in the National Institute of Neurological and Communicative Disorders and Stroke (NINCDS) Stroke Data Bank and others, based on more thorough investigation with Doppler ultrasonography and magnetic resonance imaging (MRI) technology has further lowered the incidence of high-grade carotid stenosis or occlusion as a cause of ischemic stroke while they have simultaneously raised the frequency of embolism, specifically cardiac embolism, even further.

With the greater application of modern technology came the requirement to create a category known initially as infarct of undetermined cause, now renamed *cryptogenic* stroke (see Ch. 35). This category was used when conventional studies such as brain imaging suffice to diagnose an infarct but when Doppler or angiography does not disclose extra- or intracranial stenoses, cardiac evaluation does not reveal a cardiac source, and search for systemic disease yields no signs of prothrombotic states. Far from being uncommon, a negative outcome for conventional testing is rather common, and cryptogenic stroke may account for as many as 30 percent of cases or even more. Another category was also created, tandem arterial pathology, which refers to infarcts with more than one site of disease (i.e., in tandem, from the Latin for pair) along the course of arteries supplying the region of brain infarction. Instead of raising the frequency of large-artery atherosclerotic stroke, these two categories further reduced the frequency with which large-artery atherosclerotic stroke was recognized, down to a low of 6 percent in the NINCDS Stroke Data Bank prospective study of 1,805 patients with acute stroke (Table 5-1). Findings such as these, with an emphasis

on embolism and the worries of recurrence, helped add pressure to the growing trend to diagnose stroke subtype. Emerging therapies might differ by subtype in their ability to arrest the stroke in the acute stage, prevent worsening, and prevent recurrence.

Comparable data are slowly appearing from other countries, but too little is known to date of the worldwide frequency distribution of stroke subtypes to permit useful conclusions. One lasting effect has been greatly to increase interest in arriving at a diagnosis of ischemic stroke subtype in the as yet not fully realized hope that the therapy would prove specific to the subtype. Another effect has been eclipse of the former willingness to consider stroke a single entity by the view that stroke, like infectious disease and neoplasm, is a family of disorders.

Decline

There has been a widely reported claim of a gradual and steady decline in stroke since records first became available after 1900. Stroke at that time was thought to account for 40 percent of all recorded cardiovascular deaths. As recently in 1950, strokes accounted for approximately 20 percent of all cardiovascular deaths and have remained roughly constant. The major issue is whether there has been a decline in *incidence*, or simply the now well recognized decline in the *mortality* of stroke (see below).

Factors Contributing to Incidence Data

Overdiagnosis of stroke in contrast to other vascular events has been offered as one possibility for those populations that have shown a decline in incidence. This source of misdiagnosis is steadily shrinking with the widespread use of angiography, computed tomography (CT) scanning, and now MRI and the application of more modern definitions of stroke subtypes.

The initial hopes that a decline could be attributable to better management of risk factors have proved illusory. Identification of risk factors has no doubt played some role but proof has been lacking. Control of hypertension was expected to have an impact on the incidence of parenchymatous hemorrhage, but its frequency has remained fairly stable for decades. The Framingham study, along with the 1960 study of a Rochester, Minnesota cohort, reveals that an individual with coronary heart disease has a threefold increased chance of developing a stroke than a person without this disorder. Cigarette smoking has been clearly correlated with the development of coronary heart disease, but it has been less clear that it correlates directly with the incidence of stroke. Diabetes mellitus is well known factor in accelerating the atherosclerotic process but varies depending on the presence of other risk factors. The Framingham study estimated that diabetes increased the relative stroke risk twofold after adjustment for differences in associated cardiovascular risk factors. Transient ischemic attacks (TIAs) occur prior to stroke in 10 to 15 percent of cases. It has been shown that the risk of subsequent stroke is 10 percent in the first 6 months after onset, followed by an average of 6 percent per year. This is an approximate sixfold increase over the normal population of comparable age.

Better care of the stroke patient does not seem to explain those populations showing decline, since case fatality rates have not changed (see below).

Definitions of Decline

As noted above, what is in decline is also subject to argument: for some it is mortality (shown to have declined in several populations over a 15-year period); for others the decline refers to incidence; for still others, it is severity. Population-based studies in Rochester, Minnesota, indicated that the mortality rates from stroke declined 76 percent during the period 1950 to 1975. The National Center for Health Statistics also showed some decline in mortality but not to this degree. These observations spawned a large number of studies to determine whether such effects occurred in other populations and whether an explanation for the effects could be discovered. Among the studies was a more recent report from the same Rochester population, showing an end to the decline in the decades since 1975 with a rise in event rates, especially for those in the older age groups. Worldwide, no study has addressed this subject in detail. In some populations an actual increase has been described, while in others there are only some suggestions of decline, varying according to definition.

The Framingham study, in a retrospective review of the incidence, severity, and mortality of TIA and completed stroke over the life of the study, now measured in several decades, showed no overall decline in incidence of stroke but some decline in the severity of the strokes documented in men (mainly because of the dilution effect of a higher frequency of reporting of TIAs) and in the incidence of completed stroke in women. The effects seemed quite modest.

Thirty-Day Case Fatality Rates

Lumping together all types of cerebral infarction, the 30-day case fatality rates currently range from a low of 15 percent to as high as 33 percent. Within a year of stroke, between 30 and 52 percent of ischemic stroke patients will be dead, but stroke will be the cause of death only in some of these cases, many being due to myocardial infarction. Despite major advances in therapy, these rates have remained approximately the same for the past 20 years.

Although the overall rates for ischemic stroke lumped together provide a rough guide to outcome, they mask striking differences in the mortality among ischemic stroke subtypes. Recent data, derived from studies in which special efforts were made to diagnose the mechanism of the ischemic stroke, show that the low frequency of certain types of ischemic stroke hides the high associated mortality. In the NINCDS Stroke Data Bank, those strokes attributed to large-artery atherosclerosis were associated with an 18.8 percent mortality in the first 30 days. By comparison, those due to lacunar infarcts produced much lower mortality. Similar data were obtained in the Framingham study, in which the case fatality rate from atherothrombotic infarction was 15 percent. These statistics are especially sobering when it is realized that the large-vessel arteriosclerosis cases include those from carotid stenosis and occlusion, possibly subject to prophylactic surgery (see Ch. 35). The high mortality figures associated with large-artery stenosis and occlusion provide a very different data base for comparing natural history outcome for stroke against the results of various therapies than is obtained by using crude mortality data from infarcts of all types.

Mortality does not appear to be a function of the major territory involved. In the NINCDS Stroke Data Bank project, there was very little difference in mortality between supratentorial (12.2 percent) and infratentorial (13.5 percent) infarction.

Many of the factors actually identified with mortality are easily understood. Thus, a decreased 30-day survival associated with a depressed level of consciousness and history of prior stroke surely indicates large infarction. Death directly attributable to stroke generally occurs within the first week, often with transtentorial herniation (see Chs. 17 and 25), the effects being applicable for both cerebral hemorrhage and cerebral infarction.

It is perhaps somewhat surprising that no correlation has been found with the greater number of medical illnesses and outcome. After the first week, most stroke deaths are non-neurologic in nature. Cardiac complications are encountered very often in conjunction with stroke and occur throughout the 30-day period after stroke. Other complicating factors include congestive heart failure, hypertension, diabetes mellitus, and older age. Relative immobilization due to the depressed level of consciousness and motor deficits are reflected in the high frequency of pneumonia, urinary tract infection, sepsis, and pulmonary thromboembolism occurring between the second and fourth week. From this scenario one would expect that prevention and/or treatment of brain edema in the hyperacute stage, followed by early mobilization, will improve the case fatality rates. These predictions cannot be tested adequately since as yet no effective treatment for ischemic stroke has been developed.

All told, caution is advised before setting aside stroke as a problem that is on the wane.

CEREBRAL INFARCTION

For brain tissue to die from infarction, there must be either (1) an interruption in the supply of nutrients that is of sufficient duration to cause failure of cellular metabolism or (2) a restriction in the egress of the acid end products of brain metabolism that is sufficient to lower the tissue pH and to set in motion the huge cascade of neurochemical events that damage the cellular cytoskeleton. What is discussed below can be considered a rough guide to current understanding but may well soon be outmoded by the pace of discoveries.

Gross and Microscopic Pathology

From the earliest days of neuropathology it has been appreciated that at autopsy performed within a few days after a stroke the damaged brain regions are soft to the touch. In some countries infarction is still termed "softening." On naked-eye inspection the cut brain shows a loss of the distinctive difference in appearance between gray and white matter. When examined months or years after the stroke event, the same regions have become cavitated and filled by cerebrospinal fluid (CSF), reflecting the removal of the infarcted tissue.

When the infarct affects the brain surface, it leaves a dent or depression, seen on brain imaging as a gap in the brain surface (see Ch. 10). In the least affected cases the cortical surface is only slightly shrunken and the underlying white matter still seems firm, while in the more severe instances the entire affected cerebral region is gone, leaving a deep cleft, with a thin layer of the pia overlying the cleft and and the ventricular wall separating it from the ventricle below. When the deep structures are affected alone, the reabsorbed areas leave a hole or space, known as a lacune (from the Latin for hole) when small or a cavity when large. In many cases the sharp margin of the infarct has conformed enough to the region of supply of a single branch of a major cerebral artery that the source of the infarct can be assigned to occlusion of that branch. Microscopy of the softened tissue performed days to weeks after the infarct typically shows that the infarct zone is devoid of neurons and the tissue is edematous and scattered through with macrophages.

The process of infarction seems, in most cases, to be highly circumscribed: cell counts show a sharp separation between the infarct and the normal brain, the margin being as small as a few micrometers. This evidence argues against an effect of infarction that spreads like some stain into the tissue. Instead it indicates a highly circumscribed process, one tied to the tissue suffering the failure of blood flow, and not spreading, as does an infection or tumor, from the site of first involvement to affect adjacent tissues.

Pathoclysis Versus Morphostatic Necrobiosis

The usual type of infarction, in which the pathologic process has led to lysis of the cerebral structures, has been described by Lindenberg as pathoclysis (Greek: *path*, disease; *lysis*, dissolution), a term separate from the more widely used pathoclisis (Greek: *path*, disease; *klisis*, tendency toward) popularized by the Vogts to refer to tissues thought to have selective vulnerability to disease. The term *pathoclysis* is little used currently but was coined to indicate a form of infarction in which liquefaction of tissue is the predominant finding. Because it is the most common type of infarction, it is used here only for contrast with other types of histologic abnormalities, described below.

In rare cases the architecture of the tissue may be remarkably well preserved. The neurons appear shrunken in size, are eosinophilic, and take stains poorly. The tissue is devoid of macrophages and shows little sign of edema. This appearance, labeled morphostatic necrobiosis (from the Greek for preserved appearance but dead tissue), differs from the usual appearance of pathoclysis. The best explained examples occur in a setting of occlusion of the feeding arteries, where virtually no collateral flow retrograde into the zone exists, indicating that access to the circulation through some means of reperfusion plays a role in the necrotizing process. This state occurs in cases of occlusion of small, deep, end arteries, in some cases of occlusion of the basilar artery, and in occlusion of the internal carotid if there is no collateral through the circle of Willis or over the border zones linking the cerebral surface arteries. In cases in which there is no recirculation, the lesion appears to undergo a kind of mummification.

The fact that such cases are rare is less important than the observation that total tissue dissolution is not an obligatory effect of lack of circulation. It raises the hope that some form of rescue therapy might prevent total tissue dissolution and perhaps spare function.

Timetable of Infarction

In experimental animal models, cell counts on consecutive specimens have shown that cell loss and pallor, markers of developing necrosis, gradually spread over hours from a central site in a centrifugal manner, peaking at 72 hours, and eventually reach the geographic limits of the zone of the eventual infarct. The timetable of pallor is well documented in animal models. Its onset after neuronal death can be used to document the course of the development of an infarct in such settings.

The shorter the time of occlusion, the less widespread is the area of pallor and the smaller the size of the infarction. Arterial occlusion lasting less than 1 hour in animal models results only in selective neuron necrosis or laminar necrosis without leukocyte infiltration, and no tissue cavitation occurs. Occlusion lasting 72 hours or longer is associated with infarction involving both the gray and white matter (full-thickness in-

farction), leukocyte infiltration into the affected area, and eventual tissue cavitation of the infarct zone.

These findings suggest that the process of infarction is not complete from the first instant and also hold out the hope some degree of tissue rescue could occur if the occlusion could be relieved early enough.

Collateral Blood Flow

When an occlusion occurs in a pericerebral artery, the ischemic zone has a chance to receive collateral flow from neighboring major cerebral arteries via retrograde flow through the border zone vessels shared between the major cerebral territories (see Ch. 35).

The collateral flow available to an occluded artery is almost entirely end-to-end in type (e.g., a branch of the anterior cerebral artery may collateralize via the borderzone with a branch of the middle cerebral artery) (Fig. 5-1) (see also Ch. 36). Virtually no side-to-side collaterals occur between adjoining branches within the same major cerebral arterial territory. For this reason, no rescue can be expected within a territory (e.g., the ascending frontal branch of the middle cerebral artery does not link to the rolandic branch of the same middle cerebral artery territory).

For the small deep arteries (i.e., the lenticulostriate branches of the middle cerebral artery, the thalamoperforant branches of the posterior cerebral artery, and the paramedian and long and short circumferential branches of the basilar artery, as well as the pene-

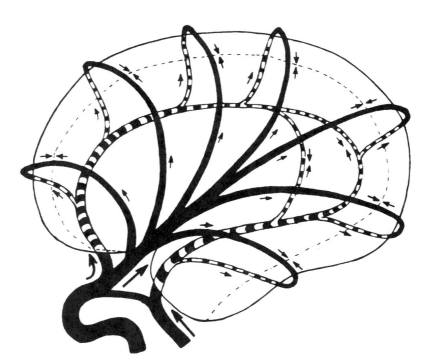

Figure 5-1. Conceptual sketch of the meningeal anastomoses over the brain. (From Heubner, 1872.)

trating arteries into the central white matter from the cerebral convexity) there are no sources of collateral flow. As soon as these arteries enter the brain tissue, they behave as end arteries. (Although anastomoses can be demonstrated histologically, they are too tiny to be significant.)

The extent of the available collateral blood flow is a major determinant of brain infarct size. For the arteries over the surface of the brain (e.g., the convexity branches of the anterior, middle, and posterior cerebral arteries and the three major arteries of the cerebellum), the infarct resulting from occlusion of a single branch may vary greatly in size. It may be so large as to span the site from the occlusion to the end of the occluded vascular territory in the border zones, where there is no retrograde collateral flow, or it may be as small as a few millimeters adjacent to the site of occlusion, where the border zone collateral is readily available. The deep arterial territories are end arteries with no collateral, thus allowing no chance for rescue from infarction by collateral flow when ischemia develops (Fig. 5-2).

There is only limited knowledge of what governs the size of these collateral vessels and whether they will respond to the hemodynamic flow demands by prompt vasodilation. The low pH of ischemic tissue spontaneously brings about vasodilation, but the timing of the full development of the collateral remains unpredictable. No therapy has yet been developed that is known to dilate them maximally in the acute phase, when they are most needed. The common ob-

servation that well developed collateral flow is found weeks to months after an infarct gives little insight into the acute process. When late, development of collaterals serves mainly to bring macrophages to digest the necrotic tissue.

Submicroscopic, Cellular, and Chemical Events

Work in recent decades has helped explain the basis for the tissue injury seen by visual or light microscopic inspection of the gross tissue and can account for the evolution of the lesion.

Ischemic Penumbra

First in animal models and later in human studies (see below) it has become appreciated that for a period of time after arterial occlusion, there is no predictably uniform zone of tissue formerly dependent on the now occluded artery that is destined for infarction. Tissue closest to the site of occlusion is the most likely to suffer infarction, but the farther a site is from that zone, the more collateral flow could reduce the risk of infarction. Studies with animal models have demonstrated the existence of a zone of tissue, adjacent to that destined for infarction, blood supply to which is inadequate to maintain clinical (or electrophysiologic) function. This zone, still intact morphologically, may be still be viable and have some chance for rescue and functional recovery. This tissue, called the ischemic penumbra (Latin: *paene*, almost; *umbra*, shadow), has been shown to remain viable for a few hours from the onset of arterial occlusion. The events associated with its existence, potential for reversal, or eventual conversion to infarction comprise much of the following discussion.

Cerebral Blood Flow and Oxygen Metabolism

For brain tissue to survive, the regional cerebral blood flow (rCBF) must be above 12 ml/100 g/min (normal being > 100 ml/100 g/min). When occlusion produces a fall in rCBF toward this critical value, the brain attempts to extract more than usual amounts of oxygen from the circulating blood.

An increase in the oxygen extraction fraction (oxygen tension in arterial blood reaching the brain relative to that in venous blood draining the brain) indicates an approaching state of ischemia, called "misery perfusion" (see Ch. 14 for more details). Its presence is a sign of a risk for infarction, which generally lasts no more than minutes to hours in experimental stroke models. Studies have shown that values of cerebral metabolic rate for oxygen ($CMRO_2$) below 65 ξmol/100 g/min correlate highly with subsequent brain infarction. In animal models the energy metabolism in the penumbra zone is unstable, at times showing normal energy and at other times showing fluctuating

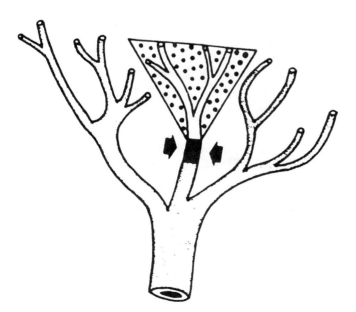

Figure 5-2. Conceptual sketch of an infarct in an end-arterial territory. (From Zülch, 1981, with permission.)

failure. This unsteady state may last up to days, suggesting that tissue rescue could possibly be achieved even late in the course after the onset of illness.

Once critical levels of rCBF have been breached, an orderly pathophysiologic process is set in motion, which plays itself out over minutes to days. Within 15 to 20 seconds of the fall of rCBF to critical levels, intracellular pH falls, and lactic acid levels rise owing to cessation of aerobic metabolism. These changes are reflected in the occurrence of clinical deficits, loss of power in the electroencephalogram, and fall in cerebral evoked potentials when rCBF falls to 20 ml/100 g/min. These events are better understood than are the means to reverse or prevent them.

Acidosis

Within seconds the brain, having no endogenous energy stores and relying on the circulation for a continuous supply of oxygen and glucose, shifts the glycolytic pathway to the production of acid end products of metabolism instead of the normal oxygen-dependent production of carbon dioxide and water. The intracellular pH plunges to an acidotic level thought to be sufficient to damage cell membranes. If the duration of occlusion is insufficient to cause infarction, the downward, ischemic shift in pH is reversed, with the pH returning almost as quickly to normal after reperfusion.

There was concern based on some animal models that the presence of large amounts of glucose could greatly exaggerate the process of acidosis, which would mean that physicians should withhold parenteral therapy with glucose in acute stroke. Based on current data, this concern appears to have been exaggerated and is not a major factor for normal blood sugar levels and normal infusion glucose concentrations (e.g., 5 percent dextrose in water), but physicians are still advised not to use large amounts of high-concentration glucose (e.g., 50 percent in water) in the early hours after ischemic stroke.

Sodium Pump Failure

Within minutes, failure occurs in the Na^+/Ca^{++} exchange pump, the dominant exchange mechanism for the regulated entry of Ca^{++} into brain cells. The Na^+ pump may be damaged by exposure to free radicals, which are released by the process of ischemia (see below).

Unregulated Calcium Entry

Over a period of minutes to hours of ischemia, Ca^{++} enters cells in unregulated amounts. There are currently known to be four voltage-dependent Ca^{++} channels, one presynaptic (N channel) and three post-synaptic (P, L, and T channels) (Fig. 5-3). In addition, there is one chemically-dependent channel, mediated by N-methyl-d-aspartate (NMDA). The T, L, and NMDA channels are all Ca^{++}-dependent and all are postsynaptic.

Glutamate and aspartate are the principal compounds that open the NMDA channel, glutamate having been subject to the greatest amount of study. The release of glutamate into the extracellular space in abnormally large amounts, opening NMDA channels to excess, has been held to be one of the major causes of unregulated entry of Ca^{++} into cells in ischemia. More than mere glutamate release seems to be involved in the ischemic process, since release of glutamate into the extracellular space can be documented in all ischemic brain zones, but as yet there has not been a clear correlation between the occurrence of glutamate release and the sensitivity of the given region to cell damage. Presumably, regions vary in their sensitivity to NMDA channel opening, and Ca^{++} entry via the other channels also plays an important role.

As was recently reviewed by Globus, entry into the cell of excessive amounts of calcium is the major factor setting in motion the cascade of events that leads to tissue injury. Unregulated Ca^{++} entry causes eventual membrane breakdown by release of intracellular phosphorylases, which activate lipases; th activation of proteases, causing proteolysis; and activation of protein kinases, leading to protein phosphorylation and hypofunction of receptors and ion channels.

Free Radicals

Within minutes of the onset of ischemia, free radicals are formed in the ischemic zone. Although superoxide radicals have been known for more than a decade, their role in brain infarction is still not entirely clear.

Hydroxyl radicals are formed by ischemia and reperfusion but the major issue is how important they might be. Superoxide ($O_2^-\cdot$) and nitric oxide ($NO\cdot$) free radicals (see below) form peroxynitrite anion ($ONOO^-$), which decomposes to form hydroxyl radical and nitrogen dioxide. Peroxynitrite can only diffuse over a distance of a few millimeters from its site of formation, which makes its biologic effects extremely limited in a spatial sense. It directly oxidizes sulfhydryl groups and reacts with the enzyme superoxide dismutase and with Fe^{+++}, Cu^{++}, and other multivalent ions.

Macrophages and neutrophils can make $ONOO^-$ directly, which interacts with Ca^{++}, Zn^{++} and superoxide dismutase. Nitroarginine given intravenously will gradually lower rCBF and reduce infarct volume by up to 80 min after ischemia, but it offers no protection when given beforehand. A new agent currently

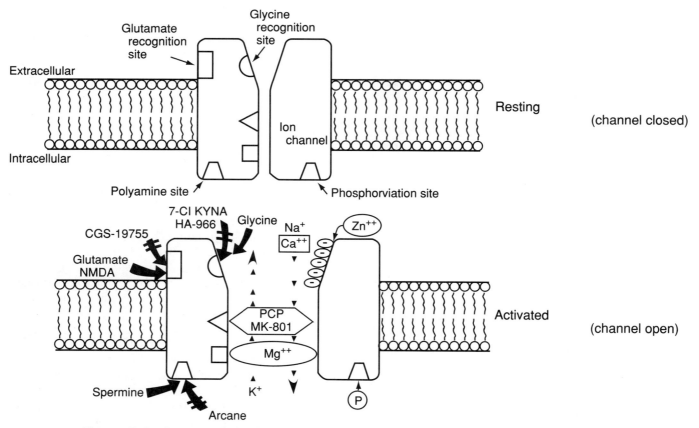

Figure 5-3. Conceptual sketch of the processes of calcium-related mechanisms in ischemia.

named Dismutec, a form of superoxide dismutase, is just entering clinical trials planned for 1995.

Nitric Oxide

Another recently recognized source of tissue injury via free radicals promptly produced in excessive amounts by ischemia is the nitric oxide radical (NO·). Normally, NO· combines with the iron center of many enzymes to either inactivate them, as it does for enzymes that stimulate cell division, or to activate them, as it does for an enzyme that allows L-arginine and oxygen to combine to generate citrulline and NO·. This reaction is a short circuit of the urea cycle metabolic cascade. Intracranially, NO· is made in the cerebellum and in macrophages. Studies of cerebellar neurons have shown that the presence of calcium and calmodulin is also required, and thus the unregulated entry of calcium into neurons could greatly increase NO· production. For macrophages, arginine and reduced nicotinamide adenine dinucleotide phosphate (NADPH) are required, the latter being available in a setting of ischemia. The enzyme, nitric oxide synthetase has a high electron affinity, which makes it an ideal electron transfer device.

NO· is a neurotoxin, as it is a free radical capable of direct neuronal damage. Although no NO· appears to exist within neurons, it is available from extraneuronal sources in a setting of ischemia. The NO· released by endothelial cells induces vasodilation. In a normal setting the NO· produced by endothelium is thought to prevent adhesion of neutrophils. Extracellular glutamate, also released by ischemia, activates receptors for α-amino-3-hydroxy-5-methyl-4-isoxazolepropionic acid (AMPA), which in turn activate hemoglobin oxygenase, which generates NO· and carbon monoxide, also leading to vasodilation.

In astrocytes and macrophages (the latter migrating into the infarct site from circulating blood), glutamate activation of the NMDA receptor allows unregulated Ca^{++} entry into these cells binding of the Ca^{++} with calmodulin activates the enzyme nitric oxide synthetase, which converts intracellular arginine to citrulline, liberating NO· in the reaction. The NO· then quickly bonds with oxygen ions to form NO_2 and NO_3.

The activation and deactivation of many enzymes involving their heavy metal centers is related to the formation of peroxynitrite from NO·. A relationship between the roles of superoxides and the iron center of many enzymes involve the reactions between superoxides and NO˙ to form peroxynitrite, which decomposes to form hydroxyl radicals and nitrogen dioxide. Peroxynitrite directly oxidizes sulfhydryl groups and reacts with Fe^{+++} and and Cu^{++} ions, which could serve to disrupt cellular chemical reactions and contribute to the necrotizing process.

NO˙ blockade has produced a variety of effects, from decreased rCBF to no effect, in animals. While this field continues to occupy the energies of molecular biologists, it remains uncertain what, if any, implications the studies will have for human disease.

Postischemic Events

Some postischemic events may bring about neuronal damage that is delayed in onset by hours to days. These include activation of genes, breakdown of the blood-brain barrier, and the inflammatory response.

Altered Excitatory-Inhibitory Balance

The release of excitatory transmitters such as glutamate changes the normal balance between excitation and inhibition, which appears to activate changes in gene expression of glutamate receptors (see below). It also activates genes, among them jun B messenger RNAs (mRNAs) and heat shock protein (hsp70 mRNA), which results in altered gene expression and protein synthesis, causing dysfunction of receptors in the ion channels and so leading to membrane breakdown. The appearance of mRNA in damaged tissue within minutes to hours has given hope that growth factors could play a role in he healing process. Thus far it appears that days pass before the growth factors generated by these mRNAs begin to emerge in the brain.

Blood-Brain Barrier

Breakdown of the blood-brain barrier allows the development of vasogenic edema, which increases vascular permeability to active substances in the damaged regions. The inflammatory response involves the infiltration of polymorphonuclear leukocytes (PMNs) and macrophages, both cell types being large enough to block the local microvasculature while they are in the circulation; their entry into the microvasculature reduces local blood flow. Polymorphonuclear leukocytes are a potent source of free radicals (see below), and macrophages also release active substances, aggravating tissue injury.

Inflammatory Response

The infiltration of polymorphonuclear leukocytes and macrophages, leading to reduction in blood flow, itself leads to release of active substances (see above), contributing to delayed injury.

Other Factors

Once hailed as important factors in ischemia, the prostaglandins seem less important in current studies. Leukotrienes, a subject of interest in the last decade, are not much studied currently. Kinins, tachykinins, and other substances in this group have received little study, but what is known has not shown a major role in the ischemic process. At least 15 different chemokines are known; they are endogenous cytokines, which produce a chemical gradient that attracts leukocyte by chemotaxis and activates leukocyte infiltration. Cytokines may play a role in cell toxicity, as may adhesion molecule and white blood cell adhesion regulators and factors involved in matrix remodeling. These effects would make their appearance some time after the first 12 hours. Thus far too little is known of their function, whether therapies would modify their effect, and whether such modification would be important in treatment of stroke. They are mentioned here mainly as potential areas of future research.

Imaging Stroke in Humans

The cascade of pathophysiologic events outlined above is known from tissue culture studies and animal models of stroke. For the human, the current evidence corroborating the timetable of these events is to be seen in brain imaging. In humans, the first evidence of infarction seen on CT or MRI may not appear until about 3 to 6 hours. Once the lesions appear, few are seen to enlarge, which suggests that the process of infarction is limited to the volume of imaged change in tissue density and does not spread relentlessly over the brain.

By using newer imaging techniques such as echoplanar MRI equipment, capable of producing diffusion-weighted imaging, evidence has been found for impaired perfusion reflecting the arrested arterial circulation in the area of infarction. This technique has also shown impaired diffusion images, seen as early as 1 hour or so, before there is tissue change indicative of infarction.

The diffusion abnormality is thought to represent cytotoxic edema released by ischemia, neurochemically associated with failing Na^+,K^+ adenosine triphosphatase (Na^+/K^+-ATPase) activity. In animal models the diffusion-weighted abnormalities can be blocked by NMDA antagonists, which suggests that these abnormalities represent the events of ischemia; they can also be reversed by early reperfusion which indicates that they need not be permanent. The geographic limits of the early lesions can be documented by the perfusion deficit and correlate well with subsequent infarct size. Although the geographic limits of the perfusion abnormality do not enlarge in most cases, the degree of diffusion abnormality may greatly intensify over time, filling in the veins defined by the initial perfusion deficit, arguably the evolution of infarct over time.

In positron emission tomography (PET) studies, those patients who experienced recanalization of an occluded middle cerebral artery within 18 hours showed only an infarction in the lenticulostriate branches of this artery (a vessel lacking collateral flow), while the cerebral surface was spared. These data further indicate that the process of infarction has a time course for development and ischemia can be subject to reversal if the occlusion is relieved early enough.

Functional Reorganization

All the foregoing notwithstanding, it is the clinical improvement after stroke that is of first importance to patients and clinicians alike. It remains entirely unclear what basic biologic processes are at work in reducing the initial neurologic deficit over time.

Functional Effects of Edema

For years, the simplistic explanation for later improvement was the subsidence of edema. It was inferred that some of the initial clinical deficit was not from primary tissue injury but from functional deactivation of healthy tissue by short-lived edema formation, analogous to the limitation of movement of a sprained ankle by postinjury edema. The subsidence of the edema would be expected to allow reemergence of function of always healthy tissue, making the improvement nothing more than subsidence of some of the effects of the injury. For such effects, the term "recovery" would seem entirely proper.

Some evidence of a reversible syndrome attributable to edema has been found clinically. Studies of acute stroke have used this concept to explain the worsening that occurs in about 25 percent of patients suffering infarction. For those with infarcts explained by occlusion of small, deep arteries, improvement occurred within 4 days, while for those with larger infarcts, no such improvement occurred. The findings suggest that reversible edema explained the worsening in the former while extension of the infarct was responsible for worsening in the latter group.

Postinfarct Functional Improvement

For almost as long as the principles of cerebral localization have been practiced, there have been examples of patients whose initial neurologic disturbance suggested destruction of areas whose health was crucial to the performance of a particular neurologic function but who regained the lost function. Examples include the fading toward normal of the initial mutism following focal infarction of the inferior frontal region, the

reappearance of speech and language after infarction of Broca's area and even after infarction in Wernicke's area (see Ch. 17 for more details), and the more recent demonstration of improvement in motor function toward normal despite infarction of the sensorimotor cortex. Some clinicians initially set these observations aside as exceptions or signs of infarcts too small to have a lasting effect on brain function. It was even speculated in some cases that the embolus thought to be the cause of the occlusion had broken up and allowed revascularization before the brain was injured, the process occurring in a TIA or reversible ischemic neurologic deficit (see Ch. 36). But too many examples with autopsy correlation exist to allow such a simple explanation, facing current clinicians with the realization that some degree of functional reorganization is at work in reducing the severity of the clinical picture following brain lesion.

Diaschisis

Originally introduced by C. von Monakow (Swiss neurologist, 1853–1930), diaschisis (from the Greek for splitting or separation) was a notion introduced to explain the short-lived suspension or disturbance in function following focal brain lesions. Von Monakow inferred that some functional derangement in internal cerebral linkages occurred beyond those of the permanent lesion and that these functionally deactivated systems could be reestablished, explaining some of the improvement that occurs as time passed after a focal lesion. In addition to the reappearance of the function lost through diaschisis, his concepts also provided for a change in the character of some of the symptoms over time, not simply their subsidence. This last concept raised the possibility of a degree of compensatory capacity that is not simply restoration of initially suppressed function.

In modern times the term has been applied to reduction in metabolic activity documented in brain regions connected by efferent pathways from the site of a lesion. The most frequently documented of these reductions, shown by PET imaging, has been cerebellar hypometabolism contralateral to a large hemispheral infarct (an effect known as *crossed cerebellar diaschisis*) (see Ch. 14). This modern application of the term is a sharp limitation of the broader concepts theorized by von Monakow. The functional significance of crossed cerebellar diaschisis is still subject to debate. It appears to have no direct clinical correlate and may simply reflect the loss of descending neurotransmitter function.

Studies using single-photon emission tomography or PET in a small number of patients after small thalamic or capsular genu lesions have shown clinical signs suggesting cerebral hemispheric dysfunction for higher cerebral functions and an associated reduction in rCBF and glucose or oxygen utilization. These studies suggest that injuries to cortically bound pathways can blunt cerebral activity and produce a clinical effect mimicking lesions of the cerebral convexity. This too is the simple remote functional loss of the first phase of von Monakow's diaschisis.

Postinjury Compensatory Activation

The recent development of techniques to image cerebral metabolism has allowed the investigation of brain activity after a focal injury. In studies of aphasics, comparison of the resting rCBF values with those during the performance of language testing has shown some evidence of activation by the contralateral hemisphere, indicating a degree of compensatory activation from regions that show little or no such activity in nonlesioned normals subjects.

In recent PET studies, contralateral activation has also been seen in the homologous sites in the sensorimotor cortex following unilateral injury on the opposite side, the activation spreading over a larger area than expected in normal subjects. Furthermore, electrophysiologic mapping in patients after leg amputation over the regions of the hemispheres assumed formerly to have served the legs have shown that these areas are involved in activation of the upper extremities, suggesting shifts in functional assignments.

These observations point to a capability of the brain to undergo some degree of compensatory activity, possibly providing a better explanation of the improvement after a lesion than the former concepts of edema or diaschisis. Thus far few insights have been made obtained as to how this process occurs or as to whether it can be made to accelerate or occur in a more complete manner than occurs naturally. Further studies may give more insight into the character of the improvement and separate true recovery of function from compensatory effects that ameliorate acute syndromes, a process still very poorly understood.

Therapeutic Windows and Ischemia Modification Therapy

Any therapy to prevent disaster from the cascade of ischemic events must be administered rapidly enough to be ahead of the timetable of infarction, a process measured in minutes or hours at most. Therapeutic benefits are difficult to bring about because the same occlusion that prevents normal blood flow prevents any bloodborne therapy from reaching the same site. If the occluding particle could be broken up quickly enough, the tissue could be saved or suffer only scattered foci of infarction. Despite great advances in the understanding of the process of ischemia, it remains unclear whether a definitive therapy will emerge or

whether these processes, once set in motion, occur in a sequence inexorable as that of a collapsing building and the results of the studies simply clarify the events as they develop.

The drugs reviewed below are discussed here since none of them have either come into general use or yet passed the stage of clinical trials to ensure their benefit.

Vasodilators

The simplest attempts to achieve improvement by vasodilation are based on the hope of relaxing the occluded vessel and in so doing encouraging the more distal migration of an occluding particle. This approach might work with embolism but is not likely to help in thrombosis. Agents such as nitroglycerin can achieve this effect, but no studies have been made to determine if this simple gambit is successful. General relaxation of the vasculature could lead to improved retrograde flow into the infarct through collaterals. At present, little is known of the factors that acutely alter the caliber of border zone collateral vessels, but many of the so-called neuroprotective agents, including the calcium antagonists (see below), act in part by increasing arterial flow through the border zones, in some studies achieving much of their therapeutic value through this mechanism.

Thrombolytics

Thrombolytics are under active investigation but it remains uncertain whether their administration will rescue ischemic tissue or lead mainly to hemorrhagic complications. A high frequency of intracranial occlusive disease is found on angiograms obtained within the first few hours of a brain infarct, but the frequency is much lower if studies are done after the second day. These angiographic findings indicate that natural recanalization of intracranial occlusion is a common occurrence, and it has been documented as early as minutes after the occlusion. Attempts to speed this process with tissue plasminogen activator have met with success in surface branches but thus far have been disappointing in the major arterial trunks of the circle of Willis and the carotid.

Hypothermia

Mild hypothermia (temperature reduction from 37° to 33°C) in an animal model is able to reduce infarct size to a substantial degree, but mainly when the cooling occurs coincident with or just before arterial occlusion. Cooling delayed for several hours could have considerable therapeutic benefit, given the ease with which patients can be cooled down to such levels, but thus far there seems little reason to believe that the desired effects can be achieved with delayed cooling.

Calcium Antagonists

In the experimental setting, uncontrolled calcium entry into cells is associated with cell injury (see above and Fig. 5-3). Glutamate, a mediator of the NMDA channel (see above), given in a setting of ischemia, greatly increases the number of damaged cells above that found with either ischemia or glutamate alone. These findings provide an obvious rationale for calcium antagonists in general and for glutamate antagonists in particular.

For some years, attention has been focused on the postsynaptic calcium channel blockers. These agents are of two types. The open channel blockers are those that block an NMDA channel that has been opened by an agonist (e.g., glutamate). The best known of these agents is MK-801 (see below). The closed channel blockers are those in which the inhibitor enters the NMDA ion channel in the absence of agonist stimulation and blocks the channel. Some new agents that achieve this effect have been developed but have not yet been well tested.

The greatest amount of laboratory and clinical experience has been obtained with the postsynaptic voltage-dependent calcium-channel antagonists (i.e., those working through the N, L, or T channels). These agents, widely used in cardiology, share many structural features but differ considerably in their effects on systemic blood pressure and in brain penetration. Poor brain penetration, with both chronotropic and negative inotropic cardiac effects and hypotension, however modest, have made verapamil (Calan, Isoptin), diltiazem (Cardiazem), and nifedipine (Procardia) unattractive as agents for clinical trials. Two others (Sandoz PY 108-068, Nicardipine) underwent some clinical trial exposure in stroke but the small patient population tested prevented any clear results. Nimodipine, a well tolerated compound available in oral form, has been extensively tested in acute ischemic stroke both in animal models and in humans and appears to provide a benefit (see Ch. 35).

Despite the success with nimodipine, researchers still strive for even better results with newer agents. For the NMDA calcium channel system, the glutamate recognition site is blocked by cis-4-phosphonomethyl-piperidine-2-carboxylic acid (CGS-19755) and by the unsaturated analogue D-(3-[C+]-2-carboxypiperazine-1-phosphonic acid) (D-CPPene), and the glycine recognition site is blocked by 1-hydroxy-3-aminopyrrolid-2-one (HA966). Within the NMDA channel one competitive site is blocked by dizocilpine (MK-801), Ceretsat (CNS-1102), and dextromethorphan, while the other is blocked by Mg^{++} and Zn^{++} ions. A polyamine site is blocked by Ifenprofil. No agents have yet been developed to attack the phosphorylation site.

Initial experience with the one of the earliest NMDA channel antagonists, MK-801, led to it withdrawal owing to the occurrence of (reversible) psychotic behavioral effects. Neuroprotective effects could not be assessed in the small clinical experience. Several hundred people have been treated with dextromethorphan without major negative side effects, but at the higher doses somnolence has been seen. A small clinical trial of CGS-19755 showed some success but also some psychiatric side effects, all reversible, during the treatment period. The difficulties in regulating the blood pressure effects of Mg^{++} and Zn^{++} ions and the psychotomimetic effects of the street drug phencyclidine (PCP or "angel dust") have made them unsuitable. Other agents passing from animal to human testing include Cerestat, whose effects are similar to those of MK-801; Remacemide, a drug with low affinity for the NMDA receptor but showing modest reduction in infarct volume in animal models and few behavioral side effects; and Eliprodil, which has shown high affinity at the polyamine site and reduction in stroke volume in an animal model, few or no behavior effects, but prolongation of the cardiac Q-T interval. Glycine site inhibitors are still in the animal testing phase but have shown major reduction in infarct volume in an animal model and and no gross behavioral effects in animals.

Antioxidants

The information available for superoxides indicates that their role in the process of ischemia is brief, mandating a treatment that must be given in minutes or hours. One clinical study of very early therapy is currently underway with 21-aminosteroids. Most of the studies with these compounds using animal models of focal ischemia have involved pretreatment, but some success has been obtained in studies done up to 1 hour after occlusion. Superoxide dismutase, an enzyme with a good record in reducing ischemia in the gut, does not cross the blood-brain barrier, which limits its usefulness in its current form for brain ischemia.

Nitric Oxide Blockers

Enzymatic inhibition of nitric oxide synthetase can be achieved by the use of N-nitro-L-arginine. Blocking arginine conversion is neuroprotective, but the same blocking effect also affects mitochondrial reactivity, which can be a result as undesirable as blocking NO· formation. In animals, brain infarct volume can also be reduced by use of Allopurinol, an agent that blocks superoxide dismutase. Allopurinol can limit the size of intestinal infarction in animals. For the brain, the doses needed far exceed that required for blocking superoxide dismutase, and therefore it is suspected that the drug has its own separate effect.

AMPA Antagonists

The AMPA receptor-mediated channel is involved in Na^+, water, and Ca^{++} exchange. AMPA antagonists reduce infarct volume in focal ischemia in animal models and work better than NMDA antagonists in global ischemia. The well studied AMPA antagonist NBQX (6-nitrosulfamoylbenzoquinoxalinedione) shows more benefits in a global ischemia model than in focal ischemia. The nephrotoxicity of the current AMPA antagonists currently limits their usefulness.

Other Therapeutic Approaches Still in the Stages of Preclinical Testing

Presynaptic calcium antagonists (N channel blockers) exist, mostly being obtained from crustacean and spider venoms, ω-conopeptide MVIIA (known as compound SNX-111) having received especially attention. After its use, failure of the extracellular glutamate to rise to the degree expected indicated that the agent succeeded in reducing some of the release of glutamate. Infarct volume has also been reduced by 50 per-

Table 5-2. Current Status of Neuroprotective Therapy

Proposed Mechanism	Agent
Calcium antagonists	
Voltage-dependent channels	
Presynaptic N and postsynaptic T,L	Pertussis toxin
	Nimodipine[a]
	+ <18 h USA trial
	+ <12 h meta-analysis
	Nicardipine[a]
	PY 108-068[a]
Presynaptic N, postsynaptic L	Cd^{++}
Presynaptic only	
N, P channel	ω-Grammotoxin SIA (from tarantula)
	ω-Conopeptide GVIA
N channel	ω-Conopeptide MVIIA SNX-111
	Holoena curta venom
P channel	Funnel web spider toxin
Postsynaptic only	
L channel	PN 200-110 (a dihydropyridine)
	BAY K8644 (a dihydropyridine?)
NMDA channel (Postsynaptic only)	
Competitive NMDA antagonists	
Glutamate and NMDA site	Ciba Geigy CGS 19755[a]
	D-CPP-ene
Glycine site	HA-966
	7-Cl KYNA
Polyamine sites	Ifenprodil
	Eliprodil[a]
Noncompetitive antagonists	
Ion channel	Zn^{++}
	Mg^{++}
	MK-801 (dizocilpine)
	Phencyclidine (PCP, angel dust)
	Dextromethorphan[a]
	Ramecemide[a]
Phosphorylation sites	None
Sodium channel and NMDA antagonism	Lubeluzole
AMPA & kainate antagonists	NBQX
Antioxidants	
21-Aminosteroids ("lazaroids")	Tiralazide[a]
PEG-SOD	

Abbreviations: NMDA, N-methyl-*d*-aspartate; AMPA, α-amino-3-hydroxy-5-methyl-4-isoxazole-propionic acid.
[a] Compounds that have undergone some clinical trials.

cent in rat models, but a drop in mean arterial blood pressure was also evident. Since hypotension is known to exaggerate the effects of ischemia, this blood pressure drop would not be welcome in a clinical setting. Work is just beginning with sodium channel blocker, neutrophil inhibitor, growth factor, and fibroblast growth factor therapy.

Evidence exists from patients with homocysteinurias of a higher rate of strokes and other vascular events than that expected from s control population of similar age. The issue is unsettled as to whether it is the level of homocysteine that contributes to the vascular risk through some form of direct vascular injury. Regardless of the uncertainty, it is worthy of note that many elderly patients, modestly deficient in folate or cobalamine (see Ch. 71), have elevated homocysteine levels, which could be contributing to an age-related risk for vascular disease. Further studies may shed light on the value of therapy with folate or vitamin B_{12}.

For all the proposed therapies discussed above, it remains uncertain what implications these studies of ischemia mechanisms will have in human disease. It seems enough to suggest that one single agent will suffice to block the many pathways that lead to cell damage in a setting of ischemia. Calcium antagonists have reached the stage of clinical trials (see above), but agents that block the development of or take up superoxides and those that alter nitric oxide concentration have not yet reached the stage of human trials. Which approach will prove the most useful is impossible to determine. The reason is in part that it has yet to be understood which of the many compounds offering promise on the basis of animal models will prove tolerable to humans. Despite these uncertainties, the principles are now well established that ischemia modification can be achieved. Table 5-2 lists the current neuroprotective agents.

HEMORRHAGE

Parenchymatous Hemorrhage

Parenchymatous hemorrhage is characterized by a mass of blood (hematoma), liquid and then clotted, which spreads in a concentric fashion from its site of origin, distorted in shape somewhat by the density of tissue and the planes it encounters.

Pathoanatomy and Histology

The hemorrhage typically arises from a very small artery from which blood is released into the brain parenchyma in a steady fashion until either the hemorrhage stops or the patient expires. Although there is a rent in the artery responsible for the bleeding, the violence of bleeding suggested by terms such as rupture, commonly applied to aneurysms (see below), is less applicable to parenchymatous hemorrhages, which require minutes or hours, not seconds, to accumulate a mass large enough to make a diagnosis of stroke evident.

In the vast majority of cases, active bleeding occurs for only some minutes, rarely as long as 1 hour. The bulk of the hematoma is formed by a compact mass of red blood cells, histologically consisting of collections of platelets admixed with and surrounded by concentric lamellae of fibrin. The mass may act to tamponade the rent in the vessel wall. When successful, the tamponade brings the bleeding to a halt. Bleeding typically continues, however, when the rent in the artery is too large or in states of compromised thrombosis (e.g., anticoagulant therapy).

When the hematoma is arrested, the microscopic characteristics remain unaltered for many days until the first signs of a reparative process are observed, about 3 weeks from the onset. A rim of hemosiderin-laden macrophages appears at this time, marking the beginning of a process of clot removal that proceeds slowly from the periphery into the center of the hematoma. While this process is occurring at its periphery, the center of the hematoma undergoes changes that transform it, on gross inspection, into a soft, spongy mass. After many months of progressive phagocytosis, the hematoma is reduced to a collapsed cavity lined by reddish orange discoloration reflecting the hemosiderin-laden macrophages.

Aneurysm

Aneurysm, a disorder of vessels, derives its name from the Greek for widening. In most cases of concern to neurologists, however, aneurysms are bulges in the walls of arteries and not mere widenings. Aneurysms may occur in the extracranial or intracranial space. It is the intracranial site that occasions the most clinically important disorder and is the subject of this discussion.

Rupture and Vasospasm

Most aneurysms lie in the subarachnoid space and are part of the wall of the larger arteries. In contrast to parenchymatous hemorrhages, when aneurysms bleed, the event qualifies for the dramatic term *rupture* because blood under full arterial pressure is released into the subarachnoid space, where tamponade is difficult to achieve and large amounts of blood accumulate instantly. It is believed that an aneurysm typically bleeds actively only for a few seconds; if it continues much longer, the patient has accumulated so much intracranial free blood as to compress the brain with the fatal results (see Ch. 37).

After the bleeding has halted, the consequences of the blood in the subarachnoid space lead to a vascular process termed vasospasm, one of the feared complications that explain many examples of delayed ischemic stroke.

Proposed Mechanisms for Vasospasm. It is the persistence of the large subarachnoid clot that is most associated with vasospasm. Within the clotted blood are a large number of vasoactive substances that may cause vasospasm. They include serotonin, prostaglandins, catecholamines, angiotensin, and histamine, as well as whole blood, a hemolysate of fresh whole blood, erythrocyte breakdown products, hemoglobin, oxyhemoglobin, and even bilirubin but not platelet-rich plasma alone. The role of the adventitial layer of pial vessels innervated by adrenergic fibers, whose norepinephrine-synthesizing capabilities appear to be compromised by subarachnoid hemorrhage, is still unsettled. Neuropeptide Y has also been found in CSF in a setting of spasm.

The presence of the clotted blood is thought prevent the spasmogens from being carried off by the CSF and allows them to be absorbed by the pial vessels. The coating of blood has also been postulated to lead to local tissue acidosis and an anaerobic state, with inhibition of arterial wall synthesis of prostacyclin and overproduction of thromboxane A, resulting in vasospasm and platelet hyperaggregation.

At the cellular level a reciprocal interaction has been shown between calcium and magnesium, in which increased calcium or decreased magnesium causes constriction of myofibrils while increased magnesium causes relaxation. In subarachnoid hemorrhage, the calcium magnesium ratio is increased from the usual 1:1 to 3:1, providing another mechanism for vasospasm.

Timing of Vasospasm. Two phases of vasospasm have been recognized, the first rarely documented in humans, the second considered responsible for most of the ischemic complications. The first phase of vasospasm occurs within seconds or minutes of vessel rupture, causing TIAs rare cases of transient focal syndromes identified as TIAs (see Ch. 35). This phase lasts only minutes and is usually gone within hours. The vast majority of cases show evidence of delayed vasospasm, occurring only after the third day and lasting up to 3 weeks from the time of hemorrhage. Once established, vasospasm may extend beyond 3 weeks. Very late appearance of spasm (7, 14, and 52 weeks after initial subarachnoid hemorrhage) has been described in rare instances.

Distribution of Vasospasm. The process of vasospasm usually affects the circle of Willis and the stems of the major cerebral arteries, in almost all cases beginning in the proximal vessels and spreading distally along the major CSF cylinders, passing over the convexity in the general direction of the superior sagittal sinus. There has as yet been no ready explanation of the predilection for involvement of the larger vessels. Spasm far out over the hemispheric surface is rare, and spasm of the deep vessels has proved difficult to demonstrate. Some evidence suggests that this proclivity for involvement of the larger vessels results from the differential responsiveness of larger vessels to sympathetic stimulation. This mechanism would not explain the spread of vasospasm through the arterial tree in a centrifugal fashion, which seems to be the effect of chemical spasmogens working their way through the CSF cylinders over the brain surface.

Predictors of Vasospasm. It is the total amount of the subarachnoid blood that appears to be the best predictor of spasm. A high incidence of cerebral vasospasm severe enough to produce symptoms has been found when the early CT scan shows globular subarachnoid clots larger than 5×3 mm in the basal cisterns or layers of blood 1 mm or more in thickness in the cerebral fissures. The occurrence of vasospasm is also significantly correlated with increased intracranial pressure.

The clinical consequences of vasospasm are discussed further in Chapter 37.

ANNOTATED BIBLIOGRAPHY

Al Rajeh S, Awada A, Niazi G, Larbi E. Stroke in a Saudi Arabian National Guard community. Analysis of 500 consecutive cases from a population-based hospital. Stroke 1993;24:1635–9.

Stroke incidence is lower in Saudi Arabia as compared with industrialized countries, but this is probably explained by the predominance of young age groups in the former.

Aring CD, Merritt HH. Differential diagnosis between cerebral hemorrhage and cerebral thrombosis. Arch Intern Med 1935;56:435.

Early study of a hospital population, implying a high rate of stroke due to thrombosis.

Bae HG, Lee KS, Yun IG et al. Rapid expansion of hypertensive intracerebral hemorrhage. Neurosurgery 1992; 31:35–41.

Occurred in only 3 percent of 320 patients.

Barnett HJM, Mohr JP, Stein BM, Yatsu FM (eds): Stroke. 2nd Ed. Churchill-Livingstone, New York, 1992.

Standard text.

Bonita R, Syewart A, Beaglehole R. International trends in stroke mnortality: 1970–1985. Stroke 1990;21:989–92.

Generally downward.

Brainin M, Seiser A, Czvitkovits B, Pauly E. Stroke subtype

is an age-independent predictor of first-year survival. Neuroepidemiology 1992;11:190–5.

Better vital prognosis for lacunar strokes.

Castaigne P, Lhermitte F, Gautier JC. Role des lesions arterielles dans les accidents ischemiques céréraux de l'athérosclerose. Rev Neurol (Paris) 1965;113:1–32.

Cerebral infarcts correlated with thorough postmortem of cerebral arteries.

Chang CC, Chen CJ. Secular trend of mortality from cerebral infarction and cerebral hemorrhage in Taiwan, 1974–1988. Stroke 1993;24:212–8.

Hemorrhage and infarction follow different trends.

Chollet F, DiPiero V, Wise RJ et al. The functional anatomy of motor recovery after stroke in humans: a study with positron emission tomography. Ann Neurol 1991;29: 63–71.

Studies in six patients showed actiavtion of ipsi- and contralateral brain regions over time. Ipsilateral pathways appear to play a role in mediating recovery.

Crompton MR. Cerebral infarction following the rupture of cerebral berry aneurysms. Brain 1964;87:263.

Pathology studies, some consistent with local embolism.

Demeurisse G, Verhas M, Capon A. Remote cortical dysfunction in aphasic stroke patients. Stroke 1991;22: 1015–20.

Activation of brain areas remote from the primary injury.

Fisher CM. The arterial lesions underlying lacunes. Acta Neuropathol (Berl) 1969;12:1–19.

The histopathology of lesions in the small, deep arteries.

Fisher CM, Ojemann RG. A clinico-pathologic study of carotid endarterectomy plaques. Rev Neurol 1986;142: 573.

Report of 34 cases studied in detail includes only 3 involving where embolism from ulceration in minor stenosis. Persistent neurologic deficits correlated best with severe stenosis or occlusion.

Fisher CM, Ojemann RG. Basal rupture of cerebral aneurysm—a pathological case report. J Neurosurg 1978;48: 642.

Few cases reported but many may exist, adding to surgical burdens to place the clip proximal to the rupture site.

Forbus WD. On the origin of miliary aneurysms of the superficial cerebral arteries. Johns Hopkins Med J 1930; 47:239.

A classic article.

Foulkes MA, Wolf PA, Price TR et al. The Stroke Data Bank: design, methods, and baseline characteristics. Stroke 1988;19:547–54.

Large artery atheroma an infrequent cause of stroke.

Garcia JH, Yoshida Y, Chen H et al. Progression from ischemic injury to infarct following middle cerebral artery occlusion in the rat. Am J Pathol 1993;142:623–35.

Evolution of infarction studied from 30 minutes to 7 days in a rat model. Ischemia lasting less than 6 hours did not produce necrosis.

Gautier JC. Cerebral ischemia in hypertension. In Ross Russell RW (ed). Cerebral Arterial Disease. Churchill Livingstone, London, 1978, pp. 181–209.

Discussion of the neuropathology and pathophysiology.

Gautier JC, Hauw JJ, Awada A, et al. Artères cérébrales dolichoectasiques. Association aux anevrysmes de l'aorte abdominale. Rev Neurol (Paris) 1988;144:437–46.

Clinical picture and literature review.

Ginsberg MD, Globus MY, Dietrich WD, Busto R. Temperature modulation of ischemic brain injury—a synthesis of recent advances. Prog Brain Res 1993;96:13–22.

Current status of hypothermia.

Globus MY. Overview of ischemia. In Hartmann A, Hearse D, Kuschinsky W (eds). Cerebral Ischemia and the Heart. Proceedings of symposium, June 12–16 1994. Timmendorfer-Strand, Germany (in press).

Thorough review of current concepts of neurochemical events in ischemia.

Gorelick PB, Alter M (eds). Handbook of Neuroepidemiology. Marcel Dekker, New York, 1994.

Many useful chapters on stroke epidemiology.

Gruener N, Gross B, Gozlan O, Barak M. Increase in superoxide dismutase after cerebrovascular accident. Life Sci 1994;54:711–13.

Superoxide dismutase levels were normal 24 hours after ischemic stroke but increased two to three times normal thereafter, to a peak at after 1 week.

Harmsen P, Tsipogianni A, Wilhelmsen L. Stroke incidence rates were unchanged, while fatality rates declined, during 1971–1987 in Goteborg, Sweden. Stroke 1992;23: 1410–15.

Fatality rates, not incidence, declined.

Heiss W-D. The ischemic penumbra. In Current Trends in Neurology and Neurosurgery, 1994.

Ful review, with many annotated references.

Huebner O. Zur Topographie der Ernährungsgebiete der einzelnen Hirnarterien. Zentralbl Med Wiss 1872;10: 817–21.

Humphrey P. Stroke and transient ischaemic attacks. J Neurol Neurosurg Psychiatry. 1994;57:534–43.

Review, with data, from the United Kingdom.

Kamii H, Kinouchi H, Sharp FR et al. Prolonged expression of hsp70 mRNA following transient focal cerebral ischemia in transgenic mice overexpressing CuZn-superoxide dismutase. J Cereb Blood Flow Metab 1994;14: 478–86.

Oxidative stress limits the expression of hsp70 following temporary focal ischemia.

Kistler JP, Crowell RM, Davis KR et al. The relation of cerebral vasospasm to the extent and location of subarachnoid blood visualized by CT scan. Neurology 1983;433:424.

The thicker the clots, the more the spasm.

Kondziolka D, Bernstein M, Spiegel SM, terBrugge K. Symptomatic arterial luminal narrowing presenting months after subarachnoid hemorrhage and aneurysm clipping. J Neurosurg 1988;69:494–9.

Some unexplained cases with very late spasm.

Kriegstein J, Oberpichler H (eds). Pharmacology of Cerebral Ischemia. Wissenschaftliche Verlagsgesellschaft, Stuttgart, 1992.

Details of superoxides.

Lhermitte F, Gautier JC, Derouesne C, Guiraud B. Ischemic accidents in the middle cerebral artery territory. A study in 122 cases. Arch Neurol. 1968;19:248–56.

These cases include a group of infarcts whose cause was undetermined.

Lindenberg R. Patterns of CNS vulnerability in acute hypoxaemia, including anaesthesia accidents. In Schade JP, McMenemey WH (eds). Selective Vulnerability of the Brain in Hypoxaemia. Blackwell, Oxford, 1963; pp. 189–210.

Pathoclysis and morphostatic necrobiosis explained.

Masuda J, Yutani C, Waki R et al. Histopathological analysis of the mechanisms of intracranial hemorrhage complicating infective endocarditis. Stroke 1992;23:843–50.

Pyogenic arteritis found with and without aneurysm formation distributed in the small cortical arterial branches.

Mendelow AD. Mechanisms of ischemic brain damage with intracerebral hemorrhage. Stroke 1993;24(suppl.): I115–7.

Some evidence that the brain surrounding an intracerebral hematoma develops ischemia.

Mohr JP, Caplan LR, Melski JW et al. The Harvard Cooperative Stroke Registry: a prospective registry of patients hospitalized with stroke. Neurology 1978;28:754–62.

Embolism the most frequent form of stroke.

Molinari GF, Smith L, Goldstein MN. Pathogenesis of cerebral mycotic aneurysms. Neurology 1973;23:325–32.

Experimental models.

Moyer DJ, Welsh FA, Zager EL. Spontaneous cerebral hypothermia diminishes focal infarction in the rat brain. Stroke 1992;23:1812–16.

No benefits when cooling was delayed by some 40 minutes.

Nedergaard M, Vorstrup, Astrup J. Cell density in the border zone around old small human brain infarcts. Stroke 1986;17:1129–37.

Sharp border between normal and infarct zones, arguing against a large penumbra outside the infarct zone.

Pearce JM. Von Monakow and diaschisis. J Neurol Neurosurg Psychiatry 1994;57:197.

Historical review.

Philip AW, Janet LC, Ralph BD: Epidemiology of stroke. In Barnett HMJ, Mohr JP, Stein BM, Yatsu FM (eds). Stroke: Pathophysiology, Diagnosis, and Management, 2d Ed. Churchill Livingstone, New York, 1992, pp. 3–27.

Overview of studies of stroke epidemiology.

Schneider M. Durchblutung und Sauerstoffversorgung des Gehirns. Verh Dtsch Ges Herz Kreislauf-forsch 1953;1:19.

The seminal paper describing perfusion failure.

Stegmayr B, Asplund K, Wester PO. Trends in incidence, case-fatality rate, and severity of stroke in Northern Sweden, 1985–1991. Stroke 1994;25:1738–45.

Less severe but little decline in incidence.

The tPA-Acute Stroke Study Group: An open multicenter study of the safety and efficacy of various doses of r-tPA in patients with acute stroke: preliminary results. Stroke 1988;19:134.

Hemorrhagic transformation of tissue recanalized by tPA therapy.

Von Monakow C. Gehirnpathologie. A. Holder, Vienna, 1905.

Original description of diaschisis.

Wilkins RH. Aneurysm rupture during angiography: does acute vasospasm occur? Surg Neurol 1976;5:299–303.

Literature review showing that acute spasm occurs.

Wolf PA, D'Agostino RB, O'Neal MA et al. Secular trends in stroke incidence and mortality. The Framingham Study. Stroke 1992;23:1551–5.

No clear sign of decline in stroke incidence.

Yang GY, Chen SF, Kinouchi H et al. Edema, cation content, and ATPase activity after middle cerebral artery occlusion in rats. Stroke 1992;23:1331–6.

Immediate decline in activity after occlusion.

Zülch K-J. The Cerebral Infarct. Springer-Verlag, Berlin, 1981.

Zülch K-J, Hossmann V. Patterns of cerebral infarction. In Toole JF (ed). Vascular Diseases, part I. In Handbook of Clinical Neurology. Vol. 53. Elsevier Science Publishers, Amsterdam, pp. 175–98.

Infarct size and availability of retrograde collateral via the border zones.

6
Trauma

J. C. Gautier and J. P. Mohr

Trauma to the central nervous system (i.e., the head and spinal cord) is common in civilian life and warfare. To the leading cause, the awful toll of the roads, must be added the ongoing wars, violence in cities, transport accidents, earthquakes, typhoons, and the like that result in huge numbers of casualties. In recent decades, thanks to progress in rehabilitation, the outcome of nervous system trauma has greatly improved the length of life, but advances in functional recovery have not progressed abreast. Large numbers of patients, often young, still live a gloomy life as a result of the severe sequelae. Although neurologists cannot alter the primary consequences of trauma, they can alter their consequences and, in many cases, prevent secondary damage (see also Ch. 83).

For the sake of clarity head and spinal cord trauma are considered separately, but it is stressed throughout this chapter that they are often associated and that, at the trauma site, it must be presumed that they are associated.

HEAD

A sizable part of a busy neurologist's practice is made up of the sequelae of head trauma when an opinion is sought for therapy, prognosis, and evaluation of disability for insurance companies and the courts, but neurologists must also be prepared to examine acute severe cases, either in consultation or as they happen in sudden large civilian catastrophes (e.g., plane crashes or wartime). This chapter chiefly considers blunt (synonymous with closed, nonpenetrating, or nonmissile) trauma. Open injuries caused by missiles or injuries with depressed vault fractures require prompt neurosurgical care, making the neurologist's role more limited. It is convenient to distinguish the consequences of impacts (i.e., fractures of the skull and contusions and lacerations of the brain) from

those of movements imparted to the head (i.e., diffuse axonal injury).

Epidemiologic Considerations

Head trauma is of prime importance because injury to the brain most often causes severe and permanent disabilities. Trauma is common at all ages and in both sexes and is the leading cause of hospital referrals in young and adult men. Probably many more cases do not enter hospital statistics.

In Western countries, about one-half of the cases are due to road accidents, with falls, accidents at work, and assault ranking high among the other causes. Major accidents such as disasters of air, rail, road, and sea transport, riots, explosion with the collapse of buildings, and the like frequently bring up large clusters of cases.

Pathologic Findings

When the soft, jellylike brain tissue is subjected to quick and often forceful multidirectional movements of translation, the rotation and swirl of the cerebral hemispheres around the axis of the fixed brainstem produce tearing and shearing of the brain tissue, termed diffuse axonal injury.

Diffuse axonal injury has two major features. First, there are focal lesions involving mainly the corpus callosum and the dorsolateral quadrants of the rostral brainstem in the region of the superior cerebellar peduncle. They probably result from impaction on adjacent free dural edges of the falx cerebri and tentorial notch. Lesions of the corpus callosum are often several centimeters long and predominate on the splenium. Second, there are diffuse lesions with rupture of axons in all regions of the brain with a high predominance in the parasagittal white matter, corpus callosum, medial lemnisci, and corticospinal tracts in the brainstem. Such lesions are particularly frequent in road accidents, and they are the chief pathologic basis of post-traumatic coma in the absence of an expanding intra-cranial lesion (see Hematomas and Brain Edema below). They are also the main underlying lesion for the vegetative state. In minor concussion with an apparent complete clinical recovery, they can be present to a minor degree.

Other characteristic features of severe blunt head injury are hematomas, high intracranial pressure, and hypoxic brain damage. Hematomas can be epidural or subdural (see below). Intracerebral hematomas are associated with frontal or temporal contusions and lacerations or are deep in the thalamus or striatum. They probably result from tearing of the intraparenchymatous vessels, which can also be responsible for diffuse petechial hemorrhages. High intracranial pressure can result from hematomas or from brain swelling; it can develop very early after severe head trauma. In adults, it usually involves one cerebral hemisphere, is nearly constant beneath a subdural hematoma, but can occur in isolation. Hematomas and brain swelling act as acute expanding lesions with mass effect and consequent herniations of the cingulate gyrus under the falx cerebri or the uncus and parahippocampal gyrus into the tentorial notch (tentorial herniation). In fatal head trauma, presence in the cortex of βA4-amyloid protein (similar to that found to be associated with neuritic plaques in Alzheimer's disease) has been reported. Moreover, in mild head injury (loss of consciousness for 5 minutes or less), amyloid precursor protein (precursor of βA4), a marker of fast axonal transport, has been found in the brain, particularly in the fornices.

Concussion

The word *concussion* (from the Latin *concutere*, to shake violently) applies to an immediate loss of consciousness, be it short or long, that results from a blow to, or violent motion of, the head.

Blows on the head can produce complex effects. In a car accident, for example, the head and body often move in many successive directions, causing several different blows to occur, some so rapidly that even high-speed photography of impact dummies used in crash tests has not permitted full analysis of the changes in position and points of contact. Moreover, the consequences of a blow can differ depending on whether the skull is fixed (e.g., the head is resting against a wall or floor) or the head is free to move under the impact. Another factor is whether the head ends the movement by swinging around the axis of the neck or impacts on a resistant plane, such as the floor or ground, the resistance of which provides yet another factor in the outcome.

Despite the many circumstances in which the head strikes or is struck by objects, for loss of consciousness to occur, the head must undergo an acceleration-deceleration movement. Over a sufficient range and speed, consciousness may be lost in experimental animals and humans even without impact on the head. Conversely, where the head is propped up on a hard surface, such as a wall or tree, and submitted to a progressive crushing force, consciousness is not lost until much severe damage to the brain has occurred. (The French word for concussion is *commotion*, which conveys even better the idea of movement. In this instance, however, it should be noted that the words cannot be swapped, for "commotion" in English means civil unrest while *concussion* in French means embezzlement.)

Complex mechanical phenomena occur during acceleration and deceleration movements of the head, which have been amply confirmed in high-speed films of prize fighters whose loss of consciousness more often occurs from a combination of punches (sometimes not very powerful) that rotate the head repeatedly in opposite directions (the one-two punch or a flurry of punches) rather than the powerful smash on the front of the face.

Fractures

Falls or blows vary in their effects, from a simple crack of the skull, which cause no underlying tissue injury and is seen only as a hairline on a skull radiograph, to gross open wounds with hair, skin, and bone fragments driven into brain tissue, herniating it out onto the surface of the head.

Linear fractures are generally unimportant, but they signify an increased risk of intracranial bleeding, especially when they run across the bony grooves of the middle meningeal artery (see Epidural Hematoma below). They can be difficult to distinguish from the lucencies of veins and sutures, their straight course being their main characteristic. The use of the time-honored skull radiograph for every head trauma has been questioned, and a recent study recommended that it be omitted in low-risk patients, namely those who are asymptomatic or who have only one or more of the following: headache, dizziness, scalp hematoma, laceration, contusion, or abrasion. To skip the plain skull radiograph in a given patient is always a difficult decision in the authors' view. It is reasonable to obtain a plain skull radiograph when there has been loss or there is alteration of consciousness, amnesia at any time, a possible neurologic disorder, foreign body in the skull, clinical evidence of a basal fracture (see below), evidence of social isolation that precludes supervision of the patient during the ensuing weeks, or inadequate clinical assessment as a result of associated injuries or intoxication.

Basal fractures of the skull, sometimes all but invisible on inspection of skull films, can cause injury through impingement on cranial nerves, the pituitary stalk, or the cavernous sinus. They can also create a communication between the subarachnoid space and the cranial cavity and the outside world, with leakage of cerebrospinal fluid (CSF) or blood and access for entry of air (and bacteria) into the skull and intracranial cavity.

Basal skull fractures can also damage cranial nerves (see Ch. 29) and allow CSF leaks to occur. Fractures through the anterior fossa can cause loss of smell (anosmia), usually permanent, from tearing of the slender first nerve bundles as they cross through the cribriform plate. Contusion and laceration of the basal aspect of the frontal lobe (see below) could also play a role in anosmia. Leakage of blood into the soft tissues of the orbit from fractures of the floor of the frontal bone or orbital bones gives the raccoon or panda appearance of bruises around the eyes. Contusions of the forehead may smash the frontal branch of the trigeminal nerve in its subcutaneous course, setting the stage for later pain in the upper orbital ridge across the forehead as the nerve regrows.

When the fracture line runs across a nasal sinus or the ethmoid bone, there can be rhinorrhea (i.e., leakage of CSF with its attendant risk of meningitis). In the acute stage, CSF is generally mixed with blood, and because clotting is delayed, a drop on a piece of linen gives a diagnostic double-ring pattern of the blood as it separates from the CSF. Many such cases stop spontaneously within 1 week. Patients should be instructed not to blow their nose, and antibiotic prophylaxis is mandatory. Later, the discharge is clear and often intermittent. CSF can be distinguished from a nasal discharge because it contains glucose. In cases in which the diagnosis is uncertain, lumbar introduction of fluorescein, metrizamide, or radioactive substances can detect a leak by their presence in nasal pledgets.

Fractures across the sphenoid bone can damage the optic nerve with generally permanent blindness. There is an afferent loss of the pupillary reaction to light. The pituitary stalk can be severed, with consequent diabetes insipidus, loss of libido, impotence, and amenorrhea. Ocular motor nerves can be damaged from their origin to their termination in the orbit. A third nerve palsy can be due to tentorial herniation, in which case mydriasis is usually the first sign to appear. Ocular motor palsies must be distinguished from trauma to the orbital content. A fracture can tear the internal carotid artery in the cavernous sinus. After such a tear, arterial blood passes forcefully in the sinus and distends afferent veins, causing a severe pulsatile exophthalmos, a harsh bruit over the eyeball, and ocular motor palsies. In severe cases, amblyopia and glaucoma may develop as a result of retinal circulation disorders. Either the fistula can be obliterated by embolization, or the internal carotid artery must be ligated. The trauma that precipitates a carotid-cavernous fistula can be trivial in patients with defective connective tissue, such as Ehlers-Danlos syndrome.

Fractures across the middle fossa can impinge on the branches of the trigeminal nerves with consequent numbness and later pain in the corresponding territories. This is a separate but similar problem to the frontal nerve contusion described above.

Fracture of the petrous pyramid can cause an immediate or delayed paralysis of the facial nerve. The latter type has a better prognosis. Similarly, deafness can be due to lesions of the inner and/or middle ear. When the eardrum is disrupted, there can be leakage of CSF and blood from the external ear, with an attendant risk of meningitis and an indication for antibiotic prophylaxis. Auroscopy carries the risk of precipitating meningitis. After 24 to 48 hours, the skin over the mastoid process appears bluish and boggy (Battle's sign).

Major fractures, usually compound and depressed fractures, result from sharp blows that drive bone fragments into the skull. The dura is often torn by the force of the fracture, and brain lesions of variable extent occur beneath the fracture site. The overlying scalp is bruised or boggy, sometimes misleading the examiner into thinking the only lesion is in the scalp. The communication between the subarachnoid and brain tissue and the outside produces an immediate risk of infection. The late risks are focal deficits and epilepsy. Prompt neurosurgical repair is mandatory to elevate the depressed bony fragments and establish a watertight seal of the dura.

The presence of air that has entered the skull by way of the fracture through direct openings in the skull or through fractured sinuses is visible on horizontal plain radiographs. Air can be subdural or subarachnoid and appear in the ventricles or in the brain itself (aerocele). The appearance of air in the ventricles from missile wounds in World War I gave several leading neurosurgeons of the day (including Walter Dandy, American neurosurgeon, 1886–1946) the idea of deliberately instilling air through a lumbar puncture to outline the ventricles and subarachnoid space, soon to be known as pneumoencephalography, a popular test until it was eclipsed by computed tomography (CT) and magnetic resonance imaging (MRI). Air in the head carries the a risk of meningitis and requires surgical repair of the leak sites.

Contusions and Lacerations of the Brain

In its strict meaning, the word *contusion* means damage without disruption of the pia while the term *laceration* implies that the superficial brain tissue has been disrupted. However, both types of lesions occur in the same regions of the brain and are often associated. Both are hemorrhagic in nature and predominate on the crest of gyri. They result from the acute shaking of the brain at the moment of the impact and reflect the effects of two main mechanisms. First, they occur in the area of the impact, known as the coup lesion (from the French for a blow), and also in the brain area diametrically opposite (contrecoup lesion) where the lesions are often more severe, particularly with blows on the temporal region. The reason the contrecoup lesion is often larger is unclear but could relate to the expansion of the shock wave from the point of impact across the cranium. Second, the acute shaking of the brain makes its soft tissue glide or grate across the rough inner surfaces of the skull, the most prominent being the floor of the anterior fossa, or over prominent bony reliefs, such as the lesser wing of the sphenoid bone. These two effects explain the finding that lesions are chiefly found on the brain poles and on the inferior aspects of the frontal and temporal lobes, and they often extend along the sylvian fissure. The symptoms and signs specific for these contusions are not known. Postmortem examination often discloses definite old lesions in patients with no history of trauma. Such lesions are occasionally seen using MRI in patients whose histories of head injuries may be quite remote (Fig. 6-1). That they may be asymptomatic only means that such lesions can occur without gross permanent disorders of nervous function. From their location, one could easily surmise that they play a role in post-traumatic anosmia and post-traumatic epilepsy.

Gliding contusion also explains the hemorrhagic parasagittal lesions that are more particularly related to settings of acceleration and deceleration and, thus, are often associated with diffuse axonal injury and deep cerebral hematomas (see Concussion above).

Clinical Situations

Four main clinical situations are considered: acute severe blunt head trauma, complications after a lucid interval, minor concussion, and outcomes of nonmissile head trauma according to their degrees of severity.

Acute Severe Blunt Trauma

The patient usually remains comatose for minutes, hours, or a few days after severe closed-head trauma. The depth and evolution of the coma toward improve-

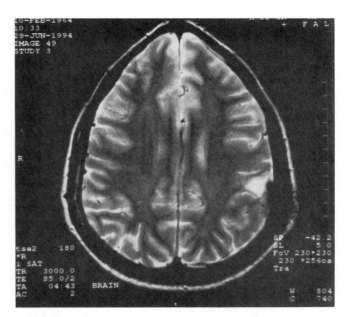

Figure 6-1. Remnant of a contusion from a fall over ten years before. The patient was briefly unconscious but had no symptoms or focal signs then or subsequently. The collapsed gyris is evident adjacent to the site of the thickened section of skull.

ment or worsening are the main indices of prognosis. The Glasgow Coma Scale (Table 6-1) has become a practical convenient bedside tool for estimating coma based on whether the eyes are open and what motor and verbal responses occur to simple testing. In light degrees of coma, patients can put their tongue out and can wiggle their fingers and toes, which gives a rough measure of the function of the brain and cord.

Table 6-1. The Glasgow Coma Scale

Eyes opening	
Spontaneous	4
To speech	3
To pain	2
Nil	1
Best motor response	
Obeys	6
Localizes	5
Weak flexion	4
Abnormal flexion	3
Extensor response	2
Nil	1
Verbal responses	
Oriented	5
Confused conversation	4
Inappropriate words	3
Incomprehensible sounds	2
Nil	1
Total	3–15

(From Teasdale and Bennett, 1974, with permission.)

INITIAL CARE IN SEVERE BLUNT HEAD
    TRAUMA
        Airway free
        Cervical cord control
External-internal (chest, abdomen)
        Bleeding, hypovolemic shock control
Depth of coma (Glasgow scale)
        Pupils
        Focal nervous system dysfunction
        Depressed or basal skull fracture
        Fractures of chest, pelvis, or limbs
        Associated intoxications

Several points in the diagnosis and management apply to all cases of acute severe head injury in the early minutes and hours. The airway must be free or freed and ventilation unimpaired. In severe head injury, especially when intubation is needed, the cervical spine must be considered to be fractured until proved otherwise. No traction must be exercised on the neck, which must be stabilized (e.g., with a rigid collar). Because the size of the pupils must be monitored, mydriatic drops are prohibited. A flaccid paralysis of one upper limb may be a sign of avulsion of the brachial plexus, not injury to the cord; such a limb is susceptible to more nerve injury by its being moved excessively by attendants. Bloody and CSF discharges from the nose or ear imply antibiotic prophylaxis (see basal fractures above). Blood testing should include levels of alcohol and drugs. Except when the level is more than 2 g/L, coma should not be ascribed to alcoholic intoxication and even then, only with reservations. Trauma to the neck can cause dissecting aneurysms of the internal carotid artery. Such cases occur in severe, complex traumas, as in road accidents, but are also known to be associated with minor head trauma. Some hours after the blow, a more or less devastating infarction develops abruptly in the territory of the dissected artery. With fractures of long bones, there can be fat embolism within 2 or 3 days after the fracture, sudden acute dyspnea, and coma with or without focal deficits. Secondary complications such as these are obviously difficult to diagnose in comatose, ventilated patients.

Events After a Lucid Interval

In patients who have regained a clear mind, disorders of consciousness can begin anew after a more or less protracted period, termed the *lucid interval*. It is usually measured in hours to days but may be prolonged for weeks, rarely months. The occurrence of a lucid interval is of utmost significance because it raises the possibility of an intracranial bleeding with consequent high intracranial pressure and tentorial herniation, which is a neurosurgical emergency. However, many alterations in consciousness after a lucid interval do not result from lesions amenable to neurosurgery; on the other hand, bleeding that requires urgent surgical operation can occur in comatose patients who never regain consciousness. Moreover, CT in severely head-injured patients can reveal bleeding that has not yet brought about clinical symptoms or signs. Nevertheless, decline in the level of consciousness after a lucid interval still has a great clinical value in minor head trauma and should prompt CT or MRI scanning when such tests are available and other actions when they are not available. On no account should the occurrence of a lucid interval be taken as a favorable sign that requires no action. The leading cause of disorders of consciousness after a lucid interval is bleeding.

Epidural or Extradural Hematoma

In this setting, blood is collected between the dura and the calvarium. In adults and less often in children, there is usually a skull fracture with dissection or rupture of a major meningeal artery, most commonly across the bony groove of the middle meningeal artery. The artery is torn off so that the hematoma generally expands quickly with a resultant short lucid interval. The secondary loss of consciousness progresses rapidly to coma with signs of expanding intracranial mass and the classic clinical picture of transtentorial herniation: ipsilateral paralytic mydriasis, extensor plantar response, and death. The diagnosis should be made before evidence of herniation. The CT scans shows the high-density lens-shaped clot. Emergency neurosurgical evacuation of the collected blood then carries an excellent prognosis. Most extradural hematomas are temporal, some can occur at other sites, and some are bilateral. Again, it should be stressed that a fracture of the skull is not always present, especially in children. Nor is an initial loss of consciousness ever present. In practice, all patients with a recent skull fracture should be admitted for supervision and CT or, where available, MRI.

Subdural Hematomas

Cortical veins move with the brain during trauma; the dural sinuses are fastened to the calvarium. These bridging veins are subject to disruption during violent head movements. The blood leaking from the veins tends to spread largely in the subdural space. As already mentioned, swelling of the underlying hemisphere is frequent.

In acute subdural hematomas, there may or may not be a short lucid interval. Subdural bleeding is associated with contusions and lacerations. When consciousness has been regained, obtundation and stupor

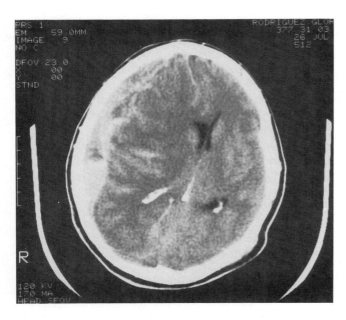

Figure 6-2. Noncontrast CT scan showing a large, acute subdural hematoma separating the surface of the brain from the inner table of the skull, displacing the brain structures well across the midline.

quickly reappear, and signs of transtentorial herniation would appear. CT shows the hyperdense crescent-shaped clot and the shift of midline structures (Fig. 6-2). When CT is not available, the inward displacement of the cerebral arteries over the hemispheral convexity seen on carotid angiography is sufficient to make a diagnosis of such a clot. Neurosurgery is indicated, although brain lesions can be responsible for part of the disorders. The term *burst lobe* has been applied to cases with intracerebral hemorrhage, contusions, lacerations, and a subdural hemorrhage.

The clinical setting is different in chronic subdural hematoma because the pathologic process is also different. The blow on the head can cause a loss of consciousness, but more often it is mild and trivial (e.g., bumping the head on a shelf or against the frame of a door of the car or merely a sudden jarring motion). In some cases, no significant trauma can be found in the patient's history. Tearing of the bridging veins after such minor traumas could be accounted for by a degree of brain atrophy because the patients are often aged or by a condition that favors bleeding, such as alcoholism or taking anticoagulant drugs. Chronic subdural hematoma can be bilateral. The interval between the blow and the appearance of symptoms is commonly several weeks, which suggests that the hematoma expands slowly. That could be due to minor bleeding or, as the blood becomes encapsulated by connective pseudomembranes, by additional fluid en-

tering the hematoma from the thin-walled vessels of the pseudomembrane. The content of the hematoma is a dark, turbid fluid with various quantities of fresh blood. This accounts for the variable degrees of density, from high density to isodensity, on CT. MRI offers the possibility of observing the separation of the subdural hematoma itself from the brain below and the skull above (Fig. 6-3). Rebleeding appears to be the more likely cause than does the long-favored hypothesis that, because of a high osmolarity in the hematoma, CSF seeps into the pouch, thus bringing additional volume.

The clinical diagnosis is often difficult because the blow on the head might be forgotten and there has been no loss of consciousness, only some stunning or commonplace transient pain. The symptoms are rather vague: a dull headache, some slowness in ideation, drowsiness, giddiness, confusion, and poor sphincteric control. In this extracerebral slow compressive lesion, focal signs are distinctly rare, except for a slight degree of hemiparesis. This evolution would lead, sometimes by fits and starts, to tentorial herniation and death. CT shows the crescent-shaped, more-or-less hyperdense hematoma with often considerable shift of the midline structures to the opposite side. This shift is absent in bilateral chronic subdural hematomas. When CT is not available, the diagnosis can be made by carotid angiography. The presence of an ipsilateral hematoma without a brain shift would

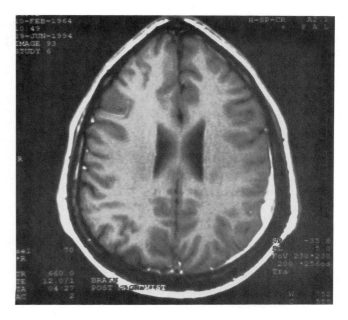

Figure 6-3. Old subdural hemorrhage visible on gadolinium-enhanced T₁-weighted MRI, shown as a thin membrane separating the brain from the inner table of the skull. This lesion was asymptomatic.

suggest a contralateral hematoma and indicate contralateral angiography.

Delayed Intracerebral Hemorrhage

In some patients who have regained consciousness or in others who have remained comatose since the blow on the head, acute, generally massive, intracerebral hemorrhage can occur 1 week or so later (popularized in German by the term *spät apoplexie*, late stroke). The clinical picture is that of hemiplegia, deep coma, and signs of tentorial herniation. The diagnosis is easy with CT. The pathophysiology is not well elucidated.

Delayed Acute Swelling

Patients who lost consciousness at the time of the blow and then improved, but rarely to the point of a really clear mind, can relapse rapidly into stupor or coma. An intracerebral late hemorrhage is feared (see above) but CT shows only diffuse swelling of the brain.

Delayed Hemiplegia or Coma

As previously mentioned, trauma to the neck can cause a dissecting aneurysm of the carotid or vertebral arteries, and fractures of the long bones can cause cerebral fat embolism (see above). Both accidents, of course, can occur after a lucid interval.

Vasovagal Syncope

After a brief loss of consciousness or after having been only stunned or dazed, the patient walks about a few seconds or minutes, only to fall unconscious again. There is pallor, low blood pressure, and a small and slow pulse. This is vasovagal syncope caused by emotional upset or pain. Recovery occurs within a few minutes.

Minor Head Trauma With Concussion

This is by far the most common type of blunt head trauma. After the blow, there is instant loss of consciousness, collapse to the ground, a brief arrest of breathing with a slow pulse, and hypotension. The respiratory and circulatory disorders clear within seconds. The return to normal is of variable length, minutes or hours, and follows several steps. First, patients open their eyes and next withdraw their limbs from painful stimuli. Simple orders are obeyed, and then simple questions are answered in a confused fashion and finally correctly. The return of speech does not signify the end of the concussive disorders. The landmark of recovery is the ability to form clear ongoing memories, and this can occur much later, hours or days, during which the patient can walk around and carry on a simple conversation. The length of this anterograde or post-traumatic amnesia, which extends from the blow to the recovery of a functioning memory for events, is a good marker of the severity of the concussion and, thus, of high clinical import. There is also a retrograde amnesia of variable length that can shrink during the following weeks or months.

The loss of consciousness is the hallmark of concussion, but transient amnesia is common in patients who are only stunned or groggy and can later complain of disorders that, in the aggregate, are labeled as post-traumatic nervous instability (see below). Skull fracture is or is not associated with minor concussion. The rationale for skull radiographs has been mentioned.

Other Syndromes

A concussive blow can trigger an attack of migraine. When it is the first migrainous episode in a child or young patient, the diagnosis can be difficult. A normal CT scan is a great help.

Some people (e.g., prizefighters, steeplechase jockeys, and some soccer players) might undergo repeated concussions. There is evidence that the effects of these concussive episodes are cumulative. In severe cases (punchdrunk syndrome or dementia pugilistica), there are pyramidal, extrapyramidal (parkinsonian), and cerebellar signs with poor memory and slow thinking. Characteristic lesions are atrophy of the fornices, with destruction of the septum pellucidum, lack of large pigmented neurons in the substantia nigra, lesions of the undersurface of the cerebellum and around the foramen magnum, and the presence of neurons with tangles similar to those in Alzheimer's disease, although lacking neuritic plaques. These clinical disorders can appear years after retirement from the ring.

Outcomes of Blunt Head Trauma

In patients who do not die on the scene of the accident or later fall into the category of brain death, the outcomes vary widely over a range of disability. The four main problems in neurologic practice are persistent vegetative state, severe sequelae of long-standing comas, the postconcussion syndrome, and post-traumatic epilepsy.

Persistent Vegetative State

Some severely brain-injured patients never regain consciousness (see Ch. 17). They open their eyes but do not look and do not give evidence that they recognize their close family. Brainstem reflexes are preserved. They make no movements or only very rare and small ones. They can be fed because food put into the mouth is chewed and swallowed. The pathologic basis of this persistent vegetative state is severe diffuse axonal injury plus, generally, diffuse hypoxic brain damage. Such patients can survive months and years. When the persistent vegetative state occurs, it raises diagnostic and ethical problems, and several descriptive definitions have been proposed (see Ch. 17).

Severe Sequelae of Injury

A large group of patients, after being comatose for weeks or months, slowly recover. The duration of the post-traumatic and retrograde amnesia accordingly covers weeks or months. Various degrees of memory dysfunction and slow information processing usually persist. In many patients, deep reflexes are brisk with a bilateral extensor plantar response, incoordination, and dysarthria. Post-traumatic hydrocephalus is possible. Psychosocial maladjustment often hampers return to a normal family and vocational life.

The postconcussion syndrome (synonymous with post-traumatic nervous instability) is a common sequela of minor head injury with concussion. Patients complain of headache, giddiness (often with vertigo), poor memory, poor sleep, irritability, inability to concentrate, and intolerance to noises. Headache is of variable type, throbbing, or tension type (see Ch. 24). There is often paroxysmal positional vertigo that, in the authors' view, is likely to be due to post-traumatic cupulolithiasis (labyrinthine concussion) (see Ch. 29), although it sometimes results from fracture through the labyrinth. The neurologic examination is generally normal. In most cases, there is associated anxiety or depression and litigation problems. A psychological component can be present. Although these factors are acknowledged, the authors hold the view that, from human and animal data, it is likely that, in many cases, there are indeed some lesions of diffuse axonal injury. It is possible that MRI will shed some additional light on the common and worrisome question of the postconcussion syndrome.

Post-Traumatic Epilepsy

Seizures can appear on the site of the accident, usually aggravating any coexistent cerebral hypoxia (see Ch. 79). They can appear in the first week (early epilepsy), in which case this symptom is a good predictor of late epilepsy. The latter affects about 10 to 15 percent of those with severe blunt trauma, but the toll is much higher with brain wounds. The seizures are of the grand mal type, with a possible focal onset or purely focal. In most cases of late epilepsy, they appear within 6 to 12 months. Patients without seizures 2 years after the trauma are at a low risk (about 5 percent). Phenytoin reduces the risk of early seizures during the first week after severe head injury. The question of preventive therapy against late epilepsy is still not settled. Alcohol intake has a definite ill effect on the appearance or reappearance of seizures and, thus, should be clearly discouraged.

SPINAL CORD

Traumatic injuries to the spinal cord are frequent, mostly in young males, which reflects their usual causes: road accidents (about 50 percent), sports injuries (e.g., football, rugby, hockey, water skiing, horseback riding, and diving, not necessarily, contrary to common belief, in shallow water) and of course war casualties. There is also direct trauma from stab wounds, bullets, and shotgun pellets. Falls in middle-aged and aged, tottering people carry a special risk of damage to the cervical cord (see Ch. 31).

Spinal cord damage, especially cervical, is commonly associated with severe head trauma. In the initial management and assessment of severe head injuries, it is good practice to consider the cervical cord damaged until it is proved otherwise, and appropriate caution is mandatory in handling the patient (see below).

Direct Injuries

The wound is usually obvious in direct injuries but bullets, shotgun pellets, or shell or bomb fragments can enter the spinal canal through the interlaminar spaces, with minimal obvious skin or spine lesions. The cord is crushed partially or completely or lacerated. Bone and disc fragments can compress the cord. There are generally associated lesions of the nerve roots and spinal ganglia and of spinal arteries and veins. Severe swelling and hemorrhages of the cord can thus be associated with epidural and subdural hemorrhage. Later, a glial and connective tissue scar is present.

Clinically, in severe cord injury, there is acute tetraplegia or quadriplegia, with usually severe sequelae. The spinal laminae prevent blades, usually knives, from entering the spinal canal directly from behind. When they penetrate, it is from a direction lateral to the midline, and they are thus apt to cause a hemisection of the cord. In Brown-Sequard's seminal article, three cases indeed were due to stab wounds. Cases have been described with transsection of both posterior columns. CT and MRI have greatly improved the analysis of the lesions (see Ch. 31).

Indirect Injuries

In accidents, forces that cause fractures of the spinal column are nearly always complex, and they correspond to three basic mechanisms.

First, forced flexion chiefly causes an acute compression of the vertebral bodies with wedge-shaped fractures or, in extreme cases, explosion-fragmentation of the vertebral body. There can also be fracture of the posterior arch of the spinal canal, including pedicles, articulations (dislocation), and laminae. Simultaneously, the annulus fibrosus is ruptured with extrusion of disc fragments into the spinal canal where, together with possible bony fragments, they can compress the cord and its vessels. Akin to this flexion mechanism are the wedge-shaped fractures of the vertebral bodies that result from falls from high scaffoldings, windows and so forth onto the heels or buttocks. Considerable violence is generally needed, but less force is required when the patient is a frail, osteoporotic, aging woman or a patient who is ill with vertebral metastases.

Second, forced rotation can cause a unilateral dislocation. When there is dislocation, the upper part of the spine tends to bump or glide forward, thereby menacing the cord because the spine is now unstable.

Third, forced extension or hyperextension is a frequent cause of cervical cord damage. The problem is of special interest to the neurologist because the diagnosis is often difficult. Normal hyperextension of the neck reduces the sagittal dimensions of the cervical canal by 50 percent. In addition, contrary to the thoracic and lumbar spine, which are made up of big vertebrae supported by strong muscles, the cervical spine is a slender flexible bamboolike stem, approximately 15 cm long, to which is attached the head; the latter is a heavy weight of approximately 4 kg. Normally, the neck remains stable on the shoulders, and the head is stabilized on the neck through the action of the relatively weak neck muscles. Moreover, this implies alertness, as shown by dozing and intoxicated people who wag their head. Forced hyperextension of the cervical cord is most important in accidents such as road accidents, in which patients first lose consciousness and then are subjected to violent forces that act on the head. In this case, the momentum of the head allows extreme hyperextension because the anterior longitudinal ligament can be ruptured. Further reduction of the spinal cord and, thus, damage to the cord is due to inward bulging of the ligamentum flavum in forced hyperextension. In such accidents, the cervical spinal cord can be lesioned without fracture of the spine, or the fracture is reduced to a tiny bony flake or osteophyte, which is detached from the anterior lower margin of a lower cervical vertebra. The fractured or detached particle can be absent or not detectable on usual radiographs. Therefore, the absence of a visible fracture does not exclude the traumatic origin of a tetraplegia. After such a trauma, there may be no pain in the neck, or the patient may be unconscious from associated head trauma. However, the cervical spine is unstable, and further damage to the cord could result from unconsidered movements that must be prohibited by the use of a preventive rigid collar and the utmost caution in the assessment and transport of casualties. Finally, the trauma can be trivial, such as falling downstairs or tripping on a mat. This is well known in old people in whom the dimensions of the spinal canal have been previously greatly reduced by spondylosis, particularly those of the cervical canal. Here sudden hyperextension, without fracture, can cause traumatic tetraplegia.

Pathologically, the cord lesions that result from indirect trauma are characterized by acute swelling with varying degrees of hemorrhage and destruction of tissue. High-dose methylprednisolone given within 8 hours of the onset improves the patient's neurologic recovery, presumably because it suppresses the breakdown of the membrane by inhibiting lipid peroxidation and hydrolysis at the site of injury. In the cervical spinal cord, lesions often predominate in the central part, just behind the central canal. There can be associated lesions of the nerve roots and spinal ganglia. After some months, the destroyed tissue is replaced by a glial and connective tissue scar.

In acute and chronic lesions, somatosensory-evoked potentials and magnetic stimulation help to evaluate the severity and prognosis. MRI provides excellent imaging of the spinal cord and spinal column lesions.

The clinical course may vary. Immediately after violent trauma to the cervical or thoracolumbar spinal cord, there is a state of acute paralysis termed *spinal shock* (see Ch. 31). All motor, reflex, sensory, and autonomic functions of the cord are in suspense. In some patients, recovery occurs within minutes or hours. This has been termed *spinal concussion* from the similarity to cerebral concussion (see above). Such comparison is supported by the clinical picture of the sudden loss of function followed by rapid recovery and not by a clear knowledge of the pathophysiology of the reversible spinal shock. In patients who recover slowly, a minimal reflex activity reappears within months in the lower limbs and sphincteric and genital reflexes. This is followed by exaggerated flexor activity (i.e., the triple flexion or involuntary withdrawal of the big toe, leg, and thigh in response to plantar stimuli (basically, the Babinski sign) (see Ch. 22). After months or years, extensor reflexes may reappear, allowing spinal standing. This classical course is rather variable from case to case.

Early Management Considerations

At the scene of the accident, if the patient is conscious, the main points to consider are as follows. Is there spinal pain, with a root radiation or with a motor or sensory deficit? When there is a suggestion of spinal cord injury or the patient is unconscious, the head and neck are placed in a neutral position with a gentle longitudinal traction. Whenever possible, especially for those trapped in a vehicle, a cervical splint (e.g., a Hines' splint with a foam collar or sandbags) should be used to prevent neck movements. The patient should be carried supine to a firm stretcher by four people, which avoids spinal movement as far as possible. In tetraplegic patients, the sympathetic system is paralyzed, and in cold climates, the risk of poikilothermia must be prevented by thermal blankets.

Acute Clinical Syndromes

At the acute stage, several clinical syndromes can be distinguished. Although there is much overlapping, they are useful for the clinician to surmise where the main brunt of the disorders lies.

Damage to the conus medullaris and cauda equina determines a flaccid paraplegia with paralysis of the pelvic floor, areflexia, sensory impairment in the saddle region, bladder and rectum paralysis, and failure of erection and ejaculation.

Lesions of the lumbar and thoracic cord result in paraplegia with, in some cases, the mentioned successive periods of exaggerated flexor and then extensor activity and sphincteric, sexual, and autonomic disturbances. At a given level, the whole cord is not necessarily deprived of function by trauma. Therefore, some syndromes suggest that lesions predominate on the anterior, posterior, or central cord (see Ch. 31). This is mostly true in cervical cord injuries. In the anterior cord syndrome, there is paralysis with wasting, areflexia at the level of the lesion and below it, and impairment of thermal and pain sensation. Position and vibration sense are spared. This syndrome is often associated with a protruding ruptured disc and could be due to anterior compression of the cord. It is, however, also characteristic of occlusion of the anterior spinal artery (see Ch. 35), which could result from compression by the protruding disc.

In the posterior cord syndrome, there are paresthesiae in both arms, sometimes also on the neck and trunk, Lhermitte's sign (shooting electric paresthesiae spreading down the spine on flexion of the neck), and impairment of position and vibration sense. This posterior syndrome could be due to the mechanical impact of the laminae and bulging ligamentum flavum on the posterior columns.

The central cord syndrome, in which lesions lie predominantly just behind the central canal, is characteristic of cord damage caused by hyperextension of the spine. The clinical picture could be misleading because paralysis predominates in the upper limbs with relative sparing of the legs. There may or may not be an extensor plantar sign, and lower limb reflexes can be brisk but, in some patients, near normal. This is due to the medial position of the corticospinal fibers to the upper limbs in the lateral corticospinal tract in the spinal cord. There is bladder dysfunction and varying degrees of sensory loss. In old people, as pre-

viously mentioned, this can result from a trifling fall forward. Facial bruises are a clue to such a fall.

Laboratory Testing

It is mandatory to have a good lateral radiographic view of all seven cervical vertebrae in which the shoulders, which could obscure the view of the lower vertebrae, should be gently pulled down. This allows the clinician to see the telltale flake of bone referred to above. MRI, when feasible, would provide the best views of the cord, but here again, the risks of an unstable spine and unconsidered movements imparted to the neck must be stressed. In a good number of cases, the central cord syndrome is associated with signs that suggest larger lesions of the cord or, not rarely, with features of the Brown-Sequard syndrome.

Outcome

The outcome is often good. Good hand function, hyperpathia, Lhermitte's sign, and normal perianal sensation on admission would indicate a favorable prognosis. Post-traumatic syringomyelia (see Ch. 65) occurs in a few patients with severe injury of the spinal cord. Years after the trauma, loss of motor and sensory function with the features of syringomyelia ascend upward. There can also be a downward progression of the central cavity, which usually forms in the aftermath of severe central cord lesions, but this lower part of the syrinx is clinically silent as a result of the preexisting cord lesion. MRI provides excellent imaging of this process. The pathophysiology is unclear.

ANNOTATED BIBLIOGRAPHY

Head

Adams JH. The autopsy in fatal non-missile head injuries in neuropathology. In Berry CL (ed). Current Topics in Pathology. Springer-Verlag, Berlin, 1988.

A clear and concise account of current pathologic views.

Blumbergs PC, Scott G, Manavis J et al. Staining of amyloid precursor protein to study axonal damage in mild head injury. Lancet 1994;344:1055–56.

Amyloid precursor even in mild concussion.

Corsellis JAN. Boxing and the brain. BMJ 1989;298:105–9.

The neuropathology of the punchdrunk syndrome.

Denny-Brown D, Russell WR. Experimental cerebral concussion. Brain 1941;64:93–164.

A seminal article on the role of movement in concussion.

Driscoll P, Skinner D (eds). ABC of major trauma. Br Med J 1990;300:1265–7, 1329–33, 1575.

A review of basic emergency measures.

Foster JB, Leiguarda R, Tilley PJB. Brain damage in National Hunt jockeys. Lancet 1976;1:981–3.

Concussion is cumulative.

Gennarelli TA, Thibault TE, Adams JH et al. Diffuse axonal injury and traumatic coma in the primate. Ann Neurol 1982;12:564–74.

Concussion occurs without impact. Diffuse axonal injury is the main basis of prolonged traumatic coma.

Jennett B. Head trauma. In Asbury AK, McKhann GM, McDonald WI (eds). Diseases of the Nervous System. Clinical Neurobiology. Vol. II. 2nd Ed. WB Saunders, Philadelphia, 1992, pp. 1229–37.

A review of the Glasgow studies.

Jordan BD. Neurologic aspects of boxing. Arch Neurol 1987;44:453–9.

Acute and chronic ailments of prizefighters and prospective views.

Masters SJ, McLean PM, Azcareses JS et al. Skull x-ray examination after head trauma. Recommendations by a multidisciplinary panel and validation studies. N Engl J Med 1987;316:84–91.

Skull radiography can be skipped in low-risk patients.

Roberts GW, Gentleman SM, Lynch A, Graham DJ. βA4 amyloid protein deposition in brain after head trauma. Lancet 1991;338:1422–4.

βA4 a concomitant of head trauma.

Spudis EV. The persistent vegetative state-1990. J Neurol Sci 1991;102:128–36.

An update with ethical issues.

Symonds Sir C. Concussion and its sequelae. Lancet 1962; 1:3.

Classical article.

Teasdale G, Bennett B. Assessment of coma and impaired consciousness: a practical scale. Lancet 1974;2:81–4.

Trunkey D. Initial treatment of patients with extensive trauma. N Engl J Med 1991;324:1259–63.

Brain and spinal cord injuries, a major problem, among other ones.

Spinal Cord

Bracken MB, et al. A randomized, controlled trial of methylprednisolone or naloxone in the treatment of acute spinal cord injury. N Engl J Med 1990;332:1405–11.

High-dose methylprednisolone within 8 hours of acute injury improves recovery. No benefit was seen with the use of naloxone.

Cook JB. The diagnosis of traumatic tetraplegia. In Garland H (ed). Scientific Aspects of Neurology. ES Livingstone, Edinburgh, 1961, pp. 240–8.

An excellent account of hypertensive injuries to the spinal cord.

Hughes JT. Pathology of Spinal Cord. Lloyd-Luke, London, 1978.

A concise classic.

Kulhani MV, Bondurant FJ, Rose SL, Narayana PA. 1.5 Tesla magnetic resonance imaging or acute spinal trauma. Radiographics 1988;8:1059–82.

MRI is the choice imaging method for spinal cord lesions in acute spinal trauma.

Merriam WF, Taylor TKJ, Ruff SJ, Phah MJM. A reappraisal of acute traumatic central cord syndrome. J Bone Joint Surg [Br] 1986;68:708–13.

Variations in signs and mechanisms of traumatic central cord syndrome. Outcome generally good.

Newton MR, Greenwodd RJ, Britton KE et al. A study comparing SPECT with CT and MRI after closed head injury. J Neurol Neurosurg Psychiatry 1992;55:92–5.

Single-photon emission CT showed more lesions than either CT or MRI. The number correlated with the Glasgow Coma Score. Four or more lesions showed a poor score and poor outcome; two per patient had a better score and better outcome.

Olsen WL, Chakeres DW, Berry I, Richard J. Traumatismes du rachis et de la moelle. In Imagerie du Rachis et de la Moelle. C Manelfe (ed). Vigot, Paris, 1989.

A thorough update of CT, MRI, and ultrasound imaging in spinal injuries.

Swain A, Grundy D, Russell J et al. ABC of spinal cord injury. BMJ 1985–86;291–292:1558–1705, 44–609.

A comprehensive series from emergency to late management.

Section II
Techniques of
Investigation

7
Autopsy and Brain Biopsy

J. C. Gautier and J. P. Mohr

Whatever the advances of investigations during life (e.g., computed tomography [CT], magnetic resonance imaging [MRI], or sophisticated biochemical tests), autopsy (which is synonymous with postmortem examination or "postmortem") is the ultimate audit of medicine, the yardstick of clinical care and research. To dispense with autopsy is an unfortunate trend in many institutions and one that certainly endangers the value of clinical research. Together with its natural continuation, microscopic pathology, autopsy is irreplaceable to ascertain cause(s) of death, unravel often unrecognized associated pathologic conditions, understand images from CT and MRI, clarify pathophysiologic processes, and finally, provide material for research and teaching. Postmortem of the nervous system should be part of a general autopsy that allows nervous lesions to be put into the perspective of internal medicine and general pathology and frequently reveals a non-neurologic immediate cause of death, such as pulmonary embolism, in nervous diseases. It is the firm belief of the authors that pathology is to clinical neurology what foundations are to a building. Only through acquaintance with macroscopic and microscopic pathology will symptoms, signs, and imaging of nervous lesions be properly understood. For all neurologists, a significant part of their experience should include the neuropathologic laboratory, where invaluable first-hand experience can be acquired in autopsy and pathology.

When special circumstances require it, every neurologist should be able to perform an autopsy to secure potentially important material. The present chapter is not a short account of neuropathology; rather, it aims at providing the clinician with guidelines to postmortem examination and the general principles of sampling the central nervous system. Biopsy of nerve and muscle is considered in Chapter 8.

Except in very unusual settings, knowledge of the clinical history is a prerequisite to autopsy. A postmortem can have one or several points of interest, including diagnosis, evaluation of clinical care (with drugs or surgery trials, research (rare diseases that imply taking samples for biochemistry or electron microscopy), and even medicolegal implications. The last consideration may involve appropriate photographs of skull and/or spine. Experience with such studies can be crucial to later attempts to understand the cause of death.

BRAIN AUTOPSY

Initial Steps

The delay between death and postmortem is recorded. Where unconventional infectious agents are suspected (e.g., in Creutzfeldt-Jakob and Gerstmann-Sträussler-Scheinker diseases and the acquired immunodeficiency syndrome [AIDS]) special procedures preventing contamination are to be followed. These can be found in the references at the end of this chapter. Plans for embalming impose particular procedures, well known by the mortuary assistants. Face, scalp, eyes, and neck are first inspected.

The incision to reflect the scalp from the skull is from mastoid to mastoid just posterior of the vertex, which allows the scalp to be reflected half forward almost to the the supraorbital ridges, the rest rearward to the occiput. A large part of the vault of the skull has to be removed to ensure full access to the brain. Waterproof electric saws with fan blades, specially designed for postmortem, are generally used. A hand saw can be used when needed. The temporal muscle is scraped where the saw will cut across the temporal bone. The cut begins about 1 cm above the supraorbital ridges for those not to be viewed later in a funeral home. To avoid the visible line of the saw under the forehead of the repositioned scalp, a higher cut can be made along the hairline, but this cut often makes it difficult to gain access to the undersurface of the frontal lobes and is to be avoided if possible. Posteriorly, the cut continues horizontally on each side to the coronal plane of the mastoid processes. The temporal bone is thin, as thin as 2 to 3 mm in some people, so care must be taken not to cut the dura with the temporal bone. From their rear end the cuts are prolonged to the midline just above the palpable external occipital protuberance.

After the skull cap has been loosened all around, it can be levered off with a chisel. In infants and old people, skull and dura can be adherent and may have to be separated by using a supple spatula. With careful technique, the dura remains intact. Extradural hematomas generally remain attached to the dura. The superior sagittal sinus is now opened along its full length, beginning posteriorly. Next the dura must be cut along the edge of the sawed skull. To avoid brain damage, the dura is retracted with a toothed forceps and cut, step by step, preferably with curved scissors, which are at each step kept close to the forceps, beginning anteriorly near the midline. The superior sagittal sinus should not be transected. Both halves of the dural cap are then retracted to the midline. Except for chronic subdural hematomas, any blood present on the subdural space usually flows out. The falx cerebri must now be cut close to its insertion on the ethmoidal midline. The scissors are introduced between the frontal lobes, and by small cuts, beginning anteriorly, the falx is freed off. The entire dural cap together with the superior sagittal sinus is gently retracted backward and left hanging loose from the torcular. During the retraction small bridging veins from cortex to sinus usually have to be cut out. If there is evidence of meningitis, it is better to sample exudates than to take specimens with sterile swabs. The same applies for meningitis at the base of the brain and around the spinal cord.

Taking Off the Brain

To separate the brain from the skull, one must clearly see the base of the brain. As the brain tissue is a soft, jellylike substance, it can well be—and too often is—damaged at this point in the autopsy. The key to success is to use gravity as much as possible to deliver the brain; to make the best use of gravity, one needs simply to push as far as possible toward the shoulders the block that was under the nape of the neck during removal of the skull cap. The neck is now fully extended and the brain is "ready to leave" the skull. The fingers of the left hand (in a right-handed person) are gently inserted under the tips of the frontal lobes, and the olfactory bulbs are manipulated so as to be removed with the brain. With curved-on-the-flat (Mayo) scissors, which are preferable to straight scissors or a scalpel, careful sectioning cuts away the optic nerves, internal carotid arteries, pituitary stalk, and oculomotor nerves, each being cut off as close as possible to its entry into or exit from the skull. The insertion of the tentorium cerebelli along the petrous part of the temporal bone must now be cut, by using the scissors and commencing medially. The cut should proceed by small steps, a few millimeters long, with care taken not to damage the superior aspect of the cerebellum.

Now the brain is almost delivered, and its weight must indeed be supported with the left hand in order to avoid stretching or tearing of the midbrain. A clear view of the anterior wall of the posterior fossa, including the clivus, petrous, and occipital bones, is obtained. The fifth through twelfth cranial nerves and the vertebral arteries are cut as close as possible to their exit from or their entry into the skull. The last and most important step is to separate the medulla from the spinal cord. This is done by using a scalpel, cutting transversely at the junction of medulla and cord. One should not try to cut as low as possible simply "to get more cord," as this results in tapering wedges of cord, unsuitable for study. The brain is finally delivered, the dura being left with the skull.

The extra steps next described should be delayed until the fresh brain has been inspected and properly placed in fixative. To remove the pituitary gland the posterior margin of the diaphragma sellae is first incised and the dorsal sella is removed. The diaphragm is then incised on each side and gently lifted with a forceps held in the left hand, which allows the right hand to dissect the pituitary from the fossa. The gland should be fixed at least 24 hours prior to further dissection. Eyes are not routinely removed (for that special technique, see Adams and Murray, 1982). If a fracture of the temporal or occipital bone is suspected, the dura should be incised on the clivus and pulled and stripped off, which also allows the examiner to look for any abnormality of the bone over the middle ear and the mastoid cavity.

Handling the Fresh Brain

As soon as the brain is delivered, it is examined by the pathologist, weighed, and put into a fixative. Two basic principles are (1) the fresh brain should not be cut; and (2) the brain should not be placed lying on a hard surface, as in a few minutes irreparable distortion would appear. The only exception to this is when blood is present around the brain, mostly at its base, in cases of subarachnoid hemorrhage. To look for a ruptured aneurysm the fresh blood should be gently washed with saline to expose the circle of Willis and its main branches, as fixation transforms the leaked blood into a tight and hard material, prohibiting useful dissection of the arteries.

The usual fixative is 10 percent formol in saline, filling three-quarters of a 10-L bucket. The brain is immersed and suspended by a string passing between the basilar artery and the pons. The fixative is changed 3 days later and then at weekly intervals. Usually correct fixation is achieved after 1 month.

In certain cases the whole brain is not placed in formol saline. Parts are spared for special techniques provided that postmortem takes place within a few hours of death. For electron microscopy (e.g., in virus or storage diseases) small blocks of brain tissue, 3 mm × 3 mm × 3 mm, sampled at appropriate sites are fixed in glutaraldehyde and later embedded in epoxy resin. For histochemistry (e.g., determination of neurotransmitters), blocks of tissue are frozen at −80°C. Immunocytochemistry currently tends to be preferred to histochemistry, as it allows identification of proteins such as virus particles and their location through specific antibodies. The morphologic features of the tissue must be preserved; therefore during freezing, formation of ice crystals must be avoided. To achieve this, the fresh tissue is snap-frozen in nitrogen-cooled isopentane. Laboratories of molecular biology may also be provided with 1 mm³ of fresh tissue frozen in nitrogen.

The Heart and Extracranial Cerebral Arteries

Since cardiac embolism is a major cause of cerebral infarction, examination of the heart is a routine part of autopsy in neurologic cases. Valvulopathies and ischemic heart disease are looked for, and attention should be given to abnormal communications between cardiac chambers, particularly to a patent foramen ovale, as transcardiac embolism now appears to be a fairly frequent cause of cerebral ischemia or infarction. The aortic arch, also a source of cerebral embolism, can be easily examined and its lesions recorded. Whenever possible, the extracranial arteries should be examined throughout their length. Dissecting them as high as possible in the neck carries the risk of damage to the vessel wall and to intraluminal mural or occluding material. Moreover, such a dissection is hardly feasible for vertebral arteries and leaves out the part of the internal carotid artery that traverses the base of the skull and the cavernous sinus. Injecting water into the proximal part of the carotid and vertebral arteries cannot properly evaluate stenoses and can dislodge mural or occluding material. The best is to remove the extracranial arteries en bloc with the cervical column and the base of the skull. This can be done in less than 10 minutes and provides the material necessary for sound diagnosis and research in cerebrovascular disease. Arterial lesions can be reported on a sche-

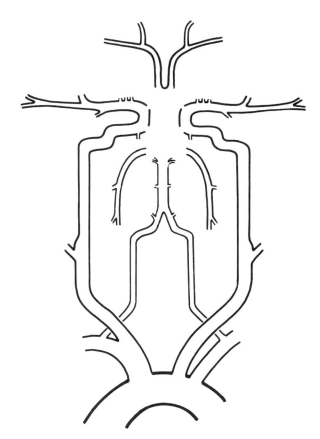

Figure 7-1. A chart for recording lesions on the cerebral arteries as seen postmortem. The variable segments of the circle of Willis are depicted by the examiner in each case. (Courtesy of Prof. J. J. Hauw, Laboratory of Neuropathology, La Salpêtrière, Paris, France.)

matic chart, which in addition allows recording of individual variations of the circle of Willis (Fig. 7-1).

Dissecting the Brain

After fixation, the brain is first inspected and gently palpated and is then placed, base upward, on a nonslippery surface, usually a corkboard.

Attention is usually directed first to the basal arteries (i.e., those of the circle of Willis and the brainstem). These vessels can be dissected out and the individual variations of the circle of Willis and basilar artery recorded (Fig. 7-1). Samples of arteries for histologic studies must be precisely labeled inasmuch as several samples are taken on the same artery and their location on the artery is noted on special sketches. Notes taken at this time about the macroscopic appearance of the artery and its contents (color, texture, etc.) as observed with a hand lens will be invaluable for interpreting the histology of the arteries later. The end of the arterial sample to be used for slides is cut transversely while the opposite end is cut obliquely, thus

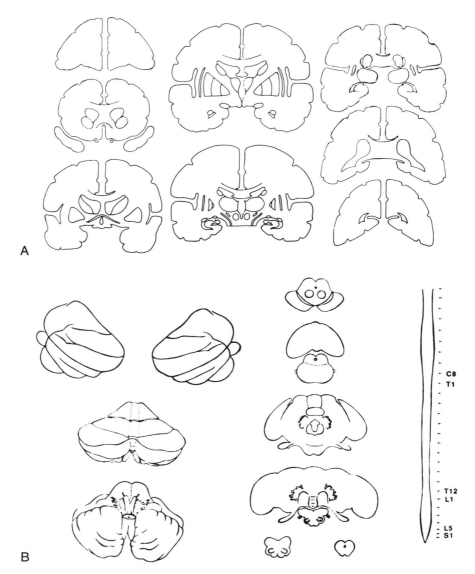

Figure 7-2. **(A)** Eight drawings of coronal slices of the cerebral hemispheres for recording postmortem lesions. **(B)** External views and horizontal slices of the cerebellum and brainstem and a general view of the spinal cord (on the right) for recording postmortem lesions. (Courtesy of Prof. J. J. Hauw, Laboratory of Neuropathology, La Salpêtrière, Paris, France.)

allowing embedding (see below) with a correct orientation. Whenever possible the macroscopic appearance of the arteries should be compared with angiograms, carefully noting the delay elapsed between angiography and postmortem examination, because intra-arterial material can change with time. This approach of separating the arteries from the brain is to be undertaken only if there are no plans to study the relationship between brain surface arteries and deep infarction. For the latter studies, the vessels should be left on the brain and the tissue cut and processed with the vessels still in place.

Now the brainstem and cerebellum must be sepa-

rated from the rest of the brain. This is a delicate step, as the midbrain is both short and often important for histologic study. The cut across must be precisely transverse. The brain being base upward, the left hand (of a right-handed person) holds it in place while the thumb and index finger gently grip the pons. With a large-blade scalpel, the cut is begun on the upper lateral surface of the pons, just caudal to the oculomotor nerve, and is extended across in one sweep, without stopping the right hand. The left hand can then lift up the brainstem and cerebellum. The next cut is made through the rostral midbrain, parallel to the previous one. This provides a block containing the oculomotor nerves, the substantia nigra, the motor, sensory, and cerebellar pathways, and the red nuclei. Now the medial parts of the temporal lobes can be easily examined, particularly for herniation.

The cerebral hemispheres can be sliced in several ways, according to the known or presumed pathology. Sagittal sections are suitable for midline lesions such as pituitary tumors. Horizontal sections show nicely the internal capsule, the lateral ventricles, and the basal ganglia. For correlations with CT or MRI, the sections can be slanted accordingly. However, the usual procedure is to cut coronal slices that display internal capsule, cerebral peduncles, basal ganglia, hippocampus, lateral geniculate bodies, arterial territories, brain shifts, and herniations. The first cut is carefully symmetrical across both hemispheres, beginning at the junction of the anterior two-thirds and posterior one-third of the mammillary bodies. The hemispheres are cut in slices of equal thickness, about 1 cm. To ensure equal thickness, cutting angles can be used. Thus 8 to 12 or more slices are obtained. Macroscopic lesions can be recorded on chart's (Fig. 7-2A).

The brainstem and cerebellum can be cut in either of two ways. First, cuts can be made transversely through the pons and cerebellum and through the medulla and cerebellum (Fig 7-2B). Second, the cerebellum can be detached by sectioning the six cerebellar peduncles. Cuts across the cerebellum should be at right angles to the folia, and slices should be about 1 cm thick. The first cut is at the junction of the lateral two-thirds and the medial one-third of the hemisphere to display the dentate nucleus. A cut is made on the midline through the vermis. For study of the arterial supply to deep infarcts, it has been found convenient to trim away the sides of the brainstem and then to make long and thin slices from the posterior side of the brainstem toward the front, being careful to avoid disturbing the basilar artery and its immediate branches as they penetrate the brainstem on the frontal surface. When the site of infarction is reached by these thin sections, the specimen can be trimmed transversely and the entire block containing the infarct and its vascular supply embedded as a single piece.

Blocks of tissue for microscopy are selected according to clinical data and macroscopic appearance. They are dehydrated and embedded either in paraffin wax (most often) or in celloidin. Blocks of paraffin can be cut in 5 to 20-μm sections and can be stained by many of the usual stains, (e.g., hematoxylin and eosin, hematoxylin-van Gieson, Masson's trichrome, phosphotungstic acid-hematoxylin, periodic acid-Schiff), with impregnation of neurone bodies and processes by silver. Thus, these sections provide a good display of the main nervous structures and vessels. With experience, much information can be gained from hematoxylin and eosin staining. A disadvantage of paraffin embedding is about a 30 percent shrinkage of tissue during dehydration. Celloidin embedding makes it possible to obtain slides of the whole hemispheres, but embedding lasts several weeks and the sections are thicker, 15 to 20 μm and in some cases as thick as 35 μm. They are chiefly used for low-power microscopy and myelin stains, such as Loyez, or cell body stains, such as cresyl violet (Nissl).

Nervous tissue, either fresh or post fixation, can be frozen. This bypasses the process of embedding and allows slides to be prepared quickly. In particular, freezing avoids the processing of tissue in alcohol, thus leaving lipids in place. Therefore, frozen sections are used to display fat. They are also used for histochemistry or for the Holzer stain, which displays astrocytic gliosis. Of course, there are many more stains with particular applications. The reader is referred to Weller (1988) and to textbooks of neuropathology.

THE SPINAL CORD

Removal of the spinal cord is a required part of postmortem examination in patients who have died of a neurologic disease. It should be part of autopsy practice but rarely is the whole vertebral column removed en bloc so that after fixation, the cord, roots, and posterior root ganglia can be dissected. The anterior approach, advocated by Adams and Murray (1982), allows a good dissection of the posterior root ganglia, proximal nerves, and, where necessary, the brachial plexus. The classic approach is posterior. A midline incision is made from the nape of the neck to the sacrum, and the muscles are reflected from the spinous processes and laminae. The latter are cut as laterally as possible, and the long posterior cap of the spinal canal is then lifted, leaving the dura intact. Representative posterior root ganglia can be dissected out. This requires experience, particularly in the cervical region, where the ganglia are situated far laterally from the cord. By proceeding from the base of the skull and using a scalpel, the dura is freed from the foramen magnum. By lifting back up the dural sac with an artery forceps placed in the lower lumbar region, so that the cord is not damaged, the entire cord with its dural sac is removed. Successive rostral cuts are used for the nerve roots, while the left hand holding the forceps maintains the cord as straight as possible to avoid artifacts. When the dura is intact, the cord can be fixed in the bucket, along with the brain (see above). When the dura has been opened, it is better to open it from top to bottom by a midline incision, anteriorly and posteriorly.

After proper fixation and opening of the dura, the anterior aspect of the cord is identified by the presence of the anterior spinal artery. An irregular venous plexus marks the posterior aspect. Segmental levels can be identified by identifying the first thoracic segment, which bears the last large roots of the cervical enlargement. Segments above and below can be identified by counting the posterior roots. The cord is usually cut into horizontal slices. Embedding and processing are similar to those for the brain (see above), except that because the blocks are much smaller, embedding is a matter of days (with paraffin) or a few weeks (with celloidin).

CEREBRAL BIOPSY

Removal of a fragment of brain tissue in a patient defines cerebral biopsy. This does not include the routine extemporaneous examination of a fragment of tumor in neurosurgical operations. As central nervous tissue does not regenerate, cerebral biopsy implies permanent damage and a risk, albeit slight, of perioperative complications (e.g., hemorrhage or infection) and postoperative complications (e.g., epilepsy). Obviously, the indications for cerebral biopsy must be considered on the basis of strict guidelines. Of course, biopsy should be performed only where every modern diagnostic modality can be used to examine the tissue. In every case the decision to perform it is a consensus involving the neurologist, pathologist, and neurosurgeon, and an informed consent must be obtained from the patient or relatives. Where there is room for doubt, the opinion of the ethics committee of each particular institution should be sought.

The more straightforward indications are those diseases (e.g., lymphoma or viral encephalitides) that are very severe and impossible to diagnose with certainty by other methods and for which there is a treatment of reasonable effectiveness. Where efficient therapy is still not available but preventive measures exist, as may be the case in familial, purely cerebral diseases (e.g., adult ceroid lipofuscinosis, Alexander's or van Bogaert and Bertrand's disease), cerebral biopsy can also be considered. Research per se is not an indication, although, to be sure, parts of the tissue obtained can be used in research that implies hope for better knowledge and treatment of the disease under scrutiny.

Cerebral biopsy must be performed according to strict technical guidelines. Under general anesthesia (or local anesthesia for stereotactic biopsy) through a trephine hole, the biopsy is taken generally on the convexity of the frontal lobe of the nondominant hemisphere. Occasionally other sites are possible. For deep-seated lesions, stereotactic and MRI-guided stereotactic biopsies are possible. In the usual way, one or several fragments of frontal lobe are cut off with a scalpel. Diathermy is not used, as that would damage the edges of the incision. The pathologist and a technician are present in the operating theater with a supply of suitable sterile material. Special protective rules apply to diseases such as Creutzfeldt-Jakob, Gerstmann-Sträussler-Scheinker, AIDS, herpes zoster, cytomegalovirus, varicella-zoster virus, and hepatitis. Where tissue culture is planned, a small fragment is first cut off and immediately placed in a sterile box and sent to the laboratory. The main fragment must include leptomeninges (for vessels, see Ch. 38) and gray and white matter and should be a cube with sides about 15 mm long. The pathologist quickly divides the block into small fragments for electron microscopy, histochemistry, immunocytochemistry, parasitology, and flux cytometry. A good representative part of the block is fixed in buffered 4 percent formol for embedding in paraffin wax.

Examination of the cerebral biopsy allows either of three possible conclusions: (1) the biopsy is diagnostic (i.e., abnormalities that definitively confirm the diagnosis have been found); (2) the tissue is abnormal but not diagnostic; (3) to evidence of abnormality has been found. With the advances in clinical investigation techniques, the indications of cerebral biopsy have become more accurate, and provided that the sampled block is of sufficient size and correct orientation (particularly with respect to providing enough white matter), the positive diagnostic yield is fairly satisfactory, with well over 50 percent of examinations being diagnostic in most laboratories.

ANNOTATED BIBLIOGRAPHY

Adams JH, Murray MF. Atlas of Post-mortem Techniques in Neuropathology. Cambridge University Press, London, 1982.

A remarkable booklet, with wise advice and photographs on each step of the autopsy.

Blackwood W. Cerebral biopsy. In Bruyn, Vinken PJ (eds). Handbook of Clinical Neurology. Vol. 10. Elsevier, Amsterdam, 1970.

A concise and fairly complete account.

Hauw JJ, Henin D, Duyckaerts C et al. Autopsie et SIDA. Le risque infectieux en anatomie et cytologie pathologiques. Med Mal Infect 1989;4:230–33.

Special precautions for autopsy and handling of unfixed specimens in AIDS (SIDA in French).

Weller RO. A general approach to neurological problems. Berry CL (ed). In Neuropathology, Current Topics in Pathology. Springer Verlag, Berlin, 1988.

Many details and a list of stains.

8
Muscle and Nerve Biopsies

J. J. Hauw and B. Eymard

Muscle and nerve biopsies are often considered in the diagnostic approach of neuromuscular disorders or for exploration of systemic diseases. They can provide valuable diagnostic information provided that indication and technique are good.

INDICATIONS AND CONTRAINDICATIONS

Indications and contraindications depend heavily on the usual practices of the country and of each neurologist. The following points should be considered.

1. A biopsy (i.e., an invading technical diagnostic procedure) must be performed only when no other investigation can provide the same data. This means that a careful clinical examination, biochemical analyses, and electrophysiologic recordings have to be performed and their results evaluated before biopsy. The muscle that is undergoing biopsy must be spared by the electrophysiologist to prevent the "needle myopathy" (i.e., necrotic and inflammatory areas induced by needle punctures) that may be misleading.

2. A biopsy usually adds little when there is neither clinical nor electrophysiologic involvement of the sampled organ. With a few exceptions, when there are no sensory symptoms or signs, a nerve biopsy specimen involving a sensory nerve is likely to be normal.

3. A biopsy must be performed only when it can be fully processed with every technical procedure needed to answer the questions asked of the pathologist. For example, looking for a necrotizing angiopathy may be an emergency and requires simple techniques. On the contrary, there is usually some time to study a metabolic or degenerative neuropathy, and this needs optimal and complete processing. A full examination of a specimen from a muscle or nerve biopsy is a complex time-consuming procedure.

4. A biopsy in the lower limbs should be avoided in diabetes mellitus, after deep venous thrombosis, in the case of venous ulcer, when there is any trophic disorder, and especially in arteriosclerotic occlusive disease. Muscle or nerve biopsy should not be performed in patients with blood dyscrasias. Anticoagulant therapy has to be stopped on the day preceding the biopsy and can be resumed on the same day or the day after.

5. A muscle biopsy is a well-tolerated short surgical procedure. A nerve biopsy is slightly longer and may result in some dysesthetic sequelae.

CLINICAL REASONS FOR MUSCLE AND NERVE BIOPSY

Muscle Biopsy

From a clinical point of view, a muscle biopsy may be part of the investigation of a suspected neuromuscular disorder (Table 8-1). It may distinguish denervation from primary muscle disease when other data are doubtful and may recognize primary muscle diseases, namely, inflammatory myopathies; muscular vasculitis and cholesterol emboli; muscular dystrophies; congenital myopathies; mitochondrial and lipid myopathies; and some toxic, metabolic, and drug-induced myopathies. A muscle biopsy may also be performed for the histologic diagnosis of a systemic disease, for instance, vasculitis or sarcoidosis, without muscle symptoms being present.

Nerve Biopsy

Nerve biopsy is usually performed in suspected neuromuscular disorders. It may help to distinguish axonal degeneration from segmental demyelination when

Table 8-1. Muscle and Nerve Disorders in Which Muscle and/or Nerve Biopsy May Be Useful

Condition	Muscle	Nerve	Combined
Myopathic disorders			
Inflammatory	+ + +	−	−
Toxic and drug-induced	+	−	+
Endocrine	−	−	−
Genetically determined	+ + +	−	−
Myasthenia gravis	−	−	−
Myasthenic syndromes	+	−	−
Neurogenic disorders			
Anterior horn cells disorders	+ +	+	+
Motor nerve roots disorders	−	−	−
Peripheral neuropathies			
Metabolic and toxic polyneuropathies	−	±	±
Inflammatory polyradiculopathies	−	±	±
Collagen vascular disease	+ +	+ + +	+ + +
Infectious and malignant diseases	+	+ + +	−
Genetically determined	−	+ + +	+ +
Mononeuropathies and mononeuritis multiplex			
Entrapment and trauma	−	−	−
Collagen vascular disease	+ +	+ + +	+ + +
Diabetes mellitus	−	−	−

clinical examination and electrophysiologic tests give doubtful results. It can also find causes of neuropathies that are not found by other means (e.g., vasculitis, amyloidosis, leprosy, sarcoidosis, lymphomas, and other malignant blood diseases). Finally, in a few cases, a nerve biopsy may be performed in the absence of nerve symptoms or signs, for example, for investigation of an infantile metabolic encephalopathy or inherited disorder with mild or no peripheral expression and, for some authors, for suspected vasculitis. Combined nerve and muscle biopsies can be performed together with the same skin incision. This is especially easy when the superficial peroneal nerve and peroneus brevis are taken together. Combined biopsies of the sural nerve and the gastrocnemius can also be performed through an incision at midcalf level, but this is a less common procedure. This is useful for analyzing a mixed sensory motor polyneuropathy. When a proximal muscle biopsy has to be performed together with a nerve biopsy, two separate incisions have to be done. In the authors' experience, this procedure is not easily accepted by the patient when local anesthesia is used. This can be performed with general anesthesia, for example, for exploration of a metabolic disorder in a child.

SELECTION OF TECHNIQUE

Open biopsy is the most frequently used method for muscle biopsy. It gives the best material for muscle fiber typing and is mandatory for vasculitis detection. Needle biopsy is a simple, minimally invasive, and fast technique that may be repeated if negative results are found or to assess the evolution of a disease, but it can miss patchy lesions. It cannot be used for nerve sampling. Ideally, a choice should be available between both techniques. In fact, most teams use one or the other technique.

SELECTION OF SITE

Muscle Biopsy

When a neuromuscular disease is explored, especially to detect lesions of the muscle fiber proper (e.g., denervation atrophy, myopathic changes, and some inflammatory myopathies), the muscle to sample has to be affected, but severely atrophic muscles should be avoided because the changes may then be nonspecific. When the purpose of the biopsy is to find a systemic disease, a nonaffected muscle can be sampled. The deltoid muscle or the biceps in the upper limb, the quadriceps, the gastrocnemius, or the tibialis anterior in the lower limb are usually chosen because of their size and their well-known normal appearance. The peroneus brevis is also sampled together with the superficial peroneal nerve. In case of symmetric involvement, the biopsy should be performed on the nondominant side (i.e., on the left side in a right-handed patient).

Nerve Biopsy

The choice of the nerve for biopsy is restricted for practical reasons. In the lower limbs, only two nerves are readily used. They are similar, as far as the density and diameter histogram of myelinated fibers and the frequency of pathologic alterations are concerned. The sural nerve is commonly sampled in North America and the United Kingdom. This is a cutaneous sensory nerve, the distal part of which supplies the skin of the lateral aspect of the heel and the distal side of the foot and fifth toe. Biopsy is performed at the ankle level. The patient lies prone on the operating table, with the ankle slightly everted and the foot at 90 degrees with the leg. Compression of the calf distends the saphenous vein, which lies immediately adjacent to the nerve in the trough between the external malleolus and the Achilles tendon. The incision is made along the course of the vein. The nerve is found beneath Scarpa's fascia, most commonly on the medial side of the vein. A long segment can be removed. The superficial peroneal (musculocutaneous) nerve is commonly sampled in France and some other European countries. It is a cutaneous sensory nerve the distal territory of which consists of the skin of the lateral part of the dorsum of the foot and the dorsum of third and fourth toes. The patient lies curled up. Biopsy is performed 1 cm ahead of a line joining the head of the fibula to the external malleolus at the junction of the upper two-thirds with the lower one-third of the line. The nerve is seen when it becomes subcutaneous at the level of the intermuscular septum between peroneal and extensor muscles. Fragments 3- to 4-cm long can comfortably be removed. A concomitant biopsy of the peroneus brevis (lateral to the intermuscular septum) can be easily done. Other nerves that have been sampled are the saphenous nerve and the intermediate cutaneous nerve of the thigh.

Upper limb nerve biopsies are seldom performed. The superficial radial nerve at the junction of the middle and distal thirds of the forearm or other small cutaneous nerves enlarged at clinical examination can be chosen, especially for the diagnosis of leprosy. Other nerves, such as the greater auricular nerve, may also be sampled, especially when enlarged.

A skin biopsy can be performed at the onset of the dissection when a metabolic or degenerative disease is explored. Samples of skin are taken for light microscopy, electron microscopy, and cell culture. Removal of two symmetric thin and long fragments, including the dermis, allows an even scar.

TECHNIQUE OF OPEN BIOPSY

First, close cooperation between clinician, pathologist, and surgeon is required for open muscle biopsy and nerve biopsy, maybe more than in any other branch of pathology, and this is best achieved when two or even three of these partners are the same person.

Who Should Perform the Biopsy?

When an open biopsy is scheduled, it may be done by a surgeon or by the pathologist, which is the best solution when possible. In the first case, the surgeon has to be informed of the technical care needed to prevent artifacts (see below). When clinicians do not read the biopsy themselves (or together with the pathologist), they must provide detailed information on the patient.

Precautions

Open biopsies are performed in an operating room with the same technical precautions as in any general surgical procedure. When the biopsy is performed by a surgeon, a technician or a neuropathologist must provide indications concerning the fragments to sample and receive the specimen in the operating room for immediate handling. When the neuropathologist personally performs the surgical procedure, the nurse can handle the samples.

Technique

A local anesthetic is typically used, except for children. Infants can usually be managed with preanesthetic sedation, and older children can be reasoned with. General anesthetic has to be avoided in patients with malignant hyperthermia and those diseases that may be associated with secondary hyperthermia, such as Duchenne's dystrophy, myotonia congenita, or central core disease.

Drawing a skin mark for the incision is useful. Ten milliliters (2 to 5 ml in children) of 1 percent lidocaine, without epinephrine (in the authors' experience) is gently infiltrated into the skin and subcutaneous tissue. Precautions are taken not to infiltrate the muscle or the nerve.

After incision of the skin, dissection can be carried out with few sections, with the operator using a swab and thin rounded-end scissors to push a way through the subcutaneous tissue. Autostatic retractors are helpful to move apart the lips of the incision and locate the fragments to sample. After incision of the fascia, any surgical trauma, and especially any traction to the muscle or the nerve, is avoided. Thin forceps allow the surgeon to hold the perimysium or the perineurium gently. Some authors perform the biopsy under the microscope.

Muscle Biopsy

For muscle biopsy, no anesthesia of the muscle proper is performed because it would induce histologic artifacts. After the thin connective sheath covering the muscle with fine scissors is cut, four or five well-dissected muscle fascicles 1- to 2-cm long and a few millimeters wide are sampled. This is a slightly painful procedure. Some authors use specially devised forceps to keep the muscle bundle at resting length. On rare occasions, larger fragments are removed for biochemical purposes (e.g., analysis of a mitochondriopathy).

Nerve Biopsy

For nerve biopsy, before longitudinal dissection and section of the nerve, some authors anesthetize the proximal exposure by injecting 0.2 ml of lidocaine into the nerve (a slightly painful procedure), but some do not. In either case, the patient must be forewarned that a short (a few seconds) but severe flash of pain will probably be experienced at the time of the section. A fragment 2- to 4-cm long (whole nerve biopsy) or several fascicles of the same length are sampled. Some authors prefer longer fascicles up to 8 to 10 cm.

After the biopsy, hemostasis is obtained by firm pressure for a few minutes on the site of sampling and sometimes ligating a few remaining bleeding points. The fascia is reapproximated with an absorbable suture and the skin, with a Teflon suture. Three to five stitches are left for 8 to 10 days. Some authors use an absorbable subcutaneous running stitch. A dry dressing applied by an elastic bandage is applied for 10 to 15 days. The patient is told to use the limb gently (without walking or strong movements, such as cutting meat) during the next 2 days.

Complications

Complications of the operation (bleeding, infection, and opening of the scar) are rare.

Should Sampling of the Full Thickness of the Nerve or Only a Few Fascicles Be Done?

The answer to this question depends on two main factors: the habits of the surgeon/neuropathologist and the reason for the biopsy. The full thickness of the nerve must be removed for the diagnosis of vasculitis because the vasa nervorum, including the middle-sized artery adjacent to the nerve, have to be examined. Other reasons for a full biopsy are a shorter procedure, a greater chance to find scanty lesions such as amyloidosis deposits, a more accurate study of quantified parameters of the nerve (morphometry), and a better assessment of fascicular or other focal lesions. In contrast, a fascicular biopsy leads to a smaller area of anesthesia. Although opinions are varied, inquiries have shown that patients do not complain of more discomfort when the nerve has been fully sectioned.

Histopathologic Techniques

These largely depend on the purpose of the biopsy and of the habits of the neuropathologist. When a vasculitis or any focal lesion is sought, large fragments of muscle and/or nerve should be examined, which is best done when paraffin-embedded samples are semiserially cut. For the thorough study of an unexplained or degenerative neuropathy, a number of different techniques are commonly used, such as measure of the density and assessment of the distribution of diameters of myelinated fibers and unmyelinated axons and analysis of teased nerve fibers.

In the authors' laboratory, for muscle biopsy after sampling, special efforts are made to avoid stretching the muscle fibers. A thin fascicle is immediately fixed in 2.5 percent glutaraldehyde (Sörensen buffer) for electron microscopy. Cross- and longitudinal sections are epoxy embedded and stored or processed for semithin sections. Ultrathin sections are made only if electron microscopy is needed, which is rare in adult patients. Two short muscle fascicles are removed for histochemical and immunohistochemical analysis. They are put on a saline-moistened gauze swab in a Petri dish or in a small tube and kept 10 to 15 minutes before the carefully oriented cross sections are frozen in isopentane chilled in liquid nitrogen. Staining with hematoxylin-eosin, periodic acid-Schiff, modified Gomori's trichrome stain, and oil red O and histochemical testing with succinic dehydrogenase, nicotinamide adenine dinucleotide tetrazolium reductase, phosphorylase, and adenosine triphosphatases at various pHs are performed.

In some adult patients, a reduced set of histoenzymologic techniques is used. It is performed on the same day and allows a fast report (in 80 to 90 percent of cases, examination of other samples does not significantly modify the diagnosis). The other frozen fascicle is kept at −80°C for further histochemical and immunohistochemical analysis or in situ hybridization with polymerase chain reaction testing if needed, but they are seldom used (10 to 20 percent of the cases for diagnosis and also for research purposes). A large and longer fascicle (or a few fascicles) is fixed with 3.7 percent neutral formaldehyde (10 percent of the commercially available formaldehyde solution kept in a container together with powdered calcium carbonate). It is carefully oriented for cross section and longitudinal paraffin embedding. Two to four sections are stained by hematoxylin and eosin. When looking for focal lesions, 6 to 10 semiserial sections are prepared. Another fragment is dry cooled and stored at −80°C for biochemical analysis.

For nerve biopsy, a 1 to 2-cm-long fragment (or three to four fascicles of the same length) is immediately fixed with 5 percent glutaraldehyde (Sörensen buffer) followed by 1 percent osmium tetroxide (without suspending the nerve, a procedure recommended by some authors). It is dissected under a binocular microscope to separate long segments. These are epoxy embedded (without dimethylaminomethyl-phenol) and kept at 80°C until use for the preparation of teased nerve fibers. They are transferred to a slide covered with by epoxy (with dimethyla-minomethylphenol) that is coverslipped and polymerized by baking at 60°C. Short segments are epoxy embedded for examination of cross sections by light microscopy (semithin sections). Electron microscopy can be performed when needed. A fascicle is frozen for immunohistochemical analysis, as described for muscle biopsy, and kept at −80°C. Other fascicles are used for biochemistry (dry frozen at −80°C) or for cell cultures.

MAIN FINDINGS FROM MUSCLE BIOPSY

Normal Muscle

The normal muscle is composed of muscle fibers organized into fascicles. Each mature muscle fiber is a multinucleated very long cell lined by a basement membrane that also surrounds the so-called satellite cells (small immature cells that can differentiate into muscle fibers). Most of the numerous muscle cell nuclei are peripherally located and may be difficult to recognize from satellite cell nuclei. Muscle cells contain the usual organelles and central myofibrils. Histochemical techniques allow the recognition of different types of fibers on the basis of their content in oxidative enzymes, phosphorylase, and adenosine triphosphatase, which depends on the innervating neuron.

Normally, there is a mixture of different fiber types, and they are distributed at random in a mosaic pattern (Fig. 8-1A). The fascicles are separated by epimysial connective tissue (or epimysium), containing blood vessels of various diameters (arteries are typically 100 to 200 μm, and small vessels of the microcirculation and venules are also seen) and nerves. Endomysial connective tissue (or endomysium) is composed of inconspicuous fine strands of connective tissue, including capillaries and a few larger vessels of the microcirculation, and some nerve fibers go to motor end-plates (neuromuscular junctions) and to muscle spindles and other sensory terminals. Large bundles of fibrosis or the presence of adipocytes are pathologic features.

Histopathologic Analysis and Main Techniques

Both conventional techniques and histochemical stains should be routinely performed. Hematoxylin and eosin and Gomori's trichrome stains demonstrate pathologic changes concerning the following.

1. Fiber size (atrophy and/or hypertrophy). Schematically, fiber atrophy can affect isolated fibers (this is not very specific); it can be distributed in small or large groups either inside a fascicle or involving a whole fascicle (this indicates denervation atrophy, see below); it can occur in foci (this is usually of vascular origin); or, lastly, it can be perifascicular in dermatomyositis.

2. Number, morphology, and distribution of nuclei.

3. Fiber necrosis (necrotic fiber are either very stained or pale and liquefied, undergoing phagocytosis), often coexisting with regeneration (small basophilic fibers when seen with hematoxylin and eosin, with vesiculated nuclei).

4. Splitting, corresponding to the partial division of the fiber.

5. Granular staining in the periphery of the fiber or disrupting their myofibrillar content, usually indicating an abnormal accumulation of mitochondria.

6. Increase in connective tissue (collagen and fat).

7. Presence of cellular infiltrates in the endomysium and/or perimysium, in the vicinity of necrotic-regenerating fibers or around the vessels. The characterization of cell infiltrates may be performed by immunostaining.

Histochemical techniques are commonly used.

1. Oxidative enzyme reactions are used such as reduced nicotinamide adenine dinucleotide-tetrazolium reductase, or succinic dehydrogenase to stain the intermyofibrillary network. They reveal structural changes that may be overlooked with conventional techniques, such as cores, which are zones devoid of oxidative activity or whorled fibers; target fibers; or lobulated or moth-eaten fibers characterized by various disruptions of intermyofibrillar network. Oxidative stains also show readily accumulations of mitochondria.

2. Adenosine triphosphatase reactions stain the myosins, characterizing the myofibrils. Furthermore, such reactions, preincubated at different pHs, distinguish different populations of fibers: type 1 (slow twitch, oxidative) and type 2 (fast twitch), which is subdivided into 2A (oxidative and glycolytic), 2B (glycolytic), and 2C (fetal type, present in case of regeneration). Abnormalities in distribution (grouping), type predominance, selective involvement of one fiber type for atrophy, or hypertrophy are considered. A detailed analysis of fiber diameter as a function of the type can be made by preparing a histogram of 200 fibers.

3. Specific reactions are routinely used to show glycogen (periodic acid-Schiff reaction), phosphorylase activity, lipids (oil red O and Sudan black). Other complementary histochemical techniques

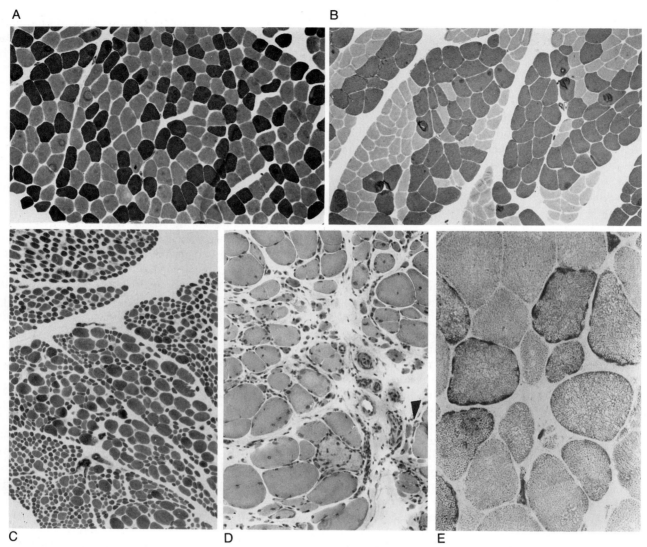

Figure 8-1. (**A**) Normal biopsy showing a mosaic pattern with interspersed type 2 fibers (staining dark) and type 1 fibers. The nuclei are peripherally located. No variation in fiber size is present. (Adenosine triphosphatase, pH 9.4; ×160.) (**B**) Denervation atrophy. Note type grouping of fibers. (Adenosine triphosphatase, pH 9.4; ×160.) (**C**) Severe spinal muscular atrophy, Werdnig-Hoffmann disease. The biopsy of the deltoid shows a large group atrophy, involving type 1 and type 2 (staining dark) fibers. Enlarged fibers are uniformly type I in histochemical reaction. (Adenosine triphosphatase, pH 9.4; ×80.) (**D**) Dystrophic pattern. Gastrocnemius biopsy revealing a major variation in fiber size, with coexisting enlarged and atrophic fibers, fiber splitting, increased connective tissue proliferation. Distal myopathy. (Hematoxylin-eosin, ×160.) (**E**) Mitochondrial myopathy. With the oxidative reaction, a subsarcolemmal aggregation of mitochondria is evidenced in many fibers. (Succinic dehydrogenase, ×400.)

are used if necessary, such as acid phosphatase to ascertain the lysosomal origin of vacuoles and assess the distribution of mild infiltrates of phagocytes, and cytochrome oxidase if a respiratory chain myopathy is suspected.

Electron microscopy, a time-consuming technique, is limited to those cases in which ultrastructural features are specific and needed for the diagnosis (see above). Other techniques can be performed. Methyl-ene blue or silver stains to assess the subterminal and terminal nerve fiber pattern, which can show reinnervation, and acetylcholinesterase or immunohistochemical analysis to study motor end-plates are today less used than are immunocytochemical tests for dystrophin or other proteins or in situ hybridization and polymerase chain reaction techniques for viral identification. In addition, biochemical study of a sample is frequently useful, particularly when a metabolic disorder is suspected.

Main Varieties of Muscle Lesions

Schematically, the following points must be ascertained in the study of muscle biopsy: Is there a pathologic process? If so, is this due to denervation ("neurogenic atrophy"), to an inflammatory disease (inflammatory myopathy), to a metabolic myopathy, to a muscular dystrophy, or to a congenital myopathy? What is the meaning of those mild nonspecific changes that are frequently found? What is that of a normal biopsy result?

Denervation Atrophy

Whatever the cause of denervation, muscle lesions display a common pattern that depends heavily on the stage and evolution of the motor neuropathy and on the degree of regeneration (Fig. 8-2). In the acute stages, muscle fibers have a normal appearance for days or even weeks. Then, atrophy of some fibers scattered throughout the fascicles occurs. They exhibit an angular appearance, dense staining, and high oxidative enzyme activity, whatever their type. When there is reinnervation, type grouping occurs. Groups of fibers of the same histoenzymologic type (Fig. 8-1B) result from the formation of giant motor units. Ten adjacent fibers of the same type, at least, should be seen, and groups of both main subtypes of muscle fibers should coexist to establish the type grouping, especially when disproportion of fiber type is high in the sampled muscle. This can be seen without any changes found by conventional stains. Then, target fibers are seen (this is best done with oxidative enzymes preparations), and small groups of atrophic angular fibers occur in the center of fascicles.

In long-standing denervation (months and years), especially in motor neuron diseases, whole fascicles are made of very atrophic fibers that contain numerous nuclei, contrasting with other less affected fascicles. In acute denervation, necrotic and basophilic fibers, indicating regeneration and sometimes associated with an inflammatory cellular infiltrate, can be seen. This may be confusing in a primary inflammatory muscle disease (polymyositis). In chronic denervation, muscle fiber hypertrophy, numerous centrally located nuclei, and muscle splits are found. This may be confusing in a primary degenerative muscle disease ("pseudomyopathic changes"). Usually, however, interstitial fibrosis is less marked in denervation atrophy than in primary muscle disorders.

Spinal Muscular Atrophies

In severe spinal muscular atrophy (SMA, Werdnig-Hoffmann disease) with early infancy onset and fatal outcome before the age of 1 year and in intermediate SMA with onset between 6 and 12 months and non-progressive weakness, the histologic features are large group atrophy, interspersed with a variable amount of markedly hypertrophic fibers (see Ch. 82). Hypertrophic fibers have type one features, and atrophic fibers show a mixed pattern of types 1 and 2 fibers (Fig. 8-1C). There is no necrosis or degeneration. In the beginning of the disease, the muscle biopsy specimen may be nearly normal, apart from a small size of all fibers, without marked denervation-reinnervation characteristics.

In mild SMA (Kugelberg-Welander disease), the pattern is different. Smaller clusters of atrophic fibers, grouping of the large fibers of both types, and type 2 predominance are found. Architectural changes within the fiber are common, such as target and whorled fibers. Splitting and internal nuclei can occur. It may be difficult to distinguish mild SMA from muscular dystrophy. Focal groups of atrophied fibers are often present in Becker's disease. Type fiber grouping is more likely in SMA. Results from other investigations, such as creatine kinase and electromyography, and molecular genetics are useful.

Muscular Dystrophies

These are a heterogeneous group of long-standing muscular disorders, related to a primary defect of a muscle protein or glycoprotein (generally unknown), which induce a progressive degeneration of muscle fibers (see Ch. 82). Classification of dystrophies relies on clinical data, inheritance pattern, and when possible, molecular grounds. We first review the main histopathologic features and then the contribution of biopsy results to the diagnosis.

Main Histopathologic Features

All the varieties of muscular dystrophies display a common "dystrophic" pattern (Fig. 8-1D), including the following.

1. A degeneration-regeneration process with muscle fiber necrosis and regeneration, resulting in fiber loss.
2. Variation in fiber size, usually with enlargement and atrophy of fibers.
3. Increase in endomysial and perimysial connective tissue.
4. Fiber splitting.
5. Changes in the architecture of the intermyofibrillar network.
6. Increased number of internal nuclei.
7. Impaired types 1 and 2 distribution. Special features may be found in some muscular dystrophies. However, they are not pathognomonic.

Duchenne's Muscular Dystrophy. In Duchenne's muscular dystrophy, foci of degeneration with necro-

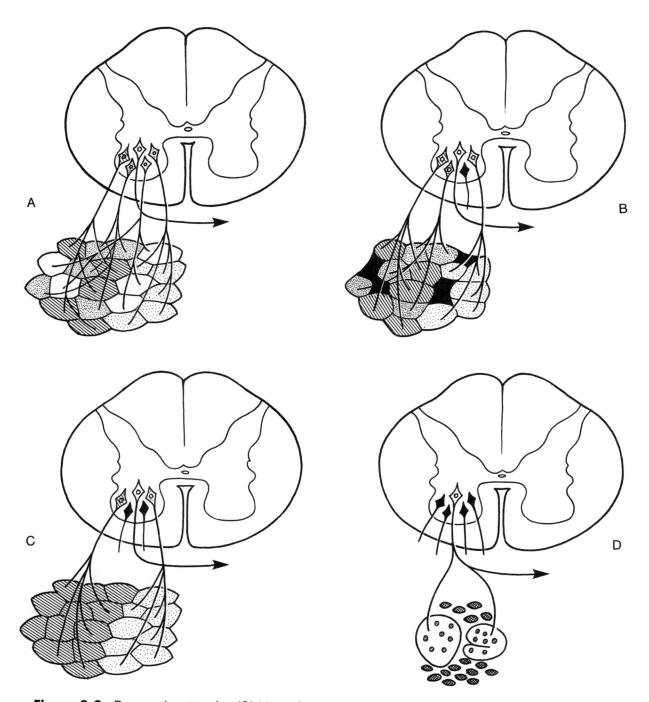

Figure 8-2. Denervation atrophy. (**A**) Normal appearance of a muscle fascicle innervated by spinal cord anterior horn neurons. (**B**) The death of one of the neurons leads to atrophy of some fibers scattered throughout the fascicle. They exhibit an angular appearance and dense staining. (**C**) When there is reinnervation, type grouping occurs. (**D**) Chronic denervation, with muscle fiber hypertrophy, numerous centrally located nuclei, and muscle splits (pseudomyopathic changes). Note that the reinnervation of the muscle fascicle is extremely deficient, and is provided by an axon that was initially (Figs. A, B, C) directed to another fascicle.

sis and phagocytosis and of small basophilic (regenerating) fibers are numerous. There are cellular infiltrates of mononuclear cells (lymphocytes and macrophages) in relation to necrotic fibers. Enlarged densely stained fibers are present, fiber type differentiation is impaired, and type I predominance is found. The endomysial and perimysial connective tissue is abundantly increased and occurs early in the disease. In preclinical cases, the muscle biopsy specimen is usually already pathologic, with variation in fiber diameter, increased cellularity, and presence of degenerating and regenerating fibers. Except for necrotic fibers, the intermyofibrillar network is preserved.

In female heterozygotes, the muscle biopsy may show unequivocal changes even when the serum enzymes levels are normal (30 percent of definite female carriers). There are focal changes with a "dystrophic" pattern, that is, variation in fiber size, including hypertrophic fibers, split fibers, occasional basophilic fibers, internal nuclei, and phagocytosis, and proliferation of endomysial connective tissue. In some cases, only minimal or borderline changes are seen.

Becker's Muscular Dystrophy. In Becker's muscular dystrophy, fibrosis and inflammatory reactions are not as prominent as in Duchenne's muscular dystrophy. Group atrophy and angulated fibers, similar to those seen in denervation, can be found. In both, a dystrophin deficiency is in evidence, as emphasized below.

Fascioscapulohumeral Dystrophy. In Fascioscapulohumeral dystrophy, the biopsy specimen is often normal if it is performed in the deltoid, which is usually mildly affected on clinical grounds. The biceps is a better muscle for analysis. In contrast with many other dystrophies, there is usually an increase in the mean diameter of all types and the presence of small isolated angulated fibers. Necrotic fibers scattered throughout the biopsy are common. One of the usual features of this disorder is the inflammatory response, which may be profuse on occasion. It can then be differentiated from polymyositis by the presence of hypertrophic fibers, which are seldom seen in polymyositis. Fibrosis, fiber splitting, and type one predominance are usually present in the late stages.

Limb-Girdle Dystrophy. In Limb-girdle dystrophy, there is a great variation in the size of fibers, with many large fibers. Fiber splitting is very marked, and internal nuclei are common. Abundant moth-eaten and whorled fibers are also common. Phagocytosis and inflammatory response is less marked in limb-girdle dystrophy than in other dystrophies. Type one predominance is frequently found.

Myotonic Dystrophy. In myotonic dystrophy (Steinert's disease), the following features are characteristic: (1) type one fiber atrophy and type 2 hypertrophy; (2) high density of internal nuclei, which are more numerous in myotonic dystrophy than in almost any other disease, and form chains of internal nuclei in longitudinal section; and (3) the presence of numerous ring fibers with peripheral myofibrils running at right angles to the normal axis of the fiber.

Congenital Muscle Dystrophy. In congenital muscle dystrophy, the striking feature is the replacement of muscle by adipose tissue, and connective tissue proliferation.

Oculopharyngeal Dystrophy. In oculopharyngeal dystrophy, small angulated fibers and vacuoles rimmed with material that stains red with Gomori's trichrome stain and blue with hematoxylin-eosin are found. Moth-eaten fibers are prominent. This is the only variety of muscular dystrophy that justifies the use of electron microscopy for definite diagnosis. Intranuclear tubular filaments with a 8.5 μm outer diameter make the diagnosis.

Other muscular dystrophies (distal dystrophy, Emery-Dreifuss dystrophy) are rare disorders. Severe childhood autosomal recessive myopathy is seen in North Africa.

Contribution of Muscle Biopsy to the Diagnosis of Muscle Dystrophy

Histologic and histochemical features of muscle are not sufficient to characterize the varieties of muscular dystrophy. Clinical data are essential, such as X-linked transmission, onset in early childhood, hypertrophy of calves, cardiomyopathy, and severe evolution, which suggests Duchenne's muscular dystrophy. A later onset and milder course characterize Becker's muscular dystrophy, and autosomal dominant inheritance and characteristic distribution indicate fascioscapulohumeral dystrophy. Myotonia, cataract, and autosomal dominant inheritance are characteristic of myotonic dystrophy; autosomal recessive transmission without facial involvement suggests limb-girdle dystrophy. Dominantly transmitted ocular myopathy beginning after 50 years is likely to be oculopharyngeal dystrophy. However, clinical data may be poor, some case are nonfamilial, and weakness may be absent. Evidence of the molecular defect responsible for the muscle dystrophy is now the crucial piece of information, allowing a definite classification. The most significant example concerns Duchenne's and Becker's muscular dystrophies, which result from genetic mutations within the dystrophin gene. Dystrophin testing on muscle, using immunohistochemical tests and immunoblots, is the most convenient method to identify these dystrophies and to differentiate them from unrelated disorders (Fig. 8-3). In Duchenne's muscular dystrophy, dystrophin is absent in most muscle fibers, except for some "reverting" fibers (Fig. 8-3C). This pattern results from an "out of frame" gene deletion, which creates a translational stop codon (see Ch. 4). By contrast, in Becker's muscular dystrophy, an "in frame" deletion permits the synthesis of truncated dystrophin, leading to a reduced overall amount of dystrophin. Western blot shows dystrophin of abnormal quality (usually of a smaller size) and of reduced amount. Immunostaining at the surface membrane is patchy and discontinuous.

Dystrophin abnormalities have also been found in patients with clinical phenotypes differing from Becker's muscular dystrophy, as shown for familial X-linked myalgia and cramps, or late and/or mild myopathies. In female heterozygote with Duchenne's muscular dystropy patients, dystrophin expression may display mosaicism, which is characterized by immunostaining of interspersed dystrophin positive and negative fibers. This phenomenon is not constantly found, even in obligate carriers. Besides dystrophin abnormalities, a selective deficiency of the adhalin component of the glycoprotein complex associated with dystrophin has been demonstrated in severe childhood autosomal recessive myopathy, mimicking Duchenne's muscular dystrophy on clinical and histologic grounds. In myotonic dystrophy, the DNA mutation (an abnormal repeat sequence) can be easily evidenced in a blood sample, confirming the diagnosis in poorly symptomatic patients and facilitating genetic counseling. Because protein deficiency in muscle has not been demonstrated so far in Steinert's disease, the usefulness of muscle biopsy is questionable.

Congenital Myopathies

Congenital myopathies are muscular disorders characterized by a very early onset of the condition, at least pathologically, if not always clinically (floppy baby); a nonprogressive course; a defined pattern of inheritance; a high incidence of associated dysmorphic features; and a characteristic histopathologic pattern. Muscle biopsy is the only way of making an accurate diagnosis. It differentiates congenital myopathy from other similar diseases such as spinal atrophy or muscular dystrophy. It is also the main clue for classification. A full analysis of the muscle, including histochemical techniques and electron microscopic analysis is essential, because many of the abnormalities are readily missed with routine stains and sometimes with histochemical tests.

Central Core Disease

With most oxidative preparations, the core appears as a well-defined rounded unstained zone, occupying a large area of the muscle fiber. Although typically described as "central," running along the whole length of the muscle fiber, it is often found in an eccentric position. The cores affect type I fibers selectively. Electron microscopy shows that these areas contain densely packed myofilaments that are not segregated into normal myofibrils (Fig. 8-4A). The filamentous architecture of the core is variable. Sarcomeric organization may be preserved, with sarcomers being shorter than normal and an altered ratio of thick to thin filaments and zigzag appearance of Z lines (structured cores), or it may be disrupted, with the myofilaments being in complete disarray (unstructured cores). The two types of cores may coexist in the same biopsy. A type 1 fiber predominance is frequent. Core density may vary from one muscle to another and from one member of a family to another. In a same individual, the pathologic process may increase with age, without progression in clinical severity. There is no clear correlation between the density of the cores and the clinical severity.

Minicore Disease

The muscle may look normal on standard staining, apart from some variability in fiber size and an increase in internal nuclei. With histochemical techniques, muscle fibers show small defects and irregularities in the intermyofibrillar network. In contrast to cores, minicores are focal and do not run along the length of the fiber. On electron microscopy, the minicores are focal circumscribed areas (running over two to six sarcomeres) with disruption of the myofibrillary pattern, Z-band streaming, and zigzagging.

Nemaline Myopathy

The term "nemaline myopathy" refers to the thread-like undulations produced in the muscle by accumulation of minute rod-shaped granules. Rods can be demonstrated by light microscopy with Gomori's trichrome stain; they do not stain by any histochemical technique. By electron microscopy, the rods are dense structures, usually of rectangular shape (Fig. 8-4B), with a lattice pattern of constant periodicity, in continuity with the Z lines. They form aggregates at the periphery or in the center of the muscle fiber. The main component of the nemaline bodies is α-actinin. There is no correlation between the clinical severity and the degree of involvement of fibers. Type 1 fibers are predominant and small, and they are selectively involved by rods.

Centronuclear Myopathies

These are defined by the high proportion of central nuclei. Different entities have been described: early-onset centronuclear myopathies, late-onset centronuclear myopathies, centronuclear myopathy with type 1 fiber atrophy, and severe X-linked myotubular my-

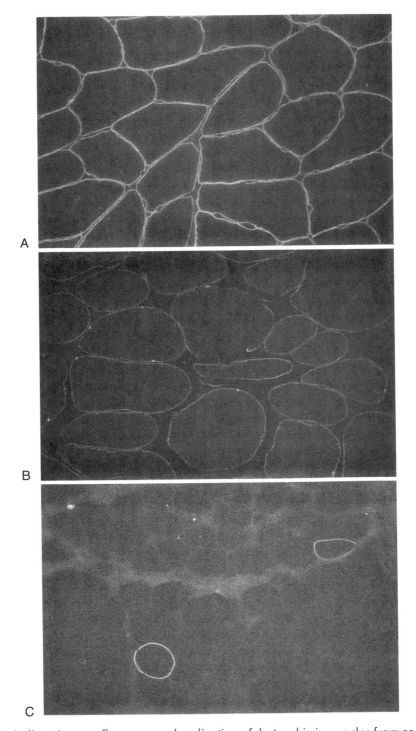

Figure 8-3. Indirect immunofluorescence localization of dystrophin in muscles from control and patients with Duchenne's and Becker's muscular dystrophies, using anti-T marmorata dystrophin antibodies. (**A**) Even distribution of dystrophin in the sarcolemma of all muscle fibers in a control case. (**B**) Weak labeling of the sarcolemma in a patient with Becker's muscular dystrophy. (**C**) Absence of dystrophin in all but two ("reverting") muscle fibers in a patient with Duchenne's muscular dystrophy. (×235.) (Courtesy of Professor M. Fardeau and Dr. F. Tome.)

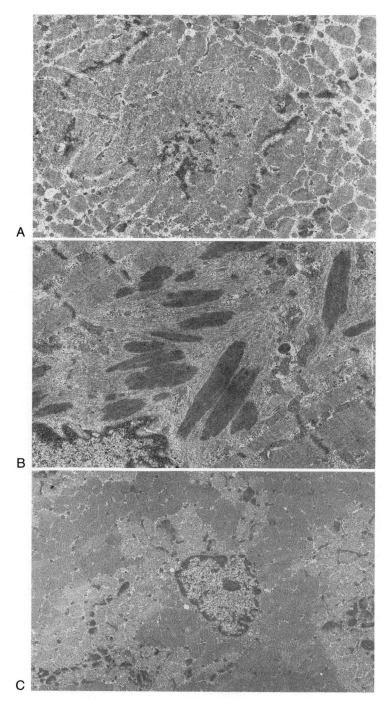

Figure 8-4. (**A**) Central core disease. Electron micrograph. Transverse section showing a circular area of myofilament disarray, corresponding to the core. (×7,400.) (**B**) Congenital nemaline myopathy. Electron micrograph. Longitudinal section showing numerous rods of rectangular shape. (×14,000.) (**C**) Centronuclear myopathy. Electron micrograph showing the centrally placed nucleus. (×6,000.) (Courtesy of Professor M. Fardeau and Dr. F. Tome.)

opathy. In the early- and late-onset types, the lesions are similar. Central nuclei are seen in 25 to 95 percent of muscle fibers, with the intermyofibrillary network being radially arranged around the central nucleus. The nucleus, which is surrounded by a small area devoid of organelles, is normal by electron microscopy (Fig. 8-4C). Type I fiber predominance is always found and type I fiber atrophy may be present. X-linked myotubular myopathy is a well-defined disease, with very severe involvement in boys, leading to death from respiratory failure in the early neonatal period. There is a uniform myotubular pattern in every fiber of every muscle. Female carriers often exhibit some myotubes or mild type 1 fiber predominance.

Congenital Fiber Type Disproportion

Muscle biopsy is characterized here by small type 1 fibers compared with type 2 fibers. Type 1 predominance is frequently associated. The limits of this entity are uncertain and raise the question of specificity of the histologic features. The clinical condition may vary considerably (benign and severe forms in neonates), and a similar pattern is found in various disorders (congenital myotonic dystrophy or nemaline or centronuclear myopathies).

Congenital Myopathies With Intracytoplasmic Inclusion Bodies

These are rare, ultrastructurally characterized, entities. They include fingerprint, reducing-body, and sarcotubular myopathies. In some patients with presumptive congenital myopathy, no specific ultrastructural finding is present. A type 1 predominance is the only feature.

Metabolic Myopathies

Muscle biopsy is a fundamental clue in the accurate diagnosis of metabolic myopathies. Histochemical techniques characterize abnormal features, namely glycogen or lipid storage or piled up mitochondria. Electron microscopy may give further indications, such as the presence of a lysosomal membrane circumscribing vacuoles. Finally, the enzymatic deficiency is proved, sometimes by histochemical tests, always by biochemical analysis.

Glycogenoses

In most muscle glycogenoses, whatever the deficient enzyme or the clinical condition (exercise intolerance and myoglobinuria or progressive weakness), muscle biopsy shows an excessive storage of glycogen. This appears as vacuoles that are positive with periodic acid-Schiff stain. Electron microscopy reveals an excessive accumulation of glycogen granules. Histopath-

ologic particularities are associated with the different varieties of diseases.

Myophosphorylase Deficiency. In myophosphorylase deficiency (type 5 glycogenosis, McArdle's disease), the most frequent glycogenosis, which induces exercise intolerance and myoglobinuria, there are subsarcolemmal vacuoles, and focal necrotic and regenerating fibers (indicating myolysis) may be present. A histochemical method is used to demonstrate enzyme deficiency. Histologic changes similar to those of McArdle's disease are found in other glycogenoses with a similar clinical pattern such as phosphofructokinase deficiency (type 7 glycogenosis, Tarui's disease) and phosphorylase kinase (type 8 glycogenosis). A few cases of glycolytic enzymes presenting with exercise intolerance have been identified: phosphoglycerate mutase I, phosphoglycerate kinase, and lactic dehydrogenase. A vacuolar myopathy with an increased periodic acid-Schiff reaction is found in phosphoglycerate mutase I but is absent in phosphoglycerate kinase. Decreased enzyme activity is shown in muscle.

Acid Maltase Deficiency. In acid maltase deficiency (type 2 glycogenosis), the deficient enzyme, 1-4α-glucosidase, is lysosomal. Vacuolated fibers are highly reactive for acid phosphatase, a lysosomal enzyme. By electron microscopy, excessive accumulation of glycogen is present in two different locations. Much of it is in a freely dispersed state; in addition, some appears in lysosomes, which may contain also heterogeneous cytoplasmic degradation products. In the infantile form (Pompe's disease), virtually all muscle fibers have large glycogen-containing vacuoles. In the adult form, only a few or even no fibers display vacuoles in the clinically unaffected muscle. Acid phosphatase reactivity is found, however, in the few vacuoles. Acid maltase deficiency is ascertained in leukocytes and in muscle.

Branching Enzyme Deficiency. In branching enzyme deficiency (type 4 glycogenosis), vacuoles are located mainly in type 1 fibers and contain periodic acid-Schiff-staining material that is diastase resistant. Electron microscopy shows normal glycogen and abnormal filamentous material, corresponding to unbranched, amylopectin-like glycogen.

Debranching Enzyme Deficiency. In debranching enzyme deficiency (type 3 glycogenosis), there are deposits of glycogen in liver, striated muscle, and to a lesser extent, in cardiac muscle. Biochemical studies show the absence of debranching enzyme in muscle and liver.

Mitochondrial Myopathies and Cytopathies

These are a complex group of neuromuscular and other disorders associated with respiratory chain dysfunction. The clinical presentation is heterogeneous, depending on extension of the disease (only muscular involvement or multisystemic disorders, involving the muscle, brain, heart, kidney, and liver), age of onset (from infancy to late adulthood), severity, and evolution. Muscle biopsy provides useful diagnostic clues in most cases. On routine histologic stains, the fibers are disrupted by accumulation of mitochondria, appearing as purplish blotches on Gomori's trichrome stain (ragged red fibers) and as dark red-staining material with hematoxylin and eosin. With oxidative reactions, increased enzyme activity (corresponding to mitochondrial aggregates), usually subsarcolemmal in distribution, is found (Fig. 8-1E). The number of abnormal fibers is usually higher with oxidative techniques than with routine stains. Excessive lipid and glycogen on the corresponding stains are also demonstrated in the abnormal fibers.

When examined by electron microscopy, the following changes are found: large aggregates of mitochondria under the sarcolemma or less frequently between myofibrils and structural modifications of mitochondria with enlargement and elongation, increase or conversely paucity of cristae, and presence of crystalline inclusions and osmiophilic globular bodies.

Ragged red fibers are present in most mitochondrial disorders, namely, in chronic progressive external ophthalmoplegia, Kearns-Sayre syndrome, associating juvenile chronic progressive external ophthalmoplegia, pigmentary retinopathy, and heart block, and in other well-characterized encephalopathies such as mitochondrial encephalomyopathy with lactic acidosis and strokelike episodes (MELAS) and myoclonus epilepsy and ragged red fibers (MERRF). However, ragged red fibers may be absent in other respiratory chain disorders such as infantile mitochondrial myopathies, Leigh's encephalopathy, or Leber's hereditary optic neuropathy. Lipid storage myopathy and ultrastructural evidence of abnormal mitochondria are often present, particularly in infantile cases. However, mitochondrial abnormalities are nonspecific lesions. In old patients, some ragged red fibers are common and not significant. They have also been occasionally found in Duchenne's muscular dystrophy, myotonic dystrophy, neurogenic atrophy, and inflammatory myopathies.

If a mitochondriopathy is suspected, further investigations should be performed on the muscle sample. A deficient activity of cytochrome oxidase, corresponding to the fourth complex of the respiratory chain, may be shown by a simple histochemical reaction in most mitochondrial disorders. A parcellar defect with presence of cytochrome oxidase-negative fibers is found in all cases in which ragged red fibers are present, whatever the primary respiratory defect. Most ragged red fibers are cytochrome oxidase nega-

tive. In addition, apparently normal fibers are deficient in this enzyme, helping in the diagnosis of mitochondriopathy when mitochondrial accumulation is mild. The absence of cytochrome oxidase staining in all fibers is found in infantile mitochondrial myopathies. In this group, cytochrome oxidase deficiency, confirmed by biochemical techniques, is the primary molecular defect. Infantile forms of such a deficiency may be lethal or benign. In the latter, muscle cytochrome oxidase activity, initially negligible, is progressively expressed, in parallel with clinical improvement, which indicates a replacement of a fetal defective subunit of cytochrome oxidase by an adult isoform.

Polarographic and enzymatic studies may be performed to specify the affected complex of the respiratory chain. Finally, the detection of a mutation of mitochondrial DNA in muscle is very useful; single deletions are found in all cases of Kearns-Sayre syndrome and in one-half of chronic progressive external ophthalmoplegia, and various characteristic point mutations are evidenced in MELAS, MERRF, and Leber's disease, certifying the diagnosis.

Disorders of Lipid Metabolism

Muscle biopsy is an important step in the diagnosis of lipid metabolism disorders, especially those involving carnitine metabolism. This metabolite has two main functions: (1) transport into the mitochondria of long-chain fatty acids, coupled to carnitine by carnitine palmityltransferase, and (2) modulation of the intramitochondrial coenzyme A/acyl-coenzyme A ratio, depending on intramitochondrial metabolic pathways, mainly β-oxidation and respiratory chain.

Carnitine Palmityltransferase Deficiency. This is the main cause of metabolic myoglobinuria in humans. Rhabdomyolysis is triggered by fasting and prolonged exercise. Muscle biopsy in interictal periods is usually normal, in contrast with data in phosphorylase deficiency, an alternative diagnosis. If present, lipid accumulation is usually mild. Necrotic fiber and regeneration indicate recent myoglobinuria. Carnitine palmityltransferase activity is decreased in muscle, leukocytes, and fibroblasts.

Carnitine Deficiency. This affects mainly children, and is characterized by various signs and symptoms: muscle weakness and fatigue and cardiomyopathy or recurrent metabolic crises in systemic deficiency. Whether primary, as a result of a defective transport of the molecule from the serum into muscle and other tissues, or secondary because of defects of β-oxidation, respiratory chain or intermediary metabolism, or renal disorders, the main pathologic hallmark is massive muscle triglyceride storage. It is readily revealed by the presence of numerous lipid droplets, located mainly in type 1 fiber and stained by oil red O or Sudan black techniques. Under the electron microscope, the lipid droplets appear as empty round spaces, without limiting membranes. Low levels of carnitine are found in the muscle only (myopathic form) and also in the liver and serum (systemic form).

Periodic Paralysis

This group of autosomal dominant disorders is characterized by recurrent bouts of paralysis, which are relapsing and remitting. The serum potassium level during attacks may be low (hypokalemic periodic paralysis), high (hyperkalemic periodic paralysis), or normal.

Histologic features are similar in the hyperkalemic and hypokalemic forms. In recent-onset cases, muscle biopsy may show no pathologic abnormality, even at the ultrastructural level. A vacuolar myopathy is readily found in patients with a long duration of disease and persistent weakness during attacks. The vacuole is often central and unique and usually reacts for acid phosphatase, which suggests a lysosomal characteristic. Collections of tubular aggregates are also found in type 2B fibers only, reacting intensively with nicotinamide adenine dinucleotide-tetrazolium reductase but not with succinic dehydrogenase (contrary to the case in mitochondrial accumulation) or with adenosine triphosphatase. Electron microscopic studies show that vacuoles arise from local dilation of the T tubules and sarcoplasmic reticular vesicles.

Malignant Hyperthermia

In this syndrome, which is characterized by severe hyperthermia, muscle rigidity, metabolic acidosis, and myoglobinuria, cases are provoked by general anesthesia with halothane and succinylcholine. Histologic changes seen by light and electron microscopy are nonspecific in primary malignant hyperthermia transmitted as an autosomal dominant trait. If present, central cores indicate a central core disease, which may be asymptomatic (the mutation concerns the ryanodine receptor, a gene also involved in primary malignant hyperthermia). Other muscle diseases, such as Duchenne's muscular dystrophy and myotonia congenita, may also be associated with malignant hyperthermia. Susceptibility to malignant hyperthermia can be reliably detected by an in vitro provocative test, which assays contraction of excised strips of muscle in the presence of halothane and caffeine.

Endocrine Myopathies

Muscle is involved in several endocrine disorders that affect the function of thyroid, parathyroid, adrenal, and pituitary glands. Muscle biopsy abnormalities are usually mild and do not give further clues to the underlying cause. This is in contrast with the patient's signs, particularly weakness. Type 2 fiber atrophy is the most consistent change in the muscle biopsy specimen, particularly in hypercorticism.

Toxic and Nutritional Myopathies

Muscle lesions are not specific, with the exception of some drug-induced myopathies. Alcoholic myopathy may present acutely, with multifocal rhabdomyolysis, or may be more a chronic disorder, with type 2 fiber atrophy, and often, a denervation pattern. In diabetes mellitus, denervation atrophy or focal necrosis, indicating muscle infarcts, can be found. Microvasculitis can be found. Hyalinosis of small vessels is a nearly constant finding. Various types of amyloidosis can also be associated with deposits in the muscle, which usually affect vessel walls.

Drug-Induced Myopathies

Cholesterol-lowering agents (clofibrate and 3-hydroxy-3-methylglutaryl coenzyme A reductase inhibitors) induce acute/subacute painful myopathy with necrosis and regeneration and sometimes an inflammatory reaction. Necrotizing myopathy is also associated with aminocaproic acid, emetine, heroin, and vincristine. In the latter case, a denervation is also present. Penicillamine, procainamide, phenytoin, and hydralazine may induce inflammatory myositis. Eosinophilic myositis and fasciitis has been reported in patients taking the amino acid L-tryptophan. A mitochondrial myopathy, characterized by numerous ragged red fibers has been described in patients treated with zidovudine for human immunodeficiency virus (HIV) infection. A vacuolar myopathy secondary to autophagic degeneration of muscle is associated with long-standing administration of chloroquine; denervation changes may also be found. Amiodarone, perhexiline, vincristine, and colchicine are also known to cause autophagic myopathy or nerve and muscle involvement (neuromyopathy). In hypokalemic myopathy, which affects patients treated with diuretics, amphotericin B, licorice, or purgatives, vacuolation is present in association with fiber necrosis and regeneration. Besides the classic chronic steroid myopathy characterized by type 2 fiber atrophy, a more acute and severe myopathy has been reported in patients treated for status asthmaticus by high doses of corticosteroids and pancuronium. Biopsy in this latter instance showed regenerating and occasional necrotic fibers and widespread atrophy of muscle fibers. Ultrastructurally, there is disorganization of myofibrils and selective loss of thick (myosin) filaments. Immunohistologic stains for myosin isoforms confirm the decrease or absence of this protein.

Inflammatory Myopathies

These are a heterogeneous group of acquired myopathies. They can be due to known infection or to immunopathologic mechanisms, sometimes autoimmune, of still obscure origin. From a pathologic point of view, they can be divided into two groups. First, there are disorders that affect mainly (primarily?) the muscle fibers, with various degrees of necrosis ("necrotic fibers") and regeneration ("basophilic fibers"). These are associated with mononuclear cells infiltrates and sometimes with a striking perifascicular atrophy. Second, there are muscular manifestations of systemic diseases. The inflammatory lesions are seen mainly in the interstitial tissue (connective tissue, including vessels). They may be specific. In contrast, muscle fibers are less affected. In some cases, focal lesions of necrosis and regeneration may indicate infarcts from arterial occlusion. Microorganism-induced myositis is a rare disorder. Muscle lesions may belong to one or the other group of inflammatory myopathies.

Viruses

Usually, a nonspecific myositis, or rhabdomyolysis, is associated with infections by coxsackieviruses, influenza viruses (responsible for most cases of virologically studied "benign acute childhood myositis"), and some arboviruses. In HIV infection, when systematically looked for, it is frequent to find isolated perivascular cuffs (i.e., mononuclear cell infiltrates surrounding vessels of the microcirculation, such as arteries of less than 70 μm in diameter, capillaries, and venules) or genuine vasculitis, involving the walls of these vessels ("microvasculitis") without muscle necrosis or regeneration, especially in the early stages of viral infection. Iron pigment deposits are also found. These lesions are often associated with denervation atrophy. Rare cases of HIV-1-induced inflammatory myopathies with interstitial inflammatory cell infiltrates, microvasculitis, and necrotic-regenerative lesions of muscle fibers have been reported. They strongly resemble polymyositis. No HIV particles have been found, but HIV antigen gp41 has been identified in muscle macrophages in a few cases.

These disorders are difficult to distinguish from zidovudine-associated myopathies, which seem to be more frequent. In the latter, characteristic ragged red fibers are more often seen. This might be due to the toxic effect of the drug. Acquired nemaline myopathy has also been described.

Human T-cell lymphotropic virus type 1 (sometimes associated with HIV) has also been found by immunohistochemical tests or in situ hybridization in a few cases of mild inflammatory myopathies in which major histocompatibility class I determinants are expressed. In addition, cytomegalovirus has been shown by in situ hybridization in rare cases of acquired immunodeficiency syndrome neuropathies with vasculitides (see Ch. 49).

Bacterial Myositis

Bacterial forms of myositis are uncommon today in industrialized countries but still frequent in developing countries (see Ch. 39) Pyomyositis, also referred to as "tropical myositis," is mainly due to *Staphylococcus aureus*. It usually affects a single large muscle. Cell infiltrates made of mononuclear cells, followed by polymorphonuclear cells, are later associated with necrosis of muscle fibers and abscess formation. Tuberculous myositis is exceedingly rare and may be related to local extension from a tuberculous focus or to miliary tuberculosis (see Ch. 46).

Parasites and Fungi

Trichinosis (caused by ingestion of inadequately cooked meat containing *Trichinella spiralis*) is the most frequent parasitic disease of the muscle. Encysted larvae may be found on muscle biopsy. *Taenia solium* cysticerci, Echinococcus cysts, *Toxocara canis* larvae, a number of other parasites, and some fungi may be rarely found in muscle biopsy (see Chs. 40 and 43). They must be suspected when focal inflammatory infiltrates, sometimes containing multinucleated cells or calcified debris, are seen. In patients with acquired immunodeficiency syndrome, *Toxoplasma gondii* is occasionally found, sometimes without any inflammatory infiltrate (see Ch. 49).

Idiopathic Inflammatory Myopathies

Polymyositis. This is a primary muscle disease that appears to be due to a T8 cytotoxic process restricted to those muscle fibers that express class I histocompatibility antigens. The muscle biopsy specimen may be normal but usually shows scattered necrotic fibers and basophilic fibers, evenly distributed. Some non-necrotic muscle fibers are sometimes invaded by mononuclear cells that can have a characteristic central distribution. Isolated or small groups of atrophic fibers, sometimes containing central nuclei, are often seen and could suggest denervation. Inflammatory mononuclear infiltrates, principally made of CD8-positive lymphocytes and monocytes, are present in the endomysium, sometimes near necrotic fibers and in septa. The number of capillaries is usually normal. In subacute and chronic cases, enlarged ("hypertrophic") and split fibers are seen. Mononuclear infiltrates are sparse and may be lacking in some cases. There is a conspicuous interstitial fibrosis. No indication for a viral cause of polymyositis has been found. The differential diagnosis of subacute and chronic cases includes muscle dystrophies. In contrast, in acute cases, confusion may arise with rhabdomyolysis or with other idiopathic inflammatory myopathies. Systemic malignancy is not usually associated with polymyositis.

Inclusion Body Myositis. In the rarer inclusion body myositis, a similar autoimmune mechanism seems to be present. Muscle biopsy shows necrosis, regeneration, and mild inflammation, which may lead to the diagnosis of polymyositis. Partial invasion of non-necrotic fibers by CD8 + lymphocytes and macrophages may be present. In addition, angular fibers, often grouped, could evoke denervation. Rimmed cytoplasmic vacuoles of various shapes and sizes, which contain basophilic granules, are seen on hematoxylin and eosin-stained sections. However, they are seldom acid phosphatase positive and contain β-amyloid peptide and hyperphosphorylated τ protein. A red ovoid more specific inclusion of 5 to 6 μm is sometimes present among these granules. Although characteristic, rimmed vacuoles are not pathognomonic for inclusion body myositis. They can be found in cramp syndrome, in reducing body myopathy, in periodic paralysis, and in acid maltase deficiency. In addition, in inclusion body myositis, there are eosinophilic cytoplasmic and nuclear inclusions. By electron microscopy, they are made of characteristic microtubular structures 15 to 18 nm in diameter, resembling the nucleocapsids of paramyxoviruses, and antigens of mumps virus have been demonstrated by immunohistochemical tests. No definite proof of the viral nature of this disease has however been found. Although the clinical spectrum of inclusion body myositis is not determined, malignancy is not usually associated.

Dermatomyositis. This is a primarily vascular autoimmune disease with a predominant humoral mechanism. Muscle biopsy shows prominent perifascicular lesions. Fiber atrophy is the most frequent. Various degenerative, necrotic, and regenerative aspects of muscle fibers and disappearance or necrosis of capillaries are also possible. There are microvascular deposits of the C5b-9 complement membrane attack complex. Rare necrotic and basophilic fibers, single or grouped into disseminated microinfarcts, are found in the center of fascicles. However, fairly uniform involvement of some fascicles is also found. Inflammatory mononuclear cell infiltrates, which may be lacking, predominate in the interfascicular regions. They are made of a mixture of CD4, CD8, and B cells. By electron microscopy, tubuloreticular structures such as those seen in systemic lupus erythematosus are detected in endothelial cells, lymphocytes, and macrophages. No virus particles, viral epitopes or genoma fractions have been found. Inflammatory myopathy, which may accompany other connective tissue disease,

shows all the features of dermatomyositis. The differential diagnosis includes microvasculitis, nodular focal myositis (isolated perivascular cuffs seen in connective tissue disease, especially in rheumatoid arthritis and in myasthenia gravis), and especially, acute denervation of the muscle (which may induce focal necrosis of muscle fibers and microvasculitis). Systemic malignancy is associated with dermatomyositis in about 15 percent of adults.

Necrotizing Myopathy With Pipestem Capillaries. Microvascular deposition of complement attack complex and minimal cellular infiltration has been more recently described. Thickened fibrous capillaries with deposits of amorphous material and thickening of basal lamina, and decrease in capillary density, are characteristic of this disorder. This immune-mediated microangiopathy may be associated with carcinoma.

Sarcoidosis. This is characterized by focal interstitial granulomas consisting of epithelioid and a few giant cells surrounded by a crown of mononuclear cells, without caseation. Muscle sarcoidosis may be found in the absence of any neuromuscular symptoms. Similar changes have been found in patients who lack any other localization of sarcoidosis ("granulomatous myositis," which may be an unusual form of polymyositis). The differential diagnosis of muscle sarcoidosis includes needle myopathy because regenerative basophilic muscle cells may be mistaken for the giant cells of sarcoid granuloma and the localized granulomas after injections and parasites, especially trichinosis, more often than the exceedingly rare tuberculous or leprosy granulomas.

Localized Nodular Myopathy. The biopsy specimen of a localized nodular myopathy may show polymyositis-like lesions, with sometimes prominent muscle necrosis or vasculitis, inflammatory pseudotumor, or proliferative pseudosarcomatous myositis. This rare benign condition is probably a self-limiting disorder. Its mechanism remains obscure.

Eosinophilic Fasciitis. In eosinophilic fasciitis (Shulman's syndrome), sclerosis and inflammatory cell infiltrates (mainly mononuclear and containing sometimes polymorphonuclear cells, with a few eosinophils) are present in the subcutaneous fascia and may involve the muscle interstitium and the deep dermis. In some cases, sclerosis is very conspicuous (see Ch. 33).

Eosinophilic Myositis. This is characterized by an inflammatory cell infiltrate containing eosinophilic leukocytes, contrasting usually with little necrosis of the muscle fibers. This may be due to a variety of causes, including parasitic and systemic diseases and the myalgia-eosinophilia syndrome caused by L-tryptophan consumption. Rare cases of focal myositis have an eosinophilic cell infiltrate (see Ch. 33).

Vasculitic Syndromes

Vasculitic syndromes bear in common inflammation, and sometimes necrosis, of blood vessel walls. Vascular lesions are described below with nerve biopsy. Vasculitis involving large arteries (i.e., more than 70 μm in diameter when measured in a noninvolved area) is usually associated with polyarteritis nodosa or related disorders. Microvasculitis involving the microcirculation (small arteries, capillaries, and venules) is a frequent finding in muscle biopsy. The genuine leukocytoclastic vasculitis is rare, and it must be distinguished from acute lesions induced by clamping small vessels, namely polymorphonuclear leukocyte margination and crossing of vascular walls. When abundant, lymphocytic microvasculitis is called focal interstitial myositis. It must be considered a pathologic lesion, although with little specificity. This is especially true when it is found near necrotic or basophilic fibers. When in the connective tissue surrounding the muscle fascicles, it has a better diagnostic value and may be seen in any connective disease, including Gougerot-Sjögren disease; polymyalgia rheumatica; and particularly, rheumatoid arthritis, malignant disease (especially lymphomas, where it may be present long before the clinical diagnosis), mixed essential cryoglobulinemia, myasthenia gravis, and acquired immunodeficiency syndrome. It can also be seen in acute denervation atrophy. Selective type 2 fiber atrophy, denervation atrophy, and seldom muscle infarcts can be found in isolation or associated with the lesions of the vessels. It may be added that an inflammatory myopathy of varying severity can be found in hypersensitivity to drugs. Phenytoin and other antiepileptic drugs have been repeatedly considered responsible for inflammatory infiltrates in skeletal muscle (see Ch. 38).

Myasthenia Gravis

Ultrastructural studies of the neuromuscular junction have contributed highly to the understanding of the pathophysiology of this disease. The main data are the following: simplified postsynaptic regions, decreased amount of acetylcholine receptors, and deposits of immunoglobin G and complement attack complex. In most cases of myasthenia gravis, routine muscle biopsy has no place in the diagnosis. The histologic alterations are mild and nonspecific (presence of some sparse atrophic types 1 and 2 fibers or a more diffuse type 2 fiber atrophy), and other data support the diagnosis, such as the edrophonium test, electrophysiologic studies showing a decrement in muscle function, and the presence of antiacetylcholine receptor antibodies. However, in some patients, the diagnosis is more difficult because of the absence of such antibodies, an electromyographic decrement, and no clinical fluctuations. In these cases, particularly in primarily ophthalmoplegic forms of myasthenia gravis, muscle biopsy contributes by ruling out mitochondrial myopathy or oculopharyngeal dystrophy.

Meaning of Mild Nonspecific Changes

These have to be interpreted in the clinical context. Age, exercise, or lack of use of the muscle can be associated with muscular changes. In elderly patients, a type 2 fiber atrophy, presence of moth-eaten fibers, or a mild denervation can be observed. After lack of use, a type 2 atrophy is seen, whereas, in active patients, a type 2 hypertrophy is common. Mild changes, such as mild irregularity in fiber diameter, a mild increased amount of central nuclei, and rare isolated necrotic fibers, are not specific and have to be linked to the clinical data.

Meaning of a Normal Biopsy

Normal biopsy results can be due to inadequate sampling (distal muscles can be normal in inflammatory myopathy) or to early (in denervation) or late (in rhabdomyolysis) biopsies. In some genuine muscle pathologic conditions, such as myasthenia gravis, the muscle can be normal or show only mild nonspecific changes.

MAIN FINDINGS ON NERVE BIOPSY

Normal Nerve

The normal nerve consists of myelinated fibers, with each of them being made up of an axon ensheathed by a compacted rolled-up process from the membranes of an individual chain of Schwann cells (the myelin sheath), of nonmyelinated axons lying recessed within a separate cleft in the surface of cords of other Schwann cells, and of connective tissue, also named interstitial tissue or interstitium. This includes the following (Fig. 8-5).

1. The endoneurium, which directly surrounds the myelinated fibers, unmyelinated axons, and Schwann cells, and includes some fibrocytes, rare mastocytes, and a few small blood vessels from the microcirculation.
2. The perineurium, which ensheathes each nerve fascicle and is made of several layers of compactly arranged flattened cells. The cells have basement membranes and are linked by tight junctions.
3. The epineurium, which encases each fascicle, extending to the common connective tissue surrounding the nerve and adjacent vessels. These consist of the main artery of the nerve, which reaches usually a diameter of 100 to 200 μm.

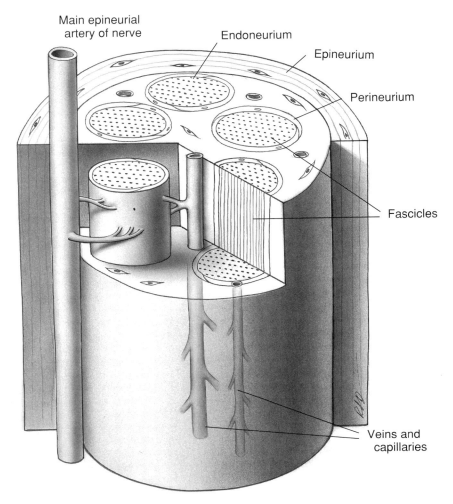

Main epineurial
artery of nerve

Endoneurium

Epineurium

Perineurium

Fascicles

Veins and
capillaries

Figure 8-5. Diagram of the different compartments, and of the blood supply, of a nerve. (Modified from Dyck, 1967, with permission.)

These elements should be systematically analyzed when a nerve biopsy specimen is examined. Myelinated fibers are first assessed on cross sections of paraffin- and/or epoxy-embedded fragments. Their overall number and the density of each class of fibers; the distribution of small and large fibers; the thickness of myelin sheaths by comparison with the diameter of its axon; and the presence of ovoids of degenerating axons and associated myelin, tomacula (focal enlargements of myelin sheaths), giant axons, and associated Schwann cell proliferation grouping into Büngner's bands or onion bulbs are noted. When lesions of myelinated fibers are seen or suspected, teased nerve fibers preparations are used. They show at best the main pathologic processes affecting the nerve (Fig. 8-6), that is, axonal (or wallerian) degeneration (Fig. 8-7) and segmental demyelination (Fig. 8-8).

The length of internodes (i.e., segments of myelin between two nodes of Ranvier and depending on the same Schwann cell), the thickness of the fibers, and the irregularities of myelin sheaths allow recognition of the following processes: axonal degeneration (myelin ovoids and spheres), regeneration after axonal degeneration (short regular internodes), segmental demyelination (paranodal or internodal), or remyelination after segmental demyelination (excessive variability of myelin thickness and short irregular internodes, (Fig. 8-9). The morphometry of cross sections of epoxy-embedded fragments or of teased nerve fibers preparations may be indicated.

Schematically, the following points must be ascertained by the study of myelinated fibers. Is the neuropathy caused primarily by axonal or Schwann cell lesions? If axonal, are the large myelinated fibers or the small ones selectively involved? Are there indications for regeneration or for a specific diagnosis? This

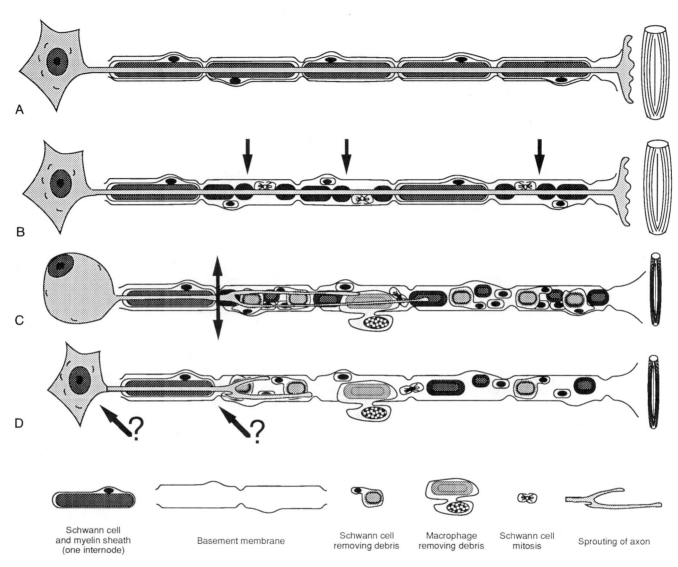

Schwann cell
and myelin sheath
(one internode)

Basement membrane

Schwann cell
removing debris

Macrophage
removing debris

Schwann cell
mitosis

Sprouting of axon

Figure 8-6. Diagram of the main processes affecting peripheral nerves. (**A**) Normal myelinated fiber; regular internodes of the same length and thickness are seen. (**B**) In segmental demyelination, there is patchy damage (*arrows*) of individual Schwann cells and/or myelin sheaths. The neuronal cell body is not affected; there is no denervation atrophy. (**C**) In wallerian degeneration, the section (*arrow*) of the axon causes central chromatolysis of the nerve cell body and denervation atrophy of the muscle. (**D**) In dying-back neuropathy, axonal breakdown may be due to a pathologic condition of the nerve cell body or axon (*arrows with question marks*). There is denervation atrophy of the muscle, and usually no central chromatolysis. (Modified from Bradley, 1974, with permission.)

is best seen on paraffin-embedded sections of formaldehyde-fixed fragments cut either in cross or in longitudinal sections. They allow a thorough study of connective tissue that can show vasculitis, inflammatory or tumor cell infiltrations, or abnormal deposits and may thus indicate the cause of the neuropathy.

Other studies include electron microscopy, which allows the morphometry of nonmyelinated fibers to be ascertained the study of myelin and storage disorders, immunohistochemical tests for identification of cell in-

filtrates and various deposits, in situ hybridization, biochemical tests, including the polymerase chain reaction, and cell cultures.

Primary Involvement of Axons and Nerve Cell Bodies

Main Axonopathies

Destruction of axons causes a concomitant degeneration of the myelin, but this does not destroy the basement membrane that outlines the myelinated fiber at the external surface of the Schwann cell.

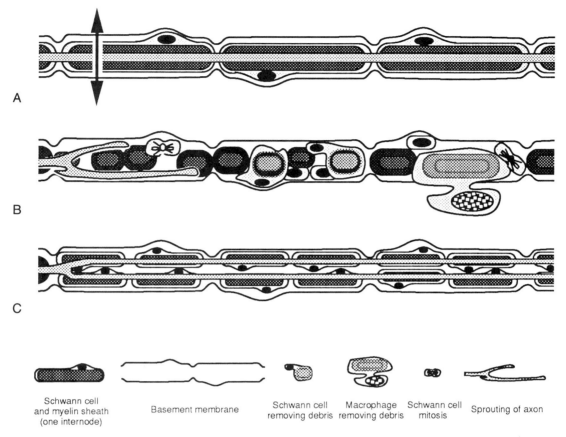

Schwann cell
and myelin sheath
(one internode)

Basement membrane

Schwann cell
removing debris

Macrophage
removing debris

Schwann cell
mitosis

Sprouting of axon

Figure 8-7. Diagrammatic representation of the course of wallerian degeneration and regeneration. **(A)** Axonal section in a normal myelinated fiber. **(B)** Distal degeneration of axons and myelin, removal of debris by Schwann cells and macrophages, proliferation of Schwann cells within the basement membrane of the previous myelinated fiber (called Büngner's bands), and sprouting of proximal portion of axon. **(C)** Regeneration of two small myelinated fibers with short internodes into the basement membrane of the previous myelinated fiber; clusters (or fascicles) of regeneration. (Modified from Poirier et al., 1990, with permission.)

Wallerian Degeneration. This is the degeneration of axon and myelin sheaths distal to the axonal section. It is followed by a fast proliferation of distal Schwann cells, which remain inside the basement membrane of the same nerve fiber, constituting Büngner's bands. Small nerve buds sprout from the injured axon at, and proximal to, the section level. These numerous small regenerating axons grow distally into the Büngner's bands and produce clusters of closely apposed small fibers, some of which become myelinated, the so-called fascicles of regeneration of Nageotte (Fig. 8-7).

Dying-Back Neuropathy. This is a slow distal axonopathy involving first the longest fibers, which are also the largest ones. Its mechanism is not fully understood. Dysmetabolism of the perikaryon, disturbances of axonal transport, lack of distal growth factors, and action of toxic factors have been suggested. Axonal

degeneration occurs concomitantly in the central processes (posterior columns of the spinal cord) and the peripheral processes of sensory neurons. In this slowly evolving processes, axonal degeneration and regeneration (distal and collateral sprouting) are similar to, although milder than, that seen in wallerian degeneration.

Neuronopathy. This is a more rapidly evolving neuronal death in which the perikaryon and its neurites degenerate simultaneously. There is often a selective vulnerability of, for instance, the small or the large neurons of the spinal root ganglia. The mechanisms of neuronopathy and the cause of the selective involvement of some neuronal populations remain unclear.

Other lesions of the axon include axonal atrophy and axonal swelling. Axonal atrophy is seen mainly in large fibers and is best shown by morphometry. The

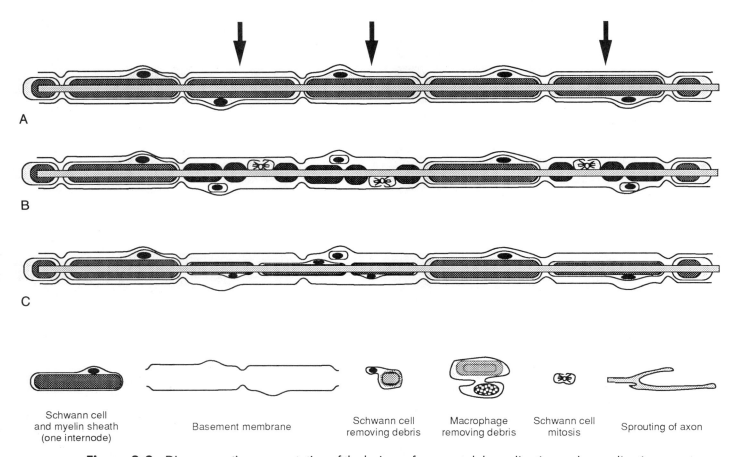

Schwann cell
and myelin sheath
(one internode)

Basement membrane

Schwann cell
removing debris

Macrophage
removing debris

Schwann cell
mitosis

Sprouting of axon

Figure 8-8. Diagrammatic representation of the lesions of segmental demyelination and remyelination. (**A**) Destruction of scattered Schwann cells and/or myelin internodes (*arrows*) along the myelinated fiber, with axon sparing. (**B**) Degeneration of myelin, removal of debris by Schwann cells and macrophages, proliferation of Schwann cells within the basement membrane of the previous myelinated fiber. (**C**) Remyelination of involved internodes leads to myelinated fibers with internodes of irregular lengths and thickness. (Modified from Poirier et al., 1990, with permission.)

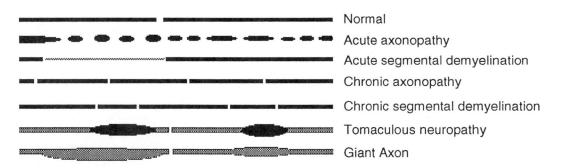

Normal

Acute axonopathy

Acute segmental demyelination

Chronic axonopathy

Chronic segmental demyelination

Tomaculous neuropathy

Giant Axon

Figure 8-9. Schematic diagram of the main lesions seen on teased nerve fibers preparations. (From Ratinahirana and Hauw, 1992, with permission.)

axonal diameter is lower than it should be in myelinated fibers of the same diameter range. This is often due to abnormalities in neurofilament synthesis. Axonal atrophy may be associated with secondary demyelination, which may be severe. Axonal swelling results from focal accumulation of neurofilaments as a consequence of abnormalities of the slow axonal transport. In proximal axonopathies, axonal swelling is seen initially in proximal axons. Axonal atrophy or degeneration occurs distally.

Biopsy Findings

Acute (or Recent) Axonal Involvement. This is indicated by ovoids and balls of degenerating axons and myelin. They are best seen on teased fibers preparations but can also be found on longitudinal sections, and even cross sections, of nerves. They must be distinguished from crush artifacts, often seen on a border of the section, and the rare tomacula and axonal swellings. Axonal sprouting of myelinated fibers is easily seen in semithin cross sections and in teased nerve fiber preparations, which show thin fibers with short regular internodes. Morphometric studies may show a higher density of myelinated fibers than normal and reveal a shift to the left of the distribution of the diameters of myelinated fibers. Büngner's bands made up by Schwann cell proliferation are usually easy to recognize. Myelin retraction on both sides of nodes of Ranvier, which indicates recent axonal degeneration, is best shown on teased fiber preparations. Chronic axonal involvement is indicated by rarefaction of nerve fibers, hypertrophy, and sometimes proliferation of Schwann cells and fibrocytes and increase in their density. Clusters of regeneration may still be seen on semithin cross sections (see Fig. 8-11B), and thin regenerative fibers are a usual finding on teased fiber preparations. Morphometric studies may indicate axonal atrophy.

Main Disorders

Most degenerative, metabolic, malignancy-associated, and toxic neuropathies are axonal in type. In addition, interstitial neuropathies induce distal axonal degeneration. Many axonopathies involve mainly the large myelinated fibers. When small myelinated fibers and amyelinated axons are preferentially involved, amyloidosis, leprosy, diabetes mellitus, acquired immunodeficiency syndrome, and Fabry's and Tangier diseases must be evoked. These are only indications, and in advanced stages of any neuropathy, no selective involvement of nerve fiber type is found.

Primary Schwann Cell-Myelin Involvement

Myelin degeneration occurs with sparing (at least relatively) of axons and of the external basal lamina that outlines the external surface of the Schwann cell.

Acute (or Recent) Segmental Demyelination and Remyelination

Destruction of normal (or apparently normal) myelin involves scattered internodes along the myelinated fiber. It usually begins in the paranodal region. When this occurs on a few scattered internodes, their remyelination may be performed by their own Schwann cells after phagocytosis of the degenerated myelin by Schwann cells and monocyte-macrophages. This leads to a thin internode of normal length. If proliferated Schwann cells remyelinate longer segments of demyelinated axons, this leads to internodes of irregular lengths and thickness. When severe, such lesions can be recognized on transverse semithin sections; numerous abnormally thin (compared with the diameter of the fiber) myelin sheaths are present. Morphometric study of the "g" factor (internal diameter/external diameter of myelinated fibers) may be helpful in milder lesions. Teased nerve fiber preparations provide the best data, however, and allow easy quantitation of the proportion of fibers affected by demyelination-remyelination and axonal degeneration.

Chronic Segmental Demyelination and Remyelination

This induces Schwann cell proliferation around the intact axon and leads to a concentric arrangement of Schwann cells and basement membranes called "onion bulbs" (Fig. 8-10). There is frequently an increase of the noncellular component in the endoneurium (collagen and proteoglycans). Onion bulbs can be seen on teased nerve fibers preparations. The lesions are best recognized on transverse paraffin-embedded fragments or semithin sections (Fig. 8-11C). The most serious diagnostic difficulty on biopsy arises from onion bulbs caused by proliferated perineural cells ("perilemumas"), which are seen in the exceedingly rare localized hypertrophic neuropathies (Fig. 8-11D). Mild onion bulbs must be confirmed by electron microscopy, however, for they may be difficult to distinguish from regenerating clusters of fibers containing a small myelinating axon.

Major Myelinopathies

Acute (or Recent) Segmental Demyelination and Remyelination

Inflammatory Demyelinating Neuropathies. These are the main acquired demyelinating neuropathies and include Guillain-Barré and Fisher's syndromes and those similar disorders that occur in the course of infection by HIV, cytomegalovirus, hepatitis virus, and other viruses. On distal biopsy samples, the mononuclear cell infiltrates of the endoneurium, sometimes grouped around small vessels, or in their walls (microvasculitis) are less conspicuous in idio-

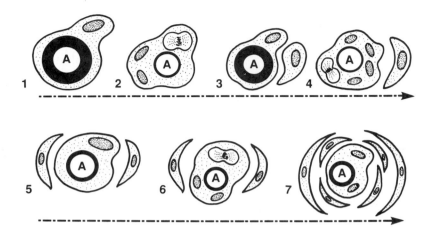

Figure 8-10. Schematic diagram of the segmental demyelination and remyelination processes leading to Schwann cell proliferation and onion bulb formation in hypertrophic neuropathy (*A,* axon). (*1*) Transverse section of a myelinated fiber. (*2*) Demyelination, phagocytosis of myelin debris by the Schwann cell, and mitosis of the Schwann cell. (*3*) Remyelination of the axon. (*4*) Demyelination, phagocytosis of myelin debris by the Schwann cell, and mitosis of the Schwann cell. (*5*) Remyelination. (*6*) Demyelination, phagocytosis of myelin debris by the Schwann cell, and mitosis of the Schwann cell. (*7*) Onion bulb. (Modified from Bradley, 1974, with permission.)

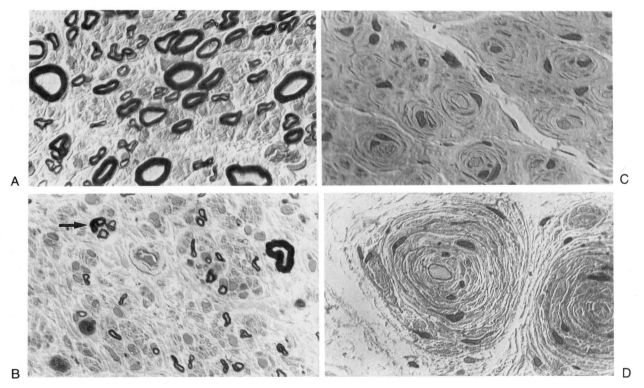

Figure 8-11. (**A**) Normal nerve. Semithin cross section. (Toluidine blue, Nomarski's optics, ×260.) (**B**) Chronic axonal involvement indicated by rarefaction of nerve fibers and proliferation of Schwann cells and fibrocytes. A cluster of regeneration composed of small-diameter myelinated fibers is seen in the upper left (*arrow*). (Toluidine blue, Nomarski's optics, ×260.) (**C**) Hypertrophic neuropathy with onion bulb formation indicating chronic segmental demyelination and remyelination. Hypertrophic form of Charcot-Marie-Tooth disease (HSMN type 1). (Toluidine blue, Nomarski's optics, ×260.) (**D**) Onion bulbs caused by proliferated perineural cells that are seen in the very rare localized hypertrophic neuropathies ("perilemnomas"). (Paraphenylene-diamine, Nomarski's optics, ×650.)

pathic disorders than in HIV infection, in which they predominate in the early stages of the disease. Electron microscopy shows macrophages surrounding and phagocytizing myelin sheaths. Some degree of axonal degeneration may be associated, which may be prominent in certain cases of Guillain-Barré disease (especially in the chronic forms) and in many cases of HIV- and cytomegalovirus associated inflammatory neuropathies.

Neuropathies Associated With Dysglobulinemia. These are often of the demyelinating type. This is especially the case for immunoglobulin M-linked polyneuropathy, associated more frequently with benign gammopathies than is Waldenström's disease. Direct immunofluorescence shows specific localization of heavy and light chains of the abnormal immunoglobulin on the myelin sheaths. In addition, some major dense lines of the myelin sheaths are frequently enlarged by electron microscopy. In the POEMS (polyneuropathy, organomegaly, endocrinopathy, monoclonal gammopathy, and skin changes) syndrome, neuropathy, uncompacted myelin, or loose myelin is found. Demyelination seems secondary to axonal atrophy.

Hereditary Neuropathy With Liability to Pressure Palsies. This features sausage-like ("tomaculous") changes of myelinated fibers. They are due to focal hypermyelination by an increase in the number of myelin lamellae, sometimes due to foldings and reversals in the direction of the myelin spiral. It is sometimes associated with demyelination or hypomyelination. Tomacula must be numerous (more than 20 percent of fibers are usually affected on teased fiber preparations) to make the diagnosis because a few tomacula are a nonspecific feature.

Toxic Demyelinating Neuropathies. These are rare and are associated with a characteristic drug-induced lipidosis best seen by electron microscopy. In the side effects of perhexiline maleate, the demyelinating and axonal neuropathy is associated with a sphingomyelinase deficit. Amiodarone induces a rare axonal and demyelinating neuropathy. The neuropathy of chloroquine-linked neuromyopathy is predominantly axonal.

Hereditary Demyelinating Neuropathies. These can be shown on biopsy specimens in recent segmental demyelination and remyelination. This is especially the cases in hypertrophic neuropathies (see below). Childhood leukodystrophies, sulfatidosis (arylsulfatase A deficiency), Krabbe's disease (galactosylceramide-β-galactosidase deficiency), and adrenomyeloneuropathy (characterized by high levels of saturated very long-chain fatty acids) are the most frequent diseases that cause segmental demyelination and remyelination, sometimes associated with axonal degeneration. Nerve biopsy is performed only in atypical cases because less invasive diagnostic techniques, such as leukocyte enzymology, biochemical analysis, or molecular genetics are available.

In sulfatidosis, nerve biopsy allows the demonstration of metachromasia after toluidine blue or cresyl violet stains, and electron microscopy shows characteristic profiles. This is also the case in Krabbe's disease and adrenomyeloneuropathy.

Hypertrophic Neuropathy by Chronic Segmental Demyelination and Remyelination

Most hereditary demyelinating neuropathies cause hypertrophic neuropathy. This is the case for the hereditary demyelinating motor and sensory neuropathies (HMSN) corresponding mainly to the hypertrophic form of Charcot-Marie-Tooth disease (HSMN type I in Dyck's classification) and to Dejerine-Sottas disease (HMSN type III), Refsum's disease (a rare inborn disorder of lipid metabolism caused by an isolated phytanic acid α-hydroxylase deficiency), and very rare other disorders, which are often familial. Molecular genetic techniques have made a recent impact on these disorders, the classification of which is in progress. In addition, every persisting demyelination, including the chronic forms of inflammatory neuropathies, can lead to hypertrophic neuropathy.

Hypomyelination

These disorders are characterized by thin myelin sheaths on fibers of all diameters. This change is seen in Dejerine-Sottas disease and in a rare autosomal recessive condition in children, presenting as congenital or early nonprogressive peripheral neuropathy. It is recognized on semithin sections and electron microscopy. Very thin myelinated fibers and onion bulbs, mainly composed of basement membranes, are present. There is evidence of persistent demyelination. The mechanism of this disorder is unknown. For the diagnosis of hypomyelination, morphometry and comparison with normal controls of the same age range may be useful in some cases because the density and the proportion of myelinated fibers of various sizes do not reach adult values before the teen-age years.

Amyelination

Absence of myelin is rare. The patients, who often present with arthrogryposis multiplex congenita, respiratory distress, and swallowing difficulties, have a total or near-total amyelination of the peripheral nervous system.

Interstitial Neuropathies

Vasculitis

An inflammatory cell infiltrate develops in the vessel walls (see Ch. 38). In necrotizing vasculitis, there is associated fibrinoid necrosis. In polyarteritis nodosa and related disorders, also called systemic necrotizing vasculitis, some middle-sized arteries (80 to 200 μm in diameter) are affected by necrotizing vasculitis. In microvasculitis, the walls of vessels of the microcirculation only (small arteries, capillaries, and venules) are affected. In the nerve, there is little or no fibrinoid necrosis. Microvasculitis has to be distinguished from mere perivascular cuffs, which are of little significance.

Polyarteritis Nodosa and Related Disorders. These are frequently recognized on nerve biopsy because the small artery lying near the nerve has the adequate diameter for diagnostic lesions. Lesions of the arteries of the nerve are similar to those of other organs, fibrinoid necrosis of the media and mononuclear and polymorphonuclear cell infiltrates, sometimes containing eosinophils, are the characteristic features (Fig. 8-12A). The lesions are focal and can be seen only after serial sectioning, which is mandatory when there is clinical or pathologic suspicion, especially if healed arterial lesions (occlusion or focal sclerosis of the wall) or an associated microvasculitis are present. When normal, a nerve biopsy does not rules out the diagnosis, which can be detected by another biopsy. Variants of polyarteritis nodosa have been described. Churg-Strauss syndrome is characterized, on pathologic grounds, by the high density of eosinophils in the cellular infiltrates and abundance of extravascular infiltrates. In Wegener's granulomatosis or Liebow's lymphomatoid granulomatosis, the finding of specific lesions by nerve biopsy is exceedingly rare. Lesions indistinguishable from those of polyarteritis nodosa can be found in some cases of severe rheumatoid arthritis, in systemic lupus erythematosus, in Gougerot-Sjögren syndrome, and in acquired immunodeficiency syndrome and are often considered to be genuine polyarteritis nodosa.

Microvasculitis. This may be seen in any connective disease (including Gougerot-Sjögren disease, polymyalgia rheumatica, and rheumatoid arthritis), in malignant disease (especially lymphomas), in mixed essential cryoglobulinemia, and in any inflammatory or infectious disorder of the nerve, especially inflammatory demyelinating neuropathies and acquired immunodeficiency syndrome. It has also be seen in the absence of a recognized cause for the neuropathy.

The consequences of vasculitis on nerve fibers are usually nonspecific axonal degeneration, which can be

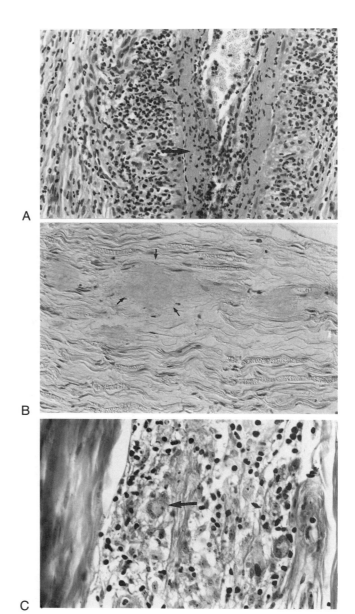

Figure 8-12. (**A**) Necrotizing vasculitis of the polyarteritis nodosa type. A middle-sized artery 150 μm in diameter is affected. Lesions are fibrinoid necrosis of the media (*arrow*) and mononuclear and polymorphonuclear cell infiltrates, containing eosinophils, extending largely into the epineural connective tissue. (Hematoxylin-eosin, ×160.) (**B**) Portuguese form of amyloidosis. The endoneural deposits of abnormal transthyretin (one of which is shown by thin arrows) pushes aside the myelinated fibers. (Congo red, ×160.) (**C**) Sarcoid granuloma. A granuloma made of epithelioid and giant cells (*arrow*) in the epineurium. (Hematoxylin-eosin, ×260.)

heterogeneous from one fascicle to another or within the same fascicle. The classic centrofascicular rarefaction of nerve fibers is unusual.

Cholesterol Emboli

They have to be systematically checked, especially when a vasculitis is suspected.

Leprosy

In tuberculoid leprosy, granulomas with epithelioid and giant cells may be seen. More often, the nerve is destroyed and enlarged by a dense fibrous tissue in which few or no myelinated fibers are recognized. This should lead to a suspicion of the diagnosis of leprosy, even if it cannot be proved. In lepromatous leprosy, classic Virchow cells (i.e., large spumous macrophages containing *Mycobacterium leprae* that can be shown by Ziehl-Hansen stain) may be found. In fact, most cases are difficult to recognize, and very sensitive stains such as auramine should be used.

Sarcoidosis

Granulomatous lesions are seldom seen in the nerve (Fig. 8-12C). When found, they do not indicate nerve tuberculosis, which is exceedingly rare. The diagnosis of sarcoidosis is better performed on a muscle biopsy.

Amyloidosis

In amyloidosis, the characteristic acellular deposits are best seen by Congo red under polarization, or after thioflavine T staining, they can be found in the endoneurium, displacing the nerve fibers (Fig. 8-12B), or in the vessels walls. Typing of various proteins that may be components of amyloidosis, especially AL or transthyretin, may be done by immunohistochemical tests. When there is a suspicion of amyloidosis, a nerve biopsy is seldom performed today because the diagnosis can also be made by noninvasive techniques (including molecular genetic techniques for Andrade's disease) or by a skin biopsy.

Tumor Infiltrates

These are occasionally found in various tumors or leukemias and may reveal the malignancy.

Other Findings

Nerve biopsy may show more or less specific lesions in a number of pathologic conditions, including ceroid lipofuscinosis and most metabolic disorders. The significance of polyglucosan bodies sometimes found in nerve fibers is discussed, especially when they are seen in elderly patients. For the assessment of a metabolic disorder, muscle and nerve biopsies are usually performed only when skin, conjunctival, or rectal biopsy findings are negative. As in muscle biopsy, the changes have to be interpreted in the clinical context (age, nutritional status, and presumed site of nerve disease).

ACKNOWLEDGMENTS

We thank Professors M. Fardeau and J. C. Gautier for helpful discussion. Mrs. H. Collin and Mr. P. Mielle provided expert technical assistance.

ANNOTATED BIBLIOGRAPHY

Bradley WG. Disorders of Peripheral Nerve, Blackwell, Oxford, 1974.
A short textbook with useful schemes.

Carpenter S, Karpati G. The pathological diagnosis of specific inflammatory myopathies. Brain Pathol. 1992;2: 13–9.
Short recent point of view on inflammatory myopathies.

Chaunu MP, Ratinahirana H, Henin D et al. The spectrum of changes on nerve biopsy in 20 patients with HIV infection. Muscle Nerve 1989;12:452–9.
The frequency of microvasculitis in the early stages of HIV-one infection is emphasized.

Dubowitz V. Muscle Biopsy, a Practical Approach. 2nd Ed. Bailliere Tindall, London, 1985.
The "gold standard" for techniques and results in normal and pathologically involved muscle.

Dyck PJ. Peripheral neuropathy. Postgrad Med 1967;41: 279.

Dyck PJ, Karnes J, Lais et al. Pathologic alterations of the peripheral nervous system of humans. In Dyck PJ, Thomas PK, Lambert EH, Bunge R (eds). Peripheral Neuropathy. WB Saunders, Philadelphia, 1984, pp. 760–870.
Precise descriptions of nerve biopsy techniques and results.

Dyck PJ, Thomas PK (eds). Peripheral Neuropathy. 3rd Ed. Vols. I and II. WB Saunders, Philadelphia, 1993.
Comprehensive textbook on pathologic condition of the nerve.

Emslie-Smith AM, Engel AG. Necrotizing myopathy with pipestem capillaries, microvascular deposition of complement attack complex, and minimal cellular infiltration. Neurology 1991;41:936–9.
A new inflammatory myopathy.

Engel AG, Franzini-Armstrong C. Myology. 2nd Ed. Vols. I and II. McGraw-Hill, New York, 1994.
Exhaustive textbook on pathologic conditions of the muscle.

Eymard B, Hauw JJ. Mitochondrial encephalomyopathies. Curr Opin Neurol Neurosurg 1992;5:909–16.
Recent review on mitochondrial encephalomyopathies.

Fardeau M. Congenital myopathies. In Mastaglia FL, Walton JN (eds). Skeletal Muscle Pathology. 2nd Ed. Churchill Livingstone, Edinburgh, 1992, pp. 237–91.
Expert review on congenital myopathies.

Harding AE, Thomas PK. Symposium on inherited neuropathies: the interface between molecular genetics and neuropathology. Brain Pathol. 1993;3:129–90.

Recent overview on inherited neuropathies.

Mastaglia FL, Walton JN (eds). Skeletal Muscle Pathology. 2nd Ed. Churchill Livingstone, Edinburgh, 1992.

Textbook on pathologic muscle conditions, including biopsy data.

Pamphlett R. Muscle Biopsy. In Mataglia FL (ed). Inflammatory Diseases of Muscle. Blackwell Scientific Publications, Oxford, 1988, pp. 17–36.

Precise description of muscle biopsy, including needle biopsy.

Poirier J, Gray F, Escourolle R. Manual of Basic Neuropathology. WB Saunders, Philadelphia, 1990.

A short introduction to neuropathology.

Ratinahirana H, Hauw JJ. Morphométrie. In Bouche P, Vallet JM (eds). Neuropathies Periphériques. Doin, Paris, 1992.

Seilhean D, Baumann N, Turpin JC et al. Neuropathology of lipidoses. In Duckett S (ed). The Neuropathology of the Developing Human Nervous System. WB Saunders, Philadelphia, 1995, 592–619.

Recent review on pathology of lipidoses.

Vital C, Vallat JM. Ultrastructural Study of the Human Diseased Peripheral Nerve. Masson, New York, 1980.

An atlas of nerve lesions found by electron microscopy.

9
Spinal Fluid Examination

Larry E. Davis

Once a mainstay of neurologic diagnosis when few other investigatory techniques existed, lumbar puncture (LP) has received less attention in recent years owing to the ascendancy of neuroimaging, Doppler ultrasonography, and clinical neurophysiology. Yet the supremacy of the LP as a basis for diagnosis of meningeal infections, neoplastic infiltrations, and subarachnoid hemorrhage remains unsurpassed, despite other challenges. Cerebrospinal fluid (CSF) examination serves a wide range of other purposes as well, and the LP even has therapeutic indications.

ANATOMY AND PHYSIOLOGY

The majority of CSF (approximately 60 percent) is produced by choroid plexuses located in both lateral ventricles and the fourth ventricle (Fig. 9-1). CSF passes from the lateral ventricles into the third ventricle and through the aqueduct of Sylvius into the fourth ventricle and exits into the subarachnoid space via the foramina of Luschka and Magendie (see also Ch. 59). After exiting these foramina, CSF travels upward in the subarachnoid space to pass through the tentorial opening, reaching the sulci of the cerebrum, where CSF is absorbed through the arachnoid villi (pacchionian bodies, named for A. Pacchioni, Italian anatomist, 1665–1726) into the superior sagittal sinus. A lesser amount of circulating CSF passes down through the foramen magnum and into the spinal cord subarachnoid space and is then recirculated upward.

The total CSF volume in adults is approximately 140 ml. The ventricles contain about 25 ml and the spinal cord subarachnoid space 30 ml, and the remaining volume is in the subarachnoid space around the brain. The production rate in adults is about 20 to 25 ml/h or 500 to 600 ml/day, resulting in a turnover of CSF about four times a day. The rate of CSF absorption is linearly related to the CSF pressure, but CSF production is independent of CSF pressure until the latter is above 450 mm CSF.

INDICATIONS AND CONTRAINDICATIONS

The time-honored indications for a diagnostic LP are to rule out infections of the meninges, cancer or leukemia involving the meninges, and subarachnoid hemorrhage and to diagnose Guillain-Barŕe syndrome. CSF examination is often helpful in the diagnosis of multiple sclerosis and encephalitis, and LP has some therapeutic indications, including lowering intracranial pressure in benign intracranial hypertension or injecting drugs for meningeal leukemia or fungal meningitis.

Increased intracranial pressure caused by an intracranial mass is the leading contraindication for LP because of the risk that CSF removal may alter intracranial dynamics, leading to a shift of intracranial structures with uncal herniation (see Chs. 17 and 25). A properly performed history and neurologic examination should rule out syndromes suggestive of mass lesion, chief among which are dilated pupil, papilledema, or major syndromes of hemiparesis, aphasia, homonymous hemianopsia, or ataxia. It is prudent in such cases to perform a neuroimaging study by computed tomography (CT) or magnetic resonance imaging (MRI) prior to performing the LP. If a space-occupying lesion is detected that has produced shifts in the anatomic positioning of brain structure, increased intracranial pressure can be inferred and the LP delayed.

Other illnesses that may increase the risk of an LP include a bleeding disorder and local cutaneous infection. Included among the bleeding disorders are exposure to anticoagulant therapy, platelet values below 50,000/mm³, and a known arteriovenous malformation in the lower spinal cord; the risk is that of developing an epidural or subdural hematoma in the lumbar

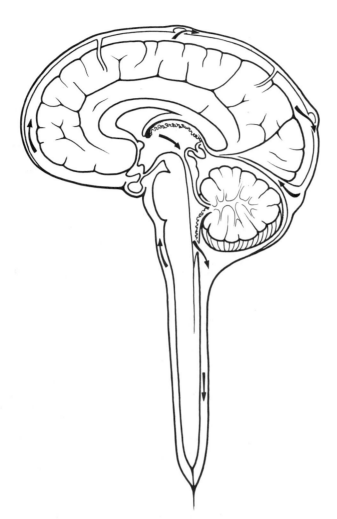

Figure 9-1. Most CSF (approximately 60 percent) is produced by choroid plexuses located in both lateral ventricles and the fourth ventricle.

region, which can compress the lower spinal cord and nerve roots. These complications usually develop after damage to Batson's epidural venous plexus, subdural vessels, or radicular blood vessels of the cauda equina. The diagnosis post-LP is suggested by flaccid paralysis, local back pain, sensory loss in the legs, or sphincter disturbances. Correction of the coagulopathy is recommended before proceeding with the LP. Performing an LP through a localized skin or subcutaneous infection runs the risk of introducing the infection into the CSF. When LP is needed in such cases, a cisternal tap should suffice to collect the CSF.

TECHNIQUE OF LUMBAR PUNCTURE

As for any procedure, written consent is recommended. For tense patients, antianxiety drugs such as chlordiazepoxide or diazepam can be given orally 1 to 2 hours before the lumbar puncture.

In adults the spinal cord descends to approximately the T12-L1 space. At that point lumbar and sacral nerve roots pass downward into the lumbar sacral regions. In small children the spinal cord may reach as low as L1 or 2, and as a consequence the safest in which to place the needle is the lower lumbar space (L3–L5).

Whenever possible, the LP should be performed in the lateral recumbent position (Fig. 9-2) to allow accurate determination of CSF opening pressure. Obese patients may have to be punctured in the sitting position. The spinous processes should form a straight horizontal line and the tips of the iliac crest should be perpendicular to this line. Flexing the back by bending knees and head together on a braced pillow expands the space between the lumbar spinous processes, making it easier to insert the needle. The skin over this area is cleaned with Betadine or alcohol. Lidocaine (1 to 2 percent) may be injected intradermally at the site for needle entry.

The needle is usually inserted at the L3-L4 or L4-L5 interspace, which is easily identified as the area in which the perpendicular line between the tips of the iliac crest cross the horizontal line formed by the spinous processes. For adults it is common to use a 20-gauge needle. Smaller-gauge needles such as 22-gauge are more flexible and may bend in passing through back muscles and connective tissues. The needle bending may be sufficient to make it difficult to find the small dural space without hitting bone. Use of a 25-gauge needle and guide does not allow measurement of opening pressure. The needle with its stylet in place should be introduced through the skin and angled slightly toward the head (as if the needle were going to the umbilicus). The bevel of the needle should be up so as to make a small hole as the needle passes the longitudinal fibers in the dural membrane. As the needle passes through the dura, one often feels a sudden change in resistance ("pop" sensation). The movement of the needle can be stopped at any time and the stylet removed to check for the presence of CSF. If blood is encountered, the needle should be withdrawn and the patient repositioned before needle reinsertion.

Once CSF is encountered, attachment of a three-way stopcock and a manometer allows measurement of the opening pressure. Next, CSF should be withdrawn in a sequential fashion. Normally, four to five tubes of CSF are collected. Each tube should be appropriately numbered. In adults, 6 to 20 ml of CSF is normally removed. The amount of CSF to be removed depends on the number of tests to be ordered. It is possible to do a cell count, glucose, protein, and culture on as little as 2 to 3 ml of CSF in hospitals that have microchemistry facilities. This becomes impor-

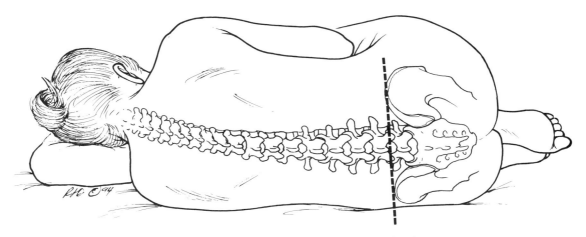

Figure 9-2. Lateral placement of the patient for lumbar puncture.

tant when lumbar punctures are performed on infants or young children. It is often helpful to collect 2 ml into an extra tube for the Laboratory to "save" in case additional CSF tests need to be ordered.

After obtaining the CSF, the needle can be removed from the back without replacing the stylette. There is no evidence that drinking a large amount of water prevents a post-LP headache, but lying prone for 1 to 3 hours may reduce its incidence. Whether use of a 22-gauge needle instead of a 20-gauge needle lessens the frequency of LP headaches is unsettled.

It is mandatory to transport the CSF quickly to the laboratory to prevent lysis of white blood cells and lowering of CSF glucose levels by WBC metabolism.

FINDINGS ON LUMBAR PUNCTURE

Opening Pressure

The normal CSF pressure in the lateral recumbent position varies between 70 and 180 mm CSF (mean 150 mm CSF). In the sitting position the CSF level rises to about the level of the cisterna magna (about 280 mm CSF). Minor oscillations in CSF pressure are synchronous with respiration and pulse rate and vary between 5 and 10 mm CSF. Visualization of these minor pressure fluctuations is helpful in ascertaining that the CSF pressure is accurate. If the CSF pressure is between 150 and 220 mm CSF, slight straightening of the patient's legs may relax abdominal muscles and lower the pressure somewhat. Forced deep breaths should be avoided because the resulting hypocapnia induces falsely low pressure readings owing to cerebral vasoconstriction.

Appearance of Cerebrospinal Fluid

Normal CSF is crystal clear and colorless when compared with a similar tube filled with water against a white background or x-ray view box. A turbulent ap-

pearance suggests a pleocytosis or fat from fat emboli to the CNS. After centrifugation to precipitate any cells, xanthochromia (faint yellow color) may be seen in CSF containing more than 200 mg/dl protein or oxyhemoglobin/bilirubin from RBC breakdown secondary to a subarachnoid hemorrhage, traumatic tap, or systemic jaundice.

Cells

The cell count should be done within $\frac{1}{2}$ hour of the lumbar puncture as cells lyse on prolonged standing. Normal CSF contains less than five lymphocytes per mm³. Cell counts between 5 and 10 white blood cells per mm³ suggest disease, while counts greater than 10 white blood cells per mm³ should warrant a presumptive diagnosis of inflammation. Neutrophils in the CSF are abnormal. Lymphocytes are less easily distinguished, sometimes thought to be present when the actual particles are talc from the examiner's gloves. The total cell count may be performed on a hemocytometer. The differential count is often done on CSF in which the cells are sedimented or centrifuged (cytospin) onto a glass slide, which is then stained with Giemsa or Wright stain. The absolute white cell count and the percentage of each cell type (i.e., lymphocytes and neutrophils) must be determined even though they can vary widely in viral, bacterial, and tuberculous meningitis.

Normal CSF has less than 5 red blood cells (RBCs) per mm³. A small number may be occasioned by a traumatic LP (see below), but a source of intracranial or intraspinal bleeding is the first consideration.

Protein

Protein in normal CSF varies with the age of the patient and the site from which the CSF was obtained (Tables 9-1 and 9-2). Low CSF protein levels have little

Table 9-1. Upper Limits of Normal Lumbar Spinal Fluid Protein

Age	Protein Limit
Newborn	100 mg/dl
2 months	60 mg/dl
4 months	25 mg/dl
Adult age <30 years	30 mg/dl
Adult age >30 years	45 mg/dl[a]

[a] In some new chemistry autoanalyzers the upper limit is 60 mg/dl.

Table 9-2. Upper Limits of Normal Lumbar Spinal Fluid Protein

Production Site	Protein Limit
Lumbar	45 mg/dl
Cisternal	25 mg/dl
Ventricular	15 mg/dl

significance. Protein in CSF may become elevated in a wide variety of diseases. An elevated protein can be thought of as an elevated erythrocyte sedimentation rate, sensitive for central nervous system (CNS) disease but not specific.

MAJOR CAUSES OF INCREASED CSF PROTEIN

CNS infections
  Meningitis
  Encephalitis
  Brain abscess
CNS tumors near ependymal or meningeal surface
  Meningeal carcinomatosis
  Brain tumor
Obstruction of spinal CSF pathway
  Froin's syndrome
Metabolic diseases
  Hypothyroidism
  Uremia
Peripheral neuropathies
  Guillain-Barré syndrome
  Heavy metal neuropathy
Blood
  Subarachnoid hemorrhage
  Subdural hematoma
  CNS trauma
  Traumatic tap

Immunoglobulin G

Most of the γ-globulins in CSF belong to the IgG class. Intrathecal IgG synthesis occurs in a variety of infectious, postinfectious, inflammatory, and demyelinating diseases.

A quantitative IgG CSF determination is usually made by nephelometry or radioimmunodiffusion. Normal ratios of CSF IgG to CSF total protein are less than 12 to 14 percent. Ratios above 14 percent are commonly found in multiple sclerosis, neurosyphilis, tuberculous meningitis, fungal meningitis, subacute sclerosis panencephalitis (SSPE) and CNS sarcoidosis. Occasionally, elevated ratios are seen in other neurologic diseases such as Alzheimer's disease, peripheral neuropathy, and stroke. The normal ratio of blood IgG to total protein is 15 to 18 percent. In patients with very high CSF proteins, the CSF IgG/total protein ratio may be elevated solely because of a break in the blood-brain barrier.

Electrophoresis patterns of CSF differ from those of serum: CSF has a greater transthyretin (prealbumin) fraction; a clear β_2 or τ fraction proportionately greater than in serum; and a γ-globulin fraction proportionately lower than in serum. Electrophoresis generally requires 5 to 10 ml of CSF. This sensitive method can be used to look for the presence of oligoclonal bands in the γ-globulin region, which are not found in normal CSF. Their presence suggests that the CSF contains a disproportionate amount of an antibody that is sufficiently similar in size and electrophoretic charge that it migrates homogeneously. Oligoclonal bands are often seen in the CSF of patients with multiple sclerosis, fungal meningitis, TB meningitis, SSPE, or neurosyphilis or during convalescence from bacterial or viral meningitis and viral encephalitis. Patients with other neurologic diseases may also occasionally have oligoclonal bands.

Glucose

Normal CSF glucose is 60 to 70 percent that of blood glucose with a normal range of 45 to 50 mg/dl CSF. Blood glucose enters the CSF from blood through the choroid plexus or meningeal capillaries via a facilitated carrier transport system and simple diffusion. This system does not require energy and can be saturated when hyperglycemia is present. Normally, 1 to 2 hours is required before changes in blood glucose alter CSF glucose levels. Ideally, an LP should be performed in a fasting patient, when a blood glucose determination taken at the time of the LP can safely be compared with the CSF glucose level. Since this is often not practical, a note of the time since food or intravenous dextrose exposure can be useful. Under these conditions the CSF/blood glucose ratio may be lower than 60 percent, especially when the blood glucose is above 150 mg/dl.

Absolute CSF glucose values below 40 mg/dl (when the blood glucose is approximately normal) are considered abnormal. Low CSF glucose levels can result from bacterial or fungal glucose metabolism, inflammatory or carcinomatous cell metabolism of glucose, or interference with blood-CSF transport due to bacterial or fungal toxins or cytokines, as well as other causes occasionally including viral meningitis and subarachnoid hemorrhage.

Cultures

CSF cultures need not be routinely performed. They should be ordered to pursue suspected systemic or meningeal infection and in immunosuppressed patients or when the CSF contains a WBC pleocytosis. Fungal and tuberculous cultures should be included if the meningitis is clinically subacute or the patient is immunosuppressed.

Bacteria

In acute bacterial meningitis, the CSF contains 10^3 to 10^9 bacteria per mm^3. Bacteria can be isolated from CSF with a sensitivity of about 95 percent and a specificity of 99 percent. CSF or CSF sediment should be placed on both liquid and solid bacteriologic media. Usually anaerobic media are not necessary. About 1 to 4 days pass before antibiotic sensitivities are available. CSF is a fairly good culture medium for bacteria, which makes it a good practice to place a tightly capped tube of CSF directly in an incubator if no ready access to special media exists.

Tuberculosis

Several weeks are required for tubercular bacilli to be cultured. These organisms are always in low titer, making it uncommon for acid-fast bacilli to be identified on CSF smear. The low bacillus count also warrants taking the culture from the precipitate of 5 to 10 ml of centrifuged or filtered CSF.

Fungi

As with tubercular bacilli, about 5 to 10 ml of CSF should be centrifuged. The precipitate should be cultured on fungal media. Cultures require 3 to 25 days to grow the fungi.

Viruses

Viruses often can be isolated from CSF in viral meningitis but only rarely in viral encephalitis. A 3-ml sample of CSF should be inoculated onto appropriate viral tissue culture cells. Enteroviruses (echovirus, coxsackievirus, and poliovirus), mumps, lymphocytic choriomeningitis, and herpes simplex type 2 are the viruses most often isolated from CSF. It is rare to isolate arboviruses, measles virus, or herpes simplex virus type 1 from CSF. CSF cultures require 2 days to 3 weeks before turning positive.

Other Tests for Infectious Organisms

Apart from direct identification from staining and later growth in culture media, many infectious disease can be diagnosed by specific tests for the proteins unique to certain organisms.

Bacteria

The Gram stain (H. C. J. Gram, Danish bacteriologist, 1853–1938) on sediment obtained after centrifugation of CSF is rapid (less than 15 minutes), simple, and will distinguish gram-positive from gram-negative bacteria. Typically, the test has a sensitivity of 75 percent and a specificity of 95 percent. The probability of visualizing bacteria depends on the number of organism present: 25 percent of smears with less than 103 colony-forming units (CFU)/ml, 60 percent with 103 to 105 CFU/ml, and 97 percent with more than 105 CFU/ml are positive. Possible causes of false positive Gram stain smears include misinterpretation of cell debris on smear or bacterial contamination of tubes from lumbar puncture trays, of glass slides, and of Gram reagents. The only disadvantages of the Gram stain are that it does not yield the bacterial strain or the antibiotic sensitivity of the infecting organism.

The detection of bacterial antigens in CSF involves use of the latex particle agglutination test, in which a specific antibody to an infectious agent is attached to a latex particle. If bacterial antigens are present in CSF, they combine with the antibodies to form a lattice, which creates a visible agglutination. Detection of bacterial antigen in culture-proven CSF varies with the bacteria studied: detection of *Haemophilus influenzae* antigen can be excellent (95 percent); that for other bacterial antigens may only be fair, (e.g., group B streptococcus 79 percent, *Neisseria meningitides* 75 percent, and *Streptococcus pneumoniae* 67 percent). Commercially available kits have a false positive rate of about $\frac{1}{2}$ to 1 percent. Gram stain of CSF sediment has a sensitivity about equal to that of latex agglutination kits in detecting bacteria. Countercurrent immunoelectrophoresis, another method to detect CSF bacterial antigens, is more difficult to perform than latex particle agglutination.

Bacterial antigen tests do not need to be ordered on every case of bacterial meningitis, particularly when the Gram stain yields typical bacteria. The antigen tests are of value in the analysis of partially treated meningitis. Their disadvantages are their failure to detect uncommon bacteria and lack of antibiotic sensitivities.

Fungi

The latex particle agglutination test suffices to detect *Cryptococcus neoformans* antigen. This antigen test is more sensitive and specific than searching for organisms using an India ink stain of the sediment. In the India ink test the polysaccharide capsule that surrounds *C. neoformans* yeast is visualized as a clear halo around the yeast outlined by adjacent black carbon particles. Since the polysaccharide capsule is difficult to see when the yeast is viewed in CSF under a microscope, *C. neoformans* organisms can be mistaken for lymphocytes. Furthermore, the polysaccharide capsule does not stain with Giemsa or Gram stain. The India ink test will not detect other fungi since they lack a capsule. A CSF complement fixation antibody test for *Coccidioides immitis* is available. The presence of CSF antibody is highly suggestive of active disease. Experimental CSF antibody tests are available for *Histoplasma capsulatum* and *Blastomyces dermatitidis*.

Tuberculosis

Bacterial antigen tests for the presence of *Mycobacterium tuberculosis* are still experimental. Detection of tuberculosteric acid (cell wall component of *M. tuberculosis*) in CSF suggests the presence of *M. tuberculosis*, but this test is not routinely available and its specificity and sensitivity are presently unknown. Another experimental but promising diagnostic test is the identification of *M. tuberculosis* DNA in CSF by the polymerase chain reaction.

Antibody Tests

Antibody tests include a heterogeneous collection of tests, many directed toward single organisms.

Neurocysticercosis

The CSF immunoblot test for neurocysticercosis appears to be highly sensitive and specific (see also Ch. 43). However, antibody to *Cysticercus cellulosae* may be present in both active and inactive disease.

Neurosyphilis

Serologic tests for syphilis (see also Ch. 41) include the CSF Venereal Disease Research Laboratory (CSF-VDRL) test and the CSF fluorescent treponemal antibody-absorbed (CSF-FTA-ABS) test. The CSF-VDRL test is the standard test recommended by the U.S. Centers for Disease Control. A reactive or positive test is normally diagnostic of neurosyphilis. This test is a nontreponemal test similar to the rapid plasma reagin (RPR) test. However, while the RPR test has many false positives in serum, the CSF-VDRL has only rare false positives. This test is quantitative. Repeat CSF-VDRL tests can be used to evaluate responses to antibiotic treatment as the titer normally falls to zero. The CSF-FTA-ABA test is extremely sensitive but has not been well standardized for use in CSF. A negative CSF-FTA-ABS test appears to rule out neurosyphilis, but a reactive CSF-FTA-ABS test does not necessarily diagnose the active disease. A reactive test may represent active neurosyphilis, old treated neurosyphilis or a biologic false-positive due to contamination with blood containing serum FTA antibodies.

Cytology

Many malignancies can spread to the meninges, and 60 percent of patients with tumor in the leptomeninges will have malignant cells detected in their CSF. Patients with malignant disease of the meninges usually have a CSF pleocytosis, which includes malignant cells and an elevated white cell count (excluding neutrophils). The CSF has a slight to marked increased protein level and a normal to slightly decreased glucose level. When malignant cells are suspected, 5 to 10 ml of CSF should be added to the fixative immediately after the CSF is collected, since malignant cells rapidly degenerate on standing. The laboratory normally concentrates the CSF by membrane filtration or cytocentrifugation and stains the cells by the Papanicolaou method. When there are few cells in the CSF, the millipore filter method recovers many more cells than cytocentrifugation.

Tests for Demyelinating Disease

It is possible to detect myelin basic proteins in CSF. Elevations of these proteins often occur during the active phases of multiple sclerosis and other CNS-demyelinating disease. The actual sensitivity and specificity of this test is not known. A 1- to 2-ml CSF sample is needed. Most laboratories do not routinely perform this test and send the CSF to an outside laboratory.

Special Tests

Under specific indications, a variety of special tests may be performed on CSF. In general, most tests that can be performed on serum can also be performed on CSF. Examples include CSF glutamine levels, usually elevated in hepatic encephalopathy, and CSF C-reactive protein, usually elevated in bacterial meningitis.

COMPLICATIONS OF LUMBAR PUNCTURE

Traumatic Lumbar Puncture

Traumatic LP occurs in 10 to 20 percent of cases. It frequently results when the LP needle hits a vein or arteriole in or adjacent to the subarachnoid space. This most often occurs when a small radicular vein of

Table 9-3. Analysis of Bloody CSF

CSF Finding	Traumatic LP	Subarachnoid Hemorrhage
Color	1st tube pink 3rd tube clearer	All tubes uniform color
RBC count	Higher in 1st than in 3rd tube	All tubes uniform
Color of supernatant fluid	Colorless	Xanthochromic
Clot	May occur on standing	Absent
Repeat LP at higher interspace	Often clear	Same as initial LP
Head CT	No blood seen	Blood possible in subarachnoid space

the cauda equina is punctured by the needle. When this happens, CSF obtained through the needle contains fresh blood, which often becomes less visible in each succeeding tube. Table 9-3 lists differences between the traumatic LP and a subarachnoid hemorrhage. Crenated red blood cells and hemoglobin and oxyhemoglobin in the supernatant may be seen in both conditions, but only CSF supernatant from a subarachnoid hemorrhage (after 2 days) may contain bilirubin.

In the traumatic tap, serum protein as well as red cells leak into the CSF, which will falsely elevate the CSF protein. A useful guide when the protein determination is made on the same tube used for the red blood cell count RBC is to subtract 1 mg/dl protein for every 1,000 red blood cells per mm^3 and 1 to 2 white blood cells for every 1,000 red blood cells per mm.^{3} Minor local bleeding after the LP seldom poses any health risk to the patient.

Post–Lumbar Puncture Headache

Headache following LP while not life-threatening, often is quite uncomfortable. The headache begins 1 to 4 hours after the lumbar puncture and can persist for up to several days. Most often the headache is frontal and occurs when the patient moves from a lying to a sitting or standing position. Return to the supine position eliminates the headache. The incidence of post-LP headaches ranges from 10 to 25 percent depending on the age and sex of the patient and the size of the LP needle use. In general, post-LP headaches are unusual in small children, uncommon in older children, and most common in adults. Women have more post-LP headaches than men. The incidence of

post-LP headaches also increases with use of larger needles.

The pathophysiology of post-LP headache appears to be persistent drainage of CSF through the hole in the lumbar dural membrane made by the LP needle. This may result in low CSF pressure and sagging of the brain on the tentorium and base of the skull when the patient assumes an upright posture.

Backache

Occasional patients develop a backache or painful paresthesias in the lower back region or legs. This usually resolves spontaneously within a few weeks and only rarely persists.

Brain Herniation

The most feared complication of an LP is shifting of the brain or cerebellum following the LP to produce an uncal or tonsillar herniation. This risk occurs primarily in the patient with increased intracranial pressure from a space-occupying lesion, especially a mass in the temporal lobe or cerebellum. Diffuse increases in intracranial pressure from meningitis or pseudotumor cerebri seldom cause brain herniation.

Despite the concern, the overall risk of brain herniation from an LP is small. In the presence of increased intracranial pressure the risk appears in about 2 percent of cases. As previously noted, if focal neurologic findings or papilledema is present, neuroimaging studies should be performed prior to the LP. If a space-occupying lesion is found, the LP should be done with extreme caution and only when absolutely necessary. Steps to reduce the increased intracranial pressure should be taken, such as administration of intravenous mannitol 1 hour before the LP.

If markedly elevated CSF opening pressure (above 300 mm CSF) is unexpectedly obtained during a routine LP, the following approach is suggested. Reflexively removing the LP needle places the patient at immediate risk for continued CSF leakage through the hole and does not yield any CSF for diagnostic evaluation. One should close the stopcock so that CSF does not leak out from the top of the manometer. Next, 2 to 5 ml of CSF should be slowly collected in appropriate tubes, which should be sent to the laboratory for emergency diagnostic testing. Following removal of the LP needle, the patient should be observed closely over the next 2 to 4 hours for any signs of neurologic deterioration. An intravenous line should be placed, and administration of mannitol (0.25 to 0.5 mg/kg) in a bolus should be considered. A neurosurgeon should be notified of the possibility of brain herniation. An emergency CT or MRI scan should be obtained to further evaluate the cause of the increased intracranial pressure. If a treatable cause is identified, emergency neurosurgical correction of the problem should be considered. If brain herniation begins, the patient should be intubated and begun on hyperventilation to reduce intracranial pressure.

ANNOTATED BIBLIOGRAPHY

Ballard TL, Roe MH, Wheeler RC et al. Comparison of three latex agglutination kits and counterimmunoelectrophoresis for the detection of bacterial antigens in a pediatric population. Pediatr Infect Dis J 1987;6:630–4.

Some difficulties but many work well.

Barrows LJ, Hunter FT, Banker BQ. The nature and clinical significance of pigments in the cerebrospinal fluid. Brain 1955;78:59–80.

Dated but still a classic.

Bell WO. Cerebrospinal fluid reabsorption. Concepts Pediatr Neurosurg 1990;10:214–34.

Review article.

Brooks JB, Daneshvar MI, Haberberger RL et al. Rapid diagnosis of tuberculous meningitis by frequency-pulsed electron-capture gas-liquid chromatography detection of carboxylic acids in cerebrospinal fluid. J Clin Microbiol 1990;:989–97.

Newer technology.

Cutler RWP, Page L, Galicich J, Watters GV. Formation and absorption of cerebrospinal fluid in man. Brain 1968;91: 707–20.

Review article.

Davis LE, Schmitt JW. Clinical significance of cerebrospinal fluid tests for neurosyphilis. Ann Neurol 1989;25:50–5.

Modern review.

Edelson RN, Chernik NL, Posner JB. Spinal subdural hematomas complicating lumbar puncture. Arch Neurol 1974; 31:134–7.

Case reports.

Fishman RA. Cerebrospinal Fluid in Diseases of the Nervous System. 2nd Ed. WB Saunders, Philadelphia, 1992.

Standard text.

Fishman RA. Studies of the transport of sugars between blood and cerebrospinal fluid in normal states and in meningeal carcinomatosis. Trans Am Neurol Assoc 1963;88:114–8.

Another clinical classic.

Glass JP, Melamed M, Chernik NL et al. Malignant cells in cerebrospinal fluid (CSF): The meaning of a positive CSF cytology. Neurology 1979;29:1369–75.

The limitations are discussed.

Herndon R, Brumback R (eds): The Cerebrospinal Fluid. Kluwer Academic Publishers, Boston 1989, pp. 131–41.

Modern standard text.

Hoban DJ, Witwicki E, Hammond GW. Bacterial antigen detection in cerebrospinal fluid of patients with meningitis. Diagn Microbiol Infect Dis 1985;3:373–9.

Techniques of investigation.

Lieberman LM, Tourtellotte WW, Newkirk TA. Prolonged post-lumbar puncture cerebrospinal fluid leakage from lumbar subarachnoid space demonstrated by radioisotope myelography. Neurology 1971;21:925–9.

Drainage may continue.

Musher DM, Shell RF. False-positive Gram stains of cerebrospinal fluid. Ann Intern Med 1973;79:603–4.

Many causes.

Petersdorf RG, Swarner DM, Garcia M. Studies on the pathogenesis of meningitis. III. Relationship of phagocytosis to the fall in cerebrospinal fluid sugar in experimental pneumococcal meningitis. J Lab Clin Med 1963;61: 745–54.

A clinical classic.

Petito F, Plum F. The lumbar puncture. N Engl J Med 1974; 290:225–7.

Standard for the details.

Ruff RL, Dougherty JH. Evaluation of acute cerebral ischemia for anticoagulant therapy: computed tomography or lumbar puncture. Neurology 1981;31:736–40.

Value of CT instead of LP.

Smith CE, Saito MT, Simons SA. Pattern of 39,500 serologic tests in coccidioidomycosis. JAMA 1956;160:546–52.

Detailed review article.

Tourtellote WW, Henderson WG, Tucker RP et al. A randomized double-blind trial comparing the 22 versus the 26 gauge needle in the production of post-lumbar puncture syndrome in normal individuals. Headache 1972; 12:73–8.

Smaller needles, less headache.

Tsang VCW, Brand JA, Boyer AE. An enzyme-linked immunoelectrotransfer blot assay and glycoprotein antigens for diagnosing human cysticercosis (*Taenia solium*). J Infect Dis 1989;159:50–9.

Available but of limited use.

10
Brain Imaging

J. P. Williams and Ruth D. Snow

METHODS OF STUDY

Computed Tomography

The term *computed tomography* (CT), earlier called computerized axial tomography (CAT) before improved equipment design allowed images in planes other than the axial, describes the basic technique used: computerized enhancement of thin-section plain x-ray beams passed through the target organ (for neurologists, most often the skull or spine). The current technology employs machines drawing on a single energy source to create a wide fan beam of x-rays. This beam passes through the head to an array of detectors, which individually measure the attenuation of the x-ray energy. A shift in the axis of the beam allows the detectors to measure another attenuation from a different angle, and the intersections of these different directions of measurement permit calculations of attenuations at different points across the paths of the beams. Manyfold multiplication, use of a curvilinear array containing as many as 2,400 detectors, and rapid rotation of the fan beam around the patient's head provide up to 800,000 individual attenuation measurements for each plane of section. The computation of all the attenuation values for each of the beams at each of the intersecting sites allows the creation of a computer-generated display of these values in planar fashion as a gray scale (or color-coded) image on a monitor.

CT is the most rapidly performed of brain imaging techniques. Each individual image can be obtained so rapidly that problems with motion may be eliminated. CT scanning allows great differentiation among normal soft tissues, particularly when used with the intravenous administration of iodinated contrast agents. Within the brain, abnormal enhancement requires breakdown of the blood-brain barrier to demonstrate a lesion. CT images clearly demonstrate acute clotted blood seen in acute parenchymal or subarachnoid hemorrhage, and CT is superior to magnetic resonance imaging (MRI) and plain radiographs (see below) for imaging bone and calcification. The disadvantages of CT are that the bony images that predominate in the posterior fossa and the floor of the middle fossa make it difficult to see the smaller volume of brain and brainstem imaged in the same planes.

The gantry housing the source and detectors of the x-rays can be tilted so that scans can be performed at a standard angle. The head angulation in the CT scan is designed to yield the most brain and the least bone. As nearly as possible, a standard imaging plane should be used (Fig. 10-1). Changing the plane will change the shape of the ventricles and other structures, possibly resulting in an angle of imaging unfavorable for diagnosis of conditions affecting the cerebral surface that lie near a bony surface. The wrong imaging plane also renders it more difficult to determine in which lobe of the brain an abnormality is located.

The thickness of each "slice" is selected to maximize the opportunity to see disease states or to ensure sufficiently thin sections to observe small changes, which could be lost in thicker sections. For routine clinical purposes, from the skull base through the sella turcica, scans should be obtained at 5-mm thickness, while 1-cm slices are adequate above the sella.

The milliamperex seconds (mAs) used in acquiring brain images should not fall below 500 mA-s (milliampere-seconds) except in emergency situations in which the patient cannot be rendered immobile even with restraints or sedation. Reducing the mAs reduces resolution, particularly in differentiating gray matter from white matter. These differences can be important in diagnosing ischemic injuries to the brain.

The unit system named after Godfrey N. Hounsfield, the EMI engineer who designed the first CT system, is based on the assumption that the attenuation value of water on the gray scale is zero HU

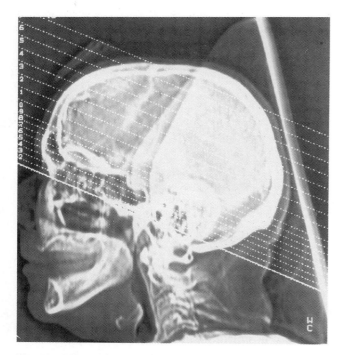

Figure 10-1. A pilot from a CT scan with the planes of the sections superimposed on the skull image at the appropriate angle. Using this particular angle will ensure that all of the brain is included on the scan. Note that the lines on the pilot from the skull base to the sella turcica are close together, representing 5-mm slices. Above this level the lines represent 1-cm slices.

(Hounsfield units). The computer-generated attenuation numbers reflecting spinal fluid are approximately +10 HU, while those of soft tissues, white and gray matter, are between +30 and +40 HU. Corresponding values for more compact and dense tissues such as liquid blood are +40 to +50 HU, for clotted blood +50 to +100 HU, and for bone well above 100 HU. The x-ray attenuation properties of fat yield negative values between −50 and −100 HU.

The range of CT numbers selected for a given display is known as the *window*. The window setting, roughly similar to the contrast knob on a black and white television set, determines the range over which the available gray-scale values will be displayed. A small or low-number window will crowd into a narrow range the available gradations of the gray scale and provide an image that is mostly black and white, with strong contrast. A wide window spreads the gray scale over a larger number of values, making an image with less contrast, one suitable for detecting subtle differences among soft tissues.

The reference CT number that represents the center of the window is known as the *level,* which can be varied over a wide scale. For a given level, those CT

numbers lower than the reference number will be displayed as increasingly dark and those above as increasingly light. At the commonly selected window levels of 40 or 50, spinal fluid appears quite dark, bone very white, and white matter slightly darker than gray matter.

We recommend that all brain scans be filmed at a window setting of 100 W (width) and 50 L (level). These settings allow for adequate contrast of all normal and most abnormal tissues within the gray scale. Attempts to improve the aesthetics of a scan by widening the window near the skull base may blur the artifacts but also may obscure most of the soft tissue anatomy and pathology. If images at other window settings are needed to discriminate between tissues at either end of the gray scale they should be obtained in addition to the standard set of pictures photographed at 100W/50L.

The modern CT scanner with spiral motion offers the possibility of CT angiography with only a venous bolus injection (Fig. 10-2).

Magnetic Resonance Imaging

Magnetic resonance imaging (MRI) has become a dominant technique because of its multiplanar capabilities and superior contrast resolution as compared with CT. MRI does not involve ionizing radiation. Images are created from the electromagnetic energy released from body tissues after they are stimulated by

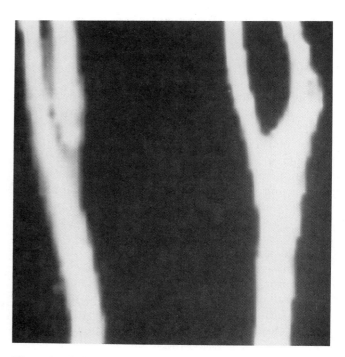

Figure 10-2. Spiral CT angiogram of the carotid bifurcations in the neck.

a radiofrequency within a magnetic field. Most MRI scanners use superconducting magnets, which must be supercooled with liquid helium and nitrogen and require careful (and expensive) maintenance.

A magnetic resonance signal can be elicited from any tissue containing mobile hydrogen protons, the most ready source of which is tissue water. Cortical bone and air have no magnetic resonance signal because they contain very few mobile hydrogen protons. Other nuclei with odd numbers of protons or neutrons, such as sodium and phosphorus, can also be imaged but with higher field-strength magnets. They occur in far lower concentration than does hydrogen, and therefore the images have lower spatial resolution.

The spatial resolution of CT is superior to that of MRI, but the contrast resolution of MRI is superior to that of CT. MRI contrast is determined by the combination of T_1 characteristics, T_2 characteristics, and mobile proton density. T_1 and T_2 are designations for tissue-specific relaxation properties, which describe each proton's behavior in longitudinal and transverse planes relative to the main magnetic field. Within the magnet each proton is aligned with the magnetic field, which is in a longitudinal plane. After a radiofrequency pulse is given to the magnetized tissue, each proton's axis of rotation is flipped into a transverse plane relative to the main magnetic field. A radiofrequency signal is emitted by the hydrogen protons as they lose transverse magnetization and resume longitudinal magnetization, known as T_2 relaxation. This emitted radiofrequency signal generates the image. The T_1 relaxation time reflects the rate of alignment of protons with the main magnetic field, also described as growth of longitudinal relaxation. The T_2 relaxation time reflects the loss of magnetization in the transverse plane.

T_1- and T_2-weighted images are obtained by changing the times of the sending and receiving of radiofrequency pulses during the scan. In T_1-weighted images, white matter is brighter than gray matter. Cerebrospinal fluid (CSF) is brighter than gray matter in T_2-weighted images. Proton density-weighted sequences fall between these tissue brightness parameters (Fig. 10-3).

Among the various standard screening protocols for brain MRI, the most useful include a combination of a T_1-weighted sagittal sequence, a multiecho axial sequence (T_2-weighted and proton density-weighted) and a T_2-weighted coronal sequence. Enhancement of the image can be achieved by use of intravenous gadolinium chelates (Gd-MRI). Imaging the brain in all three standard planes and with varying tissue signal demonstrates the anatomy and pathology to best advantage (Table 10-1).

Major problems can be encountered in patients who

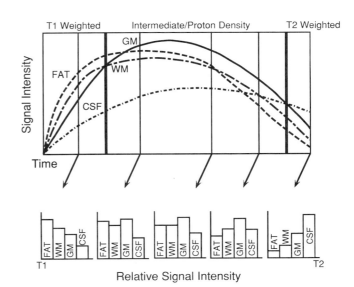

Figure 10-3. Diagram demonstrating the changes that occur in signal intensity with increasing TE and TR used in obtaining spin-echo images. The basic tissues included in the central nervous system are indicated as GM (gray matter), WM (white matter), FAT, and CSF (cerebral spinal fluid). The heavy black vertical line on the left crosses through the point at which white matter and gray matter have the same intensity. Images to the left of this line are called T_1-weighted. The heavy black line on the right crosses the point at which CSF and gray matter have the same intensity. Images to the right of this line are considered T_2-weighted. All images between these lines are considered intermediate-weighted images or proton density images.

cannot cooperate, since the examination is rather lengthy and motion renders the images useless. MRI does not visualize acute hemorrhage well. Some patients who suffer from claustrophobia and certain very ill patients may be unable to undergo this study. The patient must remain motionless for several 5- to 10-minute periods of scanning while hearing repetitive loud knocking noises. Ferromagnetic objects cannot be brought within the magnet's powerful field because they will be pulled into the magnet, potentially damaging the scanner and nearby persons. Patients with cardiac pacemakers, cochlear implants, aneurysm clips, metal foreign bodies in the eye, and certain cardiac valves cannot undergo MRI because of the risk of injury from the force of the magnetic field upon these objects. For those inadvertently studied by MRI, the desired images are usually grossly distorted because the magnetic field is bent by the ferromagnetic object.

Despite its longer acquisition time as compared with CT, MRI offers a number of advantages over CT (Table 10-2), especially in multiplanar imaging, which is easily achieved by MRI but requires repositioning of the gantry and rescanning in the CT technique.

Table 10-1. T₁- Versus T₂-Weighted Magnetic Resonance Imaging

T$_1$-Weighted	T$_2$-Weighted
Yield low signal	Yield markedly low signal
CSF	Cortical bone
Cortical bone	Calcification
Calcification	Air
Air	Deoxyhemoglobin
Edema	Hemosiderin
High flow	High flow
Yield high signal	Yield moderately low signal
Fat	Fat
Methemoglobin	Intracellular
Proteinaceous fluid	methemoglobin
Gadolinium	Yield high signal
enhancement[a]	CSF
	Gliosis
	Edema
	Extracellular
	methemoglobin

[a] Gadolinium enhancement on MRI is normally seen in the circumventricular organs, choroid plexus, intracranial arteries and veins, and dural sinuses. The blood-brain barrier can be disrupted by trauma, infarction, and inflammatory or neoplastic processes. Under these circumstances, contrast can be seen in the area of pathology. Various patterns of enhancement (solid, ring) are seen and correlate with CT patterns.

The gray and white matter differences are better defined by MRI than by CT. The lack of signal from bone gives MRI imaging an advantage over CT for infarcts in the brainstem because the images are not limited by artifacts. Signal void is also characteristic of flowing blood, which moves out of a plane of section before emitting a signal; high-resolution scans that are free of artifact allow inferences regarding vascular patency.

Magnetic Resonance Angiography

Magnetic resonance angiography (MRA) does not require injection of contrast and can be performed at the time of the routine MRI. MRA sequences involve suppression of signal from stationary background tissue and computer postprocessing of the signal emitted by flowing blood within an area of the body. The reconstructed magnetic resonance angiogram can be viewed in any three-dimensional projection. Patient cooperation is essential for MRA. Of MRAs performed at our institution, 10 percent are so severely degraded by motion that they are judged uninterpretable. Consecutive gradient echo slices in which flowing blood is bright are postprocessed by using maximum intensity projection in two-dimensional MRA. In three-dimensional MRA, consecutive three-dimensional volumes or slabs rather than slices are imaged. Time-of-flight techniques maximize the bright signal

of flowing blood on gradient echo images, which is "unsaturated" relative to the stationery tissues, which are "saturated" by multiple radiofrequency pulses. Artifactual signal loss, resulting from regions of turbulence (carotid bulb, carotid siphon) or from in-plane saturation, is well recognized as a result of comparisons with conventional angiography. Two-dimensional and three-dimensional time-of-flight techniques have proved valuable in noninvasive screening for vaso-occlusive disorders in the head and neck. Further refinement of techniques and experience with MRA are needed before it can totally replace catheter angiography.

MRA or plain T$_2$-weighted MRI has proved useful for the diagnosis of diseased arterial walls and of small (cryptic) vascular malformations. MRA is very sensitive for stenosis or occlusion of the cervical carotid arteries, the intracranial carotids and their terminal branches, and major dural sinuses. The extent of occlusive disease can be overestimated, but a negative (normal) cervical or intracranial MRA is highly accurate. MRA is less accurate in the evaluation of aneurysms and arteriovenous malformations. Arterial dissection is well evaluated by MRA and standard T$_1$-weighted MRI scans. MRA has become the diagnostic method of choice for the once uncommon diagnosis of dolichoectasia. Heavily T$_2$-weighted or echogradient sequences are very sensitive to hemosiderin and are useful for the detection of cavernous angiomas.

Angiography

Contrast angiography is indicated to answer questions that cannot be answered using noninvasive tests. Vascular stenosis or occlusion, altered circulation time, collateral circulation, and mass effect are evaluated by angiography. Digital subtraction angiography of the cerebral blood vessels is the preferred modality at this time. In order to approach the accuracy of cut film studies, a 1024 matrix unit is needed.

The modern digital subtraction unit has a number of advantages over conventional angiography. First, the time required for the study is markedly reduced, thereby limiting complications, particularly those related to the site of puncture. Second, contrast dose can be reduced, thereby limiting any potential renal toxicity. Third, with the unit mounted on a C-arm, it is possible to get multiple views without having to manipulate the patient. Fourth, the subtracted image can be viewed immediately after injection, and therefore additional views, if needed, can be obtained at that time. Finally, since only pertinent images are photographed, there is a saving in film cost when performing digital angiography.

Modern nonionic contrast agents should be used, as they are less painful to the patient and cause less nausea and vomiting. The incidence of allergic reac-

Table 10-2. Comparison of MRI and CT in Neurologic Diagnosis

Indications for MRI	Indications for CT
General	General
Iodine allergy	Intracranial aneurysm clips
Renal insufficiency	Cardiac pacemaker
Superior contrast resolution	Uncooperative patient
Subtle enhancement of inflammatory or neoplastic process	
Variety of techniques	
Standard spin-echo for anatomy	
Gradient-echo for flow, hemosiderin	
Fat suppression (FAT SAT) for improved visualization of pathology	
Short tau inversion recovery (STIR)	
Dating of hemorrhage	
Brain	Brain
CT limited by bone artifact	Acute trauma
Posterior fossa disease	Suspected acute intracranial hemorrhage
Brainstem or cerebellar disease	
Intracanalicular acoustic neuromas	
Craniovertebral junction abnormalities	
Extra-axial fluid collections	
Middle fossa disease	
Temporal lobe lesion	
Extra-axial fluid collections	
Disease at the vertex	
High frontoparietal lesions	
Extra-axial fluid collections	
CT limited by periventricular partial volume artifact	Bone detail needed
Demyelinating disease	Osseous temporal bone abnormalities
Multiple sclerosis	Fractures
Progressive multifocal leukoencephalopathy	
Deep white matter infarction	
Radiation vasculitis	
Hydrocephalus	
Elevated pressure, obstructive, or communicating	
Normal pressure	
MRI more sensitive to increased water	Visualization of calcification necessary
Small primary or metastatic tumors	Granulomatous disease
Early lymphoma	Oligodendroglioma and astrocytoma
Early infarction	Meningioma
Early inflammation	Teratoma
MRA for evaluation of	
Aneurysm	
Arteriovenous malformation	
Vaso-occlusive disease	
Ability to image directly in sagittal and coronal planes	
Sellar and parasellar masses	
Lesions adjacent to 3rd ventricle, aqueduct, and 4th ventricle	
Orbit	
Cavernous sinus	
Cranial nerves	
Spine	
Myelopathy	
Syringohydromyelia	
Tumor	
Spinal stenosis	
Infarct	
Multiple sclerosis	
Disc degeneration	
Discitis/osteomyelitis	
Metastasis	
Radiculopathy	
Disc herniation	
Facet joint arthropathy	

(Modified from Bradley, 1986, with permission.)

tions is also reduced with these agents. It is desirable to film some of the pertinent images with bones in place to serve as landmarks for the surgeon and to make these images life-size for use in the operating room.

Plain Radiography

Once the only source of information concerning the nervous system, plain films of the bony skeleton are now a distant fourth behind the more powerful imaging techniques described above. Plain radiographs may reveal evidence of the following conditions: trauma causing fractures; diseases directly involving the bony skull and skeleton, such as infections and primary or metastatic tumors; intracranial and intraspinal disease causing tissue calcification, including some parasitic or chronic infections and some tumors, especially teratomas producing cartilage or bone; and the calcific remnants of some prior hemorrhages, including the rare chronic subdural hemorrhage, aneu-

Table 10-3. Histologic Diagnosis of Brain Tumors by CT

Appearance of Unenhanced CT	Enhancement	Location	Other
Isodense			
Meningioma	Dense, homogeneous rings very rare	Adjacent to dura	Edema variable; often very little but can be extensive
Neuroma	Dense	Cerebellopontine angle	
Some metastases, lymphoma	Dense		
Hypodense			
Glioblastoma	Dense, frequently ring lesions	Deep in hemisphere (white matter)	Edema moderate, can be very large and involve both sides of brain; calcification rare; may have cysts
Metastatic, squamous carcinoma	Moderate to dense, rings less common	Periphery (gray matter)	Extensive edema of white matter; multiple, smaller
Epidermoid	Variable may not enhance	Base of brain and other cisterns	May contain calcifications
Dermoid (fat)	Partial	Base, periventricular	Fat in ventricles
Astrocytoma I & II	None to slight in adults; may be dense in children	Same as glioblastomas	Cerebellum with cysts in children; little edema
Oligodendroglioma	Moderate	Same as Glioblastomas	Dense chunks of calcium
Lipoma (fat)	None	Corpus callosum, quadrigeminal plate	Calcification
Hyperdense			
Pituitary adenoma	Dense, may be homogeneous or patchy	Sella area	Calcification rare
Craniopharyngioma	May be dense	Sella area	Calcification rare
Metastatic Adenocarcinoma	Moderate to dense, rings	Periphery of brain	May have extensive edema of white matter; multiple
Melanoma	Dense, homogeneous	Peripheral	Multiple, no edema unless large
Meningioma with calcification			
Lymphoma, leukemia	Dense, homogeneous	Dural surface	CNS positive
Medulloblastoma	Moderate to dense	Vermis	
Ependymoma	Variable density and enhancement	Calcified intraventricular tumor in children under 15	

rysm, or arteriovenous malformation. Generations of trainees measured the midline coronal position of the pineal body in cases in which it was calcified, hoping to infer from its displacement the presence of a unilateral intracranial mass. For most of the medical world, plain radiography has given way first to CT scanning and most lately to MRI and functional imaging (see Chs. 14 and 15). Pneumoencephalography, the once popular but technically difficult technique of instilling air in the subarachnoid space and following its course through the ventricular and subarachnoid spaces to seek evidence of obstruction, atrophy, or masses, has now been abandoned in most centers. Conventional angiography is being challenged by digital subtraction techniques and by entirely noninvasive techniques such as MRA and Doppler ultrasonography (see Ch. 13).

Comparison of Computed Tomography and Magnetic Resonance Imaging

CT still holds an advantage over MRI for rapid evaluation, which plays an important role in confused or agitated patients (see above) and in patients with ferromagnetic implants (clips, pacemakers) or who are surrounded by ferromagnetic equipment (respirators, stereotaxic frames, braces), and is superior to MRI in imaging acute hematomas. MRI has proved more sensitive than CT for posterior and middle fossa disease because it is free of the bony artifacts that hinder CT studies. Also because of bony artifacts on CT, MRI is also more useful for lesions on the brain surface facing the inner wall of the skull. MRI has also proved more sensitive than CT for assessment of diseases of the periventricular region, particularly multiple sclerosis, periventricular edema from hydrocephalus, and deep white matter infarcts. The multiplanar quality of MRI allows sagittal plane images whose advantages have greatly improved assessment of midline disorders, among them lesions of the third ventricle and the craniovertebral junction and cavitary lesions of the spinal cord. (See Table 10-2 for CT versus MRI comparisons).

Computed Tomography Scan

Hyperdense lesions, single or multiple, may be caused by parenchymatous hemorrhage; metastases from adenocarcinoma, melanoma, and choriocarcinoma; calcified meningioma; calcifications in aneurysms or arteriovenous malformations; or hemorrhage into primary tumors, chief among which are glioblastoma multiforme and oligodendroglioma. Hemorrhage may also occur in the sella turcica from a pituitary adenoma. Subarachnoid hemorrhage is rather transient and may not appear at all unless particularly dense.

Low-density lesions have an even larger number of sources. Leading among them are infarcts more than 1 week old, tumors, and old and recent foci of inflammation or of demyelination. Contrast is often used with CT to differentiate lesions that enhance from those that do not. Low-density lesions that show failure of contrast enhancement include very old infarctions, plaques of multiple sclerosis, progressive multifocal leukoencephalopathy, Behçet's disease, and some cases of toxoplasmosis.

Contrast enhancement is a feature of both primary and metastatic neoplasms, inflammations including granulomas, and very large acute plaques of multiple sclerosis. Ring enhancement (enhancement on the rim of a lesion, shaped more or less like a ring or an oval) is not the specific sign it was once considered to be and has been seen in gliomas, resolving infarction, resolving hemorrhage, and abscess. Contrast enhancement in the subarachnoid space occurs in meningitis and in meningeal spread of neoplasms. Radiographic characteristics of CT have been used to distinguish various tumor types (Table 10-3).

APPLICATIONS OF IMAGING

Acute Ischemic Stroke

Because of its rapidity, the imaging study of choice in acute stroke is CT, usually without contrast enhancement. The earliest sign, when present, is the hyperdense stem of the middle cerebral artery (Fig. 10-4). This finding represents the high-density sign of the blood making up the compacted embolus lodged in the stem of the middle cerebral artery, which appears as an area of focal hyperdensity and can precede parenchymal changes. Contrast enhancement can be helpful in confirming or ruling out this possibility if intracranial thrombolysis is being considered. There is a limited time frame for visualizing the clot. In many cases the mass is not dense enough to be imaged, and even when present early, the clot may later fragment and migrate distally.

Ischemic (Bland) Infarction

The essential finding that suggests infarction is of low density (reduced x-ray attenuation) involving both gray and white matter and occurring in a specific arterial distribution without significant mass effect. The earliest sign of ischemia is a subtle indication of edema. A well-known example is the disappearance of the insular ribbon (Fig. 10-5). The gray matter along the surface of the insula is of higher density than the underlying white matter and normally can be seen distinctly. When this area is involved by infarction, the decrease in tissue density caused by the edema makes the insular ribbon disappear, a finding

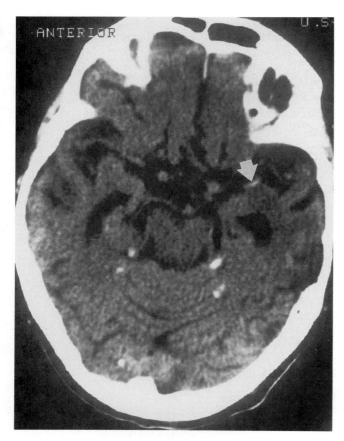

Figure 10-4. This CT section shows a hyperdense area in the left middle cerebral artery *(arrow)*. This represents a clot lodged within the lumen of the artery.

that has been reported as early as 6 hours postictus. By about 24 hours, or even earlier in large infarcts, generalized swelling of the hemisphere may occur, causing effacement of the affected cortical sulci. A mass effect reflecting the edema is at its height around the third day and is best seen by comparing the symmetry of the two sides.

MRI is very sensitive to the presence of water in an acute infarction and is superior to CT in this setting when the patient can be still enough for good-quality images to be obtained. Abnormally increased (high) signal has been seen on proton density and T_2-weighted images at 2 to 4 hours in animal models and as early as 3 hours in clinical studies. Loss of the normal flow void within a vessel indicates either slow flow or occlusion.

In the later stages of ischemic stroke, usually beginning about the seventh day, a gyriform enhancement on CT may be seen following administration of intravenous iodinated compounds (contrast agents) (Fig. 10-6). Enhancement of an infarct has no prognostic significance and simply reflects breakdown of the

blood-brain barrier and reperfusion. Occasionally contrast enhancement may show intravascular occlusion associated with the stroke.

Days to weeks later, areas of low density are seen on CT, and they appear as high-intensity signals on T_2-weighted MRI. They increase in size and frequently show no significant mass effect unless the area of ischemia is very large. As the ischemic stroke ages further, the areas of low density become more apparent and any mass effect resolves. The gradual cavitation of the lesion is reflected in the low-intensity signal that gradually emerges in T_1-weighted MRI, a reliable sign of old infarction. After weeks or months, if the loss of brain tissue is large enough, both CT and MRI may show enlargement of the ipsilateral ventricles and subarachnoid spaces, replacing the missing brain tissue volume with fluid. In cases in which the infarction is large and affects the motor pathways, it may be possible to see atrophy of a cerebral peduncle and corticospinal pathway well down into the pons due to wallerian degeneration, a finding more easily seen on MRI than on CT (Fig. 10-7). Very old infarcts may eventually calcify, occasionally producing gyriform calcification.

Hemorrhagic Infarction

In some cases of infarction, the evolution of the lesion includes a hemorrhagic phase. Classically, its occurrence was taken to be a sign of reperfusion following lysis and distal migration of an embolus, the original occlusion having allowed enough damage to the vascular intima to make it susceptible to diapedesis. It has also been seen in patients with infarction due to vasospasm (Fig. 10-8) and has been documented in the vessel distal to a persisting occlusion, where it occurred as a sign of retrograde collateral circulation. These observations provide exceptions to the older rules that hemorrhagic infarction is a sign of embolism per se and of recanalization after embolism. Heparin therapy has been considered a factor in conversion of infarcts to a hemorrhagic state, but the size of the lesion may be even more important.

The pathologic basis of hemorrhagic infarction is the diapedesis of red blood cells through damaged capillary walls. This hemorrhagic transformation of the infarct is not a frank parenchymatous hematoma. Hemorrhagic infarcts characteristically show patchy collections of blood rather than a large homogeneous area of increased density as seen with a hematoma. They will be in a single arterial distribution and frequently have minimal mass effect associated with them when compared with a true hematoma from arterial bleeding. The degree of diapedesis varies greatly in its intensity. When it is slight, the high density of the red blood cells, averaged with the low density of the

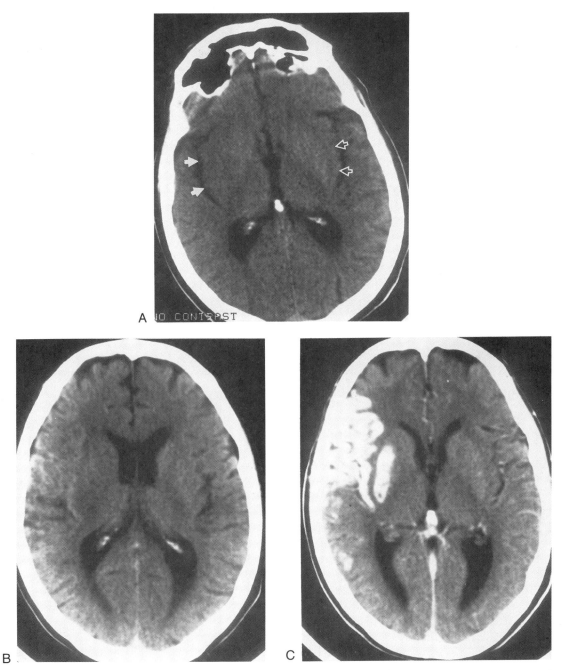

Figure 10-5. (**A**) Axial CT section demonstrates the earliest CT finding in middle cerebral artery stroke. The open arrows point to the slightly hyperdense gray matter layer over the surface of the insula on the patient's left, the normal insular ribbon. The closed arrows point to the absent insular ribbon on the patient's right. The cytotoxic edema in the gray matter has decreased its CT density so that it is now the same as the density of the underlying white matter. Low density also extends into the basal ganglia medial to this. (**B**) A similar section now shows slightly increased density in the region of the infarct so that the abnormal insular ribbon is somewhat brighter than the normal insular ribbon. This is due to reperfusion and release of blood into the infarct from blood vessels damaged by ischemia. Note that the right frontal horn is slightly smaller than the left, indicating some minimal mass effect due to the early edema seen with infarction. (**C**) Following contrast injection, gyriform enhancement is noted in the middle cerebral artery distribution and extends into the lateral portion of the basal ganglia medial to the insula. The hemorrhagic phase and enhancement indicate reperfusion.

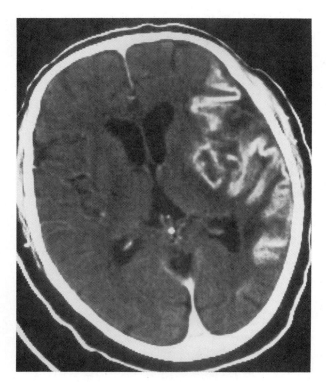

Figure 10-6. An enhanced scan shows extensive gyriform enhancement in the infarct.

edematous parenchyma, may cause the CT lesion to appear isodense with normal brain, so that the infarct is said to "disappear" temporarily on CT. Isodense infarction is usually observed around 10 to 14 days.

Venous Infarction

Venous infarction, as compared with infarction caused by arterial occlusion, has a similar appearance but typically does not show a topography explained by a specific arterial distribution (Fig. 10-9). A clinical history of postpartum state or meningitis is helpful in making this diagnosis. The diagnosis is more secure when thrombus is seen in cortical veins or a dural sinus.

Approach to Acute Infarction

Most ischemic infarcts are embolic. Since there are now techniques for lysing these emboli, it is important that not only their destination but their source be diagnosed early before permanent and massive brain damage can occur. If thrombolysis or angioplasty is to be considered, workup of the stroke, including angiography, must take place within the first 3 hours. Although the heart is the most likely source of emboli, they may originate from plaques in the carotid artery, which may be contributing to the ischemic process by nar-

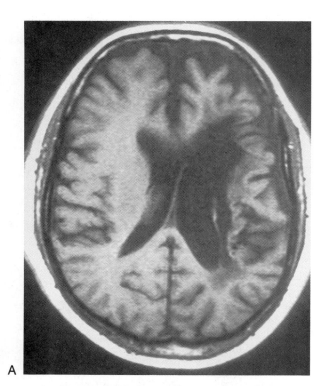

A

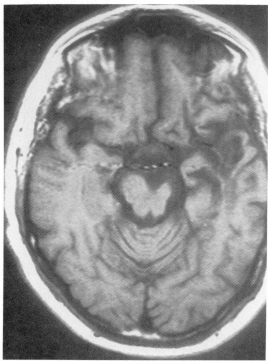

B

Figure 10-7. **(A)** T₁-weighted MRI section shows low intensity deep in the left hemisphere with enlargement of the left lateral ventricle and of the subarachnoid space over the hemisphere, indicating that this infarction is old. **(B)** A lower section through the midbrain shows marked decrease in size of the left cerebral peduncle due to wallerian degeneration. The wallerian changes can begin to show in the peduncle at about 6 weeks postinfarction.

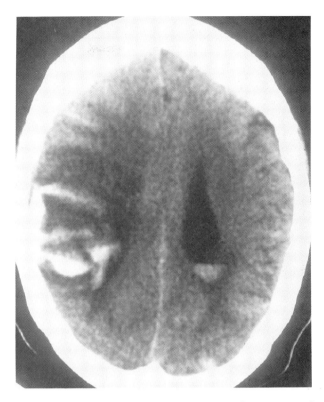

Figure 10-8. Nonenhanced CT section shows a patchy hemorrhage and low density throughout most of the middle cerebral artery distribution and a hemorrhagic infarct secondary to vasospasm induced by a ruptured aneurysm. Blood is also seen pooled in the posterior horn of the opposite lateral ventricle.

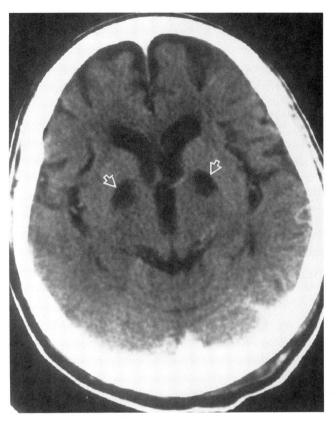

Figure 10-10. Low-density areas of the globus pallidus bilaterally represent symmetrical basal ganglia infarcts (arrows). These may be one manifestation of global ischemia.

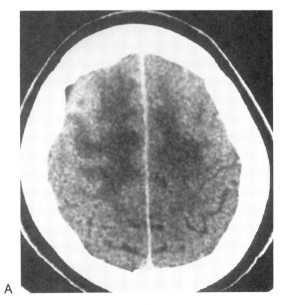

A

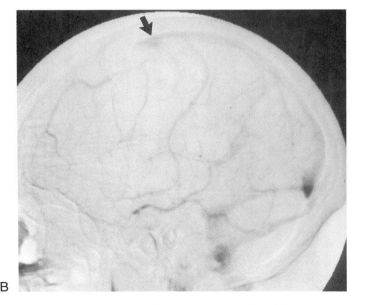

B

Figure 10-9. (A) This 16-year-old postpartum girl developed severe headache 2 days after delivery. CT scan shows a low-density area in the frontoparietal regions. **(B)** The venous phase of a carotid arteriogram in the same patient shows obliteration of the superior sagittal sinus (arrow) anterior to its midpoint.

rowing the lumen of the artery. Usually, patients with ulcerated plaques in the carotid artery, which are showering emboli into the brain, are not operated on acutely. A significant stenotic lesion may be amenable to emergency catheter angioplasty, however, if it is contributing to the problem. Occasionally an acute carotid dissection will be detected, which can be treated surgically before massive brain injury occurs. Carotid dissection is often suggested by other clinical findings such as a history of neck trauma, sudden onset of neck pain, and Horner's syndrome. Digital angiography is the best and most reliable test to examine the vessels from the aortic arch to the brain. They can also be studied with ultrasound, MRA, and spiral CT angiography. Other causes for stroke such as vasculitis and vasospasm can be diagnosed by cerebral angiography.

Hypoxemia or Hypotension

Certain situations will produce infarction outside the typical arterial distributions. Cardiorespiratory arrest or suffocation with the associated hypotension may produce symmetrical infarcts in the basal ganglia, usually straddling the putamen and globus pallidus (Fig. 10-10). Predisposing factors for infarcts in this area are that the blood supply is by small end-arteries and that the metabolic rate in this area is particularly high.

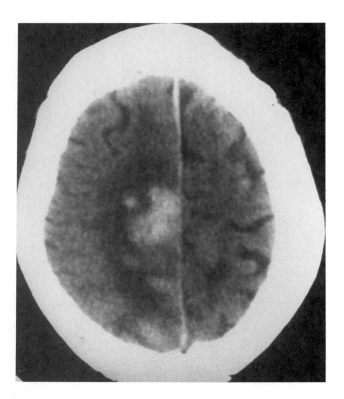

Figure 10-12. A single CT image shows an area of hemorrhage along the falx near the vertex in an elderly patient with amyloid angiopathy. The sulci are poorly seen on the right owing to effacement by the associated infarct as well as to subarachnoid hemorrhage causing the sulci to become isodense with brain.

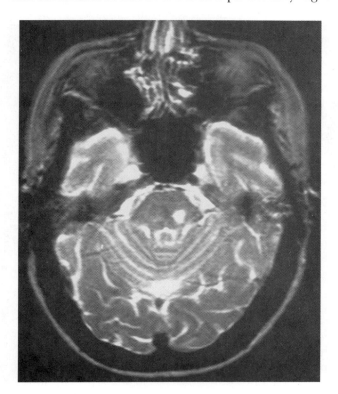

Figure 10-11. T$_2$-weighted MRI scan shows an area of high signal intensity in the left aspect of the pons, representing a lacunar infarct. These can be very difficult to see on CT.

Over the convexity, hypotension may cause socalled watershed infarcts, involving the border zone of anastomoses between two major cerebral arterial territories (see also Ch. 35). In these cases blood pressure is not adequate to supply oxygenated blood to areas in which two arterial distributions overlap, and infarction affects the border zone and contiguous distal branch territories of the arteries involved.

Small, deep, lacunar infarcts occur in the distribution of small perforating arteries, caused either by emboli or thrombi. In these cases the individual arteries have no sources of collateral circulation, and infarction is likely to affect the entire tiny arterial territory at risk (Fig. 10-11).

Ischemic infarcts may also occur in the cerebral gray matter and centrum semiovale in amyloid angiopathy. Because of amyloid deposits in the vessel wall, the weakened arterial wall may be occluded with infarction or may give way, allowing local lobar hemorrhage, with the superficial location allowing blood to escape into the subarachnoid space. Amyloid angiopathy is encountered most often in the elderly but can also occur in younger people on a familial basis (Fig. 10-12).

Another form of microvascular disease is angiopathic periventricular leukomalacia, also known as subcortical arteriosclerotic encephalopathy, a condition overlapping with Binswanger's disease. There is increasing incidence with age. The process involves the vascular system of the centrum semiovale. The most common clinical correlate is hypertension (Fig. 10-13).

Severe global ischemia will produce acute cytotoxic edema of the entire cerebrum, frequently preserving the cerebellum. In this case the CT changes include loss of gray-white discrimination, producing a "ground glass" appearance of the brain. The lateral ventricles will appear squeezed or pinched. In older patients the ventricles have been referred to as *"super ventricles,"* since they are smaller than normal (Fig. 10-14). This is the CT equivalent of brain death. As a result of the high intracranial pressure from the infarcted brain, arteriography typically shows no intracranial flow from the internal carotid artery, although the posterior fossa circulation may be preserved.

Transient Ischemic Attacks

Occasionally changes are seen on CT or MRI associated with one or more transient ischemic attacks. These changes consist of enhancement due to break-

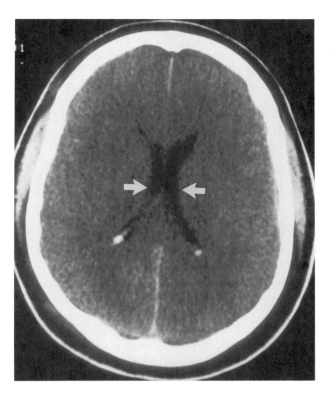

Figure 10-14. CT section at the level of the bodies of the lateral ventricles shows the squeezed or pinched appearance *(arrows)* produced by the symmetrical mass effect of the cytotoxic edema. Note there is no gray-white discrimination. This appearance is the CT equivalent of brain death.

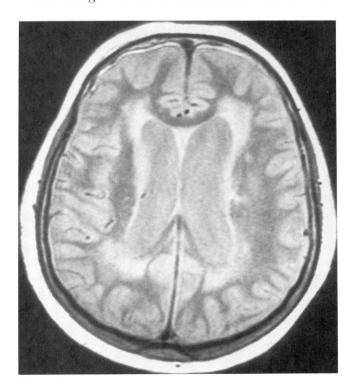

Figure 10-13. Proton density axial spin-echo image shows the hyperintensity in the periventricular region consistent with angiopathic periventricular leukomalacia.

down of the blood-brain barrier and associated edema. Even though the clinical syndrome has been brief enough to allow a clinical diagnosis of transient ischemic attack, the findings indicate some brain injury, even if transient, and have caused considerable reassessment of what is meant by the term *transient*.

Subarachnoid Hemorrhage

In general neuroradiologic practice, the most common cause of subarachnoid hemorrhage seen on CT is probably trauma (see below), the second most common in adults being ruptured intracranial aneurysm.

Aneurysmal hemorrhage into the subarachnoid space can be seen very early on CT but may be missed on MRI because magnetic resonance signal changes in acute hemorrhage are nonspecific. The majority of intracranial aneurysms occur in the area of the circle of Willis, where the associated mass of clotted blood in the dome of the aneurysm may allow the lesion to be imaged by MRI but less often by CT. In the phase of acute rupture, the blood is widely dispersed and is seen most often in the suprasellar cistern (Fig. 10-15).

Judging from the literature, a success rate of 95 per-

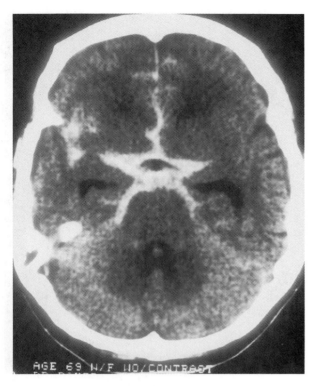

Figure 10-15. CT section without contrast shows higher-density material filling the suprasellar cistern, the anterior interhemispheric fissure, the right sylvian fissure, and the pontine and ambient cisterns. This is a fairly typical subarachnoid hemorrhage from a ruptured aneurysm. Note the bilaterally dilated temporal horns, indicating early hydrocephalus.

cent in localizing a bleeding aneurysm has been achieved by CT. Very rarely, more than one aneurysm will bleed at the same time, a finding encouraging confidence that the site of the hemorrhagic mass is the aneurysm that just ruptured.

Frequently more blood is localized in the specific region of the aneurysm, giving an indication of where the bleed has occurred. Blood in the septum pellucidum (i.e., cephalad to the third ventricle) is characteristic of anterior communicating artery aneurysms, since their location favors rupture into the overlying floor of the third ventricle. Large amounts of blood in one sylvian fissure is commonly a sign of an ipsilateral middle cerebral artery aneurysm. Hemorrhage located in the subarachnoid space of the posterior fossa is most commonly due to aneurysm of the posterior inferior cerebellar artery (Fig. 10-16). Subarachnoid hemorrhage located peripherally in the middle or anterior cerebral artery distribution should make one suspect mycotic aneurysm, which can be due to either septic or tumor emboli (Fig. 10-17). Peripheral parenchymal hemorrhage may be due to an arteriovenous malformation (Fig. 10-18). Enhanced CT and Gd-

MRI are both sensitive to arteriovenous malformations. Their chance of rebleeding acutely is less than that of aneurysms, and therefore there is more time for appropriate workup.

Atherosclerotic aneurysms occur in the intracranial carotid artery and in the basilar artery but rarely bleed. Rupture of an atherosclerotic aneurysm in the cavernous portion of the carotid artery may produce a carotid-cavernous fistula. Venous angiomas are occasionally seen coincidentally on CT, MRI, and angiography but rarely bleed.

Parenchymatous Hemorrhage

On CT an acute parenchymatous hemorrhage features a high-density appearance, which persists for at least a week, making CT a reliable method of differentiating the low-attenuation lesion typical of bland infarction from the high-attenuation lesion due to hematoma or grossly hemorrhagic infarction. The high signal of the fresh blood is lost over days to weeks owing to chemical change of the blood, which causes the CT appearance to evolve from its initial hyperdensity to an isodense (subacute) phase to hypodensity in the chronic state. Contrast administration during the subacute phase may result in ring enhancement around the hemorrhage, a pattern different from the gyral enhancement typical of infarction. In the chronic state, a hematoma is usually reduced to a slit-like cavity, and many disappear entirely into isodense tissue.

The MRI appearance of parenchymal hemorrhage varies with the age of the hemorrhage and the form of hemoglobin present. Hyperacute hemorrhage (within hours) appears *iso*intense on T_1- and T_2-weighted images. Acute hemorrhage (1 to 2 days) is T_2-*hypo*intense on high field strength scanners owing to the paramagnetic properties of deoxyhemoglobin. Early subacute hemorrhage (3 days) is *hyper*intense on T_1 owing to the paramagnetic properties of intracellular methemoglobin. Later subacute hemorrhage is *hyper*intense on both T_1 and T_2 because of the presence of extracellular methemoglobin. Hemosiderin will be seen months to years after hemorrhage, appearing *hypo*intense on T_2-weighted images.

The localization of these hematomas correlates best with the frequency and distribution of microvascular changes in brain vessels associated with chronic hypertension (see Ch. 36). The most common sites of hypertensive hemorrhage in the brain are the basal ganglia (especially the putamen), thalamus, cerebral lobes, pons, and cerebellum. Other causes are vascular malformations, coagulopathies, and amyloid angiopathy in the elderly patient.

Many of the deep hemorrhages bleed enough to accumulate a mass large enough to enter the ventricles. When the amount of ventricular blood is large,

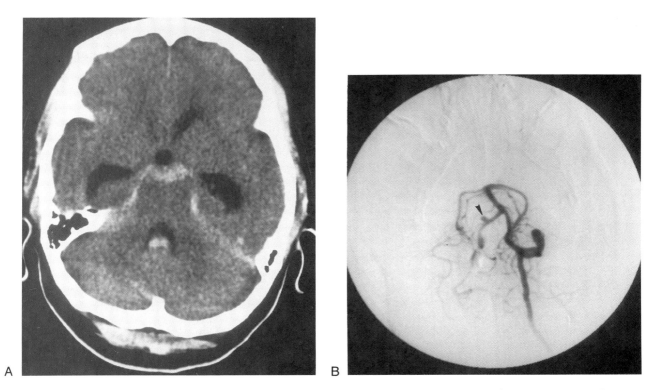

Figure 10-16. **(A)** This CT scan shows blood in the fourth ventricle and in the pontine cistern from a subarachnoid hemorrhage. The temporal horns are markedly dilated, indicating hydrocephalus. The subarachnoid hemorrhage is primarily confined to the posterior fossa. **(B)** Cerebral angiography was performed and demonstrated one small aneurysm on the right vertebral artery *(arrowhead)*.

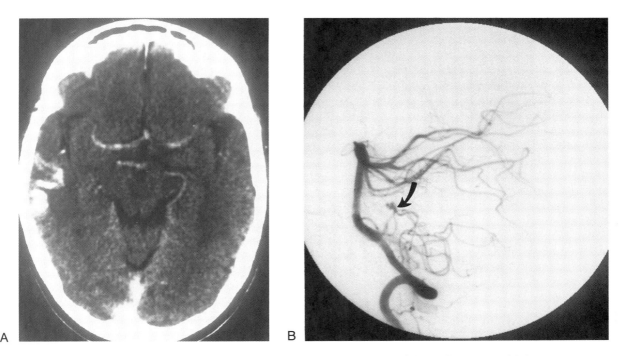

Figure 10-17. **(A)** An area of increased density on the surface of the right temporal lobe represents some hemorrhage. **(B)** An angiogram shows a mycotic aneurysm on the cranial loop of the posterior inferior cerebellar artery *(arrow)*.

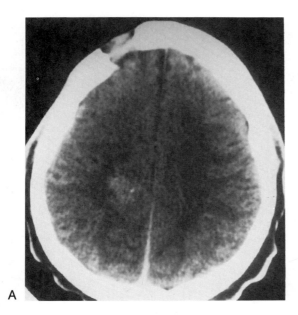
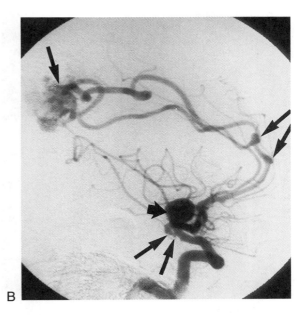

Figure 10-18. **(A)** CT section shows a small area of hemorrhage in the right parasagittal region due to an arteriovenous malformation. **(B)** Angiogram shows the arteriovenous malformation being supplied by the pericallosal and callosomarginal arteries. Proximal to the arteriovenous malformation are aneurysms *(arrows)* involving the anterior choroidal, posterior communicating, internal carotid, pericallosal, and callosomarginal arteries. In patients with an intracranial aneurysm, the incidence of a second aneurysm is 20 percent. Therefore, arteriography for aneurysms must include all the intracranial vessels. Aneurysms commonly occur proximal to arteriovenous malformations since the increased flow is probably conducive to aneurysm formation.

it may produce a noncommunicating hydrocephalus. Subarachnoid blood associated with any of these lesions may produce a communicating hydrocephalus, which is usually transient as the blood clears from the spinal fluid.

Occasionally what appears to be a stroke is an acute hemorrhage into a tumor (Fig. 10-19). In this situation, both enhanced CT and Gd-MRI are required to settle the diagnosis, the latter study often being more definitive. The Gd-MRI is frequently easier to interpret, since on CT the acute hemorrhage may obscure enhancement.

Before CT, only those patients with large hematomas causing distinctive clinical pictures were reliably diagnosed premortem. Small hypertensive hemorrhages in the lentiform nucleus and thalamus and small lobar hemorrhages still provide diagnostic dilemmas and make clinicians wary of the use of anticoagulants to treat presumed embolic stroke unless brain imaging is available to rule out small hematoma.

Trauma

See Chapter 6, for a detailed discussion of trauma.

Contusion

The sensitivity of the MRI to small lesions and the persistence of hemosiderin on the brain surface after compression of the crowns of gyri against the inner

wall of the skull permit the diagnosis by MRI of acute and chronic cerebral contusions that are usually not intense enough to be imaged on CT. Atrophy that occurs later is usually too mild to cause major changes, but in the larger lesions the missing gyral crowns and subcortical atrophy of the pathways projecting to and from the injured zone may produce local thinning of the underlying white matter, reflected in low attenuation on CT or high signal intensity on T$_2$-weighted MRI.

Subarachnoid Hemorrhage

Subarachnoid hemorrhage due to trauma is usually localized in the actual area of trauma. It is usually venous and therefore not widespread as is the arterial bleeds due to aneurysms. So-called nonaneurysmal subarachnoid hemorrhage is attributed to rupture of small veins and is not widely dispersed as with arterial hemorrhage. A characteristic pattern is hemorrhage in the posterior portion of the suprasellar cistern without hemorrhage in the anterior portion.

Subdural and Epidural Hematomas

These subdural and epidural hematomas are common lesions, which can produce focal neurologic deficits and mimic strokes. Epidural hemorrhages are a threat to life because their usual cause is arterial bleeding

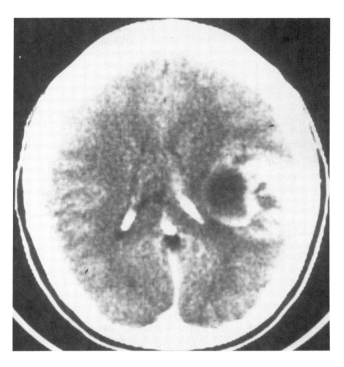

Figure 10-19. An enhanced CT section shows a mixed-density lesion in the left parietal area with high density peripherally, which is compatible with hemorrhage. Extensive enhancement shows the mixed cystic and solid glioblastoma.

striction of the ventricles. With a unilateral subdural hemorrhage, shift of the midline structures and compression of one ventricle are demonstrated.

Over time, there is dilution of the hemoglobin degradation products, leaving a subdural fluid collection with signal changes determined more by the protein and CSF content than by the hemoglobin moiety.

Tumors

Initially, there was hope that the properties of different tumors would result in tumor-specific imaging by specific pulse sequences. This hope has dimmed in the face of difficulties in distinguishing among the tumor, edema, necrosis, and hemorrhage, usually occurring together in the same lesion. (See also Chs. 51 to 58.)

Gliomas

MRI is more sensitive than CT for the diagnosis of a brain tumor. The use of contrast CT or Gd-MRI is the preferred method if the plain images are not abnormal. A glioma typically appears as a low-density, contrast-enhancing mass lesion with low density (edema) extending throughout the adjacent white matter on CT and as a hyperintense mass on T_2-weighted MRI. Plain and even contrast-enhanced CT may be negative in low-grade gliomas, especially those presenting clinically as isolated seizures. Malignant transformation of low-grade tumors is suggested by

from disruption of the middle meningeal artery, a disruption not reliably arrested by local tamponade. Subdural hemorrhages usually arise from bleeding from veins bridging the skull and brain surface and may be self-limiting. Anticoagulant therapy is among the causes. Although subdural hemorrhages are usually caused by some form of head trauma, the patient may or may not recall any such events. Occasionally aneurysms will bleed directly into the subdural space, producing a subdural hematoma and presenting an immediate surgical emergency due to the mass effect (Fig. 10-20).

Subdural hematomas are commonly first seen clinically when they have reached the subacute stage, when they may be isodense to brain on CT and difficult to see if the hematoma is bilateral. When subacute, they are easily seen on MRI as T_1- and T_2-hyperintense subdural fluid collections. Because the dura lacks a blood-brain barrier, residual hemosiderin deposits will not be seen after subdural hemorrhage. In the early subacute phase, subdural hematomas will be T_1- hyperintense owing to intracellular methemoglobin. With bilateral subdural hematomas, the CT or MRI changes in the brain that are separate from the subdural collection consist of effacement of cortical sulci and con-

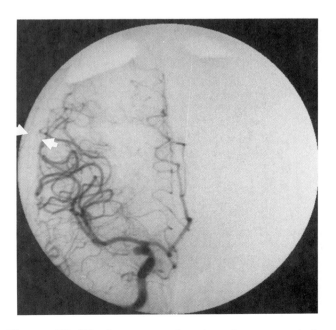

Figure 10-20. Anteroposterior view shows a posterior communicating artery aneurysm and in addition shows displacement of the vessels from the inner table of the skull by the subdural hematoma *(arrows)*.

the development of enhancement on subsequent images. Contrast CT or Gd-MRI may show a ring-enhancing lesion with glioma, but this finding is also known to occur late after hematoma and with metastatic tumor and abscess.

Pilocytic astrocytomas often have a cystic component visible on imaging and tend to show prominent enhancement on both CT and Gd-MRI. Occasionally, a mural nodule associated with a cyst is found on enhanced scan.

Meningiomas

Most *intracranial* meningiomas have an isodense or isointense appearance on unenhanced CT or T_1-weighted MRI images. The superficial location and the hyperostosis of the adjacent bone help with the diagnosis. Some meningiomas also show calcification, which is best appreciated on CT. After contrast CT or Gd-MRI, prominent, diffuse enhancement is typically seen. The suppression of bone images typical of MRI make this technique best for imaging *spinal* meningiomas, which appear as contrast-enhancing intradural extramedullary lesions.

Lymphoma

Diffuse, prominent enhancement on CT or Gd-MRI is characteristic for almost all lymphomas, a finding not alone sufficient for diagnosis. Thallium single-proton emission CT (SPECT) scans may be helpful in differentiating lymphoma from infection in acquired immunodeficiency syndrome (AIDS) patients.

Metastases

Where available, Gd-MRI is preferred to contrast CT, but both usually show a ring-enhancing lesion surrounded by edema extending into the adjacent white matter. Although a few gliomas are multicentric, multiple foci constitute a strong indicator of metastases. The majority of metastases are found along the arterial border zones: high frontal convexity, high parietal region, lateral occipital lobe, inferolateral temporal lobe, precuneus on the medial surface of the hemisphere, and posterior margin of the cerebellum. Few involve the corpus callosum, basal ganglia, pons, medulla, or spinal cord itself. Few exhibit the tendency to cross midline structures, a common property of gliomas. In contrast to most meningiomas, metastases only rarely are calcified, but this appearance can develop following radiotherapy. Spinal epidural metastases are usually diagnosed by Gd-MRI, where available, myelography being now largely replaced by MRI.

Acoustic Neurinoma

The great difficulty in imaging acoustic neurinoma by CT when it is still small has now been minimized by Gd-MRI, which usually shows the enhancing mass. CT scan, even with contrast enhancement, suffers the artifacts of adjacent bone and patient movement and presents difficulty in imaging the lesion even with contrast enhancement.

Pituitary Tumors

As with acoustic neurinomas, imaging of pituitary lesions is no longer a difficult diagnostic problem. The anatomy of the gland, chiasm and optic nerve, adjacent carotid arteries, and the cavernous sinus are all well seen with MRI, and the distinct appearance of microadenomas separates them from the adjacent healthy tissues.

Ependymomas

Gd-MRI identifies many ependymomas, which are small lesions, but the diagnosis remains difficult. Contrast CT is less successful.

Leptomeningeal Cancer

Imaging has limited value in the setting of leptomeningeal cancer but may demonstrate subarachnoid nodules from "dropped" metastases in Gd-MRI scans. Myelography has a role when MRI is not available.

Hydrocephalus

MRI detects the smaller causes of obstructions in the CSF pathway better than does CT. The sagittal view, easily imaged by MRI, shows a bulging of the anterior inferior third ventricle in hydrocephalus that is not found in atrophy and thus helps in separating ventricular enlargement in the two conditions. Pulsation studies of the CSF through ventricular pathways have created a new means of assessing the sites of obstruction. (See also Ch. 59.)

Infection

(See also Chs. 39 to 50 for detailed discussion of the neurologic aspects of infectious diseases.)

Bacterial Infection

Modern imaging techniques (MRI and CT scanning) have greatly facilitated diagnosis (see Ch. 39) of the inflamed cerebrum but have not yet permitted differential diagnosis of cerebritis, unorganized abscess, primary or metastatic malignancies, and even some cases of acute infarction. When well established, cerebritis shows as a homogeneous area of contrast enhancement. Likewise, well developed abscesses show a thin, uniform capsule on enhanced scan, a ring enhancement picture resembling that of metastasis. Meningitis from any cause generally causes a diffuse CT-enhanced appearance of the meninges, especially in the posterior fossa, where meningeal infiltrates are most heavily concentrated.

Granulomatous Infection

Most foci of granulomatous infections are seen on Gd-MRI. Individual tuberculomas have even been detected.

Parasitic Infections

In schistosomiasis, CT or myelography may detect the thickened and nodular lower spinal cord and conus from the presence of the organisms (see Ch. 44). In acute transverse myelitis, CT myelography is usually normal and even Gd-MRI shows a myelitis whose features are not diagnostic of the infection. Trypanosomiasis has been reported to show contrast-enhancing CT lesion(s) with edema, resembling tumor (see Ch. 45).

Behçet's Disease

Behçet's disease features small, high-intensity T_2-weighted MRI or contrast-enhancing CT lesions resembling infarction, clustered in the brainstem and thalamic regions (see Ch. 66).

Demyelinating Diseases

It was at first uncertain if Gd-MRI would document the lesions of multiple sclerosis, but it has become apparent that 75 percent of clinically symptomatic patients show lesions by Gd-MRI, and the number and areas of Gd enhancement correlate with the clinical progression of the disease. (See also Chs. 73 and 74.)

Degenerative Disease

See Chapters 60, 61, 75, 76, and 77 for detailed discussions of Alzheimer's disease, other dementing degenerative diseases, and movement disorders.

Atrophy

No definite diagnosis has yet been established to diagnose the brain atrophy of Alzheimer's disease as distinct from that due to other causes, including acute dehydration, nutritional deficiency, alcoholism, steroid use, and renal disease, and from that found in the neurologically normal elderly, all of which share signs of widening of the cerebral sulci and enlargement of the ventricles. Alzheimer disease has some correlation with increased size of the ventricles, especially the third ventricle, and some emphasis has been laid on the reduced size of the medial temporal lobe in Alzheimer patients under age 65. MRI has demonstrated the same findings, with higher frequency of atrophy of the amygdala and hippocampus.

Parkinson's Disease

Shrinkage of the midbrain is a feature of Parkinson's disease. When brainstem and cerebellar atrophy is seen, the diagnosis of Parkinson's disease can be considered in doubt.

Huntington's Disease

The flattening of the head of the caudate, well known to pathologists, can be seen on CT and MRI, sometimes in advance of the clinical signs that make the diagnosis of Huntington's disease obvious.

Wilson's Disease

The increased copper deposition in the putamen and globus pallidus in Wilson's disease has been reported as decreased signal intensity in some cases studied by T_2-weighted MRI.

Metabolic

In *hepatic* disturbances, T_1-weighted MRI has been reported to show increased signal intensities in the basal ganglia. In renal metabolic disorders, CT or MRI may show signs of edema. (See also Chs. 67 to 72.)

Congenital Deformities and Dysraphic States

MRI has revolutionized the ease of detection of dysraphic states including spina bifida and cavitary lesions, prominent among them being syringomyelia. Plain T_2-weighted usually suffices. Flow dynamics of the spinal fluid with parenchymatous cavities can be appreciated. (See also Chs. 31, 32, and 65.)

ANNOTATED BIBLIOGRAPHY

Bradley WG Jr. MR appearance of hemorrhage in the brain. Radiology 1993;189:15–26.

Bradley WG Jr. Magnetic resonance imaging in the central nervous system: comparison with computed tomography. p. 81. In Kressel H (ed). Magnetic Resonance Annual. Raven Press, New York, 1986.

The characteristics vary over time.

Breningstall GN, Marker SM, Tubman DE. Hydrosyringomyelia and diastematomyelia detected by MRI in myelomeningocele. Pediatr Neurol 1992;8:267–71.

Easily imaged by MRI.

Damasio H. A computed tomographic guide to the identification of cerebral vascular territories. Arch Neurol 1985; 40:138–42.

The standard.

De Coene B, Hajnal JV, Pennock JM, Bydder GM. MRI of the brain stem using fluid attenuated inversion recovery pulse sequences. Neuroradiology 1993;35:327–31.

Fine details of anatomy in normal subjects is possible with modern MRI.

Donauer E, Rascher K. Syringomyelia: a brief review of ontogenetic, experimental and clinical aspects. Neurosurg Rev 1993;16:7–13.

MRI diagnoses syrinx and other dysraphic states.

Hugg JW, Matson GB, Twieg DB et al. Phosphorus 31 MR spectroscopic imaging (MRSI) of normal and pathological human brains. Magn Reson Imaging 1992;10: 227–43.

New developments. The ^{31}P magnetic resonance spectroscopic imaging (MRSI) technique shows chemical shifts and metabolite ratios in normal subjects, which contrast with patients with neurologic disease, including those with transient ischemic attacks, normal pressure hydrocephalus, and glioblastoma.

Kase CS, Williams JP, Wyatt BS, Mohr JP. Lobar intracerebral hematomas: clinical and CT analysis of 22 cases. Neurology 1982;32:1146–50.

Distinctive syndromes.

Marion DW. Complications of head injury and their therapy. Neurosurg Clin North Am 1991;2:411–24.

Long review, including many neuroradiologic aspects.

McDowell FH, Brott TG, Goldstein M et al: stroke: The first six hours (NSA consensus statement). Stroke (Special Ed. Clin Updates) 4:1, 1993.

Early changes are detectable.

Mohr JP, Biller J, Hilal SK et al. MR vs CT imaging in acute stroke. Stroke 1992;23:142.

Both are comparable for ischemic stroke imaged in the first few hours.

Mushlin AI, Detsky AS, Phelps CE et al. The accuracy of magnetic resonance imaging in patients with suspected multiple sclerosis. The Rochester Toronto Magnetic Resonance Imaging Study Group. JAMA 1993;269: 3146–51.

Clinical and MRI assessments in 300 multiple sclerosis patients found that MRI was more accurate than double-dose, contrast-enhanced CT but was negative in 25 percent of the patients clinically diagnosed with multiple sclerosis.

Rauch RA, Bazan C III, Larsson EM, Jinkins JR: Hyperdense middle cerebral arteries identified on CT as a false sign of vascular occlusion. AJNR 1993;14:669–73.

Sometimes misleading and false.

Rautenberg W, Aulich A, Rother J et al. Stroke and dolichoectatic intracranial arteries. Neurol Res 1992;14: 201–3.

MRI clearly delineated the lesions in most of the 45 patients in this series.

Smith ME, Stone LA, Albert PS et al. Clinical worsening in multiple sclerosis is associated with increased frequency and area of gadopentetate dimeglumine enhancing magnetic resonance imaging lesions. Ann Neurol 1993;33: 480–9.

New lesion and larger areas of enhancement in old lesions seen on gadolinium MRI correlated with relapsing and worsening in nine cases.

Stehling MK, Firth JL, Worthington BS et al. Observation of cerebrospinal fluid flow with echo planar magnetic resonance imaging. Br J Radiol 1991;64:89–97.

Details of CSF flow are now possible, allowing new classifications of types of hydrocephalus.

Truwit CL, Barkovich AJ, Gean-Marton A. Loss of the insular ribbon: another early CT sign of acute middle cerebral artery infarction. Radiology 1990;176:801.

Diagnostic sign now well-recognized.

Williams JP, Joslyn JN, White JL, Dean DF. Subdural hematoma secondary to ruptured intracranial aneurysm: computed tomographic diagnosis. J Comput Assist Tomogr 1993;7:149.

Unusual example.

11

Electroencephalography, Evoked Potentials, and Magnetic Stimulation

F. Mauguière

Apart from electromyography (EMG), which is reviewed in Chapter 12 of this book, electroencephalography (EEG), sensory evoked potentials (EPs), and motor responses evoked by transcutaneous magnetic stimulation of brain or of spinal cord and roots (motor evoked potentials [MEPs]) are the currently available neurophysiologic diagnostic tests in clinical practice. This chapter is not intended as a full review of all aspects of these techniques but rather aims at providing clinicians with the essential information concerning their scope and limitations. The author is fully conscious of having been biased by his own convictions when writing this chapter. For a critical analysis the reader is urged to consult the textbooks or articles cited as references, which contain the complementary information that may be needed.

ELECTROENCEPHALOGRAPHY

Normal and Abnormal Electroencephalographic Activities

In normal adults waking EEG activity consists mainly of sinusoidal fluctuations of voltage potentials, which are recorded on the scalp as 8- to 12-Hz oscillations. As shown in Figure 11-1, these oscillations are most prominent over the occipital areas. They are blocked by eye opening and mental activity and are known as the α-rhythm. Faster activities (β-rhythms) are also present, mainly in the frontocentral regions, in the normal waking EEG activity of adults. β-Rhythms are increased and more widespread on the scalp in patients treated by barbiturates or benzodiazepines. Occasionally bursts of oscillations slower than the α-rhythm (4 to 8 Hz), which are known as θ-activity, are recorded in the temporal regions of awake adults.

Their amount and diffusion increase with age (Fig. 11-2). Slower δ-waves (1 to 4 Hz) are absent in normal awake adults.

The most common EEG abnormalities are arrhythmic slow activity; epileptiform spike or spike-wave activity; voltage attenuation; and continuous electrocerebral inactivity. Focal arrhythmic slow activity in the θ- or δ-range is highly correlated, when it is continuous, with localized cerebral lesions such as infarction, tumor, hemorrhage, or abscess. An example of this type of focal arrhythmic wave activity, also referred to as polymorphic δ-waves, is illustrated in Figure 11-3.

Generalized arrhythmic slow activity manifests as a global disorganization of the EEG, which can be seen, usually in association with impaired vigilance, in many conditions, including metabolic, toxic, or infectious encephalopathies or traumatic coma. As shown in Figure 11-4, this generalized δ-activity may be unreactive to external stimuli in deeply comatose patients.

Intermittent generalized slow waves, organized in bursts of widespread and synchronous rhythmic θ- or δ-activity, occur in various situations, including metabolic or toxic disorders or deep midline or posterior fossa lesions, that perturb the generation of EEG rhythms through a dysfunction of the thalamocortical circuitry.

Focal or generalized epileptiform spike or spike-wave activity (Fig. 11-5) may occur interictally in patients with epileptic seizures. Generalized spikes or spike waves are also observed in individuals who do not present with clinical seizures but who are predisposed to epilepsy because of an abnormally low epileptic threshold. Similarly, focal epileptiform activity can reflect a potentially epileptogenetic focal lesion in patients with no history of seizures. Seizure activity can consist of various types of epileptiform discharges, in-

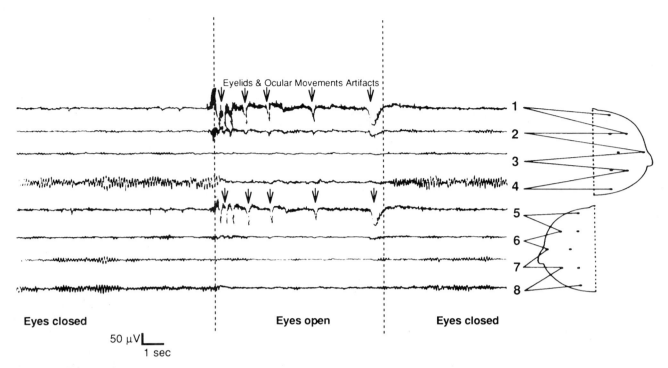

Figure 11-1. Normal α-rhythm in an adult subject. The α-activity is recorded symmetrically in the two occipital regions (leads 4 and 8) when the subject keeps the eyes closed. It is blocked by eye opening, which provokes ocular movement and eyelids artifacts recorded in the frontal regions (leads 1 and 5). Calibration: 50 μV, 1 s.

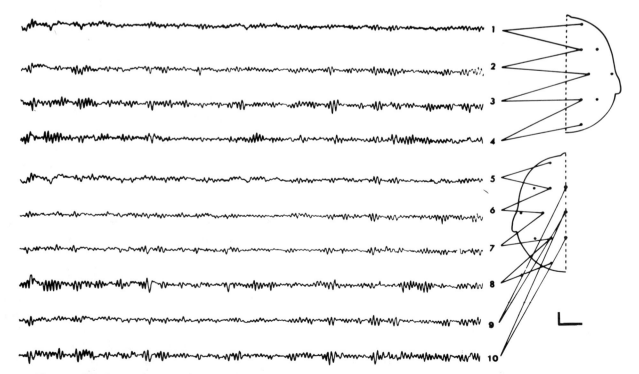

Figure 11-2. Widespread θ-activity in a 75-year-old subject. Note the lower frequency of the EEG background activity recorded with eyes closed in this subject (6 to 7 Hz) when compared with that illustrated in Figure 11-1. Calibration: 50 μV, 1 s.

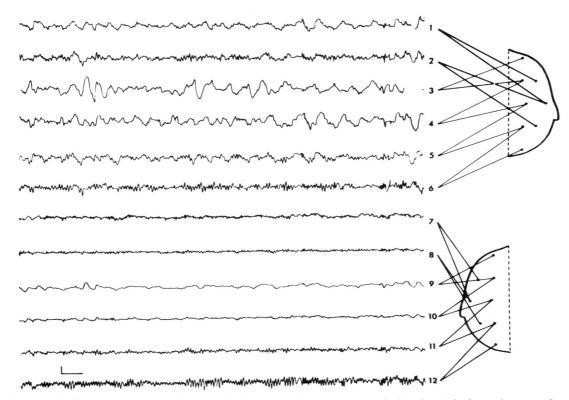

Figure 11-3. Focal arrhythmic δ-activity. Focal δ-waves are recorded in the right frontal region (leads 1, 3, and 4) in this patient with a cerebral abscess. The background activity is preserved, with a normal α-activity in the two occipital regions (leads 6 and 12). Calibration: 50 μV, 1 s.

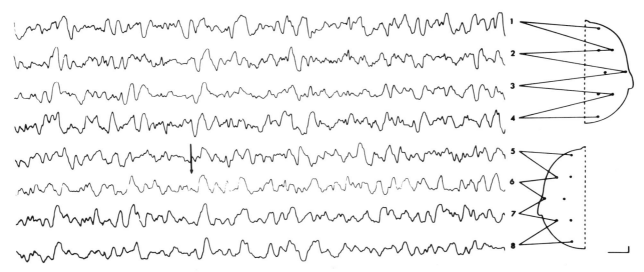

Figure 11-4. Generalized arrhythmic slow activity. The EEG activity in this head-injured comatose patient shows generalized δ-waves, which are not modified by auditory stimulation *(arrow)*. Calibration: 50 μV, 1 s.

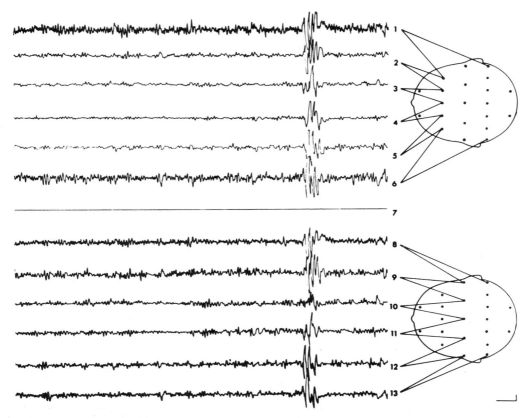

Figure 11-5. Burst of generalized spike waves. This generalized epileptiform spike-wave activity was recorded in a young adult with juvenile myoclonic epilepsy. Calibration: 50 μV, 1 s.

cluding rhythmic slow waves, spikes, spike waves, or fast activities.

Periodic lateralized epileptiform discharges (PLEDs) indicate an acute destructive focal cerebral lesion, including cerebral hemorrhage and infarction, a rapidly growing high-grade tumor, and herpes simplex encephalitis (Fig. 11-6).

Periodic generalized complexes can be recorded in severe encephalopathies such as subacute sclerosing panencephalitis (Fig. 11-7) or Creutzfeldt-Jakobs disease (Fig. 11-8). They are associated with a progressive deterioration of the basal EEG activity with disappearance of the normal background α-activity.

Focal voltage attenuation indicates either a loss of cortical neurons, as observed in porencephaly, severe atrophy or cerebral contusion, or the presence of an extracerebral space-occupying lesion that reduces the voltage of the activity picked up by scalp electrodes, such as a subdural hematoma. It can also be observed in the very acute stage of cerebral infarctions. The burst suppression pattern (Fig. 11-9) consists of occasional generalized bursts of high-voltage slow-wave and spike activities separated by intervening periods

of cerebral inactivity. It is unreactive to external stimuli and observed in deeply comatose patients. Severe hypoxia secondary to a circulatory arrest, critical brain hypoperfusion, or deep barbiturate intoxication can produce this EEG pattern, which, in postanoxic coma, is usually accompanied by massive myoclonic body jerks, synchronous with EEG bursts.

Generalized voltage attenuation usually indicates severe depression of cerebral functions, as observed in anoxia or deep comatose states secondary to intoxication by central nervous system (CNS) depressant drugs, particularly barbiturates. Brief and reversible voltage attenuation of the EEG activity can be observed, preceded and followed by a burst of generalized δ-waves, during syncopes due to cardiac arrest or extreme bradycardia lasting for more than 8 to 10 seconds (Fig. 11-10). During this phase of EEG depression, decorticate posturing and repeated clonic jerks of the four limbs are usually observed, which precede the return to normal consciousness.

Continuous electrocerebral inactivity, unreactive to any kind of stimulation, represents the most severe

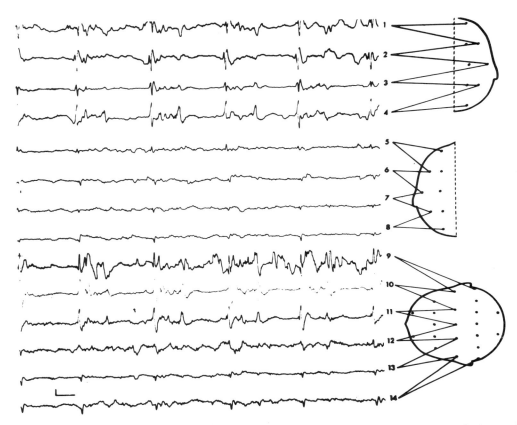

Figure 11-6. Periodic lateralized epileptiform discharges (PLEDs). PLEDs were recorded over the right hemisphere (leads 1, 2, 3, 4, 9, 10, and 11) 36 hours after an acute ischemic stroke with flaccid left hemiplegia. Calibration: 50 μV, 1 s.

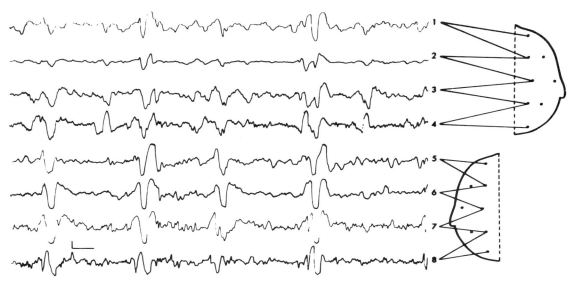

Figure 11-7. Periodic generalized slow complexes. Periodic complexes of large generalized δ-waves are associated with disappearance of α-activity in this 9-year-old girl with subacute sclerosing panencephalitis. Calibration: 50 μV, 1 s.

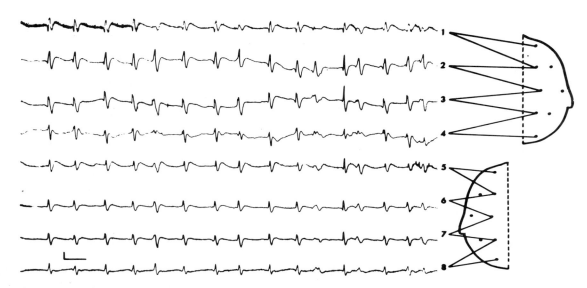

Figure 11-8. Periodic generalized triphasic waves. These generalized periodic complexes were recorded in a patient with Creutzfeldt-Jakob disease. There was no EEG activity other than the periodic triphasic waves. This aspect is observed at the preterminal stage of the disease. Calibration: 50 μV, 1 s.

form of generalized voltage attenuation and is observed in brain death (Fig. 11-11).

Recording Techniques

The EEG is recorded with scalp disk electrodes positioned symmetrically on both sides of the head in standard locations known as the International 10–20 System. Bipolar recordings in which pairs of electrodes are connected to each of the amplifier channels and arranged in different types of montages are the most widely used (see Figs. 11-1 to 11-10). Common montages include 16 to 20 channels, which can be reduced to 8 or 10 for bedside EEG recording. Sphenoidal electrodes, as well as cortical recording using grids of

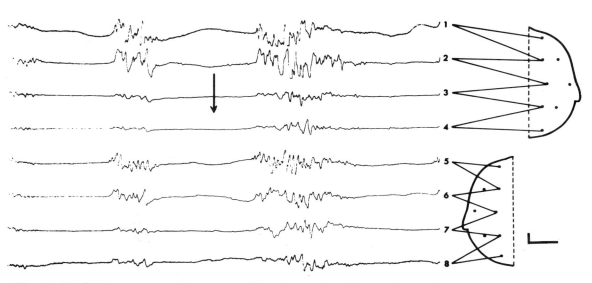

Figure 11-9. Burst suppression pattern. These intermittent bursts of θ- and δ-activity separated by periods of flat EEG lasting 5 to 8 seconds were recorded in a deeply comatose patient after an episode of severe brain hypoxia due to a cardiac arrest. Painful stimulation *(arrow)* did not modify the EEG activity. Calibration: 20 μV, 1 s.

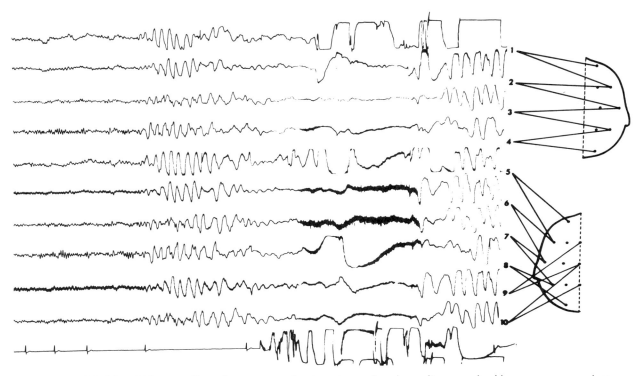

Figure 11-10. EEG recording of a syncope due to extreme bradycardia provoked by eye compression. The slowing of cardiac rhythm (bottom record, ECG) causes a flattening of the EEG accompanied by a tonic posture and clonic jerks, which are responsible for the muscle and movement artifacts recorded on the scalp EEG leads and on the ECG record. The phase of transient voltage attenuation is preceded and followed by generalized rhythmic slow δ waves. Calibration: 50 μV, 1 s.

subdural electrodes and intracerebral implanted electrodes, are used only for the presurgical assessment of untractable focal epilepsies.

In addition to the recording of spontaneous activity, hyperventilation and intermittent photic stimulation are two activating procedures routinely performed in most laboratories. These two techniques aims at provoking focal or generalized changes in activity that may be of diagnostic importance and would otherwise remain undetected. Hyperventilation and intermittent photic stimulation, respectively, prove particularly useful for precipitating spike-wave discharges in "petit mal" absence (see below) and juvenile myoclonic epilepsy (see Ch. 79).

When the waking EEG is normal, sleep recordings can be informative in some types of epilepsies in which interictal or ictal activities are increased during sleep. Conversely, the usefulness of sleep deprivation for activating epileptiform discharges is still a matter of controversy. This technique is unpleasant for the patient and cannot be considered as a routine procedure.

Ambulatory EEG and inpatient video EEG monitoring offer a double advantage over conventional EEG by increasing the duration of the recording and permitting a survey of the EEG during sleep. Moreover, video recording permits correlation in time of EEG changes with clinical ictal symptoms and particularly permits localization of the EEG discharge at clinical seizure onset. Other maneuvers can be carried out depending on the clinical context and the diagnostic aim. Vasovagal stimulation by ocular compression or massage of one carotid sinus can reproduce the bradycardia or asystolia and the related EEG changes (Fig. 11-10) that occur during spontaneous syncopes. Precipitation of EEG discharges or clinical seizures by pentylenetetrazol or Megimide is now not widely used, and these two drugs are no longer available in the United States. Apart from their vegetative side effects, mainly nausea and bradycardia, these drugs may induce seizures different from those occurring spontaneously in a given individual. Recording of spontaneous discharges or seizures by long-term EEG monitoring, even after reduction or withdrawal of the anticonvulsant therapy, is preferable to drug activation.

Frequency analysis completed by topographic map-

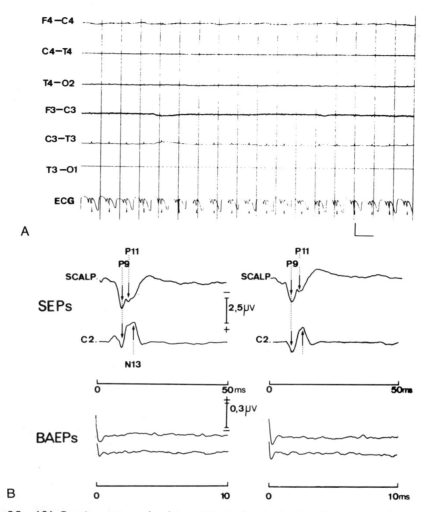

Figure 11-11. (A) Continuous cerebral inactivity in brain death, No activity other than ECG artifacts (leads C3-T3) are recordable on the scalp. Cerebral inactivity is assessed by using long-distance bipolar montages (in this case frontocentral [F4-C4 and F3-C3]; centrotemporal [C4-T4 and C3-T3]; temporo-occipital [T4-02 and T3-01] and maximal amplification (calibration: 20 μV, 1 s). By convention even and odd numbers are used to label electrodes placed on the right and left half of the scalp, respectively. **(B)** Median nerve SEPs and BAEPs in brain death. (Left: left median nerve and left ear stimulation; right: right median nerve and right ear stimulation). SEPs: After stimulation of the median nerve at the wrist, the activities of brachial plexus roots (P9), dorsal columns (P11), and cervical cord dorsal horn are picked up normally in the cervical region (C2) and on the scalp in the parietal region opposite to stimulation. The brainstem P14 and all cortical components of the response are absent. BAEPs: No responses were obtained on two runs of 2,000 stimulations on each side.

ping of computerized EEG has achieved a certain popularity, and the number of commercially available mapping systems is regularly increasing. Frequency analysis and EEG mapping can bring information unrevealed by visual inspection of the EEG record and permits display of statistical values derived from quantitative analysis. The question remains, however, as to whether this complementary information has diagnostic utility in a given individual. At present there is no firm demonstration that additional evidence of brain dysfunction, potentially useful for diagnosis and

patient care, may be obtained by computerized EEG and topographic mapping in the absence of significant changes on routine EEG testing. Spike mapping and source localization, using various types of dipolar models, represent a useful complementary technique for localizing epileptic foci. However, when functional neurosurgery is envisaged in a patient with intractable focal seizures, the information provided by spike mapping must be confronted with data provided by other noninvasive techniques, including metabolic tomographic investigations, and eventually validated by intracerebral recordings. The reader is referred to the textbook by Daly and Pedley (1990) for a recent review of all aspects of current clinical EEG practice.

Clinical Uses

Epilepsy

In spite of the advances in neuroimaging, EEG remains the most helpful test in epileptology. In most instances it is used to record in the interictal state. It then provides useful diagnostic information only when it shows epileptiform activity consistent with the clinical presentation of spontaneous seizures, since interictal EEG activity can be entirely normal on a single recording in a substantial number of patients presenting with unquestionable epileptic seizures. Moreover, spike or spike-wave EEG activity can be recorded in nonepileptic patients and is poorly correlated with the frequency or the likelihood of seizure recurrence in epileptic patients. Thus interictal epileptiform activities should be interpreted in relation to the clinical context and should not in any case be viewed as an indispensable and irrefutable sign of epilepsy or as a reliable index for drug treatment monitoring.

The major use of EEG in epilepsy is to help in the classification of a patient's seizure type and in the identification of epileptic syndromes. In that respect ictal EEG activity, especially when associated with the ictal symptoms of spontaneous seizures, is certainly more helpful than interictal EEG. Quite often anamnestic data per se are not convincing enough to classify correctly the seizure type. For instance, a clinically generalized tonic-clonic seizure can be generalized from the onset or be secondary to spread from a focus, and an ictal lapse of awareness can reflect either a generalized nonconvulsive form of epilepsy, such as petit mal or absence seizures, or a focal cerebral dysfunction in temporal lobe epilepsy. This distinction has major implications since there is usually no demonstrable cerebral lesion in primary generalized epilepsies manifesting by various types of diffuse synchronous epileptiform activities, while in most cases a focal lesion must be suspected in patients whose seizures have a focal onset, particularly adults with no past history of epilepsy. EEG is also the only means of identifying as epileptic some confusional states, known as absence or petit mal states, which could be misdiagnosed as toxic, metabolic, or psychiatric confusions. The recording of generalized rhythmic slow and spike waves makes the diagnosis, and clinical as well as EEG manifestations immediately disappear with an intravenous injection of benzodiazepine.

The concept of epileptic syndromes also has major practical implications and is based on the association of patient characteristics (age, sex, family history of epilepsy), specific seizure types, and EEG findings. The three main epileptic syndromes with a rather good prognosis are petit mal absence seizures, benign focal epilepsy of childhood, and juvenile myoclonic epilepsy. In all these syndromes the EEG background activity is normal, and fairly specific epileptic discharges are easily identifiable. Bursts of generalized 3-Hz spike and wave complexes, concomitant with brief lapses of awareness and facilitated by hyperventilation, are observed in petit mal absence seizures (Fig. 11-12). Pseudorhythmic central or midtemporal spikes, enhanced during sleep, are the sign of benign focal epilepsy of childhood (Fig. 11-13). In juvenile myoclonic epilepsy bursts of spike-wave and polyspike and wave complexes are usually recorded (Fig. 14-5), which may be facilitated by eye closure and fast intermittent photic stimulation and are often associated with myoclonic jerks.

Conversely, there are other epileptic syndromes of childhood in which a generalized slowing of the EEG activity is associated with specific EEG abnormalities and carries an ominous prognosis. The severe disorganization of the EEG activity called *hypsarrhythmia* is a key symptom of West's syndrome, which in most cases prompts a decision to administer corticosteroid therapy when observed in association with infantile spasms (Fig. 11-14). In the Lennox-Gastaut syndrome, a severe form of childhood secondary generalized epilepsy characterized by absence seizures with muscle atonia, the generalized slowing of the EEG activity mixed with interictal bursts of slow (<3 Hz) spike waves cannot be confused with the EEG aspect of petit mal epilepsy, in which interictal EEG activity is normal.

The above-cited examples illustrate the wide scope of EEG in epilepsy. What is not included in this scope can be summarized as follows: (1) EEG has been supplanted by neuroimaging techniques for localizing a focal lesion revealed by a first seizure in an adult, even though it may show some interictal focal slowing revealing a permanent cerebral dysfunction in the lesion area; (2) epilepsy should never be diagnosed on the sole basis of epileptiform EEG activities when they are not associated with clinical seizures; (3) the drug treatment of epilepsy does not aim at "cleaning" the EEG. A consequence of the last point is that in an epileptic patient who is doing well under treatment, to repeat EEG recordings and increase drug dosages in order to suppress epileptiform EEG activities represents a blamable overuse and a potentially dangerous misuse of EEG. There are only a very few cases in which antiepileptic treatment may aim at suppressing a subcontinuous epileptiform EEG activity potentially deleterious for the brain, independently of seizure control. Focal discharges observed in comatose patients after

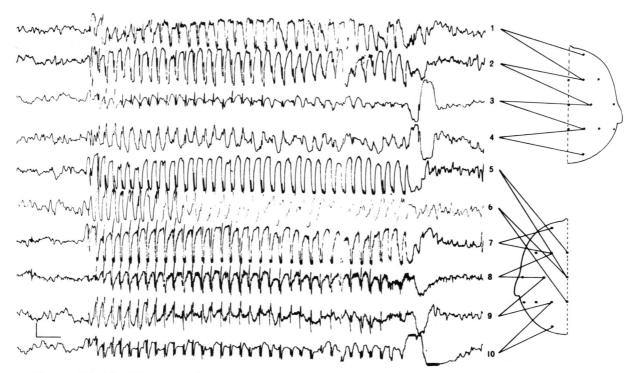

Figure 11-12. Discharge of generalized 3-Hz spike and wave complexes during a petit mal absence in a boy aged 7. Calibration: 50 μV, 1 s.

a brain injury represent the most frequent of these acute conditions in neurology and neurosurgery wards.

Focal Noninfectious Cerebral Lesions

Focal arrhythmic slow activity (see above) represents the classic EEG sign of focal cerebral lesions, which is most strongly suggestive of a structural lesion if con-

tinuously present in the EEG tracing. It has no etiologic specificity because it reflects only the local disturbance of the cerebral cortex surrounding the lesion and not the activity of the lesion itself. However, intraparenchymatous lesions are more likely to produce this type of abnormal EEG activity than extracerebral lesions, such as meningiomas or extra- or subdural hematomas. Focal epileptiform activities or dis-

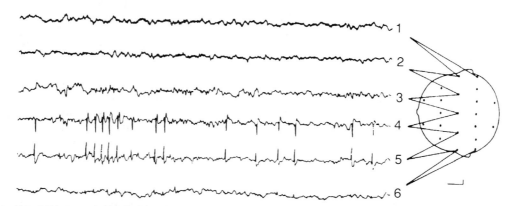

Figure 11-13. Pseudorhythmic left controtemporal spikes in a case of benign focal epilepsy of childhood. Boy aged 7 with rare tonic seizure of right arm and face during sleep. There is a polarity inversion of left pseudorythmic spikes recorded by leads 4 and 5, indicating that the spike is picked by the left central electrode, which is common to both leads. Calibration: 50 μV, 1 s.

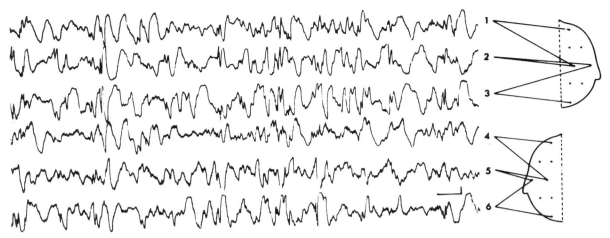

Figure 11-14. Generalized slow waves and spike waves (hypsarrhythmia) in a 9-month-old boy with infantile spasms (West's syndrome).

charges, including PLEDs, can be the only EEG manifestation of focal cerebral lesions. When observed in patients with no permanent clinical deficit, focal arrhythmic slow activity should prompt neuroimaging investigations, except when observed in the few hours or days following an acute attack of "complex migraine," including prodromic signs of cerebral dysfunction such as hemidysesthesia) hemianopia or aphasia, a condition in which focal δ- or θ-waves can outlast the acute episode. Conversely, a normal EEG does not obviate the need to carry out imaging investigations when a focal lesion is suspected on clinical grounds. There is no consensus as to whether the EEG might be predictive of post-traumatic seizures in head-injured patients showing focal arrhythmic slow activity within the few weeks following injury, although this EEG abnormality raises the suspicion of a focal cerebral contusion even when the computed tomography (CT) scan is poorly informative. In deep subcortical, midline, or posterior fossa lesions, the EEG recording may show generalized intermittent rhythmic δ-activity, which has, in fact, no specificity and can be observed in any metabolic disorders or other encephalopathies that affect the brain diffusely. The EEG activity is most often normal in single lacunae and after a transient ischemic attack outside the symptomatic period, especially in patients with no chronic cerebral hypoperfusion.

Infectious Diseases

Of all brain infectious diseases, herpes simplex encephalitis is the one in which EEG has the most determining implication for patient management, because delayed initiation of acyclovir therapy worsens the final outcome. Periodic sharp wave complexes over one or both temporal regions (Fig. 11-6) add specificity to global or focal EEG slowing or focal epileptiform discharges that may be observed in other types of encephalitis. These abnormalities may be observed as early as the second day of illness when the CT scan is often still poorly informative. Similarly, in the evaluation of patients with suspected brain abscess, focal arrhythmic slow activity may occur in the early stage, before CT scan demonstrates an encapsulated lesion. Diffuse slowing of EEG activity may be observed in many types of cerebral infectious disease, including bacterial meningitis and nonherpetic viral encephalitis, that produce an altered state of consciousness. These EEG changes are not predictive of residual brain damage or of seizures. In subacute sclerosing panencephalitis, a chronic measles virus infection of childhood characterized by dementia and myoclonus, the EEG is diagnostic when showing bilateral symmetrical and synchronous high-voltage bursts of δ-waves that repeat in regular 4- to 10-second intervals and are closely related to myoclonic jerks (Fig. 11-7).

Metabolic and Toxic Encephalopathies

In metabolic and toxic encephalopathies, diffuse EEG slowing mostly reflects level of consciousness (see below). Additional EEG features, however, increase the likelihood of a metabolic disorder with various degrees of specificity. Bisynchronous, mostly frontal, triphasic waves, which may be attenuated or blocked by sensory or painful stimulation, were first considered to be virtually specific of hepatic hyperammoniemic encephalopathy. In fact, they are now known to occur in other metabolic disorders, including uremia, hyponatremia, acute hyperthyroidism, and hyperosmolarity. Diffuse fast β-activity, when recorded in a patient with a coma of unknown origin, raises the suspicion of drug intoxication, most often by barbiturates, benzodiazepines, or both.

Dementia

A single EEG examination in the evaluation of a patient suspected of dementia is often disappointing, except when it reveals a focal slowing suggestive of a space-occupying lesion, most often located in the frontal lobes or in the temporal lobe of the minor hemisphere. However, EEG has been supplanted by CT scan and magnetic resonance imaging (MRI) in this indication as well as in the diagnosis of multiple-infarct dementia, where it may show multiple independent foci of slow-wave activity. The main justification for recording the EEG in a patient whose mental performances are rapidly declining is to detect EEG signs suggestive of Creutzfeldt-Jakob disease (e.g., periodic and synchronous sharp-wave or triphasic complexes [Fig. 11-8]), which may be absent in the early stage of the disease. In Alzheimer's disease the waking EEG shows an increase of θ-activity predominating in the temporal regions, which is associated with a slowing of the occipital α-rhythm, which progressively loses its normal reactivity to eye opening and other external stimuli. In the late stage of the disease the background EEG activity is diffusely slowed and bursts of generalized fast spikes may occur in association with myoclo-

nic jerks. The diagnostic utility of EEG is limited in the early stage of Alzheimer's disease because of (1) the problems encountered in distinguishing the early EEG changes related to the disease from the slowing of the α-activity and the intermittent temporal θ-waves observed in nondemented elderly subjects and (2) the absence of generally accepted methods to quantify and analyze statistically the EEG changes in individual patients. In spite of persisting controversy, a correlation between the increase of θ-activity and poor performances at psychometric testing is generally admitted in Alzheimer's disease.

Altered States of Consciousness: Coma and Brain Death

The EEG plays a major role in the evaluation of patients with altered states of consciousness for it permits assessment of supratentorial brain functions, particularly when consciousness is severely depressed. Apart from signaling a focal hemispheric lesion or an epileptiform activity or showing some diffuse changes in favor of a metabolic or toxic disorder (see above), the EEG helps in evaluating brain reactivity to external stimuli and thus complements clinical examination. In most cases the EEG activity is diffusely slowed in comatose patients (see Fig. 11-4). There are, however three exceptions: (1) the fast activity accompanying intoxication by barbiturates, benzodiazepines, or other de-

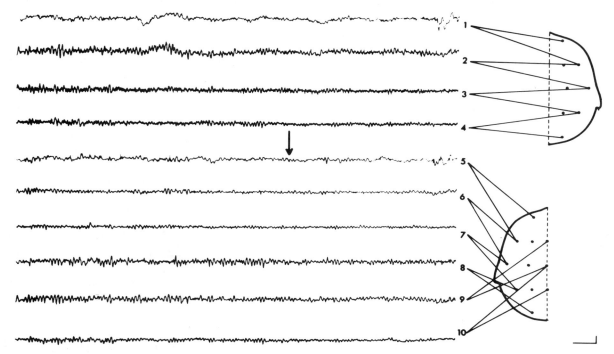

Figure 11-15. Unreactive generalized α-activity in a deeply comatose patient with brainstem infarction (α-coma). Note that this rhythmic 8-Hz activity is unreactive to painful stimulation *(arrow)*.

pressant drugs; (2) the scalp-widespread monorhythmic α-frequency activity, unreactive to external stimuli, that is observed in deeply comatose patients mainly after hypoxia or focal brainstem lesions (referred to as α-coma in current neurologic literature) (Fig. 11-15); and (3) the bursts of fast, 14-Hz spindle activity that can be recorded in reactive comatose patients. This spindle activity differs, however, from that observed in normal sleep in two main points, namely, that it is usually widespread on the scalp, while sleep spindles predominate in the central regions, and that external stimuli in these comatose patients evoke bursts of diffuse slow δ-waves instead of a return to waking EEG activity.

During coma the EEG most often shows complete disappearance of the cyclic variations of brain activity that characterize normal sleep; moreover, in reaction to external stimuli a return to a normal waking EEG activity is usually not observed. Either the EEG reactivity is lost, or it is clearly asymmetrical, or it is diffuse and symmetrical, but in any case it does not consist of a return to normal occipital α-activity blocked by external stimulations. In most cases the reaction to external stimuli manifests either by a diffuse slowing of the background activity or by a transient attenuation of a diffuse δ-activity. Both types of EEG reactivity are rather favorable as compared with complete unreactivity. Similarly spontaneous transient changes and spontaneous cyclic fluctuations of background EEG activity are usually interpreted as more favorable than a monotonous and unreactive EEG slowing. It must be remembered that comatose patients can show some motor reactions to external, particularly painful, stimuli; which are not accompanied by any EEG changes for they are not integrated at the cortical level.

The burst suppression EEG pattern (see above) usually carries an ominous prognosis provided that reversible causes of this EEG pattern primarily deep anesthesia or drug overdose, have been eliminated. The same statement applies to the permanent, unreactive electrocerebral silence observed in brain death. This is also the reason why the absence of EEG activity should absolutely be viewed not as an equivalent but only as a confirmatory sign of brain death once it has been established by clinical, biologic, and neuroimaging investigations that the coma results from irreversible structural brain damage.

VISUAL, AUDITORY, AND SOMATOSENSORY EVOKED POTENTIALS

The recording of potentials evoked by visual, somatosensory, or auditory stimuli represents a noninvasive low-cost method to assess in real time the processing of sensory information in the human central nervous system (CNS). The EP traces consist of a succession of waves or peaks, which reflect the neuronal responses at the different levels of the sensory pathways. This technique thus permits assessment of the conduction times of sensory impulses in the CNS. Most if not all of the clinically validated EP techniques concern early sensory responses and have emerged since the 1970s, when Halliday's group demonstrated that visual EPs (VEPs) could disclose clinically silent lesions of the optic pathways in patients with multiple sclerosis (MS) or a previous history of optic neuritis. Soon thereafter many other valuable applications of EPs emerged. For example, EPs proved to be helpful in (1) testing sensory functions when clinical examination is not reliable; (2) investigating purely subjective symptoms and detect whether they have an organic origin; (3) better assessing the causative mechanisms of neurologic deficits and functional recovery; and (4) monitoring cerebral functions when the patient's condition is critical or at risk in the operating theater or during intensive care.

EPs are usually classified into two categories: (1) *exogenous* sensory potentials, which are modality-specific, obligatory responses, reflecting the processing of the sensory information in afferent pathways up to cortical sensory areas; and (2) *event-related* (also called *endogenous* or *cognitive*) potentials, which are not specific for a sensory modality and reflect the task in which the subject is involved when the incoming information reaches the cortex. Current strategy for event-related EP recordings consists in using stimulation sequences in which rare target stimuli, which the subject must detect, are intermingled with frequent stimuli, which the subject must ignore ("odd-ball" paradigm). The endogenous EP components are identifiable in responses to target stimuli and are supposed to be absent in responses to nontarget stimuli. A third category of EPs, which is not yet routinely used in clinical practice, is premotor EPs, which differ from sensory EPs in that the changes of brain activity they reflect are time-locked to motor programming and efferent command and not to the processing of afferent information. Both action and postsynaptic potentials contribute to generation of surface-recorded EPs. Action potentials can be recorded as triphasic positive-negative-positive potentials by using a surface electrode placed over a nerve or as a far-field positivity when the electrode is placed at the end of a nerve or at distance from a fiber tract.

The excitatory or inhibitory nature of postsynaptic potentials cannot be inferred from the polarity of the corresponding surface EPs. Moreover, postsynaptic activity of synapses in relay nuclei can result in far-field scalp potentials, but it can also be missed by scalp recordings depending on the spatial arrangement of synaptic contacts in the nucleus. The polarity-latency nomenclature, which consists of labeling each EP component by the letter P or N according to its polarity (P for positive, N for negative), followed by its mean peaking latency in milliseconds in a control population of normal subjects, is largely used for visual, somatosensory, and cognitive EPs but not for most of the auditory EPs.

Before reviewing briefly the clinical applications of EPs in neurologic practice, the point must be clearly made that no EP abnormality can be viewed as specific of any pathology, even though it is generally accepted that demyelination causes conduction slowing and EP latency delays, whereas nondemyelinating processes are more likely to result in amplitude abnormalities. Abnormalities of short-latency EPs can reflect only three phenomena: impaired axonal conduction, abnormal synaptic transmission, and cell loss. Similarly, abnormal changes in long-latency event-related EPs reflect slowing of cognitive processes independently of the causative mechanisms. Consequently, to look for specific EP abnormalities is often fruitless, and to claim that EP changes can be interpreted out of the clinical context is misleading and potentially dangerous.

Readers will find in the books cited in the bibliography the complement of information that they may need concerning the recording procedures and clinical applications of EPs.

The Normal Evoked Potential Waveforms

Visual Evoked Potentials

Flash and pattern reversal have been used as stimuli for clinical VEP recordings. Flash VEPs present with a complex waveform, which contains up to seven distinct components peaking within the 250 ms following the stimulation. Because of their great interindividual variability, flash VEPs have been progressively replaced by pattern reversal VEPs in most clinical applications. Pattern reversal VEPs are usually obtained by reversal of a black and white checkerboard. They contain three main components, labeled N75, P100, and N140, which are recorded in the midoccipital region (Fig. 11-16). Most of the clinical interpretation of pattern VEPs is based on measurement of the P100 latency. Conversely, the amplitude of the P100 potential shows a greater interindividual variability, and interocular differences are crucial for interpreting amplitude changes in patients.

Monocular half-field stimulation causes a shift of the N75-P100-N140 waveform toward the occipital region ipsilateral to the stimulated half-field (Fig. 11-16). In the original report on the paradoxical lateralization of the N75-P100-N140 waveform obtained by half-field stimulation, it was proposed that this complex reflects the response of the cortical neurons receiving their input from the foveal part of the retina. The model of a dipolar source, with an oblique orientation toward the interhemispheric fissure and situated at the pole of the activated striate cortex, fits reasonably well with the ipsilateral predominance of the P100 potential to half-field stimulation. Readers are referred to the textbooks cited in the bibliography for a detailed description of the nonpathologic factors (age, sex, body temperature, physical exercise, stimulation parameters) that may affect the VEP waveform. Among these factors visual acuity is certainly the one whose influence on pattern VEPs is the most clinically relevant, in particular when small checks are used to evoke the visual response. It is good practice to measure visual acuity and to correct refractive errors before recording the VEPs, and patients should wear their glasses during the test. Poor visual acuity in central amblyopia may cause prolonged and reduced pattern VEPs. There is some controversy as to the possibility of provoking voluntarily a modification of pattern reversal VEPs. Abnormal VEPs can be deliberately produced by eccentric fixation or near-point accommodation and ocular convergence. In the author's practice of VEPs, however, detection of malingering does not represent a major problem in neurologic patients, and it can be solved in most cases by the control of the patient's gaze during the test.

Auditory Evoked Potentials

Brainstem Auditory Evoked Potentials. Normal brainstem auditory EPs (BAEPs) are composed of five successive waves, labeled I to V, peaking within the 10 ms following monaural stimulation by clicks (Fig. 11-17). Wave I originates from the peripheral portion of the cochlear nerve. Wave II is consistently obtained only with click intensities of more than 60 dB and reflects the activity in the proximal portion of the cochlear nerve as well as the postsynaptic responses of cochlear nucleus cells. Wave III is, with waves I and V, one of the most constant and robust components of BAEPs. It is generated by a horizontal dipolar source located in the pontine portion of brainstem auditory pathways. Waves IV and V can be clearly dissociated or combined to form a single IV-V complex. The origin of wave IV is not firmly settled, while wave V reflects both the activity of the lateral lemniscus fibers and the postsynaptic responses of midbrain auditory nuclei, including the inferior colliculi and particularly the one contralateral to the stimulated ear.

Intra- and interindividual variability of BAEPs is recognized as very low in all published series of normative values. Measurements performed in clinical

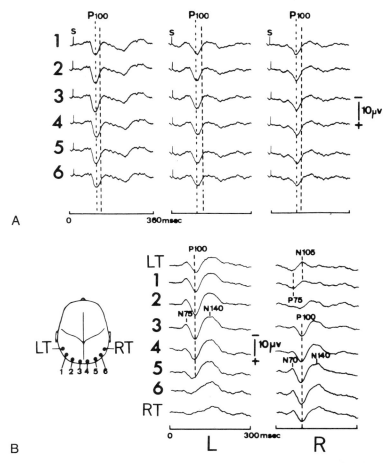

Figure 11-16. Normal pattern reversal VEPs. **(A)** The most easily identifiable component of the response is the P100 potential, which is widely distributed in the occipital regions and easily obtainable with various types of patterns. In this figure, responses obtained using black and white 100 and 20 percent contrasted checkerboards and a red light-emitting diode array are represented in the left, middle, and right columns, respectively. The dotted line on the right of that corresponding to the P100 latency indicates the upper limits of normal P100 latencies for each type of stimulus. **(B)** Pattern VEPs to half-field stimulation. Note that the P100 shifts ipsilaterally to the stimulated half-field. L, left half-field stimulation: R, right half-field stimulation.

testing include peaking latencies of waves I, III and V; interpeak latencies I-III, III-V, and I-V; and I/V amplitude ratio and interear latency differences. There is an inverse relationship between the intensity of the click and the absolute latencies of waves I to V, the latter increasing when the former decreases, but interpeak intervals are little or not at all affected by decreasing click intensities. Thus, an increased interval between BAEP peaks cannot result from peripheral (conductive or cochlear) hearing loss. Nonpathologic factors that may affect BAEPs (age, sex, body temperature, subject relaxation, stimulation rate, stimulus polarity, stimulus frequency spectrum, stimulus mode) were reviewed by Chiappa in 1990. In general, BAEPs can be considered very stable, and in particular they are not influenced by drowsiness, sleep, or

therapeutic dosages of most psychoactive drugs. Even during anesthesia or under high doses of barbiturates BAEPs persist (Fig. 11-18), and the latency changes observed are in most cases related to body temperature variations. However, high doses of intravenous diphenylhydantoin for the treatment of status epilepticus can produce a shift of latencies, and peculiar associations of depressant drugs, such as high doses of lidocaine and thiopental, used to control intracranial pressure in comatose patients can even cause complete but reversible disappearance of BAEPs.

Middle Latency Auditory Evoked Potentials. Middle latency auditory EPs (MLAEPs) are elicited within the 10- to 50-ms poststimulus latency range and consist of a sequence of five waves, of which only the peaks

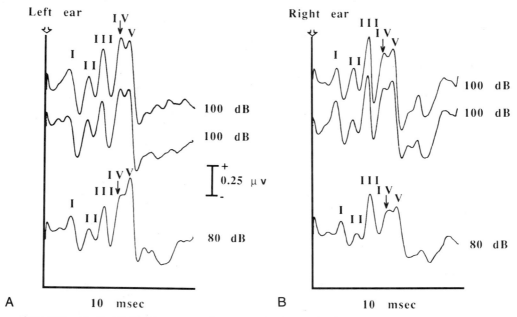

Figure 11-17. (A & B) Brainstem auditory evoked potentials (BAEPs). Illustration of the test-retest stability and the very small inter-ear differences of BAEP waves in a normal adult. Note the small increase of peak latencies when decreasing the click intensity from 100 to 80 dB (hearing level).

labeled Na and Pa, peaking, respectively, in the 16 to 20-ms and 27 to 33-ms latency ranges, are consistent enough to be clinically useful (Fig. 11-19). Because MLAEPs overlap in time with a reflex response of postauricular muscle, their origin was formerly questioned, but a muscular origin has been definitely ruled out since it was demonstrated that MLAEPs persist under curarization. Substantial changes of MLAEP waveform occur during natural sleep, and several anesthetic agents produce a severe depression of the Na/Pa deflection as well as a shift of the respective latencies of these two potentials. The detectability of the major Na and Pa components of the MLAEPs is age-dependent.

There is still some controversy concerning the origins of MLAEP waves. Most authors agree, however, that the Pa wave has a cortical origin and is generated in the primary auditory cortical areas.

Long-Latency Auditory Evoked Potentials. Long-latency auditory EPs (LLAEPs) consist of a N100 (or N1) negativity and of a P200 (or P2) positivity recorded with maximal amplitude in the frontocentral region on the midline. Neither of these two potentials can be considered entirely exogenous, and their susceptibility to nonsensory factors such as vigilance, cognitive processes, or drugs explains why they have been progressively replaced by BAEPs for routine audiometric testing. Sedative or hypnotic doses of benzodi-

azepines and barbiturates may significantly reduce their amplitudes.

The sources of N100 and P200 waves are presumed to be situated in the posterior temporal auditory and associative cortex. The auditory areas of both hemispheres are activated by monaural stimulation, which, however, evokes LLAEPs with larger voltages and shorter latencies as compared with the contralateral hemisphere.

Somatosensory Evoked Potentials

Somatosensory EPs (SEPs) differ from other EP modalities in that they are evoked by applying non-natural electrical stimulations to the skin surface, which depolarize the fibers directly and bypass the peripheral receptors. One of the advantages of SEP recording in clinical routine is evaluation of the transit time of the ascending volley from the spinal entry of the sensory fibers up to the cortex. In most studies this transit time is referred to as the *central conduction time.* Only the rapidly conducting and heavily myelinated afferent fibers are activated by electrical stimuli delivered at relatively low and non-noxious intensities. Thus, scalp SEPs elicited by nonpainful stimulations reflect activation of the dorsal columns and lemniscal fibers.

Maturation, body height, skin and body temperature, and vigilance can affect SEPs. Briefly the essential of what neurologists need concerning the non-

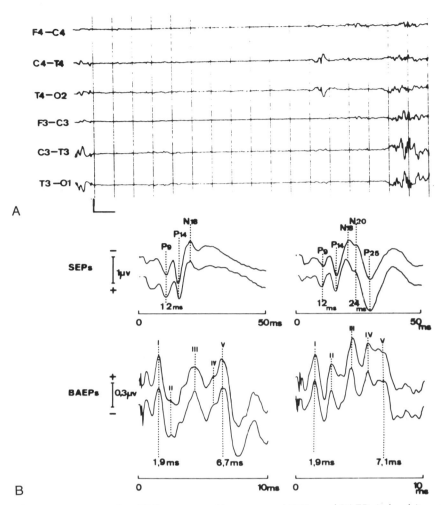

Figure 11-18. Burst suppression EEG pattern with preserved SEPs and BAEPs in barbiturate intoxication. **(A)** EEG tracing showing a burst suppression pattern with long periods of depressed activity (see Fig. 11-9 for comparison) in a deeply comatose patient. (Calibration: 50 μV, 1 s; same derivations as in Figure 11-11). **(B)** Scalp SEPs are preserved, including the cortical components after stimulation of the right median nerve (right side of figure). After stimulation of the left median nerve, only subcortical SEP components are obtained, including the brainstem P14 (compare with scalp SEP traces in Fig. 11-11); cortical components are lost because of a right hemispheric hematoma. BAEP waves are all identifiable in spite of the severe depression of EEG activity; however, the I-V interval is increased over normal limits because of hypothermia and direct effects of the drug on central conduction. Two runs of SEPs and BAEPs obtained under the same recording conditions illustrate the test-retest stability of the responses. Left: left median nerve and left ear stimulation; right: right median nerve and right ear stimulation.

pathologic variability of SEPs is as follows. Conduction velocities reach adult values before the age of 3 years in the peripheral nervous system and at the age of 5 to 6 years in dorsal columns. Later on, changes in conduction velocity related to fiber maturation begin to interact with those of body growth, and the peaking latencies progressively increase to adult values, which are reached around the age of 15 to 17 years. The central conduction time variability related to body height can be disregarded in upper but not in lower limb SEPs. Limb temperature is known to affect pe-

ripheral nerve conduction velocities, which are reduced when limb temperature decreases. Moreover, marked hypothermia (e.g., as observed in drug intoxication) prolongs absolute and interpeak SEP latencies. The very mild sleep-related changes of early SEPs reported so far are not likely to affect the interpretation of early SEPs in most patients. Consequently EEG monitoring of the vigilance state during daytime recording of SEPs can be useful only in patients with a fluctuating state of vigilance related to the disease itself or to drug sedation.

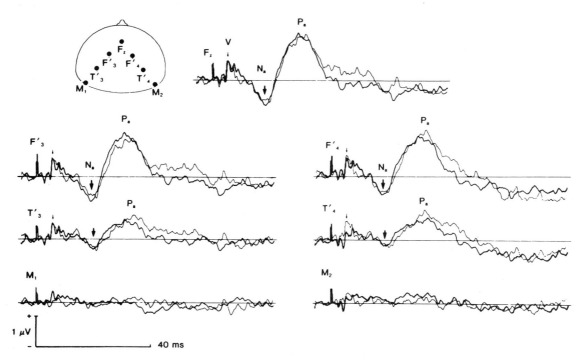

Figure 11-19. Middle latency auditory evoked potentials (MLAEPs) to monaural stimulation (normal adult wave forms). Note that the Pa wave is maximal on the midline (lead Fz), fairly symmetrical in the frontal regions (leads F'3 and F'4), decreased in amplitude in the temporal regions (leads T'3 and T'4), and virtually absent at the mastoids (leads M1 and M2). The BAEP wave V is identifiable preceding the onset of the Na wave. Note that responses to left (thick traces) and right (thin traces) ear stimulation are quite similar with regard to their amplitudes and scalp distributions. (From Ibañez et al., with permission.)

Short-Latency Somatosensory Evoked Potentials to Upper Limb Stimulation. The activity of the brachial plexus trunks (median, radial, and ulnar nerve SEPs) appears as a negative peak culminating at about 9 ms in the supraclavicular fossa of normal subjects. The response of dorsal horn neurons of the cervical cord is recorded over the spinous processes of the C4 to C7 vertebrae as an N13 potential (Fig. 11-20). Three positive potentials with mean latencies of 9, 11, and 14 ms, labeled accordingly P9, P11, and P14, can be recorded on the scalp after upper limb stimulation. These potentials reflect, respectively, the afferent volley in the trunks of the brachial plexus (P9), dorsal columns of the cervical cord (P11), and lower segment of medial lemniscus fibers (P14). Only P9 and P14 are recorded in 100 percent of normal subjects using appropriate electrode montages. There is no recordable potential on the scalp that reflects the activity of the ventroposterolateral thalamic nucleus (VPL). An N18 potential spread across the scalp has been identified following the P14 potential, which persists in posterior thalamic infarction and long after hemispherectomy and which entails retrograde degeneration of the thalamocortical neurons. Two sets of early cortical SEPs have been identified on the scalp. The

first is made of a N20-P27 complex recorded in the parietal region contralateral to the stimulation. The second is composed of the P22 and N30 potentials, which are recorded in the contralateral central and frontal regions. These potentials are also present after finger stimulation. N20 reflects the activation of area 3b in the posterior bank of the central sulcus. The origins of P22, P27, and N30 potentials are still controversial. However, data from SEP findings in patients with hemispheric lesions suggest that P27 is generated in the parietal cortex, whereas P22 and N30 could originate in the prerolandic cortical areas. Frontal SEPs are presumed to be triggered, at least in part, through direct thalamocortical connections, which are not involved in any perceptive process, but subserve the somatosensory control of motor programming (see Mauguière et al. in Barber and Blum, 1987, and Mauguière and Ibañez in Rossini and Mauguière, 1990, for a review). Experimental lesions in the monkey failed, however, to demonstrate the existence of early SEPs generated in the motor cortex.

Short-Latency Somotosensory Evoked Potentials Lower Limb Stimulation. Electrical stimulation of the tibial nerve at the ankle is adopted by most authors

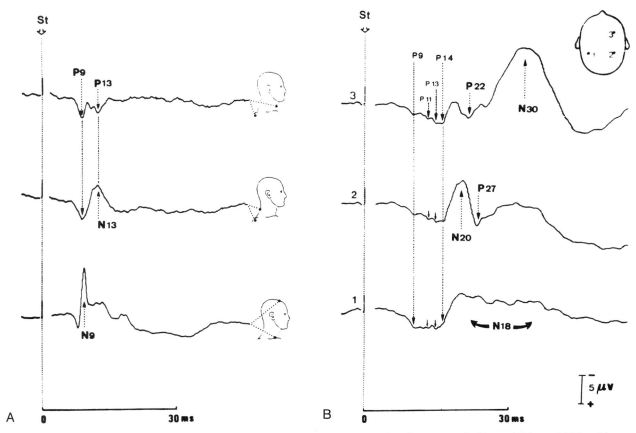

Figure 11-20. **(A & B)** Normal median nerve SEPs (see text for description). (From Lüders, 1989, with permission.)

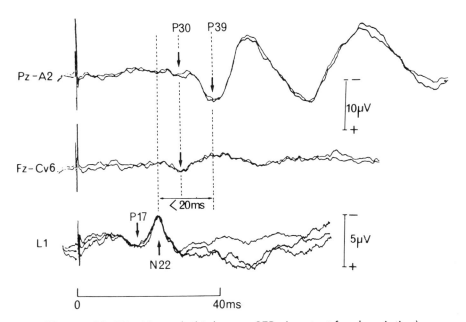

Figure 11-21. Normal tibial nerve SEPs (see text for description).

for the testing of the sensory pathways of the lower limb. It elicits three main potentials: (1) N7, which reflects the nerve action potentials in the popliteal fossa; (2) N22, usually recorded over the spinous process of the L1 vertebra, which corresponds to the postsynaptic responses of dorsal horn neurons to incoming inputs (equivalent to the upper limb N13 SEP); and (3) P39, recorded on scalp midline in the centroparietal region, which represents the earliest cortical response of SI neurons (Fig. 11–21). Electrical stimulation of the dorsal nerves of the penis or the clitoris and of the L5 and S1 dermatomes also yields consistent cortical potentials on the scalp that may be clinically useful.

Clinical Applications

Pattern Visual Evoked Potentials in Eye, Optic Nerve, Chiasmal, and Retrochiasmal Lesions

When abnormal pattern VEPs are associated with a visual loss, an already suspected eye disease will be identified by ophthalmologic examination. Major refractive errors and cornea, lens, and vitreous opacities as well as maculopathies can affect the P100 potential when they cause central scotomata. Similarly, glaucoma can be associated with delayed VEPs when there is a visual impairment in the central 6 degrees of the visual field. Pattern VEPs are also particularly sensitive to the effect of optic nerve compression. Amplitude reduction and latency shift of the P100 potential can be recorded even when clinical signs are minimal in patients with extrinsic compression of the optic nerve and chiasm. Delayed VEPs in these patients can be misinterpreted as a symptom of primary demyelination. Pattern VEPs can also be abnormal in various diseases affecting conduction in the visual pathways, such as toxic amblyopias due to alcohol-tobacco abuse, vitamin B12 and folic acid deficiency, ischemic optic neuropathy, neurosyphilis, sarcoidosis, Leber's optic atrophy, and dominant hereditary optic atrophy.

In patients with bitemporal or homonymous hemianopia, VEPs to half-field stimulation are absent when the blind half field is stimulated. Stimulation of the functional half field evokes a P100 potential, which is shifted toward the occipital region ipsilateral to the stimulated field. The detection rate of VEP abnormalities to half-field stimulation in patients with homonymous visual field defects has been estimated at 84 percent. This figure is rather low if one considers that the field defect was obvious on conventional perimetry in all patients. Thus, present VEP techniques are less sensitive than campimetry for detecting visual field defects.

Pattern Visual Evoked Potentials in Parkinson's Disease

In patients with Parkinson's disease, the P100 potential may be delayed when the eye is stimulated by the reversal of a vertical grating (see Regan, 1989). VEP delay in Parkinson's disease has been attributed to a synaptic dysfunction at the retinal level, which is related to a dopamine deficiency of the amacrine cells. Obviously, VEPs have no diagnostic utility in Parkinson's disease; they could be helpful only for follow-up studies, since their latencies were reported to parallel clinical evolution under dopamine therapy.

Brainstem Auditory Evoked Potentials in Conduction Hearing Loss and Endocochlear Lesions

BAEP abnormalities observed in these conditions usually combine (1) an increase of the latencies of all peaks as compared with those measured at the same stimulus intensity in normal subjects; (2) an increased threshold intensity necessary to obtain the wave V; and (3) relatively preserved interpeak intervals. However in severely deaf patients, all BAEP waves may be absent, and this provides no valuable information concerning the mechanism of the hearing loss. In this situation it is helpful to record the electrocochleogram using transtympanic or extratympanic electrodes in order to study the auditory EPs originating in the cochlea and the acoustic nerve.

Brainstem Auditory Evoked Potentials in Lesions of the Acoustic Nerve and Brainstem

In a patient presenting with uni- or bilateral deafness, identified as being of retrocochlear origin by audiometric testing, the BAEP abnormality that is the most evocative of a conduction defect in the acoustic nerve is an abnormal increase of the I-III and I-V intervals after stimulation of the deaf ear(s), often associated with a reduced wave V. Absence of all peaks after wave I as well as complete disappearance of all BAEP waves can also be observed in cerebellopontine lesions. Any of these BAEP abnormalities, except the absence of all waves, can occur in brainstem lesions affecting the auditory pathways, with the difference that audition is preserved in a large majority of these cases. The sensitivity of BAEPs in the detection of acoustic neuromas is excellent, and the percentage of acoustic neuromas with normal BAEPs is about 2 to 5 percent in most series. The recording of BAEPs suggestive of a retrocochlear dysfunction in a patient whose conventional CT scan is normal should prompt complementary neuroimaging investigations of the cerebellopontine angle and internal auditory canal (CT scan or MRI).

The most frequent BAEP findings in brainstem lesions consist of latency and amplitude abnormalities of waves III and V. When observed in the absence of any hearing loss, these abnormalities are highly suggestive of lesions affecting the auditory pathways in the pons or cerebral peduncles.

Somatosensory Evoked Potentials in Lesions of Peripheral Nerves and Roots

In the evaluation of peripheral pathology SEPs can be useful (1) to measure peripheral conduction velocities when sensory nerve action potentials cannot be obtained at the periphery in severe neuropathies and (2) to explore proximal lesions of the peripheral sensory pathways that are not accessible to conventional electromyographic studies.

In brachial and lumbosacral plexus lesions, SEPs can be helpful for assessing the topography of the lesion. One of the main surgical issues in traumatic plexopathies is to know whether the lesion is proximal or distal to dorsal ganglia. Upper limb SEPs showing a preserved supraclavicular N9 potential with abolition of all subsequent components indicates a proximal root avulsion. On the other hand, the absence of all SEPs including N9 indicates a complete lesion distal to the ganglia but does not eliminate the possibility of a more proximal lesion in addition to the distal lesion. Median and ulnar nerve SEPs are normal in most patients with thoracic outlet syndrome. Consequently, the diagnostic utility of SEPs is limited to patients in whom another pathology is suspected.

SEPs complement F-wave recording for assessing conduction in proximal nerve segments and roots in the Guillain-Barré syndrome. In about half of these patients, however, all median nerve SEPs are within normal limits, while tibial SEPs are more frequently affected, showing a normal or delayed peripheral N7 at the popliteal fossa with a reduced or absent lumbar N22. SEP measurement cannot be viewed as a routine examination in Guillain-Barré syndrome and should be performed only to detect proximal conduction blocks or slowing not demonstrated by conventional electromyographic or F-wave recordings. SEPs evoked by stimulation of mixed nerves are seldom useful in radiculopathies because they explore several roots simultaneously and thus entail the risk of an undetected monoradiculopathy, since normal responses can be mediated through unaffected roots.

Somatosensory Evoked Potentials in Cord and Brainstem Focal Lesions

The clinical utility of SEPs in nondemyelinating cord lesions pertains to the possibility that they offer of assessing separately the segmental responses generated by dorsal horn neurons (N13 and N22, respectively, for upper and lower limb SEPs) and the conduction time in the dorsal column fibers. In that respect SEPs represent mostly a functional screening test, which obviously does not compete with radiographic or MRI myelographic studies. However, SEPs give clear indications concerning the site of the functional damage to the cord, which cannot be provided by neuroimaging techniques alone. For example, when the volley of impulses ascending in the cervical dorsal columns is blocked or dispersed at the cervicomedullary junction, the P9 and spinal N13 are normal, whereas far-field P14 and later components are absent or abnormal in median nerve SEPs (see Mauguière, in Lüders, 1989). Conversely, when the dorsal horn of the lower cervical cord is infiltrated by a tumor or occupied by a syrinx, the spinal N13 is usually reduced in amplitude or absent after stimulation of the median or ulnar nerves at the wrist, while the central conduction time can be normal.

In cervical spondylolytic myelopathy, radiographs usually show multiple levels of possible cord lesions, and SEPs are useful; (1) for assessing whether there is any significant conduction slowing in dorsal columns (in this respect lower limb SEPs are more likely to be affected than upper limb SEPs; and (2) for detecting abnormalities of the segmental N13 SEP, indicating the level of cord dysfunction.

The far-field P14 is the only SEP component that reflects the activity of medial lemniscus fibers, whereas the widespread N18 is presumed to be a postsynaptic potential generated in the brainstem nuclei receiving inputs from the medial lemniscus. These two components are clearly reduced, delayed, or absent in lesions of the medulla oblongata, while they are preserved in most patients with pontine or mesencephalic lesions. Interruption of the spinothalamic tract in the medulla oblongata (Wallenberg's syndrome) does not modify P14 or N20.

Somatosensory Evoked Potentials in Thalamic, Capsulothalamic and Cortical Lesions

SEP data from the author's series of 241 patients with hemispheric lesions documented by neuroimaging (Mauguière and Ibañez in Rossini and Mauguière, 1990) show that median nerve SEPs are abnormal in more than 70 percent of capsulothalamic and in nearly 90 percent of posterior thalamic lesions. After stimulation of the affected side, the loss of both parietal (N20-P27) and frontal (P22-N30) components with preserved scalp far-field positivities, including P14, represent the most frequent SEP abnormality. Reduced or absent cortical SEPs are highly correlated with impaired touch and joint sensations. The occurrence of spontaneous pain or paresthesias in thalamic lesions can be associated with several SEP patterns, which reflect the degree of hemispheric deafferentation. Conversely, there is a fairly good correlation between SEP and CT scan (or MRI) findings. Cortical SEPs, including the N20, P22, P27, and N30 components, are consistently absent or abnormal in posterolateral infarctions of the geniculothalamic artery territory, while they are normal in infarctions in other thalamic arterial territories.

In large lesions involving the central and parietal regions, abnormal SEPs are similar to those observed in posterior thalamic lesions deafferenting the hemisphere, showing a loss of all cortical SEPs with preserved P14 and N18 components. In lesions outside the centroparietal area, early cortical SEPs are normal. When the lesion is close to the cortex, it can separately damage pre- and postrolandic cortices or thalamocortical fibers in the corona radiata and selectively abolish parietal or frontal SEPs. Patients with cortical lesions and abnormal or absent N20 or P27 potentials usually show astereognosis, often combined with hypesthesia for some elementary sensory modalities, but they do not present with major motor deficit when frontal SEPs are preserved. Conversely, sensations are preserved and motricity impaired in patients with absent or grossly abnormal frontal SEPs and normal parietal responses (Mauguière et al., 1983).

Evoked Potentials in Multiple Sclerosis

The diagnosis of MS is accepted as definite only when both the relapsing evolution and multifocal lesions can be demonstrated. Clinically silent plaques of demyelination located in optic, somatosensory, and brainstem auditory pathways can be detected, respectively, by pattern VEPs, SEPs, and BAEPs. EPs can also ascertain retrospectively a dysfunction of the central sensory pathways long after the appearance of transient and unexplored symptoms, possibly related to a demyelinating relapse. Delayed EPs in MS can be accepted as a sign of central demyelination only on the condition that a dysfunction of receptors or peripheral nerves has been eliminated. Overlooking this diagnostic step represents one of the most frequent cause of misinterpretation of EPs, the others being superficial anamnesis and unreliable neurologic examination.

Abnormal Evoked Potential Waveforms.
Visual Evoked Potentials. Flash VEPs are less sensitive to optic nerve demyelination than pattern reversal VEPs and have been abandoned in MS diagnosis. Abnormal aspects of pattern reversal VEPs in MS have been extensively described and discussed in earlier textbooks (Halliday, 1993; Chiappa, 1990) and will be only briefly reviewed here. A delay of the P100 potential represents nearly 80 percent of abnormal VEP waveforms in MS. Absent VEPs are observed either in the acute stage of optic neuritis or late in the course

of the disease in the absence of visual impairment. Exceptionally, normal VEPs can be recorded when stimulating the abnormal eye in the acute stage of optic neuritis. VEP abnormalities are bilateral in 50 to 70 percent of cases, depending on the criteria adopted for selecting patients. Abnormal interocular latency difference is a very sensitive indicator of optic nerve dysfunction, particularly in patients with a past history of unilateral optic neuritis. Raising body temperature increases the incidence of abnormal VEPs in MS while physical exercise reduces the amplitude of P100, but mostly in patients with delayed VEPs at rest. None of these maneuvers is routinely carried out, the former because of technical difficulties and the fear that it could precipitate a relapse and the latter because it does not significantly modify the hit rate of VEPs.

Brainstem Auditory Evoked Potentials. An increase of the interpeak interval between waves I and V is observed in one-third of BAEP-abnormal MS patients. In more than half of these patients peak V is reduced, with the I/V amplitude ratio high or absent, and in 10 percent the only persisting component is peak I. BAEP abnormalities are monaural in 30 to 45 percent of MS patients. Complete abolition of all BAEPs, including peak I, should lead to reconsideration of the diagnosis of MS when it has not been firmly established on clinical grounds. BAEP abnormalities similar to those reported in MS have also been observed in other demyelinating diseases such as central pontine myelinolysis, leukodystrophies, and Pelizaeus-Merzbacher disease.

Somatosensory Evoked Potentials. The most frequent SEP abnormalities in MS are the delay or the absence of the early cortical potentials evoked by tibial nerve stimulation at the ankle (P39) or by median nerve stimulation at the wrist (N20). Delayed cortical responses result in a prolongation of the central conduction time. SEP abnormalities can be uni- or bilateral and when unilateral may involve only one limb. Time dispersion of the ascending volley in dorsal columns and brainstem lemniscal fibers is reflected by an abnormal P14 potential, which is observed in 90 percent of MS patients with abnormal median nerve SEPs. SEPs may, of course, be abnormal in MS patients who have never experienced symptoms referable to the sensory system, but they are normal in nearly one-fourth of MS patients with sensory complaints. In that respect SEPs differ from other EPs, which are exceptionally normal in symptomatic patients. This most probably reflects the fact that SEPs do not explore all the somatosensory pathways but preferentially the dorsal column system.

Diagnostic Yield of Evoked Potentials in Multiple Sclerosis Patients.
In definite MS, VEP abnormalities are the most frequent, followed by SEP (including

tibial nerve EP) and BAEP abnormalities. This reflects the well-known high frequency of optic nerve lesions in patients with definite MS. The criterion for the diagnostic yield of EPs is the frequency of clinically silent lesions disclosed by EP testing. In that respect VEPs are also the most rewarding. In terms of detection of clinically silent lesions, brain MRI is superior to EPs. At present the most serious limitations of MRI are cost and limited clinical availability. Moreover, it must be remembered that the abnormal T2 signals evidenced by brain MRI scans in the white matter of MS patients can also be observed in clinically normal subjects over age 45.

Detecting a silent lesion in a mono- or paucisymptomatic MS does not necessarily indicate a spatial dissemination of the disease. For example, abnormal SEPs in MS patients presenting with clinical evidence of spinal cord disease but no sensory loss do reveal a subclinical involvement of the somatosensory pathways. However, abnormal SEPs in such cases can result from a single cord lesion and thus cannot be taken as a proof of dissemination.

Beside their utility as indicators of multifocal, clinically silent lesions, EPs are often useful to assess the organic basis of subjective symptoms. Abnormal responses then provide evidence of the lesion in the area suspected of being affected. EPs may also help to determine the site of abnormal conduction in MS and eventually to correlate it with clinical symptoms or imaging data.

In most of the clinical presentations of MS, the proportion of abnormal EPs that one can expect depends upon the time elapsed between the EP recording and the first clinical symptom. At present the notion that the percentage of EP-abnormal MS patients increases with time has been demonstrated only by actuarial studies of large populations of MS patients. The reliability of EPs as an early diagnostic test in MS can be assessed only by follow-up studies over several years. They should permit estimation of the percentages of EP-abnormal patients who will not develop MS and of EP-normal ones who will. There is, however, some evidence that among patients whose EPs are recorded early (i.e., when the diagnosis of MS can only be suspected), those in whom EPs disclose a silent lesion have more chance to develop MS than those with normal EPs.

Evoked Potential Diagnostic Strategies in Multiple Sclerosis. The most reasonable attitude toward EP investigations consists in choosing in any individual patient the EP strategy that has some chance to provide evidence that supports a diagnosis of MS based on clinical data. We will only briefly outline here the EP diagnostic strategies in two frequent clinical presentations of the disease.

Clinically Isolated Optic Neuritis. In patients with a first episode of optic neuritis or with a history of single or multiple attacks of optic neuritis, SEPs and BAEPs will be abnormal in less than 30 percent of cases, even when recorded several years after the first attack. This is in agreement with the fact that MS is diagnosed in a minority of patients 5 years after an attack of optic neuritis and in less than half of them after a 9-year follow-up. During an acute attack of optic neuritis, VEPs of the affected eye will almost constantly support the suspected diagnosis. When visual acuity has returned to normal, a delayed P100 is observed in more than 95 percent of affected eyes in adults and can allow retrospective diagnosis of a past episode of optic neuritis. In either of these two conditions VEPs may disclose a delayed response of the unaffected eye.

Clinically Isolated Brainstem or Noncompressive Cord Syndromes. In patients with no history of optic neuritis and with clinical evidence of isolated brainstem or cord lesions' EP recording has diagnostic utility when the diagnosis of MS is only possible or probable. VEPs are then the most informative and when abnormal, provide the strongest EP evidence in favor of dissemination. However, during or immediately after a single episode that may correspond to a first MS relapse, abnormal VEPs are recorded only in less than 10 percent of cases. This rate increases with time, even in the absence of other clinical relapses during the interval between onset and EP recording.

Abnormal VEPs and BAEPs are frequently observed in progressive spastic paraparesis. They should be looked for in any of these patients and strongly suggest dissemination of the lesions outside the spinal cord. There is a nonzero risk of overlooking a spinal cord compression when VEPs are abnormal in a patient with progressive paraparesis, since the association of cervical spondylotic myelopathy and MS has been reported.

Evoked Potentials in Coma and Brain Death

BAEPs and short-latency SEPs are considered to contribute to diagnosis and prognosis in comatose patients, while middle-latency auditory responses are emerging as probable good indicators of cortical function. Conversely, other modalities such as long-latency auditory or flash visual responses have been almost abandoned. The standard EP approach to comatose patients usually consists of a single recording session at a given moment of the patient's course. However, repeated EP testing is increasingly being recommended for detecting abrupt changes in the patient's homeostasis.

Several nonpathologic factors have been identified,

which may cause EP changes not directly related to the deterioration of brain function and are particularly relevant for EP interpretation in deeply comatose patients. Hypothermia increases BAEP and SEP central conduction times. Short-latency EPs and BAEPs, although more resistant to CNS depressants than spontaneous EEG activity (Fig. 11-18), may be substantially distorted by the high dosages of anesthetics sometimes used to reduce brain metabolic demands and intracranial pressure. Barbiturate levels needed to abolish short-latency SEPs including the N20 potential, largely exceed those currently employed in intensive care units, while potentials peaking later than 25 ms, as well as the middle-latency auditory responses Na and Pa, are much more affected by barbiturate anesthesia. Phenytoin, at the high loading doses employed in status epilepticus, affects the amplitudes and latencies of early SEPs and BAEPs. Finally, as already mentioned, high doses of lidocaine can severely distort BAEPs in comatose patients when combined with thiopental. A careful analysis of the possible influence of the above factors is mandatory in each individual case before any EP interpretation is made. Moreover, comatose patients may show SEP or BAEP abnormalities related to pre-existing pathologic conditions, including degenerative diseases or MS, which may be misleading when the patient's past history is unknown.

Coma. About 90 percent of head-injured comatose patients with neuroimaging evidence of hemispheric lesions have a fatal course or remain in a persistent vegetative state when no N20 potential can be recorded with preserved peripheral and spinal SEPs. This statement does not hold for primary brainstem lesions interrupting ascending pathways. In postanoxic coma bilateral N20 loss, when associated with preserved BAEPs, heralds a persistent vegetative state much more frequently than in head-injured patients. Increased central conduction time has been considered a reliable predictor of poor outcome. However this view, although supported by statistics, is of little value when evaluating EP prognostic significance in a single patient. Sequential assessment of central conduction time during coma reflects more accurately the patient's course and allows better predictions of clinical outcome. Death or severe disability occurs in about 30 percent of comatose patients with bilaterally normal N20, and favorable outcome predictions are more reliable when based on normal cortical SEPs, including early SEPs other than the N20, rather than on normal N20 alone.

Absent BAEPs or an isolated wave I when observed bilaterally indicates poor prognosis, provided that peripheral auditory problems, primary brainstem lesions, and drug effects can be ruled out. Conversely, normal BAEPs do not warrant good outcome from coma since the average incidence of an unfavorable course (leading to severe disabilities, vegetative state, or death) is about 30 percent in patients with bilaterally normal BAEPs during the acute phase of traumatic or cerebrovascular coma.

Coma or Pseudocoma Caused by Primary Brainstem Lesions. The diagnostic approach to patients with primary brainstem lesions may greatly benefit from EP testing. In the locked-in syndrome, EPs are preserved if brainstem auditory and somatosensory pathways are unaffected. Patients in coma due to basilar artery occlusion most often show abnormal BAEPs, especially waves IV and V. Isolated alteration of waves IV and V in brainstem infarcts suggests a basilar occlusion rostral to the emergence of the anteroinferior cerebellar artery; when the occlusion is proximal to or involves this artery, which usually supplies both the cochlear nucleus and the peripheral auditory structures, all BAEPs including wave I may be abolished. This seriously hampers the usefulness of BAEPs for the diagnosis of brain death in patients with primary brainstem lesions.

Brain Death. The concept of brain death implies irreversible loss of function in cerebral hemispheres and brainstem. Consequently, the only consistent EP pattern associated with brain death is one in which no evidence of CNS activity is detected rostrally to the foramen magnum. This pattern includes (1) a bilateral absence of brainstem P14 and of all subsequent cortical potentials in median nerve SEPs (Fig. 11-11), the value of which is reinforced if peripheral and spinal N9 and N13 potentials are preserved (these potentials remain normal in brain death except in cases complicated by spinal injury); and (2) an isolated wave I, or waves I and II, without subsequent brainstem potentials in BAEPs. Complete BAEP abolition is also a pattern often seen in brain-dead patients (Fig. 11-11), but its significance is more equivocal since it may be caused by any direct damage to peripheral auditory structures.

Brain death is not the only condition leading to the above described EP abnormalities, which can also be observed in primary brainstem lesions. Consequently, EPs must be viewed as a confirmatory test to be interpreted in conjunction with clinical, neuroimaging, biochemical, and EEG data.

Testing in Neuropsychology

Short- or middle-latency EPs do not give direct access to the intimate mechanisms underlying disorders of highly integrated cortical functions such as perception, praxis, memory, attention, and language. However, neuropsychological concepts such as *neglect* or *agnosia* are based on the assumption that primary sensory cortical areas are not anatomically disconnected from the peripheral receptors. In some conditions clinical data alone may be poorly informative with regard to the sensory afferentation of the hemispheres, for example when the patient suffers from attention or vigilance disorders, or when the anatomic organization of the sensory system itself precludes separate analysis of the function of each hemisphere, as in central auditory pathways. In patients with focal hemispheric lesions and disorders of higher cerebral function, the main use of EP recordings is thus to ascertain whether the cortex receives normally sensory inputs from the periphery. This question has been successfully addressed in occipital blindness, astereognosis, and auditory troubles related to hemispheric lesions.

Occipital Blindness. Patients with occipital blindness due to bilateral occipital infarction usually show preserved flash VEPs in response to flash stimulation, probably mediated via extrageniculocalcarine visual pathways. More surprisingly, when able to keep their eyes fixed in the direction of the stimulus, these patients may also have persisting pattern reversal VEPs. This suggests that some of the central retinogeniculate fibers projecting to the primary visual areas and part of these cortical areas themselves are still functional, as confirmed by positron emission tomography studies. In such patients the surviving neuronal pool in area 17 is sufficient to generate a P100 potential but not to ensure visual perception, either because it is disconnected from the associative visual cortex or because this cortex itself has been destroyed.

Astereognosis. SEPs help in the classification of patients with astereognosis by showing that (1) early median nerve or finger SEPs (N20 and/or P27) recorded over the contralateral parietal region are reduced after stimulation of the affected side in most patients, including some of those clinically classified as having pure tactile agnosia; (2) frontal SEP components may be unaffected; and (3) SEPs are normal in patients with unilateral tactile anomia secondary to callosal disconnection. These correlations hold only for fixed vascular or post-traumatic lesions involving the parietal cortex and can be useful to assess the organic basis of alleged astereognosis in medicolegal practice. Conversely, patients with subcortical lesions, including demyelination, but intact cortex may have normal stereognosis with clearly abnormal parietal SEPs.

Auditory Troubles in Hemispheric Lesions. Patients with unilateral damage to the auditory cortex are not deaf because the normal hemisphere still receives information from both ears. However, when two different messages are delivered simultaneously to both ears (dichotic listening test), they have difficulty with repeating words delivered to the ear contralateral to the damaged hemisphere. This auditory extinction phenomenon also occurs in patients with split-brain or neglect whose cortical auditory areas normally receive inputs from the medial geniculate body. Thus, only the recording of reduced cortical AEPs over the affected hemisphere can assess the dysfunction of auditory cortical areas in such patients (see Mauguière in Lüders, 1989). It has also been demonstrated that patients with absent responses over their dominant hemisphere do not necessarily present a language deficit and that right-handed patients with left hemiplegia and anosognosia have a multimodal sensory deafferentation of their minor hemisphere as assessed by absent cortical AEPs and SEPs.

Event-related endogenous potentials, including the P300 potential, have not yet been extensively studied in patients with focal hemispheric lesions, probably because their sources remain partly unknown. Therefore these EPs provide information on the ability of the brain to detect and categorize a target but not on the circuitry involved in this function. By combining reaction time and P300 latency studies in a decision-making task, it has been shown, for example, that the reaction times of patients with ideomotor apraxia can be severely prolonged while the latency of their P300 to visual targets remains within normal limits, which suggests that only the motor execution process is impaired. Conversely, in the same type of task patients with unilateral neglect may have abnormal reaction times and P300 latencies to targets presented in the neglected half-space.

Evoked Potentials in Dementia

Both exogenous and endogenous (cognitive) EPs have been used for assessing the effect of normal aging and dementia on the processing of sensory information by the brain. Aging moderately affects BAEPs and flash and pattern shift VEPs as well as short-latency SEPs in normal subjects. However, most of these effects seem to be related more to subtle changes of peripheral conduction or input encoding by the receptors than to abnormal processing of information by the CNS. Conversely, more dramatic changes of the P300 occur from early adulthood to old age which could reflect progressive slowing of cognitive performance. The peaking latency of the P300 elicited by target stimuli in the auditory odd-ball paradigm increases by 1 or 2 ms per year of age in normal adults. Whether this increase of the P300 is linearly correlated with age remains a debated issue. P300 changes were shown to occur in several types of dementia, including Alzheimer's, Huntington's, and Parkinson's diseases, as well as multiple infarct dementia. Thus the pathologic process responsible for the mental deterioration does not directly influence the P300 changes in demented patients. However, by combining the recording of exogenous and cognitive auditory EPs, Goodin and Aminoff (1986) concluded that only cognitive components were delayed in Alzheimer's-type dementia while both types of auditory EPs were abnormal in subcortical dementias. Conclusions from other studies are less encouraging by showing that deviations in P300 latency or amplitude do occur in dementia but also in schizophrenia and depression and are not specific enough to be useful for diagnosis.

Evoked Potential Testing in Myoclonus

It is widely accepted that spontaneous or stimulus-related bilateral and synchronous jerks of the proximal muscles of the limbs and unilateral, mostly distal, muscle jerks triggered by voluntary movement (action myoclonus) represent two separate categories of myoclonus. However, these two types of myoclonus may coexist in the same patient and it is difficult on the basis of clinical observation alone to distinguish action myoclonus related to hyperexcitability of cortical or subcortical structures from major cerebellar dyssynergia, which can be observed in various conditions, including MS and heredodegenerative diseases. The first description, in 1947 by Dawson, of giant median nerve SEPs in patients with myoclonus (see Halliday, 1993) represents an important step in our understanding of myoclonic syndromes by introducing an additional criterion for separating patients with myoclonus in to two categories namely, those with and without giant SEPs. Complete electrophysiologic investigation of patients with myoclonus includes conventional SEP recordings in response to median nerve and/or finger stimulation, but also jerk-locked EEG averaging and recording of the long-latency myogenic reflex activity (C reflex), which reflects the myoclonus itself. Giant median nerve SEPs indicate cortical hyperreactivity to afferent somatosensory inputs, while the jerk-locked averaged spike indicates that myoclonus is associated with an epileptic discharge in the efferent motor system. The presence of both enhanced SEPs and jerk-locked spikes is characteristic of *pyramidal* and *cortical reflex* myoclonus.

Not all patients with myoclonus have giant SEPs. In particular, enhanced SEPs are usually not observed in benign forms of juvenile myoclonic epilepsies or in essential nonprogressive isolated myoclonus. They are inconstant in Creutzfeldt-Jakob disease and posthypoxic myoclonus. In the two latter conditions the existence of giant SEPs probably depends on the stage of the disease. Conversely, giant SEPs are an almost constant feature in the various forms of progressive myoclonic epilepsy. Giant flash VEPs can also be recorded in patients with photosensitive or progressive myoclonic epilepsies and also represent a common finding in subacute encephalopathies with myoclonus, such as Creutzfeldt-Jakob disease.

Enhanced SEPs can be observed over the damaged hemisphere in patients with focal lesions, including supratentorial tumors, post-traumatic cortical atrophies, and ischemic and hemorrhagic strokes. In these patients the response rarely reaches the extreme amplitudes observed in progressive myoclonic epilepsies and other myoclonic syndromes with giant SEPs.

Vertex and parietal EEG spikes, corresponding to high-voltage SEPs (up to 400 μV), can be evoked by a single tactile stimulation in nonepileptic children aged 3 to 13 years with normal neurologic status. The presence of these "extreme" SEPs might presage the possible occurrence of partial motor seizures with benign outcome.

Evoked Potentials in Amyotrophic Lateral Sclerosis

It is generally accepted that BAEPs and VEPs are non informative in amyotrophic lateral sclerosis. Although several authors have reported central SEP abnormalities, SEPs are not a routine diagnostic procedure in this disease. The recording of abnormal SEPs in a patient with clinical signs of motor neuron disease should suggest an immune system disorder (lymphoma, acquired immunodeficiency syndrome [AIDS], monoclonal paraproteinemia) since peripheral as well as central somatosensory pathways are more likely to be affected in these conditions than in the idiopathic form of the disease.

Evoked Potentials in Heredodegenerative Diseases

Abnormal VEPs, BAEPs, or SEPs have been reported in Charcot-Marie-Tooth disease, Friedreich's ataxia (FA), hereditary spastic paraplegia, and Huntington's chorea. At present EPs cannot be recommended as a test for detection of subjects at risk for Huntington's disease.

Evoked Potentials in Systemic Disorders and Internal Medicine

Multimodal EPs have been reported as abnormal in various diseases and dysmetabolic states, some of which may cause or be associated with clinically silent conduction abnormalities in the CNS. However, in most of these conditions the diagnosis is settled on the basis of clinical or laboratory findings and not on that of abnormal EPs. Moreover, some of the reported EP changes are statistically significant group differences between controls and patients and have poor diagnostic value in individuals. Therefore it is uncertain whether EPs should be included in the diagnostic strategies, although they may provide useful information in prospective follow-up, pathophysiologic, or drug evaluation studies. (For a complete review see Chiappa, 1990.)

Renal Failure. Multimodal EPs have been studied in untreated, hemodialyzed, and kidney-transplanted patients. As compared with controls, patients with renal failure, when recorded before the first dialysis session, have, as a group, delayed pattern reversal VEPs, delayed peripheral and central median nerve SEPs with no change of central conduction time, and a minimal increase of the BAEP I-V interval. Hemodialysis and renal transplantation were found to have beneficial effects on BAEPs and pattern reversal VEPs, respectively. The auditory P300 was also reported as delayed in more than 50 percent of patients undergoing chronic hemodialysis.

Vitamin Deficiency. Most patients with neurologic symptoms related to vitamin B12 deficiency have abnormal tibial nerve SEPs after stimulation of the lower limbs. Abnormal median nerve SEPs are less consistent and show a conduction slowing in dorsal columns. If BAEP abnormalities are uncommon, pattern reversal VEPs are usually delayed, even in the absence of visual impairment, in patients with vitamin B12 or folic acid deficiency and clinical symptoms of subacute combined degeneration. With conventional patterns the VEP abnormalities are very similar to those observed in MS. Vitamin supplementation usually restores EP latencies to normal.

AIDS and Lymphotrophic Virus Infection. EP investigations can detect subclinical lesions of the CNS in asymptomatic human immunodeficiency virus (HIV)-positive subjects and patients with minor general symptoms of the disease (AIDS-related complex) or persistent generalized lymphadenopathy. In asymptomatic HIV-positive patients BAEPs and tibial nerve SEPs have been reported to be more sensitive than VEPs and median nerve SEPs. Multimodal EP studies combining VEPs, SEPs, and BAEPs detect abnormalities in 20 to 40 percent of HIV-positive patients, whereas percentages of EP abnormalities in AIDS are 60 and 85 percent, respectively, in neurologic symptom-free and symptomatic patients (see Farnarier and Somma-Mauvais in Rossini and Mauguière, 1990.)

MAGNETIC BRAIN STIMULATION

Muscle responses (motor evoked potentials [MEPs]) evoked by percutaneous magnetic stimulation of the motor cortex represent an important advance in the study of conduction in central motor pathways and have progressively replaced the earlier method of electrical brain stimulation. The magnetic stimulation of the scalp used for MEP recording produces a current flow that is able to depolarize the underlying motor neurons and fibers. This stimulation produces a muscle twitch, which can be easily recorded with conventional skin electrodes. (The reader is referred to Chiappa, 1990 for a detailed description of the recording technique.)

Normal Responses

Muscle responses evoked by brain stimulation are high-voltage signals, the recording of which requires only simple, conventional equipment and no averaging in most cases. For the neurologist the major utility of this technique is to permit assessment of the central motor conduction time (CMCT) in motor pathways. To measure conduction time magnetic brain stimulation is usually coupled with magnetic (or electric) spinal stimulation, and the latency of the "spinal" MEP is subtracted from that of the "cortical" MEP. The clinician must be aware, however that cervical or lumbar stimulation depolarizes motor root fibers and not the α-motoneurons themselves. Consequently the CMCT measured by this technique includes, in addition to the conduction time in the corticospinal motor pathways and the synaptic delay in the ventral horn, the conduction time in a short proximal segment of the cervical roots and in a longer segment of the cauda equina roots for cervical and lumbar stimulation, respectively. Therefore a direct measurement of peripheral conduction time using F-wave recording (see EMG section of Ch. 12 and Fig. 11-22) is recommended when a proximal root pathology is suspected.

In most clinical studies MEPs are recorded at rest and under weak voluntary contraction. When the target muscles are voluntarily contracted, MEPs are increased in amplitude and decreased in latency because of a phenomenon of central facilitation. The presence or absence of background muscle contraction should absolutely be specified in view of the effects on MEP latencies; for example, the normal central motor conduction time to small hand muscles, which is of about 8 ms at rest, drops to 6 ms under voluntary contraction.

One of the advantages of MEPs is that they permit simultaneous recordings of several target muscles in response to a single brain stimulation and thus make it possible to detect the metameric level at which the conduction is slowed down in patients with a spinal cord disease.

Current clinical experience indicates that adverse effects of magnetic stimulation of the motor cortex are extremely rare. However, focal seizures during or immediately after brain magnetic stimulation have been reported in patients with ischemic cortical lesions, and epilepsy should be regarded as a relative contraindication. Implanted metal structures within

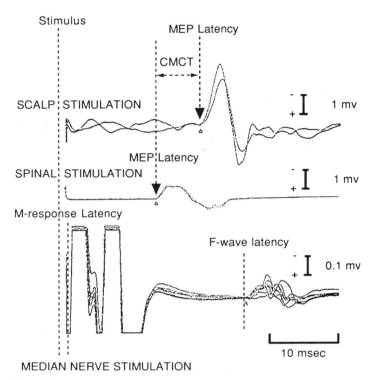

Figure 11-22. MEPs and F-wave. Two successive MEPs recorded in hand muscles (abductor pollicis brevis) after transcranial scalp and spinal magnetic stimulation in a normal adult are superimposed. Responses to scalp stimulation were obtained under voluntary contraction. The time difference between the onset latencies of MEPs to brain and spine stimulation corresponds to the central motor conduction time (CMCT) which includes the transit time in pyramidal neurons, the synaptic delay in the ventral horn of the cord, and the transit time in the proximal segment of α-motoneurons axons. The CMCT can also be evaluated by measuring the F-wave latency. The F-wave is obtained by supramaximal stimulation of a mixed nerve (in this case the median nerve at the wrist) and reflects the muscle response evoked by antidromic depolarization of α-motoneurons. Thus, the latency of the F-wave includes (1) the back-and-forth conduction times between the stimulation site and the ventral horn motoneurons; (2) the conduction time from the stimulation site (wrist) to the hand muscle (M-response latency); and (3) an additional delay of 1 ms corresponding to the depolarization time of α-motoneurons in the ventral horn. Thus the peripheral conduction time (PCT) can be derived from F- and M-wave latency as follows: PCT = [F + M − 1]/2; hence the CCT is given by subtracting the PCT from the scalp MEP latency; CCT = scalp MEP − [F + M − 1]/2. The CCT derived from F-wave latency is shorter than that derived from spinal MEP latency for it does not include any transit time in the proximal segment of ventral root fibers (see above). Note that because of the small voltage of the F-wave, amplification is 10 times as large for F-wave as for MEP recordings; this causes a saturation of the direct M-response. Superimposition of several traces is necessary to assess the consistency of the F-wave onset latency.

the brain are subject to mechanical forces from the induced current, and patients with cardiac pacemakers should not be stimulated. The theoretical risk of kindling an epileptic focus is remote owing to the low frequency of repetitive stimulation allowed by the commercially available magnetic stimulators. Safety considerations were reviewed in detail by Chiappa in 1990, and the reader is referred to that book and local safety regulations for further details on this matter.

Clinical Applications

The measurement of central motor conduction time with MEPs provides information on CNS function that

is a complement to the anatomic information provided by CT or MRI.

MS is the disease that has been the most studied. Abnormal MEPs with prolonged central motor conduction time are demonstrable in around 70 percent of MS patients and, like sensory EPs, can reveal subclinical lesions. MEP abnormalities correlate fairly well with spasticity, hyperreflexia, and Babinski's sign. Prolonged central motor conduction time may also be encountered in compressive myelopathies, degenerative ataxic disorders, hereditary spastic paraparesis, and motor neuron disease, so that the significance of the MEPs is to be interpreted with reference to the clinical context. Nevertheless, marked prolongation of central motor conduction time with relatively preserved MEP amplitudes is suggestive of slowed conduction due to central demyelination of large-diameter fibers. Conversely, MEP abnormalities in motor neuron disease are characterized by absent or severely reduced responses, with moderate prolongation of central motor conduction time. MEPs can also detect proximal conduction block in patients with Guillain-Barré syndrome who otherwise have normal motor conduction and thus represent a useful complement to conventional EMG investigation, but mostly a confirmatory test of F-wave recordings. There is no demonstrated utility of MEP recordings in patients with cerebral infarction, though abnormal responses to brain stimulation, coexisting with normal cervical MEPs, have been reported in this condition.

ACKNOWLEDGMENTS

The author is indebted to Prof. J. Courjon and Drs. M. Revol, C. Fischer, V. Ibanez, L. Garcia-Larrea, M. P. Deiber, and P. Garassus for some of the records reproduced in this chapter.

ANNOTATED BIBLIOGRAPHY

Barber C, Blum T (eds). Evoked Potentials. Vol. 3, Butterworths, Boston, 1987.

A set of review papers on the various types of sensory EPs, including mapping techniques.

Binnie C, Cooper R, Fowler C, et al. Clinical Neurophysiology: EEG, EMG, Nerve Conduction and Evoked Potentials. Butterworths, London, 1994.

Chiappa KH. Evoked Potentials in Clinical Medicine. 2nd Ed. Raven Press, New York, 1990.

A classic comprehensive and sensible book, recently updated.

Courjon J, Mauguière F, Revol M (eds). Clinical Applications of Evoked Potentials in Neurology. Advances in Neurology. Vol. 32, Raven Press, New York.

One of the earliest books on clinical applications of EPs.

Daly DD, Pedley TA. Current Practice of Clinical Electroencephalography. Raven Press, New York, 1990.

A classic in clinical neurophysiology literature, recently updated.

Goodin D, Aminoff MJ. Electrophysiological differences between subtypes of dementia. Brain 1986;109:1103–13.

A provocative article on cognitive EPs in dementia by the promoters of P300 recordings in neurologic diseases.

Halliday AM (ed). Evoked Potentials in Clinical Testing. Churchill Livingstone, Edinburgh, 1993.

A classic by the animator of the "Queen Square group," with a detailed section on VEPs. Recently updated in a second edition.

Ibañez V, Deiber MP, Fischer CM. Middle latency auditory evoked potentials in cortical lesions. Criteria of interhemispheric assymetry. Arch Neurol 1989;46:1325–32.

Lüders H (ed). Advanced Evoked Potentials. Kluwer Academic Publishers, Boston, 1989.

A critical analysis of the clinical utility and limitations of EPs.

Mauguière F, Desmedt JE, Courjon J. Astereognosis and dissociated loss of frontal or parietal components of somatosensory evoked potentials in hemispheric lesions. Brain 1983;106:271–311.

The first study of somatosensory and motor deficits associated with a selective loss of parietal and frontal SEPs in focal hemispheric lesions.

Regan D. Human Brain Electrophysiology. Evoked Potentials and Evoked Magnetic Fields in Science and Medicine. Elsevier, Amsterdam, 1989.

The most detailed book on the physiologic basis of evoked responses.

Rossini PM, Mauguière F (eds). New Trends and Advanced Techniques in Clinical Neurophysiology. Electroenceph Clin Neurophysiol Suppl, Vol. 41, 1990.

A review of all topics that were the most actively debated for the preceding two years in the clinical neurophysiology literature.

Shibasaki H, Yamashita Y, Neshige R et al. Pathogenesis of giant somatosensory evoked potentials in progressive myoclonic epilepsy. Brain 1985;108:226–40.

One of the most informative papers on the electrophysiology of myoclonus by the promoter of the back-averaging technique.

Color Plates

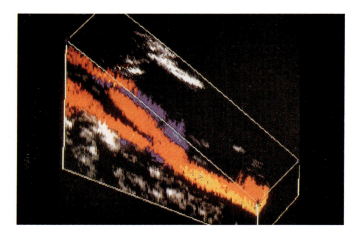

Plate 13-1.

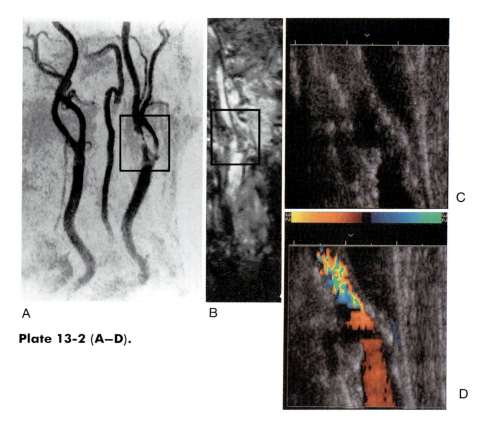

A

B

C

D

Plate 13-2 (A–D).

Plate 13-1. Three-dimensional computer-based analysis of vascular wall structure and blood flow velocity. (From Picot PA, Rickey DW, Mitchell R et al. Three-dimensional colour Doppler imaging. Ultrasound Med Biol. 1993;19:95–105, with permission.)

Plate 13-2. (A & B) Magnetic resonance angiography (MRA) and **(C & D)** color-coded duplex sonography of a subtotal stenosis of the internal carotid artery (ICA) in the neck. The stenosis at the ICA origin shadows parts of the ultrasound image from the vessel wall and intrastenotic flow condition display (Plate C); however, the diagnosis can still be made by the Doppler spectrum display (Plate B). MRA reflects the color-coded plaque image (Plate B) and also displays the entire carotid topography (Plate A).

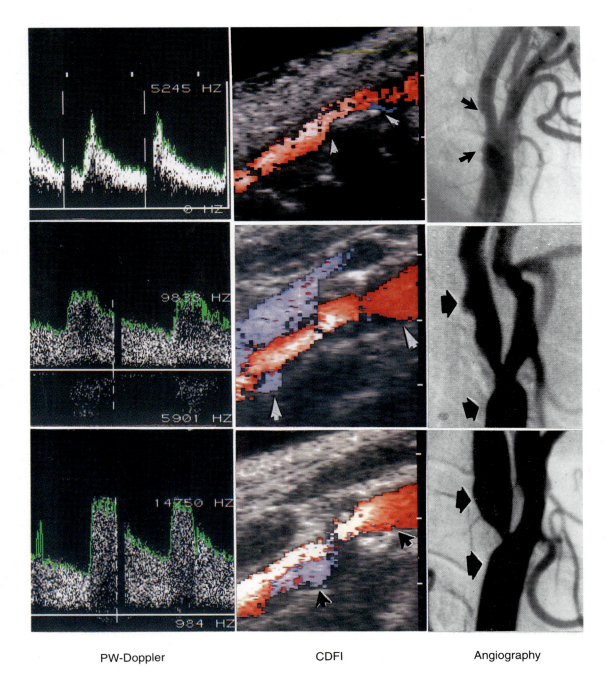

PW-Doppler   CDFI   Angiography

Plate 13-3.

Plate 13-3. Typical examples of mild (top row), moderate (middle row), and severe (bottom row) internal carotid artery stenoses *(arrows)* as shown by angiography (right-hand column), color Doppler flow imaging (CDFI, middle column), and pulsed-wave Doppler spectrum analysis (PW-Doppler, left-hand column).

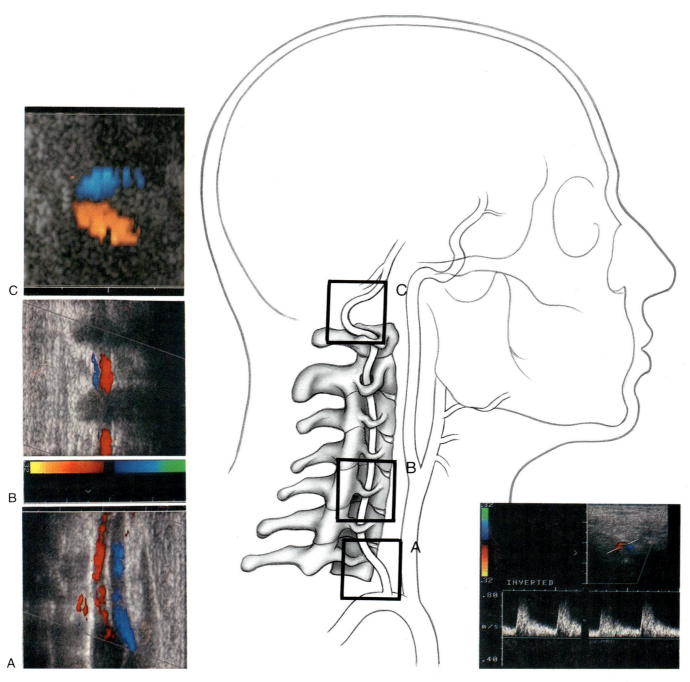

Plate 13-4.

Plate 13-4. Schematic drawing of the areas of insonation from the **(A)** proximal, **(B)** middle, and **(C)** distal vertebral artery in the neck. Typical color-coded sonograms are demonstrated with corresponding Doppler spectra.

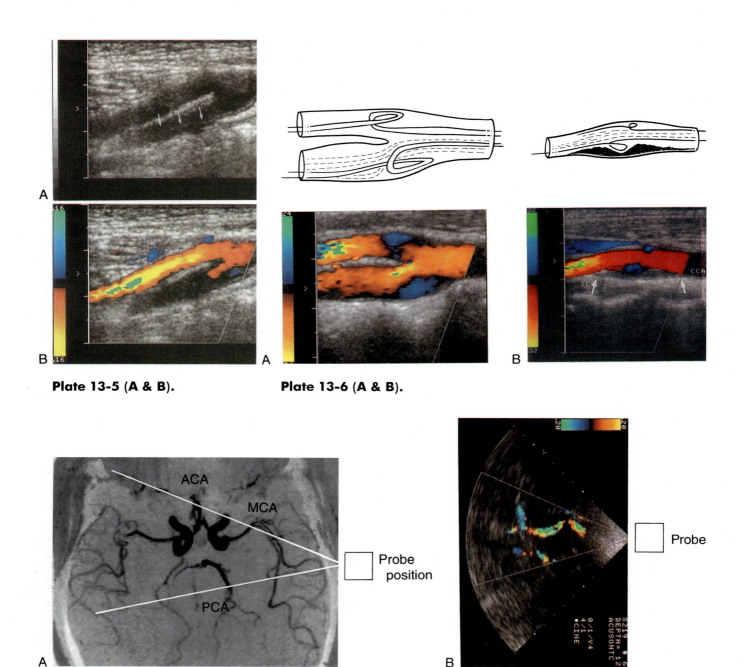

Plate 13-5 (A & B).

Plate 13-6 (A & B).

Plate 13-7 (A & B).

Plate 13-5. Characteristic features of an internal carotid artery dissection as revealed by color-coded duplex sonography and Doppler spectrum analysis. **(A)** B-mode seems to be normal but actually shows a pseudolaminar structure *(arrows)* at the interface between intramural hemorrhage and intravascular blood. **(B)** The color display shows the proximal occlusion with minimal orthograde flow within the carotid bifurcation (red and blue adjacent colors).

Plate 13-6. Demonstration of **(A)** a normal carotid bifurcation and **(B)** a small ulcerated homogeneous plaque at the common carotid artery and internal carotid artery (ICA) bifurcation, with corresponding schematic drawings of the suspected flow directions. There is no secondary vortex area at the proximal ICA where it branches from the bifurcation (Plate B) due to the mild plaque, a finding characteristic of small plaques even before the development of a detectable atherosclerotic lesion (Plate A).

Plate 13-7. **(A)** Magnetic resonance angiography and **(B)** corresponding transcranial color-coded Doppler sonography of the circle of Willis. ACA, anterior carotid artery; MCA, middle carotid artery; PCA, posterior carotid artery.

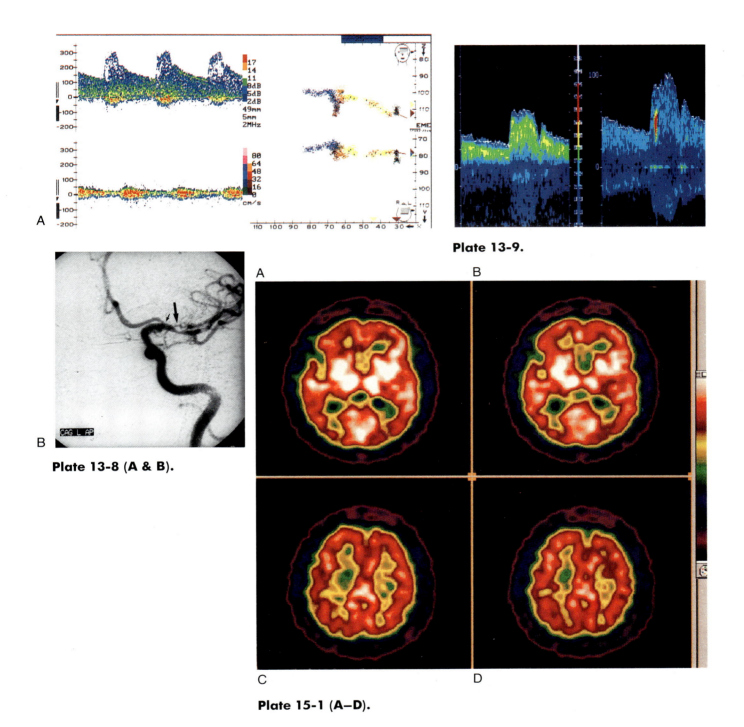

Plate 13-9.

Plate 13-8 (A & B).

A B

C D

Plate 15-1 (A–D).

Plate 13-8. Doppler spectrum at the site of and distal to a severe middle carotid artery stenosis as displayed in **(A)** the two-dimensional sagittal and horizontal sonographic projection and **(B)** the corresponding angiogram.

Plate 13-9. Flow monitoring with spontaneous high-intensity transient signal in a patient with cardiac disease, shown as a tiny red streak in the right-hand image.

Plate 15-1. (A–D) Normal technetium-99m-hexamethylpropylene-amineoxine single-photon emission computed tomograph study. Note the symmetric cortical perfusion with highest perfusion in the occipital lobes, and lowest perfusion in the deep white matter.

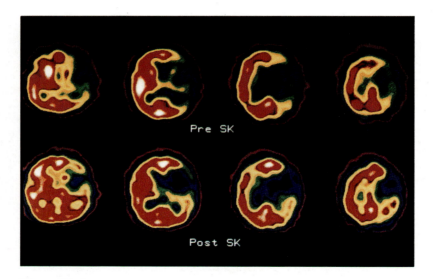

Plate 15-2.

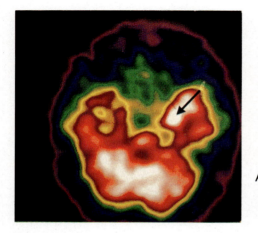

Plate 15-3.

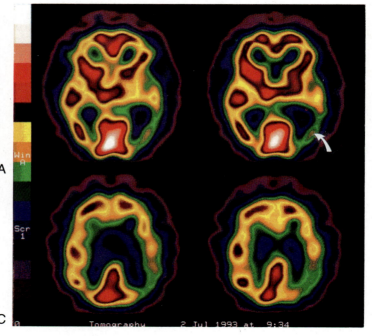

Plate 15-4 (A–D).

Plate 15-2. Marked hypoperfusion in the entire right middle cerebral territory in a patient with acute infarction.

Plate 15-3. Interictal hypoperfusion and ictal hyperperfusion *(arrow)* in a patient with left temporal lobe epilepsy. (Courtesy of Sam Berkovic, M.D., Austin Hospital, Melbourne, Australia.)

Plate 15-4. **(A–D)** Patient with Alzheimer's disease. There is marked hypoperfusion in both temporoparietal cortices *(arrow)*.

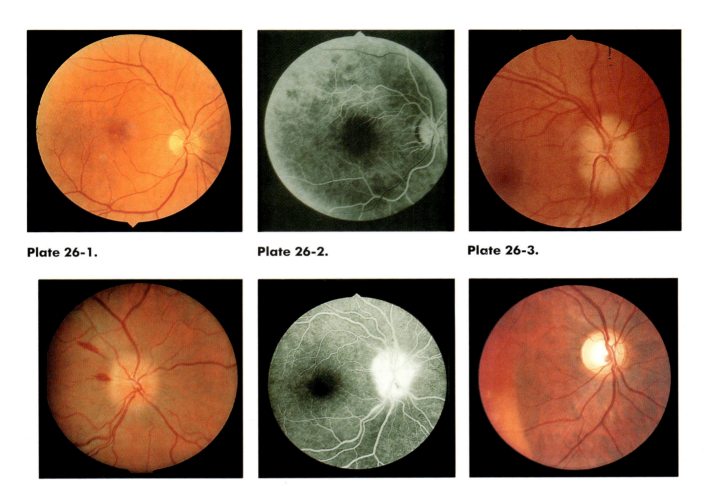

Plate 26-1.

Plate 26-2.

Plate 26-3.

Plate 26-4.

Plate 26-5.

Plate 26-6.

Plate 26-1. Normal fundus. The macula is two disks' diameters outside, on the temporal side of the disk. Veins are larger and darker than the arteries. There is a small cilioretinal artery (see text).

Plate 26-2. Normal fluorescein angiography. The arteries are injected, and the veins are beginning to fill.

Plate 26-3. Papilledema (see text).

Plate 26-4. Papilledema hemorrhages. The veins are slightly dilated.

Plate 26-5. Fluorescein angiography in papilledema.

Plate 26-6. Optic atrophy. (Courtesy Myles Behrens, M.D.)

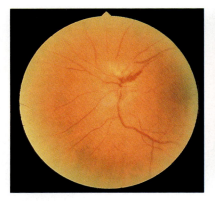

Plate 26-7.

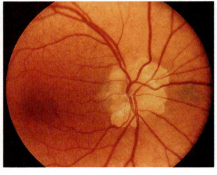

Plate 26-8.

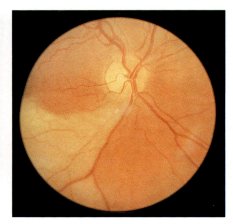

Plate 26-9.

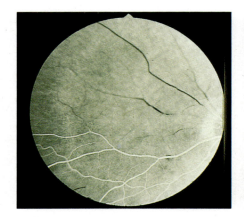

Plate 26-10.

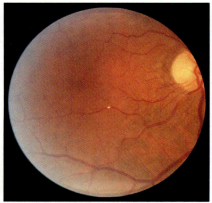

Plate 26-11.

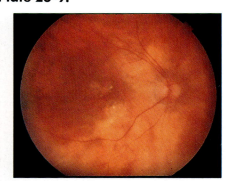

Plate 26-12.

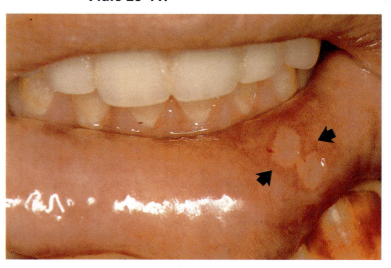

Plate 66-1.

Plate 26-7. Ischemic anterior neuropathy. The disk is swollen, and the hemorrhage present (see text).
Plate 26-8. H. Drüsen (see text).
Plate 26-9. Occulsion of the inferior temporal retinal artery by a chalk-white embolus, probably calcific, in a patient with aortic stenosis.
Plate 26-10. Fluorescein angiography revealing retinal arterial occlusion in a patient with acute disseminated lupus.
Plate 26-11. Cholesterol embolus.
Plate 26-12. Macular degeneration (see text).

Plate 66-1. Oral aphthous ulcer *(arrows)*.

12

Electromyography and Nerve Conduction Studies

Didier Cros

Electromyography (EMG) and nerve conduction studies include techniques for recording the electrical activity generated by peripheral nerves and muscles. Clinical EMG consists of analysis of the electrical signals generated by muscles at rest and during contraction. This signal is recorded with a needle electrode and displayed on an oscilloscope screen and through a loudspeaker. Nerve conduction studies are performed by using electrical stimulation of nerve trunks or of their branches and recording muscle or nerve action potentials. The abbreviation EMG is commonly used to include both electromyography and nerve conduction studies.

It is important to note that EMG and nerve conduction studies are performed to answer questions raised by symptoms described by patients or by findings on physical examination. Each EMG assessment is therefore designed during the patient's visit to the physician immediately preceding the test. The strategy used during the test may be modified by unexpected results as the test progresses. For these reasons, EMG should be considered an extension of the clinical examination rather than a laboratory procedure.

This chapter presents a description of the techniques used for nerve conduction studies and EMG followed by a brief review of abnormal findings in major pathologic entities.

METHODS

Motor Conduction Studies

Motor conduction studies are generally performed with surface recording electrodes and percutaneous stimulation (Fig. 12-1). This method is better tolerated than use of a concentric needle electrode to record the compound muscle action potential (CMAP) from the target muscle. The recording electrodes are positioned over the motor point of the target muscle (active electrode) and over one of the tendons of this muscle (tendon-belly montage). The motor fibers are then stimulated percutaneously at different levels along the course of the corresponding nerve trunk. At each site, the intensity of the electrical stimulus is gradually increased until the supramaximal level of stimulation is reached, and the stimulus is then further increased by 15 to 20 percent. This is done by monitoring the gradual increase in amplitude of the CMAP and determining the intensity beyond which no further increase in amplitude is obtained. The stimulation is then supramaximal, which means that all motor axons innervating the target muscle are excited by the electrical stimulus.

The resulting CMAP is characterized by an initial negative (upgoing) deflection and a smooth outline in normal nerves. At each stimulation site, the following parameters of the CMAP are recorded: onset latency (termed distal latency for the most distal stimulation site in any given nerve), measured in milliseconds; amplitude, usually measured from baseline to negative peak and expressed in millivolts; and duration, measured in milliseconds (in our laboratory, we routinely record the duration of the initial, negative phase of the CMAP). By using the difference in latency between CMAPs obtained at two points along a motor nerve and approximating the length of nerve separating these two points by surface measurements, it is customary to calculate a motor conduction velocity (distance in millimeters divided by latency difference in milliseconds), expressed in meters per second. This conduction velocity is, in fact, the maximum motor conduction velocity and reflects conduction in the largest, fastest-conducting motor fibers. Conduction

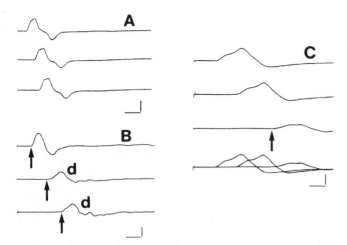

Figure 12-1. **(A–C)** Examples of motor conduction studies of the ulnar nerve (CMAP recorded from abductor digiti minimi) are shown. Stimulation at the wrist (top trace), below the elbow (second trace), above the elbow (third trace), and superimposition of traces 1 to 3 at the bottom in Fig. C. **(A)** Normal conduction study. Note that the amplitude and configuration of the CMAP remains nearly unchanged at the three stimulation sites. **(B)** Motor conduction study in a patient with chronic inflammatory demyelinating polyneuropathy (CIDP). Note by comparison with Fig. A (same calibration) the prolonged latencies at all stimulation sites (arrows) and the dispersion of CMAPs obtained with stimulation below and above the elbow (d). This study shows evidence of partial conduction block of the ulnar nerve in the forearm. **(C)** Motor conduction study of an ulnar nerve with focal neuropathy at the elbow. The study is normal at the wrist and below the elbow but shows marked delay (arrow) and reduction in amplitude of the CMAP elicited with stimulation above the elbow. The reduction in amplitude is easy to appreciate on the bottom trace. Calibration: Figs. A and B: 5 mV, 5 ms; Fig. C: 5 mV, 2 ms.

cording electrode should be repositioned when the CMAP amplitude is unexpectedly low or when the waveform is distorted. Pitfalls may also arise from incorrect positioning of the stimulating electrodes or from inadequate adjustment of stimulus intensity. The stimulating electrode should directly overlie the nerve to be stimulated and should be kept away from other neighboring nerves. This is to avoid inadvertent coactivation of fibers included in a neighboring nerve, which, in the example of wrist stimulation of the median nerve, may result in artifactual distortion of the CMAP recorded from the thenar region. Excessive stimulation intensity through correctly placed stimulating electrodes may also result in unwanted excitation of motor fibers in a neighboring nerve and in the collection of unsound data.

Temperature is also a possible cause of error in nerve conduction studies. Low temperature can result in significant prolongation of motor distal latencies and in marked slowing of sensory conduction velocity, particularly in superficial nerves such as the digital and the sural nerves. It is therefore essential to measure skin temperature prior to conduction studies in each extremity. Low temperatures should be corrected by warming the extremity before the conduction studies are performed. This method is preferable to correction of conduction velocities according to skin temperature.

Finally, certain patterns of anomalous innervation may create difficulties in the interpretation of findings in commonly examined nerves. A common anomaly (found in up to 10 percent of nerves) is the Martin-Gruber anastomosis, which is a crossover of motor fibers from the median to the ulnar nerve in the forearm. Another is the accessory deep peroneal nerve anomaly, in which part of the extensor digitorum brevis muscle is supplied by a motor branch arising from the superficial peroneal nerve in the lower leg.

Sensory Conduction Studies

Sensory conduction studies are easily carried out in superficial cutaneous nerves. Stimulation and recording are performed by using surface electrodes in most instances. Orthodromic or antidromic recording techniques (relative to the transit of physiologically evoked sensory impulses) can be used. Antidromic techniques tend to generate sensory nerve action potentials (SNAPs) of larger amplitude than orthodromic techniques because the recording electrodes are closer to the sensory fibers; this was an advantage before averaging techniques became readily available.

The SNAP is a biphasic (negative-positive) or a triphasic (positive-negative-positive) waveform. The latency of this potential is measured as the onset of the negative (upgoing) deflection that corresponds to con-

velocities in consecutive segments of the same nerve are commonly compared to assess focal compression neuropathy, which is often (but not always) accompanied by focal slowing in the involved segment of nerve. Side-to-side comparison of conduction velocities in corresponding segments is often useful to assess mild pathology.

Persons performing nerve conduction studies should be aware of the pitfalls that may be encountered in clinical situations. Correct placement of surface recording electrodes is essential. Positioning the active electrodes outside the motor point of the target muscle may result in artifactual reduction of the CMAP amplitude, which may be clinically misleading, or in distortion of the waveform, often causing an initial positive deflection. To remedy these potential problems, the anatomic landmarks for motor points should be very familiar to the operator, and the reduction in the fastest-conducting myelinated sensory fibers. Some laboratories measure SNAP latency to the negative peak. This method dates back to the preaveraging era, when the peak was the easiest part of the SNAP to distinguish from electric noise. The SNAP amplitude is the amplitude of the negative peak and reflects the number of large myelinated sensory fibers.

Pathologic abnormalities of SNAPs may include a decrease in amplitude (or in severe cases an unobtainable response) and/or a prolonged latency (often expressed as slowing of conduction velocity). These findings should always be assessed with respect to the normal values provided by the laboratory in which the study was performed. One should also recall that SNAP recording is greatly influenced by limb surface temperature because the cutaneous nerves are superficial. Cooling causes slowing of conduction velocity and increased SNAP amplitude. It is also important to keep in mind that an unobtainable SNAP only means that the subpopulation of sensory axons with the largest diameters is compromised, and provides no information on sensory axons of smaller diameter. Information on these smaller axons can be obtained with near-nerve recording techniques (which are beyond the scope of this chapter), in vitro conduction studies, or histopathologic evaluation of a nerve biopsy.

On occasion, studies of mixed nerve action potentials are clinically useful, such as palmar stimulation of the median nerve while recording at the wrist to document focal pathology due to carpal tunnel syndrome. These studies are technically very similar to sensory studies.

Late Responses

Late responses include F responses and the H reflex, which are both evoked by stimulation of a mixed nerve. Their onset latency is longer than that of the direct M (motor) response evoked by stimulation of the same nerve at the same point—hence the term "late" responses.

F responses are small motor responses following the direct M response with a latency of 25 to 30 ms in the hand muscles and 45 to 55 ms in the intrinsic foot muscles. Usually, 10 to 20 consecutive recording trials are performed in each muscle and the results are displayed in a raster or superimposition format (Fig. 12-2). F responses are generated by the largest α-motor neurons, which are connected to the fastest-conducting axons. They result from backfiring of motor neurons in response to antidromic depolarization and do not depend on synaptic connections in the spinal cord. The morphology of F responses characteristically changes from trial to trial (Fig. 12-2) because the subset of motor neurons backfiring in re-

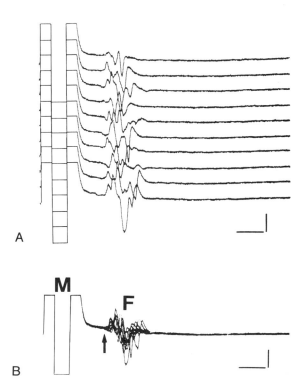

Figure 12-2. F responses recorded from abductor digiti minimi in a normal individual. **(A)** Raster of 10 consecutive F responses elicited by supramaximal stimulation of the ulnar nerve at the wrist; **(B)** superimposition of the 10 trials. Note the minimal F latency (*arrow*) and the changing configuration of F responses from trial to trial. M, m-wave. Calibration: 0.2 mV, 10 ms.

sponse to antidromic depolarization varies with each trial. F responses are useful in the detection of mild, generalized abnormalities of motor conduction, such as that seen in the early stages of an axonal peripheral neuropathy. They are also useful in the assessment of proximal demyelinating lesions, such as those seen in Guillain-Barré syndrome. In this syndrome, abnormalities of F responses (e.g., absent responses or marked delay of onset latency) may be the sole neurophysiologic finding indicating proximal demyelinating lesions undetected by conventional motor conduction studies. F response studies also provide an easy means of confirming the pathologic significance of mild focal slowing of motor conduction velocity, because their normal values are expressed as a function of the subject's height and are not biased by inaccurate measurement of conduction distance.

The H reflex is the electrical correlate of deep tendon (monosynaptic) reflexes. It is elicited by electrical stimulation of the Ia afferent fibers originating in the muscle spindles and projecting monosynaptically on the homonymous α-motor neuron. The appropriate

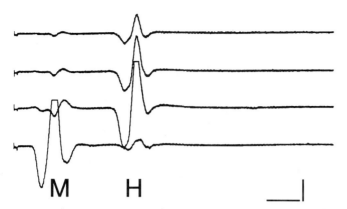

Figure 12-3. H reflex recorded from soleus in a normal individual. The intensity of electrical stimulation in the popliteal fossa is gradually increased from top to bottom. The H reflex is at first of low amplitude; its amplitude increases, reaches a maximum (truncated waveform), and then decreases markedly as the CMAP increases. M, m-wave. Calibration: 0.5 mV, 10 ms.

stimulus is submaximal so that the Ia fibers and few or no motor fibers are activated (Fig. 12-3 shows details of the effect of stimulus intensity on the H reflex). The H reflex provides information on the motor fibers and on the large afferent fibers, which are especially vulnerable to pathologic alterations. Unfortunately, in adults the H reflex can consistently be obtained only in calf muscles. Its clinical usefulness is therefore limited to the assessment of pathology affecting the distribution of the first sacral spinal root (such as polyneuropathy, lumbosacral disc disease, sciatic neuropathy, and lumbosacral plexopathy).

Proximal Stimulation

One of the limitations of conventional motor conduction studies is that only the distal segments of the main mixed nerves (e.g., the median nerve in the forearm and the peroneal nerve in the lower leg) are evaluated. Late responses provide an indirect insight into motor conduction in proximal segments (see above). In recent years, attempts to develop reliable techniques for stimulation of the proximal segments of the motor fibers have been made. Ideally, such stimulation should be supramaximal and excite the motor axons as close to their emergence of the spinal cord as possible. Research is this area is prompted by the need to be able to recognize proximal conduction block in motor fibers, since multifocal conduction block is seen is some demyelinating neuropathies, which may mimic amyotrophic lateral sclerosis clinically but have a more indolent course and may respond to therapy.

Three techniques are available to stimulate the cervical motor fibers at or very near the intervertebral

foramen: transcutaneous electrical stimulation, needle root stimulation, and magnetic stimulation. Transcutaneous electrical stimulation requires a high-voltage stimulator, a device that is not licensed for clinical use by the Food and Drug Administration in the United States. Needle stimulation of the cervical roots reaches supramaximal stimulation levels consistently but has the disadvantage of being invasive. Magnetic stimulation of the cervical region is noninvasive and well tolerated, but supramaximal levels are not reached in about one-third of recordings. These techniques are still undergoing improvement, require advanced training in clinical neurophysiology, and are presently available only in a few centers.

A conventional method of proximal stimulation of the motor fibers consists of transcutaneous electrical stimulation of the supraclavicular region (Erb's point), which stimulates the brachial plexus. Limitations of this method are discomfort and the inability to reach supramaximal levels of stimulation in more than 30 percent of trials. The latter makes Erb's point stimulation inadequate to document proximal conduction block.

Needle Electromyography

Needle examination may be conducted with several types of needle electrodes. Monopolar needles are used by some to record a signal referenced to an indifferent surface electrode. These electrodes are not accurate for assessment of the configuration of individual motor unit potentials but may be used for detection of active denervation or study of recruitment pattern. In most cases, electromyographers use concentric needle electrodes, in which the active electrode is the exposed tip of an insulated metal wire placed in a conventional needle. The shaft of the needle is the reference electrode. The area corresponding to the active electrode is about 0.1 mm², and is constant from needle to needle. At present, many electromyographers tend to use disposable needle electrodes. This responds to the concerns of patients and physicians alike regarding the risk of transmission of retroviral disease or hepatitis B and also provides a sharp new needle for each patient, which reduces the discomfort associated with punctures.

The concentric needle electrode inserted in muscle has a pickup area of 1 mm diameter including 5 to 12 muscle fibers. Because muscle fibers belonging to a motor unit are scattered throughout the muscle, in any given position the needle picks up activity from many motor units.

At rest, there is no electrical activity in normal muscle outside the endplate zone. Activity present at rest is termed *spontaneous activity* (by contrast with voluntary activity elicited by contraction of the muscle) and is always pathologic outside the endplate zone. Spontaneous activity includes fibrillations and positive sharp waves, which are single muscle fiber action potentials; myotonia, which is a high-frequency single muscle fiber activity; fasciculations, which represent involuntary activity in a motor unit or part of a motor unit; and high-frequency discharges. Fibrillations and positive sharp waves develop when muscle fibers are deprived of their motor innervation. This occurs in denervating diseases when motor axons degenerate but also in primary muscle diseases causing segmental necrosis. Segmental necrosis results in "functional" denervation of the muscle fiber segment disconnected from its motor supply. High-frequency discharges (occasionally termed "bizarre" high-frequency discharges) are complex potentials representing activity from many muscle fibers connected by ephapses. These discharges fire regularly at 5 to 100 Hz and start and stop abruptly. They are seen in chronic denervating processes as well as in some primary muscle diseases such as muscular dystrophies and inflammatory myopathies.

The configuration of motor unit potentials is studied at low levels of voluntary contraction, during which the discrete, repetitive activity corresponding to the first motor units recruited can be observed on the oscilloscope screen. The changes in configuration of motor unit potentials characteristic of neurogenic or myopathic disorders reflect the architectural changes caused in the motor unit by denervation or primary muscle disease (Fig. 12-4). In primary muscle disease the total number of motor units is normal but there is random loss of muscle fibers affecting all motor units (i.e., the number of fibers per unit volume corresponding to any motor unit is decreased). Conse-

quently, a motor unit potential, which is the summated activity of all muscle fibers belonging to that motor unit within the pickup area of the electrode, is of lower amplitude and shorter duration than normal. Additionally, it typically shows an increased number of phases (polyphasia) and an increased number of turns due to the reduction in the number of contributing generators (muscle fibers). In denervating conditions, a gradual decrease in the number of motor units occurs owing to axonal degeneration or neuronal death. The denervating process is partially compensated by reinnervation of denervated muscle fibers resulting from axonal sprouting of intact axons. Reinnervation leads to enlargement of surviving motor units, which now contain more muscle fibers than normal. The architecture of muscle is altered as a result of the reinnervation process: the muscle fiber scatter characteristic of normal motor units is lost, and small groups of fibers innervated by the same motor neuron replace the normal pattern. As a result of muscle fiber grouping, there are fewer motor units in the pickup area of the EMG needle electrode, but more fibers belonging to the same motor unit make up individual motor unit potentials. These changes in microscopic anatomy closely correlate with the abnormal configuration of motor unit potentials, which have large amplitude, prolonged duration, and an increased number of phases and turns.

Needle EMG also provides information on the pattern of recruitment of motor units. The mechanisms responsible for the generation of force by muscle rest on a process of orderly recruitment of motor units (spatial recruitment), combined with modulation of the firing frequency of individual motor units (temporal recruitment). In normal muscle, any increase in force involves recruitment of additional motor units and increase in the firing frequency of the motor units that are already active. The recruitment pattern is assessed at low levels of contraction, which provides an insight into the firing frequencies reached by the first recruited motor units, and at maximum voluntary contraction, during which a full interference without recognizable individual motor unit potentials is seen in normal muscle.

The normal recruitment pattern is altered in primary muscle disease and in denervating conditions. Primary muscle disease is characterized by a normal number of motor units but with a reduction in the total number of muscle fibers affecting all motor units. As a result of the myopathic process, the twitch generated by individual motor units is markedly reduced in amplitude, which correlates with clinical weakness. The regulation of motor unit recruitment operates through neural mechanisms that remain intact in primary muscle disease. At low levels of contraction, the

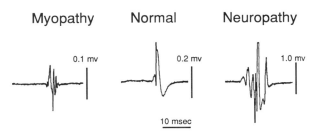

Figure 12-4. Motor unit potentials (MUPs) recorded with a concentric needle electrode. A normal MUP (*middle*) is shown for comparison. (*Left*) A myopathic MUP characterized by brief duration, increased number of phases and turns, and low amplitude: (*Right*) a neuropathic MUP indicating denervation-reinnervation, characterized by high amplitude, prolonged duration, and increased number of phases. Note that the amplitude calibration is different for each of the three MUPs. The MUP on the left is truncated owing to its high amplitude.

recruitment pattern is usually full interference in myopathic muscle. This is the physiologic means available to generate mild to moderate force using the weakened twitches of myopathic motor units. In denervating conditions, the total number of motor units is reduced within a given muscle and in the pickup area of the electrode. Early recruitment shows motor unit potentials with abnormally high firing frequencies. Maximum voluntary contractions generate a reduced interference pattern, since there are fewer motor units in the electrode pickup area.

ELECTROMYOGRAPHY AND NERVE CONDUCTION STUDIES IN DISEASE

Neuropathy caused by Compression and Trauma

Focal damage to peripheral nerves is a common problem in neurologic practice, yet human pathologic material is scarce for obvious reasons. Therefore, an understanding of the pathologic changes in these situations has been gained essentially from animal models. Experimentally, the physiologic effect of pressure is to provoke a conduction block (e.g., a reversible interruption of conduction) in the segment of nerve actually compressed, whereas nerve conduction remains normal distally. The respective roles of pressure gradient and ischemia in the genesis of conduction block are unknown. The Schwann cells and myelin sheaths are very susceptible to pressure. Ochoa and his colleagues have shown that the earliest structural change that develops following tourniquet paralysis affects the nodes of Ranvier under the edges of the compressive agent (where the pressure gradient actually takes place). When compression is maintained longer, focal demyelination develops. If compression is more severe or applied still longer, some axons may be irreversibly damaged and undergo wallerian degeneration. Large myelinated fibers are more susceptible to compression than thin myelinated fibers, and unmyelinated fibers are relatively spared. Finally, it should be added that release of chronic compression (e.g., in carpal tunnel syndrome or ulnar neuropathy at the elbow) may cause immediate improvement of conduction across the lesion (25 to 33 percent of cases) through immediate reversal of a chronic conduction block.

Neurophysiologically, compression neuropathy is characterized by a combination of the following electrophysiologic abnormalities: (1) focal conduction block; (2) focal slowing of maximum conduction velocity; (3) evidence of denervation-reinnervation in the distribution of the affected nerve by needle EMG; and (4) decrease in CMAP amplitude and in SNAP amplitude in the distribution of the affected nerve distal to the site of compression. The first two of these abnormalities reflect the consequences of demyelination and perhaps of other unidentified factors causing alterations of nerve conduction, whereas the latter two document axonal loss distal to the site of compression.

Acute nerve injuries include partial or complete division of a nerve, stretch injuries, or ischemic damage to a nerve trunk (ischemic mononeuritis). Demyelination is not a feature of these disorders, and the alterations documented by nerve conduction studies and EMG are essentially the consequences of motor and sensory fiber degeneration. In many of these cases, clinical neurophysiologic assessment may help to determine whether the affected nerve is in continuity, which may influence management decisions.

Radiculopathies and Plexopathies

Root pathology may be caused by many pathologic processes. However, the most common clinical pattern, radicular pain affecting the cervical or lumbosacral root distribution, is due to root compression by herniated disc material or by osteoarthritic degenerative changes (see Ch. 32). Neurophysiologic testing is often ordered in an attempt to obtain objective documentation of subjective sensory disturbances when muscle power and reflexes remain normal. The most sensitive technique to evaluate radiculopathy is needle EMG. Nerve conduction studies are useful to rule out peripheral nerve or plexus pathology that could mimic the symptoms of radiculopathy but do not contribute to the positive diagnosis of radiculopathies. Late responses, particularly the H reflex, may occasionally contribute to the evaluation of S1 radiculopathies. Needle EMG may reveal denervation-reinnervation in the distribution of the affected spinal root and in the corresponding paraspinal muscles. The sensory conduction studies are always normal in root lesions, even when there is dense sensory loss (as in traumatic root avulsion). This is because the fibers are damaged proximal to the dorsal root ganglion, and the distal process of the peripheral sensory neuron remains connected to its cell body and does not degenerate. For example, this feature is useful in distinguishing traumatic cervical root avulsion from traumatic brachial plexopathy, in which the SNAPs are abnormal. Needle EMG reveals changes in muscles in the distribution of the damaged root or roots. In limb muscles, the pattern of EMG changes localizes the affected root. The paraspinal muscles supplied by the dorsal ramus of the spinal nerve are commonly denervated in root pathology. However, denervation in the paraspinal muscles cannot be used to localize the affected root because of the marked overlap between consecutive myotomes.

Plexopathies, regardless of their etiology, cause degeneration of the peripheral motor and sensory neurons. Sensory conduction studies are abnormal. Needle EMG of the paraspinal muscles shows no abnormalities. An exception to this rule is provided by the radiculoplexopathies often seen in diabetic patients with the clinical syndrome known as diabetic amyotrophy.

Generalized Peripheral Neuropathy

Axonal and demyelinating neuropathies (see Ch. 80) can often be readily distinguished by nerve conduction studies. Therefore, nerve conduction studies usually are the first test ordered when planning the workup of a newly diagnosed peripheral neuropathy. Axonal peripheral neuropathies are more common and include heterogeneous disorders causing primary damage to peripheral nerve fibers. Many of these neuropathies tend to affect the longest and the largest nerve fibers within the peripheral nerves, which explains the usual distal and symmetric pattern of motor and sensory deficits. Overt axonal peripheral neuropathy causes reduction in CMAP amplitudes, mild slowing of motor conduction velocities, and prolonged distal motor latencies. Abnormalities of CMAP amplitude and latency affect foot muscles earlier than hand muscles. Slowing of maximum motor nerve conduction velocities is mild. This slowing may be due to the predilection of the pathologic process for the largest motor fibers or perhaps to development of alterations of the myelin sheath secondary to the axonopathy. SNAPs may be of low amplitude or unobtainable (the sural nerve action potential is often affected early in the course of generalized axonal neuropathy). Needle EMG reveals chronic denervation-reinnervation changes and active denervation. The EMG changes are more marked in distal muscles. In mild axonal peripheral neuropathy, the conduction abnormalities may be limited to prolongation of F response latencies (which are very helpful to document incipient axonopathy) and absence or delay of the H reflex.

Demyelinating neuropathy includes inherited and acquired disorders (see Ch. 80). A relatively common variant of inherited demyelinating sensorimotor neuropathy, which is usually transmitted as an autosomal dominant trait, is Charcot-Marie-Tooth disease (hereditary motor and sensory neuropathy type 1). This is a chronic sensorimotor neuropathy characterized by bilateral steppage gait, wasting of lower leg and distal thigh muscle, and pes cavus with hammer toes. In this disorder there is morphologic evidence for diffuse changes that indicate demyelination-remyelination affecting the entire course of the peripheral nerve fibers. As a result, conduction velocities are markedly slow. However, the CMAPs remain well synchronized and there is no evidence for focal conduction block as in the acquired demyelinating neuropathies (see below and Lewis and Sumner, 1982). The median

motor conduction velocity is commonly used to distinguish between the axonal and the demyelinating range of conduction slowing, the cutoff velocity being 33 m/s. Sural nerve action potentials are usually not obtainable. Conduction studies may be used to screen possible carriers of the gene who are clinically unaffected. Marked reduction of conduction velocities is present as early as in the first year of life.

Acquired inflammatory demyelinating polyneuropathy includes an acute variant, the Guillain-Barré syndrome, and a protracted form, chronic inflammatory demyelinating polyneuropathy (see Ch. 80). The Guillain-Barré syndrome has a rapid onset, and the patients reach peak deficits within 3 to 4 weeks of the first symptom. Initial progression is slower in chronic inflammatory demyelinating polyneuropathy, and the general course of the disease may be monophasic progressive, relapsing-remitting, or characterized by stable neurologic deficits. Both the Guillain-Barré syndrome and chronic inflammatory demyelinating polyneuropathy are predominantly motor neuropathies; the sensory deficits, when present, are limited to large fiber modalities in the distal lower extremities. Areflexia is almost invariably noted in both forms of acquired inflammatory demyelinating polyneuropathy, and an increase in cerebraspinal fluid protein with a normal cell count is usually documented. The pathology underlying the Guillain-Barré syndrome and chronic inflammatory demyelinating polyneuropathy consists of foci of mononuclear cells causing focal breakdown of myelin sheaths but sparing axons. Focal demyelination is the primary pathologic process, and axonal degeneration, when present, is thought to be secondary to severe inflammation. Focal inflammation and the resulting demyelination are found throughout the peripheral nervous system and are characteristically patchily distributed. Nerve conduction studies reveal evidence of demyelination-remyelination in more than 90 percent of Guillain-Barré cases. Nerve conduction findings documenting demyelination-remyelination include marked prolongation of motor distal latencies, slowing of maximum motor conduction velocities within the demyelinating range, and conduction block (see Fig. 12-1). In some cases conventional nerve conduction studies are entirely normal, and the sole abnormalities are unobtainable F responses, suggesting proximal conduction block. Direct evidence of proximal conduction block has been documented with needle cervical root stimulation in the Guillain-Barré syndrome. Needle EMG shows reduction in recruitment pattern in weak muscles in the acute phase of the Guillain-Barré syndrome. The configuration of individual motor unit potentials is normal in the early phase of the disease. Fibrillations and positive sharp waves can be seen in acquired inflammatory demyelinating neuropathies. They indicate secondary degeneration of motor axons and are classically an indicator of poor prognosis in Guillain-Barré syndrome.

Amyotrophic Lateral Sclerosis

Pathologic abnormalities in amyotrophic lateral sclerosis (see Ch. 63) include lower motor neuron loss and associated degeneration of the corticomotoneuronal system. These lesions cause muscle wasting and weakness in the distribution of spinal and cranial nerves, as well as bilateral spasticity. Supportive EMG evidence for a diagnosis of amyotrophic lateral sclerosis includes demonstration of motor denervation in upper and lower extremity muscles and in muscles innervated by the cranial nerves. Motor and sensory conduction studies are normal, apart from low CMAP amplitudes due to motor unit loss. Focal conduction block should be ruled out by conventional studies and proximal nerve stimulation techniques (see Methods, above), since pure motor neuropathies with multifocal conduction block may mimic the clinical picture of amyotrophic lateral sclerosis.

Primary Muscle Disease

Muscle diseases vary widely in severity from the relentless progression of Duchenne dystrophy to the non-progressive weakness of some congenital myopathies (Ch. 82). Nerve conduction studies and late responses are normal. Fibrillations and positive sharp waves are not synonymous with denervation and can be seen in primary muscle disease. They are common in Duchenne and Becker muscular dystrophies and in polymyositis and dermatomyositis. They are usually not seen in congenital myopathy, mitochondrial myopathy, or facioscapulohumeral dystrophy. Myotonia is characteristic of myotonic dystrophy and of congenital myotonia. High-frequency discharges are nonspecific findings (see Methods, above). Myopathic motor unit potentials are characteristically brief, polyphasic, and of slow amplitude, and an interference recruitment pattern is reached with minimal effort. This early interference may render analysis of single motor unit potentials difficult. The amplitude of the maximum interference pattern is also reduced in florid myopa-

thy. It is important to keep in mind, however, that mild myopathic changes may be easily overlooked.

ANNOTATED BIBLIOGRAPHY

Albers JW, Kelly JJ. Acquired inflammatory demyelinating polyneuropathies: clinical and electrodiagnostic features. Muscle Nerve 1989;12:435–51.

This article review the features of acute and chronic demyelinating neuropathies. It offers an excellent survey of the electrophysiologic criteria for demyelination in the peripheral nervous system.

Berger AR, Busis NA, Logigian EL et al. Cervical root stimulation in the diagnosis of cervical radiculopathy. Neurology 1987;37:329–32.

A description of the needle stimulation technique useful to stimulate the proximal segment of the axons of the lower motor neurons.

Cros D, Chiappa KH, Gominak S et al. Cervical magnetic stimulation. Neurology 1990;40:1751–6.

This paper provides information on the different methods of proximal stimulation of the motor fibers in the cervical region.

Cros D, Gominak S, Shahani B et al. Comparison of electric and magnetic coil stimulation in the supraclavicular region. Muscle Nerve (in press)

This study shows that electrical stimulation at Erb's point is submaximal in more than 30 percent of trials and that magnetic stimulation of the supraclavicular region is less effective than electrical stimulation.

Kimura J. Principles and pitfalls of nerve conduction studies. Ann Neurol 1984;16:415–29.

An excellent review emphasizing technical factors and anomalous innervation patterns, and providing a good discussion of newer techniques and of their practical value.

Lewis RA, Sumner AJ. The electrodiagnostic distinctions between chronic familial and acquired demyelinative neuropathies. Neurology 1982;32:592–6.

A series study differentiating motor conduction abnormalities in the two main types of demyelinating neuropathies.

Parry GJ, and Clarke S. Multifocal acquired demyelinating neuropathy masquerading as motor neuron disease. Muscle Nerve 1988;11:103–7.

A short series describing patients with a clinical syndrome suggestive of amyotrophic lateral sclerosis and with multifocal motor conduction block.

13
Ultrasonography

M. G. Hennerici, W. Rautenberg, and
W. Steinke

Ultrasonography was introduced into clinical neurology only in the early 1970s. For extracranial carotid artery disease, current instrumentation spans the technically simple continuous-wave Doppler sonography. More sophisticated instruments use a single-channel pulsed-wave Doppler technology (duplex system). The most modern instruments have color-coded duplex displays for simultaneous two-dimensional interrogation of vascular wall structures and blood flow velocity (Fig. 13-1). Pulsed-wave Doppler techniques are also used to assess intracranial large-vessel disease, cardiac dysfunction, and cardiac sources of embolism.

Technical improvements and investigator experience have spread ultrasonography beyond diseases affecting the vessels alone into problems of head trauma, epilepsy, infections, and degenerative and even metabolic disorders of the central nervous system.

GENERAL PRINCIPLES

Hemodynamics are assessed by continuous-wave and pulsed-wave Doppler sonography using the principles of the Doppler shift. This effect bears the name of Christian Andreas Doppler, who in 1842 described the effect of moving objects on the change in frequency of emitted light. The Doppler effect is familiar to anyone who has stood in one place and listened to a source of sound passing by: the pitch rises as the passing movement of sound rushes toward the listener and drops equally as the source departs. The first practical application of Doppler theory in medicine was made in 1960 by Satomura and Kaneko, who used it to measure the velocity of flowing blood.

This Doppler frequency shift ranges within the audible spectrum from 200 to 20,000 Hz, and the shift is proportional to the velocity of the source from which it is reflected (mainly the blood cells and vessel walls). When the ultrasound beam is directly in line with the blood flow (i.e., zero angle), the velocity of the flowing blood (expressed in centimeters per second) can be measured directly from the Doppler shift frequency. Under normal physiologic conditions, the angle is usually greater than zero, depending on the individual slope of the arterial segment and its accessibility to the Doppler probe, which makes the measurement of flow velocity more of a qualitative than a strictly quantitative measurement. Arterial wall movements and flow velocity alterations across the diameter of the artery being studied and nearby branching arteries may also interfere with the Doppler frequency spectrum analysis.

At the extreme of severe arterial stenoses, the actual flow may be so reduced that no Doppler shift is detected, while in states of only modest plaque formation, the changes in velocity caused by the small amount of plaque may cause so small a Doppler shift that little abnormality is found. This sort of analysis of blood flow velocity has successfully been used for the diagnosis of obstructive lesions and the associated compensatory pathways of cerebral circulation; however, additional data reflecting the amplitude of the Doppler signal would be of enormous value for interpreting the cerebral circulation with regard to cerebral blood flow volume, which is usually estimated from single-photon emission computed tomography (SPECT) and positron emission tomography (PET) data (see Chs. 14 and 15).

Despite these limitations, for a large number of disorders and over a wide range of velocity profiles, Doppler studies provide useful information about the presence of stenoses and relative changes of cerebral blood flow in response to a variety of challenges.

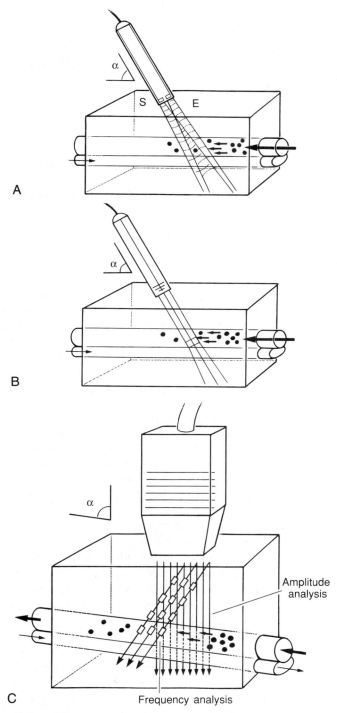

Figure 13-1. Schematic drawing demonstrating different ultrasound methods. **(A)** Pulsed-wave Doppler uses separate piezo crystals, one emitting *(E)* and one receiving *(S)* ultrasound waves. This allows a topographic diagnosis of the sample volume. **(B)** Continuous-wave Doppler sonography uses a single piezo crystal for both transmitting and receiving ultrasound signals. **(C)** Color-coded duplex sonography combines B-mode echo tomography and flow velocity signals for structural and hemodynamic analysis.

Both continuous-wave and pulsed-wave Doppler techniques are used for the assessment of normal and abnormal blood flow velocities in extracranial cerebral arteries, for which they have different advantages and disadvantages (Fig. 13-1). Because continuous-wave Doppler examination yields no images, it does not provide any information about the topography of the ultrasound-reflecting source. However, the Doppler shift that it detects applies to all moving targets in the path of the beam, regardless of velocity, and thus it allows the detection of even high blood flow velocities, which cannot be evaluated by pulsed-wave Doppler systems (Fig. 13-1). Pulsed-wave Doppler has the added advantage of providing an estimate of depth from the probe to the site being interrogated and thus can be used transcranially for the evaluation of intracranial cerebral arteries when the examiner takes into account the tissue depth from which the signal is derived.

While continuous-wave or pulsed-wave Doppler sonography provides information about intravascular hemodynamics, brightness-modulated (B-mode) echotomography images tissue and vessel structures in a two-dimensional gray- or color-scaled display. The modification of the sound waves by tissues having different acoustic impedances allows the amplitude of the reflected sound waves to be used to generate the images. Sophisticated computational algorithms can be used to reconstruct three-dimensional images from longitudinal and cross-sections.

Advanced Doppler technology uses three-dimensional reconstruction of hemodynamic parameters to estimate the spatial topography of blood flow variations and alterations adjacent to vessel wall plaque formation and nearby structurally normal segments (Plate 13-1). This technique may be applied for extracranial examination and can be used for diagnosis of different stages of evolution and causes of cerebrovascular diseases.

B-mode and Doppler-mode technologies are used in combination for subsequent imaging of both tissue and flow characteristics, adding the fourth dimension (i.e., time) to the system (Fig. 13-1). Such real-time ultrasound imaging, known as color Doppler flow imaging (CDFI), may be compared with magnetic resonance imaging (MRI) and magnetic resonance angiography techniques (Plate 13-2).

The noninvasive nature of these techniques has led to their increasing application in clinical neurology.

DOPPLER SONOGRAPHY

Indirect and Direct Tests

Even without B-mode echotomography, continuous-wave Doppler can be used to estimate direction of blood flow in the insonated vessels and to estimate

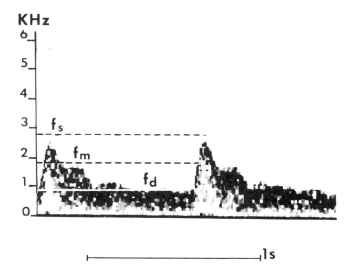

Figure 13-2. Spectrum analysis of an internal carotid Doppler signal: the signal intensity is coded gray. The characteristic parameters include F_s (systolic peak frequency), F_m (mean frequency), and F_d (diastolic frequency).

Doppler shift in frequency-spectrum analysis (Fig. 13-2). Indirect tests of the branches of the ophthalmic artery usually supplied by the internal carotid artery have been used since the initial period of ultrasonography in the study of cerebral atherosclerosis. This method can still be useful today when combined with additional direct assessment of blood flow velocities in the carotid system (direct test). Documentation of the existence of collateral pathways, with retrograde blood supply from the external carotid artery via the ophthalmic artery anastomosis, in the presence of severe stenosis or total occlusion of the internal carotid artery may be easily found with high validity. However, this test fails to detect hemodynamically significant ipsilateral carotid artery obstructions in up to 20 percent of patients if the collateralization from the contralat-

eral carotid artery or via the vertebrobasilar system is sufficient. Thus, one should be aware that detection of a retrograde flow in the fronto-orbital branches of the ophthalmic artery is a very strong indicator of an underlying pathology within the extracranial carotid system, but a negative result of this test does not exclude such an abnormality.

In most laboratories, diagnosis of extracranial arterial disease is directed at the evaluation of Doppler spectra obtained directly from the carotid artery below, at, and above the bifurcation of the common carotid artery. They depend on the appropriate interpretation of several features of the Doppler flow velocity pattern (Fig. 13-2): peak systolic velocity, which is the highest velocity during systole in the cardiac cycle; end-diastolic velocity, which is the maximum velocity value at the end of the diastole; and mean velocity a term often used for the time-averaged maximum velocity during the cardiac cycle, which is usually calculated automatically and by various but not necessarily identical algorithms in most instruments.

Carotid Artery Stenosis and Occlusion

The diagnosis of carotid stenosis (see Ch. 35) can be made with a high degree of accuracy when compared with angiographic results (Table 13-1). Mild stenosis (40 to 60 percent), moderate stenosis (60 to 80 percent), severe stenosis (>80 to 95 percent), and subtotal stenosis (>95 percent) can be reliably diagnosed and separated from total occlusion of the internal and common carotid artery in all but a tiny number of cases (Plate 13-3).

Extremely severe obstructive lesions are characterized by reduced diastolic blood flow velocities in both proximal and distal segments and may be separated from minor obstructions. Local turbulences, alterations of secondary flow zones in the carotid bulb, and the appearance of abnormal vortex flow directed toward the vessel wall within or distal to the obstruction represent other characteristic features, which may be

Table 13-1. Criteria for the Classification of Carotid Arteries by Means of Pulsed-Wave Doppler Sonography (4 to 5 MHz)

Diameter Stenosis (%)	Peak Systolic		End Diastolic		Systolic Ratio (ICA/CCA)
	Frequency (kHz)	Velocity (cm/s)	Frequency (kHz)	Velocity (cm/s)	
0–40	<4.0	<120	<1.2	<35	<1.5
40–60	>4.0	>120	<1.3	<40	<1.8
61–80	>4.0	>120	>1.3	>40	>1.8
81–95	>8.0	>240	>3.3	>100	>3.7

Abbreviations: ICA, internal carotid artery; CCA, common carotid artery. (Modified from Zwiebel and Knighton, 1990, with permission.)

demonstrated even in the presence of small plaques (<30 percent lumen narrowing). In addition, multivessel involvement can be diagnosed with high accuracy provided that the individual hemodynamic situation and collateralization are carefully considered. Obstructive lesions of the external carotid system are rare but may also be accurately diagnosed with the additional use of compression tests for identification of the external carotid artery.

In lesions above the easily insonated (submandibular) sections of the carotid, special features of the Doppler profile may prove helpful in diagnosis. Carotid artery dissections are typically high in the neck near the skull base and are not suitable for direct insonation (see Ch. 35). When they are present, the distinctive bi- or triphasic to-and-fro signal recorded throughout the course of the carotid system allows inference of this diagnosis. Acute, severe intracranial obstructions within the carotid siphon or in the middle cerebral artery may lead to blunted waveforms (reduced spectra) in the ipsilateral extracranial internal carotid artery. Intracranial arteriovenous malformations and dural arteriovenous fistulas (see Ch. 37) typically cause increased flow velocities in the extracranial arteries feeding the malformation.

Vertebral Artery Stenosis and Occlusion

Obstructions in the vertebral system are most frequently located at the origin at the subclavian artery or at the distal end at the atlas loop (see Ch. 35). Criteria for classification of their degree are similar to those for the carotid artery system; however, insonation is more difficult owing to the intrathoracic position of the lower vertebral artery, and the deep course of the vertebral artery through the spine limits assessment to those short portions that can be insonated in the interosseous course between the vertebral bodies. B-mode and color-coded duplex sonography help to identify these points along the course of the vessels. (Plate 13-4) Obstructive lesions may be separated from anatomic variations, such as hypoplasia and deep cervical pathways serving as major collaterals in the presence of focal blockage of the vertebral artery. In addition, occlusion may be differentiated from hypoplasia and aplasia with reasonable validity. Dissections of the vertebral arteries, although less common than in the carotid system, may be detected by a to-and-fro signal and by spontaneous recovery from an obstructive lesion during follow-up investigations.

Subclavian and Innominate Artery Stenosis and Occlusion

In patients with severe lesions of the proximal subclavian or the innominate arteries (see Ch. 35), Doppler sonography represents an excellent tool for the detection of characteristically associated flow abnormalities, such as the subclavian steal phenomenon and especially its variety of intermediate flow conditions in the ipsilateral (and sometimes also in the contralateral) vertebral artery (Fig. 13-3). Different stages can be separated in this most often clinically benign condition, which may lead to complex hemodynamic alterations and puzzling collateral pathways if combined with other obstructive lesions in the major extracranial cerebral arteries.

Advantages and Limitations

Continuous-wave Doppler sonography represents a reliable method for the diagnosis of hemodynamic alterations due to obstructive lesions within the extracranial carotid and vertebral artery system, although no information concerning the morphology and surface of a plaque is available. However, this hand-held, technically simple, and less expensive method provides reliable detection of carotid lesions producing a greater than 40 percent lumen narrowing.

Pulsed-wave Doppler methods offer results similar to those of continuous-wave Doppler methods provided that the Doppler sample volume is adequately positioned, which generally requires the much more expensive additional use of a B-mode system. The latter may also be used for the detection of lesions with less than 40 percent lumen narrowing, which cannot reliably be detected by hemodynamic methods only.

The diagnostic accuracy of either method is rather limited in the vertebrobasilar system. Thus, Doppler techniques in this territory are used mainly for the detection of severe obstructions at the origin and atlas loop of the vertebral arteries and in the detection of subclavian or innominate steal phenomena.

DUPLEX SYSTEM ANALYSIS

B-Mode Echotomography

Assessment of small arterial plaques based on differential acoustic impedance is the major advantage of this technique provided that the arterial segment can be directly visualized. Soft plaques containing cholesterol deposits and atheromatous debris may be separated from fibrous plaques with collagen layers and hard plaques consisting largely of calcifications. In addition, echotomography seems to be unique for a clear distinction between normal vessel wall characteristics and abnormal conditions and was recently introduced for the evaluation of minuscule intra-arterial wall changes in the range of 100 μm as possible indicators of early atherogenesis (Fig. 13-4). Whether or not this is beyond the capacity of the system is a matter of

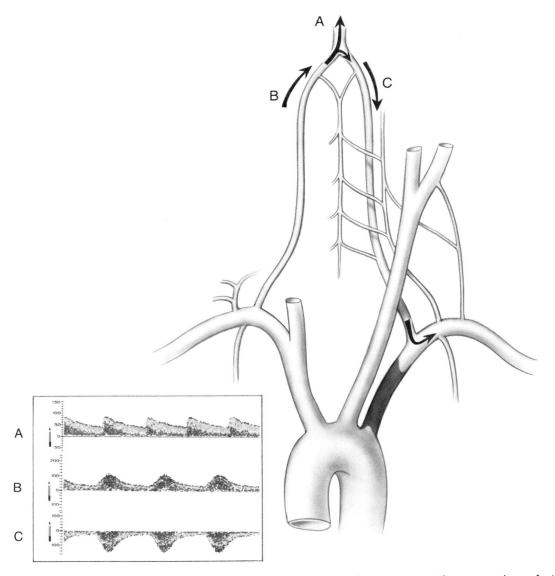

Figure 13-3. (A–C) Schematic drawing of a subclavian steal phenomenon with retrograde perfusion of the left vertebral artery (Fig. C) distal to total occlusion of the proximal subclavian artery. Blood flow from the right vertebral artery (Fig. B) supports orthograde circulation in the basilar artery (Fig. A) sufficiently.

discussion; however, this technique can follow atherogenesis development in vivo more appropriately than any other method yet available despite some still existing limitations.

However, B-mode imaging has proved to be inadequate for accurate assessment of plaque extent and luminal narrowing. Large multicenter validation studies of B-mode alone showed a poor correlation with angiography if Doppler sonography was disregarded. The overall accuracy for classifying different degrees of stenosis was only 71.8 percent and was even worse for the identification of carotid occlusion (41 percent). The additional use of Doppler measurements and

spectrum analysis now is recognized as a requisite for investigation.

Duplex Sonography

The combination of high resolution B-mode imaging studies with pulsed-wave Doppler sonography has been found to extend diagnostic reliability and is now the most widely used method for diagnosis of cerebrovascular diseases. Originally introduced for investigation of the extracranial system, duplex-system analysis in its most recent form (CDFI), has also been applied to the study of intracranial vascular branches, but its validity and accuracy have not yet been established.

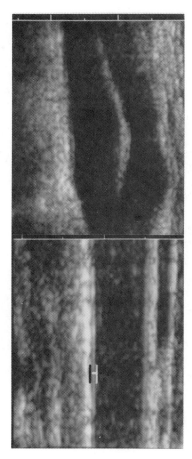

Figure 13-4. Intima media thickness measurements shown in typical B-mode imaging below the carotid bifurcation.

Duplex scanning has also been shown to be useful for assessment of carotid artery dissection (Table 13-2). When the dissection is low enough in the arterial tree to be visualized, the typical intimal flap can be imaged so as to separate both lumina using different Doppler profiles, sometimes accompanied by retrograde flow in the pseudoaneurysm. When the lesion lies above the reach of the Doppler probe and the artery is occluded (Plate 13-5), high-resolution echotomography may demonstrate only a tapering lumen while the Doppler flow spectrum shows the characteristic low-frequency, high-resistance pattern typical of occlusion above the probe.

Duplex visualization of the vertebral arteries has only occasionally been performed because display of the vessel wall and assessment of intravascular flow velocity have been limited to the origin of the vertebral artery, its proximal pretransverse course, and the intertransverse segments (C3–C6). Although retrograde or intermediate flow can be interpreted with reasonable accuracy as a hemodynamic result of a steal phenomenon in the presence of innominate or proximal subclavian artery obstructions, this approach does not add any further information to that provided by the less time-consuming and less expensive continuous-wave Doppler test.

Color Doppler Flow Imaging

CDFI represents the most recent advance in sonographic techniques. In addition to the conventional duplex system technology, CDFI provides two-dimensional information about intravascular blood flow coded in color and superimposed on the gray-scale image of the vessel anatomy. The B-mode image generated from echo amplitude analysis of stationary targets is combined with the Doppler signal as determined by phase changes between successive echoes that indicate the velocity and direction of moving targets. Rather than displaying the different fast Fourier spectra of the Doppler shift, a mean value representing an autocorrelation coefficient of the mean flow velocities in a particular segment is coded by either red or blue. The degree of color saturation correlates with the flow velocity, with saturation decreasing at higher flow velocities.

Table 13-2. Characteristic Features and Criteria of Duplex Sonography for the Evaluation of the Carotid System

Feature	Criteria
Visualization	Good, fair, poor
Sections	Longitudinal, transverse
Vascular course	Regular, variant, tortuosity (kinking, coiling)
Vessel motion	Transversal, axial, systolic-diastolic
Vessel size (diameter)	Intima-media thickness, inner diameter, outer diameter
Flow direction	Orthograde, retrograde, intermediate, flow separation, transmural
Flow velocity pattern	Axial, asymmetric, local acceleration, turbulence
Plaque morphology	Homogeneous, heterogeneous, echolucent, echointense, flat surface, ulceration, irregular surface

The result is a panel of color pixels, each representing the approximate mean frequency shift in a given space and time. The constant modification of the velocity profiles and directions creates the impression of a real-time display of flow within the lumen. At sites of flow disturbance such as stenoses, broadening of the Doppler spectrum decreases the mean frequency and with it decreases the color-coded frequency shift. Since some frequency shifts exceed equipment competence for proper display, aliasing that is fundamental to pulsed-wave Doppler sonography also occurs with color-coded Doppler signals.

In some commercially available systems with CDFI, aliasing is characterized by an abrupt change from pale red to pale blue signals with interposed black lines. In contrast, green or yellow may be mixed with red or blue to indicate spectral broadening of frequency shifts, which result in a mosaic pattern if turbulence occurs in severe stenosis.

CDFI increases the capability of conventional ultrasound for the detection and characterization of small, nonstenotic plaques and facilitates the differentiation of normal versus abnormal flow dynamics even in the absence of structural abnormalities (Plates 13-5 and 13-6). Characterization of plaque surface is improved with regard to the detection of ulceration and differentiation of smooth and irregular surfaces. Echolucent components of a plaque, such as fresh thrombotic material, can be identified indirectly by the absence of the color flow signal, and thus thromboembolic sources can be better displayed. Despite these advantages, classification of the grade of stenosis remains based on the Doppler spectrum analysis according to established criteria. The additional features from color-coded duplex sonography to characterize carotid obstructions (e.g., intensity, extent, and duration of color fading; presence of poststenotic flow reversal or turbulence) make analysis of the site and severity of the stenosis easier than with conventional duplex sonography and also improve the difficult but therapeutically useful differentiation of total occlusion from pseudo-occlusion in the presence of a very tight carotid stenosis.

Experience with CDFI in the vertebral system is limited. However, in a series of presumed normal subjects, not only could the origin and intertransverse segments of the vertebral arteries be regularly identified but also the atlas loop and the size of the vessels could be displayed, which is a major advantage of this technique for distinguishing between frequent caliber abnormalities. This is to some extent due to the better visualization of the flow stream within the small, deep vertebral arteries in the neck.

Advantages and limitations of CDFI are summarized below.

ADVANTAGES AND LIMITATIONS OF COLOR DOPPLER FLOW IMAGING FOR CAROTID ARTERY DISEASE

Advantages
- Simultaneous real-time image of blood flow and vessel anatomy
- Ease of vessel identification
- Faster data acquisition and shorter examination time
- Improved estimation of plaque surface structure and residual vessel lumen
- Facilitated localization of the point of maximal intrastenotic frequency shift
- Display of the morphologic-hemodynamic interaction
- More reliable differential diagnosis of neck masses
- High intra- and interobserver reproducibility

Limitations
- Variable interpretation of blue-coded signals as
  - Reversed flow
  - Undisturbed flow toward the transducer
  - Turbulence
  - Aliasing phenomenon
- Suboptimal angle of insonation for B-mode imaging
- Detection of very slow flow velocity
- Limited temporal resolution of color-coded flow patterns
- Shadowing of color signals due to calcified plaque

TRANSCRANIAL DOPPLER SONOGRAPHY

Methods

Since the early 1980s, high-energy pulsed-wave Doppler systems have proved feasible for flow velocity measurements in intracranial cerebral arteries. While this is in principle similar to application of Doppler measurements to the extracranial arterial system, initially hand-held probes providing only crude information about the position of the sample volume were used for the intracranial arteries. This methodology was followed by application of one or two probes in a hel-

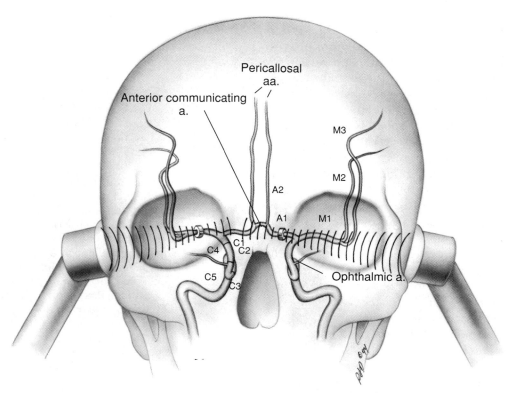

Figure 13-5. Schematic illustration of the position of the sample volume inside the skull, using the transtemporal approach.

met for mapping the signals recorded with regard to their origin in two-dimensional planes and finally by the use of color-coded duplex instrumentation. However, no appropriate resolution of either the anatomic structure, the adjacent brain tissue, or the vessel wall is available. Normal values are given in Table 13-3. Blood flow velocities vary with age, hematocrit, blood sugar and carbon dioxide concentrations, and other variables.

Given the lack of a B-mode image, interpretation of the transcranial CDFI data relies mainly on hemodynamic information such as peak velocity and direction of flow. An extracranial noninvasive study should always precede the transcranial investigation.

Three different approaches allow recording of intracranial flow velocities for routine examinations: transtemporal, transorbital, and transnuchal. Identification of intracranial vessels depends on flow direction and the distance between the signal recorded and the position of the sample volume (Fig. 13-5).

Intracranial Stenosis and Occlusion

The narrowing of intracranial vessels (see Ch. 35) produces changes similar to those occurring in the extracranial system: local increase in mean and peak flow velocities; the appearance of low-frequency, high-amplitude signals; and disturbed reversed flow phenomena. Not only the detection but even the grading of intracranial stenosis for the larger basal cerebral arteries has become possible. The combination of transcranial Doppler (TCD) sonography and magnetic resonance angiography seems to be superior to conventional angiography and has the advantage of being completely noninvasive (Plate 13-7). Occlusion of the stem (M1) segment of the middle cerebral artery

Table 13-3. Aggregated Mean Values and Standard Deviations of Transcranial Doppler Measurements in Normal Subjects

Vessel	Peak Velocity (cm/s)	Mean Velocity (cm/s)	End-Diastolic Velocity (cm/s)
MCA n = 291	89 ± 17.6	60 ± 11.25	42 ± 8.3
ACA n = 201	73 ± 16.7	50 ± 12.4	34 ± 8.5
PCA n = 201	55 ± 12.8	37 ± 9.4	27 ± 6.5
VA/BA n = 201	57 ± 13.8	35 ± 10.25	28 ± 7.5

Abbreviations: MCA, middle cerebral artery; ACA, anterior cerebral artery; PCA, posterior cerebral artery; VA/BA, vertebral artery/basilar artery.

can be assumed if no signal is detectable in this artery despite signals from the ipsilateral siphon of the internal carotid artery and the anterior cerebral artery (proving that the temporal bone allows transmission of the Doppler signals). Reduced peak and mean frequencies can be seen in vessel segments proximal to the occlusion, and distal branches sometimes show reversed flow direction, indicating activity of leptomeningeal anastomoses. In the largest reported series of 476 patients, the sensitivity for the detection of middle cerebral artery stenosis/occlusion by TCD was 79 percent with a specificity of 100 percent. Cases of early recanalization have been documented by continuous monitoring after detection of the initial acute occlusion.

The detection of obstructive lesions in the vertebrobasilar territory has proved less reliable than in the anterior circulation. The main causes are the anatomic variations and increasingly frequent slopes and kinks as well as difficulty in insonating the total length of the vertebrobasilar system.

Vasospasm

Stenosis reflecting vasospasm in subarachnoid hemorrhage (see Ch. 37) is among the most important TCD applications. Analysis of the time and course of a vasospasm in subarachnoid hemorrhage is easily managed by continuous monitoring of the large cerebral artery blood flow velocity. Correlation between the angiographic appearance of a vasospasm and TCD measurements has been reasonable, and TCD may be more sensitive in detecting early spasm. The findings guide adjustments in the medical treatment of those patients with high blood flow velocities to reduce the risk of a late ischemic stroke.

Intracranial Collateralization of Extracranial Obstructive Lesions

TCD provides noninvasive assessment of the intracranial hemodynamic collateral pathways in the presence of severe obstruction in the extracranial carotid or vertebral systems (Table 13-4). The efficacy of collateral flow can usually be assessed. Flow velocities in the middle cerebral artery distal to significant stenosis and occlusion reflect the adequacy of collateral vessels (Plate 13-8): normal peak and mean flow velocities are findings indicating adequate collateralization, while reduction of flow velocities and pulsatility indices suggest exhaustion of vascular compensatory mechanisms. However, alterations of flow velocity parameters do not carry any clinical predictive value, although several attempts have been made to evaluate the individual prognosis by responses to manipulation of the intracranial vascular reserve capacity (e.g., carbon dioxide reactivity tests).

COLLATERAL CHANNELS: TRANSCRANIAL DOPPLER CRITERIA

Anterior communicating artery
   Retrograde flow direction in the ipsilateral anterior cerebral artery
   Increased peak and mean velocities in both anterior cerebral arteries
   Increased velocities and low-frequency signals in the midline (75–85 mm), anterior communicating artery, functional stenosis
   Middle cerebral artery velocity decrease during contralateral common carotid artery compression

Posterior communicating artery
   Increased velocities in the ipsilateral (P1) posterior cerebral artery
   Increased velocities in the basilar artery
   Low-frequency signals in the region of the PCoA (60–70 mm depth)

Leptomeningeal anastomosis
   Increased velocities in proximal and distal vessel segments (e.g., PCA: P1 and P2)
   Partly retrograde flow signals in distal vessel segments (e.g., retrograde flow direction in distal middle cerebral artery branches), ophthalmic collateral retrograde flow direction of the ophthalmic artery

---

TCD also allows assessment of blood flow alterations within the basal arteries in patients with proximal lesions of the subclavian and innominate arteries resulting in various degrees of intracranial steal phenomena. The majority of patients with subclavian obstructive lesions reveal orthograde flow in the basilar artery associated with retrograde or intermediate flow conditions in the draining ipsilateral vertebral artery. Retrograde flow in the basilar artery is an extreme rarity and only present in patients with multivessel disease and/or abnormalities of the circle of Willis. In contrast, about 40 percent of the patients show minor to moderate alterations of flow velocity in the basilar artery during hyperemia of the ipsilateral arm in the absence of any clinical signs or symptoms. In principle, similar findings can be demonstrated in patients with obstructions of the innominate artery; however, abnormal flow patterns may additionally be recorded from the ipsilateral middle and

Table 13-4. Application of Different Ultrasound Tests for the Diagnosis of Various Extra- and Intracranial Vascular

	Carotid Lesions					
	Small Plaques	Fresh Thrombus Ulcer	Stenosis	Occlusion	Dissection	Dilation
CW Doppler	—	—	+ +	+ +	+ +	—
PW Doppler	—	—	+	+	+	—
B-Mode	+ +	+	+	—	—	+ +
+ PW mode	+ +	+	+ +	+	+	+ +
+ Color mode	+ +	+ +	+ +	+ +	+ +	+ +
Monitoring	—	—	—	—	—	—
Echocontrast	—	—	—	—	—	—
Functional	—	—	—	+	+	—

Abbreviations: CW, continuous-wave; PW, pulsed-wave; HITS, high-intensity transient signals.
[a] Diagnostic significances: —, none; (+), limited; +, reasonable; + +, excellent.

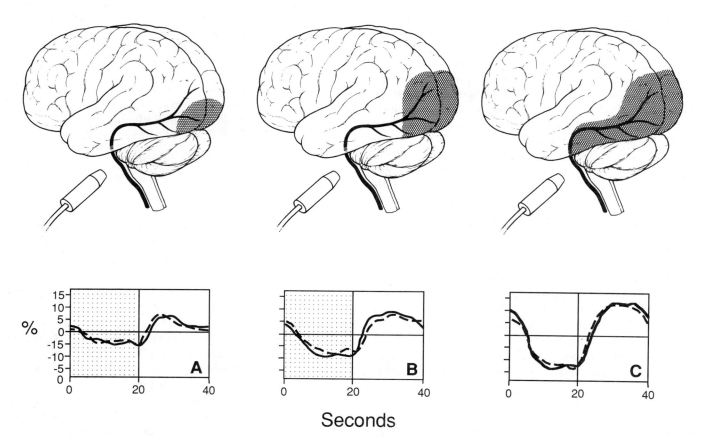

Figure 13-6. Functional analysis of vascular and metabolic coupling. Baseline signal velocity shown in the left sides of the graphs. **(A)** Increase in signal velocity caused by exposure to white light (right side of graph). **(B)** Changes in exposure to checkerboard pattern. **(C)** Changes in exposure to color film. The portions of brain regions activated by a given procedure are indicated by the hatched areas shown in each brain figure (top).

Diseases[a]

Supra-aortic Submandibular Lesions	Vertebral Lesions			Intracranial Processes			
	Stenosis	Occlusion	Steal	Vasospasms Collateral Flow	Raised Pressure	HITS	Neurovascular Dysfunction
—	+	(+)	+ +	(+)	(+)	(+)	—
+ +	—	(+)	+	+ +	+ +	+ +	+ +
—	—	—	—	—	—	—	—
—	(+)	(+)	(+)	(+)	(+)	(+)	—
+	+	+	+	+	+	+	—
—	—	—	—	—	+	+ +	—
—	—	—	—	—	—	+ +	+
—	—	—	+	—	—	—	+

anterior cerebral arteries and in some patients even from the contralateral arteries depending on the actual pathways of collateralization. In patients with innominate artery obstructive diseases, intracranial steal phenomena seem to be more often associated with the occurrence of symptoms and have a less favorable prognosis.

Dilative Arteriopathies

In patients with intracranial dolichoectatic arteries (see Ch. 35), significantly reduced peak and mean velocities can be recorded. They are of clinical importance, since such arteriopathies give rise to thromboembolism into branching small vessels within remote vascular territories with subsequent tissue infarction. These arteriopathies also lead to the development of cranial nerve and even parenchymatous compression and probably contribute to the pathogenesis of subcortical dementia.

Functional Tests

Provided the vascular-metabolic coupling ratio is normal (e.g., 1:1), investigations of both the vascular and metabolic reserve capacities are appropriate for an estimate of the hemodynamic reserve capacities in patients with extracranial arterial disease. An example is given in Figure 13-6, showing that stimulation with a complex video tape signal, which will normally include neuronal activity not only in the primary visual cortex (V1 and V2) but also in the extrastriate temporal and parietal territories (V3, V4, and V5), all supplied by the posterior cerebral artery, produces a large alteration of cerebrovascular flow velocity. In the presence of a totally occluded internal carotid artery, the absence of this response recorded from the posterior cerebral artery, directly branching off the carotid artery, indicates exhaustion of the hemodynamic reserve ca-

pacity (i.e., normal brain function results from increasing oxygen extraction and preservation of the metabolic reserve capacity). A similar test has recently been introduced for the diagnosis of patients with uncharacteristic migraine attacks; even in the migraine interval, this test reveals a hyperactive cerebrovascular regulation during neural activity.

Functional tests may also be used to evaluate the prognosis of patients in the hyperacute phase of ischemia and could eventually be reliable predictors of the most advantageous treatment. A particular example of recent investigations in patients with subcortical lacunar infarctions and severe motor deficits shows that the absence of motor evoked potentials can be used as an indicator of a poor prognosis if associated with the absence of simultaneously recorded magnetic evoked cerebral blood flow volume responses (Fig. 13-7). Despite the presence of a severe clinical deficit, however, preservation or only mild reduction of either the motor evoked potentials or the magnetic evoked cerebral blood flow volume response characterizes central neuropraxia and anticipation of good recovery from another small lacunar infarction.

Monitoring

Monitoring cerebral autoregulation hemodynamics during orthostatic maneuvers allows noninvasive assessment of function of the autonomic nervous system, which is useful in patients with multisystem degenerative diseases and central and peripheral dysautonomia. In these patients, abnormal decreases of blood flow velocities within the basal cerebral arteries can be detected during orthostatic stress (Fig. 13-8). This TCD test defines the regulatory mechanisms maintaining a constant flow over a range of systemic perfusion pressure, which allows the small arteriolar vessels to vary their size with resistance as a result of

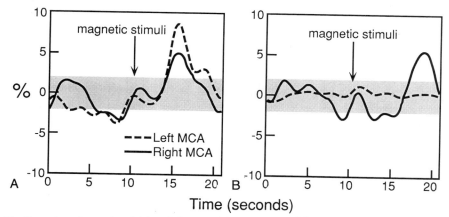

Figure 13-7. Functional cerebral blood flow volume assessed by transcranial Doppler and evoked potentials after transcranial magnetic stimulation in **(A)** a normal subject and **(B)** one with left middle cerebral artery territory stroke (right). The gray areas represent normal fluctuations. The stroke patient showed little response to magnetic stimulation.

changing perfusion pressure for maintenance of constant cerebral blood flow conditions. Hyper- and hypoventilation, as well as drugs such as acetazolamide sometimes introduced for the same purpose, do not directly reflect autoregulatory responses but interfere with this mechanism. The major difficulty in the assessment of cerebral autoregulation derives from the possibility that vessel diameter and compliance within

a variable cerebrovascular territory may change and hence hide regular blood flow velocity adaptation because the signal intensity can still not be taken into calculation.

The advantage of TCD for detecting high-intensity transient signals (HITS) within a certain range of frequencies in discrete events during a cardiac cycle has attracted increasing interest, since HITS have

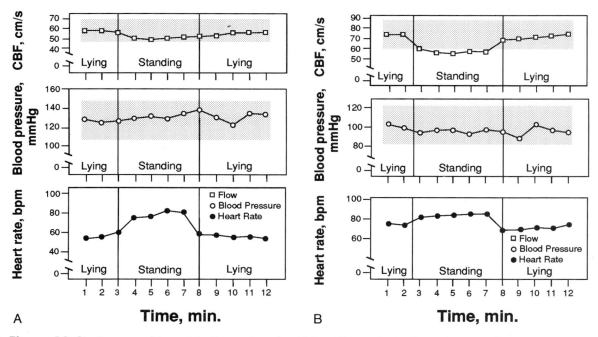

Figure 13-8. Topographic registrations of cerebral blood flow velocity, heart beat, and blood pressure during orthostasis. **(A)** Normal response of cerebral blood flow value to orthostasis. Normal intervals are shaded in gray. **(B)** Distal cerebral blood flow value in the middle cerebral artery without pathologic changes of blood pressure and heart rate in a patient with syncope.

been suggested to represent embolism to the cerebral circulation from the heart and/or the proximal extracranial arteries (Plate 13-9). Injection of microspheroidal air bubbles proved that intravenously injected cellular and coagulative material could introduce HITS in an experimental setting as well as echo reflecting microbubbles identifiable in patients with abnormal right-to-left cardiac shunts (e.g., in the presence of a patent foramen ovale). This test is now widely used to further diagnose patients with an otherwise undetectable origin of cerebral ischemia.

Experimental data suggest that blood constituents also give rise to HITS although at a considerably smaller amplitude, but they have failed so far to provide reliable parameters, which would be useful for an estimate of the constituents of particular HITS. Thousands of such clinically silent phenomena may be recorded during cardiopulmonary bypass surgery or carotid endarterectomy or spontaneously in patients with heart valve prostheses. The important question of whether a continuation of HITS is associated with an increased risk of cerebral tissue damage or functional deterioration needs to be resolved. This is of particular interest in the pathogenesis of white matter disease, which obviously occurs more frequently in older patients, who also more frequently reveal HITS, since the mechanism has been suggested to involve reduced perfusion in the end territory of very small (200 to 600 μm), deep-penetrating brain vessels. Patients with microspheroidal particles of the same size (100 to 600 μm) detected by TCD could be likely candidates for the development of white matter lesions.

ANNOTATED BIBLIOGRAPHY

Bernstein EF. Noninvasive Diagnostic Techniques in Vascular Disease. 3rd Ed. CV, Mosby, St. Louis, 1992.

Standard textbook references.

Daffertshofer M, Diehl RR, Ziems GC, Hennerici M. Orthostatic changes of cerebral blood flow velocity in patients with autonomic dysfunction. J Neurol Sci 1991;104: 32–8.

Utility of Doppler in autonomic insufficiency investigations.

Dauzat M, Laroche J-P, De Bray J-M. Ultrasonographie Vasculaire Diagnostique: Théorie et Pratique. Editions Vigot, Paris. 1991.

Clear and thorough text in French.

Di Tullio M, Sacco RL, Vendetasubramanian N, Mohr JP. Comparison of diagnostic techniques for the detection of a patent foramen ovale in stroke patients. Stroke 1993; 24:1020–4.

Bubble infusion technique.

Fieschi C, Argentino C, Lenzi GL et al. Clinical and instrumental evaluation of patients with ischemic stroke within the first six hours. J Neurol Sci 1989;91:311–21.

Utility of Doppler in the acute setting.

Hennerici M, Daffertshofer M: Imaging in cerebrovascular disease. Curr Opin Neurol Neurosurg 1992;5:49–57.

Review of recent advances in Doppler imaging techniques.

Hennerici M, Mohr JP, Rautenberg W, Steinke W: Ultrasound imaging and Doppler sonography in the diagnosis of cerebrovascular diseases. p. 241. In Barnett HJM, Mohr JP, Stein BM, Yatsu F (eds): Stroke: Pathophysiology, Diagnosis and Management. 2nd Ed. Churchill Livingstone, New York, 1992.

Textbook chapter.

Hennerici M, Neuerburg-Heusler D: Gefässdiagnostik mit Ultraschall. Thieme, Stuttgart, 1995.

Recent textbook and atlas in German.

Hennerici M, Steinke W, Rautenberg W. High-resistance Doppler flow pattern in extracranial carotid dissection. Arch Neurol 1989;46:670–2.

First description of high-resistance Doppler flow patterns in carotid dissection in the literature.

Hennerici M, Steinke W. Accuracy of high-resolution ultrasound imaging for quantitative assessment of early carotid atherosclerosis. Cerebrovasc Dis 1994;4:109–13.

An editorial issue on a B-mode controversy.

Mull M, Aulich A, Hennerici M. Transcranial Doppler ultrasonography vs. arteriography for assessment of the vertebrobasilar circulation. J Clin Ultrasound 1990;10: 539–49.

TCD proved less useful in the posterior circulation than in the anterior.

Müller HR, Casty M, Moll R et al. Response of middle cerebral artery volume flow to orthostasis. Cerebrovasc Dis 1991;1:182.

Changes in TCD velocities during orthostatic testing.

Newell DW, Aaslid R: Transcranial Doppler. Raven Press, New York, 1992

Recent text.

Padayachee TS, Gosling RG, Bishop CC et al: Monitoring MCA blood velocity during carotid endarterectomy. Br J Surg 1986;73:98–100.

The earliest descriptions of phenomena later considered as "microembolic" events detected during TCD insonation.

Rautenberg W, Schwartz A, Hennerici M. Transkranielle Doppler-Sonographie während der zerebralen Angiographie. p. 144. In Widder B (ed): Transkranielle Doppler-Sonographie bei zerebrovaskularen Erkrankungen. Springer-Verlag, Berlin, 1987

TCD studies carried out during angiography.

Ricotta JJ, Bryan FA, Bond MG et al: Multicenter validation study of real-time (B-mode) ultrasound, arteriography and pathologic examination. J Vasc Surg 1987;6:512–20.

This multicenter trial studied the reproducibility of duplex scan measurements in patients with atherosclerotic lesions.

Rother J, Wentz K-U, Rautenberg W et al: Magnetic resonance angiography in vertebrobasilar ischemia. Stroke 1993;24:1310–15.

The first study comparing magnetic resonance and conventional angiography with transcranial Doppler in 41 patients with acute cerebellar and/or brainstem ischemia.

Schwartz A, Rautenberg W, Hennerici M: Dolichoectatic in-tracranial arteries: selected aspects. Cerebrovasc Dis 1993;3:273.

Review of diagnostic significance of ultrasound, MRI, and MRA.

Steinke W, Hennerici M: The carotid bifurcation: haemodynamic aspects and three-dimensional lesion reconstruction. p. 292. In Labs KH, Jager KA, Fitzgerald DE et al (eds): Diagnostic Vascular Ultrasound. Edward Arnold, London, 1992.

Recent detailed chapter.

Zweibel WJ, Knighton R. Duplex examination of the carotid arteries. Semin Ultrasound CT MRI 1990;11:97–135.

Review on duplex technology and clinical application.

14

Functional Neuroimaging

R. S. J. Frackowiak

PRINCIPLES OF FUNCTIONAL SCANNING

Functional neuroimaging includes the techniques of planar brain scanning, which is now essentially obsolete, single-photon emission computed tomography (SPECT) with conventional nuclear medicine radionuclide tracers, and positron emission tomography (PET) with positron-emitting radioisotopes. SPECT is readily available in nuclear medicine departments, is relatively inexpensive, and is now capable, by means of specially designed scanners dedicated to imaging of the brain, of achieving spatial resolutions of $8 \times 8 \times 12$ mm in routine clinical imaging. PET has a number of advantages over SPECT, which include an image resolution of $6 \times 6 \times 4$ mm, but a major disadvantage for routine clinical use is the higher cost of the equipment.

SPECT (see also Ch. 15) uses traditional nuclear medicine radioisotopes such as technetium-99m, (^{99m}Tc), xenon-133 (^{133}Xe); and various isotopes of iodine to trace molecules of biologic interest. These large isotopes do not occur naturally, so it is often unclear whether, or how, they alter the biochemical properties of molecules to which they are attached. However, good tracers of perfusion are readily and commercially available, for example, ^{99m}Tc-d, 1-hexamethylpropylene-amine oxime (HMPAO). Isotopes used in PET, such as oxygen-15 (^{15}O), carbon-11 (^{11}C), and nitrogen-13 (^{13}N), are radioactive components of natural elements and can be substituted for their stable counterparts, leading to no modification of the properties of the labeled molecules. Fluorine-18 (^{18}F) is frequently used as a substitute for hydrogen because no positron-emitting isotope of this element exists. Even this substitution is capable of altering the transport and behavior of simple molecules to which the ^{18}F atom is attached. For example, the transport of ^{18}F-deoxyglucose (FDG) is definably different from that of ^{11}C-deoxyglucose or ^{11}C-glucose, which necessitates the introduction of correction factors in the calculations of glucose uptake rates when using each of these tracers.

The half-lives of the PET isotopes are very short, for example, ^{15}O has a half-life of 2.1 minutes, and the half-life of ^{11}C is 20 minutes. The longest-lived PET isotope in common use is ^{18}F, with a half-life of 110 minutes. In contrast, SPECT isotopes are much longer-lived, for example, ^{99m}Tc has a half-life of 6 hours. This means that a cyclotron is necessary in the proximity of a PET camera to generate the positron-emitting isotopes, while SPECT tracers can be prepared in easily usable, commercially available kits and stored for relatively long periods of time before use. However, the longer half-life of SPECT tracers is disadvantageous in other respects. The radiation dose per study is larger; for example, the effective dose equivalent of a PET blood flow scan with $H_2^{15}O$ is 0.8 millisievert, and that of an HMPAO scan is 6 millisievert (mSv) for a conventional dose of 500 millibecquerels (mBq). The shorter half-life of the PET tracers means that several scans can be performed in the same scanning session because the isotope decays to background within four half-lives of administration (about 8 minutes or so for ^{15}O-labeled tracers). Thus, 6 to 12 cerebral blood flow (CBF) scans can be accommodated in one session when using $H_2^{15}O$, whereas at most two estimates of CBF can be accommodated with HMPAO. With the latter tracer, subtraction of sequential scans is necessary to derive the two estimates of blood flow distribution when two injections of tracer are used in the same session because residual radioactivity persists from the first administration.

Although the ease of production and manipulation of SPECT tracers is undoubted, the armamentarium for useful clinical brain imaging is remarkably small to date. Recent advances have produced very promising new compounds for imaging the dopaminergic pathways, in particular the D_2 receptors (iodine-123 [123I]-benzamide) and nigrostriatal nerve terminals by tracing re-uptake sites (carboxymethoxy iodophenyl tropane-123 [123I-CIT]). On the other hand, the range of PET tracers is impressive with many available for various aspects of physiologic, biochemical, and neurochemical imaging of the brain.

The fundamental difference between PET and SPECT imaging is the quantitative nature of the former. For clinical purposes an image of a physiologic variable such as CBF may often suffice. It may be that the relative distribution of CBF is of particular interest, and in that case normalization of local CBF values to whole brain mean values is a standard and acceptable technique frequently used in SPECT. On the other hand, if absolute functional values are required, the quantitative potential of PET makes it the only imaging modality capable of making measurements that can be compared across laboratories and between and within patients. This capacity resides in the physical process of radioactive decay by positron emission, resulting in the production of two photons, which are detected simultaneously on opposite sides of the brain by the scanning apparatus. This property is exploited in such a way that it renders the problems of correction for attenuation of the emitted radiation by the tissues of the head, collimation, and definition of a precise field of view resolvable in a manner that can only be approximated by SPECT.

The interpretation of a functional image is not easy. The image obtained after the administration of a radioactive tracer does not usually reflect the functional process directly, (although this is the case with FDG, HMPAO, $H_2{}^{15}O$, $C^{15}O_2$, and ^{11}CO). Many physicochemical and biologic properties contribute to the image, including the distribution of the tracer; the uptake and release into and from nonspecific sites such as whole body stores; the permeability across the blood-brain barrier; the distribution and washout within and from the brain tissue and its various physical and physiologic compartments; and the affinity and specificity of binding to relevant sites in the brain. The calculation of a parameter of functional significance may therefore necessitate the frequent sampling of arterial blood (which is very safe from radial cannulation if appropriate caution and care are exercised), the analysis of the blood for metabolites of the tracer, and the collection of frequent brain images as a function of time. These biologic complexities limit in practice the range of functional variables that can be easily imaged and measured with PET. In the clinical context, the variables that have provided most information and are most widely used in functional imaging are energy metabolism (monitored as glucose uptake or oxygen consumption), CBF, and cerebral blood volume (CBV). The dopaminergic system has been most extensively imaged, but opiate and benzodiazepine binding sites have also been successfully investigated.

THE ROLE OF FUNCTIONAL IMAGING IN CLINICAL NEUROLOGY

The degenerative diseases of the cortex and basal ganglia, cerebrovascular disorders, epilepsies, and brain tumors have undergone the most extensive clinical investigation, as have the neuropsychiatric disorders. The remainder of this chapter will concentrate on an analysis of the results of these studies by disease category. It is often difficult to make judgments about the diagnostic use of functional imaging or its exact influence on the management of individual subjects or patients. Much of the clinical research has been of an investigative nature, concerned with identifying group characteristics and describing disease mechanisms. Some of the ensuing discussion is therefore a personal view predicated on preliminary reports in small groups of patients. Suggested readings substantiating these views and documenting larger bodies of data relevant to clinical usefulness are provided in the annotated bibliography at the end of this chapter.

Alzheimer's Disease and the Dementias

Our clinical and pathologic understanding of the dementias and their pathogenesis has made the search for more precise diagnostic criteria in life all the more pressing (see Chs. 60 and 61). Magnetic resonance imaging (MRI) provides a highly sensitive means of determining the vascular component of dementia (see Ch. 10), which may be predominant or may coexist with other degenerative processes. None of the multifocal, scattered metabolic changes described with functional imaging in multi-infarct dementia contain the information that a good MRI scan provides.

The first reports of characteristic changes on functional tomographic imaging were reported over a decade ago with PET. These have since been confirmed on numerous occasions with tracers of oxygen metabolism, glucose consumption, and CBF. Exactly similar patterns have been described with SPECT CBF scans. A pattern of parietal and posterior temporal cortical hypometabolism is found in early, mild, or moderate stages of the disease. The later stages are characterized by additional prefrontal hypometabolism of a similar degree. There is relative sparing of pre- and postcentral gyri and occipital regions as well as the basal ganglia. The degree of impairment of metabolism correlates with the determined clinically severity of dementia.

The changes are usually bilateral, but asymmetric defects may occur early in the disease. These are associated with a clinical presentation of memory deficit, with a relatively restricted cognitive or behavioral deficit that is appropriate to the hemisphere and cortical localization of the metabolic abnormality. It can be difficult to distinguish such patients from those with a focally progressive degenerative disorder such as focal progressive aphasia, progressive occipital blindness, progressive apraxia, etc., who show anatomically restricted regions of hypometabolism on their scans. One indicator that a more generalized degenerative process underlies the cognitive deficit can be obtained from the metabolic rates in areas of cortex distant from the focal deficit. Although the metabolic changes in Alzheimer's disease have a characteristic distribution, they occur in the context of a generalized decline in metabolism, whereas the progressive focal degenerations are notable in that, at least initially, unaffected areas of the brain have normal metabolism. The heterogeneity of pathology underlying progressive focal degenerations cannot be distinguished by functional neuroimaging at present. Focal spongiform change and Pick's disease may resemble each other in producing a similar clinical deficit and focal scanning abnormality. The pattern of hypometabolism correlates with cognitive deficit rather than pathology. However, other PET tracers can be used to provide at least some pathologic information. ^{18}F-dopa can be used as an in vivo tracer of viable nigrostriatal nerve terminals, and hence the integrity of nigrostriatal neurons. In Parkinson's disease the uptake of this tracer is markedly diminished in the striatum. In Alzheimer's disease the uptake of ^{18}F-dopa appears normal even in the presence of clinical abnormalities of muscle tone.

The functional images are not diagnostic in themselves and must always be interpreted in the clinical context. Thus a patient with Parkinson's disease (see Ch. 75) and dementia has been described, who at postmortem examination was found to have only the pathologic changes of idiopathic Lewy body Parkinson's disease but who demonstrated a hypometabolic pattern resembling that of Alzheimer's disease. The motor signs and history in such a patient would clearly indicate that the patient was not suffering from Alzheimer's disease, but the observation raises questions about the nature of the process leading to dementia in Parkinson's disease. A similar Alzheimer-like metabolic pattern has been suggested in Creutzfeldt-Jacob disease, although recent reports indicate a more uniform impairment of metabolism throughout the cortex. Parietotemporal defects have been reported, not surprisingly, in patients with bitemporoparietal infarctions, with local radiation therapy to these regions, and with bilateral subdural hematomas. In the last setting the distortion of the brain outline is a good indicator of the diagnosis, which in any event should not escape good neuroradiology.

In the context of the dementias in general, other patterns of relative focal hypometabolism have been observed in various diseases. In dementia related to the acquired immunodeficiency syndrome (AIDS), there is uniform hypometabolism affecting most cortical and subcortical structures in the brain, but a second pattern of increased basal ganglion metabolism has also been described. In Pick's disease (see Ch. 61) there is a pattern of frontotemporal hypometabolism, which also affects the basal ganglia. In corticobasal degeneration (neuronal achromasia) the changes are very asymmetric and focused on the premotor, inferior parietal and superior temporal regions. The pattern is essentially normal in the (pseudo) dementia of depression, although recent PET studies suggest dorsolateral and medial prefrontal hypometabolism, the latter being specific for the cognitive component of the disorder. Prefrontal hypometabolism of a more generalized nature is consistently reported in progressive supranuclear palsy. There is predominant striatal hypometabolism in Huntington's disease and lenticular hypometabolism in Wilson's disease, sometimes against the background of more diffuse cortical hypometabolism.

The reports in the rarer dementing disorders allow little to be stated concerning specificity and sensitivity in formal terms. In Alzheimer's disease, over 430 patients have been reported, among whom the number who have had postmortem or biopsy confirmation of the diagnosis is approaching 20. One preliminary report on 26 subjects recruited prospectively because of isolated memory defects addresses the issue of sensitivity. Of these patients 18 (69 percent) demonstrated biparietotemporal hypometabolism, and all of them also had normal structural scans. Patients were studied longitudinally and all had progressive extension of hypometabolic zones to those characteristic of Alzheimer's disease. The progression was mirrored by clinical deterioration and development of dementia within about 1 year of presentation. Biopsy or postmortem confirmation of Alzheimer's disease has been obtained in six of these patients. These data suggest a considerable degree of sensitivity.

There are a number of SPECT reports suggesting that in certain cases dementia may be accompanied by a predominant frontal hypometabolism early in the course of the disease. These SPECT scans may be difficult to interpret because of the attenuation correction problem, especially with low-resolution imaging and because the distinction from frontal dementias is not always made. The metabolic correlates of frontal dementia with and without amyotrophy, which not surprisingly affect the frontal lobes, have been described with PET and SPECT using HMPAO.

The accuracy of functional scanning in predicting preclinical disease has been studied in dominantly inherited Huntington's disease (see Ch. 77). Carriers of this disorder reach reproductive age, and presymptomatic diagnosis is possible in certain circumstances when the families are genetically informative. PET scanning with FDG appears to give significant information on carrier status in asymptomatic individuals also. Thus, in one report 58 at-risk subjects were studied, all of whom had normal structural scanning and normal or equivocal clinical findings. Of these subjects, 18 (31 percent) showed abnormal caudate metabolism, compared with the 20 (34) percent who were predicted to carry the gene from genetic concordance studies. Four at-risk subjects have subsequently developed the disease. There has been some debate about the sensitivity of predictive FDG scanning, although the consensus is that with modern methods and high-resolution scans the caudate glucose consumption rate if it is low, provides very valuable information.

Movement Disorders

There has been a rapid increase in information from functional neuroimaging on the integrity of the dopaminergic system in the last years. The information has been virtually exclusively provided by PET scanning. The findings in Parkinson's disease, as in Alzheimer's disease, are based largely on correlations with the clinical diagnosis, which can be erroneous in up to 10 percent of cases if the presence of striatonigral degeneration and Lewy bodies is taken as the defining pathologic characteristic. In early disease, there is an increase in striatal CBF and metabolism, most marked on the side opposite to the more affected limbs. Limitations of resolution make it difficult on present evidence to ascribe this to the putamen or pallidum. There are also reports of frontal hypometabolism, which is mild but possibly correlated with cognitive performance. The uptake of ^{18}F-dopa is decreased by at least 35 percent in the striatum. There is regional specificity, with the posteroventral parts of the putamen affected initially and the remainder of the putamen subsequently. Although the caudate is also affected, it and the ventral striatum are relatively spared. These findings are consistent with pathologic observations on the evolution of the disease. There is now evidence that preclinical nigrostriatal degeneration can also be detected. This comes from studies of subjects exposed to the nigral poison methyl phenyl tetrahydropyridine (MPTP) who have not developed the disease; from family studies, especially in twins; and from studies in some patients with akinetic rigid syndromes caused by neuroleptic exposure and in patients with isolated rest tremor. The results in these

groups remain preliminary but support the notion that preclinical diagnosis, perhaps eventually leading to primary preventive treatment or neuroprotection, is a possibility if not yet a reality.

The course of the disease can be followed by the rate of progression of the nigrostriatal pathology. There are suggestions from serial studies in patients who have undergone mesencephalic fetal cell implantation that the unimplanted striatal structures show a progressive decline in ^{18}F-dopa uptake. Correlations between disability scores in motor performance and striatal ^{18}F-dopa uptake have also been reported, but these seem relatively insensitive and do not replace careful clinical monitoring using structured and validated rating scales.

^{18}F-Dopa scanning is presently the only way to demonstrate functional engraftment of the human striatum by implanted fetal mesencephalic cells. This experimental therapy continues to be evaluated, but the demonstration of tracer uptake by PET and the correlation with clinical and electrophysiologic measures of improvement constitute clear evidence that this form of treatment may be useful in diseases that target widely distributed neuromodulatory transmitter systems.

^{11}C-Nomifensine is a blocker of the dopamine reuptake site and is a tracer of presynaptic nerve terminals. The results with this tracer are substantially the same as with ^{18}F-dopa. The clinical interest in functional neuroimaging with tracers of the dopaminergic system lies in the differential diagnosis of the akinetic rigid syndromes. This is not always an easy matter, even when L-dopa responsiveness is used as a clinical criterion. Multiple system atrophy, which includes progressive autonomic failure, striatonigral degeneration, olivopontocerebellar atrophy, and Shy-Drager syndrome, is characterized by brainstem pathology different from that in idiopathic (Lewy body) Parkinson's disease. A decrease of energy metabolism by one-third to one-half has been demonstrated in the corpora striata of patients with probable striatonigral degeneration. Cortical metabolism is also appreciably diminished by about one-fifth and in a diffuse manner. There is a decrease in frontal areas and in the cerebellum in those patients with ataxia. Patients with multiple system atrophy show a decline of putaminal ^{18}F-dopa uptake similar to that in patients with IPD, but there is also an equivalent decrease in the caudate. This is the area of principal projection of the medial substantia nigra, which is affected in addition to the lateral parts that are characteristically affected in IPD. In progressive autonomic failure, however, the striatal ^{18}F-dopa uptake is normal more often than abnormal. Indeed, an abnormal scan in the context of autonomic failure may be predictive of a more widespread degeneration such as multiple system atrophy. Three patients studied with clinical olivoponto cerebellar atrophy (OPCA) have shown normal ^{18}F-dopa uptake but abnormal cerebellar and brainstem glucose metabolism.

The Steele-Richardson-Olszewski syndrome of progressive supranuclear palsy (see Ch. 77) is characterized by frontal hypometabolism, which is accompanied by more general cortical hypometabolism in more severe disease. This pattern, seen in isolation, is not specific for this disease, as noted above. However, in the clinical context there is usually little difficulty in distinguishing such patients from those with Huntington's or Pick's disease or the other frontal dementias, although the former two will also show the characteristic caudate and temporostriatal features. Caudate and putamen ^{18}F-dopa uptake are reduced by almost half.

It seems reasonably clear that functional neuroimaging provides helpful information for the clinical differentiation of the parkinsonian syndromes in life. The pattern of ^{18}F-dopa uptake distinguishes idiopathic Parkinson's disease from other disorders. Differentiation of the multiple system atrophy from the PSP group can be helped by the different metabolic patterns in cortical and cerebellar structures, although clinical evidence provides as much, if not more useful information. The role of D_2- and D_1-receptor binding is still being evaluated. It is known that there is substantial damage to spiny neurons in the striatum in Huntington's disease, which might therefore be expected to show alterations in dopaminergic receptor tracer binding. The binding of postsynaptic tracers of the dopaminergic system may therefore add specificity to the differential diagnosis, and indeed there are two case reports indicating greatly reduced tracer binding to D_2 receptors in this disease.

Studies in other movement disorders (see Chs. 76 and 77) are as yet too sparse for any meaningful clinical interpretation to be based on them. Chorea is generally associated with caudate hypometabolism, but it is not specific for Huntington's disease. Patients with neuroacanthocytosis and benign familial chorea have shown caudate hypometabolism, but in contrast, tardive dyskinesia and the chorea associated with systemic lupus erythematosus are associated with elevations of caudate metabolism. Chorea is therefore not invariably associated with functional inactivation of the caudate. There are also differences in D_2-receptor-tracer binding between Huntington's disease, neuroacanthocytosis, and tardive dyskinesia, the first two being associated with severe depression of relative binding and the latter with none.

In summary, the use of specific tracers of various aspects of neurotransmission makes the description of pathologic patterns in life and their correlation with clinical syndromes a possibility. The validation of these findings for clinical use will take time because large collections of homogeneous patient populations with these uncommon diseases are rare, and pathologic diagnosis cannot be ascertained with certainty until death.

Cerebrovascular Disease

The role of functional imaging in the assessment and management of patients with cerebrovascular disorders has become much clearer in the last decade. At the basic level, a number of physiologic mechanisms are better understood. These range from the focal uncoupling of flow and metabolism in the acute stages of cerebral ischemia to the homeostatic mechanisms protecting the brain from the effects of perfusion failure.

It is often said that the brain does not contain stores of energy substrates. In fact the blood, which comprises about 5 percent of the brain volume, carries 8 to 10 times the amount of glucose required for the maintenance of normal cerebral metabolic requirements and twice as much oxygen as is necessary. This means that a twofold fall in perfusion can be accommodated before the metabolism and hence the function of the brain are compromised. Perfusion is normally maintained over a wide range in the face of falling perfusion pressure, a phenomenon known as *autoregulation*. This is dependent on the arteriolar component of the cerebral vasculature, which determines the resistance to flow in the cerebral vessels. This component can be monitored by reference to the state of vascular dilation reflected in the CBV. There are thus two reserve mechanisms protecting the brain against ischemia: the capacity to autoregulate, also known as *hemodynamic reserve,* which can be quantified by the CBF/CBV ratio; and the *oxygen carriage reserve,* which can be quantified as the oxygen extraction fraction. This latter variable is normally constant throughout all brain tissues, reflecting the usual coupling of blood flow to metabolic needs. These mechanisms act in series, and their sequential impairment characterizes the severity of decompensation that follows arterial stenotic and occlusive disease. SPECT scanning is able to image relative CBF and CBV and the hemodynamic reserve by monitoring relative CBF in response to a vasodilator challenge. The threshold for ischemia cannot be ascertained, as this can only be monitored with reference to oxygen metabolism.

Clinical studies have shown that the hemodynamic reserve is progressively exhausted by stenotic disease, but chronic states of impaired oxygen reserve supervene only with the most severe stenoses and occlusions, which are almost invariably multiple (see Chs. 5 and 35). There is an as yet imprecisely defined clinical role for such measurements in patients who are candidates for secondary or perhaps even primary preventive surgical therapy. This role is clearer since the results of the recent North American Symptomatic Carotid Endarterectomy Trial (NASCET) study on the efficacy of carotid endarterectomy have become available.

Revascularization operations undoubtedly improve the physiology in a vascular territory in which there is locally compensated hemodynamic compromise. Studies of patients before and after endarterectomy and other revascularization operations has shown clear evidence of the restitution of reserves in all cases. What is less clear is whether these compensated states render the patients less liable to stroke. Prospective studies have been few, and no definitive answer is presently available.

Ischemia is characterized by perfusion failure, which manifests as local hypoperfusion associated with exhaustion of the oxygen reserve as reflected in a maximal oxygen extraction fraction (close to 100 percent) (see Ch. 5). In this state the brain uses all the available oxygen delivered by the impaired flow. In humans the ischemic phase is short-lived. By 12 hours there are clear signs of local cell death, with a fall in oxygen extraction, which almost invariably is subnormal by 24 hours. The combination of low flow (and hence low oxygen delivery) with subnormal oxygen extraction is clear evidence of the loss of functional integrity of the tissue and is the pathophysiologic hallmark of infarction. Perfusion imaging has demonstrated that many infarcts reperfuse spontaneously. Various patterns of perfusion have been demonstrated in infarcted tissue for the first 2 weeks or more after an acute ischemic event. Unfortunately, this means that imaging of perfusion alone is of no use in assessing tissue viability in the acute ischemic phase and in the subacute stages of infarction. However, in practical terms the need for such assessment is currently limited because of the lack of any proven tissue salvage therapy by drugs or surgery in acute cerebral ischemia. If such treatment were available, perfusion imaging during the reversible ischemic phase would be adequate despite uncoupling, but after the first hours of the ictus, oxygen consumption would be the only measurement likely to provide objective evidence of efficacy. A general implication of these studies is that therapy of acute ischemia must be urgent if it is to prevent cell death.

Epilepsy

Functional imaging has been extensively evaluated for the management of difficult epilepsy (see Ch. 79), refractory to standard medical treatment. The main clinical interest is in the use of metabolic imaging for the assessment of patients with focal epilepsy who are can-

didates for surgical therapy in general and temporal lobectomy in particular. In partial epilepsy, interictal FDG scans show a variety of hypometabolic patterns. There is often focal, unilateral, temporal lobe hypometabolism, which corresponds to the probable site of origin of the seizures. The area of hypometabolism is invariably larger than any associated structural damage or lesion that can be shown by computed tomography (CT) or magnetic resonance imaging (MRI). FDG scanning involves imaging the distribution of radioactivity in the brain after accumulation of tracer for 30 to 45 minutes following intravenous tracer injection. In partial epilepsy, patients scanned during the ictal phase may demonstrate hypermetabolism in the same areas that show depressed metabolism interictally. HMPAO SPECT scanning may be a good way of capturing these focal ictal events, which are often short-lived, because the tracer acts as a chemical microsphere and is distributed and trapped in the tissue, as a function of CBF, in the first passage through the brain. Thereafter the distribution changes little, and the patient can be scanned at leisure in the interictal phase, at which time the scan will continue to reflect the relative distribution of perfusion during the seizure at the moment of tracer injection. The tracer can be prepared in anticipation of a seizure and will not decay rapidly, which makes this a practical investigation.

Seizure localization determined by ictal PET has a 90 percent concordance with that determined by surface and depth electroencephalography (EEG). Patients with lateralized discharges on surface and depth EEGs show ipsilateral glucose hypometabolism in 60 to 90 percent of cases. Interictal PET shows a 60 to 80 percent concordance with pathologic examination of the resected temporal lobes. A review by Engel et al. (1990) describes studies in 153 patients with partial seizures of temporal lobe origin. In 37 with congruent hypometabolism and scalp or sphenoidal EEG recordings, depth electrode studies failed to reveal any additional epileptic foci and three patients had nondiagnostic depth electrode studies. In patient's with focal hypometabolism, depth EEG mislocalized in three cases, each of which could be explained by previous structural lesions outside the temporal lobes. In two other patients, differentiation between frontal and temporal seizure foci could not be made on the basis of the scans alone. The conclusion is that if scalp and sphenoidal EEGs show findings congruent with the site of hypometabolism as indicated by interictal functional imaging, depth electrode studies can be avoided. Functional imaging should be carried out before placement of depth electrodes, as these may themselves induce damage sufficient to cause spurious asymmetry in glucose metabolism.

Information from functional scanning is of little use

in the assessment of generalized epilepsy. The precise metabolic pattern depends on the type of epilepsy. The greatest increases occur diffusely throughout the brain in absence seizures, whereas little or no increase is usually seen with primary generalized convulsions, possibly because of the occurrence of postictal depression. Reports showing uncoupling of flow and metabolism at sites of epileptic foci in frontal lobe seizures, periodic lateralized epileptiform discharges, and epilepsia partialis continua have been described and have been used to direct surgical therapy.

Seizures in infancy have also been studied by functional imaging with FDG. In Sturge-Weber syndrome, cortical hypermetabolism can be seen in the affected hemisphere in an area that is larger than any lesions seen on structural scanning. There is a temporal evolution of the findings with functional imaging, which when interpreted in conjunction with structural scanning, may help to plan the timing and extent of surgical resection. On the other hand, in Lennox-Gastaut syndrome no less than four patterns of metabolic abnormality have been described, which although interesting in suggesting a marked heterogeneity of the condition, render the clinical usefulness of functional scanning doubtful. In patients with infantile spasms and hypsarrhythmia, unilateral parieto-occipitotemporal hypometabolism has been found at times. In the absence of abnormalities on structural scans, the functional images have been used to guide curative surgery in at least one group of four young patients. In this regard, PET FDG scans appear much more sensitive at detecting subtle cortical architectonic abnormalities than structural scans. Finally, results in some patients with intractable epilepsy of infancy indicate that hemispheric hypometabolism in the appropriate clinical setting is predictive of highly successful treatment by hemispherectomy.

Cerebral Tumors

The use of functional imaging in the management of cerebral tumors (see Chs. 51 to 58) has undergone extensive examination. Over 400 patients have been studied with ^{11}C-methionine, which is a tracer of amino acid metabolism, and with D$_2$-receptor antagonist tracers. Comparisons of functional and structural imaging suggest that ^{11}C-methionine accumulation distinguishes between viable pituitary tissue and cysts, hemorrhage, or fibrosis in the gland. The D$_2$-receptor status imaged with ^{11}C-methyl spiperone may be of help in predicting the response rate to bromocriptine therapy.

FDG uptake into cerebral gliomas and astrocytomas is correlated with the degree of malignancy estimated histologically from autopsy or biopsy specimens. The initial optimistic results have been tempered some-

what by further experience. Nevertheless, in general, the more malignant the tumor the higher the metabolic rate, and this is quite independent of any breakdown of the blood-brain barrier. The sequential study of patients is particularly useful in assessing malignant transformation. Of particular clinical benefit is the functional scanning of patients following tumor resection or radiotherapy. In such cases the distinction between radiation necrosis and recurrent malignancy can be made with some confidence. However, the clinical situation does not arise very often with modern radiotherapy. Some reports have suggested that even in areas thought by FDG uptake to be necrotic as a result of radiation, biopsy shows viable tumor cells in the necrosed tissue. Recent reports evaluating the usefulness of ^{11}C-methionine suggest that this tracer can also be used to describe areas of tumor regrowth better than FDG alone.

CONCLUSION

This review of the clinical aspects of functional imaging has concentrated on those areas that are now of relevance to clinical diagnosis and management or are likely to be so in the near future. Much work with PET is currently focused on the mapping of brain systems associated with normal cerebral function and on how the breakdown of such integrated and interconnected systems by disease causes specific symptoms. Work in the field of functional mapping will have major relevance to the understanding of neuropsychiatric syndromes and to the analysis of cognitive and sensorimotor deficits associated with focal brain injury and perhaps also to the analysis of the brain mechanisms responsible for their functional restitution. Functional mapping may also provide acceptable tests of hemispheric dominance in preoperative assessments and help functional neurosurgical planning in individuals.

ANNOTATED BIBLIOGRAPHY

Bergstrom M, Muhr C, Lundberg PO, Langstrom B. PET as a tool in the clinical evaluation of pituitary adenomas. J Nucl Med 1991;32:610–15.

Can PET provide information in addition to structural scanning of the gland?

Brooks DJ. Detection of preclinical Parkinson's disease with PET. Neurology 1991;41(suppl. 2):24–7.

A review of intriguing preliminary data suggesting strongly that another degenerative disease might be detectable in a presymptomatic phase.

Chadwick DJ, Whelan J (eds). Exploring Brain Functional Anatomy With Positron Tomography. Ciba Foundation Symposium 163. John Wiley & Sons, Chichester, England, 1991.

An up-to-date book describing functional mapping of the human brain. For those interested in the potential of PET for the clinical investigation of cognitive function, neuropsychiatric syndromes and behavioral neurology.

Chollet F, DiPiero V, Wise RJS, et al. The functional anatomy of motor recovery after stroke in humans: a study with positron emission tomography. Ann Neurol 1991; 29:63–71.

Functional mapping of recovery following striatocapsular infarction.

Chugani HT, Shewmon DA, Peacock WJ, et al. Surgical treatment of intractable neonatal-onset seizures: the role of positron emission tomography. Neurology 1988;38: 1178–88.

Hemispheric hypometabolism and the appropriate clinical context are good indicators for the early surgical treatment of intractable seizures of childhood by hemispherectomy.

D'Antona R, Baron JC, Samson Y et al. Subcortical dementia: frontal cortex hypometabolism detected by positron tomography in patients with progressive supranuclear palsy. Brain 1985;108:785–800.

The frontal lobes in "subcortical dementia"—the first description of the distant metabolic effects of brainstem disease.

Engel JJ, Henry TR, Risinger MW et al. Presurgical evaluation for partial epilepsy: relative contributions of chronic depth-electrode recordings versus FDG-PET and scalp-sphenoidal ictal EEG. Neurology 1990;40:1670–7.

Recent review of the optimal ways of assessing patients before surgical treatment for epilepsy with a critical review of the role of depth electrode recording.

Fox PT, Burton H, Raichle ME. A technique for pre-operative mapping of cortical function with PET CBF imaging. J Nucl Med 1987;28:646–649.

Testing for hemispheric dominance with functional mapping.

Frackowiak RSJ. The pathophysiology of human cerebral ischaemia: a new perspective obtained with positron tomography. Q J Med 1985;57:713–27.

Review of the pathophysiology of cerebral ischemia and hemodynamic decompensation.

Frackowiak RSJ, Pozzilli C, Legg NJ et al. Regional cerebral oxygen supply and utilization in dementia. A clinical and physiological study with oxygen-15 and positron tomography. Brain 1981;104:753–78.

The first description of the characteristic metabolic changes associated with Alzheimer's and vascular dementia.

Francavilla TL, Miletich RS, DiChiro G et al. Positron emission tomography in the detection of malignant degeneration of low-grade gliomas. Neurosurgery 1989;24:1–5.

Longitudinal scanning can be a useful adjunct to clinical assessment of patients with low-grade tumors in determining malignant transformation.

Franck G, Salmon E, Sadzot B, Maquet P. Epilepsy: the use of oxygen-[15] labeled gases. Semin Neurol 1989;9: 307–16.

Another approach to localizing sites of focal seizure onset by using uncoupling of cerebral blood flow from oxygen metabolism.

Lindvall O, Brundin P, Widner H et al. Grafts of fetal dopamine neurons survive and improve motor function in Parkinson's disease. Science 1990;247:574–7.

Clinical, physiologic, and functional imaging data providing the first convincing evidence of the viability and engraftment of fetal mesencephalic cells in the striatum of patients with Parkinson's disease.

Mazziotta JC. Huntington's disease: studies with structural imaging techniques and positron emission tomography. Semin Neurol 1989;9:360–369.

Review of functional imaging in Huntington's disease.

Neary D, Snowden JS, Northern B, Goulding P. Dementia of frontal lobe type. J Neurol Neurosurg Psychiatry 1988; 51:353–61.

SPECT scanning in frontal lobe dementia.

Phelps ME, Mazziotta JC, Schelbert HR. Positron Emission Tomography and Autoradiography: Principles and Applications for the Brain and Heart. Raven Press, New York, 1986.

The definitive textbook on the subject of functional imaging. Now a little out of date, but a must for those wishing to understand the scientific fundamentals of the subject.

15

Single-Photon Emission Computed Tomography

Stephen M. Davis

Single-photon emission computed tomography (SPECT) enables three-dimensional imaging and measurements of brain function, which provide information about cerebral pathophysiology in a range of neurologic disorders. Far simpler and less expensive than positron emission tomography, it has become widely available in nuclear medicine departments in recent years. Its development has been greatly facilitated by newer radiopharmaceuticals and imaging instrumentation. The radionuclides used in SPECT scanning are single-photon γ-ray emitters, in contrast to the positron emitters used in positron emission tomography (PET) scanning, which produce two photons in coincidence after the annihilation reaction with the tissue electron.

In many centers SPECT is now finding clinical application in an increasing number of neurologic diseases. A variety of receptor SPECT techniques, using novel radionuclides, have also been introduced. Thus far SPECT scanning has been mainly applied to the imaging and evaluation of cerebral perfusion, which is termed perfusion SPECT. However, unlike PET (see ch. 14), SPECT scanning cannot currently be reliably used to measure cerebral metabolism.

SPECT TECHNIQUES

Perfusion SPECT

Perfusion SPECT utilizes either the clearance of inhaled xenon-133 (^{133}Xe) or radiopharmaceuticals that are fixed in the brain in proportion to regional cerebral blood flow (rCBF). Three major perfusion techniques are currently used. The first involves inhalation of the inert gas ^{133}Xe with imaging and measurement of rCBF using specialized detection devices. This technique was an outgrowth of the earlier two-dimensional ^{133}Xe CBF method, which used extracranial probes to estimate flow in cerebral gray matter at multiple sites in each hemisphere, the radiopharmaceutical being delivered via inhalation or by intracarotid or intravenous injection. The technique allows rCBF quantitation in units of milliters per 100 grams per minute without arterial sampling. As ^{133}Xe is rapidly cleared, multiple studies can be performed on the same day. However, spatial resolution is poor because of the rate of clearance as well as the low photon energy of the tracer. More recently, radiotracers have been developed that cross the blood-brain barrier, distribute within the brain in proportion to rCBF, and fix in the cerebral tissues for sufficient time to allow tomographic imaging of γ-emissions.

The two other rCBF techniques chiefly used involve intravenously injected iodine-123 (^{123}I)-isopropyl iodoamphetamine and technetium-99m (^{99m}Tc)-hexamethylpropylene-amine oxime (^{99m}Tc HMPAO). Both agents have high first-pass cerebral extraction, and the brain activity images correlate well with cerebral perfusion over a wide rCBF range. However, neither technique currently allows precise quantitation of rCBF. ^{123}I requires cyclotron generation, and its use is therefore more restricted than the technetium technique. In addition, owing to its rapid redistribution, cerebral imaging has to be performed within 1 hour of injection, and image quality is slightly inferior to that obtained with the various technetium-labeled ligands.

^{99m}Tc HMPAO SPECT

The ^{99m}Tc HMPAO SPECT technique was introduced in the mid-1980s and is now in widespread use (Plate 15-1). This technetium-labeled lipophilic agent is rapidly taken up and fixed in the brain in proportion to perfusion with virtually constant maintenance over several hours. Steady-state conditions are reached approximately 2 to 3 minutes after injection. This allows the rCBF study to be performed up to a few hours after injection of the agent while providing a "snapshot" of rCBF at the time of injection. The method therefore lends itself to the study of hyperacute stroke and the ictal blood flow changes associated with complex partial seizures. Currently, precise quantitation of rCBF is not possible, as the biodistribution and kinetics of ^{99m}Tc HMPAO are unclear, but analyses of regional activity ratios and volumetric hypoperfusion are clinically useful.

Neuroreceptor SPECT

Neuroreceptor SPECT involves the use of a range of ligands, including those developed for muscarinic cholinergic receptors, the dopamine D_2 receptor, the serotonin-2 receptor, and the benzodiazepine receptor. Only a limited number of clinical studies have been reported to date using neuroreceptor SPECT imaging. These include the application of the benzodiazepine antagonist ^{123}I-iomazenil in temporal lobe epilepsy and of the dopamine D_2 receptor antagonist ^{123}I-iodobenzamide in Parkinson's disease.

Instrumentation

The imaging systems used in SPECT utilize either camera-based techniques or dedicated cerebral systems with fixed or rotating detectors. γ-Camera techniques are more widely used than the dedicated cerebral detector systems, because they can be used for body as well as head scanning. The recent introduction of multihead cameras has provided higher resolution with shorter scanning times than the earlier single-head systems. These modern SPECT techniques can produce a spatial cerebral resolution of 6 to 9 mm, with imaging times of only 10 to 20 minutes (Plate 15-1). Perfusion imaging using ^{133}Xe SPECT currently requires a dedicated cerebral imaging system, such as a rotating detector array or a fixed detector system.

CLINICAL APPLICATIONS

Cerebrovascular Disease

Increased understanding of underlying mechanisms of disease have come from measurements with perfusion SPECT in a range of cerebrovascular disorders, including hemodynamic carotid disease, transient ischemic attacks (TIAs), cerebral infarction (see Ch. 35) and subarachnoid hemorrhage (see Ch. 37). More precise diagnosis and previously unavailable prognostic information have accrued. Furthermore, SPECT

can be used as a template for the assessment of interventional therapy for acute stroke.

Cerebral infarction studied by rCBF SPECT typically shows focal hypoperfusion, the extent of the abnormalities correlating with clinical stroke severity. While hypoperfusion is invariable early in cerebral ischemia, the structural tissue changes imaged by computed tomography (CT) scanning and the increases in tissue water content detected by magnetic resonance imaging (MRI) take longer to develop, so that these two popular neuroimaging techniques show no abnormalities in some cases studied early. However, despite the diagnostic sensitivity of SPECT in acute stroke, it is unlikely to have a major role in routine stroke diagnosis, mainly because SPECT does not reliably differentiate between hemorrhage and infarction and may fail to exclude nonvascular pathologies.

The limitations of acute CT scanning (see Ch. 10) prompted interest in SPECT in the hope that it might provide early prognostic information that could be valuable in guiding the type and intensity of acute therapy. Despite initial disappointments, recent studies have shown a good correlation between the severity of acute regional hypoperfusion and functional recovery. However, the perfusion data only improve the prognostic value of clinical determinants to a small degree. Subacute SPECT scans, obtained days to a few weeks after stroke onset, show variable rCBF changes, including hyperemia in some cases. This has been attributed to non-nutritional flow.

In patients with acute infarcts, measurements of hypoperfusion with SPECT can provide a template for the evaluation of experimental stroke therapies that increase perfusion. Thrombolytic therapy, aimed at acute recanalization of occluded vessels with reperfusion of ischemic cerebral tissue, is currently being investigated in several large multicenter, randomized trials. Early reports suggest improved reperfusion with thrombolytic therapy monitored by SPECT (Plate 15-2).

In some patients with TIAs and carotid artery disease, hemodynamic mechanisms are important. The distal hemodynamic effects of extracranial carotid stenosis can be evaluated by SPECT. Vascular reserve, assessed by measuring the augmentation of rCBF with the vasodilator acetazolamide, is reduced in a significant proportion of patients with severe stenosis or occlusion of large arteries. The reversal of these perfusion abnormalities with carotid endarterectomy suggests that SPECT may help in therapeutic decisions. Following TIAs in some patients, prolonged disturbances of rCBF have been shown. Persistent reduction of rCBF by more than 30 percent after a TIA has been associated with a higher risk of infarction over the subsequent few weeks. In patients with TIAs,

SPECT can therefore aid in delineation of a higher risk group.

Subarachnoid hemorrhage is associated with delayed neurologic deterioration in approximately 30 percent of patients. Spasm, usually leading to ischemia caused by impaired perfusion, is the most important cause of morbidity after subarachnoid hemorrhage. Transcranial Doppler ultrasonography has facilitated the noninvasive diagnosis of large-vessel vasospasm, particularly in the middle cerebral artery, but does not directly provide information about perfusion in the microcirculation. The sensitivity of transcranial Doppler is particularly limited by the poor correlation with vasospasm in arteries other than the middle cerebral and its inability to insonate the smaller intracerebral arteries and arterioles. The demonstration of regional hypoperfusion with SPECT has proved to be a more specific indicator of cerebral ischemia than the diagnosis of vasospasm with transcranial Doppler. The severity of hypoperfusion correlates with delayed ischemic deficits and has prognostic value. The two hemodynamic techniques provide complementary information in subarachnoid hemorrhage concerning the state of the large intracerebral vessels and microvascular tissue perfusion. The finding of tissue hypoperfusion with SPECT in patients with delayed deficits, at a time when the CT scan is normal, can influence the type and intensity of therapy for vasospasm. For example, the demonstration of focal hypoperfusion can be used to evaluate new and potentially invasive therapies for vasospasm, such as balloon arterial dilation, in patients who are unresponsive to medical treatment.

Head Injury

A number of studies have shown that SPECT imaging of rCBF after head injury provides information in addition to that obtained by CT scanning. Focal rCBF disturbances, not seen on CT scanning, can be detected by SPECT. Perfusion deficits in excess of CT-demonstrated changes predict a worse prognosis. Patients in a persistent vegetative state after head injury and with a global reduction of cortical blood flow on SPECT have a particularly poor long-term prognosis.

Epilepsy

It is estimated that up to 35 percent of epileptic patients have partial seizures, of whom 25 percent are refractory to medical therapy. A significant proportion of these patients are candidates for surgical excision of the seizure focus. Temporal lobectomy is the most commonly used surgical technique in patients with intractable complex partial seizures of temporal lobe origin (see Ch. 79).

Electrophysiologic techniques including electroencephalographic (EEG) videotelemetry, depth electrode EEG, and surface electrocorticography are all valuable diagnostic modalities, but seizure localization often remains difficult. In patients with refractory complex partial seizures, SPECT imaging now has an established role in seizure localization as a prelude to surgery for epileptic foci and has reduced the need for invasive investigations. Interictal PET studies can be used to demonstrate both focal hypoperfusion and hypometabolism and provide a valuable guide to seizure localization in temporal lobe epilepsy. Interictal SPECT has also been used in the evaluation of complex partial seizures, often demonstrating focal hypoperfusion that corresponds to EEG foci. However, interictal SPECT is less reliable than PET and is considered to localize the seizure focus in only 50 percent of cases in some series.

There is marked focal hyperperfusion associated with a focal epileptic discharge. Although perfusion SPECT at the precise time of a seizure is technically very difficult to achieve, early postictal SPECT, within a few minutes of the seizure, is highly reliable in localization of a temporal lobe focus, with a diagnostic accuracy approaching 100 percent. A postictal perfusion "switch" in temporal lobe seizures has been described, with a change in 1 to 5 minutes from unilateral temporal hyperperfusion to relative mesial temporal hyperperfusion and lateral temporal hypoperfusion. This may reflect the underlying metabolic processes of neuronal activation and recovery (Plate 15-3).

Neuroreceptor SPECT may also be useful in the analysis of seizure foci, demonstrating reduced benzodiazepine receptor density with ^{123}I-iomazenil SPECT. The HMPAO SPECT technique lends itself to seizure analysis, as the agent can be injected during or very closely after the event in the monitoring ward, providing a snapshot of perfusion changes at that time, and yet allowing up to a few hours for subsequent imaging. In experienced centers it has led to a reduced need for invasive investigations, particularly depth electrode recordings for lateralization of temporal lobe foci.

Alzheimer's Disease

The prevalence of dementia is approximately 5 percent of the population aged 65, rising to 20 percent of those aged 80 years. The two chief causes are the common Alzheimer's disease (dementia of the Alzheimer type) (see Ch. 60) and the rare multi-infarct dementia (see Chs. 35 and 61). Structural neuroimaging methods such as CT or MRI are useful in excluding structural cerebral lesions that might be potentially treatable, such as hydrocephalus, subdural hematoma, cerebral abscess, or brain tumor. In some dementia patients, CT and particularly MRI scanning may demonstrate focal infarcts or white matter lesions suggesting multi-infarct dementia, while hippocampal atrophy favors a diagnosis of Alzheimer-type dementia.

Functional neuroimaging with SPECT (Plate 15-4) is likely to have a future major impact on the diagnosis of this common, progressive, and currently untreatable condition. In Alzheimer-type dementia PET scanning demonstrates characteristic metabolic abnormalities, with glucose hypometabolism and associated hypoperfusion in the temporal and parietal lobes, correlating with the clinical severity of dementia. The typical distribution of hypoperfusion is also demonstrated by SPECT, correlating with the temporoparietal functional depression shown by PET and the clinical pattern and degree of the dementia. The occipital lobes and cerebellum tend to be spared, and frontal involvement only occurs late in the course of the disease.

These changes have been demonstrated by using both the isopropyliodoamphetamine SPECT and the HMPAO SPECT technique, distinguishing the patients from normal controls and from those with multi-infarct dementia. Furthermore, the degree of hypoperfusion tends to correlate with the severity of the disease, and its regional emphasis correlates with the pattern of the neuropsychological deficits. For example, greater hypoperfusion is evident in the dominant hemisphere in patients with early speech involvement, while nondominant hypoperfusion predominates in those with early spatial and constructional deficits. In contrast, frontal lobe hypoperfusion on SPECT in dementia patients has been associated with Pick's disease and progressive supranuclear palsy.

The pattern of temporoparietal hypoperfusion has been thought to be related to the loss of projection neurons in the parahippocampal gyrus that innervates these regions of the neocortex. For some authors, the severity of the regional hypoperfusion abnormalities has proved to be a reliable measure of cognitive functional deficits. Although bilateral posterior cortical rCBF deficits are highly predictive of Alzheimer-type dementia, unilateral temporoparietal deficits are not diagnostically specific and can be due to vascular lesions.

While Alzheimer's disease is currently untreatable, the identification of this characteristic hypoperfusion pattern on SPECT allows more accurate diagnosis in vivo, with important implications for early diagnosis and evaluation of new therapies. Trials of experimental therapies for Alzheimer's disease can be conducted to determine whether there is any improvement in the regional hypoperfusion, using the SPECT findings as a guide.

Multi-Infarct Dementia

The diagnostic distinction between dementia of the Alzheimer type and the far less frequent multi-infarct dementia depends mainly on clinical criteria and structural neuroimaging methods, particularly MRI (see Chs. 10 and 35). Imaging with SPECT can yield additional diagnostic information. Cortical temporoparietal hypoperfusion favors Alzheimer's. In contrast, focal areas of hypoperfusion in both the cortex and deeper structures, correlating with infarcts, are more frequent in multi-infarct dementia patients.

Primary Brain Tumors

SPECT imaging with thallium-201 (^{201}Tl), which localizes in brain tumors, has been shown to help differentiate low-grade from high-grade gliomas (see Ch. 52). Dual-isotope SPECT with ^{201}Tl and ^{99m}Tc HMPAO can be used to distinguish between radiation necrosis and recurrent glioma. Tumor recurrence is suggested by high ^{201}Tl uptake and preserved or increased perfusion on HMPAO SPECT in the tumor bed. These findings should have important applications in the assessment of cerebral tumors and in the evaluation of their response to therapy.

Parkinson's Disease

Specific PET abnormalities are present in Parkinson's disease (see Ch. 75), with glucose hypometabolism in the basal ganglia and depressed uptake of fluorine-18 (^{18}F)-fluoro-L-dopa in the caudate regions. There have been some reports of hypoperfusion in the basal ganglia when using SPECT, but other investigators have found no consistent abnormalities. It has been estimated that dementia occurs in 10 to 40 percent of patients with Parkinson's disease. There have been consistent reports of temporoparietal hypoperfusion in such patients, similar to the pattern in Alzheimer-type dementia and contrasting with normal perfusion in nondemented subjects.

Neurotransmitter SPECT of dopamine D_2-receptors has been performed with ^{123}I-iodobenzamide, which localizes primarily in the basal ganglia. This technique holds promise for clinical studies of the dopaminergic system in Parkinson's disease.

Huntington's Disease

Studies using ^{18}F-deoxyglucose PET have demonstrated glucose hypometabolism in the caudate nuclei in patients with symptomatic Huntington's disease (see Ch. 77), as well as in some patients who are at risk for this dominantly inherited disorder. These functional abnormalities can be detected earlier than the characteristic caudate atrophy and increased intercaudate separation shown on CT or MRI scans in patients with more advanced disease. Similar changes have been reported with use of perfusion SPECT. Hypoperfusion on both isopropyliodoamphetamine and HMPAO SPECT has been found in the caudate nuclei and adjacent structures, preceding the morphologic changes identified by the structural imaging techniques. Nonspecific patchy or diffuse cortical hypoperfusion has also been reported in patients with advanced disease. These findings may complement the genetic testing of at-risk subjects and facilitate trials of experimental therapies.

AIDS-Dementia Complex

While CT and MRI scanning are used to diagnosed various neurologic diseases associated with the acquired immunodeficiency syndrome (AIDS) (see Ch. 49), including cerebral infections, tumors, and progressive multifocal leukoencephalopathy, perfusion SPECT has been shown to be useful in diagnosis of the AIDS-dementia complex. This has been characterized as involving multifocal cortical and subcortical areas of hypoperfusion, particularly affecting the frontal, temporal and parietal lobes, which are not usually demonstrated by CT or MRI scans. While these abnormalities are not specific for AIDS encephalopathy, the pathophysiologic changes are present at the early stages of the disease. The technique appears to be very sensitive, with a good correlation between the severity of the rCBF abnormalities and the stage of the dementia. Potentially, early interventional therapy in AIDS patients may be administered on the basis of these SPECT changes, particularly given the high prevalence of cerebral involvement in the disease.

Psychiatric Disorders

Cerebral imaging with SPECT is likely in the future to aid in the diagnosis and assessment of treatment in a variety of psychiatric disorders. For example, frontal lobe hypoperfusion has been demonstrated in patients with depression, which resolves with therapy. This rCBF pattern could be useful in differentiating patients presenting with organic dementia from those with depressive illness presenting as a pseudodementia. In schizophrenia, reported findings have included frontal lobe hypoactivity and increased perfusion in the basal ganglia.

ANNOTATED BIBLIOGRAPHY

Baird AE, Donnan GA, Austin MC et al: Reperfusion after thrombolytic therapy in ischemic stroke measured by single-photon emission computed tomography. Stroke 1994;25:79–85.

Measurement of reperfusion with thrombolytic therapy after stroke.

Berkovic SF, Newton MR, Rowe CC: Localization of epileptic foci using SPECT. p. 251. In Luders H (ed): Epilepsy Surgery. Raven Press, New York, 1991.

Review of SPECT in the epilepsies, including analysis of interictal, ictal, and immediate postictal studies.

Bogousslavsky J, Delaloye-Bischof A, Regli F, Delaloye B: Prolonged hypoperfusion and early stroke after transient ischemic attack. Stroke 1990;21:40.

A study of prolonged perfusion abnormalities in some transient ischemic attack patients, with adverse prognostic implications.

Carvalho PA, Schwartz RB, Alexander E et al: Detection of recurrent glioma with quantitative thallium-201/technetium-99m HM-PAO single-photon emission computerized tomography. J Neurosurg 1992;77:565.

The value of SPECT techniques in the differentiation of recurrent glioma from postradiation necrosis.

Cordes M, Henkes H, Ferstl F: Evaluation of focal epilepsy: A SPECT scanning comparison of 123-I-Iomazenil versus HM-PAO. AJNR 1992;13:249.

Benzodiazepine receptors in focal epilepsy.

Davis SM, Andrews JT, Lichtenstein M et al: Correlations between cerebral arterial velocities, blood flow, and delayed ischemia after subarachnoid hemorrhage. Stroke 1992;23:492.

Correlations between tissue perfusion abnormalities using SPECT, arterial blood flow using transcranial Doppler, and clinical manifestations of delayed ischemia after subarachnoid hemorrhage.

Davis SM, Chua MG, Lichtenstein M et al: Cerebral hypoperfusion in stroke prognosis and brain recovery. Stroke 1993;24:1691–6.

SPECT in prognosis and brain recovery after stroke.

Fayad PB, Brass LM: Single photon emission computed tomography in cerebrovascular disease. Curr Concepts Cerebrovasc Dis Stroke 1991;26:7.

General review of SPECT in cerebrovascular disease.

George MS, Ring HA, Costa DC et al: Neuroactivation and Neuroimaging with SPET. In Clinical Use of SPET Imaging in Psychiatric and Neurological Disease. Springer-Verlag, London, 1991, pp. 51–120.

Clinical applications.

Habert MO, Spampinato U, Mas JL et al: A comparative technetium 99m hexamethylpropylene amine oxime SPET study in different types of dementia. Eur J Nucl Med 1991;18:3.

SPECT in different types of dementia.

Holman BL, Devous MD: Functional brain SPECT: the emergence of a powerful clinical method. J Nucl Med 1992;33:1888.

Diagnostic probability of Alzheimer disease based on perfusion SPECT patterns.

Holman BL, Johnson KA, Gerada B et al: The scintigraphic

appearance of Alzheimer's disease: A prospective study using technetium-99m-HMPAO SPECT. J Nucl Med 1992;33:181.

Current techniques and clinical applications.

Kung HF, Alavi A, Chang W et al: In vivo SPECT imaging of CNS D$_2$ dopamine receptors: initial studies with iodine-123-IBZM in humans. J Nucl Med 1990;31:573.

Dopamine receptors.

Masdeu JC, Brass LM, Holman BL et al. Brain single-photon emission computed tomography. Neurology 1994; 44:1970–7.

Recent review article.

Nagel JS, Ichise M, Holman BL. The scintigraphic evaluation of Huntington's disease and other movement disorders using single photon emission computed tomography perfusion brain scans. Semin Nucl Med 1991;21:11.

Clinical review.

Roper SN, Mena I, King WA et al: An analysis of cerebral blood flow in acute closed-head injury using technetium-99m-HMPAO SPECT and computed tomography. J Nucl Med 1991;32:1684.

SPECT vs. CT after acute head injury.

Rowe CC, Berkovic SF, Austin MC et al: Patterns of postictal cerebral blood flow in temporal lobe epilepsy: qualitative and quantitative analysis. Neurology 1991;41:1096.

Immediate postictal SPECT and seizure location.

16
Evaluation of Autonomic Reflexes

E. Oribe and O. Appenzeller

The basis for function of the autonomic nervous system (ANS) will be described in Chapter 34, to which the reader is referred for introduction of the clinical semiology. In the present chapter the testing of ANS function is detailed.

The integrity of autonomic reflex pathways can be explored through autonomic tests. The objectives of autonomic testing are to demonstrate the presence of autonomic dysfunction (at the bedside or in the laboratory) and to determine the extent of involvement and the site of the lesion. Afferent and efferent limbs and the central structures involved in different autonomic reflexes can be studied. Tests that evaluate the overall integrity of ANS reflex pathways require normal afferent pathways. Other tests provide an indication of the integrity of efferent pathways independently of afferents. Few test central autonomic structures. As tests of autonomic function rely on measuring endorgan responses, it is important to ensure that effector organs are functional.

Most autonomic tests are simple and straightforward to perform but often difficult to interpret. Multiple factors should be taken into account, including patient anxiety and degree of effort, habituation of the response after repeated tests, dehydration, use of medication, metabolic status (e.g., hypoglycemia), time after meals and type of meal, circadian rhythms, smoking, and an age-related decline in autonomic function. Ambient temperature, the position of the patient when performing the tests, and the patient's sex may alter autonomic results. It is important, therefore, that each laboratory develop a range of normal test values taking the above factors into account. The clinician should be reluctant to conclude that a patient has autonomic dysfunction based on a single abnormal test result, and it is best to perform several tests all pointing to one lesion before deciding on the significance of the results. Ultimately, the diagnosis of autonomic dysfunction depends on the presence of abnormal test results in a clinical setting suggesting autonomic dysfunction.

Most autonomic tests use relatively simple equipment. As cardiovascular autonomic tests rely on measurement of heart rate and blood pressure responses to different stimuli, usually an electrocardiograph (ECG) machine or monitor and a manual blood pressure cuff are sufficient. Several simple and useful bedside tests, which have been shown to be reliable and reproducible, are summarized in Table 16-1. Continuous beat-to-beat heart rate and blood pressure data, which can now be acquired noninvasively with photoplethysmographic or tonometric devices (Ohmeda Finapres, Colin CBM 3000), permit assessment of complex beat-to-beat autonomic responses in a laboratory setting. More sophisticated testing that involves statistical or frequency analysis of heart rate, blood pressure, and respiratory parameters relies on the use of electronic data acquisition and computer-assisted analysis.

CARDIOVASCULAR AUTONOMIC TESTING

Cardiovascular autonomic tests provide an indirect indication of the integrity of autonomic pathways by measuring reflex changes in heart rate, blood pressure, and plasma concentration of neurotransmitters and hormones in response to maneuvers that activate (load or unload) baroreceptors.

Sympathetic function can be assessed by determining the reflex changes in plasma norepinephrine concentration or the degree of vasoconstriction elicited by reductions in blood pressure or venous return (e.g.,

213

Table 16-1. Simple Bedside Tests of Cardiovascular Autonomic Nervous Function

Test	Measurements	Normal Response[a]	Abnormal Response	Site of 'Lesion'[b]
BP and HR supine and standing	BP and HR supine after 20 min and standing after 2 min	↑ HR <30 bpm ↓ SBP <20 mm Hg	= HR ↓ SBP	Sympathetic efferents
	HR at beat 30/beat 15 after active standing	> 1.03	< 1.00	Vagal efferents
HR variability (deep breathing)	Maximum − minimum HR	> 10 bpm	< 8 bpm	Vagal efferents
	Maximum R-R during expiration/minimum R-R during inspiration (E/I ratio)	> 1.10	< 1.05	Vagal efferents
HR variability (Valsalva's maneuver)	Longest R-R after maneuver/shortest R-R	> 1.15	< 1.10	No rebound bradycardia during phase IV: vagal efferents No tachycardia during phase II: sympathetic efferents

Abbreviations: BP, blood pressure; SBP, systolic BP; HR, heart rate; R-R, ECG R-R intervals; bpm, beats per minute; =, unchanged; ↓, decreased; ↑, increased.
[a] Values are for normal subjects of both sexes under 60 years of age.
[b] Site of lesion if afferent and central baroreflex pathways are intact.

by standing, head-up tilting, lower body negative pressure, or administration of vasodilator agents). Increases in sympathetic efferent activity can also be induced independently of baroreceptor afferent pathways by cortical arousal (e.g., mental stress) or by direct stimulation of cholinergic postganglionic sympathetic neurons with the cholinesterase inhibitor edrophonium. Efferent sympathetic outflow to muscle and skin blood vessels can be measured directly by intraneural microneurography (recording of muscle and skin sympathetic nerve activity) in a research setting.

Evaluation of parasympathetic autonomic cardiac control is based on measuring changes in heart rate in response to maneuvers that either inhibit or stimulate parasympathetic efferent activity. Examples of reflex inhibition of parasympathetic efferent activity include the initial responses to maneuvers such as isometric exercise, standing, or head-up tilting. Maneuvers that enhance parasympathetic outflow include deep breathing and production of blood pressure increases by the Valsalva maneuver or by administration of pressor drugs. The integrity of efferent parasympathetic pathways can also be assessed independently of baroreceptor afferent pathways by massaging the carotid sinus (not recommended in elderly subjects), by eye-ball pressure, by performing diving or simulated diving tests, or by infusion of atropine.

TESTS OF OVERALL BARORECEPTOR REFLEX INTEGRITY

Hemodynamic Responses to the Upright Posture

Measuring the reflex autonomic responses to assumption of the upright posture (see also Ch. 34) provides information on the integrity of the afferent, central, and efferent baroreflex pathways. The ANS responses to active standing and passive tilting are different. Standing produces an immediate fall in cardiac output due to gravitational blood pooling below the heart. This is accompanied by an increase in heart rate, mediated through reflex vagal withdrawal, which is maximum at about the fifteenth heart beat. Upon active standing, contraction of limb and abdominal muscles produces a transient increase in venous return and a blood pressure overshoot, which peaks at about the thirtieth heart beat and results in a slowing of the heart rate due to reflex parasympathetic activation (Fig. 16-1).

The ratio of the maximum and minimum heart rates at about the fifteenth and thirtieth beats after standing therefore is used as a measure of vagal function. The initial vagally mediated heart rate response to standing is followed by progressive increase in heart rate due to an enhanced sympathetic tone acting together with continued vagal inhibition. The normal blood pressure responses to standing are a minimal

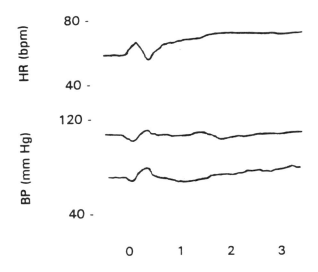

Figure 16-1. Normal blood pressure (BP) (upper trace, systolic pressure; lower trace, diastolic pressure) and heart rate (HR) changes induced by active standing in a healthy control subject. An initial increase in HR is followed by a relative slowing in response to a rebound in BP produced by contraction of muscles during active standing. These initial changes in HR are vagally mediated.

decrease in systolic and an increase in diastolic pressure accompanied by an increase in heart rate. A symptomatic fall of systolic pressure of more than 30 mmHg is abnormal.

Passive head-up tilt results in a more gradual and less pronounced increase in heart rate, and a blood pressure overshoot is absent. During head-up tilt the initial transient fall in blood pressure is followed by a rapid restoration of values within 2 minutes.

Lower Body Negative Pressure and Neck Chamber Devices

Lower body negative pressure and neck chamber devices, presently used in research applications, provide an assessment of the overall integrity of the baroreflex pathways. By applying negative pressure to an airtight frame placed over the lower body and sealed at the level of the umbilicus, lower body negative pressure "suctions" part of the circulating blood into the lower body (i.e., produces pooling), simulating the effects of gravity and hemorrhage on circulating blood volume.

With lower body negative pressure, low-pressure cardiopulmonary baroreceptor function can be tested selectively, as central venous pressure can be decreased without affecting arterial blood pressure. Neck chamber devices apply either negative or positive pressure at the level of the carotid baroreceptors

and allow manipulation of the arterial baroreflex environment without affecting low-pressure baroreceptors.

Baroreflex sensitivity testing with pressor agents (e.g., phenylephrine or angiotensin) provides measures of the reflex decrease in heart rate mediated predominantly by the vagus nerve in response to rises in blood pressure.

Valsalva Maneuver

The response to the Valsalva (A. M. Valsalva, Italian anatomist, 1666–1723) maneuver assesses the integrity of the afferent, central, and efferent pathways of the baroreflex and allows measurement of sympathetic and vagal function. To perform this test, subjects exhale forcefully through a mouthpiece with a small leak (to prevent cheating) against a 40 mmHg resistance for 15 seconds.

Blood pressure and heart rate changes induced by the Valsalva maneuver are divided into four phases. During phase I, at the onset of straining, there is a rise in arterial pressure due to mechanical compression of the aorta, accompanied by a reflex reduction in heart rate. During phase II, while the subject is exhaling against resistance, there is reflex tachycardia in response to the fall in cardiac output and blood pressure produced by increased intrathoracic pressure, which decreases venous return. During this phase tachycardia is due to reflex parasympathetic withdrawal and increased sympathetic outflow. During phase III, when forced exhalation ceases, the fall in intrathoracic pressure produces a transient rise in pulmonary venous capacitance. This causes a fall in venous return, further reducing systemic blood pressure while heart rate continues to increase. During phase IV there is a rebound increase in blood pressure (i.e., overshoot) due to continued vasoconstriction and increased cardiac output, which in turn results in increased vagal efferent activity, with consequent bradycardia and a return of blood pressure to baseline.

The Valsalva ratio is calculated as the ratio of the longest ECG R-R interval during phase IV (bradycardia due to vagal activation) to the shortest interval during phase II (tachycardia due to vagal withdrawal and sympathetic activation).

In autonomic failure, abnormal sympathetic outflow leads to defective peripheral vasoconstriction, blood pressure decreases markedly during phase II (by > 20 mmHg systolic), and there is no blood pressure overshoot and no bradycardia during phase IV of the Valsalva maneuver. In this situation the circulation behaves according to mechanical laws without the modulating effects of the ANS. Degrees of autonomic dysfunction can be recognized through detailed analysis of responses during the different phases of the maneuver by using beat-to-beat recording techniques.

TESTS OF EFFERENT SYMPATHETIC PATHWAYS

The Cold Pressor and Mental Stress Tests

The cold pressor test assesses the integrity of a reflex arc, which includes afferent sensory nerves (pain), spinothalamic tracts, suprapontine and intrathalamic relays, and efferent sympathetic pathways, peripheral sympathetic nerves, and vascular receptors. In this test immersion of the hand in ice water produces arteriolar vasoconstriction and an increase in blood pressure and cardiac output. The rise in blood pressure in response to emotional stress accompanying mental tasks (mental stress test) indicates the integrity of efferent sympathetic pathways. Such stressful mental tasks as mental arithmetic or tests during which the subject is pressed to make choices are among the stimuli that result in a reflex increase in blood pressure and heart rate. The lack of an adequate blood pressure response indicates a lesion of efferent vasoconstrictor fibers. Standards for these tests are difficult to establish and there are large intra- and interindividual variations in responsiveness.

Plasma Norepinephrine Levels

Plasma norepinephrine levels, which reflect the balance from the spillover of norepinephrine from postganglionic sympathetic neurons and norepinephrine clearance, can be used to investigate the capacity of baroreceptor-mediated stimuli to activate efferent sympathetic neurons. Blood is sampled with the subject supine and again after at least 10 minutes in the upright position. The normal response is an increase in norepinephrine over 100 percent of supine values.

Measurements of plasma norepinephrine concentration following an injection of edrophonium, a short-acting cholinesterase inhibitor, can be used to test the responsiveness of sympathetic postganglionic neurons independently of baroreceptor afferent pathways. This test can be used to differentiate between central (i.e., preganglionic) and peripheral (i.e., postganglionic) sympathetic neuronal damage. As released NA is eliminated mainly by re-uptake into neurons, where it is metabolized to vanillylmandelic acid and 3-methoxy-4-hydroxyphenylglycol, measurement of ratios of norepinephrine to metabolites provides an estimate of the activity of sympathetic neurons.

Other Tests

Some pharmacologic tests determine if a lesion produces denervation supersensitivity or if it is pre- or postganglionic. Denervation supersensitivity is shown by the increased response of a denervated organ when it is stimulated. This upregulation is thought to result in part from the increased quantity and sensitivity of denervated endorgan receptors. For example, infusion of a low dose of phenylephrine produces an increase in blood pressure (which is absent in normal subjects) in patients with autonomic failure and denervation supersensitivity. The amount of norepinephrine released into plasma following graded boluses of tyramine, which increases norepinephrine release, indicates if a lesion is pre- or postganglionic.

TESTS OF PARASYMPATHETIC CARDIOVASCULAR CONTROL

Several tests permit assessment of parasympathetic cardiovascular control. The presence of respiratory sinus arrhythmia (RSA) (i.e., beat-to-beat heart rate variation accompanying breathing) depends on the integrity of efferent vagal neurons. RSA is modulated by cardiothoracic afferent pathways, including those from the stretch receptors in the lungs and chest wall and from cardiac and aortic baroreceptors. Inspiration results in an increase in heart rate and expiration results in a slowing of the heart rate. These changes are mainly mediated through the vagus nerve. Statistical analysis of ECG R-R intervals, such as the standard deviation and the mean square of the successive differences while the subject breathes quietly, provide time domain measures of RSA.

The expiratory/inspiratory (E/I) ratio and the maximum-minimum heart rate difference provide an index of RSA during deep breathing. The E/I ratio is calculated as the ratio of the longest R-R interval during expiration to the shortest R-R interval during inspiration while the subject is breathing at a rate of six breaths per minute (10-second cycle, 5 seconds of inspiration). The difference between the maximum and the minimum heart rate during deep breathing should be more than eight beats. Both the E/I ratio and the maximum-minimum heart rate difference during deep breathing are effort (tidal volume)- and age-dependent.

Frequency domain analysis allows further characterization of heart rate (or blood pressure) variability by breaking down segments of continuous heart rate (or blood pressure) signals into their constituent frequencies. Power spectral analysis techniques provide frequency domain analysis that reveals periodic components within a time series that would otherwise go unnoticed with time domain analysis methods. Power spectral analysis of heart rate and blood pressure variability shows that the resulting spectra are distributed around two main frequency bands, a low-frequency band at 0.03 to 0.15 Hz and a high-frequency band at 0.15 to 0.4 Hz. Spectral power in the low frequency band reflects mainly sympathetic activity as it increases with postural tilt and is reduced by, β-adrenoceptor blockade. Spectral power in the high-frequency band reflects parasympathetic activity, as it correlates with respiration, is reduced by atropine, and is abolished by vagotomy. Thus, power spectral analysis allows simultaneous assessment of sympathetic and parasympathetic influences on the sinus node.

Analysis of the heart rate variability power spectrum has demonstrated decreased high-frequency components in, among other conditions, aging, autonomic neuropathies, primary autonomic failure, ischemic heart disease, hypertension, and fetal distress, suggesting the presence of a diminished parasympathetic outflow to the heart. Such analysis has also shown a total (high- and low-frequency) decrease in heart rate variability with advancing age, following cardiac transplantation (disconnected hearts), and in autonomic failure. While the technique is currently a simple, non-invasive research tool, more complicated power spectral analysis may prove to be of clinical value in the future. Efferent parasympathetic neurons can be tested independently of the afferent part of the baroreflex.

The cold face test explores the integrity of trigeminal-brainstem-vagal pathways. In this test, the maximum bradycardia elicited by application of a cold compress to the ophthalmic divisions of the trigeminal nerve reflects vagal function. The isometric exercise test (sustained handgrip, for example) assesses the integrity of vagal pathways by measuring the initial heart rate increases due to parasympathetic withdrawal in response to sustained muscle contraction. Tachycardia in response to graded doses of intravenous atropine assesses vagal efferents and their influence on heart rate. The integrity of efferent parasympathetic pathways can be tested independently of baroreflex afferents by massaging the carotid sinus (not to be done in the elderly or in those with extracranial carotid disease).

SUDOMOTOR TESTING

Sudomotor testing permits evaluation of sympathetic innervation of eccrine sweat glands. The integrity of central and peripheral sympathetic pathways to sweat glands can be determined by analyzing the sweating response to increasing the body temperature by heating and to intradermal injections or iontophoresis of cholinergic drugs.

Thermoregulatory sweat tests assess pre- and postganglionic sympathetic pathways indicating the surface area of the body that sweats in response to raising the central body temperature by 1°C. Indicators that

change in color (e.g., iodine with starch, 25 percent alizarin red, and 25 percent calcium carbonate in corn starch) when in contact with sweat are spread on the body. Some methods of testing postganglionic sweat gland innervation rely on counting sweat droplets imprinted into Silastic or other matrices that are applied to the skin. In these tests sweating is induced in response to intradermal injections of acetylcholine or iontophoresis of acetylcholinesterase inhibitors. In general, impregnation and imprint methods are laborious, and results are difficult to interpret as there are interindividual variations in sweat gland distribution.

The quantitative sudomotor axon reflex test (QSART), which assesses the integrity of postganglionic sympathetic sudomotor axons by quantifing the amount of sweat induced by iontophoretic stimuli, has been standardized in some autonomic laboratories.

The site of the sudomotor pathway lesion can be inferred by combining thermoregulatory sweat tests with tests that assess postganglionic pathways (i.e., QSART). For example, with postganglionic sympathetic sudomotor lesions, themoregulatory sweat test and QSART responses are absent, whereas with preganglionic lesions QSART responses are normal. Because of its variability, the sympathetic skin response, which measures the electrical activity from dermal sweat glands via surface electrodes, usually is of value only when absent.

GENITOURINARY FUNCTION

The urologic evaluation of patients with autonomic failure should include measurement of the urinary residual volume. Measuring the volume of urine remaining in the bladder after voiding discerns if retention of urine is present and helps in guiding treatment. Cystometrography, when urinary retention is present, quantifies bladder filling and emptying volumes, pressures, and times, giving an indication of detrusor function. Sphincter electromyography of the periurethral striated muscle (or anal sphincter activity, which correlates closely with the external urinary sphincter activity) can be helpful in differentiating primary autonomic failure from Parkinson's disease with bladder involvement.

Erectile function can be assessed by intracorporeal injection of papaverine, which discriminates between neurogenic or psychogenic and vascular causes (in this instance there is failure to achieve erections). The blood supply to the penis can be investigated by duplex ultrasonography.

GASTROINTESTINAL FUNCTION

Gastric emptying can be assessed by measuring the emptying of radiopaque pellets and meals containing radioactive tracers. Plain and barium-contrasted radiographs may suggest intestinal pseudo-obstruction by revealing small bowel dilation (common in chronic intestinal pseudo-obstruction) and excluding mechanical obstruction. Manometry studies, which rely on measuring intraluminal pressures at different sites of the gastrointestinal tract, help differentiate neuropathic from myopathic causes of pseudo-obstruction. Neuropathic lesions produce uncoordinated (dysrhythmic) but normal-amplitude phasic pressure peaks, whereas myopathic lesions (as with amyloidotic infiltration) result in low-amplitude phasic pressure peaks. Blood flow can be measured by Doppler ultrasound techniques through the mesenteric artery.

PUPILLOMOTOR TESTING

Pupillomotor testing allows assessment of the autonomic innervation to the pupil by measuring its responses to illumination or to drugs. The pupillary diameter at rest in darkness is a function of the balance between parasympathetic inhibition and sympathetic activation. Dilation of the pupil results from inhibition of preganglionic parasympathetic neurons from the Edinger-Westphal nucleus, which causes relaxation of the iris sphincter, and from activation of the sympathetic efferents to the dilator pupillae. Conversely, constriction results from stimulation of parasympathetic and inhibition of sympathetic efferents.

The pupil cycle time is a simple method of testing pupillary autonomic function. A slit-lamp is used to focus a narrow beam of light on the pupillary margin. As the pupil contracts in response to light falling on the retina, the stimulus is blocked by the constricting iris sphincter, and the pupil again dilates. The pupil cycle time is calculated as the average length of a cycle based on 100 cycles measured with a stopwatch. The upper limit for a normal cycle time is 1,150 ms.

In the autonomic laboratory, pupil diameter is tested in darkness with use of either infrared photography or television. The amplitude of change in diameter of the pupil with illumination is a good measure of parasympathetic response, and the latency to three-fourths of maximum dilation is a good measure of sympathetic activity.

Pupillary responses to conjunctival instillation of drugs indicate if sympathetic and parasympathetic pupillary innervation dysfunction is present and can identify if a lesion is pre- or postganglionic. A constricted pupil will dilate with cocaine (2 to 10 percent) eyedrops if sympathetic innervation is functional, as cocaine interferes with norepinephrine re-uptake. Phenylephrine (1 to 2 percent) dilates a constricted pupil if denervation supersensitivity is present owing to a defect in sympathetic innervation. If the defect is postganglionic, a constricted pupil will not dilate with instillation of drugs such as hydroxyamphetamine (0.5 to 1 percent) that release norepinephrine but do not act directly on norepinephrine receptors. Dilute pilocarpine solutions (0.125 percent) will constrict a pupil that is dilated as a result of a parasympathetic lesion (where denervation supersensitivity is present); constriction is absent if the pupil is damaged or under the effects of anticholinergic agents. Instillation of a dilute solution (0.01 percent) of the synthetic atropine analog tropicamide results in dilation of supersensitive pupils and may be of diagnostic value identifying patients with Alzheimer's disease.

THE FLARE RESPONSE

Intradermal injection of histamine (0.1 ml of a 1:1,000 solution) produces a response that includes local cutaneous vasodilation (a flare) surrounding the injection site. The presence of the skin flare is used to indicate the integrity of dorsal root ganglia and their peripheral axons which mediate the response through the release of vasoactive neuropeptides.

Skin flare responses may be diminished with peripheral unmyelinated sensory fiber dysfunction and plexus lesions distal to dorsal root ganglia. Anatomic evidence of afferent branching of the main sensory axon, on which the hypothetical axon reflex flare response mechanism rests, is, however, still lacking.

ANNOTATED BIBLIOGRAPHY

Appenzeller P, Wood S, Appenzeller O. Testing autonomic function; clinical effects of age and stress. In Yoshikawa M, Uono M, Ishikawa S (eds): New Trends in Autonomic Nervous System Research. Elsevier Science Publishers, Amsterdam, 1991, p. 196.
Review chapter.

Bannister R, Mathias CJ (eds). Autonomic Failure. A Textbook of Clinical Disorders of the Autonomic Nervous System. 3rd Ed. Oxford University Press, Oxford, 1992.
Textbook.

Canal N, Cohi G, Natali Sora MG, Cerrutti S. Etude par analyse spectrale de la variabilité de la fréquence cardiaque des anomalies du système nerveux autonome en pathologie neurologique. In Serratrice G, Pellissier JF, Pouget J, Blin O (eds): Le Système Nerveux Autonome: Acquisitions Recentes. Expansion Scientifique Française, Paris, 1991, p. 32.
Review.

Low PA (ed): Clinical Autonomic Disorders. Evaluation and Management. Little, Brown, Boston, 1993.
Textbook.

Section III
Clinical Semiology

17
Coma

J. P. Mohr and J. C. Gautier

Coma leads the list of clinical states that test the skills of the physician in diagnosis and management. Its causes span a whole range of conditions, temporary and permanent, reversible and fatal, and the spectrum of physical and neurologic findings make its study a continuing source of insight into brain function. The urgency for a diagnosis of the cause of the depressed state of consciousness has brought brain imaging, blood and spinal fluid testing, and other laboratory assessments to the fore. Advances in brain imaging have been so rapid that the insights into brain physiology that are dependent on careful clinical observation are still lagging behind. The following discussion reflects some of these large gaps in knowledge and attempts deliberately to stress many concepts of coma that were all but taken for granted until recently. Although understood well enough to be treated successfully in some cases, much of the neurology of coma remains unsettled.

The term *coma* is derived from the Greek *komas*, deep sleep. On cursory evaluation coma shares some features of sleep in normal subjects. Clinical observations disclose very little difference in the early states of drowsiness and stupor in naturally developing sleep and in an evolving brain disturbance that will eventually cause coma. It is neither clinically useful nor an insight into physiology to note that disease states usually make the subject less readily rousable while a persistent state of full alertness can be achieved from the drowsiness before ordinary sleep. Depending on the seriousness of the illness or the severity of the sleep deprivation, this observation may also apply to patients sinking into the state known as coma.

The major differences between coma and sleep are in the observable behavior after the subject loses voluntary activity. In natural sleep, the voluntary activity is replaced by another kind of activity, which with its various stages and cyclic behavior is in its own way as regular as an awake state.

Several features are distinctive for sleep and are not seen in diseases that cause loss of consciousness. Sleep and coma both feature the absence of periodic lid contractions known as blinking, and the absence of swallowing. Sleep is characterized by the presence of sudden jerks at the onset, a rapid eye movement (REM) phase, frequent changes of body posture, regular breathing, and fully or partially closed eyelids. By contrast, the subject passing into coma typically shows no cyclic activity and remains immobile, and in a fully developed state of coma, all spontaneous activity is lost and the eyelids remain ajar with the eyes conjugate forward as in death. When the cause of the evolving coma is a major brain injury, focal signs of the primary disease may appear with limb posturing, sweating, dramatic changes of respiratory patterns, and alteration in pupillary sizes.

Once fully in coma, the victim is totally inactive, fails to show even the slightest response to the most vigorous stimuli, and requires assistance from a ventilator for breathing and from parenteral medications to maintain blood pressure. More often, the state is less extreme and stimulation produces some form of arousal.

TERMINOLOGY

Many systems of classification are based on the level of alertness in response to a specified form of stimulation, as it is this single state that is still believed to be basic to issues of coma.

In the most widely used classification the term *alertness* refers to an individual in a normal awakened state. *Drowsiness* describes a state of reduced activity, from which the subject rouses spontaneously or can be roused with a minimal stimulus, such as a spoken word. Although the dictionary definition of *stupor,* the next lower level of alertness, refers to a dazed state, the term is used by neurologists interchangeably with *somnolence* to describe a subject who is persistently inactive unless roused but carries the implication that the subject will become inactive once again when the arousal stimulus is withdrawn. Once that state of inactivity seems persistent, not subject to fluctuations and resistant to simple vocal stimulation, terms describing deep sleep seem more appropriate. *Sopor* (Latin for deep sleep) is used in some countries, mainly Germany, to describe the deep depression of consciousness in disease just above the level of coma.

When *coma* is used as the term describing the clinical state, no evidence is found for alertness, and the sufferer is said to be unconscious. *Semicoma* refers to a subject who is unconscious but able to show some reflex activity, limb movement, or change in respiration or pupil activity after stimulation. Coma is reserved for the state of complete unresponsiveness to any form of stimulation.

Although appealing in their simplicity and seeming self-definition, many of the commonly used terms classifying coma have proved rather unhelpful in the rapidly changing clinical environment in which most patients are found. However, the terms have become fixed in use in medical practice. (See Ch. 6 for the Glasgow Coma Scale.)

PATHOPHYSIOLOGY

Coma and Specific Lesion Sites

Of all the locations in which a discrete lesion may occasion loss of consciousness, it is in the pathway of the reticular formation or reticular activating system (RAS) where the greatest effect occurs from the smallest and most circumscribed lesions. As its name implies, this network of plurisynaptic cells, which stretches through the brainstem from the lower pons through the midbrain in its central portion to the thalamus and inferomedial frontal lobes, plays an essential role in arousal from sleep and maintenance of response to stimuli. Depending on the extent of its injury, the expected degree of arousal from a given stimulus is reduced or blocked altogether. The effect of a given lesion on the RAS depends mainly on how much of the RAS pathway is damaged.

The fairly compact course of the RAS through the narrow region of the upper pons, midbrain, and medial thalamus makes these regions especially vulnerable to fairly small lesions, while far larger lesions are required to affect the RAS more rostrally, where the pathway gradually diverges and fades into the cerebrum.

In the small space of the upper brainstem, coma or

profound reduction in activity may occur from arterial occlusions of the upper basilar or paramedian branches of the posterior cerebral artery territories, in vessels whose territory of supply in the midbrain and thalamus is too small to produce much clinically evident damage to major motor or sensory pathways. The shearing effects from sudden violent rotations of the head in trauma may disrupt the RAS from movement and cause slitlike hemorrhagic or ischemic lesions of the midbrain. Masses from the cerebrum can push, distort, and bend the upper brainstem directly downward through the axis of the midbrain or indirectly through uncal or tentorial herniation. Inflammatory or necrotizing lesions of the brainstem can also involve the RAS. Injuries in this region from whatever cause are usually accompanied by disturbances in ocular motility and pupillary reaction, but again, they may be small enough and located posterior enough to the main motor pathways that no major weakness appears in the limbs or face.

By contrast, most degenerative disorders (e.g., Alzheimer's disease or multisystem degeneration) either spare the RAS or only lightly affect it. Even when the effects are widespread and involve even the midbrain or thalamus, disorders of consciousness rarely occur.

Injuries to the thalamus and inferior frontal region often produce a state of greatly reduced activity. In the first hours and even days, the inactivity resembles sleep in the regular breathing and lack of focal findings but resembles coma in the great difficulty in arousing the patient and the promptness with which the inactive state reappears when the stimuli are withdrawn. Few disturbances in eye movements or pupillary activity are found. The state is termed *akinetic mutism* (see also Ch. 28).

The lower pons and medulla contain too little of the RAS for coma to result from lesions here even when quite large. Lesions large enough to wreck the motor pathways may so severely limit the patient's capacity to move (locked-in state) that coma is entertained as a diagnosis on quick examination, but more thorough study settles the issue. When lesions are large enough to cause coma, the motor system is typically greatly damaged with bilateral weakness or paralysis of limbs, and striking changes occur in respiratory patterns. These latter changes take several forms. The most striking is bursts of hyperventilation, which may last seconds or minutes before abruptly subsiding. The term *central neurogenic hyperventilation* is used to separate it from hyperventilation in response to metabolic acidosis. Rarely, following a deep inspiration the breath is held for as long as 1 minute or more. During this period, described as apnea (from the Greek for breathless), the patient is usually quite inactive, only to become more active when breathing reappears. Cycles in which crescendo hyperventilation is followed by decrescendo to apnea, lasting from 15 seconds to more than 1 minute with one extreme state gradually merging into another, have been called *Cheyne-Stokes respiration*. This state, once considered ominous, is rarely a sign of danger unless the cycles are as short as about 10 seconds. Profound disturbances of sweating, either drenching sweats or dry skin on a hot day, also may occur with major lesions of the pons.

Although discrete lesions of the lobes of the cerebrum rarely produce coma, stupor or coma may develop if the inactivated territory is quite large. Temporary balloon occlusion of the origin of either of the two middle cerebral arteries during treatment for arteriovenous malformations has been found to produce transiently such global inactivation of cerebral function that the issue of damage to the RAS cannot be determined. At the least, these findings indicate that the loss of activity makes it possible that some aspects of consciousness require some function in the cerebral hemispheres. They also indicate there may not be a dominant hemisphere for consciousness. When extensive bihemispheric infarction of the cerebrum occurs following bilateral carotid occlusion, the patient is immediately plunged into a state of inactivity, which is not coma. Examination of the patient days later can show cycles of blinking lasting minutes to hours, alternating with similarly long periods without blinking, which suggests that some sleep-wake cycles are occurring. This may be the only evidence that the RAS has been spared. Major trauma to the convexities may cause a state of inactivity for days or weeks, which is often called coma, but usually the patient is observed to pass through sleep-wake cycles, which argues that some of the initial inactivity is explained in part by the injury to the major motor pathways. The deeper structures such as the thalamus and brainstem are usually spared, and any disorders of eye movements are in the horizontal plane, with deviations of both eyes usually to the side of the lesion away from the weak limbs opposite.

A surprisingly large number of areas of the brain tolerate even large lesions without an effect on the level of alertness. Coma is rare and drowsiness uncommon from any but the largest suddenly occurring lesions of the individual lobes of the cerebrum, including those from infarction, the most common cause. Penetrating wounds from gunshot and missile fragments do not alter consciousness even when the missile has crossed the brain or carried away half of one side of the head, until the mass effect from bleeding evolves or unless the force of the missile striking the head torques the head on the neck to injure the upper brainstem, as occurs in boxing with the knockout punch (see Ch. 6). Consciousness is also not disturbed by infarcts or small hemorrhages of the centrum semi-

ovale, the individual basal ganglia, corona radiata, or internal capsule or even by posterior or laterally placed lesions of the thalamus.

It has been inferred that the RAS itself is the site of the depressive effects of drugs, anoxia, hypotension, and metabolic derangements.

MASS EFFECTS WITH BRAIN TISSUE HERNIATION AND COMPRESSION

Any cause of brain swelling can produce the syndrome of herniation and displacement. There seem to be no special features of the origin of the mass that separate one cause from another except by temporal profile or special location. The syndrome from a mass from active bleeding evolves faster than that from an indolently growing brain tumor. A location near the midbrain favors earlier appearance of coma for a given lesion size than does one remote in the frontal pole.

When coma is caused by brainstem displacement from an evolving mass in the cerebral hemisphere above, there is always abundant clinical evidence of focal or lateralizing signs before depression of consciousness occurs. The wide range of clinical findings prior to brainstem distortion are varied and prominent enough to make it difficult to decide what focal symptoms merely accompany and which are caused by the displacement effect. Once the midbrain compression has begun in earnest, although events proceed rapidly, special clinical study shows that the effects of herniation over dural edges can be separated from the effects due to brainstem compression.

Herniation Over Dural Edges

A mass developing in the cerebrum expands asymptomatically so long as there is sufficient compliance of the cerebral tissue. Once this compliance is exceeded, the tightly squeezed tissue, forced against the broad and unyielding inner table of the skull, continues to expand only by extruding itself under, over, and around the equally unyielding dural membranes that partition the skull cavity and keep the individual cerebral hemispheres in their proper place.

Subfalcial Herniation

Along the falx cerebri, the medial frontal region first pushes the corpus callosum across the midline and then follows with the medial surface of the frontal lobe, which folds under the lower edge of the falx (Fig. 17-1). Although the compression may crimp veins and arteries that run along the medial surface of the frontal lobe, frank infarction is rare. The clinical syndrome of subfalcial herniation is not well documented, in part because the extensive motor deficits already obvious from the large mass in the frontal lobe make it difficult to find those elements specific to the herniation. It

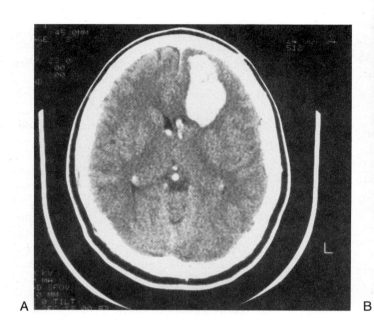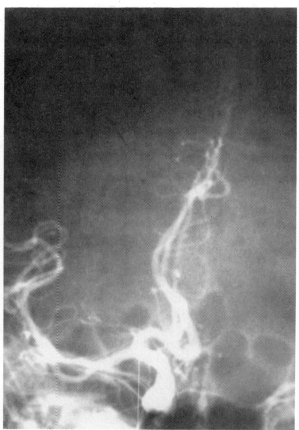

Figure 17-1. **(A)** CT scan and **(B)** angiogram showing subfalcial herniation in a setting of frontal hemorrhage. The CT scan shows the medial surface of the frontal lobe displaced across the midline under the falx cerebri, while the angiogram also shows the anterior cerebral artery displaced under the falx across the midline. (Courtesy of Dr. A. Khandji.)

is remarkable that even severe degrees of subfalcial herniation seem well tolerated and consciousness is rarely lost.

Uncal Herniation

When an expanding mass forces cerebrum over the other major dural ledge (Fig. 25-16), the notch of the tentorium cerebelli (Pacchioni's foramen ovale), the local anatomy results in a distinctive syndrome. As in subfalcial herniation, consciousness is not altered by the mere medial displacement of the uncus. In rare instances of diseases confined to the anterior temporal lobe, such as abscess, metastatic tumor, or encephalitis, the full syndrome of uncal herniation has been documented in patients who remain alert. The uncus, the most medially situated of the anterior temporal lobe components, is intimately associated with the third cranial nerve, whose fibers are embedded in the arachnoid of the uncus. A small movement of the uncus suffices to stretch these fibers, with resultant wide dilation of the ipsilateral pupil and paralysis of

some or all of the peripheral motor nerves of the ipsilateral eyeball. Mydriasis is the first sign to appear because the parasympathetic fibers of the third cranial nerve are superficial (see Ch. 28). In the initial stages of the herniation, the opposite eye shows normal pupillary reaction and ocular motility. If the mass recedes, the function may be restored. If the mass continues to enlarge, enough of the medial temporal lobe may bend over the hard-edged tentorium to kink the posterior cerebral artery and adjacent veins attached to the temporal lobe, with a wide swath of infarction along the inferomedial temporal and occipital regions. Numerous patients have been studied who have survived uncal herniation and are left with a contralateral hemianopia from the posterior cerebral territory infarction and with impairment of ipsilateral pupillary and ocular motility, but no permanent damage to the opposite pupillary function or ocular motility and no permanent impairment of consciousness. Respiratory changes may be difficult to detect but may take the form of cyclic respirations. They are usually not a prominent feature of the syndrome and require careful observation for their detection.

Because the most common form of mass that causes uncal herniation also displaces the midbrain, the syndrome of evolving uncal herniation has rightly been long regarded as a sign of impending disaster. Yet the uncal herniation is only the sign of the mass in the cerebrum above and behind it. It is the continued growth of the hemispheric mass that ultimately causes the devastating effects from compression of the midbrain, not the uncal herniation itself.

Compression

Brain tissue compression without frank herniation over a dural membrane involves reduction of tissue compliance followed by bending and other distortion of tissue, with resultant ischemia, hemorrhage, or direct tissue necrosis. Such processes require time. Once the tissue is fully compressed, however, signs may then evolve in rapid succession. In two special settings, the state of alertness rather abruptly gives way to coma.

Brainstem Compression from Cerebellar Mass

The most familiar of the syndromes occurs from compression of the lower brainstem from a cerebellar mass, most often with hemorrhage but also with large infarction. The initial syndrome features vomiting, inability to stand and walk, occasional ipsilateral facial palsy, and paresis of ipsilateral conjugate gaze, which are all signs of the cerebellar mass compressing the brainstem, during which the patient typically remains alert. Within a time frame varying from as little as 1 hour to as long as 3 days, and heralded by as little as the sudden appearance of diplopia or unilateral weakness, stupor appears, followed within minutes by coma—changes so dramatic that there is scarcely time to act before all is lost. A similar compressive syndrome may affect the upper pons when the mass is midline and in the superior vermis of the cerebellum. In these cases, within minutes the eyes typically become arrested in the conjugate forward position or directed slightly downward, with unreactive pupils in midposition. This condition, often mislabeled *upward herniation,* is really a transverse compression of the upper pons from a mass located in the cerebellum directly behind. The dramatic transition in these cases seem rather like the extremely rapid evolution of findings in severe spinal cord compression, where adequate function may give way to paralysis within minutes. With this background description, the pathophysiologic issues raised by syndromes that occur from midbrain compression may be better understood.

Midbrain Compression

Midbrain compression takes several forms, depending on the main direction of the vector forces acting on the upper brainstem. The most common vector produces compression with medial displacement from an enlarging cerebral hemisphere. This side-to-side compression results in an anteroposterior elongation of the midbrain with medial displacement, which may cross well beyond the midline and lead to death before any important amount of downward displacement occurs. In fatal cases, stupor is usually present when the midline has been displaced by 6 mm and coma when by 8 mm, but in very slowly developing mass lesions, displacements in excess of these values have been seen in patients still awake (Fig. 17-2). The evolving mass most commonly disrupts the function of the tectum of the midbrain before its more ventral portion, paralyzing upward gaze in some cases, while some sufferers have still been able to walk around. The pupils may show the same abnormalities on both sides, but if asymmetry occurs, it is usually the pupil ipsilateral to the mass that is first affected, and pupillary enlargement occurs before loss of reactivity. Even at the advanced stage of paralyzed upward gaze and pupillary inactivity, the patient may yet respond to commands. Frank loss of consciousness, when it occurs later, is rather abrupt. With rapidly declining consciousness comes paralysis of the limbs, which had still been moving minutes before. If the mass continues to enlarge, the entire medial temporal edge of the hemisphere eventually curls over the long anteroposterior edge of the tentorium cerebelli, producing the properly named tentorial pressure cone, by which time most of the devastation from the compression and medial displacement of the midbrain has long since reached its clinical climax.

Unusual vector forces from the middle portion of the temporal lobe may displace the ventral portion of the midbrain before the tectal portion, rotating the anterior portion around the axis of the tectal portion. The anterior edge of the peduncle may be pressed into the narrow, bladelike edge of the tentorium cerebelli, causing weakness of the limbs contralateral to the notched peduncle before other major signs occur.

The simplest, if least frequent, vector forces are exerted directly downward from the midline and are due to a symmetrically placed mass immediately above the midbrain. This condition may arise when severe bleeding enormously enlarges the cerebral ventricles, adding to the volume of the existing ventricular fluid to form a hemocephalus, or when bilateral subdural hemorrhage or a mass crossing the corpus callosum produces mass effects that balance in the two hemispheres. A few striking examples have been published, showing a concentric ring or doughnut appearance of the mass bulging over the tentorium cerebelli along its entire length, squeezing and displacing the midbrain directly downward (Fig. 17-3). As compared with the

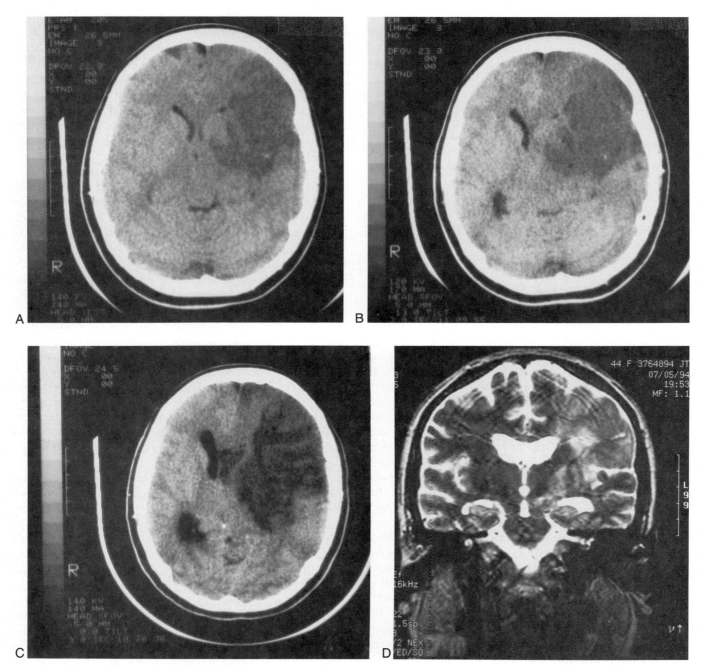

Figure 17-2. Four stages of midbrain compression. **(A)** Viewed from an axial CT scan, the large middle cerebral artery territory infarction has just begun to produce slight displacement a few hours after the acute stroke. **(B)** By the second day, edema and "mass effect" have displaced the midbrain and thalamic structures slightly across the midline. **(C)** By the fourth day, at the height of compression, the midline structures have been rotated and displaced considerably, during which time the patient appeared in a state of uncal herniation. **(D)** A week later, a coronal T$_2$-weighted MRI scan shows the midline structures back at their normal position, and no lasting damage is evident from the displacement.

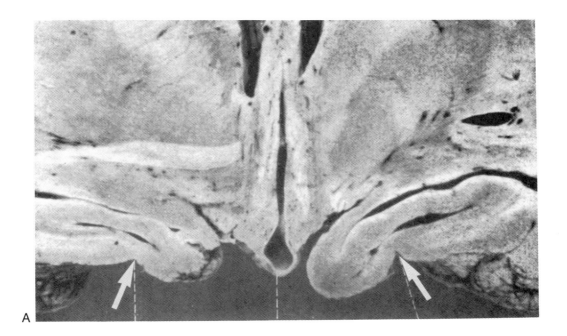

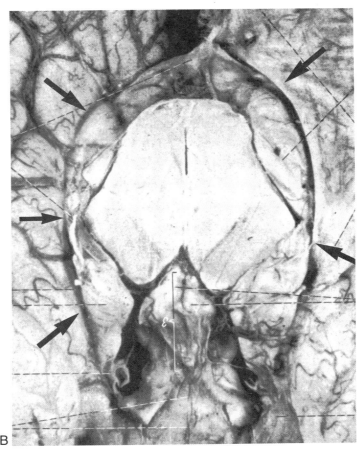

Figure 17-3. Concentric downward displacement of both unci from a large hemorrhage filling the ventricles above. **(A)** The herniation through the tentorial notch is demonstrated (*arrows*) in the coronal plane and **(B)** in a view from below. (From Spatz and Stroescu, 1934, with permission.)

rigid, densely compacted medulla and lower pons, the more compliant and gelatinous midbrain is shortened along its vertical axis and the brainstem buckles backwards, compressing and paralyzing the midbrain tegmentum. In such instances it is surprising how much downward displacement can be tolerated by the midbrain before stupor and coma intervene. In some cases of a downward mass from extracerebral hematoma (subdural or epidural), surgical evacuation has allowed nearly full recovery in patients initially unresponsive, with immobile eyes and unresponsive pupils.

In the authors' experience, it is in this uncommon form of compression that the syndromes attributed to rostrocaudal deterioration apply. Rostrocaudal compression often begins with reduced activity and stupor before many signs of focal dysfunction are seen: Cheyne-Stokes respiration, a cycle of increasing then decreasing hyperventilation lasting some 30 to 45 seconds followed by apnea of some 15 to 20 seconds; conjugate eye movements, easily elicited by even small passive rotations of the head, and small pupils, which react sluggishly to bright light. These signs are accompanied by little weakness of the limbs in the early stages. The authors have found that the concept of rostrocaudal deterioration in function from mass effect in the cerebrum does not account for many of the clinical findings in the therapeutically vital early phase of midbrain compression, but they fully agree that the concepts apply to those unfortunate patients who have passed through the stage of frank tentorial herniation and are in the final agonal stages of lower brainstem compression.

In all comas with syndromes of mass effect due to parenchymatous disease, when coma has occurred with paralysis of pupillary and ocular motor function, the probability of reversal to a normal state is remote. However, it is common practice to try to minimize the effects of the mass in the hope that the syndrome is not fully established.

EXAMINATION FOR COMA

The clinician brought to the bedside of a comatose patient must act to preserve brain tissue while simultaneously seeking a readily reversible cause. Thorough observation of the details of clinical examination is acceptable only after readily recognizable life-threatening causes of coma have been eliminated. Accordingly, the first steps in examination involve a quick palpation of the pulse and sternal thumping if no pulse is found. If a pulse exists and is in an adequate range, any sign of cyanosis should prompt intubation and artificial ventilation, with immediate restoration of skin color unless poisoning has damaged the oxygen-carrying capacity of blood. If breathing is de-

tected and the skin is not cyanotic, it is advisable to defer intubation initially. The distinctive odor of acetone helps to make a diagnosis of diabetic acidosis, while alcohol, of course, suggests drunkenness.

If inspection of the body and scalp yield signs of trauma, the cause may be brain contusion or extracerebral hematoma (hemispheric or posterior fossa), evacuation of the latter possibly being life-saving if done promptly. Prompt computed tomographic (CT) scanning should help settle this diagnosis. Fracture of the neck could also exist, prompting caution in passively turning the head on the neck for testing of eye movements (see below). Cutaneous hemorrhages suggest anticoagulant excess; cerebellar hemorrhage is slightly more common than brain hemorrhages in other locations in this condition. Needle tracks suggest drug overdose. Signs of excoriations suggest pruritis and perhaps chronic renal failure or hypertensive encephalopathy. The cutaneous signs of cirrhosis suggest hepatic encephalopathy or ethanol excess. Gingival hyperplasia, rhinophyma, acne, and hypertrichosis suggest prior phenytoin therapy and raise hopes of a postictal state.

A large-bore intravenous line should be inserted and blood drawn off for determination of electrolytes, including calcium, blood sugar, osmolality, creatinine, prothrombin time, partial thromboplastin time, and drug screening tests including anticonvulsant levels. Thiamine, 50 mg IM, should be given to ward off precipitation of Wernicke's encephalopathy in a vitamin-depleted patient, but infusion of 50 ml of 50 percent glucose should produce prompt restoration of consciousness if the cause was hypoglycemia. If inspection of the skin reveals needle tracks to suggest drug addiction and the pupils are found to be tiny and reactive, intravenous nalaxone hydrochloride, 0.4 mg in 10 ml of saline, should result in dilation of the pupils and prompt arousal. A Foley catheter should be inserted and urinalysis performed for signs of dehydration, water intoxication, ketones, fast-acting narcotics, and barbiturates. If osmotic agents are given, the subsequent diuresis at least will not create bladder distension with secondary hypotension.

Arousal or some sign of improvement usually occurs within hours in those who are postictal from a generalized seizure or who have been plunged into coma from subarachnoid hemorrhage. For other causes of coma, the delay in response to therapy may entail hours or a day or more, too long for treatment effect to be used as a diagnostic point in the hyperacute stage.

NEUROLOGIC FINDINGS

Simultaneously with the rapid assessment of medical disorders that may cause coma, a neurologic examination should be carried out to assess the extent of the injury. Experienced neurologists make a quick survey of limb positions, movements, and responses to reflex testing. Quick inspection of the position of the eyes and pupil size and symmetry is to be followed by assessment of the response of the eye movements to tests of head position and pupillary reaction to light and to a pinch on the neck. Respiratory patterns and major autonomic changes such as profuse sweating or dryness are also noted. In emergency clinical practice, these observations are made so close to one another that the sequence in which they are described below is almost arbitrary.

Limb Position and Reflexes

Limb position or movements, either spontaneous or in response to reflex testing, have more value in localizing the side than they do in estimating the exact site of the lesion. In an evolving lesion of the cerebrum, some forms of spontaneous movement of the limbs can be seen. These movements, known as *release signs,* take various forms, including pedaling movements of the leg originating at the hip, running movements of the legs involving the hips and knees, and scratching or polishing movements of the arms originating at the shoulders.

When an arm is found flexed at the elbow and the ipsilateral leg extended, the name given to this syndrome is *decorticate posture.* A term carried over from animal experiments, decorticate posture reflects an injury high in the neuraxis—often in the cerebrum, not the brainstem—but may be seen in lesions of the brainstem itself if the lesion is not large. To some observers it is a sign of lesser injury in the neuraxis than that producing adduction and extension.

Obvious and persistent extension and adduction of the limbs, known as extensor posturing or *decerebrate posturing,* reflects a far more severe injury to the motor pathways, usually of the deep parts of the hemisphere or brainstem and is most commonly seen as a result of severe disruption of the pons.

When the pons or midbrain is damaged to an almost fatal extent, none of these findings occur. Instead, all four limbs are limp, reflecting the destruction of all descending motor pathways, leaving the spinal cord below in a state of shock. This areflexic state lasts only a few days in the survivors, but when present in the hyperacute state it may be so severe as to suggest to many a clinician that the patient is suffering from drug overdose or neuromuscular block.

Eye Movements

The most striking spontaneous movement of both eyes occurs when both cerebral hemispheres have been severely damaged and the surviving brainstem releases horizontal (misnamed "roving") eye movements. They have a distinctively metronomic character, requiring 1 to 2 seconds for full horizontal excursion, followed by a moment of hesitation, then a swing back to the opposite extreme, and then back again and again. Passive movement of the head may arrest the metronomic feature for a few seconds, but it then becomes reestablished. The condition lasts a few days and then dies away even if the patient lives.

When the horizontal eye movements have a downward vertical component, which occurs when the eyes approach the midline (pendulum eye movements), the explanation is usually a mass compressing the tectum of the midbrain, causing Parinaud's syndrome of impaired upward gaze plus release of the brainstem horizontal eye movements.

In less severe bihemispheral injuries from cardiac arrest, anoxia, and the like, the eyes may not be actively roving, but on passive head movement the conjugate movements of the eyes seem excessively free (ball-bearing eye sign).

If the eyes are not actively moving, are positioned off the midline, or seem not to be aligned, reflex testing of eye movements can give much information on the status of the brainstem. The easiest test to perform is passive head rotation (oculocephalic response), looking for evidence that the eyes turn together (conjugately) in the opposite direction from the head movement. When this test fails to yield any satisfactory response, as it often does even in some normal subjects, it may be necessary to perform the more complicated test of irrigating the external ear canal with ice water (vestibulo-ocular reflex or ice water caloric response).

In this test the thermal effect of the ice water against the eardrum activates the labyrinth, producing a turning of both eyes (ipsilateral tonic deviation) in the horizontal plane to the side of the ice water. The ice water stimulus is supramaximal but has the advantage that the temperature of the water is readily known. This supramaximal stimulus may precipitate sudden gasping, shivering, ipsilateral piloerection, facial grimacing, and tearing of the eyes if the afferent pathways and motor functions mediating these responses are intact. In an awake patient, each time the ipsilateral tonic ocular deviation turns the eyes far beyond the midline, a rapid jerk occurs, attempting to correct the tonic deviation. Since the deviation is a persistent effect, a cycle is set up of slow lateral deviation followed by rapid midline correction, creating a rhythmic movement known as *nystagmus.* In unilateral hemispheric dysfunction, the eyes are often deviated to the side of the insult; ice water in the opposite ear is followed by tonic ipsilateral deviation, but the phasic correction mediated by the cerebral hemisphere does not occur and the eyes stay deviated for many seconds after the irrigation stops. In major unilateral cerebellar hemorrhage, the ice water may fail to bring the eyes past the midline ipsilaterally. In disease of the brainstem itself, the ice water precipitates dysconjugate movements of the eyes, revealing those pathways to have been put out of inactivated (see also Eighth Cranial Nerve in Ch. 29).

In severe states of metabolic coma, especially that caused by hypnotic drugs, leading among which are barbiturates, the eyes are usually paralyzed and no movements occur, even in response to ice water, although in a few cases a vertical nystagmus has been seen.

Pupils

If coma is from displacement of the major brain compartments, one or both pupils may be very large and unreactive to light. If only one is large, the cause is usually in the ipsilateral hemisphere. If the pupils are midposition and irregular in shape, fatal midbrain displacement is usually the cause unless the patient has had prior cataract extraction. The irregular shape of previously normal pupils reflects damage to the midbrain origin of the nerves controlling the ciliary muscles.

Tiny pupils usually mean suppression of sympathetic function, either from drugs dripped into the eye as treatment for glaucoma, from the systemic effects of drugs (especially narcotics), or from such extensive damage of the pons or medulla that only the parasympathetic responses remain. Under such conditions, a further constriction to light can be achieved by using a bright light source shone directly at the pupil.

When the hemispheres are damaged but the midbrain and lower brainstem are preserved, firmly pinching the skin anywhere will produce a transient pupillary constriction. The side of the neck has been traditionally the site pinched, hence the term ciliospinal response. Although the cervical ciliary ganglion mediates the response, the midbrain must be intact for the response to occur, and its absence with brain lesions means that the midbrain has been heavily damaged.

Respiratory Cycles

Respiratory cycles have long been the subject of interest, but only limited diagnostic value has been obtained from their careful study. Apneustic breathing and central neurogenic hyperventilation are signs of extensive brainstem injury, usually even more obviously revealed by disturbances in limb and ocular movements. The Cheyne-Stokes respiration has been seen prominently in such non-neurologic states as congestive heart failure. Grossly irregular breathing rates with striking alterations in respiratory depth are signs of major injury to the lower brainstem. Feeble openings of the mouth with tiny gasping movements of the chest resembling those of landed fish are agonal movements.

TEMPORAL PROFILE OF EVENTS

Once the patient is in coma, areflexic and unresponsive, all hope must be abandoned of using clinical findings alone to determine lesion side, site, and size. Access to the history of onset can be crucial to arriving at an accurate diagnosis of the cause of the coma. A clue to the cause of the coma is often found in the rapidity with which coma occurs. There are at least four large time categories of clinical significance.

Sudden Loss of Consciousness

Sudden loss occurs only in a limited set of circumstances. Grand mal epilepsy may leave a period of coma in its wake lasting as long as many hours. As in the unresponsive state after closed head injury, although the patient typically does not respond with arousal to stimulation, respiration is preserved and pupillary reactivity is normal. During this period, unless the seizure or head injury was witnessed, diagnoses often range from drug overdose to massive stroke. Inspection of the tongue may reveal that it was bitten during a seizure, and the skin may show the acne common in patients receiving phenytoin therapy. When arousal begins after seizure, there may be signs of dysfunction in the cerebral region (Todd's paralysis) giving rise to the seizure, which may last up 1 to week before improvement.

Cardiac arrest results in loss of consciousness within seconds, as the limited reserve of brain nutrients is quickly exhausted. Patients developing arrest have been observed suddenly to become silent while actively speaking and almost immediately lose all tone and collapse limply to the ground. An identical appearance has been seen in the initial phase of a syncope from severe aortic stenosis. The authors have witnessed a few cases of *basilar occlusion* with a major brainstem syndrome, which in one instance prompted an erroneous call to the emergency cardiac arrest team. In contrast to these states, explainable by loss of delivery of nutrients, syncope from subarachnoid hemorrhage, explained in part by the sudden flooding of blood into the subarachnoid space with massive increase in intracranial pressure, can also precipitate immediate coma. In all these states, at the height of the attack examination discloses no pupillary reactions, eye movements, reflexes, or muscle tone.

Stupor or Coma Developing Within Seconds to Minutes

Stupor or coma may develop very rapidly in other conditions causing dramatic metabolic derangement or reduction in the circulation without complete interruption. The most widely recognized is an attack of hypoglycemia. A state of coma can develops over periods from as short as a half minute to as long as a half hour. The wide variety of possible focal disorders at first appear as if the patient is in the throes of a minor stroke, immediately following which responsiveness is lost within minutes, rarely seconds. The patient is frequently known to be diabetic.

Ventricular tachycardia precipitates sudden reduction in voluntary activity, from which the patient can only be slightly aroused by vigorous stimulation. Similar to the brainstem tamponade from a ruptured aneurysm but less dramatic is the ventricular hemorrhage occurring when a large arteriovenous malformation ruptures. This causes an acute hemocephalus, which can exert pressure on the ventricles to such a degree that consciousness steadily diminishes over minutes to a level of coma.

Few toxins are sufficiently potent to produce coma within minutes, but one that is, *tetrodotoxin* (TTX), is numbered among the most potent of the nonpeptide neurotoxins. These toxins usually occur in reef fish in tropical waters. Within minutes after ingestion of fish, raw or cooked (TTX is not destroyed by heat), emesis, diarrhea, and paresthesias occur, events usually obvious to all. In a few striking cases, extremes of global paralysis with apnea and dilated pupils have made some observers believe the victim dead.

Stupor or Coma Developing Over Hours to a Day

Either a steadily expanding mass or a steadily developing toxic state is required to produce coma gradually. The most important life-threatening cause of steadily declining consciousness occurs from an enlarging intracranial hematoma, whether affecting the brain parenchyma itself or exerting pressure on the parenchyma from a mass enlarging in the subdural or extradural space. Meningitis and encephalitis cause a toxic state with reduction of consciousness early in the clinical course. The exact toxin and the brain regions affected by it are still unknown, but the depth of the loss of consciousness reflects the rate of advance of the disease. Headache and fever may be the only clinical clues to the diagnosis. Difficulties in finding words in conversation have been observed before the headache and fever, which argues that the the toxic effect is not simply systemic. Lumbar puncture is still the mainstay of the diagnosis of meningitis but should be undertaken with caution if any signs of raised intracranial pressure are found, such as papilledema on funduscopic examination. Early brain imaging by CT or magnetic resonance imaging (MRI) scanning, where possible, often detects the developing focus of encephalitis.

Drug Overdose

The course of drug overdose is rarely witnessed from its onset to coma. Most often, the patient is found only unconscious, at which time the lack of focal findings on examination, normal cerebrospinal fluid (CSF), and normal brain images are the only clues, by default, that drug intoxication may be the problem. The gradual depressant effect of sedatives and hypnotics produces a wide variety of release signs as stupor gives way to coma, including shivering, hyperreflexia, clonus, hypothermia, and hypotension. When coma has occurred, however, respiratory depression is usually complete, requiring support from a ventilator; the patient is immobile, limp, and lacking in any motor reflexes, with the eyes immobile and fixed in the conjugate forward position. Despite a comatose state, the pupils still constrict directly and consensually in response to light and dilate slightly in response to pinch on the face, neck, or trunk, which indicates that the drug effects do not depress all autonomic function at a time when they have suppressed all voluntary motor function. Small but reactive pupils are commonly encountered in barbiturate intoxication; pinpoint but reactive pupils occur with opiates; and dilated pupils occur with *glutethimide* intoxication and overdose of atropine-like compounds. Such compounds are contained in a large number of plants. Some—including such exotics as burdock root, catnip, hydrangea, jimson weed, juniper, wormwood and even nutmeg—if ingested in large enough doses, can precipitate the expected dry mouth, urinary retention, blurred vision, dilated pupils, hallucinations, and high fever but only rarely coma.

Metabolic Disorders

Numerous chronic metabolic disorders may cause a slowly evolving coma, leading among which are renal failure and hepatic encephalopathy. In hepatic encephalopathy, the patient may show remarkably focal signs, including decerebrate posturing, rigidity, cogwheeling, downward deviation of the eyes, and focal seizures, before the development of coma. The etiology of these focal signs remains uncertain, as there is rarely evidence of a prior or recent focal brain lesion on brain imaging tests. A syndrome suggesting brain herniation has even been described.

Hypertensive Encephalopathy

Hypertensive encephalopathy (see also Ch. 35) features a depressed consciousness, which evolves smoothly over several hours. The typical clinical setting is acute hypertension in a previously normotensive patient (e.g., acute nephritis in children or eclampsia). Hypertensive encephalopathy is rare in chronic hypertension, although it can occur in uncontrolled or poorly treated hypertension. The initial complaints of headache, poor appetite, and generalized malaise mimic the symptoms of meningitis. When headache, vomiting, delirium, focal signs, and seizures occur, the diagnosis is less difficult. When coma is present, there are usually no specific focal signs. The blood pressure is high, systolic pressure often topping 300 mmHg. Both CSF pressure and protein are elevated. The CT scan is normal or shows brain edema. When creatinine is elevated, a differential diagnosis between hypertensive and uremic encephalopathy is not a simple matter, and response to therapy that lowers the blood pressure is used as a diagnostic point.

Postanesthetic Coma

Postanesthetic coma occasionally confronts the neurologist. The syndromes attributable to anoxia and hypotension are similar to those that occur in a nonanesthetized state, with the exception that the metabolic protection provided by the anesthetic may limit the ultimate brain injury (although the acute effects frequently appear as severe as those without anesthesia) and some of the deficit may be attributable to the residual effects of the anesthetic agent. In patients free of complications, full alertness occurs within minutes or hours at most after cessation of anesthesia. In those exposed to skeletal muscle blocking agents or large doses of sedatives, eye movements may be paralyzed (with preserved pupillary reaction) for up to 3 days.

Malignant hyperthermia is a condition with dramatic rise in temperature, tachycardia, tachypnea, and respiratory and metabolic acidosis following exposure to *succinylcholine* (especially when given after atropine). Halothane anesthesia suffices to precipitate the syndrome in susceptible individuals. When myoglobinuria and rigidity occur, the patient's condition may be mistaken for coma. Prompt treatment with dantrolene aborts the development of the syndrome, which otherwise may pursue a fatal course. It has autosomal dominant inheritance, which may permit its detection from family history of difficulties with gaseous anesthetics.

The rare syndrome of atypical pseudocholinesterase occurs only in those exposed to succinylcholine. Because the atypical pseudocholinesterase fails to metabolize the succinylcholine promptly, the effects of the drug persist for an abnormally long period. The apnea and total flaccid paralysis of all muscles, including the ocular muscles, several hours after anesthesia is discontinued are cause for alarm, but the severity of the neuromuscular blockade may help suggest the

diagnosis. No treatment is necessary apart from maintaining respiration until the drug effect fades.

LABORATORY STUDIES

At present, brain imaging by CT or MRI scan, where available, has become the major source of information for the diagnosis of structural brain disease. An extradural or epidural hematoma shows as a high-density or high-signal lentiform mass over the convexity. Subdural hematomas, however, may have both high- and low-density components, reflecting old and recent hemorrhage (Fig. 17-4). When old subdural hematomas are present bilaterally, they may compress the brain ("balancing" subdurals) and yet appear isodense on CT because the time since their formation may have been long enough that the high-density attenuation characteristics of acute blood accumulations have been lost. Absent or tiny ventricles and absence of the usual surface convexity patterns suggest this diagnosis but will still be seen on MRI. High densities from brain contusions will fade to an isodense appearance within days but are usually evident on T_2-weighted MRI indefinitely and may be a clue to an unrecognized seizure disorder. Widespread high densities in the subarachnoid space suggest an acute subarachnoid hemorrhage. Masses from tumors and abscesses should appear as isodense or low-density lesions on CT and as variegated high-signal lesions on T_2-weighted MRI, with varying degrees of displacement

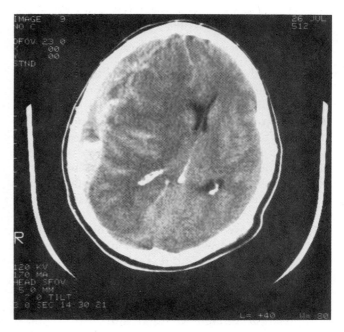

Figure 17-4. Axial CT scan showing large subdural hemorrhage displacing the midline.

of adjacent brain on either test; CT scan enhancement following infusion of contrast usually occurs. Encephalitis and large infarcts may precipitate coma before the lesion shows as a low density or enhances following infusions of contrast, and in such cases the CT scan appears essentially normal. Contrast enhancement of the subarachnoid space on CT scan suggests meningitis but may not be present as an early sign.

The mainstay of neurologic diagnosis until the 1980s was the lumbar puncture, now relegated to a minor role for patients in coma except those with fever and a stiff neck, in whom infection is a possible explanation. Meningitis and subarachnoid hemorrhage are the main diagnoses pursued by lumbar puncture. In meningitis, the degree of cellular reaction may be slight in the early stages, but in tuberculous meningitis the CSF can be bloody, raising the possibility of subarachnoid hemorrhage. Treatment based on a presumptive diagnosis is more prudent than insistence on a classic formula of elevated white cell count, low sugar, and normal or elevated protein. CSF must be sent for culture, and stains for bacteria and fungi are expected.

In subarachnoid hemorrhage the CSF is uniformly bloody. A bloody tap due to poor technique or bad luck may mimic subarachnoid hemorrhage but a spun down aliquot should show xanthochromia in subarachnoid hemorrhage and be clear in a "blood tap." In parenchymatous hemorrhages of small size, the fluid is usually clear, but if the hemorrhage is sufficiently severe to have precipitated coma, the fluid is usually bloody.

CLINICAL SYNDROMES AND ETIOLOGY

Trauma

Injuries from falls and collisions with large objects cause loss of consciousness mainly from the effect of the rotational forces acting at the midbrain, which produce immediate and distinct effects. Trauma can also directly injure the cerebrum with resulting brain swelling, sometimes great enough to displace brain structures (herniation, see below), or can cause bleeding into the brain or into the extraparenchymatous brain spaces, producing the same mass effects. Loss of consciousness with wounds from missiles that penetrate into the brain usually comes instantly from direct injury to the RAS or within seconds to minutes from accumulation of blood from active bleeding or from edema, in the same way as with blunt head trauma. Rotational forces are often minor.

The importance of the torsional effects in causing coma in injuries with head displacement is reflected in the surprisingly high incidence of little or no signs of major external injury. Many famous prize fights have ended not with a spectacular knockout punch, lifting the victim off his feet or flattening his nose against his face, but in the wake of a flurry of alternating horizontal blows, which torque the head rapidly back and forth, dazing the victim enough that he no longer braces his head against such torsion as he was taught so to do in training. This effect, known from the neurophysiology laboratory for decades, is thought to disrupt the RAS with small midbrain lesions from the shearing effects. In a few striking cases, prolonged coma has followed falls that produced little external indications of injury. The same torsional effect occurs from falls or from sudden decelerations as in automobile accidents. When the head is braced, surprisingly large injuries, even with half the head carried away by cannon fire, have been reported with consciousness initially preserved.

Few victims have been examined instantaneously, but in prize fights there is no doubt the loser has been knocked out as he lies immobile with eyelids open and does not blink until arousal begins seconds to minutes later. The respiratory cycles, pupillary signs, and responses to special forms of stimuli have not been well described in this group of injuries (see also Ch. 6).

Focal Infarction

Occlusive disease in the brainstem and thalamus is the most frequent source of the circumscribed lesions that have formed the basis for so many of the concepts of coma. In the pons, infarction must be extensive and bilateral for coma to occur; unilateral lesions even of large size have no effect on consciousness even in the hyperacute stages. Unilateral midbrain occlusive disease is commonly associated with ipsilateral infarction in the thalamus above because of common blood supply arising from the top of the basilar artery. Sudden coma has occurred in embolism that occludes the top of the basilar artery, producing bilateral midbrain and thalamic infarction. Some of these patients have shown clinical signs of rather limited infarction, sparing the main motor and sensory pathways but involving ocular motility on one or both sides, and have been affected by a state of drowsiness prolonged for days to weeks. Sleep-wake cycles are biased toward the sleep state, the patients often falling into what seems like a deep state of sleep even when being examined. Reversals of sleep patterns also can occur, with the patient awake much of the night. After some weeks the normal cycles of sleep reappear and there is no long-term disorder of consciousness. Some instances of this syndrome have been seen from infarction circumscribed enough that conventional CT scans have been normal and only on MRI or autopsy has a small lacune-like unilateral infarct been found. Insufficient numbers of cases exist to say that a map has been made of the regions whose lesions reliably cause or spare such changes in consciousness.

The accompanying signs all reflect the pathways serving motor, sensory, and ocular motility and have no special features that occur in those left awake or those made comatose from the same lesion. In the midbrain, the oculomotor nerve seems especially vulnerable, and its unilateral action has been abolished by an infarct small enough to be accompanied only by ataxia of the limbs, while larger infarcts additionally cause supranuclear gaze palsy, bilateral ptosis, and pupillary abnormalities with a stuporous state.

Infarction above the midbrain has produced unilateral partial oculomotor palsy with contralateral impairment of elevation, sparing pupillary function, and in one case produced only weakness of upward gaze. In those patients who are comatose from reversible balloon occlusion of the middle cerebral artery stem, coma develops within seconds, accompanied by comparable evolution of conjugate eye deviation and hemiparesis; coma does not precede or follow these signs. Coma that develops after established hemispheric infarction is explained by midbrain displacement (see above). (See also Ch. 35.)

Hemorrhage

Parenchymatous hemorrhage is discussed in detail in Chapter 36 and subarachnoid hemorrhage in Chapter 37.

The effects of released blood depend chiefly on the site and volume of the release. Coma is precipitated when blood occupies something approaching half of the pontine tegmentum and straddles the midline. Surprisingly enough, small brainstem hemorrhages cause loss of consciousness only infrequently, especially when they remain unilateral and lie more in the tegmentum. Hemorrhages affecting the cerebellum cause coma only when they are large enough to compress the pons (see above). In the posterior and lateral thalamus, even large hemorrhages usually leave the patient wide awake. The midbrain is rarely affected by primary hemorrhage.

In massive subarachnoid hemorrhage, increase in intracranial pressure sufficient to produce something approaching temporary tamponade causes sudden coma, which fades as the tamponade effect subsides. In the moments after the violent hemorrhage, patients have been found completely comatose, a completely limp, and areflexic, with lids ajar, pupils in midposition and unreactive, no respirations, and extreme bradycardia. The state gradually passes over some minutes. In less severe cases patients suffer violent headache with vomiting but not loss of consciousness.

When a large arteriovenous malformation bleeds heavily into the ventricular system, hemocephalus (i.e., enlargement of the ventricular system as it fills with blood) causes rapidly evolving stupor, which may reach the point of coma if a large enough volume of blood accumulates. The eyes are found deviated slightly downward from the effect of the midbrain compression. The level of consciousness usually is restored over the succeeding days, with no permanent coma, which suggests that the stretching effect is itself not a permanent lesion.

Anoxia and Hypotension

The clinical syndromes from anoxia and hypotension indicate that neurons are not uniformly affected but instead suffer in an orderly and predictable manner, depending on how severe the deprivation of oxygen or blood is and for how long it lasts. The principles of selective vulnerability (hippocampus) and distal insufficiency (high frontoparietal and posterior temporo-occipital regions) explains the spectrum of findings. Over the surface of the cerebrum the most sensitive areas are the parieto-occipital regions supplied by the longer cortical branches of the middle cerebral artery, while the least sensitive are the sylvian vessels in the proximal fields of flow. Patients suffering minor effects from cardiac arrest may thus have no loss of consciousness but show striking difficulties in the interpretation of complex thematic pictures, reading, drawing, and reaching into space. Those more affected act as if blind from an occipital lesion and have weakness of the upper limbs with preservation of the ability to make sounds, even repeat aloud, and to move the face and oropharynx. Those most severely affected are comatose and paralyzed in the limbs and make only grimacing movements with the face and oropharynx. Among those damaged extensively enough to be in coma, efforts have been made to determine who is likely to die. This subgroup typically lack contralateral conjugate eye movements in response to special reflex testing (see below). In the most profound lesions, the tectum of the midbrain has also been injured, and no pupillary response is found tc bright light.

PROGNOSIS

Irreversible Brain Death

The criteria for brain death, first suggested by Mollaret and Goulon (1959), were subsequently formalized in the now old Harvard criteria. The essence of these criteria is that no evidence of brain activity can be found under the most strenuous of test circumstances. The patient must have no evidence of response to any form of stimulus, including no reflex responses. There is no breathing when off a respirator for 3 minutes (apnea test). To ensure that the reason for no breaths is brain destruction, the carbon dioxide tension must be normal at the start of the apnea test. An electroencephalogram must show no evidence of cerebral activity. Because greatly reduced temperature or barbiturates can cause a flat electroencephalogram, the study can only be made in a patient whose core temperature is within a few degrees of normal (not below 32°C), and the history of onset and laboratory blood levels must exclude any exposure to barbiturates.

These criteria were established in the days before adequate brain imaging allowed proof of the extent of the brain injury in cases of stroke or cardiac arrest. Although causes such as gunshot wounds and the like were always evident over the years, the devastating effects of brain hemorrhage, brain infarction, or damage from cardiac arrest, only inferred by clinical judgment earlier, are now subject to adequate brain imaging and even assessment of metabolic activity.

It has more recently been suggested that brainstem death is the crucial point of brain death, so that the absence of five brainstem reflexes is reliably correlated with brain death and can be used in the decision to justify discontinuation of treatment. Transcranial Doppler ultrasonography is being suggested as a tool for the rapid assessment of the brain dead state, as such patients show extreme resistance to arterial blood flow from the occluded circulation or extremely high intracranial pressure.

With organ transplantation now an active branch of medicine, worldwide access is available for organs of the irreversibly brain dead but only if the organs are removed and taken to the donor in a timely fashion. Powerful pressor therapies or stimulants given in the hope of maintaining life in the irreversibly brain-injured patient may irreversibly damage potentially transplantable organs, making it practical and humane for criteria to be created to ensure that the proper actions are taken.

Persistent Vegetative State

A particularly difficult management problem has been the condition known as the persistent vegetative state. The essence of this disorder is that the victim has suffered severe bilateral disease of the cerebral hemispheres and yet has survived and lives a life that appears to the observer to be devoid of voluntary activity, even though observations over an entire day or more show that the patient's eyes close and the pattern of breathing suggests a period of sleep, after which the eyes open, blinking occurs, and the patient seems, in this way, awake. This condition is most often encountered after trauma, resuscitation for cardiac arrest, or severe respiratory or blood pressure depression from intoxication or drug overdose. The issues raised by

this state have become more legal than medical, and guidelines developed for the diagnosis have been drawn more carefully than have recommendations for treatment.

The American Academy of Neurology has defined this state as ". . a form of eyes-open permanent unconsciousness in which the patient has periods of wakefulness and physiological sleep/wake cycles but at no time is the patient aware of him- or herself or the environment." This definition is intended to convey the notion that sleep-wake cycles in themselves do not constitute evidence of awareness of the environment. The belief that clinicians may assume the patient to have no such awareness is based on inferences drawn from autopsy findings of extensive bihemispheral infarction and findings in some studies by positron emission tomography that metabolic utilization of glucose is greatly reduced in such patients. These clinical definitions, intended to provide a rationale for discontinuation of therapy in a person showing no signs of interaction with the environment and evidence of extensive brain injury, do not really settle the question of awareness of the patient. The further description of the Academy of Neurology's position is based on the assumptions that such a state has existed for at least 1 to 3 months and that the cause is hypoxia or brain ischemia.

The issue of life support would never have been possible were it not for a few spectacular cases of seeming resurrection from the dead, as has been witnessed after drug intoxication, usually from barbiturates, in some cases of tetrodotoxin poisoning, and in rare instances of recovery from drowning, usually in very cold water.

The wording is as strict as that intended in the original Harvard criteria: the patient is to show no signs of interaction with the environment. The time has not yet arrived when those showing feeble signs of response are also abandoned as incapable of being salvaged, but with further research, the issue of the criteria for a functional recovery should be approached.

ANNOTATED BIBLIOGRAPHY

Adams JH, Graham DI, Lang LS. Diffuse axonal injury in humans: an analysis of 45 cases. Ann Neurol 1982;12: 557.

Naked eye inspection often seems surprisingly normal. Extensive small lesions can occur with little or no evidence of fracture or major surface injuries.

American Academy of Neurology Executive Board. Position of the American Academy of Neurology on certain aspects of the care and management of the persistent vegetative state patient. Neurology 1989;39:125.

When it is clear that the course is stable and there is no behavioral response whatsoever, withdrawal of treatment may be considered.

American Neurological Association (ANA) Committee on Ethical Affairs. Persistent vegetative state: report of the American Neurological Association committee on ethical affairs. Ann Neurol 1993;33:386–90.

The current position of the ANA.

Beecher HK. A definition of irreversible coma: report of the Ad Hoc Committee of the Harvard Medical School to examine the definition of brain death. JAMA 1968; 205:85–88.

Blum K, Manzo L (eds). Neurotoxicology. Marcel Dekker, New York, 1985.

Informative surveys of a large field, including plant and fish toxins.

Cohen SI, Aronson SM. Secondary brain stem hemorrhages. Arch Neurol 1968;19:257–63.

Hemorrhages were found in 199 of 7,100 autopsies with secondary brainstem herniation. None were found with supratentorial subdural lesions whose volume was less than 25 ml; they occurred in 42 percent when the subdural hemorrhage was 76 to 100 ml and in 80 percent when it was more than 100 ml.

Edgren E, Hedstrand U, Kelsey S, et al. (The BRCT I Study Group's) assessment of neurological prognosis in comatose survivors of cardiac arrest. Lancet 1994;343:1055–8. Commentary by Saltauri L, Marosi M. p. 1052.

Large modern series.

Fisher CM. Acute brain herniation: a revised concept. Semin Neurol 1984;4:417.

Displacement across, not downward.

Fisher CM. The neurological examination of the comatose patient. Acta Neurol Scand 1969;36 (suppl):1–56.

A clinical classic.

Goldie WD, Chiappa KH, Young RR, Brooks EB. Brainstem auditory and short-latency somatosensory evoked responses in brain death. Neurology 1981;31:248.

Guides to interpretation.

Henschel EO. Malignant Hyperthermia. Appleton & Lange, East Norwalk, CT 1974.

A bit dated, but nothing this good has appeared since, and clinical cases are well described.

Howell DA. Longitudinal brain stem compression with buckling. Arch Neurol 1961;4:572–9.

First description of the syndrome with neuropathological correlation.

Johnson RT, Yates PO. Clinicopathological aspects of pressure changes at the tentorium. Acta Radiol 1956;46:242.

Side-to-side compression with anteroposterior elongation of the midbrain by medial movement of the posterior temporo-occipital lobes.

Kemper T, Romanul F. State resembling akinetic mutism in basilar artery occlusion. Neurology 1967;17:74.

Protracted coma from a ventral and tegmental pontine infarct.

Kinney HC, Korein J, Panigrahy A et al. Neuropathological findings in the brain of Karen Ann Quinlan. N Engl J Med 1994;330:1469–75.

Extensively studied famous case of persistent vegetative state, showing at autopsy typical example of anoxic-hypotensive brain injury with extensive biparietal-occipital and thalamic findings.

Malone M, Prior P, Scholtz CL. Brain damage after cardiopulmonary by-pass: correlations between neurophysiological findings and neuropathological findings. J Neurol Neurosurg Psychiatry 1981;44:924.

No brain damage if intraoperative electroencephalographic monitoring showed no abnormalities. Brain damage in the high cerebral convexities, the vascular "distal fields," occurred in patients with more than 7 minutes' worth of abnormalities.

Meythaler JM, Varma RR. Reye's syndrome in adults. Arch Intern Med 1987;147:61.

Hepatic findings and typical clinical evolution and neurologic picture.

Mohr JP. Neurological complications of cardiac valvular disease and cardiac surgery including systemic hypotension. In Klawans HL (ed). Neurological Manifestations of Systemic Diseases, Part I. In Vinken PJ, Bruyn GW (eds): Handbook of Clinical Neurology. Vol. 38, North-Holland, Amsterdam; 1979, pp. 143–71.

Full review of the literature of the syndromes up to that time, detailing the history of the concepts of neurologic damage in cardiac arrest and open heart surgery.

Mollaret P, Goulon M. Le coma dépassé. Rev Neurol (Paris) 1959;101:3–15.

Seminal paper.

Morruzzi G, Magoun HW. Brain stem reticular formation and activation of the EEG. Electroencephalogr Clin Neurophysiol 1949;1:445.

The classic description of a brain region stimulation of which produces arousal.

Mueller-Jense A, Neunzig H-P, Emskötter T. Outcome prediction in comatose patients: significance of reflex eye movement analysis. J Neurol Neurosurg Psychiatry 1987; 50:389.

In 81 cases tested, absence of vestibulo-ocular reflex eye movements and of pupillary light reaction allowed prediction of negative outcome in all. Absence of oculocephalic response was less useful, as 31 percent of those with absent oculocephalic response had intact vestibulo-ocular reflex.

Multisociety Task Force on PVS. Medical aspects of the persistent vegetative state. N Engl J Med 1994;330: 1499–1508.

Review article.

Oswald I. Sudden bodily jerks on falling asleep. Brain 1959; 82:92–103.

The sudden loss of tone with violent contraction of the affected parts is a distinctive feature of the onset of sleep.

Petty GW, Duterte DI, Mohr JP et al. Transcranial Doppler findings in coma and cerebral death. Neurology 1990; 40:300–3.

Peaked waveforms were diagnostic.

Plum F, Posner JB. The Diagnosis of Stupor and Coma. 3rd Ed. FA Davis, Philadelphia, 1980.

The current classic on the subject, filled with references.

Ropper A. Neurological intensive care. Ann Neurol 1992; 32:564–9.

Current trends in management.

Ropper A. Lateral displacement of the brain and level of consciousness in patients with acute hemispheral mass. N Engl J Med 1986;314:953.

CT showed displacement in the horizontal plane, not downward herniation.

Scheinker IM. Transtentorial herniation of the brain stem. A characteristic clinicopathologic syndrome; pathogenesis of hemorrhages in brain stem. Arch Neurol Psychiatry 1945;53:289–98.

Scheinker introduced this term, which he contrasted with older terms.

Spatz H, Stroescu GJ. Zur Anatomie und Pathologie der fässeren Liquorume des Gehirns. Nervenartz 1934;7: 481.

Example of concentric herniation producing a ringlike effect (bilateral subdural) but no Duret hemorrhages.

Tatemichi TK, Duncan CM, Moser FG et al. Syndromes of paramedian thalamopeduncular arteries: clinical and MRI correlations in infarctions of the upper midbrain and thalamus. Ann Neurol 1992;22:159.

Infarcts were imaged by MRI. Those above the midbrain produced impairments of upward gaze, some without oculomotor disturbances; some in the midbrain produced very circumscribed oculomotor dysfunction without involvement of the opposite side. None produced the pictures typical of midbrain compression in evolving mass.

18

The Aphasias

J. P. Mohr and J. C. Gautier

References to a sudden acquired disorder of speech or language can be found in the Bible, and such observations have been recorded down through the centuries. For more than a century, insights into language-brain relationship were based on the study of cases of acquired brain disease determined by autopsy. Lacking modern imaging in living patients, clinicians had to rely almost entirely on careful clinical examination to make a diagnosis of the disease process and, using the same observations, attempt to make inferences of the function of the healthy brain and guess the lesion site and size. Despite a large number of observations, made at varying times and in varying degrees of completeness, clinicoanatomic correlations were made on but a small number of patients, with autopsy findings done on formalhehyde-fixed brains weeks to years after the onset of the syndrome. When the hardships imposed by these limitations are considered, it is remarkable how useful the insights have been into brain function and how well they have stood the test of time and still daily serve clinicians.

From this set of correlations, some general principles emerged (see below) that attempted to provide a conceptual framework for the syndromes. It is perhaps no surprise that the same set of observations was explained by different theories. In recent years, the high quality of current brain imaging technology has provided a more efficient means to discover brain lesions and, for the first time, an opportunity to identify during life and track prospectively the course of the syndrome and the brain lesion in larger numbers of patients. The insights provided by these observations have shown some degree of variation in the range of syndromes for a given lesion and lesions for a given syndrome. Other stresses on previously rigid traditional notions of brain-behavior correlations have been generated by observations from the emerging field of functional imaging. Far from overturning all prior observations, the new studies are providing, for the first time, a chance to resolve some of the long-standing ambiguities that have plagued the original theses of aphasia.

THEORIES OF SPEECH AND LANGUAGE DISORDERS

Historical Aspects

The details of historical reviews no longer affect other sections of the field of neurology to the degree that they do the aphasias for reasons cited above. However, without definitive studies to validate one or another theory, the diagnosis and management of the aphasias in many centers worldwide is still based on one or more of these theories reviewed below, despite the thin veneer of data on which they are based.

Speech Laterality

The notion that one side of the brain is dominant for speech and language function dates back to the middle of the nineteenth century and has stood well the test of time. Pierre P. Broca (French surgeon and anthropologist, 1824–1884) put his exposure to phrenology to use in trying to infer the basis for the loss of speech that followed brain lesions. Phrenology (Greek: *phrenos,* mind; *logos,* discourse), a now-discredited field, postulated that distinct regions of the brain defined behavior functions whose proportions were reflected by the external shapes or reliefs of the skull (Fig. 18-1). In the heyday of this approach to brain function, certain elevations and depressions of the skull were thought to correspond to the likes of instinct of reproduction; love of offspring; self-defense and courage; caution and forethought; satire and witticism; religion; and such more readily testable functions as vision, movement, and hearing. At its zenith, Kleist, having studied the survivors of head

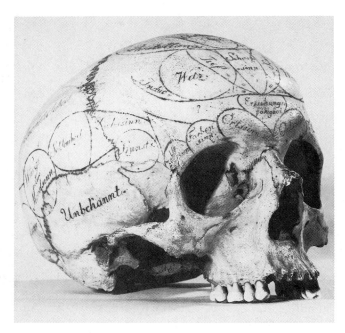

Figure 18-1. Skull with phrenological labels. *Unbehannt,* "unknown"; *Witz,* "jokes." (After Franz Joseph Gall; courtesy of Michael Brainin, M.D.)

wounds from World War I, offered, in his major book on the subject in 1934, localizations not only for the now-familiar movements, sensation, hearing, and vision but also for functions such as motor sequences, plans to undertake everyday activities, and ethical standards. From this peak, there has been something of a retrenchment of strict functional correlation, and it is safe to say much of the basic conceptions of phrenology are past. However, some of the basic notions of motor and sensory functional-structural correlations implicit in phrenology have powerful influences on present-day understanding of functional physiology (see Ch. 25 for the notions on the homunculus).

One of the basic tents has long since been discarded, that is, that brain regions responsible for certain functions would become large if overused or be large in persons highly competent in that function and would be reflected in the shape of the skull, accounting for the variations among individuals. This belief may have arisen from the everyday observations on the relationship between muscle size and exercise. Now considered foolish, the importance of head shape has nonetheless become thoroughly embedded in most societies who assume high intelligence in those with large foreheads ("high brows," i.e., large frontal lobes).

Phrenology played a major role in aphasia theory. Some phrenologists had noted that talkative people seemed to have large eyes and suggested the overdeveloped brain parts responsible for excessive talking must have been just above the eyes, causing them to bulge forward. One of Broca's teachers, the French physician J. B. Bouillaud (1796–1881) suggested that patients deprived of speech would have bilateral inferior frontal lesions. Primed with this prediction, Broca sought out such cases on his ward and reported two cases later to become famous. In both, he found the predicted inferior frontal lesion but made his great contribution by noticing that, in both cases, the lesion was not bilateral but was confined to the left hemisphere, the hemisphere that serves the dominant right hand. These two cases offered the first evidence of dominance of one hemisphere, the left for right-handed persons, a concept that has survived many challenges since then. The correlation of speech loss with a focal lesion of the inferior frontal region that was later to bear his name was another issue (see below).

More than 95 percent of individuals use the right hand preferentially and experience some form of disturbance in speech and language function from a lesion in the left hemisphere. Speech dominance and handwriting are not, however, simply correlated. Left-sided brain lesions in left handers usually cause speech disorders, although the severity of the syndrome is usually less than that seen in right-handed patients. Right-sided lesions in left handers are more liable to cause speech disorders than are right-sided lesions in right handers. Speech and language disorder from right hemisphere lesions in a right-handed patient are rare, with scarcely more than two dozen reported.

The *Wada test* (J. A. Wada, Japanese-Canadian neurologist) was developed soon after the discovery that resection of the hippocampus for intractable epilepsy could result in severe memory disorders. It was possible by intracarotid injection of amobarbital sodium to determine which side of the brain was dominant for speech and language. The usual response is the sudden appearance of contralateral paralysis of the limbs, ipsilateral eye deviation, and in the hemisphere dominant for speech and language, either arrest of speech, failure to reply to dictated commands, or loss of consciousness. Return to normal occurs within a few minutes. (The test was performed only after a conventional angiogram first demonstrated the patency of the carotid artery. The test itself carries few risks apart from that attending any injection of contrast material into the carotid artery. The proprietary home for amobarbital is Amytal.)

As a gross test of hemisphere dominance, the Wada test shows a high degree of reliability. Those patients with left dominance in the test are found to be so during subsequent cortical mapping in the operating room. However, some of those who seem right hemisphere dominant show left-sided language function by cortigraphy.

There has been less reliability for memory testing, prompting some workers to inject the amobarbital under microcatheter control directly into a posterior cerebral, testing each side separately. Left-sided injections more reliably induce reversible short-term memory disorder.

Less satisfactory have been the attempts to infer the anatomicofunctional correlations within the hemisphere fed by the amobarbital injected into the ipsilateral carotid artery. Radiolabeled amytal studies have shown wide variations between the distribution of the drug and the arterial branching patterns seen on conventional angiography, which makes it clear the material does not permeate uniformly throughout the vascular territory. Furthermore, patients who remain awake often respond to dictated commands with the nondominant limbs, a performance at variance with acute syndromes of major dominant hemisphere injury in which, typically, no response occurs to dictated commands. Superselective injection of amytal into individual branches of the major cerebral vessels in patients with arteriovenous malformation (see Ch. 37) is becoming a popular means to determine whether occlusion of the vessel will be tolerated without symptoms, but the predictions of success based on no symptoms after amytal injection are not yet fully validated.

Theories of Cerebral Organization

Separate Centers of Limited Function

Apart from his contribution to laterality for speech, Broca also started interest in the notion that a brain injury in a single area could alter speech and language function. Each of his two famous cases had large infarcts that affected the left sylvian region, yet he was drawn to the inferior frontal region as the most important site for reasons of phrenologic teachings (see above). Finding at least a portion of the lesions in the inferior frontal region, Broca reasoned that the remainder of the large lesions had developed only later, as is true for tumors, infections, and other disorders that begin as a small focus and spread outward. Although seen in retrospect as having been in error in greatly underestimating the size of the lesion, Broca was a sufficiently skillful debater as to overcome the objections of others in establishing his principle of an inferior frontal lesion causing a "motor aphasia" or "aphemia." He seems also to have been in error in coining the term aphasia, which he cited as Greek in origin, as a loss of language and aphemia as a loss of speech. Greek scholars at the time objected that no such terms existed, yet these objections also fell by the wayside. Efforts to substitute terms such as "alogia"

(from the Greek for lack of word or discourse) and the like all failed. Eventually, aphasia superseded all other appellations.

Barely a decade later, Karl Wernicke (German neurologist, 1848–1905) offered a supplement to Broca's theses. Drawing on the teaching of Theodor H. Meynert (Austrian neurologist, 1833–1892), in whose neuropathology laboratory he spent some 6 months as a visiting fellow, Wernicke used Meynert's principle that motor function originated forward of the fissure of Rolando and sensory behind it to explain what he saw as different syndromes of speech and language from different lesion sites. He proposed the notion that a lesion in the posterior half of the brain could cause a "sensory aphasia," which was to comprehension of language what Broca's lesion was to speech (Fig. 18-2). Using other notions popular in psychology at the time, Wernicke speculated that the brain region responsible for hearing was central to all language functions; that is, the child first hears, then learns to repeat, and then learns to associate sounds with visual forms in reading, in so doing gradually acquiring the skills of speech and language, which functions are then mediated by the original posterior brain region through which these skills were acquired.

These early efforts laid the groundwork for much of what was to follow. The initial formulations for localization seemed all the more convincing as work by others proceeded apace on the notion of a "homunculus" for sensorimotor function (see Chs. 25 and 35). With the use of these principles, lesions at the foot of the rolandic fissure seemed to cause paralysis of the face and tongue, which made it easy to understand how lesions in Broca's area, just ahead, could affect

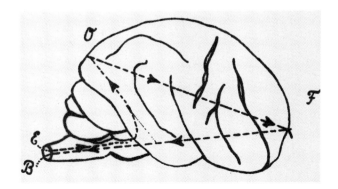

Figure 18-2. The first conceptual diagram suggesting sensory and motor speech areas are connected by a subcortical pathway. O, sensory speech center; F, motor speech center; O–F, association pathway between the two centers; E–O, pathway for audition; FB, pathway to the speech musculature. (From Wernicke, 1874.)

skilled movements of the oropharynx and disturb speech. Likewise, Heschl's auditory gyrus, in the temporal lobe, was the site of discrimination of sounds, which made Wernicke's area, thought to be just behind, a strong candidate for the region where such sounds were understood as language.

Once the notion was proposed of separate centers, each serving their unique function, linked together by fiber pathways, the way was paved for the elaboration of syndromes predictable by this model. Syndromes of brain lesion were interpreted as disruption of specialized cortical surface "centers" or of white matter pathways, separately or in various combinations. Several authors (L. Lichtheim, German physician, 1845–1928, the best known) drew complex wiring diagrams by which they sought to predict the lesion for various clinical syndromes (Fig. 18-3). Included among them were "subcortical sensory aphasia" (also known as pure word deafness), "cortical sensory aphasia" (Wernicke's aphasia, from a lesion involving the posterior temporal region described by Wernicke where the "engrams" for speech comprehension were deemed to be), "conduction aphasia" (a lesion in the white matter pathway that link the cortical sensory and cortical motor speech areas), "cortical motor aphasia" (Broca's aphasia, from a lesion of the inferior frontal region, Broca's area) and "subcortical motor aphasia" (a lesion between the frontal lobe and the brainstem nuclei that controls vocalization).

In all of these syndromes, damage to some part of an afferent-efferent loop, whether the afferent pathway, the main cortical areas (also known as centers), or the efferent pathway, in some way, would interfere with repeating aloud, a central clinical test for these paradigms. When the simplistic nature of these concepts is considered, examples of the syndromes crudely satisfying the major criteria were found that seemed to support the theories.

Patients were soon encountered who could repeat aloud yet who had poor comprehension or poor speech formulation, findings that taxed the simple model. To accommodate these cases, speculation was made that words heard or seen were understood by an anatomic link between the main sensory cortical regions (those that serve auditory function are Heschl's gyri and those for vision, the calcarine sulci) and the rest of the brain, where the memory for the correlations were thought to be stored. The term "transcortical" aphasia was created to explain how a patient could repeat and speak well but understood little, with the latter failure being explained by a lesion of the fiber pathways that connect the speech centers to the rest of the brain (i.e., transcortical pathways). For those patients whose comprehension was impaired, "transcortical sensory aphasia" might be the term applied. For those with adequate comprehension who could repeat aloud but who were unable to formulate spoken responses, "transcortical motor aphasia" might be considered to exist.

The great appeal of this connectionist model was the chance to relate disordered behavior to specific lesions of white and gray matter. For these reasons, it retains its place as a basis for investigations. Unfortunately, considerable difficulty has been encountered in finding good autopsy-documented examples of the major syndromes. Few examples of a lesion to explain the transcortical syndromes have been found. Many exceptions have also been found, even to the original major syndromes. Especially troublesome to theory were those cases with a syndrome but no lesion appropriately situated to cut off the cortical centers from the remainder of the brain and those with a lesion but no syndrome or one different from that predicted.

Although confidence has faded that the disconnection hypothesis could explain the aphasias, the syndromic terms coined by the early workers have passed

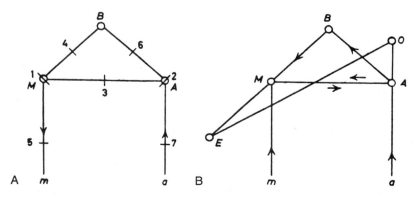

Figure 18-3. (A&B) Scheme of connections and disruptions that could account for syndromes of aphasia. A, verbal auditory center; B, concept center (German: *Begriffscentrum*); O, visual language center; E, writing center. (From Lichtheim, 1885, with permission.)

into common use, taxing the memory of students to learn the elements even though they may not predict the clinical correlations. Proponents of their use point to the long history of the terms, their grossly accurate brain correlations, and their utility in teaching trainees to analyze syndromes in an orderly manner. However, this model has thus far been insufficient to explain the developing literature in brain metabolism studied by the newer brain images methods such as positron emission tomographic (PET) scanning.

One Major Center

From these same observations grew another notion, that of a master region, through which words heard and seen were passed en route to comprehension and through which some preverbal thought (a concept never proved to be correct) was conveyed en route to being formulated into words to be spoken or written. This cerebral region, situated in the posterior portion of the sylvian fissure and roughly straddling Wernicke area, which was described as the sensory speech center, would thus be crucial for language behavior, and other cerebral regions would mainly serve to bring speech forms to and carry them from this central zone.

In its simplest forms, syndrome analysis from this viewpoint was directed toward discovering evidence of damage to this central language mechanism, irrespective of the input or output channels involved in the behavior being tested. Damage to the former was true aphasia, which, once acquired, could be detected to even the subtlest degree; any damage to centrifugal or centripetal pathways was incidental to the main effects on the central mechanism.

This emphasis on the essentially unitary nature of aphasia has had great appeal to those studying the linguistic effects of the lesion but has been dissatisfying to others because of its inexact predictions of the cause, site, and size of the lesion.

Speech Versus Language

Any discussion of the aphasias carries with it the problem of separating disorders of the systems that mediate language and motor acts (i.e., speech) from those involved in pure language functions. Speech and language are separate terms intimately associated with one another, and the term "aphasia" traditionally covers both disorders.

Speech

By the general term *speech,* (or the more specific terms speech behavior or discriminations of speech forms), are meant the activities of the brain, peripheral nerve, and muscles that serve vocalization, writing or drawing, hearing, seeing, and searching the shapes and sounds that are used in interpersonal communication. By definition, only those disorders of speech that result from a cerebral lesion are included in the study of the aphasias. These behaviors are the most amenable to bedside and laboratory testing, and their deficiencies have been those most readily related to brain lesions large and small. The clinician often gleans clues as to the locus and size of the lesion first by the occurrence and type of the disturbed use of speech forms by the patient.

Disturbances in speech have been most frequently encountered from lesions grouped around the sylvian fissure, with some from lesions as high as the midportion of the sensorimotor cortex on either side of the rolandic fissure. Speech arrest has occurred from electrical stimulation at many sites along the sylvian fissure and even from stimulation on the surface of the medial frontal lobe, in the supplementary motor area, remote from the sylvian fissure.

Focal epileptic discharges in the posterior temporal region have caused the hallucination of words heard, with some sounding as though they are spoken by persons familiar to the patient. Lesions in these areas certainly produce difficulties in reading and hearing speech, which in some instances, can be explained by faulty discrimination, such as failure to discriminate clusters of stimuli arrayed on a line or certain sequences of sounds. Such errors appear to the observer as errors in language usage (aphasias), which raises the possibility that some of the behavior thought to involve language goes on at the sites where the stimuli are discriminated or produced.

In general, disorders of speech production usually are termed *dysarthria* (i.e., difficulty in articulating writing disorders, which does not simply result from paralysis of muscles that serve limb movements are known as *dysgraphias*).

Language

By the term *language* is meant those less easily specified behaviors that permit individuals to communicate by using certain sounds and shapes that have a semantic (i.e., meaningful) value and are learned, used singly or in groups according to syntactic rules, and subject to change with training. To some neurologists, the term language refers simply to the use of the rules of grammar and the selection of single words or sets of words based on meaning. Disordered use of language is what is meant by aphasia, and when used, aphasia refers to disorder speech or language caused by a cerebral lesion.

Far less is known of the effects of brain lesions on language, per se, because the speech behaviors are usually also affected from brain disease. The efforts to design experiments to study language alone have foundered on difficulties about the certainty that the instructions were understood or the response was reliable. Unhelpfully, most schools of psychologists and linguists, from pavlovian to skinnerian, have also imposed their own theoretical structure on the study of the aphasias. Despite these burdens, data appear to support a clustering of one form of linguistic behavior from left frontal lesions, with another form from left temporoparietal lesions, arguing against the unified nature of aphasia that was the dominant view through much of this century. These observations provide a background against which to contrast the clinical features of speech and language disorders found in focal brain disease.

SYNDROMES OF APHASIA

Because theories of aphasia arise from observations in living patients, a review of these clinical sources of insight into higher cerebral functions appears useful, if only to stress the biases and limitations that future studies, it is hoped, will overcome. After more than one century of effort, much of the disturbances known as aphasia remain poorly understood, in part because of limitations in the database.

The bulk of information concerning disturbances in speech and language comes from studies of patients with acquired focal brain lesions. The most frequent causes of brain lesions are such disturbances as stroke, with infarction far more frequent than hemorrhage. Brain tumors and masses from local abscess formation are another source, but it has been known for one century that this source of material produces a lesion that gradually expands and, with the expansion, comes worsening or a change in the original syndrome. The giant abnormality often found at autopsy has been difficult to try and relate to the original syndrome, which makes this source of information less popular for the study of clinicoanatomic correlations. The same reasoning applies to trauma, in which the lesion, although easily found, is rarely focal and often passes rather deep into and sometimes across the brain. Encephalitis infrequently affects the brain regions most sensitive to speech and language disorders when injured. Atrophy affects wide regions of the brain and was difficult to study by the only methods available until recent decades: the autopsy and light microscopy. Metabolic derangements have not been easy to relate to specific regional disturbances in brain function.

These observations should not be taken to mean that, only through the study of stroke, is insight into speech and language obtained. Instead, they are intended to indicate the limitations that studies of one disease state may have imposed on understanding of higher cerebral function. Electrophysiologic studies, described below, have given rise to a somewhat different formulation of speech and language function than that obtained from studying brain lesions. It is hoped that metabolic studies in living patients will provide even more valuable insights.

Total or Global Aphasia

Massive destruction of either hemisphere produces a dense paralysis of the opposite limbs, with forced extreme deviation of the eyes to the side of the injury, and suppresses response to stimuli presented by vision, touch, and even sound to the affected side of space. In some right-handed people, an initial loss of consciousness occurs acutely after destruction of the sylvian regions of the left hemisphere (Fig. 18-4).

In the acute phase, for those who remain awake, all communication by language seems to be lost. The patient obeys no gestures or spoken or written commands, however simple; repeats no words; and is usually mute. Spontaneous gestures, sighs, frowns, tears, and self-help activities such as grooming and feeding with the uninvolved left-sided limbs give the impression that the patient is attempting to communicate with the world. Surprisingly, a handful of spoken single words or phrases such as simple expressions in common use for greetings and initial conversational banalities such as "How are you?," "Fine," OK," "Sure," and "Thank you," examples of utterances known as verbal stereotypes, may be uttered and spoken in the recognizable voice characteristic of the patient before the syndrome occurred. Careful testing shows such utterances are not reliably related to any subject matter heard or seen. Their occurrence often creates in lay observers the misleading option that patients "know what they want to say but cannot say it." Although the verbal stereotypes might be thought to arise from undamaged parts of the left hemisphere, the same syndrome has also been documented in the rare instances of hemispherectomy of the dominant hemisphere for brain tumor and in the extreme massive injuries in which the left hemisphere of a healthy young soldier has been carried away by shot or shell in battle.

The subsequent course varies considerably. In most cases of nonfatal infarction, hemorrhage, and successfully treated abscesses and encephalitis, the initial picture of total aphasia often improves to varying degrees over weeks to months, which presumably reflects the reactivation of surviving portions of the left side of the brain.

In the case of infarction, most of the lesions that cause total aphasia involve the frontocentral regions surrounding the sylvian fissure and also commonly

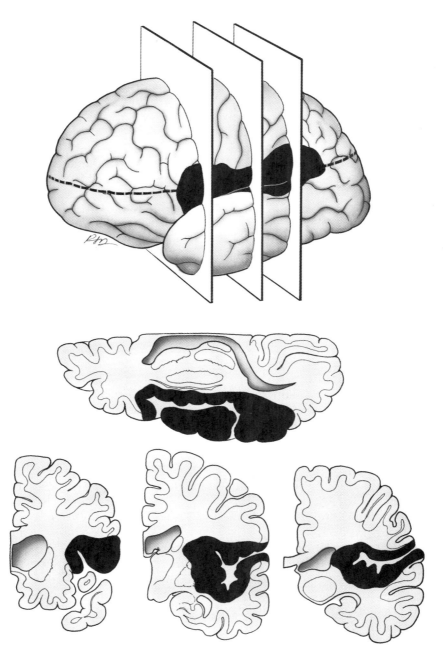

Figure 18-4. Diagram showing the usual topography of the infarction causing total or global aphasia. The lesion extends from and includes the inferior frontal region (Broca's area), the insula and operculum, inferior portion of the supramarginal gyrus, Heschl's transverse auditory gyri, the posterior superior temporal plane (Wernicke's area by some definitions), and the angular gyrus. Subinsular structures usually affected include the extreme capsule, claustrum, outer portions of the putamen, corona radiata, and the temporal isthmus. Larger lesions also exist, but this topography is sufficient to cause the syndrome.

affect some parts of the posterior half of the brain. The inferred (but as yet metabolically unproved) reactivation of this surviving posterior region is what is believed to account for the slight to moderate improvement in comprehension or words seen and heard.

The comprehension that seems so satisfactory in simple conversational contacts (in which the patient can use visual and auditory cues unwittingly provided by helpful relatives anxious to show the patient's improvement) is easily shown to be more profoundly affected when testing is done with more control of the stimulus presentations. In this setting, patients often show a comprehension of simple words and pictures, less often of nonpicturable words, and least often of relations between words based on rules of grammar (e.g., "In this picture, who is giving what to whom?"). The relatively better comprehension of words seen and heard contrasts with the persisting mutism, verbal stereotypes, or severely limited repertoire of spoken words; to the causal observer, the patient's speaking and writing are more disturbed than are listening and reading, a syndrome also known as major motor (Broca's) aphasia, described in more detail below.

For many, improvement does not occur. The verbal stereotypes often fade in variety, number, and frequency over the ensuing weeks, to the despair of observers who take it as a sign that the patient is getting worse. The reason for the decline is not clear nor whether it represents gradual loss of speech skills by the language-inefficient right hemisphere. Only the simplest form of interpersonal communication based on language develops in those whose left middle cerebral artery territory is totally destroyed; the right hemisphere has little, if any capacity to "take over" the function of the left, even given extensive training.

Total aphasia with mutism (or, at most, a few verbal stereotypic utterances) is frequently present in the first minutes after a major epileptic seizure and may occur early in the course of herpes simplex encephalitis, whether from the infection, seizure, or both. Only the rapid restoration of function in the succeeding minutes or hours helps the physician guess that the acute state was merely postepileptic (postictal). Masses from brain abscesses and tumors almost never cause this global disturbance in function as a first sign, usually yielding the syndrome only very late in the course of the illness when the diagnosis is all too clear.

Broca's Aphasia

Total aphasia is a concept easily grasped, with its implication that the entire speech and language mechanism has been put out of action. With the lesser but still major syndrome or motor (Broca's) aphasia, the distinctions are not as clear. In this disorder, the first of the syndromes of aphasia to receive an eponym, the main emphasis is placed on the disproportionate difficulties shown by the patient in speaking aloud. This difficulty in speech skills, with little impairment in comprehension, was the main disturbance emphasized by Broca himself and the feature attributed by him to a focal lesion in the inferior frontal region, the third frontal convolution that now bears his name. Revisited in the light of current knowledge, it seems evident that the clinical picture of Broca's aphasia requires a far larger lesion than that of Broca's area alone (Fig. 18-5) and calls into question exactly what

is meant clinically by the term Broca's aphasia. In this book, the authors mean the syndrome that is described below and emerges from an earlier clinical picture of total aphasia (see above).

In its fully developed form, the speech disturbance is a difficulty in accomplishing motor movements that is not explained merely by weakness of the muscles to be used (i.e., a dysarthria that can be looked at a dyspraxia of speech). In the initial years of the field of aphasiology, dyspraxias were explained by the lesion having caused the loss of memory for the movements of speech, which had earlier been acquired through practice. It is easy to understand how this refreshingly simple hypothesis, frowned on today as inelegant, occurred to those observing the unskillful, uncoordinated breathing; crude vocalizations; and mispronunciations and difficulties shifting to the next syllable that characterize the speech of such patients. Whatever the cause, oral dyspraxia (i.e., dyspraxia for complex oropharyngeal movements apart from these of speaking, see Ch. 19) is usually associated with Broca's aphasia.

In the years that followed Broca's first reports, the meaning of Broca's aphasia enlarged to a syndrome that also featured a disturbance in the language content of the spoken speech. The disturbance became known by the early years of this century as telegraphic speech and agrammatism. The former term was used because the sentences uttered by the patient had the laconic structure typical of telegrams, in which the high cost per word dictated a then-familiar short, pithy style that lacked filler words and modifiers. Agrammatism as a term came into general use when it was shown that these laconic utterances were also simplified by the omission of many word endings, changes in the form of tenses, and other modifications required by the rules of grammar for a given language. The utterances thus contained a high frequency of roots and stems of words and words with high informational content, mainly predicative words, but few modifiers. Severely disturbed patients have language abilities little better than the verbal stereotypes observed in total aphasia; those less affected utter predicative word clusters such as "stroke. . . ambulance. . come hospital." The agrammatism and effortful speaking combine to produce a reduction in speech and language responding that has been characterized as "nonfluent aphasia." This term, while accurate in characterizing the disturbance of such patients, is not sufficiently precise to stand alone as a term because it could be used just as well to describe patients without aphasia who stammer, those who fill gaps in speech with vocalized pauses (e.g., "er," "uh," and "hmm"), or those who hesitate while groping for a word not easily recalled.

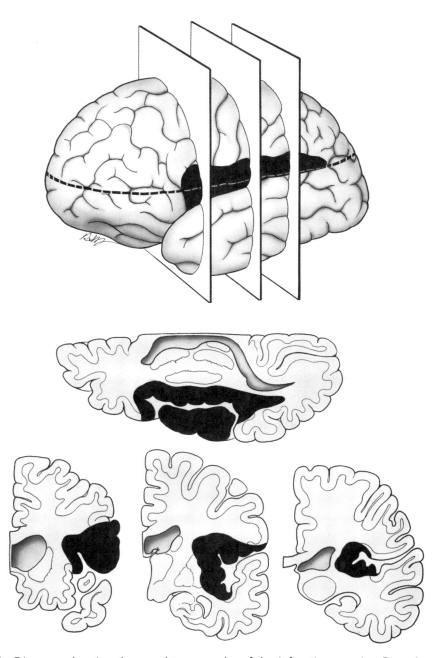

Figure 18-5. Diagram showing the usual topography of the infarction causing Broca's aphasia. The lesion is similar to that causing total or global aphasia but is somewhat smaller and affects fewer of the deep structures.

As a further indication there is more to Broca's aphasia than a difficulty limited to skills in speaking, a similar type of language disturbance has also been found to be present when such patients are tested for comprehension: reading comprehension is poor for sentences with a high frequency of grammatical words such as "he showed it to her, not to them." This disorder, which does not require the patient to speak aloud, reflects a disturbance in language processing of lexical stimuli and has been called deep dyslexia.

As a syndrome, the language disturbance in self-initiated speech and in auditory and visual language comprehension suggests that the responsible large lesion of the sylvian region has some effect on the brain's ability to apply the rules of grammar both in speech formulation and comprehension of word strings seen and heard.

The full extent of the disorder and its implications for the theories of language are rarely tested in detail in the busy clinical setting. Instead, sympathetic loved ones learn quickly to avoid the passive voice, complex word order, or too many indefinite articles and possessives. The patient's satisfactory comprehension of simple declarative sentences, one-step commands, and picturable nouns makes comprehension seem superior to the obvious faults both in vocalizing and in formulating sentences. Thus tested, the syndrome seems so aptly described as motor aphasia (i.e., emphasis on the difficulty in speaking) that this term has shown a remarkable resilience over the last century and every effort to replace it has fallen by the wayside. A few synonymous terms are still in use, among them dysfluency (akin to nonfluency, see above), which is used to characterize the dyspraxic speech and dysfluent aphasia. The unfortunate term "expressive aphasia" has also been used but is not recommended because this term also does not convey the distinction between the disorders of speech or language and that of poor education or poor social graces.

The most frequent of the causes of Broca's aphasia is a major infarction that involves most of the insula, upper and lower operculum, and adjacent regions surrounding the sylvian fissure (Fig. 18-5). The diagnosis of the lesion's location is made more easy by the accompanying disturbances in motor, sensory, and visual function, elements often minimized when the lesion is confined to the insula and operculum alone. The initial case from which the syndrome drew its name had the large infarct that involved the whole of the sylvian fissure and its surrounds. For many years, through repeated refinement of the dogma based on Broca's original thesis (but not on his actual observations), the lesion thought to explain this complex was taken to be the third frontal (Broca's) convolution, which was envisioned to contain the lost engrams. Although upward of a dozen examples exist in which this small a lesion has caused the syndrome in the acute phase, only the case of Van Gehuchten, kindly sent to the authors by the interested grandson of the original author, has remained unimproved as long as 1 year; the details in this case are slight. Indeed, the syndrome of Broca's aphasia usually arises in the wake of what was initially total aphasia and is rarely seen in an acute setting. It may gradually emerge as a tumor enlarges or an abscess grows but is rare in postictal states, encephalitis, acute head injury, degenerative states (such as Alzheimer's disease), or symptomatic metabolic brain disease.

Broca's aphasia prognosis is poor. After initial improvements in the first few months, it tends to persist for months and years with little subsequent change.

Variants of Motor Aphasia

The arrangement of branches of the upper division of the middle cerebral artery favors their individual occlusion from embolism, providing frequent opportunities to assess the speech and language effects of highly circumscribed lesions in the region of the sylvian fissure. Most of the observations of the following syndromes arise from brain infarction because few other causes allow such limited lesions.

Pure Mutism

Also known as anarthria, this syndrome, with normal or near-normal auditory and visual comprehension, is the usual acute syndrome seen with focal infarction in the inferior frontal regions (Fig. 18-6). Often, the infarct focus is in Broca's area, but the same syndrome has been recorded from infarction at the foot of the rolandic sulcus in the sensorimotor region and even, in some instances, from infarction in the inferior parietal lobule. All these sites abut one another along the insula and upper operculum. Thus far, no definite rules have been established to predict which site will be affected nor to explain why this same lesion has no effects on speech behavior in other patients.

During the time the patient is mute, even right-handed subjects can write properly with the unaffected left hand, a point that argues against a major aphasia and against the act of writing depending, in some way, on the act of speaking. The mutism usually fades promptly, sometimes within hours, giving rise to speech dyspraxia typical of, but milder than, that encountered in Broca's aphasia. However, the utterances rarely contain evidence of the grammatical condensation and simplified sentence structure typical of the language disturbance in Broca's aphasia. In addition to the speech dyspraxia, some degree of dyspraxia is often found for the act of swallowing and moving the face and oropharynx into certain positions on command, but the dyspraxia for movements other than speech is surprisingly mild (see also Ch. 19).

The site of the lesion in the insula or upper operculum usually also suggested clinically by the accompanying weakness of the opposite face and arm or hemiparesis that includes the leg. In a few instances, the involvement of the face and limbs was totally absent, a point that favors this mutism as having its unique origin and not merely being part of a larger syndrome.

Focal infarction due to embolism is the only reliable cause for this syndrome because of its capacity to occlude one branch only; larger infarcts produce the bigger syndrome of total or Broca's aphasia. A few freak penetrating brain injuries (examples include the point of an umbrella through the orbit, a fall in which the head struck a stone, and a penetrating shell fragment

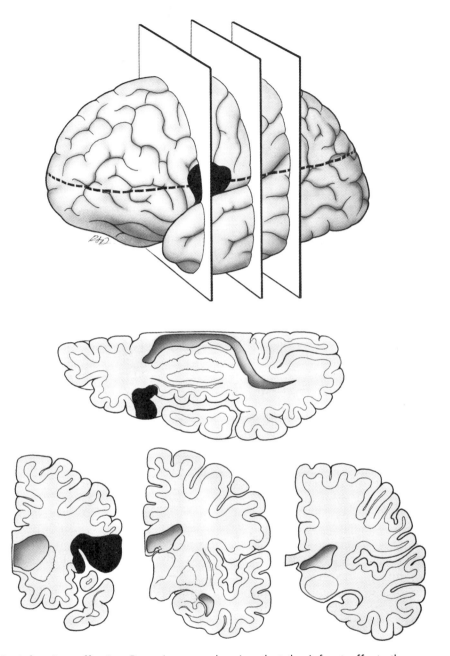

Figure 18-6. Infarction affecting Broca's area, showing that the infarct affects the gray matter and subjacent white matter but spares the basal ganglia and the cerebrum posterior to the inferior frontal region, including the insula.

in battle) and one instance of focal hemorrhage from an arteriovenous malformation have occurred. Other etiologic factors such as tumor, abscess, encephalitis, epilepsy, and toxic states cause larger lesions and a different syndrome. Although some cases persist indefinitely, most patients are usually normal within weeks, and many have returned to vocations that demand high-level speaking skills.

Subcortical Lesions With Mutism

Fewer than a dozen instances have been reported in which the mutism was caused by an infarction deeper in the brain, in the pathway to or at the level of the internal capsule. In such instances, infarction has usually occurred in the opposite capsule, and the new infarct sweeps away the control that one hemisphere can exert over bifacial and oropharyngeal movements, producing a syndrome of mutism. However, this one is accompanied by a severe disturbance in swallowing (dysphagia).

The severity of the dysphagia is evident from the beginning and helps diagnose the deeper site of the infarct. Although known by the classic formulation as subcortical motor aphasia, this latter syndrome scarcely justifies the term aphasia. However, a handful of instances have been reported in which the lesion was in the dominant hemisphere and lay between the surface and the internal capsule. One was an instance of small hemorrhage and another, an occlusion of a very lateral branch of the lenticulostriate branches of the middle cerebral artery. Improvement in this syndrome is very slow, with months and even years passing before satisfactory improvement occurs for speaking and swallowing alike. Once testable, the voice has a heavy nasal quality, which reflects the persisting weakness of the soft palate, and has none of the dyspraxic features typical of the surface infarction.

Cortical Dysarthria

Rarely, a small infarct that involves the sensorimotor cortex can alter the rhythm of speaking and cause a shift from the usual cadence and dialect. Only a few instances of this disorder have been reported; so the full range of the syndrome is not well understood. The voice is noted by others and by the patient to be changed in the pronunciation and melody (prosody) of speech, which alters the distinctive characteristics that enable a person to be recognized by voice over the telephone. The voice, described in most reports as sounding "foreign," usually has this distinctive lilting quality. To Europeans, the speaker sounds Scandinavian or Swiss. To Japanese ears, patients have been reported to sound Korean. No disturbance in language is evident. The syndrome has a good prognosis; full recovery within weeks is the rule.

Literal Paraphasia

This syndrome has a distinctive disturbance in speaking, featuring errors known as literal paraphasias. Paraphasias are errors in speech or language, in which the syllables or words uttered are different from those intended. The form here discussed is termed literal paraphasia, being some approximation to the correct response in form or sound. This term is intended to convey the notion that the error is a substitution of a unit of the word (e.g., "peshure" instead of the intended word "pleasure"), which is analogous to typographic errors in poorly trained typists. These errors are also known as phonemic paraphasias because it is inferred that they represent replacement of one sound set (i.e., letter or syllable sound or phonema) by an-

other with too many replaced phonemes, the utterances may have so little resemblance to the target phonemes as to be rendered incomprehensible jargon to the listener. However, some such errors may yield recognizable words (e.g., "measure" instead of "pleasure") that occur occasionally in normal discourse, with the meanings of some of them labeled as freudian slips by those seeking a hidden purpose behind the mispronounced word. An uttered word or fragment of a word that is a recognizable word has also been described as a "verbal" paraphasia (see below, Wernicke's aphasia).

The syndrome of literal paraphasia was long thought to be explained by postrolandic infarction that involved the sensory cortex controlling the kinesthetic settings of the oropharynx. The effect of the lesion was thought to impair the kinesthetic feedback that was considered to be important in the precise positioning of the oropharynx to form the desired syllables. The resulting speech was marred by inaccuracies, which to those familiar with the sounds produced by minor changes in position of the tongue, lips, and palate, would be recognizable as close approximations of the desired positions but would strike the ear of the uninitiated as unrecognized sets of syllables. When the syndrome was mild, mere slips of the tongue would seem to have occurred, but when severe, the neologisms would approach incomprehensible jargon.

That the causative lesion in literal paraphasias may be frontal, rolandic, or the expected postrolandic parietal focus has defied easy explanation. That terms like aphasia or paraphasia would apply to such utterances is largely an opinion formed by the listener, especially should the listener have little knowledge of the anatomy of speech sound production. Patients are usually acutely aware of the errors. They quickly learn to speak more slowly and to keep the word content of the sentences shorter, sometimes creating the false impression that their voluntary telegraphic speech is obligatory. Tests involving the comprehension of words seen or heard ar usually flawlessly completed, and the acted of speaking is performed skillfully, save for the mispronunciations, which sometimes are so annoying they interrupt the flow of speech. It can be argued this is a disturbance of articulation and not a true aphasia.

Embolism is almost the only cause, but one instance of an extremely small superficial hemorrhage has been reported. The duration of the syndrome is usually short, and rapid improvement takes place in the days after the lesion occurs.

Wernicke's Aphasia

This is the syndrome considered by many to be "true" aphasia. Lesions beginning in the posterior end of the sylvian fissure and spreading varying distances across

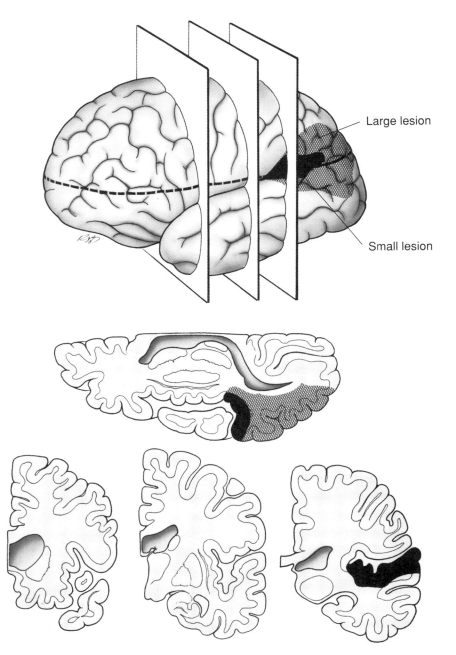

Figure 18-7. Lesions causing Wernicke's aphasia. The small lesion, limited to the posterior sylvian region, involved the superior temporal plane and often has a good prognosis. The larger lesion, spreading along the posterior temporoparietal region, has a poorer prognosis for clinical improvement.

the posterior half of the brain (Fig. 18-7) appear to produce not only an incapacity to repeat aloud and such a deranged content of words as to make the uttered speech incomprehensible but also a disturbance in the comprehension of words heard and seen disorganized writing, and a distinctly disturbed grammar.

Early clinical studies suggested that the phonemic and verbal paraphasias that contaminate the patient's speaking and writing were a sign of a deranged use of language that also interfered with the patient's comprehension of spoken and written language. Furthermore, such patients often seemed poorly organized and unskillful in their daily activities, performing practiced but complex tasks in the wrong order like some preschool children.

In the days before brain imaging in living patients,

the crude estimates of the site and size of the lesion were made especially difficult by the lack of weakness or sensory disorder of the face or limbs and by difficulty in determining whether defects in vision for contralateral space were present. It was little wonder that many inferred the lesion might be small and that, when functioning normally, this slim region had a powerful influence on language function. A small number of autopsies suggested the region was just behind Heschl's transverse auditory gyri, which is essential for the discrimination of sounds.

It required little theory to envision that this region served to select, from the sounds heard, those that are unique for language. Working with the long-popular minimalist view of seeking the smallest lesion that could explain the largest clinical disturbance, maps of lesions were produced, seeking the site of their overlap, in a Venn diagram paradigm. It was concluded by many that it was the site of the intersection, not the extent of the lesions, that explained "Wernicke's area" as lying just behind Heschl's transverse gyrus in the posterior superior temporal plane or planum temporale (see Ch. 30). The notion of a small site also suited the then-popular connectionist view of definable cortical centers linked to one another by white matter tracts (see above).

This unitary view was not supported by much data. With the small number of cases of infarction studied by autopsy, it was difficult to decide what lesion was responsible for the syndrome. Most of the lesions had their anterior border at the posterior end of the sylvian fissure and spread posteriorly from that site, as would be predicted by the vascular anatomy of the branches of the middle cerebral artery. Because embolism into these branches most often caused the syndrome, the anatomy of the syndrome was explainable at least by the cause as by the brain organization in the tissues supplied by these branches. Many cases with only a small lesion limited to the superior temporal plane showed only a modest disturbance in language, with little or no difficulty reading or writing, that often rapidly improved toward normal. Wernicke's own cases do not settle this point. Even S. E. Henschen (Swedish neuropathologist, 1847–1930), who devoted his retirement to the assembly of the reported autopsy literature up to 1920, found 35 well-studied cases and concluded that a superior temporal plane lesion did not cause the full picture of Wernicke's aphasia. In the years since, small lesions that are said to have the full clinical picture have actually been shown by autopsy or imaging to be infarcts that spread well beyond the superior temporal plane. Others were examples of subcortical hemorrhage the initial large mass of which, displacing the overlying posterior cortex, acutely explained the full syndrome but at autopsy had a small

residual hemorrhage and also a much reduced syndrome. When the syndrome has been fully developed in the acute stage, and especially when it has persisted chronically, the lesion has been found to spread well beyond the superior temporal plane. Recent studies of war-wounded soldiers also found the degree of disturbance in language function to be directly dependent on the size and extent of the lesion posterior to the posterior superior temporal plane. This disparity between dogma and data continues to be reflected in the textbooks, in which the site and size of Wernicke's area tends to be depicted as large for those authors who conceptually oppose strict clinicoanatomic correlations and as small for those who follow the connectionist model of function.

Apart from the issue of lesion size, the clinical elements of the syndrome have been observed to occur in clusters, with some as isolated features. Instances of poorly organized motor skills, in the absence of the aphasia, have been found from lesions that involve the parietal region separate from the superior temporal plane, which suggests that the syndrome of Wernicke's aphasia is not unitary. When computed tomography (CT) scanning became available, cases were found in which relatively intact reading and writing skills contrasted with poor auditory comprehension and repeating aloud; this provided an argument against a unity nature for the syndrome. Recently, PET scanning during tests of reading has not shown the activation of the angular gyrus and superior temporal plane as predicted by the model but has shown activation of the occipital lobes.

The traditional connectionist formulation can now be contrasted with the alterative that Wernicke's aphasia may be a syndrome the many elements of which occur less often because of a unitary organization of all the language and praxic skills than because several different brain functions that occur in the posterior half of the brain may be affected by the lesion sweeping across all of them. It is no longer necessary to envision that all language stimuli seen or heard must pass ultimately to the posterior superior temporal plane for their translation into meaning. Instead, the posterior half of the brain appears to have some areas that are most involved in the auditory processing of language; others, in the visual; and still others, in motor skills that involve writing.

Despite these variations in sensory discriminatory function depending on site of the lesion, the clinical features of the speech and language disorder reflected in lesions that involve the posterior half of the brain still share many common elements in disturbed use of language, most of which are the opposite of Broca's aphasia. First, speech function separate from language content shows no difficulties observed in the skills of articulation; there is none of the effortful speaking as in motor aphasia; and the good articulatory skills contrast with the poor selection of words to give the syndrome the commonly applied appellation of "fluent aphasia," coined to contrast it with the "non-fluent aphasia" of the larger sylvian lesions (see above). However, this simplistic term is misleading because many of these patients show great disruption in the smoothness of speech caused by difficulties in word finding and in assembly of grammar-based word elements (e.g., selection and proper positioning of prefixes and suffixes on words, resulting in errors such as "denecessariness" instead of "unnecessary," see below). In some instances, when the lesion is acute, large, and deep, the patient may even show disorder known as logorrhea (Greek; *logos*, speak; *-rrhea*, excess), speaking freely and volubly as in agitated delirium. Many patients with logorrhea seem to have no insight or awareness of their grossly deranged language usage and can be said to be anosognosic for their deficit (see Ch. 19), a deficiency that often makes them impatient and quarrelsome (the angry aphasic patient) with the normal people around them who seem, for some reason unclear to the patient, not to understand what the patient has said.

The language content of the speech is filled with the grammatical words missing in Broca's aphasia, but the key, predicative words, so over-represented in Broca's aphasia, are under-represented here. To the observer, the lack of meaningful content may escape detection in conversational exchanges in which the patient performs well, with an easy flow of speech and high content of grammatical words. In sustained narrative, as in history taking, ample opportunity is provided for errors to be observed, and here the omission of many important verbs and nouns, the occurrence of incomplete phrases, and illogical sequences of clauses could cause some observers to think the patient is confused, psychotic, or under the influence of drugs. Some hesitancy may be evident when the expected word is omitted, but often the expected response, the target word, is substituted by a mispronunciation in the form of a similar-sounding word (literal paraphasias), as in the sylvian syndrome of literal paraphasia. Of greater diagnostic value are substitutions by other words with similar meanings (verbal paraphasias). Those that occur instead of the target word may occur as errors based entirely on meaning (semantic verbal paraphasias) or similarity in sounds (formal verbal paraphasias). Some instances of formal (i.e., errors similar to the target word in form or shape, such as "hook" for "took") verbal paraphasias are close to literal paraphasia and can be thought of as literal paraphasias the syllable clusters of which happen to form a recognizable word; others are clear examples of ap-proximations to the target word both in form and meaning (e.g., "could" for "should"). Accompanying the specific literal and verbal paraphasias are a variable number of recurrences of prior words or portions of words, the recurrences of which are known as "perseverations." The frequency of the perseverative utterances directly parallels the degree of difficulty the patient is having at the time. Typically, topics handled well show little or no perseveration; those that cause difficulty may result in a large number.

Formal bedside testing shows that repeating aloud is difficult for the patient, especially for polysyllabic and unfamiliar words. In the past, this disturbance in repeating aloud was taken to be an essential feature of the syndrome, and great stress was placed on this difficulty. The errors expected are literal paraphasias, but a surprising number of verbal paraphasias may also occur, arguing that the difficulty in repeating aloud is not merely a difficulty "connecting" the posterior sylvian region to the anterior nor merely a disorder of auditory discrimination but also a disorder in comprehension or language usage in formulating responses. Especially distinctive are errors in tests of repeating numbers aloud when the patient utters other numbers. The patient may read short phrases aloud well, making most of the errors when words of high information content appear. However, reading aloud and for comprehension appear most deranged for those words that contain the predicative elements of a sentence (i.e., the words that convey the essential elements of a sentence). In its most mild forms, reading aloud suggests that the patient does not understand the main points of the text.

In extreme cases, the patient can be said to be cut off from useful interpersonal communication. Spoken speech may be so deranged by literal and verbal paraphasias and cluttered with perseverations that it is incomprehensible, a state known as "jargon aphasia." Likewise, the impairment in comprehension may be so severe that all attempts at contact, with words and gestures, do not appear to be understood. Add the patient's anosognosia and angry mood and the preservation of full motor power, and even a frail individual can be difficult to manage in the setting of the acute lesion. In extreme circumstances, some patients may be initially misdiagnosed as acutely psychotic.

The causes of Wernicke's aphasia make up a longer list than those of Broca's aphasia. The syndrome, in its acute form, may arise from occlusion of the posterior temporal branch, the angular branch, or occasionally, even the middle temporal branch of the middle cerebral artery, together or in combination. Thrombosis of a cortical vein from infection may trigger an acute syndrome. The larger the infarct is, the more likely is the full syndrome to arise. Acute hemorrhage in the posterior half of the brain may trigger the full syndrome. Epilepsy limited to the posterior half of the brain has caused the full syndrome, even without motor movements or loss of consciousness during the ictal period. Such seizures are common in the early stages of herpes simplex encephalitis. Wernicke's aphasia may be a sign of a migraine aura. Direct brain injury from gunshot wounds or missiles requires a large wound to cause the full syndrome acutely. Although abscesses, primary or metastatic tumors, and even Alzheimer's disease may cause the syndrome, the evolution is slow in all these cases, and a severe form of Wernicke's aphasia is decidely unusual in this setting.

The prognosis is largely a function of the size of the lesion. The effects of epilepsy usually subside fully within 1 week. When the syndrome arises from hemorrhage, a great improvement occurs over months. The full syndrome from infarction or wounds has a poor prognosis because of the size of the lesion, and it may remain static for years. In cases with a favorable outcome, the usual sequelae are a mild difficulty in recalling words on formal naming tests (see below, amnestic aphasia).

Variants of Wernicke's Aphasia

These conditions are often considered to be but fractional states approximating Wernicke's aphasia, missing some major element or heavily involving another. However, two observations are important in insights into language mechanisms. First, the lesions found that cause the variants are often in the same area and roughly the same size as those that trigger the full syndrome of Wernicke's aphasia in other patients, a point never adequately explained. Second, the variants are not merely a milder stage of Wernicke's aphasia but are different enough that it may be said that some of the expected elements are not present to any degree. Such a finding could be explained as individual differences in precise cerebral organization or as evidence that no two lesions are the same and no two patients are examined in the same way at the same time in their clinical course.

Conduction Aphasia

This clinical syndrome features poor repetition with normal auditory and visual comprehension of language (see also above, Literal Paraphasia). It was a syndrome formulated early in the history of the connectionist theories of aphasia and is more a prediction than a common finding. The assumption was that a lesion in a presumed pathway that conveys instructions from the sensory language zone to the motor would prevent words heard from being repeated aloud, with all else being normal. The supposed pathway was taken to be the arcuate fasciculus, a con-

densed band of white matter medial and superiorly to the insula, in a position that connects Wernicke's area with Broca's area (Fig. 18-8).

Despite the simple requirements of the syndrome, few instances have actually been reported. In most cases in which the syndrome approximates the required features, auditory and even reading comprehension has been obviously impaired. Furthermore, the speech errors have been largely those of the syndrome of literal paraphasia, or the language content of speech has been heavily contaminated with semantic verbal paraphasias with repetition no worse than in spontaneous speech.

More disturbing to the connectionist thesis, the autopsy evidence in all the reported cases has been superficial infarction with widely varying degrees of penetration into subcortical structures, with some of the infarcts being entirely superficial. Furthermore, many of the superficial infarcts have been in the posterior temporal plane, the site usually assumed to cause Wernicke's aphasia. A single case that was reported by magnetic resonance imaging (MRI) to show a subcortical infarction has been interpreted by others as showing a superficial infarction.

The syndrome, when present in pure form, is usually transient, with the deficits fading within days. Many instances of "conduction aphasia" are merely examples of the syndromes of literal paraphasia from superficial infarction of the lower rolandic or inferior parietal region, requiring no other explanation. In others, the lesion that involves the posterior temporal plane produces a mild form of Wernicke's aphasia in which repeating aloud is the most obvious of the disturbances. In such cases, the conduction aphasia component is the persisting syndrome, but it is usually mild.

Pure Word Deafness

Also known as subcortical sensory aphasia, this rare disorder is traditionally attributed to a disruption of subcortical pathways from the brainstem by way of Heschl's transverse gyri to Wernicke's area in the posterior superior temporal plane. In its original formulation, disturbed auditory comprehension was supposed to be the only deficit. Such cases are almost unknown in an acute syndrome, because the causative lesion, either a large subcortical hemorrhage or a surface infarct, causes a syndrome that begins as Wernicke's aphasia from which the difficulty in auditory comprehension persists and other components fade.

Only eight cases have been reported from a unilateral lesion confined to the superior temporal plane in the dominant hemisphere, and in seven, paraphasic speaking was prominent. This arguing against "pure word deafness" and in favor of a mild form of Wer-

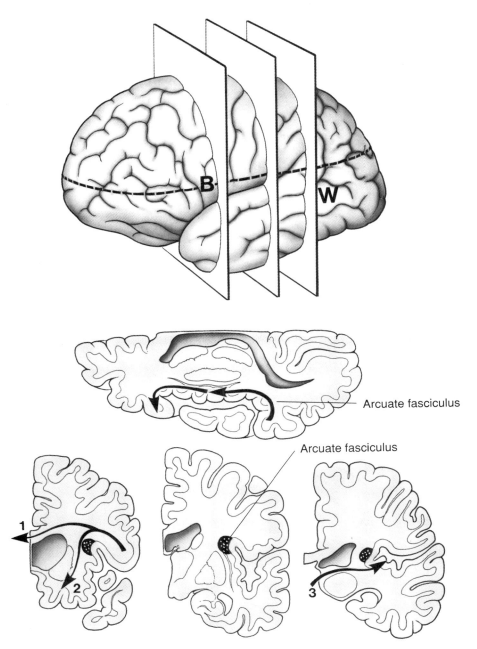

Figure 18-8. Alleged pathways mediating repeating aloud. The lesion preventing repeating aloud is considered to interrupt this fasciculus along its course between Wernicke's and Broca's areas, but many examples exist in which the lesion is not subcortical, yet repeating aloud is affected and vice versa. B, Broca's area; W, Wernicke's area; 1, transcallosal pathway from Broca's area to the opposite frontal region; 2, ipsilateral pathway from Broca's area to the oropharyngeal musculature; 3, auditory pathway from the brainstem to Wernicke's area. The position of the arcuate fasciculus is shown.

nicke's aphasia. A few instances have been reported from infarction that affected the right and left hemisphere, each involving Heschl's transverse gyrus to some degree. In these cases, the disturbances in auditory comprehension approached those of the requirements of the syndrome, but the lesion was not "subcortical" at all. Such cases conform to the definitions of auditory agnosia (see Ch. 19). Brain tumors rarely begin in the deep temporal region to cause isolated pure word deafness, and lesions such as abscesses and encephalitis usually produce a more severe disturbance.

Alexia With Agraphia

Also a rare condition, this syndrome shows little disturbance in speech skills and in repeating aloud, although auditory comprehension seems less disturbed than does comprehension of visual language stimuli such as printed words. Like many other classic syndromes, its clinical features have only rarely been observed in isolation. It is separate from the condition known as alexia with*out* agraphia (see below).

In all but 5 of the 250 cases found based on autopsy by Henschen (1920), the combination of dyslexia and dysgraphia was part of a larger clinical syndrome that also featured paraphasias in speech, which suggests it was a form of Wernicke's aphasia. The lack of major disturbance in auditory comprehension was what prompted early theorists to consider it an isolated syndrome for two major reasons: first, it was thought that adequate auditory comprehension would mean Wernicke's area was spared; and second, it was believed that the lesion that caused the difficulty in reading and writing would be in the pathways that carried visual information from the visual system (i.e., in the lateral parietal lobe, with the most prominent gyrus being the angular gyrus). The lack of an isolated syndrome is an important point against the predictions of connectionism, in which it was inferred that the angular gyrus somehow mediated the reading behavior. This view, which suggests that Wernicke's aphasia has an auditory and a visual component, was reflected in some of the diagrams of aphasia-causing lesions by French authors in the early years of this century (Fig. 18-9).

As a prominent part of a syndrome of Wernicke's aphasia in lateral and posterior parietal infarcts, it is common to find that alexia is disproportionately more severe than auditory comprehension.

A separate disorder of reading without aphasia is seen in an isolated (pure) alexia (alexia with*out* agraphia), a distinctive disorder not associated with difficulty in writing. In such patients, the lesion is usually large and usually an infarction, and it affects the posterior cerebral territory of the dominant hemisphere, wrecking the direct visual radiations from the right side of space and shutting off all transcallosal projections of all kinds. In the famous case reported

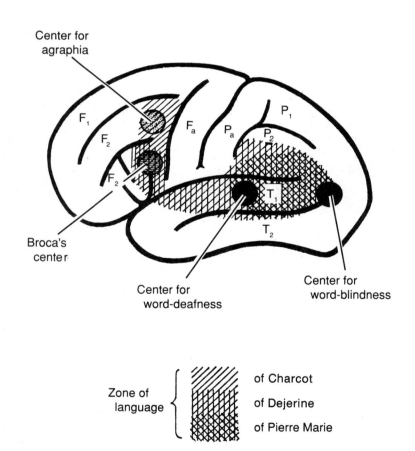

Figure 18-9. Diagram of brain regions involved in aphasia after focal lesions according to various French authors. (From Brain, 1964, with permission.)

by Dejerine in 1891, the patient could write well but was unable to read what he had written and had difficulty reading other forms of lexical stimuli, including printed words. Such patients typically treat lexical stimuli (letters or words presented in printed texts or in handwriting) as foreign forms, often offering wildly inaccurate guesses as to the names of the letters. That theirs is a problem with the meaning of lexical stimuli and not blindness or unfamiliarity with visual displays is demonstrated by their ability to name objects (e.g., faces, animals, tools, and buildings) and even words that are presented in a familiar logo form (e.g., the distinctive cursive script used by Coca-Cola). To cause the severe and persistent form of alexia, in which the patient is unable to comprehend any of the visual lexical stimuli, a lesion is required to be strategically placed or of sufficient size to disrupt the visual cortex of the dominant hemisphere and the transcallosal pathways from the nondominant hemisphere (see Ch. 25). Less complete lesions cause a right-sided hemidyslexia of varying severity, and small lesions may pose only a short-term problem in reading the right-hand end of longer words.

Semantic Aphasia

This unusual syndrome is another variant of Wernicke's aphasia that is rarely encountered in isolation. As opposed to "pure word deafness" and "alexia with agraphia," in which the major problem involves either the auditory or the visual route of language decoding in addition to the language disturbance typical of Wernicke's aphasia, semantic aphasia features the language disorder in the absence of difficulties repeating aloud and least often in disturbances related to the functions of the speech modalities such as speech skills and the capacities to discriminate words that are heard and seen. Few examples of isolated semantic aphasia have been documented.

Little is known of the exact site(s) that cause(s) this syndrome except that the lesions affect the parietal or temporal lobe. In some, the main injury was a penetrating brain wound in war that affected the deep parietal and deep temporal lobes; in others, there is atrophy (as a sign developing during the course of Alzheimer's disease) or a primary or metastatic tumor. Occasionally, the syndrome of herpes simplex encephalitis has been present. This type of aphasia has rarely been reported to be caused by an acute syndrome of infarction.

The existence of the syndrome, even as part of a larger disorder, has been of interest because, by studying such cases, insight can be gained into the most complex, abstract levels of language activity. The conceptually disconnected strings of words, which have a character like a delirium, have struck many listeners as a reflection of the disorganization of preverbal thought. Such inferences are difficult to investigate, with most having been reported as a few examples of utterances only and none with extended analysis. One feature that has been prominently observed is the occurrence of grossly neologistic paraphasias, usually uttered when a noun or other predicative word is expected, with the gross error embedded in an otherwise satisfactory sentence structure such as, "I would say that's your wapple but it could be your sadlow." Little evidence of awareness of the errors (anosognosia) has been seen, and the patient can often write such grossly neologistic responses in a satisfactory cursive handwriting, which indicates that the systems involved in writing play little editorial role in language responses.

Transcortical Sensory Aphasia

This disorder, which is easy to formulate from connectionist theory but difficult to find as clinical examples, appears to be an unusual syndrome that was postulated in the early days of aphasiology as a consequence of disconnecting the sensory language area from the centers of concepts (i.e., other cortical regions that ordinarily receive projections from the sensory language zone to arouse associations that permit the appreciation of the meaning of sounds heard and perhaps also of words seen). Few examples have emerged over the years, with fewer still having documentation by autopsy or radiologic images. The clinical examples have often been in cases of Alzheimer's disease, a state that comes closer to satisfying the anatomic requirements than most others; the lesions presumably have been of the cortical regions themselves, rather than of any putative transcortical pathways. Others were encountered from high and posterior parietal infarctions. Kertesz (A. Kertesz, Canadian neurologist) has risen to the challenge by using CT scans and the Western Aphasia Battery tests on patients that satisfy his criteria for the syndrome. The lesion was diagnosed by isotope brain scan in 12 and by CT scan in 6. The lesions were rather large, involving the posterior half of the brain from the occipital pole forward on both the medial and lateral surfaces, in many reaching far forward along the mesial occipital lobe, with most in the territory of the posterior cerebral artery. The high incidence of hemianopia, "visual agnosia," and sensory loss supports this location. The speech was described as fluent and circumlocutory, often with semantic jargon. Strings of well-articulated and acceptable English words that were semantically not relevant to the questions or to the previous sentence were frequently observed. Comprehension was poor, and repetition was intact.

So little is known of this syndrome that its status can only be said to be unclear at present.

Amnestic Aphasia

This disorder, known also by the synonyms "anomic aphasia" and "nominal aphasia," is separate from the major syndromes of Wernicke's and Broca's aphasias. It is characterized by a failure to recall the names of people and many other individual nouns when the stimuli were presented in visual or auditory form. It is a difficulty in word finding or a lack of words. Some consider the lack of words to be one of the core elements of aphasia; hence this syndrome is considered part of the syndromes of aphasia and not part of a general memory disorder. The omissions are so distinctive and so different in character from the semantic verbal paraphasias that contaminate naming efforts in the other syndromes of aphasia that the authors discourage the use of the term anomic aphasia because it does not describe the difference in the naming patterns between these two broad categories of aphasia and could mislead others as to the syndrome being described.

Instead of paraphasic errors, amnestic aphasic patients usually merely do not respond, often falling silent or hesitating as if the name is about to be produced momentarily ("tip of the tongue" effect). Often, the patient indicates familiarity with the missing name by describing attributes of the item; using circumlocutions; and occasionally, offering lame excuses for failure, testimonials of prowess in other areas, or protestations that such testing is irrelevant. Although not invariable, it is a common finding that the correct name is accepted among the choices offered. A surprising specificity of the errors may occur, with the names of same items repeatedly failing to occur, although other items in the same stimulus class (i.e., fruits), are named without hesitation.

Amnestic aphasia is considered classically to be a sign of deep temporal lobe involvement but is commonly present in posterior cerebral artery territory infarction in the dominant hemisphere. It is a usual late sequela and the last element to improve in Wernicke's aphasia.

Syndromes From Lesions of the Thalamus or Basal Ganglia

Thalamic activity appears to be important in maintaining a steady state in the cerebral structures involved in language because some thalamic lesions mimic lesions in the cerebral surface regions concerned with speech and language. Most of the few patients documented with these syndromes have had small thalamic hemorrhages, although some have been reported from infarctions. The acute clinical syndrome resembles that of a normal person greatly deprived of sleep, with wide variations in alertness and difficulty interacting with the examiner. The distinctive speech and language behavior of these patients is such that, when they are first engaged with conversation, for some seconds, the responses appear entirely normal but, after a few moments, begin to change to an incomprehensible jargon. During the normal end of the spectrum of interpersonal interaction, few observers would think the patient has any disturbance in speech and language; at the opposite end, no useful speech or language interaction is achieved. The syndrome typically improves to normal over days.

Deep lesions that affect the basal ganglia and internal capsule structures typically produce no disturbance in speech or language unless they are large. Under the latter circumstances, the clinical picture is that of global or total aphasia. There has been little insight into the site or size of the lesion that correlates the transition between little or no disturbance and a profound disturbance in speech or language.

A small number of patients with dominant hemisphere internal capsule (genu) infarction have been reported on; a picture of acute disorders with delays in responses and laconic sentences was seen in formal testing. Cerebral blood flow studies have shown widespread reductions over the frontal lobe on the same side, although MRI shows no signs of infarction. It has been hypothesized that these patients have interrupted thalamocortical projection systems, which govern cerebrovascular responsivity, and show this clinical picture from the impairment of vascular response, which secondarily limits the cerebral metabolic rates needed to sustain speech and language behavior. Modest clinical improvements have been reported, but for many patients the deficits persist.

Thalamic lesions have their own distinctive forms of speech and language disorder; these are encountered almost entirely in a setting of hemorrhage into the left thalamus in right-handed patients. The main features of this syndrome are a fluctuating performance in language function from almost normal to a profusely paraphasic fluent speech akin to a delirium. When the patient can be tested in detail, speech is fluent and well articulated, repetition is intact, naming is poor, and spontaneous speech contains many paraphasias. The basis for the disturbance remains unsettled, but it has been speculated that it reflects the loss of thalamic mediation of cerebral activity in the regions that control speech and language, similar to the accompanying disturbances in the level of alertness from damage to the reticular activating system. The syndrome occurs infrequently because most hematomas are either too small to cause any disturbance or so large as to cause stupor or coma.

Primary Progressive Aphasia

For all syndromes of aphasia except for this one, it is the clinical characteristics of the syndrome in the acute phase that allow the classification as to type. However, some patients present with an aphasia, fluent or not fluent in type, that progresses relentlessly over the years without evidence of other brain dysfunction. In particular, there is no dementia. Other patients, whose dementia begins by a prominent dysphasia, do not belong to this group.

In primary progressive aphasia, a variety of lesions have been found postmortem in the left inferior frontal gyrus and temporal cortex, that is, Pick's and Alzheimer's diseases or spongiform changes that mostly occur in layer 2 of the cortex. One case with Creutzfeldt-Jakob disease is on record.

CLINICAL ASSESSMENT

Testing for aphasia has been the subject of wide variation in methods, with each seeking information concerning the aspect of aphasia of interest.

Formal Tests

Formal tests for aphasia from personnel trained in the use of the popular standard tests are useful to clinicians for purposes of classification of the syndrome and determination of major changes in performance over time. Such tests take time, often many hours, and are not suited for efficient use at the bedside. Among the popular tests used in America are the Boston Veterans Administration Test for Aphasia (created at the Boston Veterans Hospital and spread widely from there, often referred to as the Boston Test or simply the Boston). Also in common use are the Porch Index of Communicative Ability and The Western (University of Western Ontario) Aphasia Battery. Now largely superseded are the Head (H. Head, English neurologist, 1861–1940) Battery, later changed by Halstead (W. Halstead, American psychologist, 1909–1968) to the Head-Halstead Battery and then to the Halstead-Reitan Battery (R. Reitan, American psychologist, 1922–), the Eisenson Test (founded by a psychologist at and popularized by the New York Neurological Institute), the Token Test, and others too numerous to mention. Each country has its own popular tests. All of them share the essential features of a small series of items to be named aloud, pointed to on dictated command, or written as names or drawn as figures on sheets of paper. Some tests involve the manipulation of objects to test praxis (see Ch. 19), and most of them also involve strings of words to be repeated aloud, sentences to be read aloud, and short paragraphs to be read aloud or silently, after which questions are read aloud or dictated aloud to seek answers relating to the information in the paragraphs.

The tests are typically arranged along a continuum thought to represent increasing difficulty. The number of items in each group (i.e., colors, manipulatable objects, numbers, and letters) are limited, usually 5 or so, rarely as many as 10 or 20. The limits of time and the wide range of responses sought in testing sometimes means that too small a sample of any individual performance (i.e., naming of colors) is obtained to make the case of a specific type of disorder (i.e., color dysnomia). A distracted patient with a hurried examiner may result in the shortening of the examination with interpolation of the results, outcomes to be avoided in cases in which longitudinal studies are sought. Properly performed with a cooperative patient, these tests are useful for the longitudinal assessment of the course of an illness or therapy.

Bedside Testing

Bedside testing for aphasia and for syndrome subtypes has been for one century the showcase of clinical neurology. The difficulties in correlating the syndrome with the exact site, and cause of the lesion now readily seen on modern brain images has somewhat tarnished the luster of this art. However, such testing remains important in the acute clinical setting and is becoming more important once again now that early treatment for illnesses must begin before the image becomes positive.

When a patient is approached for the interview, the initial eye contact, head- and eye-following movements, and gestures and words of greeting serve to indicate that the patient can hear, see, and interact but are not good guides for assessment of the degree of language disturbance. Even a severe patient may succeed in accomplishing ordinary greetings, using verbal stereotypes ("ready-made language") such as "How are you?," "OK," and "Fine, thanks." Unprompted narrative, that is, asking the patient to tell the story of the illness, is an excellent test of the patient's language skills. Few patients will be found to have any form of aphasia if a well-organized and succinct history is given, especially if this is accomplished without the requirement of prompts from the examiner or helpful supplements from the worried family members. The examiner will be more reassured that the patient is normal if the patient can be interrupted in the narrative with a question concerning neologisms ("Were you ever in Hajaberuppastan?") and then picks up of the narrative and continues. Introduction of neologisms may prompt the patient to repeat them, aloud ("Did you say Hajaberuppastan?"), which is a reassuring sign when repeating aloud is normal.

In most centers, it is common to request the patient

to name a variety of common objects. The authors recommend objects ready to hand, such as the parts of a pair of spectacles (lenses, frames, and side pieces), the front of a shirt (collar, button, and pocket), wristwatch (face, second hand, minute hand, hour hand, and stem), parts of a shoe (heel, sole, tongue, and laces). The purpose here is to assess the degree to which names expected to be known are not recalled and to examine whether the errors are literal or semantic verbal paraphasias and whether the responses are contaminated by perseverations. There is no exact standard set for the frequency and type of errors, but the use of such tests is so widespread in the neurological community that it is widely believed that the number and types of errors are helpful in a diagnosis of the severity and type of aphasia.

More detailed testing can be pursued with the naming of colors (6 to 10 at least), naming of line drawings shown in montage form, identifying pictures of a few famous people, describing thematic pictures, and reading a complex paragraph aloud. These items test for the rare isolated syndromes (those unaccompanied by signs of aphasia in conversational speech) of color dysnomia, amnestic aphasia, "simultanognosia" and visual agnosia (see Ch. 19), and pure alexia (see Ch. 25).

For patients who do not generate a smooth and well-organized narrative, the issue is whether the problem lies primarily with the more elemental disturbances in speech (oropharyngeal and respiratory) praxis, adequate discrimination of speech sounds, or a disorder in language usage. Repeating aloud is a useful test to determine the adequacy of auditory discrimination and correct settings of the oropharyngeal and respiratory apparatus. The test should use unfamiliar sets of syllables (anagrammic rearrangement of multisyllable words is a common method, for example, in Americans, "settsachumass" instead of "Massachusetts") with emphasis on a special syllable (i.e., "settsaCHUmass") to determine that the patient replicates not only the syllable sets but also the speech intonation and melody (prosody). Errors in these tasks usually reflect lesions along the sylvian fissure. Errors in repeating aloud that are recognizable as other words (paraphasias) (i.e., "sat for Mass") suggests an aphasic basis to the errors, not merely a disturbance in sound replication. An aphasic basis can be pursued using the names of numbers in digit sequences (i.e., "3-6-1-9-5") and is confirmed when the errors are other number names (i.e., "4-3-7-8-1"). These errors often reflect lesions posterior to the sylvian region.

These tests are needed to set the stage for more complex testing in which the responses are less predictable and harder to judge as to whether they are aphasic. To demonstrate the deficit, testing must be performed so that the patient must respond to the purely verbal content of the word seen or heard, unaided by gestures or other cues. Semantic verbal paraphasias, in particular, can confound attempts to assess the severity of aphasia. To a picture of two men shaking hands, a patient who responds, "He and she are showing his faces" clearly illustrates the aphasic basis to the semantic errors ("she" for "he," "showing" for "shaking," "faces" for "hands"), but the severity of the disorder and the site and size of the lesion are less easily estimated. The most that can be learned is that a complex disturbance is present that will require more formal study.

There is less difficulty in arriving at a diagnosis for patients who are either mute and follow no dictated or simple printed commands or who speak continuously, utter an incomprehensible set of neologisms, and also follow no dictated or simple printed commands. For the former, mute, group, the lesion is usually large and located in or around the sylvian fissure. For the latter, with logorrheic jargon, the lesion is usually large and postsylvian. That some of these patients nod to gestures and even make verbal stereotype replies such as "OK" is not the sign of adequate comprehension that it is often inferred to be by family members.

Prognosis and Treatment

A basic finding in the aphasias is that the outlook for improvement is governed by the size of the lesion. The site of the lesion may determine the elements of acute syndrome (see above), but the outlook for improvement is governed more by the size. Lesions that are a gyrus in width typically predict the disappearance of almost all acute clinical disturbances, in time frames as short as a few days to as long as a few months. It is a common observation that the normal language function of such patients, seen in the office years afterwards, surprises the examiner in the face of a brain image showing a lesion in the major speech and language areas. Even a lesion as large as half a lobe may be associated with enough clinical improvement so that return to some form of useful life is possible within 1 year or so. Those whose lesions have carried away almost the entire sylvian region typically show an obvious aphasia even after decades.

Apart from treatment of the underlying disease, there has been little medical treatment that is useful in the improvement of the specific syndromes of aphasia. A small trial of bromocriptine met with some success, but others have been discouraging. Speech therapy has been the mainstay of management for almost one century. Meta-analysis and prospective studies, however, have not shown this form of therapy to have the dramatic positive outcomes that physicians and patients seek. Few doubt speech therapy is helpful, but it remains undetermined whether it is curative or creates behavior not already available.

ANNOTATED BIBLIOGRAPHY

Alajouanine T, Ombredane A, Durand M. Le Syndrome de Désintégration Phonétique dans l'Aphasie. Masson, Paris, 1939.

The first and standard linguistic study of agrammatism.

Benson DF, Sheremata WA, Bouchard R. Conduction aphasia. Arch Neurol 1973;28:339.

The lesions were superficial infarcts.

Bogen JE, Bogen GM. Wernicke's region—where is it? Ann N Y Acad Sci 1976;280:834.

Thorough review of the problem localizing Wernicke's area.

Bonhoeffer K. Klinischer und anatomischer Befund zur Lehre von der Apraxie und der "Motorischen Sprachbahn." Monatsschr Psych Neurol 1914;35:113.

Attempts to refine the pathologic localization of speech disorders.

Brain R. Speech Disorders. Butterworth (Publishers), London, 1964.

Broca P. Remarques sur le siège de la faculté du langage articulé, suivies d'une observation d'aphémie (perte de la parole). Bull Soc Anat Paris 1861;6:330.

The first article.

Damasio H, Damasio AR. Localization of lesions in conduction aphasia, in Kertesz A (ed). Localization in Neuropsychology. Academic Press, New York, 1983.

Surprising number of superficial infarcts, some in "Wernicke's area."

Dejerine J. Sur un cas de cécité verbale avec agraphie, suivi d'autopsie. Mem Soc Biol 1891;3:197.

The first well-described attempt to define alexia with agraphia.

Dejerine J, Mirallie C. L'Aphasie Sensorielle. Steinheil, Paris, 1896.

Masterful review of the literature to that time.

Geschwind N. Disconnection syndromes in animals and man. Brain 1965;88:237–94; 585–644.

The article the far-reaching influence of which triggered much of the modern interest in aphasia and apraxia.

Goldstein K. Language and Language Disturbances. Grune & Stratton, New York, 1948.

Thoughtful analyses with some pathology.

Goodglass H, Kaplan E. The Assessment of Aphasia and Related Disorders. Lea and Febiger, Philadelphia, 1972.

The Boston test for aphasia testing used in America.

Heiss WD, Kessler J, Karbe H et al. Cerebral glucose metabolism as a predictor of recovery from aphasia in ischemic stroke. Arch Neurol 1993;50:958–64.

A major predictor was the degree of activation in the undamaged regions of the left hemisphere.

Henschen SE. Klinische und Anatomische Beitrage zur Pathologie des Gehirns. Nordiska Bokhandeln, Stockholm, 1920.

A reference work for autopsy cases to 1920. The clinical details are somewhat scanty.

Hier DB, Mohr JP. Incongruous oral and written naming. Evidence for a subdivision of the syndrome of Wernicke's aphasia. Brain Lang 1977;4:115.

Wernicke's aphasia is not a unitary syndrome.

Jeffery PJ, Monsein LH, Szabo Z et al. Mapping the distribution of amobarbital sodium in the intracarotid Wada test by use of Tc 99m HMPAO with SPECT. Radiology 1991;178:847–50.

Large differences between angiographic supply and distribution of amobarbital.

Kertesz A, Lau WK, Polk M. The structural determination of recovery in Wernicke's aphasia. Brain Lang 1993;44:153–64.

Structures posterior to Wernicke's area appear important for predicting recovery. Persisting Wernicke's aphasia correlated with a lesion affecting not only Wernicke's area but also the suprasmarginal gyrus and angular gyrus (i.e., large lesions).

Kertesz A, Sheppard A, MacKenzie R. Localization in transcortical sensory aphasia. Arch Neurol 1982;39:475.

Attempts to resurrect this syndrome.

Kirshner HS, Tanridag O, Thurman L, Wetzell WD Jr. Progressive aphasia without dementia: two cases with focal spongiform degeneration. Ann Neurol 1987;22:527–32.

Neither Pick's nor Alzheimer's disease.

Kleist K. Gehirnpathologie. Barth, Leipzig, 1934.

The standard text of the extreme localizationist viewpoint.

Lebrun Y, Leleux C. The effects of electrostimulation and of resective and stereotactic surgery on language and speech. Acta Neurochir Suppl (Wien) 1993;56:40–51.

Review article.

Lhermitte F, Desi M, Signoret JL, Deloche G. Aphasie kinesthétique associée à un syndrome pseudothalamique. Rev Neurol (Paris) 1980;136:675.

Parietal infarction with disturbed kinesthetic control over vocalizations.

Lichtheim L. On aphasia. Brain 1885;7:433.

Translation from the German of the attempt to expand Wernicke's thesis into the cortical, subcortical, and transcortical varieties of aphasia.

Ludlow CL, Rosenberg J, Fair C et al. Brain lesions associated with nonfluent aphasia fifteen years following penetrating head injury. Brain 1986;109:55–80.

The lesions are large.

Mandell AM, Alexander MP, Carpenter S. Creutzfeldt-Jacob disease presenting as isolated aphasia. Neurology 1989;39:55–8.

The one case with Creutzfeldt-Jakob disease.

Mesulam MM. Slowly progressive aphasia without generalized dementia. Ann Neurol 1982;11:592–8.

Six cases that have renewed interest in the syndrome of primary progressive aphasia.

Metter EJ, Kempler D, Jackson C et al. Cerebral glucose metabolism in Wernicke's, Broca's, and conduction aphasia. Arch Neurol 1989;46:27–34.

Little sign of hemispheral asymmetry in conduction aphasia.

Mohr JP. The vascular basis of Wernicke aphasia. Trans Am Neurol Assoc 1980;105:133–7.

The full syndrome arises from an infarction that involves much of the posterior half of the brain, not a small lesion.

Mohr JP, Pessin MS, Finkelstein S et al. Broca aphasia: pathologic and clinical aspects. Neurology 1978;28:311–24.

The syndrome does not occur acutely, and large lesions are needed for it to occur at all. A few of these cases demonstrated the evanescent features of the dyspraxia.

Mohr JP, Sidman M. Aphasia: behavioral aspects, in Arieti S (ed), American Handbook of Psychiatry. Vol. 4. Basic Books, New York, 1975, pp. 279–98.

Reference to skinnerian thesis of behavior as an explanation for aphasic responses.

Nicholas ML, Helm-Estabrooks N, Ward-Lonergan J, Morgan AR. Evolution of severe aphasia in the first two years post onset. Arch Phys Med Rehabil 1993;74:830–6.

Improvement noted on serial testing for up to 18 months with the greatest changes in the first 6 months.

Rolak LA, Rutecki P, Ashizawa T, Harati Y. Clinical features of Todd's post-epileptic paralysis. J Neurol Neurosurg Psychiatry 1992;55:63–4.

Aphasia was uncommon among 120 patients with generalized tonic-clonic seizures and postictal syndromes.

Sabe L, Leigfuarda R, Starkstein SE. An open-label trial of bromocriptine in nonfluent aphasia. Neurology 1992;42:1637–8.

The small number of patients makes assessment of the outcome difficult.

Takahashi N, Kawamura M, Shinotou et al. Pure word deafness due to left hemisphere damage. Cortex 1992;28:295–303.

The most recent case, with a literature review, using a connectionist model.

Takayama Y, Sugishita M, Kido T et al. A case of foreign accent syndrome without aphasia caused by a lesion of the left precentral gyrus. Neurology 1993;43:1361–3.

The most recent report, this time from Japan.

Tamas LB, Shibasaki T, Horikoshi S, Ohye C. General activation of cerebral metabolism with speech: a PET study. Int J Psychophysiol 1993;14:199–208.

Normal subjects in 150 studies showed strong activation of Broca's area and the medial left temporal lobe during speech.

Wernicke C. Der Aphasische Symptomen complex. Cohn & Weigert, Breslau, 1874.

The original thesis. Available in several translations.

Wernicke C. Lehrbuch der Gehirnkrankheiten. Theo Fischer, Kassel, 1881.

Whurr R, Lorch MP, Nye C. A meta-analysis of studies carried out between 1946 and 1988 concerned with the efficacy of speech and language therapy treatment for aphasic patients. Eur J Disord Commun 1992;27:1–17.

Poor data made analysis difficult.

Willmes K, Poeck K. To what extent can aphasia syndromes be localized? Brain 1993;116:1527–40.

Not to the extent formerly believed.

Wyllie E, Luders H, Murphy D et al. Intracarotid amobarbital (Wada) test for language dominance: correlation with results of cortical stimulation. Epilepsia 1990;31:156–61.

Good correlation in 88 patients between left-sided positive findings in Wada test and left-sided speech function mapped at surgery. Less for right sided.

19

Apraxias and Agnosias

J. C. Gautier and J. P. Mohr

THE APRAXIAS

Apraxia (Greek: *a,* absence or loss; *praxis,* action) traditionally means the inability to carry out gestures (i.e., movements with a meaning or purpose) correctly in the absence of severe sensory, motor, or ataxic disorders and in the absence of dementia, severe aphasia, or agnosia that would preclude the patient from performing or understanding the required task. That apraxia can also disturb even meaningless movements allows it to be regarded as a disorder of motor planning.

Their explanation and syndromic classification is based on the connectionist theory of the aphasias (see Ch. 18). The failure to formulate the plans for movement, known as ideational apraxia, has been likened to the language disorder of sensory or Wernicke's aphasia and is usually seen in parietal lesions. Simply stated, and reviewed in more detail below, failure to perform a task when the command from the examiner is fully comprehended, so-called ideomotor apraxia, has been compared with the syndrome of conduction aphasia in which repeating aloud is impaired, although the patient understands well the words to be spoken. Like conduction aphasia, many of these cases show posterior sylvian lesions, some of which may involve the arcuate fasciculus or the transcallosal pathways that link the two hemispheres. Failure to execute the movements because of impairment in the motor control itself, so-called limb-kinetic or innervatory apraxia, has been considered analogous to the disturbed speech of motor or Broca's aphasia. Many such cases show lesions in the frontal lobe.

These attractive and simply grasped principles have held sway for the better part of a century but do not stand up well to the challenges of detailed examination or carefully construed research protocols, which usually show the disorder is more complex or less eas-

ily accounted for by a single type of disturbance. Because the disturbances are rarely complete, they are more properly described as dyspraxia (Greek: *dys,* bad or difficult; *praxis,* action). Part of the reason for slow progress in this field is the difficulties in separating motor behaviors based on their level of difficulty and body parts involved. Many patients with dyspraxia show the greatest disturbance in skills involving the distal ends of the extremities (hands and feet); the component of the movements involving the axial ends (shoulders and hips) are more normally performed, making the act of throwing a ball seem normal in the shoulder movement, although the hand may be positioned in such a way that it could not grip a ball.

Apraxia is a frequent finding, even a complaint (e.g., difficulties using a fork and knife, locks, gear lever, and pedals). More often, however, it is a finding of a thorough neurologic examination.

Apraxic disorders can show great variability, depending on the situations in which the patient is examined. For instance, patients given combs in the examination room might not use them properly, although they can be seen combing their hair correctly when alone in the bathroom.

What follows is a description of the well-developed syndromes and their usual explanation by location of lesion or cause. Patients with less severe disturbances are common.

Limb Apraxia

Liepmann (H. Liepmann, German neurologist, 1863–1925), who coined the word apraxia in 1900, also proposed a scheme of willed movement realization that has been largely unchallenged since and still accounts for most patients with limb apraxia. To make a gesture on command (e.g., a military salute), one must first evoke (i.e., arouse whatever the neurophysiologic equivalent contains) the "idea" of that gesture, with "idea" meaning the nervous patterns or so-called engrams learned and stored from previous experience). The storage appears to occur in the posterior parts of the parietal lobe. Moreover, the left hemisphere, which is dominant for language, is also dominant for willed action. With rare exceptions, limb apraxia results from lesions of the left hemisphere. Apraxia and aphasia usually coexist, but instances of each without the other have been reported. Fibers likely to belong to the arcuate fasciculus (see Ch. 25) are thought to link the left posterior parietal region to the premotor area (area 6, see Figs. 25-1, 25-5, and 25-6) in the frontal lobe from which they innervate both the ipsilateral motor area and the contralateral premotor area by callosal fibers (Fig. 19-1, see also Fig. 25-8).

Such a scheme can account for the two main kinds of limb apraxia. The first is *ideational apraxia*, in which the patient, when given objects, is assumed to have lost the plan of action, the idea. The type of errors that occur are considered analogous to the literal, verbal, perseverative, and syntactic errors that characterize Wernicke's or sensory aphasia from which ideational apraxia takes its conceptual origin. To the observer, the patient gives the appearance of being naive or un-familiar with the sequence of activities that should occur. This defect is particularly obvious with sequences of gestures (i.e., lighting a candle with matches or lighter; filling and lighting a pipe; or putting a letter in an envelope, sealing, and stamping it). Often, it is obvious even with single gestures (given combs, patients might look at them with perplexity and use them as a toothbrushes; given toothbrushes, they might brush their nails with them.) Ideational apraxia affects the limbs on both sides. The syndrome is generally considered to result from lesions in the region on the left angular gyrus (see Ch. 25, Fig. 25-1).

The second kind of limb apraxia is *ideomotor apraxia.* This is separate from ideational apraxia and shows no disturbance in the plan of gestures because the lesion lies anterior to the angular gyrus, either (1) in the region of the supramarginal gyrus (see Ch. 25, Fig. 25-1), presumably involving the fibers of the left arcuate fasciculus and causing ideomotor apraxia of limbs of both sides; or (2) in the left premotor cortex, where the lesion could have the same consequences (i.e., bilateral apraxia). Most premotor lesions also involve the motor area so that right-sided weakness or paralysis usually masks the occurrence of right-sided apraxia. Alternatively, the corpus callosum causes left-sided limb apraxia (Fig. 19-1, see also Fig. 25-8 and Ch. 25), or the lesions are in the right premotor area, causing left limb apraxia, although, as in (2), an associated paresis from involvement of the motor cortex by the lesion usually masks the left apraxia.

In ideomotor apraxia, the patient has lost the ability to carry out gestures correctly that do not require an object but have a symbolic value (e.g., waving goodbye, making a fist, or a military salute). In other examples, the patient cannot mimic driving a nail with a hammer, dealing cards, slicing bread, or playing the violin. Such gestures are asked by the examiner on command or on imitation. Usually, the patient begins the required gesture awkwardly, which is then interrupted by inadequate motor sequences, arrests, errors of spatial orientation of the limbs, and generally numerous perseverative sequences. The diagnosis is most easily made when the patient shows flawless (or nearly flawless) use of the limbs or objects as part of spontaneous activities, such as shaving or brushing the teeth, before or after failing to execute these activities to dictated commands when the dictated commands are repeated aloud to show adequate comprehension. Preserved ability to select the examiner's example of the proper movements also indicates the patient's knowledge of the desired movements even though the patient does not execute them.

Ideational and ideomotor apraxia usually coexist. When ideomotor apraxia is severe, it can be difficult

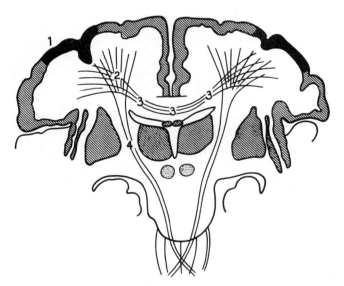

Figure 19-1. Coronal brain view showing the lesions responsible for the main forms of apraxia. (1) Left frontal lobe lesion, damaging the site of control of the right hand, which also interrupts projections to the right hemisphere, causing left-hand ideomotor dyspraxia; (2) subcortical lesion causing right hand weakness and interrupting projections to the right hemisphere; (3) callosal lesion causing left-hand ideomotor dyspraxia, with the right hand normal; (4) deep left hemispheral lesion causing right hand weakness but no left-hand ideomotor dyspraxia. (After Liepmann, 1900.)

to evidence ideational apraxia. Cases are recorded in which the latter was much more severe than the former. Ideomotor apraxia in isolation is usually a transient syndrome. Ideational apraxia, usually a sign of a large lesion is more persistent.

Limb-Kinetic, Melokinetic, or Innervation Apraxia

This condition is characterized by clumsiness of the hand that far exceeds whatever weakness or tone disorder coexists (Greek: *melos*, limb). Movements, such as quickly opposing each finger tip to the thumb, filliping, or passing a coin from the palm to the thumb and index, are maladroit, but the plan of action is not disturbed. Some authors regard innervatory apraxia as a mild pyramidal disorder and not as a true ataxia (for further details, see Ch. 25).

Oral or Orofacial Apraxia

Since the time of Hughlings Jackson in 1878, it has been noticed that patients with right hemiplegia commonly cannot put out their tongue on command while the tongue works normally in drinking and eating. Moreover, the same patients, after drinking can stuck out their tongue to lick their lips. A similar dissociation between the inability to carry out movements on command or imitation and normal movements in the real situation can be shown by asking patients to blow a kiss, to kiss the examiner's hand, to smack, to whistle, or to clear their throat. Commonly, patients cannot kiss the examiner's hand, although they can kiss their own hands. Moreover, after having kissed their own hands several times, patients can blow a kiss once or twice.

The responsible lesions involve the left central operculum and anterior part of the insula, which explains why oral apraxia usually coexists with motor (Broca's) aphasia. Callosal damage does not cause oral apraxia. Lesions of the left posterior parietal regions can, however, disturb sequences of oral movements.

Trunk Apraxia

This disorder, also known in German as *Rumpfapraxie*, is characterized by inadequate positioning of the body in a bed or chair. The term apraxia is traditionally applied to such disorders as constructional apraxia, dressing apraxia, and oculomotor apraxia, although the mechanisms are different from those of limb apraxia. They are nevertheless mentioned here because, whatever their nature, they are frequent and the student must be acquainted with them.

Constructional Apraxia

This is a defect in the ability to use two- or three-dimensional space. The patient is asked to draw on command or copy with a pencil and paper, matches,

or block designs such constructions as a square or a diamond (two dimensions) or a cube or a house (three dimensions). In the latter tasks, the lines indicating perspectives are likely to be the most inadequate. Such patients often also have characteristic difficulties in writing, forming oblique lines, which overlie or even intersect each other. Constructional apraxia results from parietal lesions on either side; right-sided lesions are probably apt to cause more specific disorders. It is generally held that it results basically from disorders of visual processing with defects in spatial organization (see visuospatial agnosia or apractagnosia later).

Dressing Apraxia

This term applies to patients who cannot put on a garment properly (e.g., shirt or coat). Left sensory or motor neglect can be the basic disorder. It can be seen as part of Balint's syndrome (see Ch. 25).

Ocular or Oculomotor Apraxia

Some alert and cooperative patients cannot initiate saccades on command to a novel target entering the visual field. Vestibular-induced saccades and opticokinetic nystagmus are less severely disturbed. The condition can be either acquired, when it results from bilateral frontoparietal lesions, or congenital, when the basic defect is unknown (see also Ch. 25).

Gait Apraxia

This term is sometimes applied to particular disorders of walking that are caused by frontal lesions ("frontal gait") (see Ch. 25).

THE AGNOSIAS

Agnosia (Greek: *gnosis*, knowledge) is a failure of recognition through a sensory channel (a synonym is modality) of a previously known stimulus, although there is no precerebral disorder of the sensory channel and the patient is alert and cooperative. There are theoretically as many agnosias as there are sensory channels, but the visual and auditory ones are the most important clinically.

Agnosia is frequent in clinical practice but often goes unrecognized or misdiagnosed outside neurologic circles because agnosic behavioral disturbances are complex and can be difficult to analyze. Therefore, it is the neurologist's duty to make the correct diagnosis with adequate therapeutic and rehabilitation decisions. Besides, apraxia provides interesting insights on the functioning of the brain and is an active field of research in behavioral neurology.

A schematic account of the treatment of information by the brain helps to grasp the pathophysiology of agnosia. When a sensory stimulus reaches a primary area, it is the final step of a sensation. For instance, the arrival of a visual stimulus in area 17 is the last part of a sensation. Destruction of area 17 causes a loss of sensation (i.e., a homonymous hemianopia). The word *perception* applies to the ensuing procedures that take place beyond the primary area to exploit the information. Adjacent to the primary areas are secondary *unimodal* areas (i.e., that process visual data only), the peri- and parastriate areas 18 and 19 and the adjoining inferolateral occipitotemporal cortex that deal with the awareness of the object (i.e., the stimulus), its shape, volume, color, movement, and so forth. This step of perception is sometimes termed the *discriminative level*. Around the secondary unimodal areas are areas of associative *multimodal* cortex in which the visual stimulus is integrated with auditory, sensory, language, and memory data, and its signification is finally recognized. This *associative level* of perception takes place in the lateral occipitotemporal cortex, perhaps as far as area 39 (the angular gyrus, see Fig. 25-1).

Agnosia, as a whole, can be regarded as a disorder of perception, resulting from lesions anywhere in the sensory and associative areas beyond the primary area. Definitions of agnosia vary. Some authors consider agnosia as both disorders at the discriminative level (apperceptive agnosia) and the associative level (associative agnosia); others term only the associative disorder agnosia. It should be noted that, in humans, verbalizing the name of an object is often considered the final step in recognition. The latter, however, can be achieved without naming the object (e.g., matching an object and its picture or pointing to the picture of a dog among a set of animals when the proposed auditory stimulus is a bark). Therefore, disorders of language, although often associated with agnosic disorders, are not part of agnosia.

Visual Agnosia

In its extreme form, patients do not recognize seen objects, although, they recognize them immediately from typical sounds or through palpation. The diagnosis of visual agnosia implies a thorough neuro-ophthalmologic assessment to detect any major visual disorder. Visual field defects often coexist but are rarely a severe hurdle to visual scanning. The lesions are usually large, injuring both sides of the occipital lobes (see Ch. 25).

Prosopagnosia

This term (Greek, *prosopon*-face) means that the patient does not recognize familiar faces of relatives and friends by sight. These persons are readily identified as soon as they speak. The disorder usually extends to recognition of familiar buildings and landscapes (so-called loss of topographic memory). A deficit in color vision is frequently associated (color agnosia or achromatopsia) not as a part of prosopagnosia but because of the vicinity of the responsible (and lesioned) cortical areas. In most cases, there is a visual field defect, commonly, a left upper quadrantanopia. In almost all well-documented cases of prosopagnosia, there were bilateral inferior parieto-occipital lesions, although there is good evidence that the lesions of the right hemisphere are the most significant. The lesions are usually infarcts in the territory of the posterior cerebral arteries.

Visual Object Agnosia

The term *object* means anything, including living creatures, that can be a visual stimulus. Patients with visual object agnosia cannot recognize any object, including faces, by sight, although they theoretically can recognize them readily from sounds (e.g., voices) or by palpation. Most patients also have alexia. Visual disorientation and optic ataxia are often present (see Balint's syndrome, Ch. 25). The disorder can be preceded by occipital blindness and resolve into prosopagnosia. Most patients have a right homonymous hemianopia. Causal lesions are more extended than in prosopagnosia (i.e., bilateral occipitotemporal damage caused generally by infarction or tumors). Left-sided lesions probably play a leading role.

Simultanagnosia

This is the failure to grasp the meaning of a picture as a whole, although parts of it are recognized. A defect in ocular scanning is the common explanation, although adherents to gestalt psychology see the disturbance as a failure of "simultaneous synthesis." Lesions of the left inferior occipitotemporal cortex are probably responsible.

Alexic Agnosia

This is alexia without agraphia (see Chs. 18 and 25).

Visuospatial Agnosia

Some patients cannot visually recognize their familiar surroundings, famous monuments, or the plans of familiar cities or countries. Usually, there are also elements of prosopagnosia (see above) or visual object agnosia. Most cases had bilateral occipitoparietal lesions. Such patients are likely to show also constructional apraxia, hence the term of apractagnosia.

Auditory Agnosia

Around the primary auditory area (area 41, part of area 42, and Heschl's transverse gyri), there are secondary auditory areas (part of area 42 and area 22,

Figs. 25-5 and 25-6). The latter are connected with occipital and parietal associative cortex and with the insula. Some parts of the auditory cortex are linked with homologous contralateral areas through callosal fibers (see Chs. 25 and 29). Auditory pathways are both crossed and uncrossed so that impulses from one ear are transmitted to both temporal regions. The destruction of auditory areas on one side has generally no clinical consequences, although some sensitive tests can be disturbed.

As a rule, auditory agnosia results from bilateral lesions and happens when the remaining normal auditory cortex is destroyed. It usually begins as a sudden deafness (so-called *cortical deafness,* which is better termed *temporal deafness* because the underlying white matter is also destroyed). The onset is sudden because it is usually due to a second embolic stroke. After a while, patients can hear sounds but cannot recognize their meaning; familiar voices, familial tunes, and meaningful sounds, such as a bleat, a bark, or a locomotive whistle, go unrecognized, although the patients readily identifies pictures of friends, singers, and animals. Amusia is a particular kind of auditory agnosia in which the perception of tones, pitch, timbre, chords, and melodies is especially impaired. Right-sided temporal lesions play a significant causal role.

Tactile Agnosia

Destruction of the primary somatosensory area (the postcentral gyrus) usually causes a contralateral impairment in the ability to identify objects by manipulation, although there are no or minor defects of elementary sensations of touch, pain, and temperature. This is traditionally termed *astereognosis* (see Chs. 23 and 25). Astereognosis must be distinguished from tactile agnosia in that it is the inability to recognize, with either hand, objects by manipulation in the absence of precerebral somatosensory defects. Such patients can tell the shape, the texture, and the nature (e.g., wood, iron, or rubber) of the manipulated object but cannot recognize it.

Cases of pure tactile agnosia are scanty. They should also be separated from left-hand tactile anomia, which is the inability to name objects manipulated by the left hand but which are nevertheless correctly matched with their image. Tactile anomia of the left hand is due to a callosal lesion (see Ch. 25).

Asomatognosias

In asomatognosia, patients have lost the notion of parts or even one-half of their body. This kind of agnosia obviously does not depend on perceptual defects in a sensory modality (see above). Instead, it depends on a disorder of the body image or body scheme. The latter is viewed as a pattern of engrams, stored in the posterior parietal region and built up during infancy and childhood by the regular influx of sensory impulses from the contralateral part of the body (i.e., sensations from the joints and muscles and kinesthetic sensations). This concept explains why, in adults, severance of a limb produces the appearance of a phantom limb (see Ch. 23) and, conversely, why the destruction of the body image causes asomatognosia. Lesions in the right and left hemisphere have no similar clinical consequences.

Unilateral Asomatognosia or Hemiasomatognosia

Asomatognosia for the left side of the body is frequent in acute right-sided posterior parietal lesions, commonly, in strokes in the territory of the right middle cerebral artery, which accounts for the usual coexistence of a left hemiplegia. As a rule, there is a severe sensory defect on the left side of the body. The patient lies with head and eyes strongly turned to the right. Asked to show the right hand, the patient shows the right hand. Asked to show the left hand, the patient shows the right hand again. The patient is impervious to this logical incongruity when the examiner asks how it can be that the right hand is also the left hand. Moreover, when the examiner takes the patient's left hand, shows it to the patient, and asks; "Whose hand is this?", the patient denies that it can be his or hers and answers commonly "yours," "a neighbor's," or "I don't know." This can be disconcerting for students, but this striking disorder only results from the disappearance of the notion of the left part of the body (see also anosognosia). Often, there is also a gross neglect for the left part of the extrapersonal space. There are degrees of severity in hemiasomatognosia; some patients, when their attention is called, can recognize that their left limbs are really theirs, although moments later they return to their inattention toward their left side.

Bilateral Asomatognosia

Lesions of the left (dominant) posterior parietal region cause somatognostic disorders different from those described above. Patients confuse the right and the left side of their and the examiner's body and cannot identify their and the examiner's fingers (finger or digital agnosia). It should be noted that right-left distinction and the identification of individual fingers is among the latest acquisitions in the body image building during childhood. Concomitant with finger agnosia, right-left confusion, agraphia, and acalculia are often present. These four elements are known together as Gerstmann's syndrome (see Ch. 25).

Anosognosia or Denial of Illness

Patients who are blind or deaf as a result of cerebral lesions can be unaware or even deny their trouble, as described by Anton in 1899. Patients who have a left hemiplegia similarly can be unaware or deny their paralysis, a state that Babinski (1914) proposed to term anosognosia (Greek: *nosos*, disease). Patients with a severe Wernicke's aphasia can have logorrhea (Greek: *logos*, speech; *rhein*, to flow) (i.e., being talkative although they are unaware that their jargon is unintelligible). Anosognosia is thus a disorder of diverse cerebral functions. Its mechanism can be approached with the examples of occipital blindness and left hemiplegia. In occipital (so-called cortical) blindness, the cortical areas and the underlying pathways of white matter that support vision are destroyed. Consequently, the notion of vision itself has, as it were, disappeared. Therefore, the notion of blindness is no longer meaningful. In left hemiplegia with hemiasomatognosia (see above) the notion of a left side of the body has disappeared. Therefore, the notion of left paralysis is similarly devoid of meaning, being, it can be said, nonexistent. More generally, when brain regions that provide the basis for a cognitive function disappear, the concept or notion of that function seems to have disappeared from the patient's mind. Admittedly, these basic data do not account for every aspect of anosognosia. For instance, in occipital blindness and left hemiplegia with anosognosia, visual hallucinations or kinesthetic hallucinations, respectively, can also play a role.

ANNOTATED BIBLIOGRAPHY

Basso A, Capitani E, Della Sala S. Ideomotor apraxia: a study of initial severity. Acta Neurol Scand 1987;76: 142–6.

No effects of the right hemisphere lesion on the initial severity of dyspraxia from a left hemispheric lesion.

Cambier J, Signoret JL, Bolgert F. L'agnosie visuelle pour les objets: conceptions actuelles. Rev Neurol (Paris) 1989; 145:640–5.

New views on visual object agnosia with a traditional basis.

Cambier J. In Sabouraud O, Masson C, Cambier J. Un trouble de la vision et du langage soudainement apparu chez un homme de 70 ans. Confrontation de la Salpêtrière, mai 1990. Rev Neurol (Paris) 1992;148:302–10.

An excellent update on visual agnosia and cerebral dominance.

Damasio AR, Eslinger P. The agnosias. In Asbury AK, McKhann GM, McDonald WI (eds). Diseases of the Nervous System. Clinical Neurobiology. WB Saunders, Philadelphia, 1992.

A review of the main kinds of agnosia.

De Renzi E. The apraxias. In Asbury AK, McKhann GM, McDonald WI (eds). Diseases of the Nervous System. Clinical Neurobiology. WB Saunders, Philadephia, 1986.

A lucid and apt update on limb apraxia.

Gazzaniga M, Bogen J, Sperry R. Dyspraxia following division of the cerebral commissures. Arch Neurol 1967;16: 606.

A modern classic for dyspraxia after surgical section of the corpus callosum.

Gerstmann J. Zur lokaldiagnoschen Verwertharbeit des Syndroms: Finger-agnosie, Rechto-Links Störung, Agraphie, Akalkulie. Jahresber Psychiat Neur. 1932;48: 135–43.

The Seminal paper on the full syndrome.

Geschwind N. Disconnection syndromes in animals and man. Brain 1965;88:237–94; 585–644.

The high point of the connectionist school.

Liepmann H. Das Krankheitsbild der Apraxie. Monatsschr Psychiat Neurol 1900;8:15–44; 102–132; 181–187.

Another neurologic classic, laying out the basis for the syndromes of apraxia.

Liepmann H, Maas O. Fall von linksseitiger Agraphie und Apraxie bei rechtseitiger Lähmung. Zeitschr Psychol Neurol 1907;10:214.

One of the few cases tested in detail.

Mesulam MM. Principles of Behavioral Neurology. 3rd Ed. FA Davis, Philadelphia, 1987.

A good review book.

20

Syndromes of the Nondominant Hemisphere

J. P. Mohr and J. C. Gautier

A century ago, the principle became established that one hemisphere, almost always the left, was dominant for language. This hemisphere also controlled the more skilled, right, hand. The designation *nondominant* refers to the hemisphere opposite the one dominant for language. In most people, the nondominant hemisphere is the right. For decades, the right hemisphere was not thought to have any such skills, and for a considerable time it was not thought to have any special high cerebral functions. It was thought to exist mainly to govern contralateral (usually left-sided) motor, somatosensory, auditory, and visual responses, similar to that done by the left hemisphere for the right side of the body and space. In the current century, however, studies exploring higher functions of the nondominant hemisphere found it dominant for many other behaviors, leading among them responses involving spatial operations and those having a high degree of emotional content. These studies helped in the acceptance of dichotomous hypotheses of brain function, which have long been popular. Taken to extremes, the left hemisphere was seen as concerned with language, writing, and calculation, but lacking in emotional attributes—a soulless computer—and the right was activated by emotionally rich experiences, including music, a sense of design and form, experiences difficult to put into words—in short, the more artistic side of the brain. Some hypotheses formulated a unitary function for the nondominant hemisphere, with all the disturbances envisioned as failure to respond to the side of space opposite to the brain lesion, loss of some internal spatial organization for the extrapersonal world, and the like.

Carefully reasoned hypotheses have been put forward of the existence of a neural network that includes a reticular element (providing arousal and vigilance), a parietal element (providing sensory and spatial mapping), a frontal element (providing the motor programs for exploration), and a limbic element (providing affective recall for emotional experiences). Measurements with the use of magnetic resonance imaging have found the right temporal lobe to be consistently larger than the left, which suggests an asymmetry that could have functional significance. No other gross asymmetries have been found that favor the right side.

Despite such attractive hypotheses, more studies have shown that the two hemispheres are not so separate in their specialized functions. Despite differences in the size of the lobes in the two hemispheres, such asymmetries do not easily translate to functional differences measured in such variables as limb size. Leg size and agility in soccer players have shown no asymmetry, suggesting that, for motor functions, the two sides could be considered equal. Recent work has also shown that the nondominant hemisphere, although not highly skilled in tasks that involve reading, writing, and spelling, plays some role in high-level language function. Poor performance has been shown on tasks that require comprehension and abstraction of content of narrative material. Furthermore, dichotic listening (a headphone on each ear receives competing auditory stimuli, usually spoken words) has shown by cortical-evoked potentials that the right hemisphere is activated in recovering aphasic patients and that motor function of the right hemisphere is involved in patients who are recovering from left hemisphere lesions and who improve in the performance of right limb movements.

Leaving aside the issues of some shared function between the two hemispheres, there are several types of disorders so often described from the nondominant hemisphere as to justify their separate consideration. The first subject, neglect, typifies the difficulties of trying to describe a syndrome (i.e., a collection of findings explained by the same causative lesions or disease) that is unique to the nondominant hemisphere.

NEGLECT FOR STIMULI FROM CONTRALATERAL SPACE

Impaired response to stimuli in contralateral space is a common finding from lesions of either hemisphere, although the bulk of the literature on this subject is from patients with right-hemisphere lesions. Some forms of impaired response can be attributed to destruction of the sensory pathway, as in deafness, anesthesia for the opposite side of the body (hemianesthesia) after destruction of the thalamic sensory nuclei, or contralateral blindness (hemianopia) from destruction of the visual radiations or calcarine cortex. Failure to respond to stimuli that occur in fields of space where stimuli cannot be detected (e.g., due to hemianopia) is not neglect. However, numerous situations exist in neurology in which the patient does not respond or shows a reduced rate or extent of response to one type of stimulus and yet responds normally to another. This situation gives rise to the impression that the stimulus that failed to elicit a response was either insufficient or neglected. The healthy nervous system has the ability to suppress a response to detected stimuli or even to fail to detect stimuli altogether. This occurs in athletes determined to catch a ball who suppress the distracting simultaneous presence of a competitor in the same field of vision, and in soldiers unaware they have been wounded until their life-threatening moments of battle have passed. Trained voluntary or untrained involuntary suppression of responses to stimuli have been feebly explained by reference to focused attention or other paraphysiologic terms, which suggests there is a system of rank ordering of stimuli of which the brain is capable and that enough "attention" directed toward one stimulus could lead to the suppression of others. How attention is activated and directed, how stimuli are rank ordered, and even what attention is or what site or sites in the brain are involved have been subjects that have occupied many neurologists for many generations. Suffice it here to say that the authors recommend adherence to the behavioral and lesion evidence and resort as little as possible to terms that are difficult to define operationally.

When the brain has suffered an acute hemispheric lesion, it is a common early finding that responses to stimuli in contralateral space are temporarily less easily evoked. There is impaired turning to the affected side of space in response to auditory stimuli, faulty reaching into space, faulty localization of an offending noxious cutaneous stimulus, and often faulty reading aloud or naming of those parts of an object that lie partly or mainly in the affected side of space.

Impaired response to stimuli from the opposite side of space occurs commonly in the hours after a focal seizure and for days to weeks after an acute frontal or parietal lobe lesion. Stroke is the most common cause, and the lesions vary from being superficial over the upper convexity or deep in the white matter or basal ganglia. There is often absent blink to a threatening movement from the affected side of space, giving the impression of a hemianopia, which is actually present in some cases when the lesion involves the visual pathways. Auditory stimuli from either side often provoke turning to the side opposite the affected side of space, giving the impression of hemifield deafness. Pinch to the affected side produces arousal, but the free hand from the normal side gropes inaccurately over the affected side, failing to localize the noxious stimulus. These signs of neglect are remarkably transient, usually fading within 1 week. They last longer only in really large multilobar lesions.

In some deep lesions, there is an underutilization of one side without defects in strength, a condition known as *motor neglect*. In most such patients, there appears to be weakness on the affected side of the body (hemiparesis), yet exhortation, strenuous prodding, and other forms of activation may suffice to show that the limbs can move with almost normal power. There is usually a lack of a spontaneous placing reaction, such as failure to place the hand in the lap or on the arm of a chair when sitting, letting it instead drag down beside the body; delayed or insufficient assumption of correct postures, resulting in heavy falls to the affected side with no attempts to minimize the effect of the fall by reaching out or correcting the balance; impaired automatic withdrawal reaction to pain; poor excursions of the limb necessary to achieve a movement, such as touching the nose, with the patient instead leaning the head forward to compensate for failure to bring the finger far enough up. This disturbance may occur in the absence of clinically detectable sensory disturbance or hemiparesis.

Lesions located in the dominant hemisphere have been shown to cause a diminished response to verbal stimuli in the opposite space. This syndrome, known as *verbal neglect*, has been shown to be separate from disturbances in vision, somatosensory function, or motor function. It was first shown in patients who, when seated before a visual display, showed errors when the choices involved words or pictures that the patient found the most difficult to name or write. In such instances, responses were made less frequently and with more errors to choices on the right-hand side of the display. When the test materials were the type easily named by the patient, such as short words, little or no evidence of neglect for the right side of space was noted. When incorrect words were placed on the unaffected side, the patients, who were aware the choices on the unaffected side were incorrect, turned to and responded to choices on the affected side, indicating the neglect effect was not obligatory but could be subjected to experimental manipulation. This form of neglect is commonly encountered when patients with aphasia are tested and most often is shown as right-sided hemidyslexia for longer words, with the patient reading short words aloud and for comprehension by misreading the right-hand end of the longer words. This hemineglect occurs even in the absence of clinically evident hemianopia. The existence of verbal neglect indicates that neglect, per se, is not a result of nondominant hemisphere lesions alone.

Impaired response to contralateral space may also be reflected in failure to touch, name, or copy all or some of those elements of a stimulus or set of stimuli that lie in the affected side of space. Known as *unilateral spatial neglect,* the defect is commonly found in right hemispheric lesions and shown by the common tests of bisecting lines far to the right of center, indicating all or part of the left-hand side is treated as not present. Some or all parts of the right-hand side may be treated as the entire line; hence, the bisection is one-half of that portion of the line. In tests of copying drawings, one side (usually the left) of a figure is not drawn. In reading or picture description, the left-hand side is not read or described. When the left-hand side of the word contains letters essential for the interpretation of the word, all or a portion of the word read may be from the right-hand end of the word and a word such as smother may be read as mother, other, her, or even er. When a thematic picture contains the important elements in the affected side of space, say, a stove whose pots are boiling, a description limited to the right-sided elements will not result in a correct interpretation of the picture. Disturbances such as these could be misinterpreted by the observer as signs of dyslexia, failure of concept formation, refusal to acknowledge threatening situations, and other misinterpretations, a warning against making too much of a few uncontrolled observations. For frontal lesions, the unilateral spatial neglect is more evident on tasks that require the patient to explore space by, say, pointing out each occurrence of the letter "f" on a sheet of lines that contain letters typed in random order. This disturbance is less evident in the bisecting lines task; the reverse appears to be the case for posterior lesions.

In large lesions of the dominant hemisphere, aphasia is so prominent that it is often difficult for the patient to perform tests that detect the presence of hemineglect. In the nondominant hemisphere, large lesions, affecting frontal and parietal, lobes at times extending into the deep white matter and basal ganglia, seem to cause a state in which the patient appears unaware of the presence of disease and sometimes unaware of the left side of the body, a state known as hemisomatognosia. In a few instances, anosognosia has been dissociated from any elementary neurologic deficits or neglect. Its course is often short, lasting at most a few months. The striking nature of the denial of illness or of affected body parts, occasionally more striking than the motor or sensory impairment, has been seen as the extreme example of hemineglect but has also fueled many imaginative views of brain function, including the loss of a putative internal concept of the body image, which resides in the right hemisphere, or as a disconnection of the right parietal from the left parietal lobe, which prevents the verbal hemisphere from describing the presence of disease in the nondominant side (see also Ch. 19).

Other syndromes that commonly accompany hemineglect include a tendency for the patient to respond to questions directed at other people, which is taken as a sign of faulty social awareness, and impersistence, a finding from lesions of either hemisphere but somewhat more common from right-sided lesions. The patient does not continue (i.e., is impersistent), in sustained motor tasks requested by the examiner, such as keeping the eyes closed, keeping the eyes turned to one side, keeping the tongue out, keeping the teeth bared, and so forth. Typically, the behavior ceases after a few seconds and ceases repeatedly despite the examiner's request that the patient continue. Its occurrence correlates with the severity of the hemiparesis, contralateral neglect, constructional apraxia, and even anosognosia, which is usually evident in the larger lesions.

DISORDERS OF SPATIAL RESPONDING

Although neglect is found from lesions of either hemisphere, and may be more or less easily demonstrated depending on the testing, some forms of disorders of spatial responding seem thus far to be more common from lesions of the nondominant hemisphere and may exist apart from the more general disorders, which is easily explained by reduced responding to the opposite side of space. They seem not merely to be subtle forms of hemineglect because they exist even when there appears to be prompt and adequate reaching into contralateral space and in the absence of faulty line bisection and other signs of hemineglect.

Disturbances in judging the position of stimuli in space have been found from lesions of either hemisphere, but the most severe have been from lesions of the posterior half of the right hemisphere. These observations apply to all of the major sensory modalities, including estimation of the position of a visual stimulus, a source of sound, or the spatial position and orientation of objects that can be palpated or found by touch on a flat or three-dimensional matrix. Disagreements still exist among investigators as to the uniqueness of the disorder in right hemispheric lesions. Some maintain that the presence of a language disorder from left-hemisphere disease prevents the full documentation of a disorder of comparable severity in left hemispheric lesions. Others are certain the right hemisphere contains special capacities for spatial responding that make right-sided lesions show a more severe disturbance.

Constructional dyspraxia is the best known of the forms of faulty spatial responding from right-hemisphere lesions. The disorder occurs in the placement of stimuli in space and under test conditions of drawing or assembly of two- or three-dimensional shapes to a dictated command ("draw a cube") or model ("copy this drawing" or "make a tower with these sticks"). A large range of tests have been used, including copying drawings of simple to complex figures, assembling puzzles and building three-dimensional models, and even tasks that involve no contact with a stimulus but a description of the effects of imagined rotations. In the simplest example, a familiar shape, such as a flat drawing of a five-pointed star, is rendered with gross asymmetry and may be missing a point, with lines that do not intersect or pass across each other, in extreme cases yielding a cluster of marks that have no resemblance to a star. In the more subtle cases, a series of building blocks used to construct a three-dimensional form from a two-dimensional picture is merely simplified and missing one or more small parts. Drawings from patients with left-hemisphere damage seem simplified and primitive, with fewer details than expected. Those from patients with right-hemisphere lesions usually show elaborate attention to detail with many duplicated lines. Although poor drawing and building of three-dimensional structures can be explained by weakness, sensory disturbance, failure to respond to the opposite side of space, and even to poor education, when such variables are taken into consideration, lesions of the right side, especially the parietal lobe and of large size, are the most constant findings. Constructional dyspraxia has been described as an isolated finding, sometimes to the surprise of the clinician, who had detected few findings in the general neurologic examination.

Apraxia for dressing, a common disorder, may be a form of constructional dyspraxia, which is brought to clinical attention because dressing is the more likely behavior to be observed in daily life than is the building of complex figures from models. The disturbance is seen as faulty positioning of articles of clothing that are to be placed on body parts, the most glaring disorder being orienting a coat so arms can be put in the sleeves. The items of clothing may be mispositioned for any of the main dimensions, top to bottom, back to front, or right to left. This disorder has been seen almost entirely from right-hemisphere lesions, usually large lesions in which both constructional and dressing apraxia appear. Dressing apraxia is rare in isolation.

A more global disorder of disorientation in extrapersonal space has frequently been described from right-sided lesions. The lesions were posterior, and some were associated with left-sided visual field disturbance. The small number of patients with spatial disturbance that seems to occur as an isolated sign have had lesions that affect the fimbria of the right hippocampus and adjacent subcallosal mesial occipital region and have even been free of visual field disturbance. Some instances of similar disorder have been found in left hemispheral infarction but in association with more global disorders of recall evident on conversational testing, a disorder not present in the right hemispheric lesions. The remarkable feature, puzzling and annoying to the victim and those in close association, is the failure to be able to recall which way to turn and what path to take for even the shortest routes, such as from the living room to a bathroom in a small apartment lived in for decades, with similar disturbance for longer routes and a failure to learn new routes, such as from the bed to bathroom in a hospital room. Patients may volunteer they do not know the way and are capable of asking others, so they are not lacking in awareness of the disturbance. In setting out, patients typically stop within a few steps of embarking from the starting point and act uncertain as to which way to walk or turn. There is rarely any plan of exploration, with the hesitancy not merely like that in someone who has forgotten but also like that in someone who is uncertain how to go about finding. What the defect represents is not certain. It is not only a failure to name or recall prior experiences at sight, a so-called agnosia, but the difficulty in making plans for exploring space and failing to turn in one direction or another has raised speculations that there may be an impairment of some form of internal spatial representation of the external world.

Prosopognosia, a disturbance in naming people at sight, could be a related condition, likened to a spatial disturbance for topography of the face. It often occurs from the same posterior right cerebral lesions. However, for some workers, it represents a loss of visual "configural processing," a loss of a learned skill that enables immediate identification of individual members of a class without conscious visuospatial analysis or remembering. Too few reports have appeared to know under what conditions it may occur in isolation.

DISORDERS OF EMOTIONAL BEHAVIOR

Perhaps it is the aphasia in left-hemisphere lesions that prevents precise delineation of other disorders that require adequate language testing to explore, but a state of pure confusion and delirium frequently occurs in right-sided lesions, especially those of the temporal lobe. Some efforts have been made to equate the disordered interaction with the environment to the illogical and semantic errors in Wernicke's aphasia from lesions of the left temporal lobe. Whether comparable to semantic aphasias or not, the deranged content of spoken responses by patients with nondominant hemisphere disease usually reflects poor immediate and retrograde memory, preoccupation with trivia and easy distractability by trivial stimuli, illogical associations, gross inaccuracies in their accounts of events, and misassessments of prowess; the most glaring examples are seen in anosognosia. More difficult to counter are delusions, compulsive preoccupations, phobias, paranoias, and fantasies, which in many cases tax the patience of the family. Emotional lability with easily provoked crying is common. Less common are hallucinations, terrifying dreams, and periods of changed sleep-wake cycles with insomnia and restless pacing around and, at other times, sluggishness. That such syndromes could be labeled confusion, inattention, and even psychosis is easily understood.

In some patients with nondominant hemisphere lesions, conversational history-taking reveals not only illogical associations and gross inaccuracies but also confabulation (i.e., statements or answers to questions that appear to be completely fabricated and inaccurate). In some instances, the responses appear to be mere exaggerations or boasts and in others, what would be considered lies from a normal person. But in the most striking cases, some of the confabulated claims are physically impossible, such as a patient with severe hemiparesis saying he climbed through the window. Confabulation has many features, some of which are part of anosognosia. Another is reduplication, usually for place, in which patients claim to be somewhere they are not, such as at home when a quick look around would convince anyone else they are in a hospital. Extreme degrees of confabulation are rare because there are usually obvious associated disorders, including major motor or sensory syndromes, anosognosia, and amnestic states.

Another common finding in conversational interaction with patients with nondominant lesions is a flat, monotonic speech, which contrasts with the expected emotional tone. In some instances, this is reversed, and the speech is emotionally labile when the content of the words would usually predict a matter-of-fact intonation. This change in speech rhythm, phrasing, pitch, and stress on words and syllables has been called *dysprosody* and has been found from lesions of either hemisphere. In left-hemisphere lesions, the disturbance is more obvious in erroneous stress on syllables, which makes the voice sound as if the speaker is unfamiliar with the rules of pronounciation of the language; crude phrasing of clauses, with misemphasis on the wrong word in a clause; and faulty intonation of questions, commands, and statements, leaving the listener uncertain whether a question or statement is being uttered. For those with right-hemisphere lesions, dysprosody affects mainly the emotional content. The emotionally deranged speech is often found associated with other signs of underlying emotional flattening or lability because such patients frequently have difficulty interpreting whether a smile or frown means happy or sad. They frequently do not detect irony, sarcasm, and emotional content in words heard and often do not repeat the emotional tone in sentences they are asked to repeat aloud, a state termed *spontaneous affective dysprosody*.

AMUSIA

This infrequently studied problem harks back to the days in neurology when highly circumscribed centers were thought to exist, each unique for mediation of certain behaviors, such as reading, writing, and musical ability. Although many patients said to show amusia have been reported who have nondominant hemisphere lesions, no clear relationship has been found between disturbances in singing or comprehension of music and a given lesion location. However, such claims keep alive the notions referred to earlier of the nondominant hemisphere as the artistic side of the brain.

ANNOTATED BIBLIOGRAPHY

Agre JC, Baxter TL. Musculoskeletal profile of male collegiate soccer players. Arch Phys Med Rehabil 1987;68: 147–50.

No significant differences were found between the dominant and nondominant legs in flexibility or strength.

Benowitz LI, Moya KL, Levine DN. Impaired verbal reasoning and constructional apraxia in subjects with right hemisphere damage. Neuropsychologia 1990;28:231–41.

Poor abstraction of information from narrative passages was as prevalent and as severe in magnitude as constructional apraxia in 41 cases.

Berthier ML, Starkstein SE, Leiguarda R et al. Transcortical aphasia. Importance of the nonspeech dominant hemisphere in language repetition. Brain 1991;114:1409–27.

Repeating aloud may be mediated by the surviving nondominant hemisphere.

Bisiach E, Cornacchia L, Sterzi R, Vallar G. Disorder perceived auditory lateralization after lesions of the right hemisphere. Brain 1984;107:37–52.

Posterior temporal lesions.

Bogousslavsky J, Regli F. Response to next patient stimulation: a right hemisphere syndrome. Neurology 1988;38: 1225–7.

Patients with major right hemisphere lesions often respond to questions directed at others.

Brain WR. Visual disorientation with special reference to the lesions of the right hemisphere. Brain 1941;64:244.

The first description.

Brust JCM. Music and language. Brain 1980;103:367.

No consistent location found with amusia.

Caplan LR, Kelly M, Kase CS et al. Infarcts of the inferior division of the right middle cerebral artery: mirror image of Wernicke's aphasia. Neurology 1986;36:1015.

Posterior right temporal lesions are more likely to produce acute confusion than posterior right parietal lesions.

Jack CR Jr, Gehring DG, Sharbrough FW et al. Temporal lobe volume measurement from MR images: accuracy and left right asymmetry in normal persons. J Comput Assist Tomogr 1988;12:21–9.

The right temporal lobe is larger.

Kleist K. Gehirnpathologie. Barth, Leipsig, 1934.

Early descriptions of constructional dyspraxia, which emphasized that the defect is in the act of the construction and is not explained by weakness or perceptual disturbance.

Landis T, Regard M, Bliestle A, Kleihues P. Prosopagnosia and agnosia for noncanonical views. An autopsied case. Brain 1988;111:1287–97.

An autopsied case with a recent large right temporo-occipital infarction in the posterior cerebral territory showed that bilateral involvement was not necessary for prosopagnosia.

Levine DN, Calvanio R. Prosopagnosia: a defect in visual configural processing. Brain Cogn 1989;10:149–70.

Prosopagnosia is a loss of visual configural processing, a learned skill that enables immediate identification of individual members of a class without conscious visuospatial analysis or remembering.

Meerwaldt JD, Van Harskamp F. Spatial orientation in right hemisphere infarction. J Neurol Neurosurg Psychiatry 1982;45:586.

The most severe disturbances come from right hemispheral damage.

Mori E, Yamadori A. Acute confusional state and acute agitated delirium: occurrence after infarction in the middle cerebral artery territory. Arch Neurol 1987;4:1139.

Acute confusion in 25 right-hemisphere cases and acute delirium in 6.

Papanicolaou AC, Moore BD, Deutsch G et al. Evidence for right hemisphere involvement in recovery from aphasia. Arch Neurol 1988;45:1025–9.

Right hemisphere is activated in recovering aphasic patients.

Ross ED. Sensory specific and fractional disorders of recent memory in man: isolated loss of visual recent memory. Arch Neurol 1980;37:193.

Spatial disorientation and prosopagnosia may represent a loss of internal spatial representation of the external world.

Roth M. Disorders of body image caused by lesions of the right parietal lobe. Brain 1949;72:89.

Dressing and constructional dyspraxia concur in right-hemisphere lesions.

Villa G, Gainotti G, De Bonis C. Constructive disabilities in focal brain damaged patients. Influence of hemispheric side, locus of lesion and coexistent mental deterioration. Neuropsychologia 1986;24:497–510.

In 185 cases, the right parietal lesion was the common finding after all other disturbances were controlled for.

Zoccolotti P, Antonucci G, Judica A et al. Incidence and evolution of the hemineglect disorder in chronic patients with unilateral right brain damage. Int J Neurosci 1989; 47:209–16.

Gradual reduction in the severity of hemineglect occurs over time, beginning at 3 months from the onset.

21

Memory Disorders

J. P. Mohr and J. C. Gautier

Memory, a term derived directly from Latin *(memoria)* is defined rather simplistically as a faculty by which prior experience is recalled. Like other faculties, such as vision, memory can be tested, but unlike other faculties, memory is not strictly bound to one sensory modality and appears to have different properties according to the task. All memories involve some form of learning, whether deliberate (trained or conditioned learning) or accidental (unplanned or single-exposure learning) and whether of an acquired skill (procedural memory) or a prior experience that is only to be described in words (declarative memory).

The term *amnesia* (from the Greek for loss of the memory) describes the loss of memory, whether of an acquired skill or the power to describe or agree with descriptions of prior experiences. In neurology, different terms are used according to the form taken by the amnestic state, an acknowledgment that procedure and declarative memory are not often lost together or to the same degree. Although a form of amnesia, the loss of an acquired motor skill is usually not described as an amnesia but rather as an apraxia (from the Greek for loss of performance) (see Ch. 19). The loss of the previous skill of recognizing objects is seen as an agnosia (from the Greek for loss of knowledge) (see Ch. 19). Among the forms of declarative amnesia, the selective loss of certain words, usually names, especially the names of persons and things, is often referred to as an amnestic aphasia because it seems to occur in the absence of a general disorder in declarative memory. It is the defective capacity to describe prior experience that has attracted the most clinical attention because so many brain diseases, acute or chronic and sudden or progressive, seem to cause a similar disorder.

How declarative memory is acquired has been difficult to investigate. Although memories are based on some form of sensory experience, and the more important would seem to be the more readily recalled, little is known as to why some passing experiences are easily recalled and some powerful and emotionally important ones are difficult to retain despite intense efforts. A better understanding of memory processes ultimately hinges on studies of patients with brain diseases. The study of surprisingly few patients, mainly in the chronic stages of an illness that began months or years before, forms the basis for much of the current hypotheses of human amnesia. As a group, these patients have shown a severe impairment in acquiring new declarative memory (anterograde amnesia) and perform far better on tasks of procedural memory. Their anterograde amnesia usually contrasts with their far better declarative memory for events before the illness. In some, there is a loss of declarative memory for events before the illness (retrograde amnesia) to a varying degree for periods from days to as long as decades before. Currently, popular hypotheses postulate the separation of immediate recall memory from recent and distant memory, based on specific anatomic substrates. As discussed below, in the acute phase of illness, the retrograde amnesia may be as striking as the anterograde, and only with time does the retrograde amnesia shrink toward the time of the onset of the illness, in many instances never fully reaching that time in the patient's life history.

BRAIN STRUCTURES AFFECTED IN MEMORY DISORDERS

Anatomy

Lesions that affect the hippocampus, its projections into the fornix, the structures near which the fornix passes to reach its precommissural bed nuclei (including the septum and anterior commissure), and the medial thalamic nuclei are the major sites of diseases that cause declarative amnestic states (see Figs. 25-1 and

25-2). Lying along the lower and inner face of the temporal lobes, the hippocampus gradually condenses into the fimbria more posteriorly and blends into the fornix. The fornix, passing over the thalamus and along the septum, ends in its precommissural (anterior commissure) bed nucleus. The fimbria of the hippocampus also projects behind and around the corpus callosum as the isthmus of the gyrus fornicatus. A final portion becomes the indusium griseum, the shrunken gray and white matter remnants that pass anteriorly along the length of the callosum. Connections also tie them to the medial thalamus and, in the lower portion, to the subthalamus (including the mammillary bodies) and anterior commissure.

These structures (see Figs. 25-1 and 25-2) share rather distinctive histologic attributes. Compared with the six distinctively differing cell layers of the convexity (neocortex, see Ch. 25), the histologic findings of the hippocampus and adjacent region differ to a degree that this area earned the Greek name of the other cortex, allocortex. Here the six layers are not so easily found. Instead, there appear almost to be three: the upper cellular layer filled with clumps of cells (islands of Calleja), a broad intermediate cellular zone, and another deeper layer with large pyramidal cells, some of which are the largest cells in the human brain. The hippocampus (from the Greek for sea horse) was named for its spiral appearance on cut section.

P. Broca (French surgeon and anthropologist, 1824–80) suggested the name, *grand lobe limbique*, for the anteroinferomedial cerebrum, including the basal olfactory region, uncus and hippocampus, medial temporal lobe, posterior inferior surface of the frontal lobe, anterior insula, supracallosal region, and anterior perforated space. Visceral responses have early been found from electrical stimulation of the medial temporal region. Lesions in animals and humans had long been noted to cause a change in behavior, especially toward a more docile state. Animals appeared to have lost their usual wariness, exploring fearlessly and seeming to fail to learn from aversive experiences, a clinical state later noted by Klüver and Bucy (see below). In 1937, J. W. Papez (American anatomist, 1883–1958) postulated that primitive emotional experiences are projected to the neocortex from the fimbria of the hippocampus, the neurons of which project through the fornix to the cingulum, forward to the precommissural bed nuclei and to the medial thalamus, and thence to the mammillary bodies. The whole forms a functionally related *limbic system,* so named because the structures were located around the edge or limbus of the medial wall of the hemisphere. Although originally conceived as mediating visceral function, amnesia became recognized as one of the effects of lesions in this "system."

Amnestic states may also include other forms of disturbed memory, apart from the more often-tested impairment in descriptive recall, and the lesions associated with these syndromes differ. Although the difficulty recalling words has some bearing on the aphasias (see Ch. 18), this disorder is one of failure to recall the experience, as reflected in conversational testing. Less is known of the anatomic lesions that underlie these disorders, but they share a loss or impairment in the exercise of a previously learned behavior, whether in naming or action. Some failures to recall what has been previously learned apply to the recall of names for people, objects, or events, a disorder termed *amnestic dysnomia*. This disorder has been reported from lesions that affect the undersurface of the temporal lobe in the dominant hemisphere without certain involvement of the hippocampus and its projections.

Other disorders involve complex motor behavior. The simplest of this type is the loss or impairment in previously acquired skills, such as the use of tools or in complex movements (*apraxia,* see Ch. 19). Dyspraxias have been most often reported from lesions near the primary motor regions over the convexity of either hemisphere, far from the limbic system.

Some forms of impairments seem to be specific, such as the loss or impairment in finding one's way along previously familiar routes, as in walking to work along city streets (*amnestic spatial disorientation*). Such disorientation has occurred from a lesion limited to the isthmus of the gyrus fornicatus (extension of the fimbria of the hippocampus) in the nondominant hemisphere.

A distinctive syndrome in monkeys (and rarely in humans) has also been described that features failure to exercise caution in situations that previous experience would have taught the animal to consider dangerous (Klüver-Bucy syndrome). Bilateral anterior temporal lobe lesions, usually on the inferior surface, is the frequently reported lesion site. Hypersexuality is also part of the picture.

In animals, cerebellar lesions produce impairment in acquiring new skills, a form of memory disorder, but such lesions have not yet been reported to produce clinically evident memory disorders in humans. The existence of these and more varieties of amnestic states clearly indicate that there is more to memory disorders than the simple impairment in declarative recall usually relied on by the clinician in assessing amnesia.

Lesion Uni- or Bilaterality

A few famous instances of memory disorder with autopsy documentation of bilateral medial temporal or thalamic lesions pointed to a clinicoanatomic correlation as far back as the turn of the century. Awareness of such effects became acute after neurosurgeons resected diseased hippocampi as treatment for intractable temporal lobe epilepsy and thereby produced several striking examples of a severe memory disorder that seemed to be present in the absence of other disorders.

At first, it was believed that bilateral lesions were necessary to produce amnesia (which was not then separated into declarative and procedural forms), but after autopsy evidence that an acute amnestic state could occur from unilateral infarction, the principle was established that unilateral lesions could cause an amnestic state. In some cases, the amnestic state partially improved after some weeks or months. From surgical experience through the corpus callosum into the third ventricle, it has also become evident that an amnestic state can result from a single lesion at one of many sites along the fornix or septum. High-quality brain imaging has even demonstrated memory disorders from small unilateral medial thalamic lesions.

Because many naturally occurring lesions such as hemorrhage or infarction, penetrating head wounds, infections, tumors, and the like are often not small or discrete lesions, much uncertainty still remains in regard to the minimum lesion size and location that may cause the maximum syndrome in declarative memory. Hemorrhagic lesions from metabolic injuries to the periaqueductal gray matter of the midbrain, the medial thalamus, and the mammillary bodies in Wernicke-Korsakoff syndrome have added these structures to the list.

CLINICAL EXAMINATION

Except for the defect in declarative memory and an annoying redundancy, the patient in an acute amnestic state would pass for normal. Reading comprehension, auditory comprehension, writing and spoken speech, simple calculation, and skilled motor acts reveal no significant abnormalities. Conversation is easily initiated, but the content is often filled with repeated remarks and questions, only to have the topic brought up again (broken-record syndrome), creating the impression the patient is preoccupied or absentminded. The ease of speaking and seeming confidence in answers may not reveal the amnesia until an answer to a simple question of recent events produces a surprising gross inaccuracy. Although recent memory seems impossible to recall, distant memories are recalled somewhat better, although not perfectly.

When tested within minutes and hours after onset, retrograde amnesia in some patients is found to extend back for decades. Those who are dead may be called on as if they were alive. Loved ones on the scene may not be recognized because of their current age

or lack of association with the patient decades before. Strikingly emotional experiences a person would never be expected to forget, such as wartime wounds, deaths of close family members, and the like, may be forgotten, even denied. Conversation usually reveals little of the concern or wariness expected from those aware they are in a test setting and often shows little insight into the existence of amnesia. Failure in testing is often shrugged off as unimportant. When pressed to explain the failures, the patient may offer circumlocutions (attempts to provide some descriptive attributes of the missing word or experience) and confabulations (fabricated responses, with some related to the subject), resort to a lame excuse, complain the testing is irrelevant, or give a testimonial of former prowess, all gambits used by normal people.

The annoying conversational redundancy eventually disappears. The time frame for the shortest syndrome (transient global amnesia, discussed later) is measured in hours, but for other states, the conversational redundancy may last days. Over weeks to months, the extreme retrograde amnesia shrinks gradually back toward the present but usually does not reach the time of onset, leaving an island of permanently lost time. Later, a general awareness of poor memory may be volunteered.

Bedside Testing

Neurologists typically rely on the accuracy of the patient's narrative history as a guide to amnestic states. It is rare for a precise, unprompted history to be given from a patient who then fails formal tests of declarative memory. Part of the general routine of examination is to test the patient's fund of knowledge, which involves the recall of the main events of importance during life (e.g., education, marriage, job) and notable events shared by the local population. Failures in recall prompt more formal testing by asking patients to recite as many items as possible in a fixed time (usually 15 seconds) that belong to an arbitrarily selected class; favorites are colors, foods, or animals. At least 10 items should be recalled within that time frame.

More formal tests in common use include the request to recall a short sentence or names. The once-familiar Babcock sentence (For security, nations require an adequate supply of wood) or the sentence used by generations of American typists (The quick brown fox jumped over the lazy dog) have given way to three arbitrarily selected names. Those favored in the Folstein Minimental Test are apple, table, and penny, which are first repeated aloud by the patient and then tested by the examiner asking later, "What were the words I asked you to remember?" A common additional test is to place three objects near the patient, hiding each while the patient watches, and then later ask the patient if there are any objects hidden that could be found.

Far more detailed testing is usually necessary to show the patient is capable of learning (i.e., a name for an unfamiliar object, a new telephone number, or a pointing response when presented with certain visual displays). This learned response can be retained for minutes unless interruptions occur, after which the patient's spoken recall for the experience is usually absent, although the nonverbalized responses (i.e., selections of visual displays or patterns of motor response) may be correctly performed after delays as long as hours or days. The relatively preserved procedural memory may have some extreme features. Painful experiences such as venipuncture or humorous experiences with a funny person may elicit a similar response on re-exposure, prompting a refusal to be touched or a smile of recognition, even though patients may not be able to explain their own refusal or reason for smiling.

DISEASES

Paroxysmal Disorders

Transient global amnesia is the prototype of amnestic states. Although its etiologic agent is still unclear and epilepsy, transient ischemic attack, and migraine are all among the possible causes, it is paroxysmal, and the features of the acute and convalescent state have been clearly defined.

The setting is an elderly individual, usually with no history of illness and sometimes immediately after an activity that causes sudden bodily changes, such as a cold shower or plunge in the ocean, a very hot day, sexual intercourse, the receipt of sudden emotionally important news, or the end of a difficult task or trip. Many such attacks have had no clearly defined precedent.

When the ictus is witnessed, some patients appear to perspire, others appear pale or frightened, and a few cry. No epileptiform activity has been noted, and none have shown any focal signs of weakness or other disturbances. The major and dramatic change is in memory. Normal just seconds before, the patient is suddenly unable to recall the events immediately preceding. Conversational testing shows a striking but patchy retrograde amnesia, which may stretch back from hours to many years. For several hours, there is often an implicit lack of awareness of the deficit, together with loss of experiences learned during the period for which the retrograde amnesia exists, such as telephone numbers, addresses, the layout of the home or place of business, and so forth. In place of normal conversation, there is a striking repetitiveness of questions or comments (broken-record syndrome)

and an inability to be satisfied with the answers given. No other abnormalities on examination are noted. Within a few hours, new memories can be acquired, and there is a gradual restoration of memory for activities before the event (shrinking retrograde amnesia) over the succeeding several hours, usually reaching a plateau by 24 hours. However, even when a stable state has been reached, the amnesia for the episode itself and for 3 or 4 hours before the episode always remains.

Laboratory studies, including computed tomography and magnetic resonance imaging, are normal. Electroencephalograms are normal, even those done during the acute period when anterograde amnesia is present. Once thought to be rare, recurrence has been documented in up to 23 percent of cases. Recent studies have shown impairment in single-photon emission computed tomography in the anterior temporal lobes.

Stroke

Both ischemic and hemorrhagic diseases commonly affect the structures that serve memory. The posterior cerebral territory supplies the posterior two-thirds of the hippocampus, and infarction in this territory may completely interrupt the fimbria and its fornix projections, with devastating effects on memory, even from unilateral infarction (when in the hemisphere dominant for language) (see Ch. 35). Visual field defects and other disturbances of higher visual function are demonstrable.

Posterior cerebral territory infarction in the hemisphere dominant for language produces an amnestic state if the infarct affects the hippocampus or its fimbria (see Fig. 25-2). This location usually ensures the infarct is large because the arteries that supply the hippocampus lie in the territory of the branches that arise just after the posterior cerebral artery has gained the surface of the brain above the tentorium. The common isolated occlusion of the calcarine branch occurs distal to the branches that supply the hippocampus, which explains the high frequency of hemianopia in posterior cerebral territory infarction and the low frequency of amnestic states. In the territories between the calcarine branch and those that supply the hippocampus lie other regions the damage of which on the side dominant for speech and language also causes dyslexia, color dysnomia, and amnestic dysnomias, making it extremely difficult for posterior cerebral territory infarction to produce an isolated amnestic state.

Like transient global and concussive amnesias (see below), the syndrome seen within hours has striking retrograde and anterograde components. Months to years may pass before the retrograde amnesia has shrunk to within hours or days of the event. The anterograde memory function remains absent for weeks, even months, before it slowly appears; even then it is often incomplete. The shrinking retrograde amnesia and improving anterograde amnesia are usually too incomplete to be able to demonstrate a "window" of permanent time loss around the ictus. The incompleteness of the improvement has made it difficult to determine whether the features of infarct amnestic states share all of those with transient global amnesia and concussion.

The *anterior choroidal artery* supplies the anterior third of the hippocampus and could cause a similar memory disorder, but thus far, no detailed clinical reports have been presented (see Ch. 35).

A few instances have been reported of amnestic states with *isolated, small, deep infarcts* (lacunae) (see Ch. 35) in the medial thalamic region. However, small vessel disease seems to be a rare cause of amnestic states. More often, deep thalamic infarcts arise from embolism that pass through the top of the basilar artery, and occlude thalamoperforant arteries. The amnestic state is not as striking as that seen from infarction of the hippocampus. The patient reveals some difficulty with recall of details but only a patchy retrograde amnesia. Improvement is slow, and a clinical picture that suggests dementia is also seen. By contrast, large infarcts from embolism at the top of the basilar artery may be as striking as those that affect the hippocampus from occlusion in the posterior cerebral artery territory, but the explanation for the difference in syndromes is not yet well understood. The assumption that the basilar cases have larger or more widespread lesions has not often been documented by brain imaging or autopsy.

Venous occlusion of the lateral sinus (see Ch. 35) may cause hemorrhagic infarction in the temporal lobe, usually producing such widespread disturbance of language and visual fields that the amnestic component is difficult to demonstrate.

Aneurysms of the anterior communicating artery (see Ch. 37) may blast blood through the lamina terminalis into the septum, anterior commissure, precommissural bed nucleus of the fornix, and even into the fornix itself. In patients who survive, the amnestic state may be the most persistent of the late neurologic effects of the rupture of the aneurysm. Aneurysms of the posterior communicating artery and those that arise at the bifurcation of the middle cerebral artery occasionally rupture directly into the adjacent medial temporal region. When the dominant hemisphere is involved, this lesion can cause a similar severe memory disorder from direct injury to the hippocampus.

Spontaneous hemorrhage into the brain in the temporal region (see Ch. 36) is not rare from hypertension or, in elderly patients, from amyloid (congophilic) angiopathy. Isolated memory loss from such lesions is decidedly rare. The authors have not encountered a single example.

Trauma

The lower and inner faces of the temporal lobe are closely opposed to the roughened floor of the temporal bone of the skull (see Ch. 6). The surface gray matter is subject to mild bruising or being squashed from falls or other blunt trauma. The damage usually turns the gray matter into a hemorrhagic pulp, which within weeks becomes flattened. The yellowed residues found at autopsy are known as *plaques jaunes* (from the French for yellow plaques). The larger lesions may cause, in addition, gross hemorrhage in the white matter. The shearing of white matter pathways in the midbrain and lower thalamus from rotational head injuries may damage the deeper projections of the structures serving memory (see Ch. 6).

When brain injury produces unconsciousness that is prolonged for days or weeks, a temporal pole contusion is expected but often is not diagnosed by computed tomographic scan because the closeness of the brain surface to the temporal bone causes the high density of the contusion to blend with the high density of the bone. A coronal magnetic resonance imaging scan poses no such problems because the high- and low-intensity hemorrhagic signals differ from the neutral bone signal. The amnesia in such states is often severe and prolonged, with incomplete remission of retrograde and anterograde components. Shrinking of the retrograde amnesia may occur for several months but remains incomplete even then. The hours before the event are forever lost.

Concussive amnesia arises from minor closed-head injury. Typically, the momentary loss of consciousness from minor head injury causes no associated amnesia. In some cases, the concussion is associated with a striking temporary amnesia with features that mimic transient global amnesia, except there is no flushing, pale appearance or other ictal features. Some patients have passed for normal; one flagged down a passing car to seek help from his minor vehicle accident and rode off for help, only to be found wandering hours later uncertain how he got to where he was dropped off. Like transient global amnesia, the remission of memory may take as long as a day and be incomplete for the events. The behavior during this period may resemble the fugue states described by psychiatrists.

Vitamin Deficiencies

An entirely preventable disorder, vitamin deficiency, remains a major problem worldwide and, with it, the amnestic states often triggered by therapy (see Ch. 71). In the days before it was appreciated that vitamin B_1 deprivation made chronic alcoholic persons susceptible to glucose loads, the damage associated with Wernicke-Korsakoff syndrome from hemorrhagic lesions in the medial thalamus and subthalamus (especially the mammillary bodies) was a common occurrence. Alcohol is not the only cause; repeated vomiting in pregnancy, stenosis of the pylorus, and other causes have also been described.

The ocular motility disorder from a midbrain lesion and the imbalance from chronic cerebellar atrophy were often less impressive in bedside testing than was the severe amnestic state. The amnestic state begins suddenly, often within hours of the administration of glucose in a setting of vitamin deficiency. The patient remains alert but displays the distinctive triad of ophthalmoplegia, cerebellar ataxia, nystagmus, and memory disorder. In conversational testing, there is little evidence of ability to describe events within the past days, even as far back as months. Confabulation can be prominent, and the patient can be led into many inaccurate remarks by an examiner who seems to be helping the patient to recall by using leading questions or comments. The severe memory disturbance persists even though the ophthalmoplegia fades and the ataxia improves.

Prevention of the lesions that cause the Wernicke-Korsakoff syndrome is accomplished easily by the routine administration of 100 mg of thiamine (50 mg intravenously or intramuscularly) before glucose intravenous therapy is instituted. No harm can arise from its use in the normal patient with adequate vitamin therapy. In the absence of this precaution, the appearance of the ocular motility disorder, usually the first obvious sign, should prompt this regimen as a medical emergency in hopes of preventing the amnestic state. Even a small dose of thiamine suffices to correct the ocular motility disorder, but delay in therapy or doses below 100 mg of thiamine may not prevent the amnesia. Reversal of established amnesia is disappointingly infrequent. Daily use of this regimen is a good plan until a balanced diet, including thiamine, is being ingested regularly.

Atrophies

In Alzheimer's disease (see Ch. 60), the neurons gradually disappear, especially in those regions that lie closest to the anterior temporal pole. The neuronal loss begins first and is especially heavy in the hippocampus. The gradual loss of memory may be the first sign of this condition, but may be overlooked in the initial stages. Memory disorder is the hallmark of Alzheimer's disease, but its features are not themselves distinctive. As opposed to the syndromes that cause acute amnestic states, Alzheimer's disease causes the slow and steady decline in memory skills that are difficult to detect early and impossible to miss later. When

the diagnosis can be made, there are also disorders of activities of daily living that indicate more than a verbally mediated amnestic state. Whether becoming lost in one's neighborhood is described as a disorder of memory or as spatial disorientation and whether failing skills in manipulating small tools is characterized as a memory disorder or as dyspraxia, the appearance of such disturbances indicates there are many sites of the brain affected. A conversationally obvious acute disorder of recent memory is rarely present until the most advanced stage of the disease, when it is accompanied by gross disorders in praxis and orientation.

Special note should be made of the common disorder in the recall of proper names. A problem for most individuals with the passage of years, however exasperating and worrisome, when it occurs in isolation, it is not a marker of impending Alzheimer's disease.

Infections

In herpes simplex virus infection (see Ch. 48), seizures and signs of brain mass usually characterize the initial phase of the illness. Only a slight amount of fever occurs. Typical accompanying signs include hemianopia, dysphasia, apathy, occasional olfactory hallucinations, hemiparesis, and even stupor. These signs reflect the edema and mass effect of the lesion that is spreading beyond the limbic structures. Many begin in a state of delirium and recover fully; for others, the bilateral lesions produce a severe and lasting memory disorder. The apathy fades in months, and many patients seem perfectly normal in their everyday behavior, except that conversational testing reveals a striking inability to describe recent events, even things they have just been doing before being distracted by the question.

Abscess formation in the temporal pole lobe is rare and usually produces a syndrome of uncal herniation in the absence of major disturbances of memory. When an abscess occurs more posteriorly, the accompanying language disorder (if the hemisphere dominant for language is affected) is more prominent than is the amnestic state, making the amnestic syndrome difficult to characterize alone.

Metabolic States

Anoxia produces its greatest effect on the cells in the Sommer sector of the hippocampus (see Ch. 25), occasionally resulting in almost pure amnestic states in the few individuals who survive pure anoxia (see Ch. 17). The setting of an anoxic brain injury is usually cardiac arrest, which brings with it hypotension, also adding lesions in many other brain regions and preventing most patients with cardiac arrest from showing isolated amnestic states.

Tumors

The temporal lobe is commonly affected by both primary and metastatic neoplasms (see Chs. 52 and 53). Other regions that serve memory, such as the thalamus and regions surrounding the septum, may be the site of the primary tumor but are only rarely affected by metastases. The syndrome caused by these slow-growing lesions does not feature isolated memory loss; the amnestic state is part of a larger syndrome. The first complaints are most often the faulty recall of names. The failure seems to occur in the absence of other disturbances in memory; it has been termed, *amnestic aphasia*. Not only proper names but nouns, adjectives, adverbs, and other parts of speech used for description or naming seem affected. Only later do elements of sensory (Wernicke) aphasia make an appearance. The rare papilloma of the choroid plexus that involves the foramen of Monro may cause an amnestic state from interruption of the fornix from the dominant hemisphere but usually only after considerable headache has occurred.

Surgery

In the decades since resection of the hippocampus first documented the sensitivity of such resections to the production of memory disorder, it has become rare for surgery to result in a memory disorder. Surgeons have learned to go no deeper than 3 cm from the temporal pole in any resections done for epilepsy or tumors, and modern surgical techniques for epilepsy produce extremely localized ablations, too small to produce a memory disorder. Operations through the corpus callosum for third ventricular tumors are now done with attention to avoid disruption of the fornix. Even when they do, the effect on memory may be transient.

Toxins

Heavy metals (see Ch. 72) lead the list of agents that can damage the hippocampal regions. These areas normally have a high concentration of zinc. Perhaps the effect is from an affinity for multivalent ions in these cells. A striking severe declarative amnestic state has been described among those who ate mussels contaminated with domoic acid, a compound that can act as an excitatory neurotransmitter. The distribution of the lesion approximated that seen with kainic acid.

Contrast reaction occurs rarely in patients who have been given large loads of dye in the basilar territory. Cardiac catheterization may be the cause, but more often, it is repeated injections of dye in the study of an arteriovenous malformation or basilar stenosis. Although the acute toxic state is inseparable from infarction, the syndrome is usually transitory.

ANNOTATED BIBLIOGRAPHY

Becker JT. Working memory and secondary memory deficits in Alzheimer's disease. J Clin Exp Neuropsychol 1988;10:739–53.

Designation of different types of memory loss in Alzheimer's disease.

Bowen BC. MR signal abnormalities in memory disorders and dementia. Am J Neuroradiol 1990;11:283–90.

Comprehensive review of brain imaging.

Duyckaerts C, Derouesné C, Signoret JL et al. Bilateral and limited amygdalohippocampal lesions causing a pure amnestic syndrome. Ann Neurol 1985;18:314.

In a setting of Hodgkin's disease. The deficit appeared suddenly and persisted for the 21 months of life.

Fisher CM, Adams RD. Transient global amnesia. Acta Neurol Scand 1964;40(suppl 9):1.

The seminal review that set forth the features of the syndrome.

Grafman J, Salazar AM, Weingartner H et al. Isolated impairment of memory following a penetrating lesion of the fornix cerebri. Arch Neurol 1965;42:1162.

Strikingly disturbed verbal learning and recall, with little or no disturbances in other higher cerebral functions, from small lesion suffered over a dozen years before, affecting both fornices.

This test is losing favor.

Mensing JWA, Hoogland PH, Sloof JL. Computed tomography in the diagnosis of Wernicke-Korsakoff encephalopathy: a radiological-neuropathological correlation. Ann Neurol 1984;16:363.

Low density bordering the third ventricle and quadrigeminal plate in a case in extremis.

Michel D, Laurent B, Foyatier N et al. Infarctus thalamique paramedian gauche. Rev Neurol (Paris) 1982;138:6.

An important case of dysmemory because the only lesion seen on the computed tomographic scan was confined to the left side, affecting the dorsomedial nucleus of the thalamus.

Miller JW, Yanagihara T, Peterson RC, Klass DW. Transient global amnesia and epilepsy. Neurology 1987;44:629.

Not even found during the acute period just after the attack when anterograde amnesia is still evident. Those with epilepsy have frequent recurrent attacks of brief duration and usually do not meet the established criteria for transient global amnesia.

Mishkin M, Appenzeller T. The anatomy of memory. Scientific American 1987;256:80–9.

Highly readable account.

Mohr JP, Sidman M, Stoddard LT et al. Right hemianopia with memory and color deficits in circumscribed left posterior cerebral artery territory infarction. Neurology 1971;21:1105–13.

One of the few autopsy-documented unilateral hippocampal infarcts.

Nichelli P, Bahmanian-Behbahani G, Gentilini M, Vecchi A. Preserved memory abilities in thalamic amnesia. Brain 1988;111:1337–53.

Full review showing differences between general breakdown in memory and disorders of specific memory functions.

Papez JW. A proposed mechanism of emotion. Arch Neurol Psychiatry 1937;38:725–43.

The article describing the limbic system.

Scoville W, Milner B. Loss of recent memory after bilateral hippocampal lesions. J Neurol Neurosurg Psychiatry 1957;20:11.

An important survey of the effects of surgical resections with the first description of H.M., the famous patient whose disordered memory after surgery has been the subject of extensive investigation.

Sidman M, Stoddard LT, Mohr JP. Some additional quantitative observations of immediate memory in a patient with bilateral hippocampal lesions. Neuropsychologia 1968;6:245–54.

The patient learned new tasks despite a poor ability to describe what he was doing. The patient is the same one reported by Scoville and Milner.

Squire LR. Mechanisms of memory. Science 1986;232: 1612–18.

Memory storage for skilled activities is believed to be localized to the specific cortical areas involved in the processing of the information to be learned and is separate from the memory storage involved in spoken recall, which is more subject to disturbance from hippocampal and medial thalamic lesions.

Tarel V, Pellat J, Naegele B et al. Troubles amnesiques après rupture d'aneurysme de l'artère communicante antérieure. Rev Neurol (Paris) 1990;146:746–51.

Thorough review of memory disorders after aneurysm rupture, showing many have none, some require testing for it to show, and a few have severe disorders.

Teitelbaum JS, Zatorre RJ, Carpenter S et al. Neurologic sequelae of domoic acid intoxication due to the ingestion of contaminated mussels. N Engl J Med 1990;322: 1781–7.

A potent excitatory neurotransmitter.

Victor M, Adams RD, Collins GH. The Wernicke-Korsakoff Syndrome. FA Davis, Philadelphia, 1971.

Full treatment of the subject in text form.

22
Disorders of Movement

J. C. Gautier and J. P. Mohr

OVERVIEW AND CLINICAL EXAMINATION

Although a gross oversimplification, the concept that the motor system is basically organized as a model made up of two kinds of neurons, upper and lower neurons (Fig. 22-1), remains crucial in clinical neurology. It is also a convenient entry to the study of the physiology and pathophysiology of movement.

The axons that form part of the peripheral cranial and spinal nerves that supply the peripheral muscles have their cells of origin in the nuclei of motor cranial nerves and in the anterior horn of the spinal cord. These lower motor neurons are controlled in part by the upper motor neurons, which descend in several tracts from cortex and brainstem to synapse with and around the dentrites and cell bodies of lower motor neurons.

Two large structures that control movements, the basal ganglia and the cerebellum, have no direct access (projections) to lower motor neurons. They are considered later.

SPINAL LEVEL

The human spinal cord is basically metameric and can be viewed as 31 separate segments that receive incoming sensory inputs from the periphery through the dorsal roots and descending motor inputs from the higher levels. For the sake of simplicity, the intersegmental connections that take part in the coordination of the activity of several cord segments are not considered here.

Outflow of the Spinal Cord

The motor outputs that control muscle contraction arise primarily from the large motor α neurons located in the ventral horn of the spinal cord. Each α neuron controls a motor unit, that is, a group of muscle fibers that can range from 10 to 20 fibers in muscles for delicate movements (e.g., eyeball muscles) to about 1,500 fibers in big muscles (e.g., hip muscles), which

are made for crude movements. When increasing force is needed, the firing rates of the motor units increase, and neighboring units are recruited. Axons of α cells make up the large A fibers of ventral roots, which constitute the main outflow tracts of the motor neurons. They are the classic "final common path" through which all messages pass from higher levels to elaborate all types of movements.

Smaller γ neurons are found among α neurons. Their axons (γ fibers) enter the ventral root en route to intrafusal fibers of the muscle spindles that record muscle stretch and are responsible for muscle tone. The rate at which these γ efferents fire determines the readiness (lowers the threshold) for muscle contraction to a stimulus, such as the muscle stretch from the tap of a reflex hammer on a tendon.

In addition to A and γ fibers, ventral roots from T1 to L2 contain preganglionic sympathetic B fibers from cells located in the intermediolateralis gray part of the spinal cord. Further down, B fibers leave the spinal nerve (see below) through the white communicating rami to enter the sympathetic trunk. Similarly, from sacral segments S2, S3, and S4, preganglionic parasympathetic fibers exit with the ventral root just as the rostral parasympathetic outflow exits with cranial motor nerves.

Finally, the ventral roots also contain afferent fibers the functional significance of which is still not clear. Some enter the spinal cord directly by way of the ventral root; others may curve back to enter the dorsal root and horn.

Gray Matter of the Spinal Cord

In the gray matter of the spinal cord, the α neurons are arranged in an orderly manner in the anterior horn. Those for the trunk and girdles are medial, and those for extremities are lateral. Cells for the extensor muscles are ventral, and those for flexors are dorsal.

283

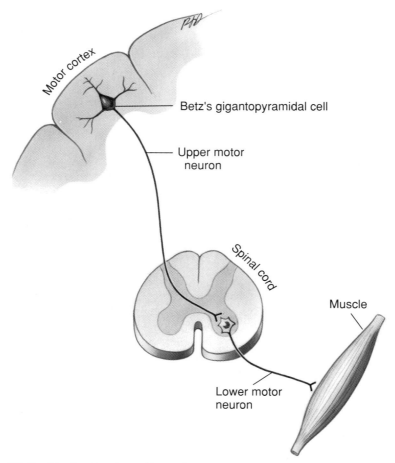

Figure 22-1. The basic, clinically useful, concept of upper and lower motor neurons.

Every muscle is innervated by a column of motor cells that extends through several spinal segments.

Besides α and γ neurons, there are numerous internuncial neurons (Latin: *nuncius,* messenger) that act as links or go-betweens for posterior (sensory) and anterior (motor) horn cells. These neurons convey messages from the Golgi tendon organs, which project on them. Other neurons (Renshaw cells) exert a feedback action on α cells. Many of the internuncial cells are inhibitory, serving to inhibit the tone and action of muscles antagonistic in action to the muscles (agonists) that carry out a given movement. This agonist-action/antagonist-inhibition is the basis of the physiologic law of reciprocal innervation. Finally, the sensory input of many one-sided stimuli (e.g., pain) is distributed to both sides of the cord through sensory input mechanisms described more fully in Chapter 23.

The spinal cord is thus endowed with mechanisms that subserve not only simple reflexes mediated by a single unit in response to a single stimulus (monosynaptic activities such as the knee jerk) but also complex synergistic activities, as exemplified by the perfor-

mance of the transsected spinal cord. Immediately after the section, spinal reflexes are absent (spinal shock), but later, the thigh and leg will flex when a noxious stimulus is applied to the foot (Babinski's sign is the first part of this movement, see below). Even in the frog, the ipsilateral or contralateral lower limb can come to the back to rub off a painful stimulus.

LOWER MOTOR NEURONS

The various cells just mentioned and their axons down to their synapses with muscle fibers (smooth muscle, heart muscle, and glandular epithelium for autonomic fibers) make up the lower motor neurons. For movements, only those fibers are considered that innervate skeletal striated muscles.

The ventral roots exit the dura and unite into the dorsal root in the intervertebral foramen. Until they have pierced the dura, the roots are bathed by cerebrospinal fluid disturbances of which can affect the functions of these segments of the roots. As they emerge from the dura, the ventral and dorsal roots

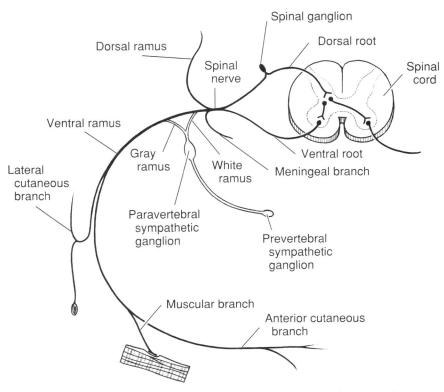

Figure 22-2. Diagram of a thoracic spinal nerve and its branches.

unite in the intervertebral foramen to form the spinal nerve (Fig. 22-2), which thus contains efferent and afferent fibers.

Each spinal nerve gives off the following four branches: (1) the dorsal ramus to the muscles and skin of the back; (2) the ventral ramus to the skin and muscles of the limbs and trunk; (3) the ramus communicans, which connects with the sympathetic ganglia; and (4) the meningeal branch, a small recurrent branches that re-enters the intervertebral foramen to innervate meninges, blood vessels, and spine. Dorsal and ventral rami branch into cutaneous and muscular peripheral nerves, which themselves branch again many times until the terminal branch constitutes motor nerves for individual muscles. These so-called motor nerves are still mixed nerves because they contain, in addition to α and γ efferents, vasomotor efferent and afferent fibers from muscle spindles, tendon organs, and pain afferents. Finally, α fibers synapse with muscle fibers.

The lower motor neuron syndrome results from any lesion or dysfunction of the cells in the spinal cord, with motor fibers in roots and nerves down to the neuromuscular junction or motor end-plate excluded. Dysfunction of the nerve-muscle junction is, of course, a cause of dysfunction of muscle but is another category of disorders of movement (see Ch. 81).

Between spinal nerve and final muscle fibers, there are many anastomoses, chiefly between the fibers of the ventral rami. They are especially developed for fibers from the cervical, lumbar, and sacral parts of the spinal cord when they constitute the brachial, lumbar, and lumbosacral plexuses (Fig. 22-3). Plexuses and anastomoses mix motor and sensory fibers from various segments ("levels") of the spinal cord, which explains why fibers from one spinal segment can reach several muscles and why peripheral nerves contain fibers from several spinal segments (levels). Plexuses give off peripheral nerves, each of which contain fibers from two, three, or even four ventral rami (i.e., roots, spinal segments, or levels).

Clinical Considerations

For the clinician to recognize the site of a lesion, this complex arrangement of muscular innervation makes it necessary to be acquainted with several orders of innervation: (1) segmental (i.e., the motor output of spinal segments or levels), (2) radicular (i.e., corresponding to the ventral roots or spinal nerves coming off from these segments. For many muscles, there is a predominant segment and root that is of great clinical import), (3) plexical (i.e., pertaining to plexuses), and (4) peripheral (i.e., pertaining to peripheral nerves or their branches). Figure 22-4 shows the segmental in-

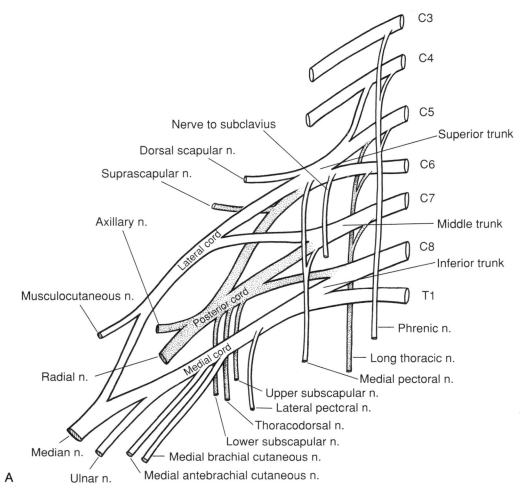

Figure 22-3. (A) Formation of the brachial plexus, indicating roots, and ventral rami from roots to peripheral nerves. Posterior divisions, cord, and peripheral nerves are shaded. *(Figure continues.)*

nervation of the muscles of the neck, limbs, and trunk. Table 22-1 gives the nerve and main root supply of the more commonly tested muscles. Whatever the site of the lesion on the lower motor neuron, the resulting fundamental disorders are weakness, hypotonia, loss of reflexes, and wasting. In some disease processes,

there may be fasciculations (see Clinical Examination and Table 22-2).

UPPER MOTOR NEURONS

Five main motor tracts that control lower motor neurons descend from higher levels: four from the brainstem and one from the cerebral cortex. Their situation in the spinal cord is shown in Figures 22-5 and 22-6.

Brainstem Tracts

The reticulospinal tract conveys messages downward from the reticular formation, chiefly from its pontine part, through the medial reticulospinal tract and medullary part, particularly from the nucleus gigantocellularis by the lateral reticulospinal tract. Both tracts carry mainly ipsilateral fibers and synapse with internuncial neurons. They control primarily muscles of the trunk and proximal parts of the limbs and mediate

Table 22-1. Nerve and Main Root Supply of the More Commonly Tested Muscles

Jaw	Sensory motor cranial nerve V
Biceps	C5–C6
Brachioradialis	C6
Triceps	C7
Pronator	C8
Finger flexion	C8
Knee	L3, L4
Ankle	S1

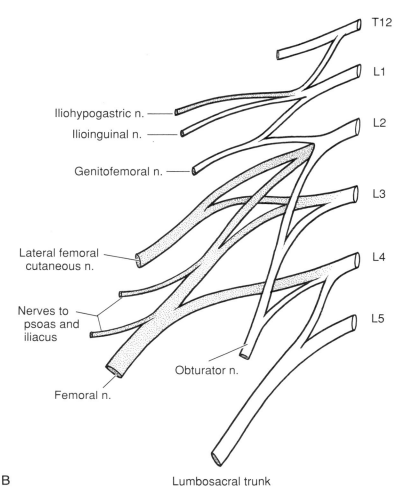

T12

L1

Iliohypogastric n.

Ilioinguinal n.

Genitofemoral n.

L2

L3

Lateral femoral
cutaneous n.

L4

Nerves to
psoas and
iliacus

L5

Obturator n.

Femoral n.

B   Lumbosacral trunk

Figure 22-3 *(Continued).* **(B)** Lumbar plexus. Nerves from posterior divisions of ventral rami are shaded. Numbers for ventral rami are similar to those for roots. *(Figure continues.)*

such basic reactions as those to sudden noise or alarm (e.g., the startle reaction).

The vestibulospinal tract, also mainly uncrossed, arises from the vestibular nuclei and projects to internuncial neurons. It plays a key role in maintaining posture and, as such, acts primarily on extensor muscles.

The rubrospinal tract (Latin: *ruber,* red) arises from the red nucleus, the highly vascularized, hence red, appearance of which gave it its name. Its fibers cross in the ventral tegmental decussation and descend in the lateral funiculus of the spinal cord. The red nucleus is an important relay on the cerebellar output and also receives projections from the precentral and

Table 22-2. Signs of Upper and Lower Motor Neurons Disease

	Upper	Lower	Remarks
Strength	↓	↓	Distribution of weakness different
Tone	Spasticity	Flaccidity	
Tendon reflexes	↑	↓	
Plantar response	Babinski's sign	Flexor or unresponsive	
Muscle size	No wasting	Wasting	See text

Key: ↓ , decrease; ↑ , increase.

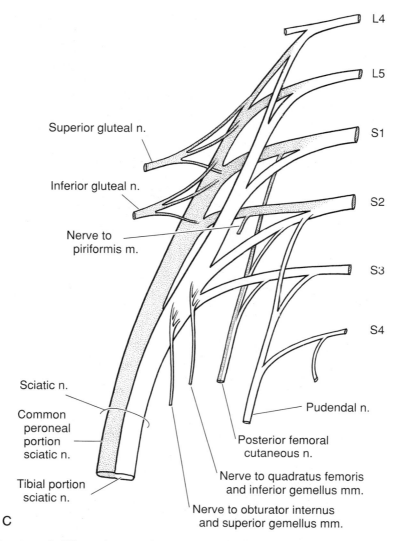

L4

L5

S1

S2

S3

S4

Superior gluteal n.

Inferior gluteal n.

Nerve to
piriformis m.

Sciatic n.

Common
peroneal
portion
sciatic n.

Tibial portion
sciatic n.

Pudendal n.

Posterior femoral
cutaneous n.

Nerve to quadratus femoris
and inferior gemellus mm.

Nerve to obturator internus
and superior gemellus mm.

C

Figure 22-3 *(Continued).* **(C)** Lumbosacral plexus. Nerves from posterior divisions of ventral rami are shaded. Numbers for ventral rami are similar to those for roots.

premotor cortex. In humans, the rubrospinal tract ends in the cervical or upper thoracic cord. It is mainly concerned with flexor muscles.

The tectospinal tract (Latin: *tectum,* roof) originates from cells in the superior colliculus, an optic relay center. Fibers cross in the dorsal tegmental decussation and can be identified down to the upper cervical segments of the spinal cord. They terminate on internuncial neurons and are concerned with orientation movements in response to visual and, perhaps, auditory stimuli.

Cerebral Tracts

The corticospinal tract is by far the largest of the descending motor pathways. Because of its large volume, long course, and frequent lesions, it also assumes the greatest significance in clinical neurology. Its traditional name is "pyramidal tract" because it makes up the pyramids of the medulla oblongata, and in common neurologic parlance, the terms "pyramidal tract" and "pyramidal syndrome" are still in use to mean corticospinal tract or syndrome. The old notion that the pyramidal tract is made up of axons or Betz giant pyramidal cells in layer V of Brodmann's area 4 (see Fig. 25-3) is wrong because there are approximately 34,000 Betz cells in humans, which thus make up only 3 to 4 percent of the 1 million fibers that pass through the medullar pyramid. The terms pyramidal tract and pyramidal syndrome are time honored but should be used with major reservations.

It is estimated that, in humans, approximately 60 percent of corticofugal motor fibers arise from area

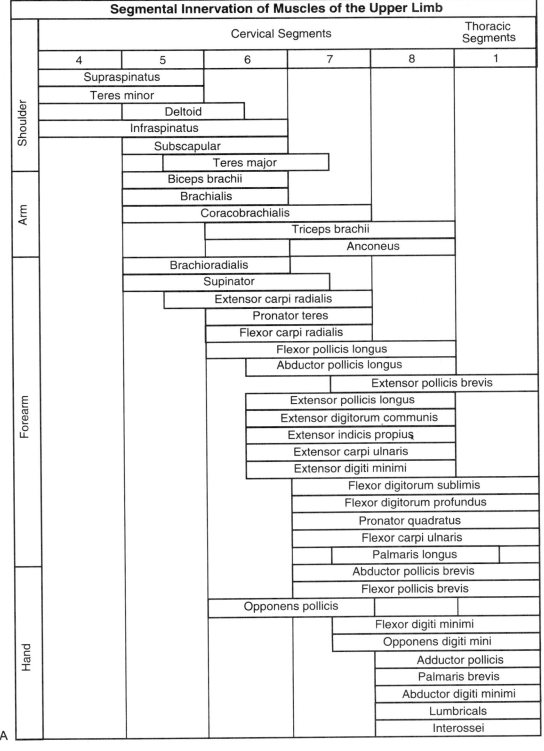

Figure 22-4. Spinal root origins for the main muscles of **(A)** the upper limb, **(B)** trunk, and **(C)** lower limb. (From Carpenter and Sutin J, 1983, with permission.) *(Figure continued.)*

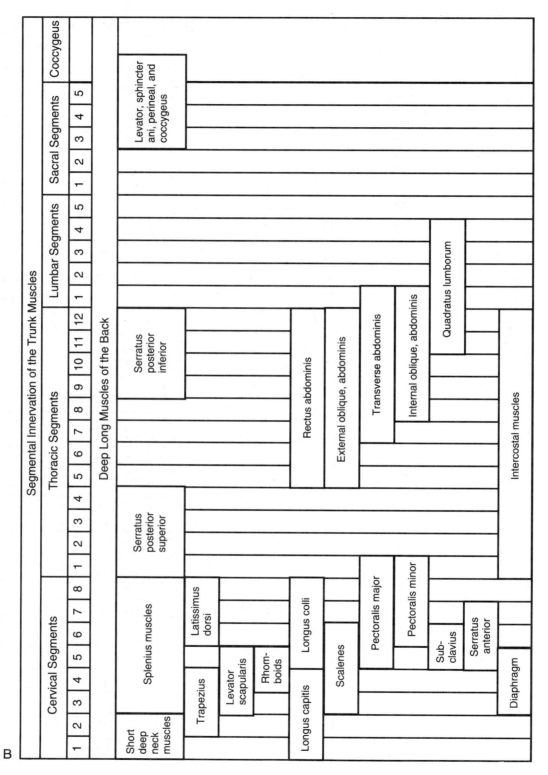

Figure 22-4 *(Continued).* **B.** *(Figure continues.)*

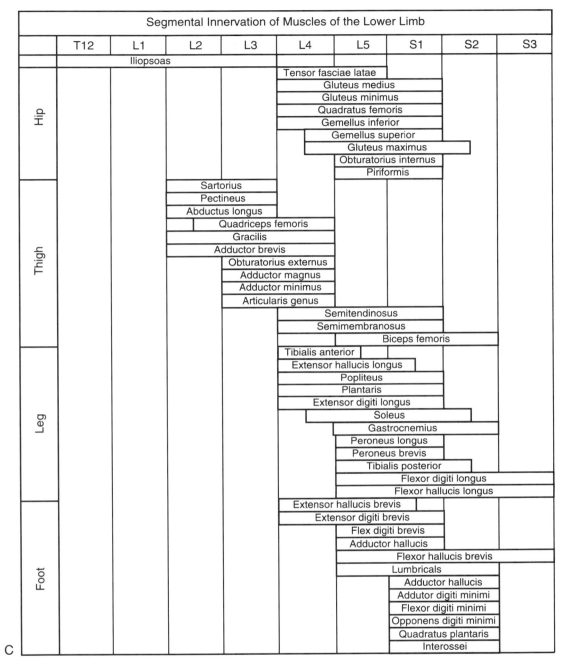

Figure 22-4 *(Continued).* **C.**

4; the remainder come from area 6 and the parietal lobe. Area 4 of Brodmann, commonly called the motor area or MI, includes the anterior wall of the central sulcus (Rolando's fissure) and adjacent areas of the precentral gyrus. The corticospinal tract is broad on the medial aspect of the brain in the anterior portion of the paracentral lobule and still broad on the upper part of the cerebral convexity, but is quickly narrows downward. In the operculum, it occupies only the anterior wall of the central sulcus. The cells of origin of the motor corticofugal fibers are arranged in columns or clusters that lay across the cortex. Discrete electrical stimulations during neurosurgical procedures, under local anesthesia, result in discrete isolated contralateral movements. Such mapping of area 4 has shown an orderly somatotopic arrangement with large areas for the mouth, tongue, and thumb. This so-called motor homunculus, lying head down, similar

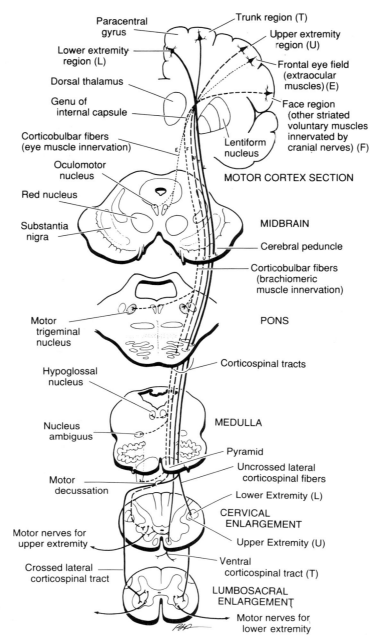

Figure 22-5. Course of the corticospinal and corticobulbar tracts in humans. Letters show the somatotopic arrangement from cortex to spinal cord. Somatotopic arrangement in the midbrain, pons, and pyramid is questionable. Uncrossed fibers to the nucleus ambiguus are not depicted.

to a trapeze artist, clinging onto the superior border of the brain (Fig. 25-9), has a somesthetic counterpart on the postcentral gyrus. Recent evidence, however, suggests multiple representations of body parts. In other words, two or more clusters of cortical cells may project on a single spinal motoneuron group that innervates an individual muscle. In addition, such cell clusters overlap clusters, controlling motor neurons for synergistic and antagonistic muscles. Studies have also shown that the exact topographic map may vary considerably from one to another individual, making the homunculus more a principle of motor organization than a reliable map in an individual patient (see Ch. 25).

Area 6 of Brodmann, also known as the premotor area, lies rostral to area 4 (Fig. 25-1). Its descending output mainly projects to the reticulospinal tract, which in turn, projects mainly on internuncial spinal neurons concerned with the axial (trunk) and proximal muscles (see above). Descending influences of the premotor area are bilateral in contrast with those of area 4, which are strictly unilateral. The premotor area seems chiefly involved in the preparation of movement and stabilization of the proximal parts to allow fine, delicate movements of the hand and fingers. Area 6 is also instrumental in motor learning, rhythm production, and spoken and written language (apractic agraphia) (see Ch. 25, Frontal Lobe). Language circuits and sequential movement circuits are lateralized (i.e., disorders result from left hemisphere lesions).

The supplementary motor area (MII) is rostral to area 4 on the median aspect of the superior frontal gyrus. Electrical stimulation in humans causes or sets the stage for contralateral raising of the arm with contralateral turning of the head and eyes. Bilateral movements of the trunk and limbs, vocalizations and autonomic responses have also been recorded. It is assumed that the supplementary motor area plays a role in the initiation of movement because lesions or excisions result in bilateral reduction of spontaneous motor activity, more severe contralaterally, and reduction of speech and of emotional behavior. Such lesions, when bilateral, probably account for much of the syndrome of akinetic mutism (see Ch. 17).

Corticofugal fibers also come from parietal areas 3, 1, 2, 5, and 7 and possibly from other regions of the brain. The role of the parietal and precentral areas in voluntary movement is emphasized by electrical recordings in humans. Unilateral movement is preceded by three cerebral potentials, namely, (1) the earlier (Bereitschaft) potential is negative and bilateral and appears at about 800 ms in parietal and precentral areas; (2) the second, termed the premotor positivity, is bilateral and appears in the parietal and precentral areas and at about 90 to 80 ms; and (3) the motor potential, the last one, is unilateral and appears in the motor cortex.

All these corticofugal fibers converge in the corona radiata in a cramped, dense bundle that must get through the narrow passage of the internal capsule.

Course of the Corticospinal Tract

Before the course of the tract is considered, some important points must be recalled. First, only one-half of the fibers in the corona radiata reach the spinal cord. Among the other half are some bundles, classically known as the corticobulbar tract, which innervate the motor nuclei of the cranial nerves indirectly (internuncial neurons) or directly (aberrant pyramidal bundles of early studies). Some components of the cortico-

bulbar tract have a clearly bilateral innervation, such as motor cranial nerves V, IX, X, and XII. The innervation of the inferior part of the nucleus of cranial nerve VII is predominantly contralateral (see Ch. 29). It appears that the oculomotor and abducens nuclei do not receive these direct cortical projections. Some elements project on subcortical structures that, in turn, project to the spinal cord (e.g., red nucleus and pontomedullar reticular formation). Some fibers project on subcortical motor structures, such as the striatum, motor nuclei of the thalamus, and inferior olive. Some fibers, contrary to historical belief, project onto subcortical sensory structures: sensory nuclei of the thalamus, dorsal column nuclei, and trigeminal nuclei. Second, cells of origin of the corticospinal tract vary greatly in size and axonal diameter and hence in velocity conduction, which on the whole, is slow. Third, all along their course, corticobulbar and corticospinal fibers make many additional contacts through collaterals: in the cortex, where recurrent fibers synapse with excitatory and inhibitory cells, with the subcortical motor and sensory structures just mentioned. This abundant collateralization holds true in the spinal cord where one fiber can send branches at different spinal levels and synapse with different spinal neurons.

In summary, the corticospinal tract (pyramidal tract) is far more complex anatomically and physiologically than was believed a few decades ago. It is really an agglomerate of subsystems, although these have an integrated activity. Many of its functions are not yet clearly elucidated. This contrasts with the simplicity of clinical concepts (see below).

The course of the tract is one of the mainstays of clinical examination, although many of the historical views have been subject to revision or are open to question. The motor homunculus (Fig. 25-9) was a major advance for clinicopathologic correlations. The advent of computed tomography (CT) and magnetic resonance imaging (MRI) has allowed the study of enough patients with such lesions in life to be done so that the accuracy of the cartoon character as the principle of the homuncular organization seems in doubt to some investigators, although it appears to be a useful explanation of the neurologic syndrome from brain injury to others. Apart from simple errors in brain lesion interpretation in some forms of brain imaging, other explanations for the variation may include multiple representation of a part of the body with possible overlap of representations of different parts and individual variations, as mentioned above.

The classic concept of the course of the pathway from the cortex through the corona radiata to the internal capsule (Fig. 22-5) shows fibers that converge with a torsional movement in the internal capsule between the caudate and thalamus medially and the lenticular nucleus laterally. Present evidence, distinct from such a view, assumes that fibers shift dorsalward in the rostrocaudal course of the internal capsule so that they are located in a compact bundle in the posterior part of the posterior limb of the capsule, at least in its caudal part. The historical notion that there is a strict somatopic rostrocaudal arrangement with cranial, cervical, and thoracic lumbar and sacral parts seems now rather crude. Several patterns of motor weakness have been documented from the same site of a lesion in the internal capsule.

To reach the midbrain, the fibers make a transition from the internal capsule to the cerebral peduncle immediately below. During this short transition, they pass below the embrace of the putamen and thalamus above and are exposed to injuries that affect the anterolateral edge of the midbrain.

In the midbrain, the corticospinal fibers occupy the medial three-fifths of the crus cerebri between frontal corticopontine fibers medially and temporal, parietal, and occipital corticopontine fibers laterally. In the basis pontis, corticospinal fibers make up a rostrocaudal system of fibers together with the corticopontine bundles just mentioned. These uncrossed corticopontine fibers synapse with cells of the pontine nuclei. The rostrocaudal system of fibers is broken up into separate pieces by the transversal axons of the pontine nuclei cells that cross to make up the contralateral middle cerebral peduncle (brachium pontis). At the pontomedullary junction, corticospinal fibers gather and come to the ventral surface, constituting the medullary pyramids.

From midbrain to medulla, the classic view of the somatopic organization of corticospinal fibers (Fig. 22-5) is a fairly reliable concept for the clinician. It shows an orderly arrangement of face, upper limb, trunk, and lower limb mediolaterally. However, there are doubts about such a precise pattern. Relatively small lesions in the very low capsule or peduncle may produce strikingly severe and long-lasting contralateral paralysis; small infarcts in basis pontis, as seen by MRI, show a striking variation in weakness profiles.

At the junction of the medulla and cord, corticospinal fibers, mainly coming from primary motor and somesthetic cortex, undergo an incomplete decussation. Although there is much individual variation, 70 to 90 percent of the fibers cross, forming three or four corticospinal tracts in the cord.

First, the crossed lateral corticospinal tract, the largest one, occupies a large area in the posterior part of the lateral funiculus, ventral to the dorsal horn, dorsal to the rubrospinal tract (Fig. 22-6). It descends down to the distal sacral segments. In three-quarters of the cords, left fibers cross the right, more cranially than right ones to the left, and there are more left fibers that cross to the right than conversely. This explains why, in three-quarters of the cords, the right side is larger than the left one, a fact not related to handedness. Fibers of the crossed lateral corticospinal tract synapse on ventral and dorsal horn cells and on cells of the intermediolateralis region. The lateral corticospinal tract is the most clinically significant part of the corticospinal tracts because lesions rostral to the decussation result in a contralateral upper motor neuron syndrome, whereas lesions caudal to the decussation result in an ipsilateral upper motor neuron syndrome (see below).

Second, the anterior or ventral corticospinal tract is made up of a relatively small number of fibers that

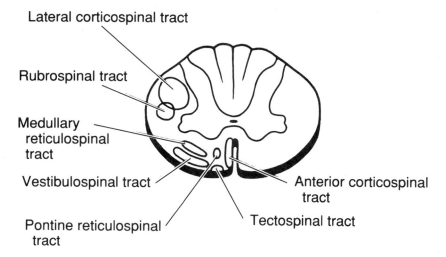

Figure 22-6. The main descending motor tracts in the spinal cord.

do not cross at the medullospinal junction. Fibers descend in the most medial part of the anterior funiculus. Its size is reciprocally related to that of the opposite lateral corticospinal tract. Depending on its size, the fibers reach to the sacral segments or only to the upper cervical segments. At each level, the fibers cross through the anterior commissure to end on cells of the medial part of the anterior horn, which innervate primarily the trunk and proximal limb muscles (see above, Spinal Level).

Third, there is an uncrossed lateral corticospinal tract, of varying size, that descends ventral to the lateral corticospinal tract. Its function is still not known.

Finally, in some cords, there is a small tract of fibers that have decussated with the lateral corticospinal tract and descend in the posterolateral part of the anterior columns in the cervical segments.

Fibers of the corticospinal tract synapse directly on α neurons, γ neurons, and excitatory and inhibitory neurons and sensory relay cells. Physiologic data show that the corticospinal fibers are important overall for the control of the distal muscles devoted to the finest movements of the hand.

Physiologic Considerations

The motor areas and their efferent pathways, the motor corticofugal fibers, are no longer considered the initiators of movement. Rather, so-called voluntary movement can be viewed as a response to external and/or internal clues. It appears that motor areas, as it were, are a final common path to various external and internal cues that call for adaptive movement. The latter can be seen as the higher level of motor reflex activity, with an afferent arm consisting of all sensory modalities, past experience, and probably programmed motor sequences, and an efferent arm, the corticofugal system, that regulates movements not only through the lower motor neurons but also by tuning the sensory feedback input from movement itself and from the external and/or internal causes that have initiated this movement.

It is generally accepted that the clinical upper motor neuron syndrome is made up of contralateral (when lesions are rostral to the corticospinal decussation) weakness, increase in tone (i.e., spasticity) increased tendon reflexes, clonus, and Babinski's sign (Table 22-2). However, it is not an easy task to transpose physiologic and experimental evidence into clinical data. Section of the pyramids or pes pedunculi causes little permanent disturbance in primates and has caused only a mild motor weakness in the few reported human cases. The most significant and lasting deficit is difficulty in handling objects (i.e., manipulation involving discrete, fine movements of the fingers and hand). This is different from the dense, spastic hemiplegia that results in humans from large convexity or internal capsule lesions. In such cases, in addition to the damage to the corticospinal tract, many other systems are destroyed, and the activity of released structures (see below) can be prominent. Thus, once again, the terms pyramidal syndrome, corticospinal syndrome, or upper motor neuron syndrome are mainly justified by tradition. However, pending new knowledge, they retain their practical value.

CLINICAL EXAMINATION IN WEAKNESS AND WASTING

Weakness means a lack of strength. It can be complete, with no muscle contraction whatever, which is called paralysis (synonym, palsy), or incomplete, which is called paresis. The paresis can be slight, mild, or severe. When a whole limb or more than one limb is involved, the term plegia (from the Greek for to strike) is used instead of paralysis. Monoplegia or monoparesis affects one limb, and hemiplegia or hemiparesis affects one-half of the body. The face may or may not be included in the latter two. Quadriplegia or quadriparesis refers to weakness of all four limbs, whether the face is included or not. Paraplegia or paraparesis describes involvement of both lower limbs.

A precise diagnosis of motor disturbances is always vital in clinical neurology because the distribution of the weakness is, in most cases, a key to the site of the lesion, whether in the nerve, cord, brainstem, or cerebrum. The range of conditions varies enormously from trauma to a distal branch of a motor nerve, when one muscle can be weak, all the way to paresis or paralysis of all, or nearly all muscles, as occurs in the Guillain-Barré syndrome. Thus, the approach to motor examination varies largely according to the patient's complaints and previous history. Nevertheless, even when there are no motor complaints, all clinical neurologic examinations include a substantial survey of motor performances.

The clinician must obviously be prepared to test the functions of individual muscles. Techniques for the most common muscle tests are depicted in Chapter 32. As a point of departure, it must be accepted that the action of the tested muscles differs from their natural or normal action. In normal movements, it is rare, if ever, for a single muscle to be called into action in isolation. Instead, in even the simplest actions (e.g., picking up an apple on a plate or pushing the button of an elevator), whole groups of muscles are involved. Some are "prime movers" that achieve the final required movement (e.g., small muscles of the hand to grasp the apple). Others are "fixators" that fix the wrist so that the hand muscles can exert their strength.

Still other muscles of the forearm, arm, and shoulder act synergistically or antagonistically.

Testing an individual muscle, therefore, requires that the examiner takes care to eliminate as far as possible the action of the usually "associated muscles."

Limb Muscles

Muscles of the shoulder and hip are tested with the patient sitting or lying on a table. For distal limb muscles, the position of the examiner's hand that immobilizes the limb is crucial. Limb muscles, in general, are tested at the midpoint of the range of their movement (e.g., 90 degrees for triceps and biceps brachialis, see Ch. 32). However, with the strength of a muscle being at it lowest when its belly is fully extended, advantage can be taken to detect small degrees of weakness. Some muscles can normally be overcome (e.g., flexors of the neck); others are normally too strong to be tested in the ordinary way. For example, calf muscles are best tested by having the patient tiptoe first on both feet and then on either foot; the quadriceps, by having the patient squat as deeply as possible; and the iliopsoas and quadriceps, by having the patient get up from sitting with either thigh crossed over the opposite one. In patients with normal builds, the muscle belly and/or its tendon can be seen and felt during contraction. Perhaps because movements of single muscles are unusual, many patients do not understand at once what is expected of them. Therefore, the examiner should first put the muscle and joint in the proper position and use simple commands such as "Pull," "Push," or "Resist" and be prepared to demonstrate the required movement. Pain, chiefly joint pain, anxiety, and old age, of course, must be taken into account.

For follow-up, the results can be recorded according to a scale. The widely used British Medical Research Council system has a 5-point scale: 0, no contraction; 1, flicker or trace of contraction; 2, active movements with gravity eliminated; 3, active movement against gravity; 4, active movement against gravity and resistance; and 5, normal power. This scale is not sensitive enough in grade 4, which many divide into 4−, 4, and 4+ for movements against slight, moderate, and strong resistance, respectively.

Trunk Muscles

Some muscles cannot be tested in the usual way. Muscles of the trunk are globally assessed by asking the lying patient to sit up. Attention is directed to the navel, the upward shift of which suggests weakness of part of the anterior abdominal wall. This can also be shown by asking the lying patient to sit up while one of the examiner's hand is placed on the patient's forehead to oppose the movement.

The diaphragm is innervated by the phrenic nerve (C3, *C4*, and C5). It is responsible for abdominal inspiration, which is distinct from thoracic inspiration, with the latter being chiefly due to intercostal muscles. Normally, the upper part of the abdomen protrudes in deep inspiration as the diaphragm pushes down on the upper abdominal viscera. Paralysis of one-half of the diaphragm can go unnoticed. Bilateral paralysis results in respiratory insufficiency, at least on exertion. Unilateral and bilateral paralyses are best seen under fluoroscopy. Diaphragmatic paralysis can be due to spinal disease involving C3, C4, or C5; trauma; myelitis; tumors; or damage to the phrenic nerve on its thoracic course. It can result from polyneuropathy of various causes and must always be looked for in the Guillain-Barré syndrome. It may be part of muscle weakness in spinal muscular atrophy or limb-girdle muscular atrophy. A safe clinical rule indicates that, when the deltoid and/or biceps muscles (innervated by C5–C6 and hence close to the spinal segments of the phrenic nerve) are paralyzed, paralysis of the diaphragm must be looked for.

Patterns of Weakness

Upper and lower motor neuron weaknesses are generally well contrasted. In lower motor neurons, weakness is either distal (e.g., in polyneuropathies) or affects the territory of roots, plexuses, or nerves. It is attended by flaccidity, loss of tendon reflexes, and wasting. In upper motor neuron lesions (e.g., in hemiparesis caused by stroke), weakness shows a unique distribution. On the upper limb, shoulder abduction, elbow extension, and finger extension are the most impaired. A useful test to detect small degrees of upper motor neuron weakness at the shoulder is to ask the seated patient, with eyes shut, to hold both arms outstretched with spread fingers. Even slight, upper motor neuron weakness determines a degree of dropping and drift out of the upper limb with sometimes a tendency to pronation.

On the lower limb, hip and knee flexion, dorsiflexion, and eversion of the foot are the most impaired. Spasticity or hypertonia (see below), the second feature of upper motor neuron lesions, predominates on the antagonists of the weak muscles, which explains the characteristic posture and walk of the hemiplegic patient, that is, shoulder adducted, elbow flexed, fingers flexed in the palm, hip and knee extended, and foot dropping with the paralyzed leg half circling at each step to prevent dragging of the toes on the ground. Testing of strength is not the sole method of clinical evaluation of the upper motor neuron. As mentioned before, the core of the function of the corticospinal tract is to control fine individual movements of the fingers. This can be tested by asking the patient to touch successively the tip of the thumb with the tip of each finger quickly and precisely, that is, filliping.

In upper motor neuron lesions, increased tendon reflexes and a Babinski's sign are also present (Table 22-2). Upper and lower motor neuron syndromes can coexist, which is characteristic of amyotrophic lateral sclerosis, also termed "motor neuron disease" for that very reason.

Motor neglect or pseudohemiplegia can be part of a unilateral neglect syndrome together with sensory, auditory, and visual neglect. It can also be "pure," that is, characterized by the underutilization of the affected limbs on one side, although there is no weakness, no disorders of tendon and plantar reflexes, and no sensory disorders. Hypotonia is often present. On verbal stimulation from the examiner, the neglected limb, for a time, is able to carry out normally the usual tasks. Motor neglect is contralateral to frontal, parietal, or thalamic lesions, more often in the right hemisphere. Apraxia is a disorder of movements in which muscle strength is normal (see Ch. 19).

Weakness as a result of disorders of the neuromuscular junction (e.g., myasthenia gravis) involves primarily the eyes, face, and oropharyngeal muscles. Episodes of acute weakness that affect muscles of the trunk and limbs are the major clinical features of the periodic paralyses with hypo-, hyper-, or normokalemia. The weakness caused by muscular dystrophy, in principle, affects the proximal muscles of the limbs, girdles, neck, and face.

Severe acute sensory disturbance impairs movements (e.g., in migraine), and it can be difficult retrospectively to differentiate disorders of movement of sensory origin from those of motor origin. Usually, disorders of sensory origin are attended by numbness and pins and needles.

With experience, it is generally easy to differentiate weakness caused by neurologic disease from chronic lassitude or fatigue. In the latter case, the complaints are less specific, vague, and indefinite, which often suggests neurosis and/or depression. The neurologic examination is normal. It must be remembered, however, that fatigue of recent onset can result from a systemic illness (e.g., anemia, malignancy, and inflammatory disorders such as giant cell arteritis). Hysterical paralysis can mimic monoplegia, hemiplegia, or paraplegia. In hysterical monoplegia, paralysis can be limited to the movements of one joint, which is very rarely, if ever, seen in organic pathologic conditions. Attempts at movements of the paralyzed part typically provoke simultaneous contractions of agonists and antagonists, with resulting bizarre movements. These attempts are made with a florid demonstration of great effort that achieves little success. Hypertonia can coexist, but contrary to organic hypertonia, it increases as

the examiner tries to overcome it. In 1984, C. M. Fisher listed many symptoms and signs of the neurology of hysteria. The neurologic examination, as far as organic signs are concerned, is normal.

Muscular Tone

In the normal subject, muscles are neither taut nor floppy; they offer a smooth, gentle resistance to passive stretching. Hypotonia or flaccidity is characterized by flabby muscles that do not resist passive movements and an exaggerated range of movements of the joints. This flaccidity is a major feature of lower motor neuron paralysis (Table 22-2).

In upper motor neuron lesions, there can be an initial flaccidity. For instance, after large sudden lesions of the corticospinal tract (e.g., in cerebral infarction), there is hypotonia caused by neural shock, just as there is flaccidity immediately after spinal transsection (see below). However, after some time, weeks, days, or hours in some cases, muscular tone reappears and rapidly increases so that the muscles become hypertonic or spastic. Passive movements meet abnormal resistance, and the quicker the movement is, the higher the spasticity. This is true up to a certain point because, presumably as a result of afferences from the Golgi tendon organs, at the acme of hypertonia, an inhibitory reflex intervenes and resistance suddenly gives up. This is the clasp knife phenomenon, which is highly characteristic of corticospinal spasticity.

Clinically, muscular tone can be tested in several ways. By pushing alternately on each hip of the standing patient, the examiner can compare the dangling and swinging arms. Passive elbow and wrist flexion-extension, passive pronosupination, the maximum range of flexion-extension of the wrist can be felt and seen. On the extended forearm, the wrist drops more on the hypotonic side. In the lower limb, in the recumbent patient at rest, the hypotonic thigh is more abducted than the normal one. With the knee semiflexed, when the thigh is flicked 10 to 15 cm up, normally, the heel remains on the bed and gently slides back down to the former position. In spasticity, because of the increased stretch reflex of the quadriceps, the heels come off the bed for a few seconds.

Spasticity must be differentiated from rigidity in which resistance to passive movements is uniform without the clasp knife phenomenon and is, for that reason, compared to the resistance of a lead pipe. Rigidity is a feature of extrapyramidal disorders (e.g., Parkinson's disease). Gegenhalten or counterholding is an intermittent resistance in which the patient appears to oppose passive movements unwittingly. It is a feature of frontal lesions.

In hypertonia, there is a "positive" disorder. The distinction of positive from negative neurologic disorders was first made by J. Hughlings Jackson (British neurologist, 1835–1911) and is a far-reaching concept in many fields of clinical neurology. It is based on the processes of encephalization, whereby in the course of evolution or phylogeny, structures have been accrued to the nervous system to reach the human brain. Each new structure exerts a new function, controls superseded structures, and is eventually controlled by newer structures, if any. Thus, the brain and spinal cord are a hierarchic, normally integrated system with the most recent pieces at the highest levels. Therefore, any lesion, particularly lesions of the highest levels have two consequences: first, a loss of function caused by the destruction of nervous tissue by the lesion (e.g., weakness or loss of the fine movements of the fingers); and second, the appearance, resurgence, or release of abnormal and more primitive activities (e.g., hypertonia or the extensor plantar response).

Although these general principles hold true, the precise causes of spasticity are not entirely clear. The examination of several kinds of spasticity, or rigidity as they are still traditionally labeled, is appropriate here. It has been mentioned above that transsection of the spinal cord causes an immediate spinal or neural shock that results in flaccidity and absence of reflexes. After a time, muscular tone reappears up to the point of hypertonia with an autonomous activity of the cord in response to painful stimuli (triple flexion of the foot, knee, and hip).

In another experimental preparation, the brainstem is transsected between the colliculi, just caudal to the red nucleus. In such an animal, there is decerebrate rigidity, namely, a state of diffuse muscle stiffness of hypertonia that predominates on the extensors. This is strictly dependent on the vestibular nuclei because the hypertonia is abolished by the destruction of the lateral vestibular nuclei. It is also abolished by section of the dorsal roots because the immediate cause of hypertonia is an overactivity of γ efferents. In humans, decerebrate rigidity is a frequent accompaniment of coma when there is damage to the upper brainstem. The arm is adducted and extended, the forearm is pronated, the leg is extended, and the foot plantar is flexed. The condition can be bilateral. Painful stimuli may provoke or reinforce these postures. Passive movements of the head that alter vestibular inputs can modify them.

Another kind of hypertonia is called decorticate rigidity, which can be bilateral. In animals, it results from supratentorial lesions that affect the internal capsule, corona radiata, and thalamus. The arm is adducted, with the forearm flexed and leg extended. Painful stimuli reinforce this posture. It is thought to be due, in a great part at least, to the release of excitatory influences of the upper reticular formation (the lower or bulbar reticular formation has an inhibitory influence). It is apparent that decorticate rigidity has much in common with the corticospinal spasticity of common hemiplegia.

The quest for cortical areas the destruction of which would determine spasticity has yet remained inconclusive. It would appear presently that lesions that involve both area 4 and 6 are likely to be followed by spasticity. The supplementary motor area may also play a role.

Reflexes

For clinical purposes, the term "reflex" means a visible motor response to a sensory stimulus delivered by the examiner. Reflexes allow the precise testing of those parts of the nervous system that are mediated by a reflex arc and influenced by descending pathways from the brainstem and brain. A reflex arc has an afferent (sensory) arm, a spinal relay controlled by descending pathways, and an efferent (motor) arm. Lesions of the reflex arc diminish or abolish the reflex (i.e., the motor response); dysfunction of descending pathways either increases or decreases it.

Tendon Reflexes

These reflexes are the visible response, as a movement, of a part of the body that result from the contraction of a muscle provoked by its elongation. Tendon reflexes are monosynaptic stretch reflexes. Lesions of the arc (muscle spindles, fibers Ia in nerves and dorsal root, spinal relay, ventral root, and motor nerves) decrease or abolish the response. This is a feature of lower motor neuron disease (Table 22-2), although it results as frequently from lesions of the sensory arm (e.g., in polyneuropathies). In severe disease of the muscles (e.g., advanced myopathies), the response, of course, may be abolished. Descending influences are either inhibitory (e.g., from the corticospinal tract) or facilitatory (e.g., from the cerebellum). Consequently, upper motor neuron dysfunction results in increased reflexes, whereas cerebellar lesions result in decreased reflexes. Hypertonia is concomitant with increased reflexes and hypotonia, with decreased ones.

The normal response of a tendon reflex (e.g., the knee jerk) is a brisk contraction of the quadriceps muscle, with a quick extension of the leg. This movement is followed by a brief sustained contraction (plateau contraction) and then the leg comes back smoothly to its initial position. The length of this relaxation can be increased in hypothyroidism and amyloidosis. When reflexes are decreased or lost, there is no or a weak response. In severe flaccidity, with complete loss of reflexes, the blow of the hammer on the hypotonic tendon elicits a characteristic dull thud. In increased reflexes, the blow of the hammer can be slighter, the muscle contraction is brusque and strong, the range of extension of the leg is greater, the sustained contraction is longer, and the relaxation of the quadriceps is slower and often irregular. The leg returns normally to its initial position because the quadriceps no longer contracts and also because the antagonists, the hamstring muscles, which have been elongated, contract reflexively. In cerebellar diseases, stretch reflexes of both the quadriceps and the hamstrings are in abeyance. A strong blow on the patellar tendon is needed to get a contraction of the quadriceps, and both agonists and antagonists react poorly to stretch. Therefore, the leg makes several to-and-fro successive movements of extension and flexion. This is called a pendular reflex, a characteristic feature of cerebellar dysfunction.

Tendon reflexes show a wide range of normal responses from very weak or apparently absent to very brisk. The symmetry of responses on both sides is an essential criterion of normalcy. Very brisk reflexes in tense, anxious people are common. Absent tendon reflexes are extremely rare in normal subjects. Apparently absent reflexes can be usually elicited by having another group of muscles contract isometrically (e.g., the patient makes a fist with the left hand while the examiner looks for the right brachialis). Jendrassik's classic reinforcement maneuver is usually effective. Just before the examiner taps the patellar tendon, patients pull vigorously, one against the other, on their two hands, which are locked by their flexed fingers. The authors recommend that, for the knee jerk, the patient be asked to push the sole of the foot slightly against one of the examiner's hands while the patellar tendon is tapped or to place the foot flat on the floor with the patient in the seated position.

Many tendon reflexes can be elicited over the body and are useful in the neurologic examination. The muscles served by these reflexes and their spinal roots of origin are listed in Table 22-1.

The jaw jerk is evoked by tapping the chin, with the patient's jaw being relaxed and half open. The tap on the chin stretches the masseter muscles, and the response is closure of the jaw. In normal people, the reflex is not or weakly evoked. A quick and strong closure of the jaw is evidence of bilateral upper motor neuron damage above the level of the trigeminal nerve. Conversely, in patients with increased upper limb reflexes, a normal jaw reflex suggests that the lesion is in the lower brainstem or upper cervical cord. When the jaw reflex is present, there is often additional evidence of bilateral upper motor neuron damage, for example, the palmomental reflex (i.e., a contraction of the chin muscles in response to a quick scratch of the ball of the thumb) and the snout reflex (i.e., a pouting of the lips in response to a light tap

on the midline of the closed lips). These are regarded as primitive reflexes that are present in the infant and would normally disappear. Their significance is not straightforward because they can be seen in some normal subjects.

The biceps reflex is evoked by tapping on the examiner's finger, which is placed on the tendon at the elbow. The patient's forearm is resting on his or her thigh or on the examiner's forearm. The response is often better felt than seen. The reflex depends on C5–C6, but in the authors' experience, the loss of the reflex is mainly due to C6 lesions, in which case the brachioradialis is also lost.

The brachioradialis is evoked by a blow on the lower end of the radius. The response is a flexion of the forearm. When the response is fairly strong, the biceps usually also contracts. When the response is weak, the reflex can be reinforced by asking the patient to flex the forearm lightly against resistance.

The triceps reflex is evoked by tapping the short tendon on the olecranon. The patient's position is similar to that assumed for the brachioradialis jerk. The examiner abducts the patient's arm and places one hand under the patient's elbow while the forearm hangs relaxed. This is a convenient position to detect a pendular reflex. The normal response is an extension of the forearm. In some patients the blow on the triceps tendon provokes a flexion of the forearm. This is called inversion of the triceps reflex, which suggests root, or more often, cord damage at C7–C8 levels. In other pathologic cases, biceps and brachioradialis (C6) are lost, although the triceps (C7) is increased. In such cases, a blow on the biceps tendon can provoke extension of the forearm (i.e., a response of the triceps muscle or inverted biceps jerk). This again suggests cord disease at C5–C6 levels.

The pronator is evoked by a glancing tap on the lower end of the ulna, with the forearm in semipronation. The response is a pronation of the forearm. This reflex is often weak in normal people.

The finger flexion is weak or apparently absent in many normal people. The patient's fingers are flexed at the interphalangeal joint. The examiner places a forefinger across the tips of the patient's fingers and exerts a slight pressure. A blow on the forefinger stretches the patient's flexors. The response is a flexion of the fingers.

The knee jerk has been commented on above. In obese or arthritic patients, it is first necessary to palpate the patellar tendon. The blow should not be directed upward because it would not stretch the muscle. A blow on the upper edge of the patella, of course, also evokes the reflex. The ankle or Achilles jerk can be evoked on a recumbent patient when the knee is semiflexed, and slight pressure is exerted on the sole so as to obtain slight tension of the calf. When possible, the best position is having the patient kneel on a chair. The blow on the tendon stretches the calf muscles; the response is plantar flexion of the foot. Loss of one ankle jerk usually results from S1 root damage as a result of a prolapsed intervertebral disc. Loss of both ankle jerks is an early sign of peripheral polyneuropathy. Ankle jerks can also be absent in very old age.

The following reflexes are part of some examinations. Hoffmann's reflex (C8 and T1) is a finger-flexor stretch reflex. The patient's middle phalanx of the middle finger is fixed by the examiner to snaps the terminal phalanx briskly into flexion. Release of this flexion results in extension, which stretches flexors. If the reflexes are hyperactive, the response is a flexion of the fingers and thumb. The pathologic significance of the reflex is disputed. It can be of value when unilateral. Rossolimo's reflex (L5 and C1) is obtained by tapping the plantar aspect of the toes, thus stretching the flexors. The response is a flexion of the toes.

Clonus is a self-sustained reflex contraction of the muscles when there is overactivity of stretch reflexes. Clonus of the quadriceps is elicited by a downward sustained thrust of the patella; clonus of the ankle is obtained by a brisk sustained dorsiflexion of the foot. When clonus is present, two or three repetitive responses of the knee and ankle jerks after one blow are common. A few jerks of clonus are normal in people with very active normal tendon reflexes.

Superficial Reflexes

These reflexes are mostly nociceptive reflexes. They are lost in lesions of the corresponding reflex arc and also early in upper motor neuron lesions. The following are commonly used.

The corneal reflex is considered infra (see Cranial Nerve V, Ch. 29). The pharyngeal or gag reflex (cranial nerves IX and X) is obtained by gently touching the pharynx with a tongue blade. The response is a contraction of the pharyngeal muscles. The gag reflex can be absent in normal people.

The sucking reflex (cranial nerves V and VII) is a pathologic reflex in which a brisk bilateral contraction of the lips occurs in response to a quick inward sweep of the lips from the corner of the mouth with a tongue blade. The sucking reflex appears or reappears (see above snout reflex) with severe bilateral lesions of the upper motor neuron.

Superficial abdominal reflexes are elicited by gently stroking the abdominal skin inward and downward with an applicator stick. Stimuli are applied just below the costal margin (T6–T9), at the navel level (T9–T11), and in the iliac fossa (T11–L1). The response is a contraction of the abdominal wall with ipsilateral attraction of the navel. The abdominal reflexes can apparently be absent in obese people or with a very flaccid abdomen. They are commonly absent in multiple sclerosis. In amyotrophic lateral sclerosis, although there is severe upper motor neuron lesions, they are usually obtained.

The cremasteric reflex (L1 and L2) is evoked by gently scratching the inner aspect of the thigh. The response is a contraction of the cremaster muscle that pulls up the testicle. The gluteal reflex (L4 and L5) is evoked by scratching the skin of the buttock. The response is a contraction of the glutei.

The anal reflex (S4 and S5) is obtained by scratching the perianal skin, which evokes a contraction of the external sphincter of the anus.

The bulbocavernosus reflex (S3 and S4) is evoked by squeezing the glans penis. The response is a contraction of the bulbocavernosus muscle that can be palpated at the base of the penis.

The plantar response (S1) is a major reflex in clinical neurology because its inversion (Babinski's sign) unequivocally means a corticospinal lesion.

The plantar response must be evoked on a recumbent patient and on a warm foot, with the lower limb being extended. Many people are anxious or ticklish, and it is convenient to inform the patient of the test to come and ask the patient not to withdraw the leg, to be "stoical" or "impassive" for a few seconds. The plantar response is elicited (e.g., with a broken tongue blade) by stroking the outer border of the sole from the heel to the toes. Some recommend a continuation across the anterior arch of the foot up to the ball of the big toe.

After 1 year of age or so, the normal response is a plantar flexion of the big toe; the other toes flex and adduct. Joseph Babinski (French neurologist, 1857–1932) in 1896 showed that the response is inverted where there is a corticospinal (pyramidal) lesion. Then, instead of flexing, the big toe extends slowly, "solemnly," sometimes with fanning of the other toes (signe de l'éventail) and contraction of the hamstrings and tensor fasciae femoris. These concomitant contractions are due to the fact that the big toe extension is only part of a triple flexion movement or a withdrawal movement of the leg to a nociceptive stimulus, analogous to the triple flexion reflex on the spine-damaged frog's leg in response to a painful stimulus (see above).

The plantar response is not an all-or-none phenomenon. Responses can be classified as extensor (Babinski's sign), equivocal, indifferent, and flexor. In some cases, while scratching the inner part of the sole would provoke flexion, scratching the outer edge of the sole or even the outer border of the dorsum of the foot evokes extension, which is the meaningful response. Some variants of technique should be noted.

Such variants consist of running firmly down the edge of the tibia with the knuckles of the middle fingers (Oppenheim), pinching the Achilles tendon (Schäffer), and abducting the little toe slowly and maximally and then releasing it (Stransky). These variants are rarely used.

A transient extensor plantar response is present during sleep, during some toxic comas, and after epileptic fits.

Crossed plantar extension is a complex phenomenon. It has been reported mainly in infantile hemi- or diplegia and in a lesion of the paracentral lobule.

Wasting

Wasting or amyotrophy means a loss of the bulk of muscle tissue. It can result from disease of the muscle cells, as in muscular dystrophies or myopathies, or from lower motor neuron diseases (Table 22-2) because the integrity of the latter is necessary to the metabolic maintenance of muscle cells. The distribution of wasting reflects the site of the lesion: anterior horn, anterior root or spinal nerve, plexus, nerve, or nerve branch. Here again, a sound knowledge of anatomy, of course, is required.

In diagnosing amyotrophy, allowance must be made for factors such as inherited features of the body, slight asymmetry of both halves of the body (which is not rare), episodic severe diseases, and malnutrition. In old age, the muscles can become very thin, but normally, they retain strength within the normal range for a short effort. Generally, significant wasting is associated with weakness. Joint disease can determine amyotrophy (e.g., a frozen shoulder with deltoid wasting or a knee trauma with quadriceps atrophy).

Amyotrophy is not a feature of upper motor neuron disease (Table 22-2). However, in hemiplegia, after some time, there is some disuse atrophy of the paralyzed muscle, and in rare cases of parietal lesions, there may be wasting of the muscles of the contralateral upper limb. The causes and mechanisms of this unexpected wasting are not known.

In chronic lesions of the lower motor neurons, there is a tendency for neighboring nerve fibers to reinnervate denervated motor units. This results in oversized and overexcitable motor units that cause fasciculations (i.e., spontaneous twitches of groups of muscular fibers). Significant fasciculations that occur in a muscle at rest for a few fasciculations after contraction or after percussion of the muscle are not necessarily abnormal. Fasciculations of the tongue must be looked for on the tongue at rest in the mouth. Fasciculations of the calves are common after muscular effort and/or dehydration, and some fasciculations in the calves, thenar eminence, or orbicularis oculi are also common in normal people. Because fasciculations are a prominent sign of motor neuron disease, these benign fasciculations must be recognized to give reassurance to anxious people (e.g., medical students who have recently been acquainted with the disease). There is a syndrome of benign fasciculations with cramps. A sound clinical rule says that fasciculations in resting muscles with no weakness, no change in reflexes, and no wasting are unimportant.

Slow persistent fasciculations are a feature of the syndrome of continuous muscle activity. Fasciculations must be distinguished from myokymia in which incessant, spontaneous, short contractions of motor units cause a continuous undulation or rippling of the muscles. These twitches are slower and last longer than fasciculations. They may be generalized or restricted to a part of the body, such as the face, in which case they suggest brainstem disease.

INCOORDINATION, RIGIDITY, DYSTONIA, TREMOR, AND INVOLUNTARY MOVEMENTS

As stated earlier in this chapter, two chief structures, the cerebellum and the basal ganglia, although they have no direct projections to the spinal cord, exert a fundamental control on movement. This is true for all movements but especially for *posture* (the situation of the body in space) and *stability* (muscular adjustments to the ever-changing postures in standing, sitting, walking, running, and so forth). As such, these structures control mainly the axial muscles (neck and trunk) and proximal muscles of the limbs. This can be contrasted with "the pyramidal system," which controls mainly distal, discrete, and fine movements, particularly of the hand and fingers. Taken together, these structures have been termed the "extrapyramidal system" (S. A. K. Wilson, British neurologist, 1878–1937). Neurologic custom, however, has restricted the labels extrapyramidal system and extrapyramidal diseases to the basal ganglia. The *cerebellum* is considered to stand apart on its own as a regulator of all movements. Its diseases are characterized by hypotonia and incoordination of movement; diseases of the *basal ganglia* are characterized by hyperkinesia (i.e., excess of movements, dystonia, and involuntary movements) or by hypokinesia (i.e., restrictions of movement).

CEREBELLUM

Throughout its extent the cerebellar cortex shows a uniform histologic structure that suggests a functional unity (i.e., that all parts play essentially a similar role). This histologic structure is unique in the central nervous system. About 15 million *Purkinje cells* with a huge dendritic tree, resembling the head and antlers of an old stag or hart, are sagittally stacked in regular rows. They are the sole output of the cerebellar cortex, which is inhibitory in function. Inputs are brought up to the cerebellar cortex by two different afferent systems. First, they are carried by the *climbing fibers,* originating in the contralateral medullary olive, which convey signals from the cerebral cortex and spinal cord but also from the red nucleus, periaqueductal gray matter, and visual system. Climbing fibers make up the major part of the inferior cerebellar peduncle, and each of them is closely bound to one Purkinje cell on the dendrites on which it terminates in an ivy-like manner, thus making a high number of contacts. Climbing fibers exert a powerful excitatory influence on Purkinje cells. Second, inputs reach the cerebellum by way of the *mossy fibers,* which bring signals from the spinal cord, particularly from muscle spindles and cortical, vestibular, visual, auditory, and reticular sources. They synapse with granule cells of the cerebellar cortex. Axons of the granule cells bifurcate into parallel fibers (i.e., fibers that run perpendicularly through the rows of Purkinje dendrites, with each Purkinje cell having about 0.5 million contacts with parallel fibers). Purkinje cells thus have remarkably large and multimodal fields of reception. Other elements of the cerebellar cortex are *basket cells* and *Golgi cells* that inhibit, respectively, Purkinje and granule cells.

Purkinje cells project on the deep cerebellar nuclei, namely from lateral to medial: dentate, emboliform, globose, and fastigial. In their way to the cortex, collaterals from both afferent fibers and systems project on these deep nuclei.

In simple terms, the physiologic role of the cerebellum can be conceived as a control of ongoing movement, particularly the timing and strength of the co-contraction-relaxation of agonistic-antagonistic prime movers and fixator muscles (see above). Hence, most clinical cerebellar disorders appear as disorders of movement. Several mathematical models of cerebellar control have been proposed that assign a key role to the cerebellum in open loop or parametric or internal feedback control. Much of the cerebellar disorders could be explained by feedback disturbances. Currently, the cerebellum can be considered to be an adaptive controller with adaptive-learning capacities, which takes parts in movements and, probably also, in some mental activities.

However uniform its histologic structure, the cerebellum shows two kinds of spatial and functional organizations (Fig. 22-7). First, there are three parts of different phylogenic and functional significance. The archicerebellum, the oldest cerebellum, is concerned with vestibular functions and, hence, is also called the vestibulocerebellum. It receives primary and secondary vestibular fibers that come respectively from the vestibular ganglion and the vestibular nuclei. The former projects ipsilaterally and the latter, bilaterally. In addition, the vestibulocerebellum receives inputs from the inferior olive and pontine nuclei, particularly visual signals. Lesions of this part of the cerebellum can be expected to determine disorders of gait, equilibrium, and stability of the eyes. The paleocerebellum, the old cerebellum, the second part, is still called the spinocerebellum because it is mainly associated with the spinal cord. It receives the posterior spinocerebellar (Flechsig's) tract (named after P. E. Flechsig, German neurologist, 1847–1929) through the inferior cerebellar peduncle and the anterior spinocerebellar (Gowers') tract (W. R. Gowers, British neurologist, 1845–1915) through the superior cerebellar peduncle. The former tract does not cross, but the latter one crosses twice; hence both project ipsilaterally. Both bring sensory cues from the lower limb and lower trunk. The cuneocerebellar tract and rostral spinocerebellar tract are considered to be the equivalent for the upper limb of Flechsig's and Gowers' tracts. Both are also uncrossed. Lesions of the paleocerebellum can thus be expected to result in disorders of midline movements, which are particularly evident in gait and walk. The neocerebellum, new cerebellum or corticocerebellum, the third part, developed during evolution, pari passu, with the cerebral cortex. It receives fibers from the inferior olive, as already mentioned, and from the contralateral pontine nuclei, (i.e., pontocerebellar fibers by way of the middle cerebellar peduncle). Pontine nuclei receive fibers from all parts of the cerebral cortex, particularly from the motor, sensory, and visual regions. Lesions of the neocerebellum can be expected to disturb mainly the voluntary, skilled, fine, and appendicular movements. Second, the cerebellum is organized into three main sagittal bands; the first the middle or vermal (from vermis) is concerned with muscles of the midline of the body and projects onto the fastigial nucleus. The second is the lateral, including most of the hemispheres, which projects onto the dentate nucleus. The third is the intermediate or paravermal; it projects onto the emboliform and globose nuclei. This spatial organization is broadly in accordance with the phylogenetic organization, namely, midline (vermian) lesions result mainly in disorders of midline movements (i.e., disorders of gait

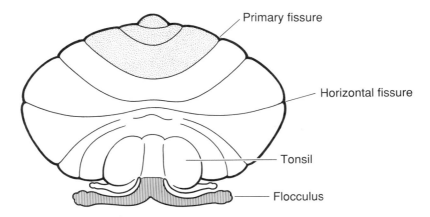

Primary fissure

Horizontal fissure

Tonsil

Flocculus

Figure 22-7. The phylogenic and anatomic subdivisions of the cerebellum. Light shading, paleocerebellum; dark shading, vestibulocerebellum; white area, neocerebellum.

and walk) and lateral (neocerebellar) lesions, mainly in appendicular disorders (i.e., limb movements).

The cerebellar output exits along three main pathways, which can be summarized as follows: (1) from the vestibulocerebellar and anterior and posterior vermis, cortex fibers project directly and ipsilaterally on the vestibular nuclei; (2) from the fastigial nucleus, crossed fibers (through Russell's uncinate fasciculus) and uncrossed fibers (by the juxtarestiform body) project on vestibular, reticular, and thalamic nuclei; and (3) axons from the dentate, emboliform, and globose nuclei enter the superior cerebellar peduncle that crosses in the midbrain (Wernekinck's decussation, named for the German anatomist F. C. G. Wernekinck, 1798–1835). A small part of the fibers of the dentate and many fibers of the emboliform and globose nuclei synapse in the red nucleus. From the latter, fibers cross in the ventral midbrain and run down the brainstem and spinal cord as the rubrospinal tract. Most of the dentate fibers go through or around the red nucleus and synapse in thalamic nuclei, chiefly in the ventrolateral nucleus. The latter, in turn, projects to the primary motor area the output of which runs down in the corticospinal tract, which decussates in the lower medulla.

Cerebellar afferents and efferents are thus either uncrossed or twice crossed. The clinical consequence is that cerebellar disorders are ipsilateral to the lesion, with the few exceptions ascribed to lesions located between Wernekinck's decussation and the red nucleus.

Ongoing movements are permanently regulated by a system of feedback sensory cues. Therefore, sensory deficits, particularly those that affect messages from muscle spindles, tendon organs, and joints, can cause movement disorders that closely resemble cerebellar disorders (sensory ataxia). The principle of the clinical diagnosis rests on the suppression of visual cues. With eyes closed, disturbances caused by sensory deficits increase; those from cerebellar dysfunction remain unchanged.

Clinical Examination

The authors think that the fundamental approach to clinical cerebellar testing is based on the disordered processing of messages between the cerebellum and the muscle spindles and tendon organs. Lost or decreased stretch signals can explain hypotonia, and many of the abnormalities seen in movements as overshooting are followed by overshooting corrections.

Hypotonia

Hypotonia is a flaccidity and abnormal extensibility of the muscles. It can be seen by the loose dangling movements of the limp arm or arms when the examiner pushes alternately on each hip of the patient. The examiner, shaking the patient's forearm, sees and feels the hand making excessively large, floppy, mannequin-like movements. Hypotonia, described earlier in this chapter, is also responsible for pendular reflexes.

The *rebound phenomenon* is another way to show delay in stretch reactions. When normal people flex their elbows against resistance and the resistance is suddenly released, the additional flexion of the elbow is quickly checked by the triceps. In cerebellar dysfunction, the triceps reaction is delayed, and the patients' hands can strike their shoulders. Similarly, if a sitting patient extends both upper limbs and pushes upward against the examiner's resistance and the resistance is suddenly released, the arm on the affected side swings upward more than that on the normal side. The loss of postural fixation of the proximal muscles also plays a basic role in the cerebellar disorders of voluntary movement.

Stance, gait, and *walking* are disordered in distinctive ways, mainly in midline lesions. When patients are standing, their legs are placed far apart. When asked to join their heels, they reel and sway unsteadily, yet falls are rare. The contractions of tendons are visible and then disappear on the patients' insteps as muscles are recruited for the struggle against instability. They are particularly obvious after the examiner has slightly pushed the patient forward or backward. When walking, the legs are wide apart, straight walking is difficult, and tandem walking is very difficult. On turning about, a characteristic cerebellar disorder, namely, *decomposition of movement* can appear. Instead of a smooth turning, the complex movement is executed piecemeal, with each part moreover being ataxic (see below). On walking, the patient tends to deviate to the affected side. In one time-honored test, the patient walks around a chair, and when turning toward the defective side, the patient stumbles over the chair. When turning to the normal side, the patient turns in a growing spiral.

Ataxia

Ataxia (Greek: *a*, lacking; *taxis*, order) refers to the lack of order of movements or of sequences of movements, literally *incoordination*. Cerebellar ataxia is made up of *dysmetria, intention tremor*, and *adiadochokinesia*. Dysmetria (Greek: *dys*, disordered; *metron*, measure) is inaccurate measurement. In the finger-to-nose test, patients are first asked to extend their arm fully to avoid the elbow being supported, with the faulty movement betraying the proximal hypotonia. Then patients are asked repeatedly to put one forefinger quickly and precisely on the tip of their nose. At the first attempt, the finger does not reach the nose (dysmetria). The limb generally overshoots the nose (hypermetria). Then, in a series of smaller and smaller approaches, the forefinger comes to rest on the tip of the nose. This series of oscillations is traditionally called intention tremor. Intention tremor, as described above, is not a true tremor, but rather, it is dysmetria with decomposition of movements. In some patients, as the finger approaches the nose, the oscillations become greater. This increasing amplitude is most probably due to lesions in the brainstem that involve, among other structures, cerebellar connections.

There are variants of this test. In the finger-nose-finger test, patients try to touch alternately their nose and the examiner's finger, with the latter being placed in varying positions. Patients can be asked to touch their earlobe, but this is a rather difficult movement with possible terminal hesitations in normal people. The authors recommend that the finger-to-nose test be done on a recumbent patient because, in addition to dysmetria, each time the hand returns rapidly to the couch, it makes a characteristic thud, probably as a result of hypotonia.

In cerebellar disease, there is no tremor at rest.

However, with lesions of cerebellar pathways in the brainstem, a vertical nodding of the head at 3 to 4 Hz can develop (titubation), and there can be a so-called rubral tremor (see below). Dysmetria in the lower limb is tested by the heel-to-knee test. The recumbent patient, with legs wide apart, is asked to touch quickly and precisely the patella of one leg with the heel, then to rub that heel quickly down the anterior edge of the shin to the ankle, and then to slide the heel back to the point of departure and repeat the movement several times.

Adiadochokinesia or dysdiadochokinesia (Greek: *a*, lacking; *dys*, disordered; *diadochos*, working in turn; *kinesis*, movement) is a disorder of alternating segmental movements. It can be tested by asking patients quickly to pat their thigh or the couch alternately with the palm and the back of their hand. The patient, with elbows semiflexed and not supported, is asked to make quick repeated movements of pronation-supination (puppet's test). Tapping the floor quickly and rhythmically with the ball of the foot can also be tested.

Dysmetria may also be evident in speech, which takes on an explosive and jerky quality; in writing, which is large, irregular, and angular; and in drawings of a spiral or of a ladder, which show similarly irregular borders. Eye movements may also show dysmetria as the saccades overshoot the target and return to it after a few approach movements. Nystagmus may be a prominent feature of acute lesions of the vestibulocerebellum (see below).

Clinical signs of cerebellar dysfunction are generally more severe in acute lesions (e.g., trauma or infarction) than in chronic ones (e.g., degeneration). In subacute lesions, they may also be severe (e.g., in the predominantly vermian alcoholic degeneration or even in olivopontocerebellar degeneration). Disorders that result from cortical lesions of the cerebellum tend to improve much more than do those caused by lesions of deep nuclei, especially lesions of the superior cerebellar peduncle.

A particular acute cerebellar syndrome results from infarction of the distal cerebellar territory of the posterior inferior cerebellar artery. Clinically, it presents as acute vertigo aggravated by motion, vomiting, unsteadiness of balance, and direction-changing nystagmus. The severe distress and the possible well-defined plane and direction of the vertigo can closely resemble acute peripheral labyrinthine disease. Within months, the syndrome may fade completely, but in some cases, it seems permanent. Surprisingly, in infarction of the cortex of the superior cerebellum, the syndrome may be so mild as not to suggest cerebellar disturbance. Although no explanation has been proposed for the difference in superior and inferior cerebellar infarction, in the authors' opinion, the striking symptoms in inferior infarction are probably explained by the acute involvement of primary vestibular fibers in the infarcted territory that are not affected when the superior cerebellum is involved.

BASAL GANGLIA

The basal ganglia are a complex constellation of big masses of cells and fibers (each human striatum contains about 110 million neurons) at the junction of the midbrain and cerebral hemispheres. They have been pushed apart in the course of evolution by the passage of the internal capsule and are scattered in a semicircle between cortex and thalamus (Fig. 22-8).

From clinical evidence, it is obvious that they play a major role in the control of movement, but in spite of recent advances in knowledge, their normal and pathologic significance remains largely elusive. Their intricate circuitry, modes of transmission, and pathologic role are presented here in a much simplified account as an introduction to the fundamentals of symptoms and signs of disturbance in their function.

The basal ganglia consist of several special nuclear groups headed by the corpus striatum, which constitute the caudate and lentiform nuclei (Fig. 22-8). The lentiform nucleus has two parts: the outer putamen and the inner globus pallidus with a lateral and a medial segment. The putamen and caudate have been nearly separated by the internal capsule, but they are still continuous and have a similar cytologic, cytochemical, and functional significance. Together, they are called the neostriatum or simply the striatum. The globus pallidus is called the paleostriatum or pallidum. The second major portion of the basal ganglia is the substantia nigra, a long, thick, black layer of cells, most prominent in humans, which extends from the upper pons to the caudal diencephalon. The substantia nigra is subdivided into two parts: the pars compacta, which is rich in cells that contain melanin, and a black pigment- and cell-poor area, the pars reticulata. The third major component is the nucleus subthalamicus (Luys' body or the corpus luysii beneath the thalamus on the inner side of the internal capsule). Just as the nearly separated putamen and caudate have the same significance, the medial pallidum and substantia nigra, pars reticulata, although wide apart, have a similar cytologic and functional significance (see below).

Besides these major structures, the exact anatomic boundaries of the basal ganglia are somewhat moot. The nucleus accumbens, an aggregate of cells at the junction of putamen and caudate, is considered to be part of the striatum. Some include the claustrum, but it seems more related to the cortex. The amygdaloid nuclear complex, which indeed is continuous with the tail of the caudate (Fig. 22-9), is involved in visceral and behavior control. The striatal part of the olfactory tubercle is rudimentary in humans.

Large afferent and efferent pathways that interconnect basal ganglia and connect them with other struc-

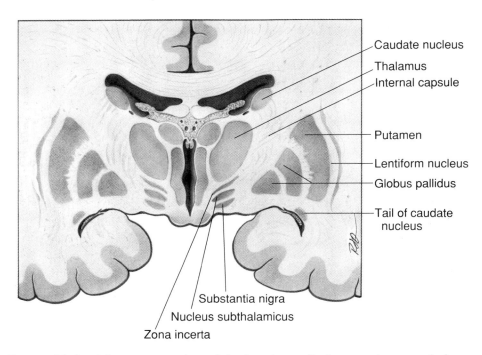

Caudate nucleus
Thalamus
Internal capsule
Putamen
Lentiform nucleus
Globus pallidus
Tail of caudate nucleus
Substantia nigra
Nucleus subthalamicus
Zona incerta

Figure 22-8. Schematic overview of the basal ganglia in a nearly coronal plane.

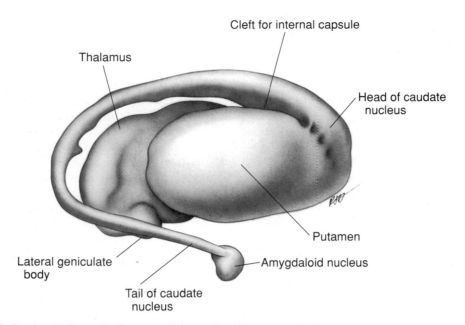

Cleft for internal capsule

Thalamus

Head of caudate
nucleus

Putamen

Lateral geniculate
body

Amygdaloid nucleus

Tail of caudate
nucleus

Figure 22-9. Semischematic drawing of the isolated striatum, thalamus, and amygdaloid nucleus showing the continuity of the putamen and head of the caudate nucleus rostrally, and the relationships between the tail of the caudate nucleus and the amygdaloid nucleus. The cleft occupied by fibers of the internal capsule is indicated. The anterior limb of the internal capsule is situated between the caudate nucleus and the putamen; the posterior limb of the internal capsule lies between the lentiform nucleus and the thalamus.

tures are known, although new essential data on fine structure accrue rapidly. On the whole, the striatum is the chief afferent; the medial pallidum and substantia nigra, pars reticulata, are the main origins of outputs.

The striatum receives afferents from most parts of the cortex, particularly the *supplementary motor,* premotor, motor, somatosensory, and associative cortex; from the substantia nigra, pars compacta; and from the centromedian-parafascicularis complex nuclei of the thalamus. It projects onto the lateral and medial pallidum and on the substantia nigra, pars compacta and pars reticulata. The pallidum receives inputs from the striatum (see above) and from the subthalamic nucleus. It projects outputs across the internal capsule through the *ansa lenticularis* and the *lenticular fasciculus* to the ventrolateral and ventral anterior nuclei of the thalamus. These nuclei, in turn, project onto the *supplementary motor area.*

Athetosis

Athetosis (Greek: *athetos,* no fixed point) describes the slow, writhing movements that predominate distally and affect mainly the limbs, neck, and head. The slow, reptilian movements flow into one another: flexion-pronation or extension-supination of the hand, adduction of the thumb-flexion of the fingers, eversion-inversion of the foot, pouting, closing-opening of the

eyes, and wrinkling of the forehead-frowning. Such involuntary movements can intrude at rest or parasitize a seemingly normal ongoing movement. Attempts to perform a discrete willed movement may set the stage for the contraction of distant muscles (synkinesia) or an en masse contraction of the muscles of a whole limb (intention spasm). Athetosis can be generalized or unilateral. Hypotonia or hypertonia may also be present, with the latter being probably due to associated lesions. Athetosis is related to both *chorea* and *dystonia* and, indeed, is rarely seen in isolation or as an acute syndrome. There are all degrees of speed between the quick movements of chorea and the slow ones of athetosis, and both chorea and athetosis often coexist in a same patient. Fundamentally, however, athetosis is closer to dystonia because both result from an excess of cocontraction of antagonists. Clinically, the very slow and sustained movements of athetosis merge into frank dystonia.

Tics

Tics are quick, brief, stereotyped, repetitive movements. They commonly involve the face, neck, and shoulders, such as blinking, pouting, smacking, and shrugging. In Gilles de la Tourette's syndrome (G. Gilles de la Tourette, French physician, 1857–1904), there are multiple tics with vocal noises such as grunting, barking, and sometimes coprolalia (Greek: *kopros,* excrement; *lalein,* to speak). Some tics could persist during sleep. Tics mimic normal movements, although they are not preceded by a Bereitschafts potential as is normal movement. The peculiar feature of tics is that they are not altogether involuntary. They occur at the height of a mounting internal tension, which the tic appears to relieve. Patients can usually delay for some time the movement at the expense of an uncomfortable rising tension. Tics are rare as a transient syndrome and are usually chronic with little change in severity over months to years.

Dystonia

Dystonia (from the Greek for disturbed tone) is characterized by involuntary, sustained, arrhythmic, sometimes repetitive cocontractions of agonists and antagonists that cause forced, distorted postures. The close relationships with athetosis have been mentioned above. Dystonia can be generalized, as in *dystonia musculorum deformans;* segmental, when it involves a limb and part of the trunk; or focal, when one part of the body is involved (e.g., in torticollis or blepharospasm). Some focal dystonias appear only during specific actions or occupations (e.g., writer's or musician's cramps). The dystonias are usually long-standing disorders not subject to great fluctuation in severity.

TREMOR

Tremor is a form of involuntary movement that is rhythmic and more or less sinusoidal. Tremors are of considerable diagnostic and therapeutic importance in neurologic practice because they are frequent and, although only a minority of them are associated with Parkinson's disease, all of them raise that fear in aging patients. A correct diagnosis provides reassurance and, including that of Parkinson's disease, in most cases, leads to efficient treatment (see Ch. 75).

The basic clinical classification of tremors simply depends on the situation in which the tremor appears, whether at rest *(resting tremor),* on maintaining a posture *(postural tremor),* or during an ongoing movement *(intention tremor).* However, this classification is a bit simplistic because some tremors do not exactly match the definition and because several kinds of tremor can coexist, at times or permanently, in a given patient. In many of these cases, electrophysiologic studies would be required to separate them.

Some knowledge of current pathophysiologic data is a sound background to clinical examination. Based on their natural history, electrophysiologic and pharmacologic characteristics, there are three main kinds of tremor: the first is an enhanced physiologic tremor; the second, essential or familial tremor; and the third, tremor at rest.

Postural Tremor

Enhanced Physiologic Tremor

The first type, enhanced physiologic tremor, is an exaggeration of the generally subclinical physiologic tremor. This tremor is postural. In normal people, enhanced physiologic tremor can emerge from time to time under the influence of emotion and fright (i.e., when there is an increase in circulating epinephrine) or after excessive xanthine (coffee or tea) ingestion. Tremors in pathologic anxiety, fear, thyrotoxicosis, and withdrawal from alcohol, among other conditions, have a similar significance. Tremor caused by stimulation of β_2-adrenergic receptors (e.g., in the therapy of asthma) has the same pathophysiologic basis.

Essential (Familial) Tremor

Essential (familial) tremor is also a postural tremor. Contrary to enhanced physiologic tremor, it is permanent, progressive, and familial in more than one-half of the cases. On movement, it does not change much, except in slow movement and at the end of movement near the target (e.g., tip of the index finger near the tip of the nose when movement merges into posture). Then the oscillations can become greater, a finding that explains why patients are socially embarrassed by drinks, soups, and noisily rattling saucers and cups.

Tremor at Rest

Tremor at rest does not occur with full muscle relaxation because a slight postural tone is necessary. It is a slow oscillation, 4 to 6 Hz, that is suspended or markedly reduced by movement. Save for exceptions, it is diagnostic of Parkinson's disease.

Tremor during maintained posture is tested by asking the patient to extend both arms with both hands outstretched, palms down. A sheet of paper balanced on the outstretched fingertips demonstrates fine tremors. In another useful test, the patient is asked to bring both index fingers close, just short of contact at the level of the nose (fencer's sign). To-and-fro or side-to-side movements of the head and a quivering voice (goat voice) result from tremor of neck and phonation muscles. Postural tremor is readily enhanced by emotion and thus generally easily demonstrated during medical examination.

Resting tremor is the rhythmic movement of the limbs when they are not engaged in voluntary activity. Typically, it appears when the patient sits relaxed with the hands in the lap or when the arms are by the side, when standing or walking. Resting tremor primarily affects the hand with oscillating flexion-extension of fingers and adduction-abduction of the thumb, activities that earned these movements the terms "pill rolling" or "bread crumbling" tremor. It can also affect the leg and jaw but rarely the head. The resting tremor combined with parkinsonian hypertonia (see below) explains the ratchet or cogwheel resistance to passive joint movements that is typical of parkinsonism. It is suppressed or reduced by movement, but often, on return to a resting position, it appears again after a few seconds. Resting tremor can be the only symptom of Parkinson's disease for long periods and can also be transient. Therefore, it can appear for a few seconds during a neurologic examination when it had been looked for in vain or during the examination of an aging patient for another problem. When Parkinson's disease is suspected and no resting tremor is apparent, it can be brought about by emotion (e.g., by asking the patient, with eyes closed, to make quick, successive mental calculations). It could be rightly argued that this brings about an additional enhanced physiologic tremor (see above), but what the clinician sees is a typical, often unilateral, resting tremor. Many patients with Parkinson's disease have, in addition, a postural tremor.

Intention Tremor

Intention tremor is the traditional term used to indicate cerebellar incoordination. As stated previously, this is not a true tremor. The existence of a pure cerebellar tremor is disputed.

Rubral Tremor

Rubral tremor is the term used to suggest the site of the lesion that causes a specific intense, complex "tremor," which occurs at rest, is increased on posture, and is still worse on movement. It probably results from lesions that involve the superior cerebellar peduncle in the region of the red nucleus, hence its name, rubral. Although it can occur as an acute syndrome from stroke, it is most commonly seen in multiple sclerosis or in chronic degenerative disorders and takes months to become well established.

Neuropathic Tremor

Neuropathic tremor is the term given to tremor seen in two different settings of peripheral neuropathies. First, a postural tremor of the essential (familial) type can be present in hereditary neuropathies (e.g., Charcot-Marie-Tooth disease). Second, a postural tremor has been observed in a variety of acquired neuropathies. It could result from a selective deafferentation. The tremor is usually less striking than are other neurologic signs.

Asterixis

Asterixis (from the Greek for lacking a fixed point), a feature of many metabolic encephalopathies, is a negative myoclonus, not a tremor. This disorder usu-

ally requires special testing for its appearance. The patient is asked to extend the arms and forcibly hyperextend the hand at the wrists. The irregularities in tone cause sudden downward deflections of the hands, giving rise to the misnomer, flapping tremor. The ease in elicitation of the asterixis is roughly related to the severity of the metabolic abnormality.

MYOCLONUS

Myoclonus (from the Greek for muscle tumult) refers to quick muscle jerks that resemble the muscular response to an electrical single shock on a motor nerve. The jerks are more or less repetitive, rhythmic or arrhythmic, and beyond voluntary control. Some of them (e.g., spinal, palatal, or epilepsia partialis continua) can persist during sleep. Myoclonus can be focal, involving one muscle, part of a muscle, or a group of adjacent muscles; or multifocal with jerks in many different muscles or generalized (i.e., a mass jerk of the whole body). Consequently, myoclonus can result in no movement, small movements of small joints such as the fingers, or large limb movements strong enough to throw the patient to the ground. The cause may be from brainstem, cerebellar, or spinal lesions. In many cases, there are diffuse lesions, or the pathologic condition is unsettled. It should be noted that myoclonus is frequently associated with cerebellar ataxia. Myoclonus is only a sign, and it has variable features. It can thus be present with widely different severity in a wide range of different diseases. Except for particular clinical settings (e.g., palatal myoclonus), the clinician is faced with two main questions: is the myoclonus symptomatic or not and is it a form of epilepsy? Table 22-3 mentions the main causes of myoclonus in young adults and adults. Table 22-4 lists the nonepileptic causes of myoclonus.

Palatal myoclonus is a rhythmic, quick (100 to 180/

Table 22-3. Causes of Symptomatic Myoclonus (Adolescents and Adults)

Storage diseases

Spinocerebellar degenerations

Basal ganglia degenerations

Dementias, e.g., Creutzfeldt-Jakob, general paresis, advanced Alzheimer's disease

Viral, e.g., subacute sclerosing panencephalitis, Creutzfeldt-Jakob (?), others (?)

Metabolic, e.g., renal, hepatic, respiratory failure, hyponatremia, hypocalcemia, alcohol or drug withdrawal, drugs

Hypoxia, e.g., Intention or action myoclonus

Myoclonus, e.g., myoclonic epilepsies, essential or familial myoclonus, or focal-segmental myoclonus, e.g., palatal, spinal myoclonus

Table 22-4. Nonepileptic Causes of Myoclonus

Physiologic, e.g., hiccup of usual duration, sneeze, hypnic jerks, periodic movements of sleep

Dystonic, e.g., in patients with chorea, athetosis, dystonia

Hypoxic, e.g., intention or action myoclonus, associated with cerebellar incoordination

Essential, e.g., sporadic or familial (can be associated with essential or familial tremor, sometimes suppressed by alcohol ingestion)

Exaggerated startle reaction, to be differentiated from epilepsy

Focal-segmental, e.g., palatal, spinal myoclonus (see text)

min), permanent jerking movement of the soft palate. It can extend to the diaphragm (fluoroscopic examination) and intercostal, pharyngeal, and facial muscles. Rarely, the patient hears a rhythmic noise in one ear. The primary lesion, usually an infarct, involves either the central tegmental tract or the vicinity of the dentate nucleus. There is gross hypertrophy of the inferior olive, probably as a result of transsynaptic degeneration, ipsilateral to the central tegmental tract lesion and contralateral to the cerebellar lesion. Palatal myoclonus is generally of little inconvenience and can be discovered serendipitously during the examination. The authors do not know of any efficient therapy. When spinal, myoclonus is usually due to infection or tumor of the spinal cord.

Myoclonus is a feature of many forms of epilepsy (see Ch. 79). A few jerks can occur at the onset of a *grand mal* seizure. Permanent, day and night, focal jerks are the basic clinical disorder in epilepsia partialis continua. In adolescents and young adults, the most common problems are *photosensitive epileptic myoclonus,* in which television screen flickering and computer games trigger bursts of myoclonic jerks, and *juvenile myoclonic epilepsy,* in which jerks of both upper limbs happen soon after awakening, often after a late night. By adolescence and adulthood, *storage* and *degenerative diseases* with myoclonus have generally been recognized.

MISCELLANEOUS
Akathisia

Akathisia (from the Greek for lacking a sitting) refers to an urge to move in parkinsonian patients. They cannot sit still and walk about to find relief, or when sitting, they jiggle and fidget. Akathisia can also occur in drug-induced parkinsonism.

Catatonia

Catatonia (from the Greek for low tonus) is a rare disorder in which the patient remains remarkably immobile and shows a waxy flexibility (flexibilitas cerea).

Even uncomfortable positions of the limbs imparted by the examiner are kept for lasting periods. Catatonia is a feature of a classic form of schizophrenia, but it may also be seen in some frontal lesions. It is important to know that it is present in malignant neuroleptic syndrome (see Ch. 83).

Hiccup

Hiccup or singultus (from the Latin for hiccup) appears to be chiefly a gastrointestinal reflex the main efferent arm of which is the phrenic nerve, which causes the clonic, repetitive jerks of the diaphragm. There is a concomitant excitation of inspiratory intercostal muscles. Rather unexpectedly, inspiration is checked within 35 ms by closure of the glottis, which causes the characteristic noise. Persistent hiccup is medically important because of the fatigue and anxiety that protracted hiccup can cause. It is by and large a male disease. The causes are numerous and different; gastric and intestinal diseases; postoperative, pleural, and mediastinal diseases; or general conditions such as uremia can be involved. Brainstem tumors, multiple sclerosis, and herpes zoster myelitis can be a cause. Hiccup is common in Wallenberg's syndrome. Epidemic encephalitis has been held responsible for epidemic hiccup. Some cases are believed to be of psychic origin, but proof is difficult to find. An organic cause is more common. Persistent or even intractable hiccup can be very disquieting and exhausting. It is often of obscure origin. In 1977, Williamson and MacIntyre reviewed the multiple and sometimes effective therapies. The authors know of two men and one woman in whom sexual intercourse interrupted a persistent hiccup for some hours. Baclofen, amitryptiline, and nifedipine have been proposed.

Hemifacial Spasm

For a discussion of hemifacial spasm and blepharospasm, see Chapter 29.

Hysteria

Hysteria can mimic tremor, chorea, athetosis, and most kinds of dystonias or present with all sorts of involuntary movements. Rarely, however, is the hysterical movements a correct replica of the neurologic organic disorder. The psychological attitude of the patient may allow the examiner to modify the disorder through suggestion. However, it must be recognized that it is not infrequent that the question of organic versus nonorganic is a difficult one, even for seasoned neurologists.

Mannerisms

Mannerisms are fragments of behavior when the patient is engaged in a task that requires focused attention (e.g., protruding the tongue when writing). They generally have no medical importance. Stereotyped gestures can be observed in schizophrenia.

AKINETIC RIGID SYNDROME

As already mentioned, inhibition of the ventrolateral and ventral anterior nuclei of the thalamus can be expected to cause restriction of movement. Indeed, several pathologic conditions that impair the normal nigrostriatopallidal circuitry, and thus normal excitation of the thalamic nuclei, result in hypokinesia. Among those conditions, the main causes are decreased dopaminergic input to the striatum caused either by loss of cells of the substantia nigra, pars compacta, in *Parkinson's disease* or by blockade of dopaminergic receptors by neuroleptics *(drug-induced parkinsonism);* less often, lesions of the striatum *(Wilson's disease* and *Westphal's rigid form of Huntington's disease);* infrequently, damage to the output pathways of the basal ganglia (i.e., medial pallidus and substantia nigra, pars reticulata, such as *progressive supranuclear palsy* and *Hallervorden-Spatz disease);* or incidental to diffuse diseases, such as advanced *Alzheimer's disease* and *hydrocephalus.*

The cardinal features of the akinetic-rigid syndrome as it is seen at its best in Parkinson's disease are akinesia, bradykinesia, rigidity, and impairment of the postural reflexes.

Akinesia (from the Greek for lacking movement) is responsible for the smooth brow, inexpressive, mask-like face with rare blinking and loss of emotional mimicry so suggestive of the diagnosis of Parkinson's disease. On walking, the arms (or one arm in incipient cases) do not swing, and speech is monotonous and mumbled. Difficulties in initiating walking are characteristic, with the patient being either totally unable to move or shuffling on the spot. Visual cues such as a stick or the examiner's foot placed before the patient's feet often determine one or two good strides. Movement is sometimes interrupted by *freezing,* particularly in narrow passages or doorways. Under the influence of strong emotions, a severely akinetic patient can sometimes recover normal motility *(kinesia paradoxica).* *Bradykinesia* (from the Greek for slow movement) is obvious in all activities, such as when the patient puts on glasses or takes up a pen or, dramatically, when, on an examiner's quip, a smile slowly arises in the patient's set face. Difficulties in sequential action are well exemplified by *micrographia* (from the Greek for small writing), when the letters become smaller and smaller. Micrographia is a reliable and early sign even in right-handed patients with an incipient, apparently left-sided Parkinson's disease. Experimental evidence points to a hyperactivity of the nucleus subthalamicus; recently, severe akinesia has been relieved by electrical stimulation of the contralateral nucleus subthalamicus.

Rigidity accounts for the characteristic flexed posture, with head forward of the chest and limbs flexed at the elbows and knees. When the examiner passively flex-extends the patient's forearm or wrist, a similar resistance is felt throughout the range of movement, as if bending a lead pipe, hence the comparison *lead pipe rigidity.* In early cases, when the diagnosis is suspected but no rigidity is felt on examination, rigidity can be brought about by asking the patient to elevate the opposite extended arm to the ceiling at medium speed (not too fast and not too slow). Meanwhile, even when there is no obvious tremor, a *cogwheel phenomenon* can often be felt. Also, in the early stages, rigidity can be more marked in the axial muscles, and difficulty in turning about in bed is suggestive of the diagnosis.

Rigidity and akinesia combine to cause the classic gait and walk of Parkinson's disease. The flexed forward patient shuffles with small steps, sometimes with increasingly fast steps, running after the center of gravity, so-called *festination* (Latin, *festinare,* to hasten). Falls are frequent because of the impaired walking or impaired righting reactions of obscure cause. Because of the poor postural reactions, patients, when falling, also do not protect themselves with their arms.

STANCE, GAIT, DIZZINESS, AND FALLS

STANCE AND GAIT

Stance, the way we stand and stay, and *gait,* the way we go, either walking or running, both require ceaseless, quick, fine adjustments of posture and movements. Such adjustments involve many sensory and motor systems, so that stance and gait are altered in most neurologic diseases. Abnormal postures and gaits can be so characteristic that they easily allow a diagnosis, but there are many subtle cases for the seasoned practitioner. Whenever possible, patients must be examined standing and walking, and wherever they may be, the good neurologist is always on the alert to spot instructive cases. Three of James Parkinson's six cases were seen in the street.

Upright stance first ensures that the skeleton does not collapse to the ground. This is made possible by an antigravity system with main inputs from pressure receptors of the feet and tonic postural reflexes from the utricle and saccule in the vestibule (see Ch. 29). A large part of the pontine and medullar reticular formation that receives these messages can be viewed as an activating descending formation the outputs of which travel along the reticulospinal and vestibulospinal tracts that control primarily axial and proximal extensor muscles. Sudden dysfunction of the pontomedullary reticular formation may account for some falls (e.g., some drop-attacks, see below). This descending activating system is under the inhibitory control of upper structures: cerebellum, basal ganglia, and corticospinal outputs, as evidenced by decorticate and decerebrate rigidity. Some of the features of hemiplegic gait can be viewed as release phenomena caused by the loss of that control (see above).

To stay upright implies that, but for short moments, the center of gravity of the body projects (lies) within the support area or basis of sustentation. The human being's bipedal erect stance is obviously a fickle one because the support area is normally narrow. Consequently, one of the characteristic abnormal stances from neurologic disease is a widening of the support area (spreading the legs apart). There is, of course, a system for postural adjustments that makes the feet move and changes the distribution of body weight so that the center of gravity keeps itself within the support area. Inputs to that system come from several collectors of signals. The best known are the muscle stretch receptors and tendon organs (i.e., proprioceptive receptors that play a prominent role). When deprived of this source of sensory intelligence, a patient cannot resist being pushed and falls immediately when blindfolded. This is the basis for Romberg's test (see below). Just as important are the vestibular receptors, including the saccule and utricle but, predominantly, the semicircular canals, that signal changes in the position of the head. Canal signals are apt to induce strong postural adaptations so that canal disease can provoke falls. Finally, vision subserves advance adaptations for situations seen ahead (possibly hearing plays a similar role for distant noises) and instantaneous adjustments to movements of the retinal image across the retina. Save for exceptional situations, this latter mechanism is of limited importance in practice. On the other hand, suppression of visual clues is also the basis of Romberg's test (see below), which thus shows the important vicarious role of vision. Clinically, poor vision is often a cofactor in imbalance. Neck movements and the position of the neck are sources of information to the vestibular apparatus receptors in the neck, joints, and muscles, which signal the position of the head relative to the body. Such signals influence the relative positions of trunk and limbs. In humans, in clinical settings, it is difficult to evaluate the significance of this source of information.

Normal walking is basically a rhythmic production of steps with a concurrent forward movement of the upper body that elicits the next step to keep the advancing center of gravity within the support area. This forward movement is the trigger of stepping. When it fails, stepping cannot be initiated. Normal stepping includes also a lateral displacement of the trunk that shifts the bulk of the body weight onto the supporting leg (i.e., when the opposite leg is lifted from the ground). Therefore, the supporting hip receives an additional weight, and hip muscles, particularly the gluteus medius, must be braced to meet that weight. When there is weakness of the girdle muscles, the patient sinks down at each step and waddles. Concomitantly with the steps, the arms swing, with the arm opposite to the advancing leg swinging forward. The neck is straight, and the trunk is erect. During three-quarters of the gait cycle, the body is supported by one limb.

During walking, contrary to running, the body is always in contact with the ground. Therefore, running and all activities that decrease contact with the ground (e.g., standing or hopping on one foot) are a challenge for the gait mechanisms.

A wide variety of styles are still within the range of normal gaits with, for example, gender differences. Moreover, stance and gait are personal and often show a surprising resemblance with that of a relative. It is well known that people can often be identified on hearing them coming. Human newborns can walk provided their weight is supported, but this ability soon disappears only to reappear 1 year or so later. In primates, walking movements can be elicited by stimulating the midbrain tegmentum or posterior subthalamus.

Gait movements are controlled by the cerebellum, basal ganglia, and motor cortex. In summary, stance and gait can be disturbed by lesions at any point of the locomotor system from muscles to cortex. To obtain full cooperation, stance and gait should be examined with a restricted medical audience and, after explaining, when necessary, that this is an important part of the neurologic evaluation. The way the patient has entered the examining room and has sat down may already have told much. Obvious cases apart (e.g., severe Parkinson's disease), complaints about stance and gait need to be analyzed carefully by examining acts of everyday life, such as getting in and out of bed, taking a bath, walking at home and on the street, putting clothes on and off, and driving a car. Disorders of movements of the upper limbs may be revealing, such as using knife and fork or a glass, buttoning clothes, and writing. The patient is next asked to walk on the toes and heels and then to squat and get up. This gives an idea of muscular strength and of joint function.

Obviously, hip and knee disease can cause stance

and gait disorder, but they can also be associated with neurologic disease. The patient is then asked to walk and turn around, first at a natural pace and then quickly. Then the patient should stand with the feet together, and the examiner looks at the instep muscle tendon (tendon dance, see below) and at the general posture of the patient's trunk and head. Next, the patient, close to a wall, is asked to close the eyes, and the examiner makes sure that the eyes remain closed. This is Romberg's test (M. H. Romberg, German neurologist, 1795–1873). It is positive when deprivation of vision makes the loss of proprioceptive signals evident (e.g., in tabes dorsalis, after a short time, the patient sways in all directions and would fall). A positive Romberg's test result is also possible with vestibular disease. With unilateral dysfunction, the patient should fall to the side of the lesion. Frequently, anxious patients standing with eyes closed state that they will never be able do it and sway. They stabilize with reassurance. Further exploration of the gait can be undertaken with more focused tests such as tandem walking, but in the authors' opinion, the tandem Romberg's test, walking backward or sideways, and hopping on one leg are liable to yield many false-positive cases and are rarely useful.

Waddling Gait

Abnormal gait is often the presenting complaint in muscular dystrophy. It reflects the weakness of the pelvic girdle muscles, which accounts also for the difficulties in climbing stairs and getting up from a low seat. The roll or waddle is due to the weak muscular bracing of the weight-supporting hip with a slump of the nonsupporting one, counterbalanced by an exaggerated sway of the trunk toward the ill-supporting side. An exaggerated lumbar lordosis and a potbelly, because of weakness of the abdominal muscles, are often associated. When patients get up from the ground, they push their trunk up with their hands along their legs and thighs (Gowers' sign). Weakness of the pelvic girdle muscles can also be demonstrated by Trendelenburg's test. When one foot is lifted off the ground, the pelvis, after a few seconds, tilts downward to that side. In the normal subject, the contralateral hip abductors brace, preventing the pelvic tilt. In patients with a waddling gait, when there is associated shoulder girdle weakness, winging of the scapulae can be noticed.

Steppage Gait

Paresis of the pretibial and peroneal muscles causes foot drop. To avoid dragging, scuffing, and tripping on curbs and stairs, the knee is lifted higher up than normal. This has been compared to the high stepping of a well-trained horse. When striking down the ground, the limp foot slaps. Steppage can be unilateral when it usually results from a compression of the common peroneal nerve. It can be bilateral in acquired polyneuropathies, heritable polyneuropathies (e.g., Charcot-Marie-Tooth disease), and motor neuron disease.

Sensory Ataxia

The patient does not know the position of the legs due to impairment of the signals from the muscle spindles and tendon organs. Therefore, the patient looks down to scan the ground and, being unsure, usually carries a cane. Even a light cane can help. The feet are wide apart. The legs are thrown brusquely higher than necessary, and they come down as brusquely pounding the floor with a characteristic stamp. Romberg's test is positive, and walking in the home in darkness is abnormally risky. The lesions can involve either nerve, posterior roots, dorsal columns, or medial lemnisci. The classic cause was tabes dorsalis. Nowadays, the causes might be chronic polyneuropathy; chronic meningomyelitis; or degenerative, compressive, or inflammatory spinal cord disease, with involvement of the dorsal columns.

Cerebellar Incoordination

With cerebellar midline lesions (e.g., in alcoholic cerebellar degeneration), the patient stands with legs wide apart. When the patient's feet are together, the instep tendons (those on the dorsum of the foot) contract and release (tendon dance). Romberg's test is negative. Steps are unequal, and turning about is performed piecemeal. In mild cases, tandem walking could be a sensitive test (see above). With unilateral hemispheric disease, the patient should deviate toward the affected side (e.g., when walking around a chair). A rubral gait ataxia has been reported with marked tilt of head and trunk and falls to the side opposite of a lesion that involved the red nucleus. There was no incoordination, tremors, widening of the base, or oculomotor paralysis.

Parkinsonian Gait

The highly characteristic parkinsonian gait results from rigidity and akinesia. Rigidity predominates on flexors, hence the stooped posture of the neck, trunk, forearms, fingers, and legs. The patient shuffles with smaller and smaller steps that can come to a halt (freezing), particularly in doorways or on stairs, or that can become more and more rapid as if the patient were running after the center of gravity, a state known as festinating gait. Initiating stepping can be difficult. The loss of arm swing is a good sign in early cases when walking might yet be near normal. During walking, one can often see a brief bout of telltale tremor.

A similar stooped posture with greatly slowed movements has been described from lesions in the medial frontal region. The rigidity seen in parkinsonism is missing.

Spastic Gait

In unilateral or bilateral corticospinal lesions, the abnormal gait results from the combined effects of spasticity and weakness. In hemiplegia, the lower limb is stiff, with spasticity predominating on the extensors. In addition, the patient cannot flex the hip and knee enough nor dorsiflex the foot. Consequently, the stiff leg is dragged in a circumduction movement, that is, compared to the course of a scythe, which minimizes scuffing. The upper limb is also paralyzed and spastic and, consequently, cannot swing. In paraplegia or paraparesis, both legs are stiff. The patient proceeds forward with great effort by small scraping steps and with exaggerated pushing movements of the trunk. In extreme cases, the legs can cross at each step (scissors gait). The paraplegic gait can result from spinal cord damage or from cerebral diplegia, usually caused by anoxia or other brain insults during the perinatal period.

Choreic Gait

In Huntington's and Sydenham's chorea, gait is disturbed by the intrusion of involuntary movements that are often exaggerated during gait examination. They involve the face and neck, limbs, and trunk in severe cases. They are brief grimaces, poutings, protrusions of the tongue, jerks of the head, extension-abductions of arms, flexion-extensions of the fingers, and twistings of the trunk. The latter, when violent, can cause falls.

Dystonia Musculorum Deformans

A gait disorder is often the presenting complaint because there is early involvement of the legs with dystonic inversion or plantar flexion of the feet. Extreme positions can be assumed, with the trunk forcibly flexed at the hips and twisted, knees flexed, and protrusion of buttocks as a result of hyperlordosis. Walking can become impossible. Such bizarre postures could raise the diagnosis of hysteria.

Frontal Gait

In frontal gait, there is no significant weakness, loss of sensation, or cerebellar incoordination, hence the controversial term of "gait apraxia." Another intriguing feature is that, although unable to walk properly, when lying or sitting, the patient can make walking movements. When standing, however, the feet are wide apart, and walking starts after a long delay. The feet look as if they are frozen to the ground, and then small, scuffing steps are obtained. They come to a halt or are followed by a few better strides, ending also in a halt. In advanced cases, patients are unable to walk and sit. When standing, the fall, generally backward. Grasping, groping, sucking, and pouting reflexes are often associated. On moving the limbs passively, one feels a variable resistance (Gegenhalten, from the German for counterreaction). Cognitive impairment is often associated. Normal-pressure hydrocephalus, tumors, and diffuse lesions are the main causes. The clinical features of the gait that separates these conditions have not been well defined. Frontal gait is poorly understood. In the authors' opinion, some of its features could be due to abulia, a basic component of frontal lobe dysfunction. Marche à petits pas (from the French for walking with short steps, first described by Jules Dejerine, French neurologist, 1849–1917) is part of the pseudobulbar syndrome together with dysarthria, pathologic crying and laughing, disturbed swallowing, sphincter disturbances, bilateral Babinski's sign, and sometimes intellectual decline. This has been ascribed to multiple lacunar infarcts or état lacunaire (from the French for lacunar state, described by Pierre Marie, French neurologist, 1853–1940). The pseudobulbar syndrome is rare nowadays. It has been proposed that it could be due to normal-pressure hydrocephalus. The authors have, however, seen the occasional case with no enlargement of the ventricles, as judged by CT or MRI.

Senile Gait

With aging, the neck and trunk become stooped, steps shorten, velocity decreases, and the percentage of double-limb support in gait increases. Running is increasingly difficult as is standing on one leg. Such changes are partly due to aging of the muscles and joints, but the neuronal loss that goes with age is basic. In addition, multiple sensory deficits: cataracts, retinal degeneration, hearing loss, vestibular decline, and mild neuropathy are often present and play a significant role in the disability. Again, normal-pressure hydrocephalus has been proposed as an important cause of disturbances of walking in elderly people.

Hysterical Gait

Rarely, hysteria causes a correct imitation of organic neurologic disease. For example, in hysterical hemiplegia, the leg is dragged as a dead piece of wood, stiffly pushed forward, or patients walk on their toes. The characteristic circumduction is absent. The arm does not assume the corresponding flexed posture. In hysterical paraplegia, every movement is abolished, and the patient is confined to bed or a wheelchair. However, tendon and plantar reflexes are normal. There may be concomitant sensory disturbances of the hysterical type. Astasia-abasia, a condition in which patients can normally move their legs in bed but cannot stand or walk is generally considered to be of hysterical origin, but some cases can be related to frontal gait (see above). Bizarre gait disorders are possible with extravagant twists and lurches but no falls, except when somebody nearby can catch the patient. When an organic disease has been initially diagnosed, it appears likely that the first examiner's mistake has been not to have the patient attempt to stand and walk. On theoretical grounds, hysteria is distinct from malingering and the Münchhausen's syndrome, but it is obviously wise to look for a gain motivation and a previous history of multiple admissions. This being so, some hysterical gaits can be difficult to diagnose and warrant a complete neurologic investigation.

DIZZINESS

Dizziness is one of the most frequent complaints in practice. Dizziness means a whirling sensation in the head with imbalance, but patients use the word in many other senses: an unsteady feeling usually without rotation, an impression "of being drunken," swaying to one particular side or not, lightheadedness, fuzzy vision, mentally unclear, woozy, or about to faint or swoon. The origin of the symptoms is likely to be vestibular if patients have experienced an impression of motion of the external world or, rarely, of themselves. Spinning of the surroundings is diagnostic, but less definite motions may point to the diagnosis (see Ch. 29). As so often happens in medicine, the previous history can be illuminating because a fair number of patients, years before, have had a frank rotatory episode. Peripheral vestibular disorders are the most frequent single cause of dizziness; among them, benign paroxysmal positional vertigo is by far the most common type of vestibular dysfunction. In the authors' experience, Ménière's disease is relatively infrequent and overdiagnosed.

The second most frequent cause of dizziness is presyncope (i.e., the discomfort, uneasiness, blurred vision, muffled sounds, salivation, and slight nausea that herald syncope, see below). Hyperventilation, caused most often by an anxiety neurosis, is the main causal factor of presyncope, which in fact, rarely goes on to a complete loss of consciousness (see below). Multiple sensory deficits (visual, auditory, proprioceptive, and autonomic) are a frequent cause in elderly people.

Other forms of dizziness are rather uncommon. Psychogenic dizziness can result from depression (by itself or from drug-induced postural hypotension), anxiety and panic (with hyperventilation being a prominent factor), hysteria, or hypochondriasis. Dizziness unaccompanied by any other symptoms is very rare in cerebrovascular disease. Dizziness, often postural, is a usual feature of the postconcussion syndrome. Many drugs, among which are anticonvulsants, tranquilizers, and of course, aminoglycoside antibiotics, which can harm vestibular cells, can be a cause of dizziness. Finally, dizziness can also come from visual dysfunction, commonly as a result of ocular disorders: acute paralysis of an extrinsic eye muscle, causing diplopia; cataract surgery with or without lens implant; and oscillopsia.

FALLS

Falls are annoying and frequent and either unattended or referred to the family doctor or general hospital. However, falls that do not result from accidental or incidental causes often come to the neurologist, and this symptom affects a fair number of outpatients.

On examination, the first step is to determine whether there has been a loss or near-loss of consciousness. When this occurs, it might be a seizure or faint; when negative, it might be unrecognized neurologic or vestibular disease or a drop-attack.

BRIEF SPELLS OF UNCONSCIOUSNESS

Brief losses of consciousness, also known as syncope (Greek: *synkope,* cut short, sudden arrest) means a brief (seconds or a few minutes) loss of consciousness as a result of a critically decreased cerebral blood flow (i.e., diffuse, short-lived cerebral ischemia). In everyday usage, syncope has come to mean fainting or swooning of all kinds of causes. It affects 3 to 4 percent of adult men and women. Faintings and blackouts are most often benign, but it is up to the neurologist to sort out cases that are a serious concern.

People who saw the patient falling or fallen can help when they are able to give a reliable and significant account. The first point is to ascertain whether there has been a complete loss of consciousness. A number of patients admit, on gentle and precise questioning, that, although they were "too weak to open their eyes and speak," they were able to hear and understand passersby. In some cases, the clinician accepts that there may have been intermittent short losses of consciousness. In both cases, there has not been a significant duration of any loss of consciousness, and a serious illness is very unlikely. Contrariwise, when there has been a definite loss of consciousness, vertigo, cataplexy, or drop-attacks are unlikely. In the rare difficult cases, associated symptoms and signs would settle the matter.

Seizures

The second point is whether the event was a seizure (fit) or a faint? The main pros and cons are the following. In an epileptic seizure, either there has been a suggestive aura or the seizure came out of the blue. Faints are preceded by a general malaise (see below). In seizures, loss of consciousness is a matter of seconds or less than 1 minute. Faints and blackouts happen during daily life; a loss of consciousness in bed at night is suggestive of epilepsy. In protracted faints, when the head remains above heart level, there can be a few jerks of the arms and twitches of the face; epileptic convulsions are generally much more violent and lasting.

A history of tongue biting during an attack serves to diagnose epilepsy. Bladder incontinence can be present or absent in both conditions and, therefore, is not a useful diagnostic point. After a seizure, the patient is confused and usually regains clear mentation within 5 to 10 minutes. Patients who have fainted are clear minded at once, although they feel washed out, sweaty, and liable to fall again if they stand up too soon. The previous history is often helpful. Years before, the fainter has fainted at school, in church, in the army, or in a hospital, when experiencing a sharp pain or simply having or looking at blood sampling. An epileptic patient may also have had a typical seizure.

The diagnosis between seizure and faint is by no means always settled. In 1979, Fisher proposed a type of seizure called "akinetic seizures," defined as nonconvulsive, transient, brief episodes of unconsciousness of cerebral origin not attributable to ischemia.

Nonepileptic Brief Losses of Consciousness

Vasovagal Syncope

Such events are commonly due to vasovagal syncope. This is due to a tendency in some people to slowing of the heart rate and peripheral vasodilation as if due to overactivity of the vagus nerve. In others, the cause is from slowing of the heart rate (bradycardia) from intrinsic heart disease. In both cases, a diffuse cerebral hypoperfusion occurs, and consciousness is lost when the systolic pressure falls below 70 mmHg or so. Teenagers and middle-aged women who have been sitting or, more often, standing for a long time at social occasions feel woozy, slightly nauseated, salivate, yawn, and have dim vision. Noises recede, and they fall limply on the ground. They are very pale. The pulse is small and slow. Injuries are typically rare, although they can happen. If the patient lies flat or, better, with the head in a low position with respect to the heart, consciousness comes about within 1 minute. Patients are sweaty and clammy and should be helped to a quiet place where they can lie down under blankets for a while and recover.

Postural Hypotension

Syncopes caused by postural hypotension, and thus by brief diffuse cerebral ischemia, are also extremely common and can be due to a variety of causes, not least among them being systemic blood volume depletion from vigorous use of diuretics in the treatment of hypertension. Micturition syncope can affect men, even young ones, who urinate during the night. Fatigue and a dinner with alcohol can favor the faint. Falling among bathroom implements can cause serious injury, but otherwise the prognosis is benign.

Cough or Tussive Syncope

Cough or tussive syncope occurs in thickset, obese, heavy smokers with bronchitis but can also happen in young people with severe bouts of paroxysmal cough. This is attributed to repeated forcible Valsava maneuvers that impede the return of the blood to the heart or severe bradycardia. By a similar mechanism, uncontrollable laughter or heavy weight lifting can cause faints. The authors know of an instance of cardiac arrest that occurred during violent laughing.

Carotid Sinus Syncope

Carotid sinus syncope is attributed to bradycardia, even to the point of cardiac arrest and a fall in blood pressure, as a result of the sensitivity of the baroreceptors in the initial part of the internal carotid artery. Impulses are conveyed by Hering's nerve, a branch of cranial nerve IX. Anecdotes report patients falling while shaving or putting a finger between their neck and a tight collar, but such cases are rare. In the authors' opinion, carotid sinus syncope is diagnosed far more often than is justifiable, and bradycardia from cardiac disease is diagnosed less often than is justifiable. In both cases, it is not a clear-cut affair. Carotid sinus sensitivity is often attributable to atherosclerosis of the ipsilateral and contralateral internal carotid arteries that must be ruled out. Auscultation of the neck and good-quality carotid Doppler insonation should do that. Prolonged stay in bed, especially in aged and debilitated patients, can weaken the pressure mechanisms that adapt to the standing position. Sitting first in bed or an armchair for a few hours or days should precede standing up.

Vagoglossopharyngeal Neuralgia

The acute pain of a vagoglossopharyngeal neuralgia can induce a faint.

Sympathectomy

Sympathectomy is a rare cause now, but on the other hand, the side effects of various drugs are frequent (e.g., antihypertensive agents; diuretics [also for their hypovolemic consequences], especially the thiazide types; levodopa; tricyclic antidepressants; and neuroleptics. Autonomic dysfunction with loss of adaptive responses to upright posture can be due to peripheral neuropathy, with the most common cause being diabetes mellitus, or to degeneration of cells of the sympathetic ganglia or lateral horn of the spinal cord. In the latter case, it can be part of *system or multiple systems degeneration* as in the Shy-Draeger syndrome or the striatonigral or olivopontocerebellar degenerations. There is also an idiopathic chronic postural hypotension (see Chs. 34 and 62). In such cases, changes in heart rate, constipation and diarrhea, loss of sweating, bladder dysfunction, and impotence in men are often associated. When the patient faints, autonomic responses such as pallor, sweating, and nausea are likely to be absent.

Other Causes

Hypoxia and acute anemia from internal (e.g., gastrointestinal bleeding) can cause faintness rather than syncope. *Hypoglycemia,* either drug induced in a diabetic patient or caused by a tumor of the Langerhans islets, would also cause faintness (or coma) rather than brief syncope. However, in doubtful cases, it is a stringent rule to draw blood for glucose level and, immediately, without waiting for the results, inject 50 g of glucose intravenously.

An isolated brief loss of consciousness is not suggestive of cerebrovascular disease. *Acute obstructive hydrocephalus,* caused by a colloid cyst of the third ventricle, can cause a faint at the acme of an intense headache. It can happen that a patient who has fainted has had a head injury. Clinical examination and imaging must decide which was cause and effect.

A long list of *cardiac diseases* can cause a sudden fall of cardiac output and syncope. Neurologists, of course, ask their patients about previous overt cardiac disease or irregular heart beats, take their pulse, and auscultate their hearts. This can detect significant *bradycardia* (Stokes-Adams syndrome), *aortic stenosis* (exertional syncope), or *dysrhythmias.* The syncope of severe aortic stenosis may resemble that of momentary cardiac arrest. Cardiologic opinion should always be sought for patients who have a pacemaker or a prosthetic valve. Congenital heart disease is generally recognized before syncope. In all cases with nonevident causes, the patient should be referred to a cardiologist who would diagnose intermittent dysrhythmia or tachycardia, silent ischemic disease, subaortic stenosis, hypertrophic obstructive cardiomyopathy, myxoma of the left atrium, or pulmonary hypertension. A ruptured dissecting aneurysm of the aorta with cardiac tamponade can present as a sudden loss of consciousness. *Hyperventilation* is probably a frequent cause of

faintness. Patients feel giddy with pins and needles in their hands and lips. True loss of consciousness is, however, rare. There is usually a background of anxiety neurosis.

Hysterical fainting also rarely, if ever, goes on to loss of consciousness. Emotional factors such as private or professional conflict can trigger the fainting spell. The patient usually lies limp. Lids can flutter, and the examiner's effort to open the eyes often meets resistance. There are, of course, no changes in the color of the face, pulse, and blood pressure. Neurologic examination, especially irrigating the ears with iced water is normal. Such faints can occur as "epidemics" in several members of a community.

In a number of cases, the syncope remains of obscure origin. With a possible significant frequency, it occurs during meals or defecation. Isolated syncope is not associated with a subsequent excess in stroke, myocardial infarction, or sudden death. This good news are generally sufficient to quench the anxiety that causes or results from isolated syncope.

Falls in Conscious Patients

Falling spells can be a feature of Ménière's disease (Tumarkin's otolithic catastrophe, see Ch. 29), although they are rarely, if ever, the presenting symptom. Falls can lead to the diagnosis of sclerosing subacute encephalitis in the young; progressive supranuclear palsy, tumor in the vicinity of the foramen magnum, and colloid cyst of the third ventricle in adults; hydrocephalus or nonspecific disease of the white matter in elderly people.

Drop-Attacks

Drop-attacks are the most common type of falling in adults, mostly in women. Falling happens suddenly with no warning in a standing or walking patient. Usually, the victim falls on her knees, sometimes flat on her face, and rarely on her back. There is no loss of consciousness. In nearly all cases, the patient rises up immediately by herself, but cases are known in which the fallen woman has been found lying down for hours. Interestingly, in some of these cases, normal movement of the legs was restored as soon as the sole could press on a wall or stair. Neurologic examination is normal. Drop-attacks can recur. Cryptogenetic drop-attacks probably mainly affect women. Three patients of Kremer (1958), who coined the term "drop-attack," were young men: one with an ependymoma of the fourth ventricle, another with fracture-dislocation of the odontoid peg, and a third with a compressive lesion that extended through the foramen magnum. Years ago, drop-attacks were considered to be transient ischemic attacks in the vertebrobasilar territory, but the authors think that no convincing evidence has accrued to support this view. Other diagnoses far exceed vascular disease as a cause. The long-term outcome of cryptogenetic drop-attacks appears to be good, with probably no increase in the stroke risk. This benign prognosis should alleviate the worries of these patients who fear the embarrassment and injuries that could result from recurring drop-attacks.

Cataplexy

Cataplexy (Greek: *kataplexis*, to strike down) is a sudden loss of muscular tone brought about by emotion. With a fully clear consciousness, the patient falls to the ground for a few seconds, rarely for more than 1 minute. Laughter is the common trigger circumstance, but surprise, anger, and all kinds of emotions (e.g., arrival of flying birds at a shooting party) can occasion a fall. Cataplexy is usually associated with narcolepsy, hence easy diagnosis. However, it can precede narcolepsy in 6 to 10 percent of the cases. There is a familial isolated cataplexy, probably unrelated to narcolepsy.

Left Hemiplegia

Left hemiplegia is a frequent cause of falls due in part to anosognosia, such patients being unaware that they are paralyzed. It is common to find left hemiplegic patients fallen on the floor near their beds when they intended to get up and walk.

ANNOTATED BIBLIOGRAPHY

Overview and Clinical Examination

Agid Y, Delevaide P, et al (eds). Revue Neurologique. Special no. 10, 1990. De la posture au mouvement. (From Movement to Posture). pp. 539–638.

Six articles in French and eight in English on the preparation and initiation of movement, akinesia, and motor neglect.

Carpenter MB, Sutin J. Human Neuroanatomy. 8th Ed. Williams & Wilkins, Baltimore, 1983.

Reference book.

Carpenter RHS. The spinal level. Higher levels of motor control, in Neurophysiology. 2nd Ed. Physiological Principles of Medicine Series. E. Arnold, London, 1990.

Clear and up-to-date account of motor control physiology.

Davidoff RA. The pyramidal tract. Neurology 1990;40:332–9.

A review update.

Fisher CM. Painful states: a neurological commentary. Clin Neurosurg 1984;31:32–53.

Thirty-one basic features of the neurologic findings in hysteria.

Freund HJ. Premotor area and preparation of movement. Revue Neurologique. Special no. 10, 1990.

An update on the physiology and pathophysiology of the premotor area.

Gastaut JL, Benaim LJ. L'amyotrophie d'origine pariétale: syndrome de Silverstein. Étude clinique de électrophysiologique. Rev Neurol (Paris) 1988;144:301–5.

Two cases and a review of possible mechanisms.

Gautier JC, Pierrot-Deseilligny E, Morin C, Awada A. Extension croisée du premier orteil. Étude clinique et neurophysiologique. Rev Neurol (Paris) 1980;136:521–9.

A case of crossed plantar extension in a lesion of the right paracentral lobule with a review of the possible mechanisms.

Itwasubo T, Kuzuhara S, Kanemitsu A et al. Corticofugal projections to the motor nuclei of the brain stem and spinal cord in humans. Neurology 1990;40:309–12.

Brainstem and spinal motor neurons seem to receive direct cortical projections, except for oculomotor and abducens nuclei and Onuf's nucleus in the sacral cord.

Jacobs L, Gossman MD. Three primitive reflexes in normal adults. Neurology 1980;30:184–8.

One or more of either the palmomental, snout, and corneomandibular reflexes were present in one-half of subjects between the third through the ninth decades.

Laplane D, Degos JD. Motor neglect. J Neurol Neurosurg Psychiatry 1983;46:152–8.

Twenty cases of pure motor neglect with the hypothesis that the left hemisphere is dominant for deliberate activity.

Medical Research Council. Memorandum no. 45. Aids to the Examination of the Peripheral Nervous System. Her Majesty's Stationery Office, London, 1976.

A precise and practical way to test muscles with their nerve radicular and segmental innervation.

Nathan PW, Smith MC, Deacon P. The corticospinal tracts in man. Course and location of fibres at different segmental levels. Brain 1990;113:303–24.

The latest news on the anatomy of the spinal part of the corticospinal tracts, including their discussion.

Rowland LP. Cramps, spasms and muscle stiffness. Rev Neurol (Paris) 1985;141:261–73.

A review of several ill-defined lower motor symptoms, signs, and syndromes.

Incoordination, Rigidity, Dystonia, Tremor, and Involuntary Movements

Agid Y, Delevaide P, et al (eds). Revue Neurologique. Special no. 10, 1990. De la posture au mouvement. (From Movement to Posture). pp. 539–638.

Six articles in French and eight in English on the preparation and initiation of movement, akinesia, and motor neglect.

Albin RL, Young AB, Penney JB. The functional anatomy of basal ganglia disorders. Trends Neurosci 1989;12: 367–75.

An update with heuristic models of basal ganglia disease.

Amarenco P, Hauw JJ, Héniu D et al. Les infarctus du territoire de l'artère cérébélleuse postéro-inférieure. Étude clinico-pathologique de 28 cas. Rev Neurol (Paris) 1989; 145:277–86.

Infarcts of the vestibulocerebellum. PICA does not supply the flocculus.

Carpenter MB, Sutin J. Human Neuroanatomy. 8th Ed. Williams and Wilkins, Baltimore, 1983.

Reference book.

Carpenter RHS. Higher levels of motor control, in Neurophysiology. 2nd Ed. Physiological Principles of Medicine Series. E. Arnold, London, 1990.

Clear and up-to-date account of motor control physiology.

De Long MR, Alexander GE. Organization of basal ganglia in diseases of the nervous system, in Asbury AK, McKhann GM, McDonald WI (eds). Clinical Neurobiology. Vol. I. WB Saunders, Philadelphia, 1986, pp. 379–393.

An update and hypotheses on functional circuitry.

Duncan GW, Parker SW, Fisher CM. Acute cerebellar infarction in the PICA territory. Arch Neurol 1975;32: 364–8.

The seminal article on infarction of the vestibulocerebellum.

Hallett M, Ravits J. Involuntary movements in diseases of the nervous system, in Asbury AK, McKhann GM, MacDonald WI (eds). Clinical Neurobiology. Vol. I. WB Saunders, Philadelphia, 1986, pp. 452–460.

An update, clinically oriented.

Ito M. A new physiological concept on cerebellum. Rev Neurol (Paris) 1990;146:564–9.

The cerebellum as an adaptive-learning controller of movements and perhaps of some mental activities.

Marsden CD. Basal ganglia and motor dysfunction in diseases of the nervous system, in Asbury AK, McKhann GM, MacDonald WI (eds). Clincal Neurobiology. Vol. I. WB Saunders, Philadelphia, 1986, pp. 394–410.

A pathophysiologic account of hyper- and hypokinetic disorders.

McKee AC, Levine DN, Kowall NW, Richardson EP, Jr. Peduncular hallucinosis associated with isolated infarction of the substantia nigra pars reticulata. Ann Neurol 1990; 27:500–4.

A milestone for the physiopathology of peduncular hallucinosis.

Pollak P, Benabid AL, Gross C et al. Effets de la stimulation du noyau sous-thalamique dans la maladie de Parkinson. Rev Neurol (Paris) 1993;149:175–6.

Severe contralateral akinesia relieved.

Revue Neurologique. Special issue: the centenary of Gilles de la Tourette syndrome. Rev Neurol (Paris) 1986;142: 801–66.

Seven articles in English and five in French on tics.

Williamson BWA, MacIntyre IMC. Management of intractable hiccup. BMJ 1977;2:501–3.

A case report with a review of multiple therapies, most without effect.

Young RR. Tremor in diseases of the nervous system, in Asbury AK, McKhann GH, MacDonald WI (eds). Clinical Neurobiology. Vol. I. WB Saunders, Philadelphia, 1986, pp. 435–451.

A clear pathophysiologic account with clinical observations.

Stance, Gait, Dizziness, and Falls

Aldrich MS. Narcolepsy. N Engl J Med 1990;323:389–94.

Advances in pathogenesis and pathophysiology.

Baloh RW, Honrubia V. Clinical Neurophysiology of the Vestibular System. 2nd Ed. Contemporary Neurology Series. FA Davis, Philadelphia, 1990.

The authoritative book on vestibular disorders.

Drachman DA, Hart CW. An approach to the dizzy patient. Neurology 1972;22:323–34.

Ménière's disease infrequent, compared with the more frequent hyperventilation and multiple sensory deficits.

Felice KJ, Keilson GR, Schwartz WJ. Rubral gait ataxia. Neurology 1990;40:1004–6.

An MRI-confirmed lesion with a new disorder of gait.

Fisher CM. Syncope of obscure nature. Can Neurol Sci 1979;6:7–20.

Analysis of 111 cases of syncope with new syndromes and hypotheses.

Fisher CM, Lacunar strokes and infarcts: a review. Neurology 1982;32:871–6.

The view that état lacunaire and partial lacunes could be due to normal-pressure hydrocephalus.

Fisher CM. Hydrocephalus as a cause of disturbance of gait in the elderly. Neurology 1982;32:1358–63.

Hydrocephalus as an important cause of disturbance of walking in elderly people.

Fisher CM. Abulia minor vs agitated behavior. Clin Neurosurg 1983;31:9–31.

Analysis of abulia.

Gautier JC, Morelot D, Gray F, Awada A. Aneurysme géant des deux artères vertébrales. Drop-attacks. Rev Neurol (Paris) 1982;138:63–7.

Drop-attacks with a compressive lesion of the lower brainstem.

Keane JR. Hysterical gait disorders: 60 cases. Neurology 1989;39:586–9.

A review of personal cases with a historical perspective.

Kremer M. Sitting, standing and walking. BMJ 1958;2: 63–127.

A splendid clinicophysiologic analysis and the seminal article on drop-attacks.

Martin JP. The Basal Ganglia and Posture. Pitman Medical Publishers, London, 1967.

A penetrating clinical analysis and a classic.

Masdeu JC, Wolfson L, Lautos G et al. Brain white-matter changes in the elderly prone to falling. Arch Neurol 1989;46:1292–6.

White matter hypodensity correlated with gait and balance impairment.

Meissmer I, Wiebers DO, Swanson JW, O'Fallon M. The natural history of drop-attacks. Neurology 1986;36: 1029–34.

Causes unknown, 64 percent; cerebrovascular disease, 8 percent; isolated, good long-term outcome.

Savage DD, Corwin L, McGee DL et al. Epidemiologic features of isolated syncope: the Framingham Study. Stroke 1985;16:626–9.

Isolated syncope not associated with later stroke, myocardial infarction, or sudden death.

Sheldon JH. On the natural history of falls in old age. BMJ 1960;2:1685–90.

An interesting study of drop-attacks.

Stevens DL, Matthews WB. Cryptogenetic drop-attacks: an affliction of women. BMJ 1973;1:439–42.

Likely due to gender differences in the mechanism of walking, good prognosis.

Sudarsky L. Geriatrics: gait disorder in the elderly. N Engl J Med 1990;322:1441–6.

A review with a reminder of the biomechanics of gait.

23

Sensation and Pain

J. P. Mohr and J. C. Gautier

Sensation is a term broadly applicable to what is seen, heard, and smelled. However, most clinicians consider vision (see Ch. 26), audition, and olfaction (see Ch. 29) as the *special senses* and use the term sensation to refer to what is felt through the skin, mucous membranes, and viscera. This *somatosensory function* encompasses a large range of experiences, including touch, temperature, sharp and dull pain, pressure, movement across the skin, location of points of contact, and position of body parts. Many experiences are uniquely detected by specialized receptors in the skin. The general direction of their sensory projections is upward or cephalad, that is, toward the brain through individual nerves and their clusters (plexi) into several pathways in the spinal cord and brainstem. Feedback loops at the spinal level provide for certain forms of reflex responding, mostly to painful stimuli. Projections ascending cephalad play on a variety of structures, some of which control fiber pathways passing downward (caudad) from the brainstem and thalamus, which also modulate the ascending signals in feedback loops. Neurotransmission is mediated by a wide variety of neurochemicals, that is, individual transmitters specific to certain types of sensation. This complex system is anything but a passive conveyer of cutaneous contact and should be thought of as an integrated system of extreme specificity.

Because pain is a subject so common to the neurologist, the material in this chapter has been organized along a conventional orderly anatomic format (nerves, roots, cord, brainstem, thalamus, and cerebrum) with separate attention paid to pain in each section.

ANATOMY AND PHYSIOLOGY

Receptors

The skin and subcutaneous and connective tissues contain histologically identifiable sensory endings (Fig. 23-1). The superficially located free (unencapsu-

lated, naked) epidermal receptors and the encapsulated Meissner's corpuscle and Merkel's disc endings exist along with the subcutaneous tissue free (unencapsulated) dermal endings and the encapsulated Ruffini organs (receptors) and pacinian corpuscles.

The free nerve terminals convey thermal and pain (nociceptive, from the Latin, *nocere*, to injure) sensation and lead to small, unmyelinated fibers. The free nerve endings respond to noxious mechanical and heat stimuli. The encapsulated endings detect mechanical displacement and feed large, myelinated fibers. Merkel's discs transmit sustained pressure. Meissner's corpuscles mediate single or oscillating weak contact. Ruffini organs are similar in function to Merkel's discs; the pacinian corpuscles are similar to Meissner's corpuscles. The area served by receptors varies, but in such high-density areas as the index finger pulp, as many as 240 mechanical receptors may be present per square centimeter. Pain fibers are more than threefold more numerous than the large myelinated fibers.

The response of the end-organs to a stimulus is graded according to its intensity and not by a simple threshold effect. Although the actual thresholds for individual sensory experiences are fairly constant, they differ for each. An electrical stimulus sufficient to produce the pinprick sensation described as *epicritic* (from the Greek for accurate judgment) by H. Head (British neurologist, 1861–1940) must be raised almost threefold to produce ill-localized, persisting, aching *protopathic* (from the Greek for crude experience) pain. The common experience of tenderness in inflamed parts has been attributed to lowering of the threshold for small myelinated and unmyelinated fibers.

Studies of single fibers have shown that those associated with pain transmission are subject to fatigue with repeated activation. The Meissner's corpuscles adapt

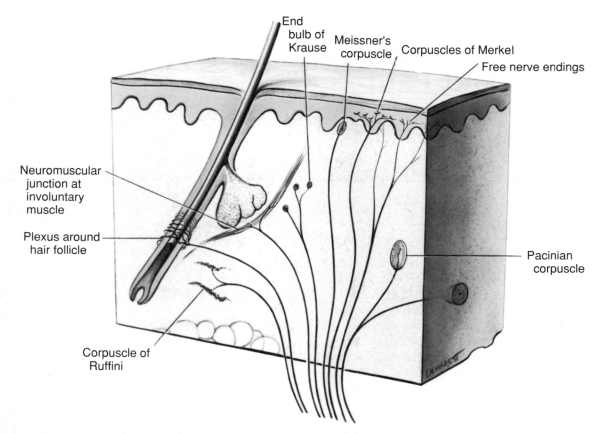

Figure 23-1. Nerve endings in the skin, showing Meissner's, Merkel's, pacinian, and Ruffini corpuscles and free nerve endings.

rapidly to stimulation, but the Merkel's discs and the free nerve terminals adapt more slowly.

Burns may lower the threshold for nociceptive and mechanical stimulation, causing discomfort (hyperalgesia) from stimuli usually not sufficient to cause pain. Age, toxins, and other diseases may reduce the number and diminish the sensitivity of nerve endings and fibers to stimulation, making the affected parts less sensitive to all forms of stimulation.

Components of Nerves

The individual peripheral nerves are made up of centrally bound (afferent) myelinated and unmyelinated sensory fibers and peripherally bound (efferent) motor fibers. Studies of individual fascicles of the peripheral nerves have shown that they individually serve specific cutaneous areas, which indicates a high degree of organization of the sensory system even at the level of the peripheral nerve. Injury to individual fascicles can produce highly focal areas of disturbed sensory function.

Small myelinated A-δ fibers carry epicritic sensation

at speeds of 4 to 30 m/s. The small, unmyelinated fibers (C-fibers) convey protopathic sensation by their slower conductions velocities (0.4 to 2 m/s), possibly mediated by substance P. A stimulus that activates both the A-δ fibers and the C-fibers produces two distinctive experiences. The first is a sharp and sharply localized sensation that is rapidly conducted to the spinal cord by the A-α (touch/pressure) and A-δ (pain) myelinated fibers, setting in motion reflex withdrawal, which serves as a mechanism for immediate escape from a noxious stimulus. The second response is delayed and polymodal (by the slower-conducting C-fibers), which produce a less well-localized and longer-lasting aching or burning sensation, which may help immobilize the part and prevent more injury while healing is initiated.

The large myelinated fibers (A-α fibers) mediate touch and skin displacement, conducting impulses as a function of the diameter of the axon and size of the myelin sheath, at speeds that vary from 30 to 72 m/s.

Pain thresholds are not uniform throughout the body or tissues. The periosteum has the lowest pain threshold among skeletal structures. The ligaments, the fibrous capsule of joints, the tendons, the fascia, and the muscles show progressively higher thresholds.

Pain in the viscera has several causes and a distinctive clinical form: rapid stretching of the capsule of solid (liver or spleen) or hollow organs in the gastrointestinal or genitourinary systems causes a rhythmic pain, often described as colic; that from anoxia of the visceral musculature causes a steady or paroxysmal pain, which is known as angina when it affects the heart.

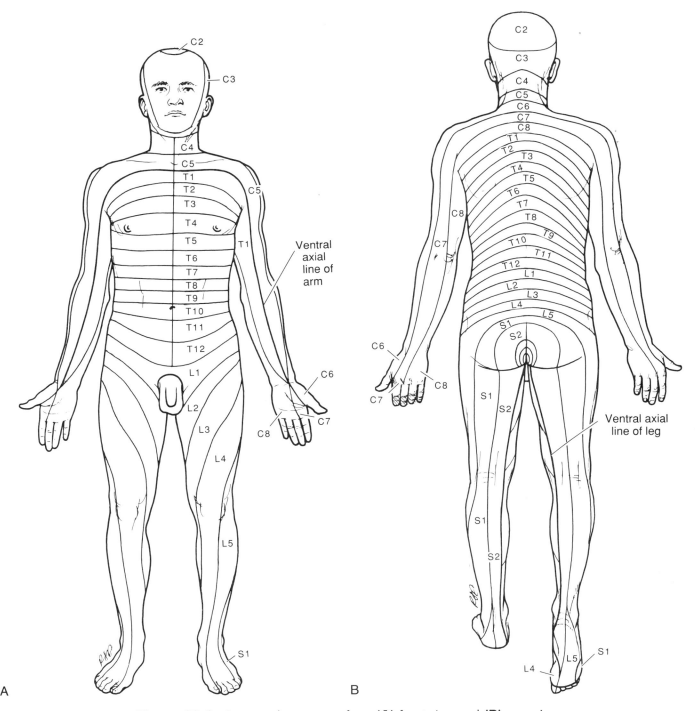

Figure 23-2. Sensory dermatomes from **(A)** front view and **(B)** rear view.

Nerves and Roots

The sensory distribution is orderly when viewed from the cutaneous segments (dermatomes) of the face, head, and trunk; each nerve supplies its own special area with little overlap (Fig. 23-2). In the limbs, the same orderly plan is evident from the fetal map of the limb bulb (Fig. 23-3), but growth during development distorts the distribution of the nerve territories in ways that has taxed the memory of generations of clinicians (see Ch. 31).

Spinothalamic Tract

The classic spinothalamic tract has been well studied. Approximately 70 percent of the C-fibers pass into the dorsal root entry zone, coursing in Lissauer's tract rostrally or caudally as high as several segments before terminating in the posterior horn. Almost all of the fibers synapse in lamina II (substantia gelatinosa) (Fig. 23-4). Although the posterior entry zone is the better known, up to 30 percent of the C-fibers reach the cord through a separate entry zone by way of the ventral root.

Opioid receptors have been found where the C-fibers and small unmyelinated fibers terminate in the superficial layers of the dorsal horn. Opioid peptides are endogenous compounds that bind to opioid receptors and mimic some of the pharmacologic properties of opiates. Opioid receptors are classified into four types: the μ receptors, which bind morphine; the δ receptors, which bind the naturally occurring opioids, the enkephalins; the κ receptors, which are found in sympathetic postganglionic neuron terminals; and the

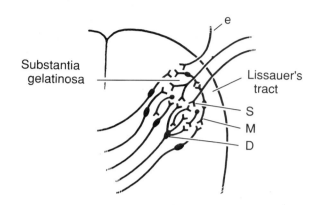

Figure 23-4. Entry of fibers into the dorsal root entry zone to synapse in the substantia gelantinosa.

σ receptors, whose functions are less well understood. There is some evidence that μ receptors can be occupied by endogenous opioid peptides. The superficial location of these receptor systems in the dorsal cord make them susceptible to the effects of morphine instilled in the subarachnoid space. The tricyclic agent, amitriptyline, blocks the uptake of biogenic amines at the dorsal horn, which may explain some of its analgesic action.

Some of the small myelinated fibers contact internuncial neurons; others make direct contact with motor neurons on the same (ipsilateral) side and on the contralateral side to mediate the rapid withdrawal of a limb after a painful stimulus, known as the nociceptive reflexes. Some of these latter neurons contain enkephalin, which may explain the value of morphine

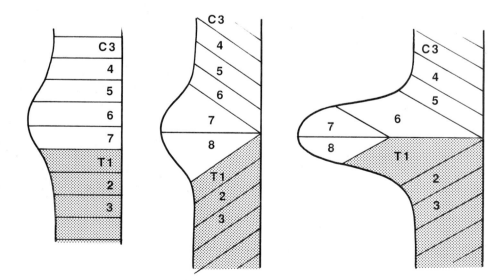

Figure 23-3. Diagram showing how the segmental patterns of sensory dermatomes become organized in the evolving limb bud.

in the reduction of the flexor spasms that reflect the nociceptive reflexes.

The axons of the spinothalamic tract originate from several laminae in the gray matter of the contralateral cord near the dorsal root entry zone, which receive both the small myelinated A-δ fibers and the unmyelinated C-fibers. None of these axons ascend in the posterior columns. From this zone, the second-order neurons project their axons to the contralateral spinothalamic tract, crossing in the white anterior commissure (i.e., just in front of the central canal). The location of the decussation explains why lesions in the region of the central canal (e.g., syringomyelia) cause a contralateral anesthesia for pain and temperature below the level of the lesion.

The spinothalamic tract has a roughly laminar organization. As the tract passes cephalad, entering fibers progressively thicken the population of the tract, with each new arrival more medially placed, so that the tract has a degree of lamination at the upper end of the cord in which fibers from the lower limb lie laterally, with those from the upper lying more medially (Fig. 23-5). Spinothalamic tract fibers stimulated in the brainstem have been found that carry information from a single limb, indicating that the pathway remains highly organized as it ascends. This organization makes it possible for surgeons to interrupt pain fibers from the leg by a laterally placed cord incision (cordotomy).

Spinothalamic fibers arising from lamina I receive projections from the peripheral nerves from the small receptive fields that respond best to noxious stimuli. Those from laminae IV to VI arise from fibers that have somewhat larger receptive fields and respond to both mechanical (innocuous) and nociceptive stimuli. Fibers from laminae I to VI terminate mainly in the ventroposterolateral nuclei of the thalamus in topographic fashion, overlying those from the posterior columns. Fibers originating in laminae VII to X have receptive fields that respond to both deep and superficial stimuli of a wide variety of types, and they have some bilateral representation. Their projections through the brainstem terminate in the brainstem reticular formation on both sides of the lower brainstem and in the midbrain reticular formation, which is thought to account for arousal after painful stimuli. They also project to the intralaminar and dorsomedial nuclei of the thalamus, which contain opiate receptors. This type of organization may provide an anatomic explanation for the highly localized response to the epicritic pain and the less well-localized protopathic pain. Interruption of the spinothalamic tract in the brainstem through stereotaxic surgery has been undertaken in rare instances to achieve pain relief.

A similar organization applies to the trigeminal system, which conveys sensation from the face through the trigeminal nucleus to the descending tract and nucleus of the trigeminal nerve down the medulla (see Ch. 28). Second-order neurons project across the brainstem to join the ascending spinothalamic tract (Fig. 23-5).

Descending pathways influence ascending sensory fibers in ways that alter nociceptive mechanisms at the spinal level. Electrical stimulation of the midbrain, especially the periaqueductal gray, has been shown to suppress the response to painful stimuli at spinal levels and also at supraspinal levels, perhaps helping to explain the suppression of pain when the subject is faced with great danger, as has been observed in life-threatening circumstances, such as on the battlefield.

These descending pathways have been traced to the medullary raphe and medullary reticular formation and thence to the dorsolateral fasciculus of the spinal cord. Along the course of the pathway, norepinephrine and serotoninergic neurons have been found. Serotonin depletion reduces the analgesic effects of periaqueductal gray stimulation. Opiate receptors have also been found in this system, suggesting that this may be another site where opiates work and that the several sites of action could have a multiplier effect on the suppression of pain. Intraventricular or subarachnoid instillation of morphine allows the drug to reach these sites easily. Ascending fibers that carry information from sharp, pinprick-type stimuli have been found to send collaterals to the periaqueductal gray en route to the ventrolateral nucleus of the thalamus. Stimulation of the nucleus of the tractus solitarius has also been found to inhibit dorsal spinal neurons.

Interactions between sensory systems have been shown to exist, suggesting that some forms of stimulation may suppress others. As mentioned earlier, large, myelinated A-β fibers have collaterals that play on and synapse with the unmyelinated incoming C-fibers. Their discharge presynaptically inhibits the C-fibers, reducing their release of the neurotransmitter substance P. Low-intensity, high-frequency stimulation of peripheral large, myelinated fibers may induce increased activity of their collaterals and suppress pain sensation; this is the basis of transcutaneous electrical nerve stimulation. Similar effects can be produced by dorsal column stimulation by reverse (antidromic) stimulation of the ascending fibers. Dorsal column stimulation also achieves activation of descending pain inhibitory mechanisms. These mechanisms are not opiate mediated. Some relief has been experienced for patients whose lesions lay in the thalamus. Deep brain stimulation in the periaqueductal gray has become a procedure that is used in humans to suppress pain.

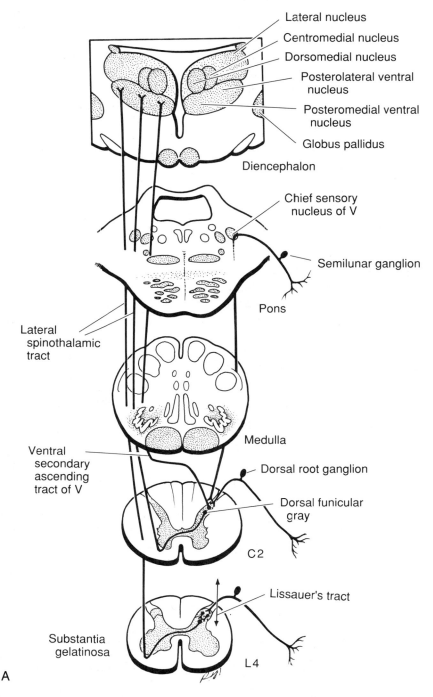

Figure 23-5. Laminar arrangement of the spinothalamic tract as it ascends though the lower, middle, and upper cord and brainstem to reach the thalamus. The fibers that join the tract near its origin are progressively displaced more laterally by those joining higher in the system. **(A)** Lateral spinothalamic tract. (*Figure continues.*)

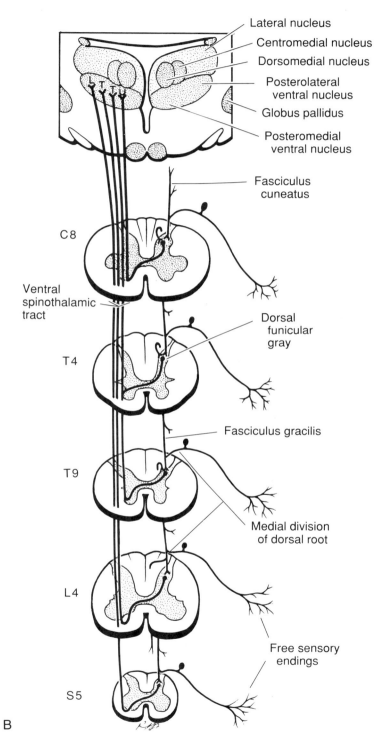

Figure 23-5 *(Continued).* **(B)** Ventral spinothalmic tract.

Acupuncture is thought by some to work through a slightly different mechanism. Low-frequency pricking stimulation may activate small, myelinated A-δ fibers that play on interneurons in the dorsal horn, which are thought to suppress incoming signals from nociceptive responses. The sites where acupuncture works best would be where A-δ fibers are closest to the surface. Naloxone, which blocks opiate receptors, would reverse the analgesic effect.

Posterior Column

The large myelinated (A-β) sensory fibers that supply the response to mechanical stimuli have their cell bodies in the dorsal root ganglia. These neurons have two large axons, one carrying the A-β information to the cell body from the peripheral nerve and the other extending up the posterior column to synapse in the medulla. Although these myelinated fibers make up the bulk of the posterior columns, some 25 percent of them are unmyelinated.

The axons that enter the dorsal root entry zone pass into the ipsilateral posteromedial portions of the spinal cord, the posterior columns, although some have segmental collaterals that synapse with the incoming C-fibers (discussed later). As the fibers enter the dorsal columns, they sort themselves naturally by their body part origins: those from the lower limbs, which reach the spinal cord at its lower point, become the first occupants of the posterior columns to which more cephalad arrivals from the trunk and upper limbs progressively thicken the population of fibers, laminating them so that, by the time the columns have reached the top of the spinal cord, the fibers from the lower extremities are in the medially situated fasciculus cuneatus and those from the upper limbs are in the more laterally situated fasciculus gracilis (Fig. 23-6).

The fibers synapse in the medulla in the nuclei cuneatus and gracilis, respectively. The output from these nuclei decussate and ascend in the medial lemniscus to synapse in the ventroposterolateral nuclei of the thalamus in topographically organized arrangement. About 75 percent of the ventroposterolateral thalamic neurons respond to cutaneous mechanical stimulation and the remainder, to movement of deeper structures (joints and muscles).

In primates, the spinocervicothalamic tract, just ventral to the dorsal horn, feeds to the ventral posterior lateral nucleus of the thalamus. Most of the cells of origin for this tract have receptive fields on hairy skin, but some from glabrous (smooth) skin have been found. A few have their fields in subcutaneous tissues. These cells share with the spinothalamic tract the wide dynamic range of responses but are low threshold and do not respond to mechanical deformation of the skin.

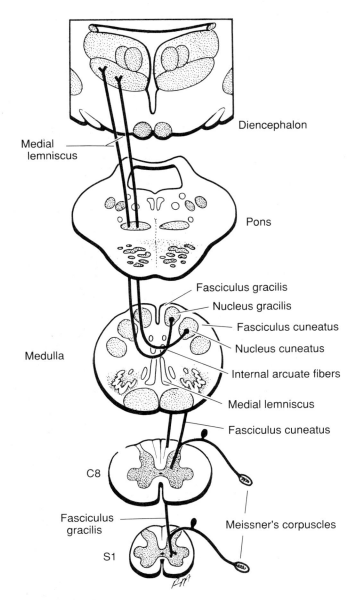

Figure 23-6. Laminar arrangement of the posterior columns as they ascend though the lower, middle, and upper cord and brainstem to reach the thalamus. The fibers that join the tract near its origin are progressively displaced more medially by those joining higher in the system.

These differences in neurophysiologic properties in tracts suggest the two pathways have different signaling properties. Approximately 50 percent of human cords studied have shown this tract, the exact function of which is as yet unsettled.

Thalamus

A well-organized topographic arrangement of the ventroposterolateral nucleus of the thalamus has been found in animals and confirmed in humans by single-

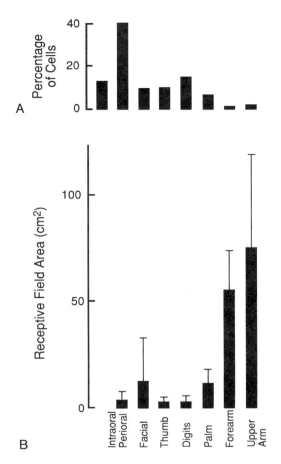

A

B

Figure 23-7. **(A & B)** The size of the receptive fields in the thalamus, showing the small area and high percentage of cells for perioral and digital sensation but the large area and small percentage for the arm alone. (Adapted from Lenze et al., 1988, with permission.)

unit studies of thalamic neurons. The location and size of the receptive field have been mapped, showing a high number of cells concentrated on perioral and digital sensation and only a few for the forearm and upper arm (Fig. 23-7). The organization of the cells is in the sagittal plane, with cutaneous and deep stimuli aligned toward one another (Fig. 23-8).

Cerebrum

From the ventroposterolateral nucleus of the thalamus, fibers reach the deeper layer of the postcentral gyrus (areas 3, 1, and 2 of Brodmann, see Figs. 25-1 to 25-6) and sensory II areas of the parietal lobes, carrying information concerning touch, position, temperature, and sharp painful experiences. Afferent projections also reach the postcentral regions from the pulvinar in some animals. Few opiate receptors have been found in the postcentral gyrus.

The intralaminar thalamic projections that carry sustained pain are widespread, mainly to the prefron-

tal region, and opiate receptors have been found in these areas. Positron emission tomographic studies have shown that painful heat stimulation activates the primary and secondary somatosensory cortical regions and the cingulum; vibrotactile stimuli only activates the primary somatosensory region. A few instances have been found in which postcentral lesions have caused severe sensory loss and persistent burning pain, at times paroxysmal, of the type encountered from thalamic lesions. Most lesions have affected the right or nondominant hemisphere. The complaints could be due to release of the intralaminar thalamic system caused by damage of the cortical region presumed to inhibit its function or to hyperactivity of the projections as a result of disconnection from the cortical lesion. Neither hypothesis has been settled. In some patients, tactile hallucinations or persistences of experiences have been described.

How the cortically bound pathways are anatomically organized in humans is still largely unknown. In earlier times, it was assumed the ascending sensory pathways paralleled those of the descending motor pathways through the internal capsule and corona radiata, a common diagram in anatomy textbooks even today. No clinical studies of patients with capsular or corona

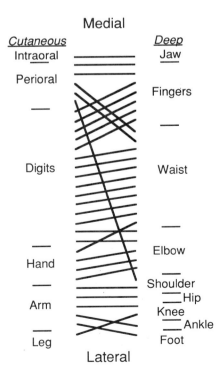

Figure 23-8. The organization of the cells in the thalamus are in the sagittal plane with cutaneous and deep stimuli aligned toward one another. (Adapted from Lenz et al., 1988, with permission.)

radiata lesions have confirmed this organization. Low and midcapsular lesions have regularly caused varying degrees of motor loss but rarely any accompanying sensory disturbance. In only one patient has a lesion caused pure sensory loss, this one from a small hemorrhage in the corona radiata above the thalamus adjacent to the ventricular wall. One patient has been described whose pain from a thalamic stroke disappeared when he had a second stroke that affected the corona radiata.

From electrical stimulation of the postcentral gyrus in conscious humans, a rough homunculus has been described, with the leg above, the hand and face intermediate, and the oropharynx below. Similar highly organized homuncular formulations have been found for every type of primate studied. In humans undergoing electrical stimulation of the surface over the postcentral convexity, considerable variation has been encountered in the exact body site that feels as though it has been stimulated. Stimulation as high as the upper third of the postcentral convexity has produced sensations in the mouth; sensations in the arm have been reported from stimulation in the lower quadrant. These variations make it necessary for surgeons to map the sensory response topography of each patient when operations are conducted around the sensorimotor cortex.

A more orderly series of findings has emerged from electrical stimulation of peripheral nerves such as the median. The evoked responses over the postcentral region, mapped in the operating room, have shown a fairly consistent locus for the hand area, usually found on the upper side of the bend in the rolandic sulcus, this bend occurring most frequently in its upper third (Fig. 23-9).

Neurophysiologic recordings in primates show that small, focal punctate stimuli at various sites on the hand activate highly circumscribed postcentral areas, suggesting a well-organized and specific system. Other cells respond to contact anywhere on a limb. Some postcentral neurons that appear to be essential have been found that respond to pain and to touch and others, to multimodal stimuli. These postcentral neurons have extensive connections with precentral neurons in guiding motor responses. Some neurons in the premotor cortex have been found to fire not only on cutaneous contact but also in the anticipation of cutaneous contact, noxious or not, so long as the stimulus approaches the animal in the space normally surveyed by the eyes. Of special interest is the discovery that some of them fire as a stimulus approaches from a portion of space even when the eyes are not specifically directed at the approaching stimulus. Such observations point to an extremely highly organized system (Fig. 23-10). Intermodal transfer training in primates before and after cortical ablations indicates that the postcentral regions play a role in learning new dis-

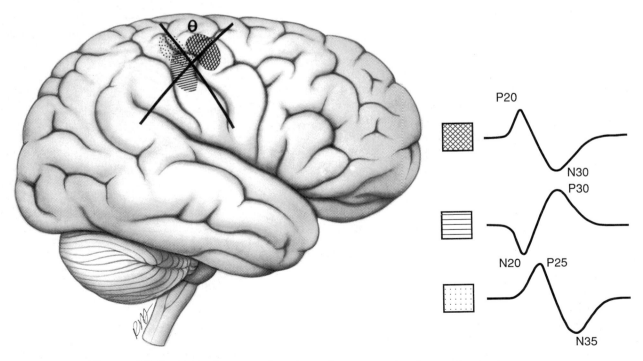

Figure 23-9. Evoked potential evidence for a postrolandic site for the hand area.

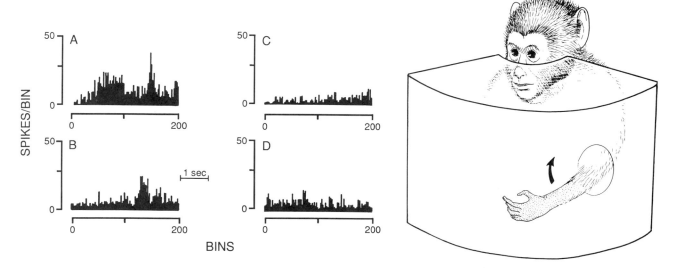

Figure 23-10. (A–D) Description of single premotor cell responding in primate facing moving targets (see text). (Adapted from Rizzolatti et al., 1981, with permission.)

criminations. Manual exploration of objects in both primates and humans has been shown to be improved by more than one property of the object (texture, shape, and size), but increases in number of elements past two or three do not greatly increase skills in object discrimination.

CLINICAL DISORDERS

Nerves and Roots

Although described in more detail in Chapter 31, passing mention is made here of various disorders that affect the peripheral nervous system. Loss of sensation or disturbances, usually pain, may occur from section of the nerve in trauma, infarction of the nerve from ischemic occlusion of a nutrient artery, direct infiltration of the nerves or their roots by cancer, or a variety of infections.

Trauma insufficient for complete disruption of peripheral nerve function may lead to a distinctive, long-term pain and dystrophic state known as *causalgia* (from the Greek for burning pain). Although any nerve or even plexus can be affected, the median nerve is the most frequently involved, and the crude trauma of high-velocity war wounds leads all causes. Herniated discs, nerve root compression in bony tunnels, inflammation of a nerve, and even venous occlusive disease can cause such pain. In the first description, S. Weir Mitchell (American neurologist, 1829–1914), drawing on his experience with missile wounds from the Civil War, offered the opinion that the pain was caused by "nutritive mischief" in the in-

completely damaged nerve trunks. Although the exact mechanism still remains incompletely understood, the components of peripheral nerves that serve sympathetic function are clearly important. Animal models have shown some C-fibers nociceptors that respond to sympathetic stimulation after (but not without) incomplete nerve injury, suggesting that activation of specific, adrenergic-sensitive fibers of the nociceptors system may explain some of the findings in causalgia and possibly the relief from surgical disruption of the sympathetic fibers in the affected parts. The trigeminal nerve has fewer postganglionic sympathetic elements than do peripheral nerves, perhaps explaining the low frequency of causalgia in the face. Damaged nerves may heal and cross their lines of transmissions, which could explain some aspects of pain after nerve injury.

Whatever the explanation, causalgia is the most dreaded complication of peripheral nerve injury. In the well-established case, abnormalities are evident in sympathetic nervous system function with increased sensitivity to catecholamines, vasomotor and other autonomic disturbances, and occasionally atrophy of the parts supplied by the nerve. The affected parts become reddened, show an increase (occasionally decrease) in sweating, and become sensitive to touch, which is perceived as pain, usually of the protopathic type. Less severe forms of the syndrome, often following myocardial infarction, have been called reflex sympathetic dystrophy (also known in some European schools as algodystrophies, post-traumatic pain syndrome, shoulder-hand syndrome, or Sudeck's atrophy).

The inflammation caused by herpes zoster may lead to a pain state known as *postherpetic neuralgia,* and here the trigeminal nerve, particularly its ophthalmic branch, is often involved. The syndrome can produce lasting discomfort, which is especially distressing in elderly patients. Grossly abnormal sensory function is the rule in the affected segments, with disturbed sensory functions of large and the small fibers. However, there is little autonomic involvement, no changes in skin temperature, and no response to sympatholysis.

The importance of neurotransmitters may be indicated by the familial disorder (*Riley-Day syndrome*), whose lack of pain sensibility has been attributed to lack of neurotransmitter.

Other conditions affect peripheral nerves. In their course through the limbs, nerves may suffer *entrapment,* especially the median nerve at the wrist (*carpal tunnel syndrome*). Other sites include the obturator foramen, the tarsal tunnel, and the lateral thigh (producing a burning discomfort in the lateral thigh known as *meralgia paraesthetica*). Nerves may be compressed against bony prominences as in the clinically controversial *thoracic outlet syndrome,* which produces pain in the neck, shoulder, arm, and hand from compression of the nerves and accompanying subclavian vessels (particularly the lower brachial plexus or ulnar nerve) by an anomalous cervical rib or by the scalenus muscle pressing the neurovascular bundle against the rib. Typists and others who engage in frequent, stereotyped, repetitive motions may suffer a variety of root and nerve syndromes, some of which are relieved within minutes by a change in activity and are not easily explained by the more obvious conditions such as disc herniation or arthritic spurs.

The involvement of single roots at or near their exit from the spinal cord causes *radicular syndromes.* Arthritic spurs or a herniated disc at the C5-6 level (sixth cervical root) cause discomfort over the trapezius ridge, shoulder, anterior arm, and radial surface of the forearm and thumb. Tender areas include the biceps regions. These are complaints not easily explained by the cutaneous distribution of the root and nerve itself. Similar disease between the C6-7 vertebrae (C7 root) changes the symptoms to the scapula, pectoral region, posterolateral upper arm, dorsal surface of the forearm and elbow, and long fingers. In the lumbar regions, most (greater than 95 percent) *lumbosacral disc lesions* occur at the L5–S1 and/or L4-5 levels.

Complete disruption of a peripheral nerve leads to loss of function. The regrowing axons appear to be preprogrammed for their eventual sites of motor and sensory supply and may disregard empty myelin sheaths in their path. In the common setting in which the nerve fascicles regrow into the wrong axis cylin-

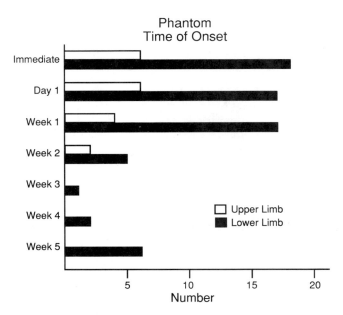

Figure 23-11. Time of onset of phantom limb symptoms in the upper or lower limb.

ders, unusual innervatory patterns appear. If the regrowth is blocked by a scar, painful lumps (neuromas) may form.

The phenomenon of *phantom limb* was first described by the French surgeon, Ambroise Paré (1510–1590) from his battlefield experiences. His description, never surpassed as clinical observation, included separation of the pain in the affected parts before and after amputation. He noted that the patient felt pain from contact with the amputation site (stump) and there was a distinction of pain and other sensations from the missing (phantom) limb, with even a described psychogenic pain. Phantom pain is also common, usually beginning shortly after the injury (Fig. 23-11). Patients experience the phantom limb for reasons Melzack (1989) theorized were due to a "neuromatrix," which imparts its own signature or all parts of the body that survive permanent injuries to neural parts.

Tracts

Studies in humans have shown that posterior column lesions cause little loss in touch or pressure sensation but cause an impairment in the detection of movement and the position of the limbs, which make manual examination of objects difficult. Major lesions of the posterior columns produce a lability of sensory thresholds for touch; some hallucinations of touch and posture; and an increased sensitivity to temperature, pain, and tickling. Although isolated lesions of the spinothalamic tract produce no specific effects on touch, when both the posterior columns and spinothalamic tracts are damaged, the effects greatly impair tactile and pressure sensation. Lesions of the anterior cord and of the anterior two-thirds of the spinal cord that leave the posterior columns intact cause no changes in tactile and position sense tested clinically.

For the spinothalamic tract, the classic clinical results of a lesion are loss of pain and temperature on the opposite side of the body. It is the spinothalamic tract that is largely being tested by the pinprick and cold tests, which shows hypesthesia below the lesion and hyperpathia in the segments near the lesion. Major lesions may bring about a dense loss of sensory function (anesthesia).

For some patients with lesions of the spinthalamic tract, whether in the brainstem or thalamus, the impaired sensation is accompanied by painful disturbances in sensation (dysesthesias) in the period immediately after the lesion, mimicking the pain of injury to peripheral receptors. Gradually, over days to months, agonizing and throbbing pain occurs (first described from thalamic lesions by Dejerine and Roussy [1906]) (French neurologists, J. Dejerine, 1849–1917, and G. Roussy, 1874–1948), a syndrome that bear their name. In some cases, the pain state may resist all therapy. Characteristically, there is hypesthesia but hyperpathia (i.e., excessive pain) when the threshold of stimulation (pinprick) has been overcome. Also, repetitive stimulation in one point causes extensive, diffuse pain. This "thalamic pain" is increased by emotion. For most survivors, it subsides slowly over many months to 1 year or more, but for a small number, it may persist indefinitely.

Thalamus

Despite the well-founded studies of somatotopic organization of the ventroposterolateral thalamus in normal subjects, highly circumscribed lesions in humans have not faithfully reflected this arrangement in the localization of symptoms. Striking variations have occurred from the extreme of impaired sensation on the entire opposite side of the body, including the genitalia, as if the patient has been split down the middle, to the other extreme of partial loss of sensation skipping areas, which would be expected to be involved in a lesion that disrupts a system organized along a topographic or homuncular scheme.

Another point at odds with the implications from animal studies has been the frequent observation that the topography of incomplete sensory loss from thalamic lesions is more sagittal than it is cross-sectional. Sensory loss is common over the shoulder, arm, axilla, lateral trunk, and lateral thigh, sparing the anterior and posterior thorax, abdomen, low back, and genitalia. It may well be that the focal lesions caused by arterial occlusions cut across the anatomic fields of somatosensory projections, causing clusters of symptoms and signs from lesions that seem at variance with the normal organization.

In posterolateral thalamic lesions, pain is infrequent, occurring in less than 20 percent of patients, but when it occurs, it can be a particularly distressing and disabling syndrome. For thalamic lesions, the Dejerine-Roussy syndrome typically affects all or parts of the contralateral body and usually occurs later (months) in the course of recovery from a thalamic lesion. Lesions of the ventroposterolateral thalamus in humans may produce contralateral anesthesia or dense hypesthesia, and even pain; those of the dorsomedial nucleus may relieve pain, suggesting a form of balance between these two great monitors of afferent input.

Cerebrum and Thalamocortical Pathways

As mentioned previously, despite the evidence of well-organized somatotopic organization of the postcentral region in animals and in normal humans, in humans undergoing electrical stimulation of the surface over the postcentral convexity for surgical removal, considerable variation has been encountered in the exact body site that feels as though it has been stimulated. Stimulation as high as the upper third of the postcentral convexity has produced sensations in the mouth; sensations in the arm have been reported from stimulation in the lower quadrant. These variations make it necessary for surgeons to map the sensory response topography of each patient when operations are conducted around the sensorimotor cortex.

In contrast with the results of highly sophisticated studies in animals, clinical correlates of postcentral lesions in humans have been something of a disappointment, taxing the clinician seeking to estimate the exact site, size, cause, and duration of a lesion. Much of the teaching concerning sensory disturbances from cortical lesions comes from the 1911 publication by Head and Holmes, who presented an overview, using as examples four patients, one with a closed head injury and three who had undergone brain surgery, two with tumors and one with a syphilitic gumma. In stable lesions, they noted no major disturbance in the appreciation of painful stimuli, temperature, vibration, and roughness. Touch with graded stimuli (von Frey hairs) disclosed a ". . . want of constancy and uniformity of response to the same tactile stimulus." Finding the affected limb with the normal hand was disturbed as was the detection of occurrence or passive movement or of its direction (now known as joint position sense). The patients usually also failed to point on a diagram to a spot touched (unseen) on the affected parts. Differences in weights of objects between the normal and abnormal limb or two weights on the abnormal limb were deranged. Detection of one versus two points of a drawing compass (*two-point discrimination*) was usually abnormal but was normal in some patients, even when passive movement detection was poor. Skillful palpation of an object to estimate its size, shape, or form and to name the object, shape, or form was usually lost, a disorder known as *astereognosis.*

The full range of symptoms from postcentral gyrus lesions is still insufficiently characterized. More recent studies in patients with highly focal lesions have described instances of pure sensory loss, with no motor disturbance. The patterns of sensory loss have varied from limited areas of sensory loss affecting the thumb, index, and middle fingers; face and hand; and hand and foot to a pseudoradicular (approximating that of a root or peripheral nerve distribution) pattern to the entire opposite side (hemihypesthesia). A few examples of disturbances to heat and cold have been described. The disturbances may persist for years but often fade within months.

CLINICAL EXAMINATION

Symptoms

Assessment of the history is essential for any diagnosis, but for the patient with symptoms of sensory disorder, it is often difficult adequately to describe the disturbed sensations. A "heavy" limb can be a weak, or a numb limb or a "sleepy" hand can be numb or paretic. No time is ever wasted in reaching a sound account of what indeed the patient feels. As for any neurologic symptoms, their characteristics should be ascertained as precisely as possible: mode on onset (sudden or progressive), course (stable, better, or worse), duration (permanent or intermittent), time table (day or night), circumstances that trigger pain (cough or change in position) or alleviate it, and drugs that help or have no effect. The topography of the symptoms aids in the diagnosis because it reflects the site of the lesions.

Some complaints are distinctive for the sensory system affected. Dysfunction of the small fibers of the peripheral nerves or the spinothalamic tract is suggested by complaints of pain, burning, or cold sensations or an impression of cold water running under the skin. Numbness (as in the sensation after a session the dentist); pins and needles (as in the tingling of extreme cold or the sensation after having slept on one's elbow); the impression of tight bands or of a vise around the ankles, wrists, or trunk; and a feeling as if walking on cotton wool individually suggest disorders of the large peripheral fibers or posterior columns of the spinal cord. An impression of an electric discharge running down the spine on flexing the neck suggests a lesion of the posterior columns in the cervical region (the sign described by Jean Lhermitte, French neurologist, 1877–1959).

Dysfunction of the sensory relay nuclei in the ventral posterior thalamus or in the sensory cortex can cause bizarre feelings, such as an enlarging hand or one that no longer belongs to the patient, one that the patient cannot properly control voluntarily. Such disturbed sensation are seen, for instance, in migraine and show how the distinction between sensory and motor symptoms can be difficult indeed. The words *paresthesiae* (from the Greek for abnormal sensation) and *dysesthesia* (from the Greek for impaired sensation) are firmly entrenched in neurologic parlance. Because they cover all abnormal sensations except pain, and for some neurologists they also describe numbness and pins and needles, they are too imprecise to be of clinical use.

Signs

Sensory examination can be a trying part of neurologic practice. There are no limits to the nuances of sensation, but experience has shown that refinements in sensory testing more often mislead than assist in the diagnosis. Therefore, most neurologists use time-honored, if admittedly rather crude and brief, procedures. No account will be given here of such devices as von Frey's hairs or Erlenmeyer's flasks, the aims of which are subtle levels of precision not practical in the realm of clinical practice.

Even with simple testing procedures, some patients, notably the most anxious ones, have great difficulties in deciding whether the sensation elicited by the stimulus test is "normal" or whether similar symmetric stimuli cause really similar sensations. Extensive sensory testing often leads to fatigue in the patient's attention. It is characteristic of clinicians lacking in self-assurance to perform endless sensory examination, only to arrive at doubtful or misleading conclusions. For clinical diagnosis, only the clear-cut differences are valuable.

Few cases require a complete sensory examination, but all cases require at least a screening examination. For the latter, the authors test touch, pinprick, sense of position of toes and fingers, vibration sense, and stereognosis. Inattention (extinction or perceptual rivalry) is also routinely tested. Both sides are symmetrically touched, and the patient is asked to report whether the stimulus has been felt on one or both sides. With cortical parietal lesions, this can be positive; there is neither sensory complaint nor deficits in sensory modalities.

Details of the Examination

In screening or detailed examinations, the following techniques are generally used.

Pain

Pinprick is tested with a safety pin. Of course, the intensity of the stimulus should not result in blood being drawn. Moreover, in a time of acquired immunodeficiency syndrome and hepatitis, the pin must be safely discarded at the end of each examination. The fingertip, not the pulp, and the nailbed are the most sensitive parts of the fingers. Where there is any suggestion of a spinal cord lesion, with a sensory level, pinprick is the best stimulus to delineate it. Continuous light scratching over the trunk is often a good choice to find a spinal level of involvement. Above the level, the pinprick is appreciated fully. Near the level, the sensation is often disagreeable. Below the level, the pinprick is felt as a dull sensation. In patients in whom the use of pinprick runs the risk of drawing blood, a satisfactory substitute for the noxious stimulus may be achieved by using light cotton wool drawn over sensitive body parts (nostril, external auditory meatus, and so forth), mimicking the march of an insect.

Touch

A wisp of cotton wool is applied, not run, along the skin. Another, thinner, wisp of cotton is used for the corneal reflex (see Ch. 28). Touch can also efficiently and easily be tested by the examiner's fingertips. When an abnormal area is found, sensation is tested by working from the insensitive toward the sensitive area, and this holds true for other modalities (e.g., pain).

Temperature

Metal (not glass, which is a poor conductor of heat) tubes or discs are used. Copper is a favorite for some; silver also has its enthusiasts. The extremes of hot and cold tap water, usually about 10°C and 43°C, are convenient. Ice water and very hot water may generate pain, interfering with temperature testing. In old patients or those with peripheral angiopathy, the hands and feet are cold, and abnormal results of temperature testing should be interpreted with caution.

Joint Position Sense

Joint position sense is tested on toes and fingers. Not infrequently, patients must be shown what "up" and "down" are before formal testing. The test is carried out with the patient's eyes closed. The examiner grasps the patient's toe or finger by the side to avoid upward or downward pressure. Just before the test, the toe or finger is moved up and down to make it difficult for the patient to recall the starting position. Some patients must be refrained from "helping" the examiner with voluntary movements. It may be necessary at times to test the proximal joint position sense.

This can be done by asking the patient with eyes closed to tell in which position is the shoulder, elbow, hip, or knee that have been positioned by the examiner. Alternatively, patients with their eyes closed can be asked to point at their big toe with their index finger after the examiner has flexed the hip or knee.

Vibration Sense

Vibration sense is tested with a 128-Hz fork. To set the fork vibrating, it is preferable to strike it on the examiner's palm or knee and not bang it on the desk because there could be confusion between feeling and hearing. The base of the tuning fork is applied on the hallux. If the vibration is not felt, it should successively be applied on the malleoli, tibial tuberosity, anterior iliac crest, lowest rib, sternum, clavicles, and then up the spine. Normal old people sometimes do not feel vibration on the hallux or malleoli. Vibration sense is helpful in the search of a spinal level.

Parietal Cortical Sensory Functions

So-called elementary modalities (touch, temperature, pain, and vibration sense) remain unaltered or very little so with lesions above the thalamus (i.e., parietal cortex or thalamoparietal projections). From a clinical standpoint, the parietal cortex subserves essentially discriminative and synthetic functions. The former is tested by two-point discrimination and the latter by stereognosia. Obviously, for clinical testing to suggest cortical dysfunction, the parts tested must not also have significant deficits for the elemental modalities that are sufficient to preclude testing. Two-point discrimination is tested with a small caliper with blunt points. These are applied simultaneously. On the pulps of the fingers, a separation of 3 to 4 mm; on the palms, of 8 to 15 mm; and on the soles of the feet, of 3 to 4 cm are normal. Astereognosis (from the Greek, *a*, lacking; *stereognosis*, knowledge of space) is the loss of ability to determine the nature of an object by handling it. When an object (e.g., a key) is placed into the hand, handling fingers can detect its temperature, its smooth or rugged surface, and its shape, with the hand acting as a template taking the cast of the object, its constituent substance (iron), from its weight, rigidity and so forth. All this information is carried to the primary sensory area in the parietal cortex and adjacent parietal, with the patient matching the test key with a set of various objects, including a key, proposed by the examiner. Clearly, as noted previously, the diagnosis of astereognosis requires that the elementary sensory modalities are not significantly disturbed. However, the power of stereognosis that remains after touch and temperature sensations are suppressed can be experienced by everyone with a glove. In paralyzed patients, the object to identify is moved about the hand by the examiner. Common objects are used in practice: a pen, the rubber ring of the reflex hammer, a car key, or coins. Normal people can name a coin by touch, but many normal subjects cannot distinguish coins of neighboring value based on size. When a patient is to be examined successively several times, it is wise to prepare beforehand objects that are different from those previously proposed. Patients with parietal lesions also have difficulties in locating cutaneous tactile or painful stimuli and in deciphering (reading) letters (minimum size, 4 cm) that are traced on their skin.

ANNOTATED BIBLIOGRAPHY

Carlen PL, Wall PD, Nadurna H. Phantom limbs and related phenomena in recent traumatic amputations. Neurology 1978;28:211–17.

Clear descriptions of these syndromes.

Cusick CG, Gould HJ 3d. Connections between area 3b of the somatosensory cortex and subdivisions of the ventroposterior nuclear complex and the anterior pulvinar nucleus in squirrel monkeys. J Comp Neurol 1990;292: 83–102.

Area 3b has somatotopically organized connections with ventroposterior thalamus and pulvinar, which contains a representation of all parts of the body, including the face. The authors believe that thalami nuclei project to several cortical sites and that cortical sites receive several different inputs.

Dejerine J, Roussy G. La syndrome thalamique. Rev Neurol (Paris) 1906;14:521.

Classical description of postinfarction pain.

Downie JW, Ferrington DG, Sorkin LS, Willis WD Jr. The primate spinocervicothalamic pathway: responses of cells of the lateral cervical nucleus and spinocervical tract to innocuous and noxious stimuli. J Neurophysiol 1988;59: 861–85.

A spinocervicothalamic tract exists that differs slightly in properties from the classical spinothalamic tract.

Fields HL, Basbaum AI. Brainstem control of spinal pain transmission neurons. Annu Rev Physiol 1978;40: 193–221.

Descending systems from the periaqueductal gray play on neurons entering the dorsal horn, mediating nociceptive responses.

Gybels J, Kupers R. Deep brain stimulation in the treatment of chronic pain in man: where and why? Neurophysiol Clin 1990;20:389–98.

Rationale and success for stimulation in the ventrolateral thalamus and periaqueductal gray.

Head H, Holmes G. Sensory disturbances from cerebral lesions. Brain 1911;34:102–213.

The clinical classic for cerebral dysfunction.

Hodge CJ Jr, Apkarian AV. The spinothalamic tract. Crit Rev Neurobiol 1990;5:363–97.

Details of spinothalamic tract origins, organization, and projections.

Inman UT, Saunders JB. Referred pain from skeletal structures. J Nerv Ment Dis 1944;99:660.

The classic article, with dermatomal, myotomal, and sclerotomal diagrams.

Keil G. Sogenannte Erstbeschreibung des Phantomschmerzes von Ambroise Paré. "Chose digne d'admiration et quasi incrédible": die "douleur es parties mortes et amputées." Fortschr Med 1990;108:62–6.

Description of the phantom limb by Ambroise Paré.

Kellgren JH. On distribution of pain arising from deep somatic structures with charts of segmental pain areas. Clin Sci 1939;4:35.

Another classic description. Hyperalgesia occurs in areas of referred pain.

Kozin F, McCarty DJ, Sims FP. The reflex sympathetic dystrophy syndrome. Am J Med 1976;60:321.

Good discussion of differential diagnosis.

Lenz FA, Dostrovsky JO, Tasker RR et al. Single unit analysis of the human ventral thalamic nuclear group: somatosensory responses. J Neurophysiol 1988;59:299–316.

Details of studies showing frequency and topographic representation of response to mechanical stimulation.

Marchettini P, Cline M, Ochoa JL. Innervation territories for touch and pain afferents of single fascicles of the human ulnar nerve. Mapping through intraneural microrecording and microstimulation. Brain 1990;113: 1491–500.

Specific areas served by individual fascicles.

Matsumoto N, Sato T, Yahata F, Suzuki TA. Physiological properties of tooth pulp-driven neurons in the first somatosensory cortex (SI) of the cat. Pain 1987;31:249–62.

Neurons can be mapped in the sensory area that may help localize the pain.

Melzack R. Labat lecture: phantom limbs. Reg Anesth 1989; 14:208–11.

The neuromatrix theory to account for phantom limb and trunk.

Michel D, Laurent B, Convers P et al. Douleurs corticales. Étude clinique, electrophysiologique et topographique de 12 cas. Rev Neurol (Paris) 1990;146:405–14.

Twelve remarkable cases of pain from cortical lesions.

Mitchell SW, Moorehouse GR, Kenn WW. Gunshot Wounds and Other Injuries of Nerves. JB Lippincott, Philadelphia, 1864.

The first description of causalgia from American Civil War experiences.

Nathan PW. The gate-control theory of pain. Brain 1976; 99:123–58.

Extensive review of the gate-control theory.

Nathan PW, Smith MC, Cook AW. Sensory effects in man

of lesions of the posterior columns and of some other afferent pathways. Brain 1986;109:1003–14.

Among the few clinical studies.

Noback CR, Straminger NL, Demarest RJ. The Human Nervous System. Introduction and Review. 4th Ed. Lea & Febiger, Philadelphia, 1991.

Rizzolatti G, Scandolara C, Matelli M, Gentilucci M. Afferent properties of periarcuate neurons in macaque monkeys. II. Visual responses. Behav Brain Res 1981;2:147–63.

Description of single premotor cell responding in primate facing moving targets.

Roland PE. Somatosensory detection of microgeometry, macrogeometry and kinesthesia after localized lesions of the cerebral hemispheres in man. Brain Res 1987;434:43–94.

Authoritative review.

Rothschild B. Reflex sympathetic dystrophy. Arthritis Care Res 1990;3:144–53.

Detailed review.

Saris SC, Iacono RP, Nashold BS Jr. Dorsal root entry zone lesions for post-amputation pain. J Neurosurg 1985;62:72.

Few helped, but best effect in those with phantom pain alone.

Sharav Y, Singer E, Schmidt E et al. The analgesic effect of amitriptyline on chronic facial pain. Pain 1987;31:199–209.

Better than placebo, requires 4 weeks for effect. Benefits not simply by improved depression scores. Doses ranged from 10 to 150 mg per day.

Soria ED, Fine EJ. Disappearance of thalamic pain after parietal subcortical stroke. Pain 1991;44:285–8.

Unique case.

Talbot JD, Marrett S, Evans AC et al. Multiple representations of pain in human cerebral cortex. Science 1991;251:1355–8.

Positron emission studies of cerebral responses to painful heat stimuli.

Wall PD, Melzack R. Textbook of Pain. 3rd Ed. Churchill Livingstone, New York, 1994, p. 1524.

Wood CC, Spencer DD, Allison T et al. Localization of human sensorimotor cortex during surgery by cortical surface recording of somatosensory evoked potentials. J Neurosurg 1988;68:99–111.

Reliable hand areas can be found.

24
Headaches and Facial Pains

J. C. Gautier and J. P. Mohr

Pains in the head or face are one of the most common complaints in clinical neurology, and skill in their diagnosis and management is acquired chiefly through experience. Because few sufferers are hospitalized, the student is encouraged to see such patients by attending outpatient clinics.

Because of the great frequency of headache, the vast span of clinical types, the known and unknown causes and mechanisms, the amount of laboratory investigations, and the number of work hours lost by those suffering headache, pains in the head are a medical and health problem of the first magnitude. National and international journals, societies, symposia, and the like are often devoted to this sole subject. Although specialized clinics exist, few patients have the means to seek their advice, so diagnosis and treatment rest on the ability of family doctors and neurologists.

Most headaches do not result from life-threatening diseases. They result, instead, from disorders of function of some part of the head (e.g., exaggerated dilation of arteries on the release of some neurotransmitter). Accordingly, this large category can be termed "functional" or "primary" headaches. Although they have material causes, these are usually not found or are hypothetical. These nonorganic, functional headaches are contrasted to "organic" cases in which a defined lesion (e.g., a tumor or arteritis) is the origin of the pain.

When patients come to the neurologist, many believe some sinister tumor or circulatory disorder is lurking somewhere in their head, especially if one of their parents died from a disease that also featured headache. In every case, even in those in which a lesion is most unlikely, a careful and thorough clinical examination is mandatory, first, not to miss a difficult diagnosis and, second, because it is the first step toward confidence and reassurance.

BASIC PRINCIPLES

Pain arises from strain or damage (caused by traction, compression, displacement, dilation, inflammation of the scalp, extracranial arteries, intracranial arteries near the circle of Willis, venous sinuses, large veins, basal dura, eye, mucosae of the nose, air sinuses, mouth, throat, ear, and joints such as the temporomandibular) or from the high cervical spine. Certain nerves, that is, cranial nerves II, III, V, IX, and X, and the three first cervical nerves can also generate pain. The bony skull, the parenchyma of the brain, most of the pia and dura over the cerebral convexities, the ependyma, and choroid plexi do not beget pain.

Painful stimuli from the anterior and middle fossa, upper surface of the tentorium, forehead, air sinuses, nose, and part of the mouth are mediated by cranial nerve V fibers and referred (felt) by the patient mostly over the anterior part of the head and forehead. This large receptive field explains why most headaches are located in the frontal and orbital regions. Painful stimuli from the posterior fossa are carried by cranial nerves IX and X and the first three cervical nerves and are referred to the occipital region, sometimes in the throat or ear. Over the scalp, the line drawn between the ears separates the territories of cranial nerve V and the cervical nerves.

EXAMINATION

The interview is pivotal for the diagnosis in most parts of medicine, but nowhere is it more important than in headache and facial pains because, in most cases, the physical examination is negative and many head pains have peculiar clinical features of their own that stamp the diagnosis. An adequate interview both gives patients time to voice their worries and, through appropriate questions, channels the history to essential points. For the sake of clarity, two sets of questions can be distinguished.

The duration of the headache is the first point (i.e., "how long?"). Acute (minutes to hours) and subacute (days to weeks) headaches raise special issues (see below) and are often seen in the emergency room in the hospital. Until proved otherwise, a recent headache is presumed to be organic. However, most patients complain of chronic pain, present for months or years, which suggests a nonorganic or nonprogressive cause. Adults who complain of recurrent headache since childhood or adolescence are likely to have migraine. The evolution of the intensity of the pain (is it worse now than 3 to 6 months ago?) is the second point, but this is not always easy to assess. Chronic unchanging pain is again suggestive of functional disease. Truly worsening pain naturally raises the suspicion of a progressing cause. Many patients seek consultation because their painful bouts have recently become more frequent, which does not necessarily mean an increase in the intensity of pain. In chronic primary headache, patients feel their pain more or less according to private and social circumstances and to concomitant anxiety or depression. Such fluctuations do not mean a progressively worsening pain. Finally, previous personal and familial medical history and concomitant diseases (e.g., migraine, trauma, or cancer) are obviously of great diagnostic significance.

To categorize the headache or facial pain, the first point is whether the pain is permanent (or near permanent) or intermittent. Pain that can be considered permanent suggests primarily a tension-type headache (see below). When it is well established that the pain is intermittent (i.e., occurs by episodes or bouts), several diagnostic possibilities arise, and some additional historical details are essential for a diagnosis. Prior to the pain, if premonitory symptoms occur, such as fatigue, elation, changes in appetite, or elements of a migrainous aura, a diagnosis of migraine is likely. If the site of the headache at its onset can be localized with the finger, migraine or cluster headache or headache from sinus disease is likely. Pain with changing sites or pain around the vertex suggests functional headache. The characteristics of the pain also help in the diagnosis. Throbbing pain, compared with the pulse beating or the heart pounding in the head, suggests arterial dilation and migraine. Dull, protracted pain, like a tight band or helmet around the head, is suggestive of tension-type headache. Short stabs of pain ("ice pick") suggest primary headache. Some patients complain of several different types of pain, which adds to difficulties in diagnosis and again suggests primary headache. The timing of the headaches is often not well defined; most episodes occur apparently at random during the day and night.

However, in one distinctive type of headache, known as cluster headache, the attacks occur almost on a predictable time table, the most distinctive being those that awaken the patient from a sound sleep around 2:00 A.M. Headache on awakening has too many causes, including migraine, for a diagnosis. The rare chronic headache that is really due to arterial hypertension (most headaches in moderately hypertensive patients are due to anxiety) has been thought to be likely to appear in the early morning, but this old notion has not been confirmed by detailed studies. Associated complaints at any time of the painful bout are common in the more severe headaches, mainly in migraine, including nausea, vomiting, seeking of a dark quiet room, and disinclination to be examined. A definite history of circumstances and factors that trigger an episode favors a diagnosis of migraine, such as menstrual periods; use of the contraceptive pill; certain foods, such as chocolate, oranges, peanuts, cheeses with "veins," such as Roquefort or Stilton; French fries; drinks, especially wine, port, or certain liquors; changes in life activities, such as new worries; lack of sleep; sudden change in stress levels, such as being away from work on the weekends (and possibly also being away from coffee).

HEADACHES

Acute and Subacute

Sudden, severe, explosive headache ("the worst headache of my life") usually reflects a stretch of pain-sensitive structures, the most life-threatening being from a subarachnoid hemorrhage. The blood floods suddenly into the subarachnoid space from rupture of a berry aneurysm or sometimes from an arteriovenous malformation. Cerebral hemorrhage, which usually arises from leakage of a small, deep artery, usually does not cause such sudden distention of the subarachnoid space and often begins without abrupt or intense headache, sometimes with no headache at all. In the now-rare hypertensive encephalopathy, headache rises steeply to a severe intensity within hours to days but is not as abrupt as that from subarachnoid hemorrhage. Generations of students have been taught about the sudden headache from acute obstructive hydrocephalus caused by sudden blockage of the third ventricle from a colloid cyst shifting forward on a change in head position, but such occurrences are rare indeed.

In meningitis and encephalitis, headache builds up rapidly in a matter of hours. The headache from lymphocytic choriomeningitis is severe and persists up to weeks with no accompanying symptoms or signs. In a patient over 50 years of age, a severe headache that is present for weeks always raise the suspicion of giant-cell arteritis. Because blindness without warning is the feared complication of this disease, its diagnosis and treatment are an emergency (see Ch. 38). Dull headache, with or without vomiting, provoked or not by changes of position, that is present for days or weeks can be due to a brain tumor. The pain may be especially severe in cerebellar tumors with accompanying hydrocephalus. The classic brain tumor headache features awakening as a result of pain in the early morning and headache worsened by laughing, coughing, or straining. The clinical examination can be negative, and computed tomography (CT) or magnetic resonance imaging (MRI) are necessary to show the space-occupying lesion.

Chronic

Some chronic headaches can be organic (i.e., after head trauma), but most chronic headaches are primary (i.e., not signs of other disease). These will be considered along the lines of the classification of primary headaches issued in 1988 by the International Headache Society.

Migraine

Migraine, a paradigm of clinical neurology, is a mysterious disease. Its definition is purely clinical (no laboratory or imaging criteria) and its boundaries, as an entity, are ill defined. Its pathophysiology involves the arteries of the head, but its precise mechanisms remain unsettled. It is a familial disease (an important feature for the diagnosis), yet its mode of inheritance is not elucidated. The word *migraine* and its old equivalent *megrim* are said to come from the Greek through old French (Greek: *hemi,* half; *cranion,* skull). In neurologic parlance, migraine is still called *hemicrania.* The word *migraineur* sounds French but is not (the French word is *migraineux*). The word *migraineur* is absent in several contemporary English dictionaries.

Migraine is an intermittent headache, mostly an affliction of women. Between the attacks, the patients are normal. The traditional view that migraine goes with a high IQ has been challenged. Certainly, in the authors' experience, most patients are intelligent women, and the condition is very rare in dull people. There are two main types of migraine: with and without aura. Both can be heralded by general changes that are well known to the patient. These include lassitude, elation, and craving for sweet foods, for example. Both can be triggered by menstrual periods, some foods, alcohol, a blow on the head, or a strong glare such as that caused by the sun reflecting on water. In other instances, there are no such warnings, and the patient awakens with a bout of migraine.

Migraine With Aura. The aura (from the Latin for breeze) typically precedes the pain. Its onset is abrupt, and visual disturbances are the most common disorder. First, a totally blank, sometimes dark, area appears near the point of fixation, a fact noticed by patients who are reading or writing. The patient may think something is wrong with the environment (i.e., the television tube has developed a defect). Soon the outer edge of the dark area is festooned by shimmering silvery or colored scintillations like flickering neon lights. Often, they have jagged contours, like herringbone tweed, zigzags, Norman arcades, or Vauban fortifications, hence the term *teichopsia* (Greek: *teichos,* rampart; *opsis,* sight). The blank or dark part is a scotoma (Greek: *skotos,* darkness). The dazzling edge spreads or drifts slowly away to the periphery of the visual field. The observant patient, occluding alternatively either eye, recognizes that the light scintillates in both eyes and can sometimes perceive that the scintillating scotoma lies in corresponding halves of the visual fields, which stamps its anatomic origin as occipital. The visual disturbances spread away from the center, reaching the edge of vision and disappearing in 15 to 30 minutes and are often the only element of the aura *(ophthalmic migraine).* In other patients, the migrainous disorder spreads from the occipital regions forward across the brain, less often arising forward of the occipital region, with sensory symptoms such as tingling and numbness in the lips, tongue, and hand. When the left hemisphere is involved, aphasia can be dramatic with jargon speech, sometimes alexia. Accompanying sensory disturbances can include somatognostic disorders, with an impression of distortion of shape and volume of the hand and arm. Several authorities state that hemiparesis can occur. The authors have found it difficult to differentiate a hemiparesis from the awkwardness due to acute sensory disturbances. Such compound auras, not limited to visual disturbances, define *accompanied migraine.*

Typically, the migraine headache appears as the aura is fading away, on the side of the cerebral disorders. It is a feature of migraine headache to begin sometimes on one side of the head and sometimes on the other side. In many patients, however, there is a preferential side, and careful questions are needed to make sure that headaches indeed begin on either side. Considering the high frequency of migraine, recurrent, unilateral headache is not unusual. However, in a small percentage of patients, the headaches are explained by an *arteriovenous malformation.* MRI or CT scan with contrast settles this diagnosis by showing the malformation.

In most cases, the pain first appears in the temporofrontal region and rapidly becomes a severe throbbing ache attended by nausea, vomiting, and dizziness. For those whose headache originates in the posterior cerebral territory, a sharp pounding pain may develop first in the lateral eyebrow, spreading after some minutes to the temple and forehead. Bright light, noises, and physical exertion exacerbate the pounding pain and general discomfort. Lying in a dark quiet room may bring relief in severe bouts. The face is pale, and the temporal artery turgid and tender. Although compression of the scalp arteries produces no change in the pain, compression of the ipsilateral carotid artery reduces the pressure in the intracranial circulation and briefly relieves the headache, only to relapse when the compression is released. The headache lasts 4 to 24 hours or even more, but fortunately, after a few hours, the sufferer usually has abandoned any plans for the day and finds refuge in slumber. For some patients, the headache can be prevented by ergot derivatives when the drug is taken at the very prodromal phase, well before the onset of pain. Those patients fortunate enough to respond, often carry a pillbox to allow them to take their medicine at the first well-known hint of the impending storm. Those already in the pain phase, before they are able to start any therapy, may respond to a new serotonin receptor agonist, sumatriptan (see below).

In the individual patient, the recurrence of bouts of migraine is somewhat regular. Many women are prone to suffer migraine around the time of menstrual periods; they may be spared them during pregnancy. The contraceptive pill can increase the severity of migraine episodes and is associated with a higher risk of stroke (see below); cigarette smoking increases that risk. In all patients, regardless of sex, with advancing age, the attacks become less frequent and, usually by age 60, migraines are a memory. This memory needs to be activated for the diagnosis in grandchildren.

Syndrome Variations. Despite the distinctive features of migraine, every clinical feature is subject to great variations.

In the rare *retinal migraine,* visual disturbances may be monocular, usually without scintillations. Although the pathogenesis is poorly understood, it exists because ischemic papillitis and retinal or optic nerve infarction (see below) have been documented. In *transient monocular blindness (amaurosis fugax),* the diagnosis of retinal migraine should be accepted with caution and stringent criteria, that is, young patients, typical migraine history, and no other possible causes. Aura without headache can occur and raises difficult issues with regard to epilepsy and transient ischemic attacks caused by atherosclerosis or cardiac embolism. The most significant characteristics of the migraine process are that the aura spreads or builds up much more slowly, in many minutes; the build-up of symptoms occurs in a few seconds in epileptic and transient focal ischemia. Scintillations and scintillating scotomata, the

hallmark of migraine, are very rare, if not absent, in epilepsy or posterior cerebral artery ischemia. In compound auras (accompanied migraine; see above) the migrainous disorder involves successively different arterial territories, such as the posterior cerebral (scintillations) and the middle cerebral (jargonaphasia). Together with an onset in childhood or adolescence, recurrence for years, and a family history, a diagnosis of migraine is generally safe. C. M. Fisher in 1980 proposed that some transient ischemic episodes in late life could be "migrainous accompaniments." Transient global amnesia has also been proposed to be a migrainous disorder, but proof is lacking in both hypotheses.

The attack can be protracted for 1 to 3 days, with such persistence raising fears of infarction (see below). The severity of the attacks is variable. Many patients, although sick, keep up their usual pursuits. However, extreme exacerbations can occur in which an attack does not end or bouts of attacks recur at a stretch, unrelenting for days, leading to utter misery (*status migrainosus*). Ergot intoxication or unrestrained use of narcotic or sedatives must be suspected in such instances. Admission to the hospital, isolation from kin and friends in a dark, quiet room, therapy with neuroleptics and/or corticosteroids usually lead to recovery in a few days.

A frequent clinical variant, nearly always in young women, features bilateral scintillations and paresthesiae. Dysarthria and staggering are common; confusion or stupor and fainting are possible. A disorder in the basilar artery territory best accounts for this syndrome, hence the term *basilar artery migraine.*

In rare cases, a hemiplegia outlasts for days or weeks the migrainous episode (*hemiplegic migraine*). In some, hemiplegia affects in succession either side of the body. Hemiplegic migraine can be a familial condition with an autosomal dominant inheritance. When the family history is lacking, an unexplained stroke in a young patient should be ascribed to migraine with caution and, of course, after consideration of all other possible causes.

Migraine Without Aura. Also termed *common migraine,* migraine without aura is more frequent than migraine with aura. A family history is often lacking. It should be kept in mind that some throbbing headaches (e.g., headaches with high fever or caused by inhalation of amyl nitrite) are not migraine. Without the stamp of the aura, migraine can be overdiagnosed. It can be associated with tension-type headache (see below).

Other Variants. In the rare *ophthalmoplegic migraine,* the oculomotor nerve is usually affected with an extrinsic and intrinsic paralysis. In most patients, the paralysis occurs as the headache is fading and is rarely permanent. Ophthalmoplegic migraine raises the possibility of a parasellar or suprasellar lesion, particularly an aneurysm of the internal carotid artery. Angiographic results are usually negative.

Migrainous infarctions are the worst complication of migraine, but they are rare. They occur mostly in migraine with aura and commonly involve the posterior cerebral artery territory, sometimes the middle cerebral territory. Retinal infarction and ischemic optic neuropathy can occur. As previously mentioned, oral contraceptives and cigarette smoking increase the risk of infarction. The precise nature of the arterial lesion is not clear. Spasm, edema of the arterial wall, and embolism caused by mitral valve prolapse (which would be frequent in migraine) are proposed mechanisms. Dissecting aneurysms have been reported. Mitochondrial encephalopathy with lactic acidosis and stroke-like syndrome is diagnosed chiefly in children or in young adults.

Migrainous infarcts appear as low-density areas on CT and it was reported at the beginning of the CT era that clinically silent low-density areas of focal or diffuse cerebral atrophy were not uncommon in severe migraine. The question is not clearly settled, but it is wise to have a CT scan in a clinically normal patient with severe migrainous bouts. Despite the temptations, migraine is not an indication for angiography. A few reports have documented a migrainous attack apparently triggered during injection of contrast medium and arterial occlusions in the wake of the study. Between attacks, the angiograms are normal; during the attacks, most are still normal. In a few cases, nonvisualization of major intracranial arteries, proximal constriction of the infraclinoid part of the internal carotid arteries, or multiple segmental narrowing of the pericerebral arteries (as in hypertensive encephalopathy) (see Chs. 35 and 38) has been reported.

In families with a strong migrainous trait, headaches usually appear during childhood when they can be quite worrying with blindness, severe vertigo, disorientation, and aggressive behavior. Sometimes, they follow a trivial blow to the head.

Pathophysiology. The pathophysiology of migraine is, at present, conjectural. Because research is very active in this field, changes in hypotheses are frequent. The following is a much simplified account of the chief available data. Two basic facts, although imprecise, appear almost certain: first, there is a familial factor, and second, paroxysmal circulatory arterial disorders are present during the migrainous attack.

After Wolff's studies during the 1940s, it was long agreed that the aura resulted from arterial constriction and the headache resulted from arterial dilation. Measurements of regional cerebral blood flow have, with exceptions, substantiated a decrease in such flow concomitant with the aura; no such decrease has been found in migraine without aura, a fact which, in passing, could question the fact that migraine with and without aura are expressions of one and the same disease. Whatever the case, the regional cerebral blood flow decrease during the aura does not simply account for the clinical data for two reasons. First, the decrease is not such as to determine ischemic symptoms. Second, however sophisticated, measurement of regional cerebral blood flow have technical and theoretic hurdles that preclude final conclusions.

The opposite view, namely that the primary disorder originates in some disturbance of brain function and the arterial disturbances are a consequence of it, has many proponents. Some underscore the resemblance between the march of the aura and Leão's spreading depression. The latter is a wave of functional inhibition that slowly (at 2 to 3 mm/min, also the pace of the clinical aura) expands from the site of various (chemical or electrical) injuries to the rabbit cortex. Leão's depression is a poorly understood phenomenon, showing much variation among animal species and not really known in humans. Other researchers hold that the primary neural disturbance involves the orbitofrontal cortex and the hypothalamus and that these structures could alter blood flow through the locus ceruleus (adrenergic) and/or the raphe nuclei (serotoninergic). Undoubtedly, and whatever their origin, there are great variations in many neurotransmitters at the time of the migrainous bout. Changes in serotonin are the best known example. A fall in plasma and platelet-contained serotonin occurs at the start of an attack; between attacks, reserpine that induces a release of serotonin from platelets can also induce an attack of migraine.

A specific agonist of the serotonin type 1 subtype receptor, sumatriptan, has been recently reported to have remarkable antimigraine properties. It produces vasoconstriction and could also alleviate neurogenic inflammation of the dura. Not all countries yet have sumatriptan available, and most data on its pharmacokinetic properties still are from young, healthy volunteers. The drug can be given subcutaneously or orally. Most patients reported decreased head pain, sometimes transitory. Adverse effects have been documented in some 10 percent, including a reaction at the injection site, tingling, hot sensation, dizziness, malaise, and fatigue. More important are reports of chest pain because sumatriptan could exert the same vasoconstrictor effects on the coronary vasculature as it does on the cerebral vessels. Asthma and cardiac arrhythmias have been reported in isolated cases. The drug is contraindicated in those with ischemic heart disease, Prinzmetal angina, or uncontrolled hypertension and in those receiving lithium or antidepressants, which are inhibitors of serotonin reuptake. Sumatriptan should not be given with ergotamine because both are vasoconstrictors.

Still, all these data do not account for a major feature of migraine (i.e., it is a one-sided headache). Interesting evidence comes from Moskowitz et al.'s experiments, supporting the existence of a "trigeminovascular system." This system is made up chiefly of fibers belonging to the first division of the sensory trigeminal nerve, that is, the ophthalmic nerve. The peripheral fibers innervate the meninges and the wall of arteries and contain many vasoactive neuropeptides (e.g., substance P, calcitonin gene-related peptide, and neurokinin A). Release of these neuropeptides causes both vasodilation with an increase in blood flow and vascular permeability. Resulting nociceptive impulses would stimulate pain receptors in the brainstem. This could explain both the throbbing character of vascular headaches and that some of them, among which migraine is included, are one sided.

Treatment for Migraine. Simple analgesics, including aspirin, indomethacin (see below), and the like are the common treatment to which most patients turn during periods of headache. Recent work on the 5-HT$_1$ agonist sumatriptan has indicated that a single 6-mg dose s.q. may relieve headache in the majority of migraine patients, whether or not their headache was preceded by aura. In these studies the treatment has been given when the headache has started. A recent placebo-controlled, double-blind trial with sumatriptan given during the aura phase neither aborted the aura nor the subsequent headache. No worsening of aura or headache occurred.

Treatment During the Aura. For a small number of patients, the aura before the headache is reliably predictive of a headache and in some patients it may be possible to abort the headache. The mainstay of abortive therapy has for years been the use of an *ergot compound.* The most commonly used is ergotamine given orally or sublingually in a dose of 2 mg at the start of the aura or headache, with this dose repeated at 30-minute intervals until 6 mg have been taken or the headache subsides. Rectal administration of a suppository of ergotamine tartrate with caffeine is an alternative for those unable to tolerate the oral compound due to nausea or vomiting; it may be repeated at 1 hour.

Prophylaxis for Migraine. For those subject to headaches whose rate of recurrence interferes with normal daily routine, attempts at prophylaxis may be useful. The *β-blocking agents* are the first to be tried,

propranolol having the most success. The majority of patients with classic or common migraine will experience a reduction in frequency or severity of attacks. Doses are begun at 80 mg per day and are doubled after 1 week. The therapy may well need to be used long-term, with some patients experiencing relapse after being off therapy for 1 month or more. *Tricyclic antidepressants,* leading among them amitriptyline, in doses ranging from 25 mg to as high as 100 mg q.d., may reduce the frequency and severity of attacks but often require up to 1 month before their effect is noted; the headache control effect seems separate from the antidepressant effect of the compounds. The *calcium antagonists* flunarazine or nimodipine, 30 mg t.i.d., have shown success in reducing migraine in a high number of cases. Nifedipine, verapamil, and diltiazem have been less successful. Treatment for several months may be required before an effect is seen. *Methysergide* in doses of 4 to 8 mg per day controls migraine in some patients. Its popularity is limited because its use carries a risk of retroperitoneal fibrosis. This risk can be reduced considerably by drug-free periods of roughly 1 month for at least every 6 months of therapy.

Tension-Type Headache

Tension-type headache is the most common headache, also called stress headache or *psychogenic headache.* It appears characteristically in adult women. It is a nonthrobbing, day and night, almost permanent headache. It can be episodic but is usually chronic. The sufferers complain of pressure on the head, especially around the vertex, as by a tight band or helmet. Anxiety and/or depression are commonly associated. There is no photophobia, but the patient often wears dark glasses because "light hurts." The neurologic examination is normal. Tension-type headache means tension of the muscles of the neck and shoulders that hold, stabilize, and move the head on the trunk. Gentle palpation of these muscle where they attach on the occipital bone often elicits pain reminiscent of the patient's headache.

Many patients ascribe their pains to spondylitic degenerative lesions of the cervical spine, which are indeed frequent, but of doubtful causal role. The authors do not encourage neck manipulations for they are not aware of significant benefits and because of the risk of damage to the vertebral arteries. It is usual to correct refractive defects of sight or phorias that could determine a misposition of the head, thus straining the neck muscles. Therapy of anxiety or depression is often beneficial. As previously mentioned, migraine and tension-type headache can coexist.

Cluster Headache

Cluster headache is a distinct clinical entity. The patient, often a middle-aged man, complains of recurrent bouts of pain that have several highly remarkable features. The pain, an intense, nonthrobbing, burning ache, is one sided in the temporo-orbital region. There is concomitant ipsilateral lacrimation and block or running of the nostril. Many patients have noticed that the eye is red and smaller (ptosis) and some, that the pupil also is smaller on the painful side. The bout of pain lasts more or less 2 hours during which, instead of lying down as do those with migraine, patients with cluster headache stride about in their rooms. Bouts of cluster headache can recur several times a day, but what is highly characteristic is that they awaken the patient about 2 hours after he has fallen asleep. Strikingly, for days or weeks at a stretch, the headache attacks appear regularly on the same side, at the same hour with the punctuality of an alarm clock. After this cluster (hence the term), the headaches typically disappear altogether for months or years. During the painful period, they are often triggered by ingestion of alcohol, which, on the contrary, has no such consequence during the free interval periods. Instead of lying in the fronto-orbital region, the pain can rarely be occipital or subauricular.

Carotidynia, a similar pain along the carotid artery in the neck, is possibly related to cluster headache. Several types of periorbital pains or neuralgias were formerly known by the nerve thought to be involved or by eponyms: petrosal, vidian, ciliary (Charlin), or sphenopalatine (Sluder). They are probably variants of cluster headache. Cluster headache has received many appellations in the medical literature, among which are erythroprosopalgia, facial erythromelalgia (because the painful region is congested), Horton's histamine cephalalgia (histamine is no longer believed to play a causal role), red migraine, cluster migraine, and migrainous neuralgia (Harris). Few probably think today that cluster headache is a truly migrainous affection. The cause is unknown, and the mechanisms are obscure. The sphenopalatine ganglion is probably an important piece in the disturbed neural network.

Oxygen inhaled in the affected nostril can cut off an attack. Methysergide, an antiserotonin drug, also is efficient, but it must be given progressively to be tolerated because the small doses administered at the beginning of the treatment do not influence pain. The drug must be stopped after some weeks because of the risk of retroperitoneal fibrosis. Lithium can be a good preventive treatment, although in many patients, cluster headaches spontaneously disappear for long periods.

Chronic paroxysmal hemicrania resembles cluster in many respects, but the bouts of pain recur many times a day for months or years. Some cases could be dramatically relieved by indomethacin.

Cluster is to be distinguished from the *hypnic headache* syndrome, a generalized, recurrent, benign headache that can regularly awaken aged patients and usually responds to lithium. There are no autonomic signs in such patients at the height of the attack.

Miscellaneous Primary Headaches

Idiopathic stabbing (ice pick) headache is common in migraine and not rare in tension-type headache. Pain comes by short series of jabbing, punchlike strikes. This is a benign condition. Some severe cases may be relieved by indomethacin.

Cold food, long gulps, or chugalugging iced drinks can produce an intense, severe stabbing pain that lasts 20 to 30 seconds (*ice cream headache*). Patients who are prone to this pain experience it generally at the same place (e.g., the internal angle of the orbit, side of the nose, or back of the eye). If the sufferer resumes drinking, the pain usually does not reappear. The cause is unknown but has been related to cold application in the oropharynx along the course of the internal carotid artery.

Some patients, on coughing (*cough headache*), laughing, blowing their nose, straining at stool, or on intense sudden physical effort, experience a bursting pain in the head for a few minutes. The cause is unknown; after some months or years, the headache subsides. In a few cases, such a headache can be related to some abnormality in the vicinity of the foramen magnum (e.g., *Arnold-Chiari malformation* so that CT or MRI are advised when the patient seeks neurologic advice for the first time.

Orgasm headache is rare but distressing to the sufferer. At the acme of intercourse, some people, almost always men, complain of a sudden explosive headache that can last minutes or hours. Pain can recur at each subsequent orgasm, thus causing much worry. There is generally no detectable cause, and the prognosis is benign. However, the first bout raises the suspicion of a subarachnoid hemorrhage, which must be ruled out (CT or cerebrospinal fluid [CSF]). In other patients, a dull tension-type headache develops during sexual arousal.

Miscellaneous Headaches With a Known Cause

After a *lumbar puncture,* headache is prevented by lying flat for 36 to 48 hours. However, a dull or throbbing headache is not rare when the patient sits or stands up, and it can last for days. The probable cause is leakage of CSF through the puncture hole(s) of the theca. It should be less frequent with fine needles, deft hands, and successful taps at the first attempt. The headache of a *hangover* has also been ascribed by some to low CSF pressure, and it has been said that it could be prevented by drinking a large quantity of water before going to bed. (For *post-traumatic headache,* see Ch. 6.)

Nerve compression headache is a rare disorder. Usually occurring in elderly persons, the sudden sharp pains, which resemble tic douloureux, are explained by traction on the trigeminal nerve by a dilated or bowed basilar artery; in some patients, surgical separation of the artery from its contact with the nerve may abolish the pain temporarily but not usually permanently.

External compression headache refers to superficial pain resulting from the compression of a cutaneous nerve (e.g., by the head appliances used in games or sports).

Various conditions have been said to be the cause of headache, including anemia; macroglobulinemia; or chronic intoxication by carbon monoxide, carbon tetrachloride, benzene, or even lead. Hypercapnia is the cause of headache in sleep apnea with morning headache in obese, snoring patients. Drugs, such as the contraceptive pill or dipyridamole, can cause headache, but the mechanism is unknown. Cured meats, frankfurters, and many wines transported from foreign countries and containing nitrites can induce a throbbing bilateral headache *(hot dog headache).* Monosodium glutamate, an ingredient of Chinese cooking, can cause headache and a feeling of facial tightness together with dizziness, abdominal pains, nausea, and diarrhea *(Chinese restaurant syndrome).*

Acute nasal *sinusitis* typically causes headache after standing up and, particularly, after stooping. There is local tenderness. *Barodepression,* as in airplane pilots or skiers, can also generate sinus pain.

Eye strain can be painful and caused by noncorrected myopia, hypermetropia, or phorias. A severe temporal or frontal, sometimes hemicranial, headache with vomiting is a cardinal feature of *acute glaucoma.* The eye is red, the eyeball is hard, and the pupil is dilated and does not react to light. It requires emergency ophthalmologic treatment. For *painful ophthalmoplegias (Tolosa-Hunt syndrome or pseudotumor of the orbit),* see Chapter 28.

Pain in or around the ear can, of course, be due to ear disease. It can also be due to throat lesions such as a nasopharyngeal tumor. *Glossopharyngeal neuralgia* causes a deep, lightning pain in the ear on swallowing. Pain in the ear and throat precedes and can outlast *geniculate herpes* (see below). Some pains around the ear are perhaps related to migraine or cluster. The pain of *Costen's syndrome* is considered below. The neurologist should never forget that pain originating from cranial nerve X can be referred to the ear (see Ch. 29).

FACIAL PAINS

Although there is no sharp border between headache and facial pains, the frequent *trigeminal neuralgia (tic douloureux)* (see Ch. 29, Cranial Nerve V) and the rare *glossopharyngeal neuralgia* (see above) are so distinctive clinically as to separate themselves from headache.

Trigeminal neuropathy may occur, but it lacks the lightning-bolt quality characteristic of trigeminal neuralgia. There is sensory loss. Some of the causes include systemic diseases, such as lupus, Gougerot-Sjögren's syndrome, or scleroderma or a lesion along the root of cranial nerve V, but many cases remain idiopathic. In *lower-half headaches* with recurrent unilateral pain in the cheek, radiating to the neck and orbit, the pain can be throbbing with nausea or vomiting. In such cases, there is typically sensory loss. Some cases are deemed to be migrainous, and some are possibly related to cluster headache. (For treatment, see Ch. 29, Cranial Nerve V.)

Costen's syndrome (J. B. Costen, American otolaryngologist, 1895–1962), once attributed to occlusal dysharmony with temporomandibular joint dysfunction, features pain felt around the temple and along the jaw, characteristically on chewing, but the pain can persist between meals. Hearing loss, ear pain, ringing in the ears, dizziness, headache, and burning on the side of the tongue and nose may also occur. On examination, patients are asked to open and close their mouth repeatedly while the examiner palpates both mandibular joints. A degree of pain can be normally elicited, and the diagnosis of Costen's syndrome, which is probably overdiagnosed, should be accepted only when pain is clearly predominant on the side of the spontaneous pain and when this provoked pain is clearly reminiscent of the patient's complaint. The treatment consists of a perfectly precise readjustment of the bite, which can be achieved by a good dental surgeon.

There is still a fairly large group of patients who complain of permanent or almost permanent pain in the face, particularly in the cheek or jaw, often after extraction of a tooth or other dental procedures. The neurologic examination is normal, and such pains are likely to be chronic.

ANNOTATED BIBLIOGRAPHY

Bateman DN. Sumatriptan—drug profiles. Lancet 1993; 341:221–4.

Succinct update.

Bates D, Ashford E, Dawson R et al. Subcutaneous sumatriptan during the migraine aura. Neurology 1994;44: 1587–92.

No benefits in aura or headache prevention.

Bickerstaff ER. Basilar artery migraine. Lancet 1961;1: 15–17.

The seminal article.

Bird N, MacGregor EA, Wilkinson MI. Ice cream headache: site, duration and relationship to migraine. Headache 1992;32:35–8.

Palatal or pharyngeal application caused ipsilateral pain within 13 seconds, lasting about 21 second, and followed by bilateral headache after swallowing the ice cream.

Blau JN. Ear pain referred by the vagus. BM J 1989;299: 1569–70.

Pain in the ear as a result of a hiatal hernia.

Blau JN. Migraine: theories of pathogenesis. Lancet 1992; 339:1202–9.

Exhaustive review.

Buzzi MG, Moskowitz MA. The trigeminovascular system and migraine. Pathol Biol (Paris) 1992;40:313–7.

Most recent review of this hypothesis.

Costen JB. Syndrome of ear and sinus symptoms dependent upon disturbed function of the temporomandibular joint. Ann Otol Rhinol Laryngol 1934;43:1–15

The original description, but etiology still disputed.

Fisher CM. Late migrainous accompaniments as a cause of unexplained cerebral attacks. In Castaigne P, Lhermitte F, Gautier JC (eds): Cerebrovascular Diseases. 2nd Conferences de la Salpêtrière: JB Balliere, Paris, 1980, pp. 293–322.

Some transient ischemic attacks in aged patients could be migrainous.

Gautier JC, Pradat-Diehl P, Loron P et al. Accidents vasculaires cérébraux des sujets jeunes. Rev Neurol (Paris) 1989;145:437–42.

In 7 of 16 migrainous patients, a dissecting aneurysm was the cause of the stroke.

Glenn AM, Shaw PJ, Howe JW, Bates D. Complicated migraine resulting in blindness due to bilateral retinal infarction. Br J Ophthalmol 1992;76:189–90.

A young woman developed blindness over a 6-year period from recurrent episodes of migraine-related occlusions of a branch retinal artery.

Headache Classification Committee of the International Headache Society. Classification and diagnostic criteria for headache disorders, cranial neuralgia and facial pain. Cephalalgia 1988;8 (suppl 7):9–96.

The latest classification with qualifications for diagnoses.

Lance JW. The Mechanisms and Management of Headache. 4th Ed. Butterworths, Sydney, 1982.

Reference book.

Lance JW. Advances in biology and pharmacology of headache. Neurology 1993;43 (suppl 3):1–47.

Recent symposium including references to the use of sumatriptan.

Mewman LC, Lipton RB, Solomon S. The hypnic headache syndrome: a benign headache disorder of the elderly. Neurology 1990;40:1904–5.

Awakens old people and responds to lithium.

Moskowitz MA, Buzzi MG, Sakes DE, Linnik MD. Pain mechanisms underlying vascular headache. Progress report 1989. Rev Neurol (Paris) 1989;145:181–93.

The trigeminovascular system and vascular headaches.

Olesen J, Edwinsson L. Migraine: a field matured for the basic neurosciences. Trends Neurosci 1991;14:3–5.

Present concepts in pathophysiology and a therapeutic prospect.

Rasmussen BK, Olesen J. Migraine with aura and migraine without aura: an epidemiological study. Cephalalgia 1992;12:221–8.

The lifetime prevalence of migraine with aura is 5 percent compared with 8 percent for migaine without aura; the latter is more frequent in women. Attacks of pain are shorter in the migraine with aura.

Schon F, Harrison MJH. Can migraine cause multiple segmental cerebral artery constrictions? J Neurol Neurosurg Psychiatry 1987;50:492–4.

A case of segmental narrowing with references.

Tatemichi TK, Mohr JP. Migraine and stroke. In Barnett HJM, Mohr JP, Stein BM, Yatsu FM (eds). Stroke. Churchill Livingstone, New York, 1992, pp. 761–86.

Review of cases and hypotheses.

Vincent D, Loron P, Awada A, Gautier JC. Paralysies multiples et recidivantes des nerfs craniens. Syndrome de Gougerot-Sjögren. Rev Neurol (Paris) 1985;141:318–21.

Trigeminal neuropathy. A case and review.

25

Disorders Due to Regional Pathology: The Cerebral Lobes and Corpus Callosum

J. P. Mohr and J. C. Gautier

There are four main cerebral lobes, named for the bones that they underlie: frontal, parietal, temporal, and occipital (Figs. 25-1, and 25-2). Two additional regions not often named as lobes are the insula (from the Latin for island) hidden in the depths of the lateral fissure at the junction of the frontal, temporal, and parietal lobes, and the limbic lobe of Broca (French anthropologist and surgeon, 1824–1880) (Latin: *limbus*, border), a conglomerate of phylogenetically related cortical areas that surround the upper brainstem (Fig. 25-3). Finally, the lobes are joined across the midline by the corpus callosum (Fig. 25-3). Before considering the individual cerebral lobes, it is convenient to have in mind the general anatomic and histologic features of the cortex.

ANATOMY

The major characteristic of the human cerebral hemispheres, as compared with subhuman brains, is the huge expanse of gray matter covering the hemispheres, the cortex (Latin for bark) or pallium (Latin for coat). Lodged in the skull cavity, the brain's roughly 1,400 to 1,500 cm^3 volume fits into this small space by the cortex being deeply folded or pleated. The extent of the folding can be estimated by reference to the fact that only one-third of the cortical mantle can be seen on the surface. Were it unfolded and flattened, the cortex would make up an area of 2,200 cm^2 (i.e., a rectangle 12 × 100 cm).

When the pia mater is stripped off the brain surface, the furrows that separate the folds can be clearly seen. Some indent the surface deeply, are rather constant in shape or pattern, and are termed the fissures. Others,

more shallow and much more numerous, are called sulci (Latin: *sulcus*, furrow). Generally speaking, the term fissure is used to describe the furrows that separate the lobes, while the term sulcus describes the furrows that separate the gyri (Latin: *gyrus*, convolution). The two hemispheres are separated by the longitudinal fissure, which harbors the falx cerebri.

Each hemisphere is divided into lobes by several fissures (Figs. 25-1 to 25-3). On the convex aspect of the brain two of the fissures, the lateral and the central, are prominent and constitute well known landmarks in neurology and neurosurgery (Fig. 25-1). The lateral of sylvian fissure (Sylvius, Dutch anatomist, 1614–1672) begins at the base of the brain on the lateral part of the anterior perforated substance (Fig. 29-1). It runs laterally to the limen insulae or threshold of the insula, where the fissure bifurcates into a short, Y-shaped anterior branch, dividing the rear part of the inferior frontal convolution into the pars orbitalis, pars triangularis, and pars opercularis. The pars triangularis and pars opercularis in the dominant hemisphere are referred to as Broca's speech area (see Ch. 18). The second, posterior branch of the sylvian fissure, some 8 to 10 cm long, runs obliquely upward and caudally, separating the frontal and parietal lobes from the temporal. The end of the fissure is capped by the supramarginal gyrus (gyrus supramarginalis), an often cited convolution linking the parietal and the temporal lobes (Fig. 25-1). The central or rolandic fissure (Rolando, Italian physician, 1770–1831) runs from the superior edge of the hemisphere, where it slightly indents the paracentral lobule, a cue to localize the fissure (Fig. 25-2). It runs in a ventral and rostral

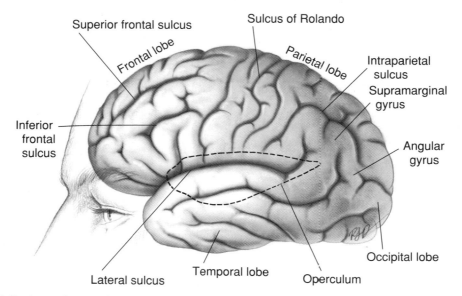

Figure 25-1. Lateral view of the cerebral convexity showing the main cerebral lobes and their anatomic landmarks.

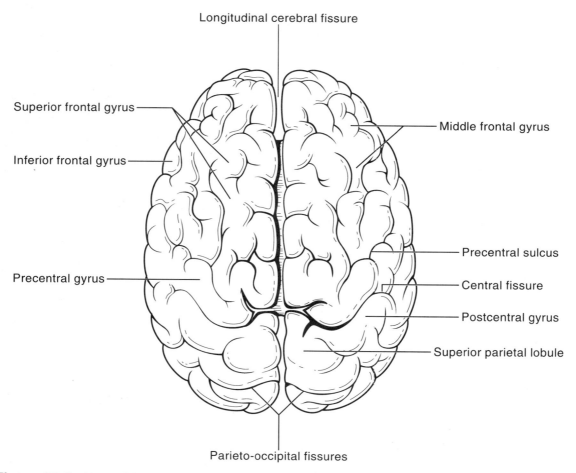

Figure 25-2. View of the brain from above, showing the main convolutions and illustrating the rather posterior location of the rolandic fissure.

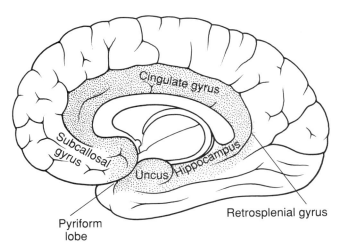

Figure 25-3. Medial view of the cerebral convexity, showing the main cerebral lobes and their anatomic landmarks. The stippled area is the limbic lobe (see text).

direction (Fig. 25-1), uninterrupted from top to bottom, with two bows along its course. Its ventral end remains separated from the lateral fissure by the operculum (Latin: *operculum,* lid), which hangs over and covers the insula in the depth of the lateral fissure. On the whole, the central fissure is more posteriorly placed than is often recognized (Fig. 25-2) and this is particularly true for its dorsal end, which can be identified on the upper cuts of CT. The left cerebrum has a larger frontal lobe than does the right, which causes the central (rolandic) fissure to be located more posteriorly in the left and more anteriorly in the right hemisphere. The other main fissures are mostly or entirely on the medial aspect of the hemisphere. They are the parieto-occipital, the cingulate or callosomarginal, the collateral, and the calcarine.

HISTOLOGY

Estimates of the number of cortical neurons in humans vary widely. Their number is currently put at about 26 billion, or about three times the number of glial cells. About 90 percent of the cortex of the human brain is phylogenetically recent; therefore it is called the neocortex or neopallium. As it is also morphologically fairly uniform, it is referred as the isocortex or the homotypical or homogenetic cortex. By contrast, the phylogenetically older regions of cortex in humans are the olfactory and hippocampal cortices, which have a dissimilar morphology and are known as *allocortex* (Greek: *allos,* other) or *archipallium* (from the Greek for old coat). The allocortex itself is divided into the archicortex (hippocampal cortex) and the paleocortex (piriform or primary olfactory area).

Histologically, there are five types of neurons, by far the most common being the pyramidal and stellate or granule cells. In the isocortex the cell bodies are arranged in six layers (Fig. 25-4). From the surface to the white matter these layers are (I) the plexiform or molecular layer, which contains chiefly synapses between dendrites and axons of cells from deeper layers; (II) the external granular layer, harboring small pyramidal and granule cells connecting with the deeper layers; (III) the external pyramidal layer, a broad band with pyramidal cells whose axons descend into the white matter as association or commissural fibers; (IV) the internal granular layer, densely packed with granular cells, the main terminal for specific sensory inputs such as the somatosensory afferents; (V) the internal pyramidal or ganglionic layer, with many large pyramidal cells, the Betz cells of the motor strip, axons of which enter the projection pathways and, for a lesser part, the corpus callosum; and (VI) the multiform or fusiform layer, which has a wide array of all types of cells, particularly fusiform cells, whose axons enter projection and association fibers.

The six-layered isocortex displays two patterns of cellular arrangement. The first is the homotypical cortex with six easily recognizable layers (Fig. 25-4A). This cortex makes up 75 percent of the surface of the brain and serves the functions of the association cortex, processing information arriving to, about to leave, or linking areas within the brain. The second type of cellular arrangement is the heterotypical cortex, in which the predominance of certain cellular types somewhat blurs the layers. When pyramidal cells are predominant and granule cells less numerous, the cortex is said to be agranular; this is a feature of efferent areas (e.g., the primary motor area [Fig. 25-4B]). Conversely, when granule cells are predominant, the main function is afferent or receptive; this granular cortex has a large number of very small cells, hence its name *koniocortex* (Greek: *konios,* dust) and is typically of the primary sensory areas serving vision, hearing, and somatosensory function (Fig. 25-4C). (The makeup of the primitive three-layered cortex is discussed below in the section Temporal Lobe.)

Within the cortex, besides the tangential lamination there is a functional arrangement of cortical cells in columns or slabs radially oriented toward the brain surface. Neurons of such columns constitute units that respond to highly specific stimuli: some columns in the visual cortex respond only to vertical or horizontal bars, to colors, or even to each 10-degree change of edge between 0 and 180 degrees. This highly specific sensitivity to stimuli of sensory cortical units is matched by a similar specificity of motor units, examples of which are discussed below in the section Frontal Lobe.

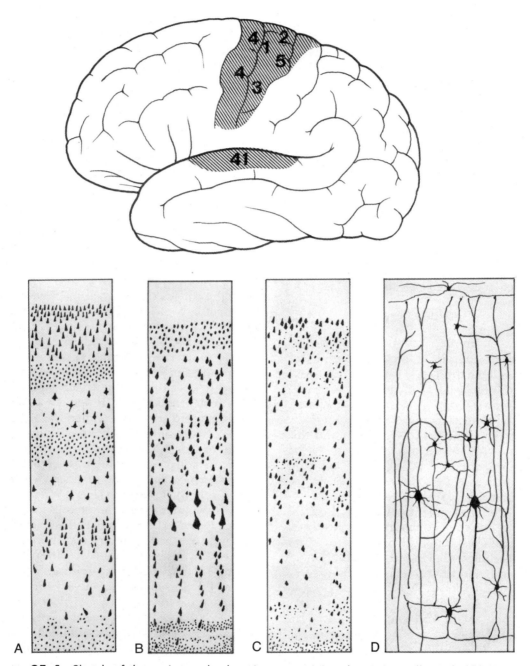

Figure 25-4. Sketch of the main cerebral regions containing the major cell types. **(A)** Homotypical cortex characteristic of most of the cerebrum. **(B)** Agranular cortex typical of Brodmann motor area 4. **(C)** Granular cortex typical of primary sensory areas such as Brodmann areas 1, 2, 3, 5, 41. **(D)** Typical arrangement of axonodendritic connections in the gray matter. (From Cobb, 1958, with permission.)

Another characteristic of this columnar organization is that from receptor to cortical units, through relays such as the thalamus, or lateral geniculate body, neighboring cortical units respond to stimuli received by neighboring receptors. A retinal functional unit (a group of photoreceptors passing information to bipolar cells, which in turn feed a ganglion cell) is anatomically and functionally linked with a group of geniculate cells, whose signals are in turn accepted by a slab or by contiguous slabs of cells in the visual cortex.

In a given functional column, cells are richly interconnected by dendritic and axonal synapses (Fig. 25-4D). It has been estimated that a cortical neuron in the rat has an average of some 8,000 synapses, which makes about 700 million synapses per cubic centimeter of cortex, and that the "wiring," (i.e., the length of axonal and dendritic processes) is amazingly developed, being up to 1 km in length per cubic centimeter of cortex.

Such specialized cellular units pass their processed information to neighbor units for still further processing. Dendritic and axonal branches, some from tangentially developed cells such as the horizontal cells, provide the anatomic basis for such functions. Some tangential myelinated fibers are prominent in the fourth and fifth cortical layers, where they are known as the external and internal bands of Baillarger (French neurologist, 1809–1890).

Several systems have been created for mapping the cortex in many areas according to local particulars of cell type layout. Brodmann's (German anatomist, 1868–1918) system of numbering cerebral surface areas has remained in general use even though the histologic distinctions on which it was based have long been recognized as inadequate in many details (Fig. 25-5). However, the nomenclature is in such wide use

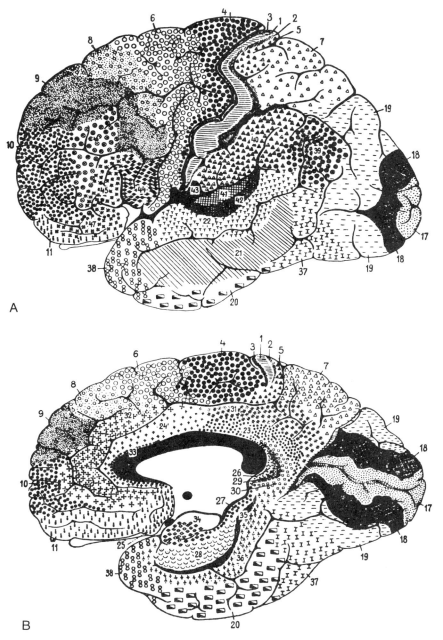

Figure 25-5. (A & B) Brodmann's original brain map, purporting to show histologically distinct brain regions (see text). (From Brodmann, 1925, with permission.)

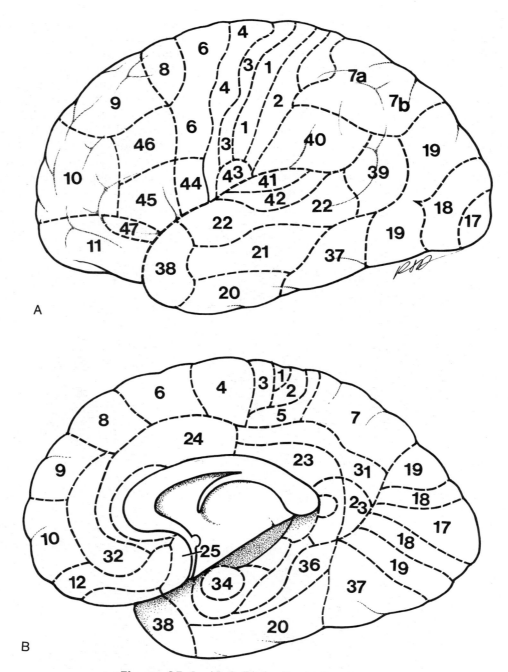

Figure 25-6. (A & B) the Brodmann areas.

that neurologists are expected to know what brain regions are meant by some numbers, especially areas 1, 2, 3, 4, 6, 8, 17, 18, 19, 39, 40, 41, 42, and 44 (Fig. 25-6).

THE LOBES

The division of the cerebral hemispheres into lobes is macroscopically obvious and hence one of the earliest observations in descriptive anatomy of the brain. However, the limits of the lobes are not clear everywhere, and moreover, they do not constitute barriers to the rich interlobar connections. Despite such limitations, the time-honored division of the cerebrum into lobes remains clinically valid, since the lobes still represent to a large extent physiologic entities (see below), and consequently their lesions bring about distinct constellations of symptoms and signs (i.e., characteristic syndromes).

In all animal species throughout the phylogenetic evolution, the cortex remains organized along similar general principles. There are primary areas, which receive specific sensory information or from which motor messages depart to lower levels. These strongly specialized areas are located in different lobes: motor in the frontal lobe, somatosensory in the parietal, visual in the occipital, and auditory and olfactory in the temporal.

The major feature of phylogenetic evolution is the development of secondary areas of unimodal cortex, which process information from (sensory) or to (motor) primary areas, and of secondary areas of multimodal or associative cortex, which process information from different sources. For example, at the boundaries of the parietal, temporal, and occipital lobes, cortical areas 40 (gyrus supramarginalis) and 39 (gyrus angularis) (Fig. 25-6) integrate somatosensory, auditory (including language), visual, and memory data. Likewise, the polar end of the frontal lobe contains secondary (premotor) areas which process motor messages prior to delivering them to the primary motor area (see also Ch. 22). The huge development of this associative cortex is unique to the human brain, which otherwise shows the same basic lobar pattern as the brains of animals.

Another token of the persisting individuality of the lobes of the human brain is that each of them has a particular connection with the thalamic nuclei (Fig. 25-7). These connections explain how lesions of thalamic nuclei can clinically mimic syndromes of the corresponding lobe. Modern imaging using positron emission tomography (PET) and single-photon emission computed tomography (SPECT) scanning (see Chs. 14 and 15) have shown functional correlation of such thalamic lesions with hypofunction of the lobes linked to that thalamic region.

In the hemispheres, the lobes are connected by ipsilateral and commissural association fibers. Among the latter, short ones (U-shaped fibers) sweep around the bottom of sulci to link neighboring gyri. Along the borders of the lobes they connect neighboring regions. Long association fibers (Fig. 25-8) comprise three main bundles: the uncinate fasciculus connects the frontal and temporal lobes; the arcuate fasciculus arches above the insula, connecting the frontal and temporal lobes; and the cingulum (not to be confused with the cingulate gyrus, beneath which it lies) con-

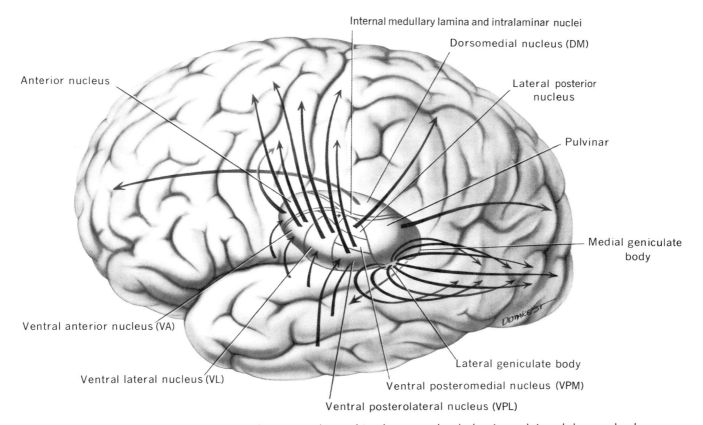

Figure 25-7. Diagram showing the main relationships between the thalamic nuclei and the cerebral lobes. (From Noback et al., 1991, with permission.)

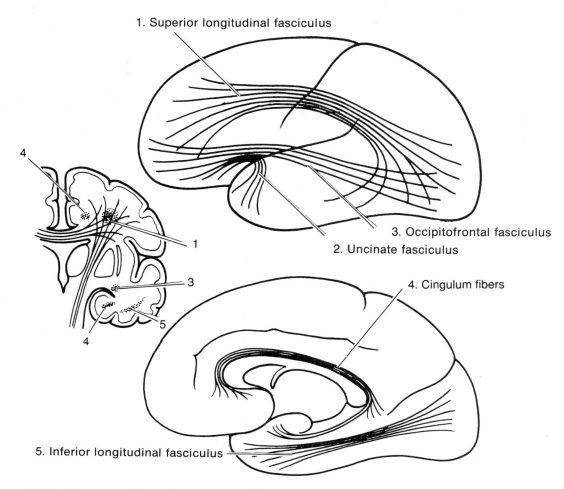

1. Superior longitudinal fasciculus

3. Occipitofrontal fasciculus

2. Uncinate fasciculus

4. Cingulum fibers

5. Inferior longitudinal fasciculus

Figure 25-8. Diagrams of the main association fiber systems in the cerebrum, seen in axial and coronal views. (Adapted from Lazorthes, 1967, with permission.)

nects the frontal and parietal lobes with the parahippocampal gyrus and neighbor temporal convolutions (see Temporal Lobe, below). Several minor fiber systems also link the lobes in the same hemisphere: the inferior occipitofrontal fasciculus runs from far back in the occipital lobe; and the superior longitudinal fasciculus connects the frontal and temporal lobes to the parietal and occipital.

Fibers termed *commissures* transfer information from one hemisphere to the other (Fig. 25-9). The corpus callosum, a broad and thick band of white matter, connects large cortical regions on one side with corresponding areas of the opposite hemisphere (see the section Corpus Callosum, below). The far smaller anterior commissure crosses the midline rostral to the columns of the fornix and connects olfactory structures and lateral parts of the temporal lobes on the two sides.

Interruption of ipsilateral or commissural connecting fibers may cause highly circumscribed distur-

bances in brain function. The best known and least disputed are the "split brain" disturbances caused by interruption of the corpus callosum, in which objects palpated by the left hand are not named, and dictated instructions heard and repeated aloud are not performed by the left hand (see the section Corpus Callosum).

The lobes are by no means isolated parts of the brain. In addition to the projection fibers referred to above, which reach or leave individual lobes, there are diffuse neurochemical systems—cholinergic, dopaminergic, adrenergic, serotoninergic, and others—that project on widespread cortical areas, generally from relatively small nuclei in the brainstem or basal brain. These projection systems affect neurotransmitter functions and are not strictly related to the "hard wiring" of the anatomic pathways seen grossly, nor are they strictly comparable in function. They constitute another form of neural networks not appreciated in the study of gross anatomy alone. It remains to be

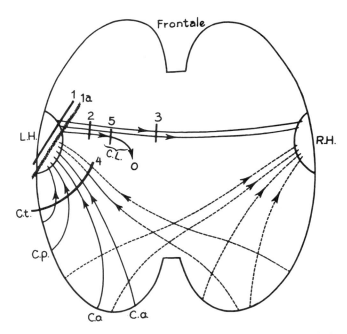

Figure 25-9. The major transcallosal pathways. LH, left hemisphere site for movement of the right hand; RH, right hemisphere site for movement of the left hand; C.o., occipital cortical association fibers; C.p., parietal cortical association fibers; C.t., temporal lobe cortical association fibers. The numerals refer to sites of lesions that interrupt the pathways: 1, destruction of the site of left hemispheric control of the right hand, which also interrupts projections to the right hemisphere, causing left hand ideomotor dyspraxia; 1a, less severe lesion, not destroying right hand function but interrupting projections to the right hemisphere; 2, subcortical lesion causing right hand weakness and interrupting projections to the right hemisphere; 3, callosal lesion causing left hand ideomotor dyspraxia, with the right hand normal; 4, subcortical lesion interrupting ipsilateral and contralateral projections from temporal, parietal, and occipital lobes, causing bilateral ideomotor dyspraxia; 5, deep left hemispheric lesion, causing right hand weakness but no left hand ideomotor dyspraxia. (From Liepmann, 1900.)

determined whether the neurotransmitter network is more important than the traditionally emphasized hard-wired network.

FRONTAL LOBE

Anatomy and Histology

The huge increase in size of the anterior parts of the frontal lobe is a feature of nonhuman primates and culminates in humans so that, from the central fissure to the frontal pole, the frontal lobe makes up two-thirds of the cerebral convexity (Figs. 25-1 and 25-2). This vast expanse and anterior location makes it the most frequent target of missile wounds of the brain. Further, by its sheer percentage volume, it is the site

most often reached by bloodborne diseases, from infections to metastases.

On the medial side of the hemisphere, the lobe extends down to the callosomarginal fissure (Fig. 25-3) (i.e., it makes contact with the gyrus cinguli and more generally with the limbic system). Its inferior aspect lies on the rough bony roof of the orbit and cribriform plate, covering the olfactory bulb. Damage to the orbital part of the lobe and anosmia are common sequelae of concussion (see Chs. 6 and 29), and meningiomas of the olfactory groove are a frequent cause of the frontal syndrome.

The gross anatomic landmarks on the convexity are its posterior border, which is the central (rolandic) fissure, and its inferolateral border, which is the inferior part of the lateral (sylvian) fissure. The precentral sulcus and two horizontal sulci demarcate the precentral gyrus and the superior, middle, and inferior frontal gyri (Fig. 25-1).

On histologic and physiologic grounds three regions—the primary motor, premotor, and prefrontal areas—can broadly be recognized from posterior to anterior (Figs. 25-2, 25-5, and 25-6). The *primary motor* area (area 4), includes the anterior bank of the central fissure and part of the precentral gyrus, since in its middle and lower parts area 4 is a narrow strip (Figs. 25-5 and 25-6). Area 4 is an agranular cortex with Betz cells. It is an excitable cortex, which means that electrical stimulation causes movements of the contralateral limbs. The *premotor area* (area 6) also an agranular cortex but without Betz cells, is also an excitable cortex. In the premotor cortex a small, ill-defined area on the medial side of the hemisphere is termed the *supplementary motor area.* In the rear portion of the middle frontal gyrus are the excitable *cortical eye fields,* part of area 8. Rostral to area 6, astraddling the superior edge of the hemisphere, mainly in the superior frontal gyrus but slightly encroaching the cingulate gyrus, is a region of control of micturition and defecation. *The prefrontal area,* made of granular, nonexcitable cortex, includes areas 9, 10, 11, 12, 32, 45, 46, and 47, to which is added the *paralimbic,* subcallosal cortex (areas 24 and 26 and parts of 32 and 12), also termed *parolfactory,* anterior cingulate and caudal orbitofrontal regions, which are transitional between granular and simple allocortex (see the section Temporal Lobe, below).

Many pathways cross the frontal white matter. The *corticofugal* pathways include corticospinal (see Ch. 22), corticoreticular, corticostriate, corticothalamic, and corticopontine fibers, and additionally, corticofugal fibers to various nuclei of the brainstem. The *corticopetal* pathways are wide projections from the dorsomedial nucleus of the thalamus (Fig. 25-7) and a widespread projection from small group cells of the basal brain and brainstem with various transmitters (see above). The *connection fibers,* either ipsilateral or commissural, include those of the corpus callosum (Figs. 25-8 and 25-9).

Physiology and Pathophysiology

Much information about the clinical consequences of frontal lesions has been gained from clinicopathologic correlations of naturally occurring lesions, from stimulation during surgery and ablation in humans and from stimulation or ablation in primates.

Basically, the frontal lobe is essential for the organization of movement and plays a key role in human behavior vis-à-vis the external world. In the present state of knowledge, the effects of lesions cause the *frontal lobe syndrome,* whose component parts are (1) disorders of movement, paralysis, disorders of the eye and head movements, apraxia, behavioral disorders, and neglect; (2) disorders of micturition and defecation; (3) vasomotor disturbances; (4) cognitive disorders; (5) reduced initiative; (6) disinhibition of behavior. In addition, the aphasias due to frontal lesions, including those of Broca's area (area 44), are traditionally considered separately from the frontal lobe syndrome (see Ch. 18).

Disorders of Movements and Theory of the Homunculus

Ablation of the primary motor area causes a contralateral flaccid paralysis, the effect being most prominent in the distal portions of the limbs and especially severe for the fine movements of the hand. At the onset, the contralateral face is paralyzed, but eventually, for reasons not entirely clear but attributed to bilateral innervation, movements of the upper part of the face reappear and seem more or less normal. The leg often improves sufficiently to support the weight of the body in standing, but the ankle, foot, and toes are often paralyzed. This clinical picture of the late results of ablation of the motor cortex has been recognized for over a century.

Since the end of the 19th century clinical observation on focal motor epilepsy, discrete stimulation and ablation in animals and humans (including soldiers acutely wounded on the battlefield), and many clinicopathologic correlations made days to years after the original lesion all have pointed to a somatotopic organization of the motor system in Brodmann area 4.

This organization has been summarized and popularized in the concept of the homunculus (Latin: little man) face down on the operculum, upper limb on the middle convexity, and leg over the edge of the hemisphere in the anterior part of the paracentral lobule (see also Ch. 22). The volume of cortex allotted to each body part is proportional to the functional

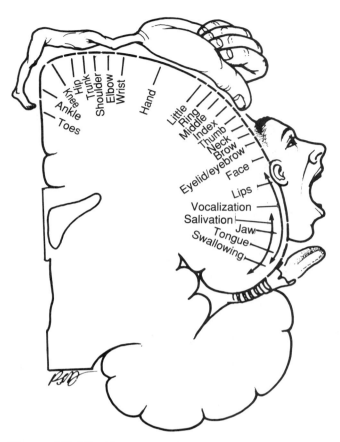

Figure 25-10. The commonly represented homunculus. (Adapted from Penfield and Rasmussen, 1959, with permission.)

importance of that part. The little man is thought to have big lips; a big tongue and thumb; and small forehead, arm, and leg (Fig. 25-10). Electrical stimulation of the exposed brain at surgery has demonstrated movements of the oropharynx, including the lips and tongue, at the lowest portion of the rolandic region and adjacent insula in the sylvian fissure; just above, movements of the face; over the midportion of the rolandic region, movements of the arm, hand and fingers; and high over the longitudinal fissure and projected onto the medial surface of the hemisphere, movements of the leg, foot and genitalia. Movements of the axial ends of the limbs or the trunk have only rarely been elicited from electrical stimulation in the rolandic region.

Reasoning from primate studies and from stimulation of the human brain dating back over a century and corroborated by some human studies, clinicians have inferred that control of movements of the axial ends of the limbs (i.e., shoulder and hip) arises from motor areas anterior to the rolandic region. The putative origins of movements of the trunk and neck have not yet been adequately explained.

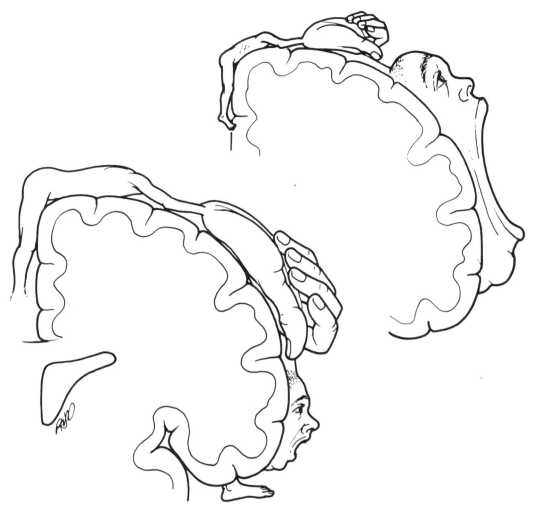

Figure 25-11. Other configurations of the homunculus drawn from the same data used to construct Figure 25-10.

Fig. 25-10 is the clinicians' tacit reference when they hypothesize about the site of cortical motor lesions. Gross correlations (i.e., face down, leg up) have proved sound, but it must be admitted that the homunculus is an oversimplification and a rather loose approximation. Support for the general concept exists, but the exact point-to-point correlations are rather weak, which suggests that there may be considerable interindividual variation, as summarized above (Fig. 25-11).

Electrical Stimulation. The movements occasioned by surface electrode stimulation have been fairly simple, such as deviation of the elbow and dorsiflexion of the wrist, and have not been highly organized or susceptible to replication from similar stimulation at a later time. In the published maps from humans, the movement of the stimulator along the

prerolandic region produced movements of different body parts in a predictable chain of the face below, arm next, and leg highest, but the sites for movements of the upper extremity in individual cases have extended as high as the longitudinal fissure and to well out in front of the rolandic cortex. Face movements have generally been elicited in the lower third of the rolandic region, but some have been produced from stimulation as high as the lower end of the upper third. The findings provide only sketchy support for a stable correlation between stimulus site and motor response. The classic studies of Penfield and Boldrey revealed considerable variation in the convexity sites that elicited movements of the major body parts, and many investigators since have remarked on the difficulties in mapping the motor region by stimulation. Such experiences have made investigators who use brain mapping for epilepsy surgery prepared for considerable variation in the exact stimulation sites at which given movements will occur.

Implanted subdural electrodes have been used to identify regions whose discharge seems correlated with a given neurologic function. There has generally been something of a ladderlike arrangement, with the finger and arm movements produced higher over the convexity than head and mouth movements. However, a rather wide variability has been seen in the size and location of the regions of the cortex that evoke speech and language and in the sites that provoke eye and head movements.

Regional Cerebral Blood Flow Studies. Studies of regional cerebral blood flow using hand activation have shown activation of large areas, spreading from the midrolandic region well back into the parietal lobe, both contralateral and ipsilateral to the moving hand. PET has only recently begun to yield evidence on areas activated in response to certain tasks. For humming and speaking aloud, both perirolandic regions have been found activated, the activation in a small series extending over a wide zone from the midportion to the upper edges of the convexity but not affecting the lower or perisylvian regions. Movement of the hand has been shown to activate a wide vertical zone of the rolandic region, also affecting the mid to upper third but not the lower area near the sylvian fissure.

The types of movements found in *focal motor seizures* have long been taken to reflect the homuncular motor organization of the motor cortex. The jacksonian march, named after J. Hughlings Jackson (English neurologist, 1835–1911), typically begin in the ends of the fingers or the corner of the mouth and spreads to involve contiguous regions, often sparing axial portions such as the shoulder or hip. The high frequency of these patterns was taken to mean the more frequently involved movements are better represented over the brain surface. Only one case of seizures limited to the abdominal muscles has been described.

In contrast to the effects of focal seizures, it has been difficult to see the formula at work in the patterns of weakness caused by brain lesions from wounds and strokes. In brain lesions from stroke, several variations of patterns of weakness have been seen: equivalent weakness in face, arm, and leg: weakness of the limbs exceeding the face, and distal weakness (hand and ankle) predominating over proximal appendicular (shoulder and hip) weakness; axial weakness exceeding that of the distal appendicular movements; faciobrachial weakness; and few examples of isolated monopareses. In particular, from infarction of the lower third of the rolandic region, weakness affecting the face, hand, and leg have been seen more often than weakness limited to the face. Infarction affecting each

of the major rolandic zones has commonly caused a formula of hemiparesis, with equivalent weakness of the hand, shoulder, foot, and hip and, less often but with roughly equal frequency; weakness of the face and arm more than the leg; faciobrachial weakness sparing the leg; or isolated weakness of the face, arm, or hand with roughly equal frequency.

Other formulas of incomplete weakness of one side (hemiparesis) have proved disappointing predictors of brain injury in specific regions of the rolandic convexity. Weakness limited to a single limb (monoparesis) has been found from sites varying widely over the rolandic region and from lesions varying in size from small to quite large. The lesion size of weakness limited to the hand has been in some cases as large as that associated with severe weakness of the face, arm, and leg (hemiparesis) in others. No precisely reliable locus and no certain general lesion size has been found for weakness of the face, the arm, the hand, or the leg. However, tongue weakness is usually an indication that the lesion is in the lower rolandic region.

After an acute lesion from stroke or trauma or shortly after a major seizure, examinations performed within minutes to hours typically find the affected parts motionless and limp. When the face is affected, the forehead is often as weak as the lower half of the face and the eyelid hangs open, mimicking a facial nerve paralysis (pseudo-Bell's palsy) (see Ch. 29). Within minutes, hours, or days the limp limbs become stiffer as tone appears in the flexor muscles of the arm and the extensor muscles of the leg. The forehead becomes active while the lower face remains weak. The tongue deviation usually disappears about the same time and swallowing become satisfactory.

These observations in patients with stroke or trauma indicate that the traditional clinical examination, based as it is on assessing the raw power of parts of the body opposing the examiner, seems a mediocre guide to the precise size and location of the brain lesion affecting the rolandic convexity. They also show how a focal brain lesion may yield a syndrome whose features differ somewhat from that predicted by the known functional organization of the brain in normal subjects.

The Premotor Area (Area 6)

Area 6 (Figs. 25-1 and 25-6) is about six times as large as area 4, but the clinical consequences of its lesions are still rather ill defined. A first vexed question is that of spasticity: we do not know precisely which lesions cause the commonly observed spasticity associated with hemiplegia. Evidence points to the anterior border of area 4 or to area 6, but no definite answer can be offered at present. Similarly, a kind of fluctuating resistance to passive stretching of muscles termed *geg-*

enhalten (German: counterholding) has no satisfactory explanation in terms of sites of the causal lesion.

Recent studies have shed some light on the physiology and pathophysiology of the premotor cortex. Area 6 can be regarded as an association cortex in which impulses from sensory regions set the stage and provide feedback control for movements. Such movements, in addition, are modulated by some physiologic trace of previous experiences of motor accomplishments (i.e., so-called memories of movements), referred to in earlier times as "engrams." The notion of such memories accounts for the beneficial effects of training for skilled movements such as vocational activities or sports. Electrical stimulation of area 6 elicits movements more complex than those elicited from area 4.

Area 6 lesions also cause impairment in rhythm production, which suggests a role in the temporal organization of movements. Single-cell electrode recordings have revealed that some neurons fire when the animal is grasping with the mouth and others when holding with the mouth, and a large "vocabulary of movements" has thus been recorded. Rather than coding for simple movements, cells appear to be coding for participation in complex actions, an effect that has led Rizzolatti and Berti (1990) to refer to "grasping with the hand neurons," "holding neurons," or "tearing neurons." Some neurons are related to axial movements, some fire on anticipation of contact, and some fire even before any obvious movement. Some respond to tactile and some chiefly visual stimuli, increasing their rate of firing as a stimulus approaches the subject. This could even happen independently of the orientation of the eyes with respect to the approaching stimulus, a fact that favors the possibility that there are premotor cells sensitive to events in the extrapersonal space independently of the position of the eyes.

There is also evidence of dominance of the left premotor cortex for the most finely tuned motor activities. Left premotor lesions cause bilateral impairment of acquired skilled movements and limb-kinetic apraxia, which is likely the same basic disturbance (see Ch. 19). There is also dominance for rhythm production (see above).

Lesions close to Broca's area usually cause apraxic agraphia, in which the acquired movements in handwriting are impaired but not the recall of the sequence of letters involved in spelling, so that selection of keys on a typewriter is usually performed correctly.

Supplementary Motor Area

Stimulation of the supplementary motor area (SMA), which has a rostrocaudal representation for face, arm, and leg, causes bilateral movements that are slower and more tonic than those elicited from area 4. Posture is the main function of the SMA. Besides posture, the SMA plays a key role in the initiation and planning of movement. Recordings using single cell electrodes have found a degree of homuncular organization, which is different from that of area 4 in that there is a larger representation for proximal muscles. One of the basic functions of the premotor cortex appears to be to subserve the postural setup of proximal, contralateral, and to some extent ipsilateral muscles to allow free movements of the hand. This bilateral influence is accounted by the bilateral projections of area 6 via the corticoreticular fibers. Clinically, such disorders can be rather crudely evidenced by having the patient make swimming or windmill movements with the arms or pedaling movements with the legs, with both sides in either the same or opposite directions.

Lesions of both SMAs and surrounding regions, as in some anterior cerebral artery occlusions or ruptured aneurysms of the anterior communicating artery, also cause akinetic mutism, a state in which the patient lies immobile and utters no words but nevertheless is not unconscious and has normal wake-sleep cycles.

Movements of the Eyes and Head

Electrical stimulation of the posterior part of the middle central gyrus (part of area 8) (Fig. 25-6) causes turning of eyes and head toward the opposite side, which is termed a *contraversive* movement. Generally, deviation of the eyes occurs prior to that of the head. Eye movements are conjugated saccades (see Ch. 28), and the cortical eyes fields are assumed to be the place where voluntary eyes movements are generated. Contraversion of eyes and head is most frequent at the onset of an epileptic fit, and the movement is then traditionally termed *adversive*. The causal lesion can involve area 8, but there are many exceptions reminding that contraversion of eyes and head can also result from stimulation of the anterior part of the frontal lobe, the SMA, and the occipital cortex.

Deviation of eyes and head toward the side of the lesion (ipsiversion) is a common observation in acute stroke ("le malade regarde sa lésion"). It is generally assumed to result from the predominance of the non-lesioned cortical eyes fields. However, when conjugate ocular deviation has been found with limited lesions, these have more often been deep in the white matter than on the surface of the convexity. Ocular and head deviation is more often associated with right hemisphere lesions and is commonly associated with reduced responses to stimuli in the contralateral side space (inattention, neglect). Thus, ocular and head deviation could be part of a more complex disorder of motor responses to environmental stimuli. The deviation tends to be temporary, lasting less than 1 week, although rare cases can persist for many weeks. The mechanism of recovery is not clearly understood.

From Reflex to Behavioral Motor Disorders

Frontal lesions from the premotor cortex to the prefrontal region can cause several similar syndromes that reflect the dysfunction of progressively more complex motor organizations. The grasp reflex of the hand is an unwitting flexion of the fingers when the examiner lightly strokes the patient's palm, particularly between the thumb and index finger, with a finger or pen. In some patients the reflex can be produced even with the eyes closed. The patient cannot release the grip, and efforts on the examiner's part to disengage the grasped object only make the grip tighter. There can also be a grasp of the sole of the foot—a stimulus to the anterior part of the sole or plantar aspect of the toes causes the latter to flex and adduct. In patients with the grasp reflex, the snout and sucking reflexes (see Ch. 22) can often be elicited. All such reflexes are normal in the newborn and normally disappear about the third to the fourth month.

In alert patients the grasp reflex is characteristic of a contralateral premotor lesion. Some patients tend to grasp every object that enters their visual field. The hand contralateral to the lesion can thus be drawn in any direction by the object held by the examiner (groping reflex or reaction). The term *magnetic apraxia* has been proposed for the tendency to grab with either hand visually or tactually presented objects. This is not an apraxia in the strict sense of the term (see Ch. 19) but rather a grasping behavior.

More complex abnormal behavior can result from a lesions of one or both frontal lobes, usually in their inferior medial and orbital parts. These include utilization behavior in which the mere presentation of objects compels the patients to use them; imitation behavior in which they imitate the examiner's gestures and behavior; and the environmental dependency syndrome in which in everyday social situations they feel compelled to engage in activities suggested by the surroundings (e.g., games or gardening). Such disorders have been interpreted as resulting from a loss of the normal balance between the functions of the frontal and the parietal lobe, the latter receiving impulses from the external world and setting up action schemes that normally are checked (i.e., accepted or delayed or suppressed) by the former.

Frontal Gait

See discussion of gait disorders in Chapter 22.

Neglect

Anterior frontal lesions can cause neglect for, or inattention to, the contralateral extrapersonal space to the point in some cases of mimicking a hemianopia (see also Ch. 26). The term *motor neglect* indicates a reduced activity in the absence of paresis, reflexes, and sensory disturbances. The patient, as it were, appears to forget one side of the body, as shown by abnormal placements of the limbs and impairment of exploratory movements into the opposite (to the lesion) space. However, when the patient is prodded into activity, strength appears normal. Lesions in the prerolandic region have been found in some cases, usually on the surface but some deep and then usually large. The disorder can vanish within days or weeks.

Two main mechanisms have been proposed for neglect: first, a disturbance in response directed toward the contralateral side (attentional spatial disturbance); second, a representational theory based on the existence of cells that would respond to events in the contralateral space independently of eye position (see above). A dysfunction of these cells could account for the neglect, inattention thus being a secondary issue.

Alien Hand

The rare disorder termed *alien hand* results from lesions that most often are large and medial, usually but not always sparing the corpus callosum. However, it is likely that involvement of the callosal fibers in the frontal lobe (forceps major) plays a significant pathogenic role. In most cases it is the left hand that patients feels to be foreign or "alien," (i.e., not belonging to them). Some patients go as far as personification, giving the hand names as if belonging to another person. There is also an "autonomous" activity of the hand with involuntary movements. A grasp reflex is frequent. Bimanual activities such as mirror movements or conflicts between the hands, such as which will lift the telephone receiver, are possible. The disorder usually fades over weeks or months.

Impersistence

In this disorder patients fail at continuing for more than a few seconds such willed acts as eye closure, breath holding, gazing on one size, tongue protrusion, or hand gripping. Most patients have a right-sided lesion. Impersistence is thought to reflect impaired attention and focused concentration. It is not a diagnostic marker of frontal lobe injury. Although a frequent finding in acute lesions, it may also persist for months after many other signs have improved.

Disturbances of Micturition and Defecation

Right, left, or bilateral medial lesions in the regions of areas 8, 9, 32, and 33 (Fig. 25-6) cause a lack of awareness of bladder (to a lesser extent of rectal) events. The normal desire to micturate and the feeling of impending micturition are absent or diminished. Retention or constipation are less frequent.

Clinically, the patient can be surprised by being wet as a result of unwitting urination. Less severe disorders cause frequency and urgency. Incontinence and retention are part of the syndrome of the anterior cerebral artery (see Ch. 35). In patients with frontal tumors, urinating in incongruous places is frequent. Because of disinhibition of the personality (see below), a common associated finding, the patient can appear indifferent to the social repercussions of such improper behavior.

Vasomotor Disturbances

Vasomotor disturbances were part of the early descriptions of the premotor syndrome. Facial, truncal, and limb vasomotor reflexes are disturbed on the side opposite to the lesion. Clinicians commonly observe that the paralyzed limbs can become edematous, bluish, cold, or abnormally warm.

Cognitive Disorders

For a long time, and especially since the end of the 19th century among the phrenologists, a high forehead was regarded as suggesting high intelligence, hence the expression "high brow." For decades, the frontal lobe has been presumed by many to be the part of the brain most responsible for intellectual capacities. However, a strong body of evidence militates against such a view; many frontal lobectomies have been performed for trauma or tumor without detectable cognitive deficit. Similarly, lobotomies or leukotomies, which were performed around the early 1940s for mental disease, particularly obsessive-compulsive neurosis, apparently did not cause cognitive disorders. Such patients retained their previous knowledge and performed reasonably well on general tests such as the Wechsler Adult Intelligence Scale.

There are, however, cognitive disorders in patients with frontal lesions, although they can vary considerably from patient to patient and from examination to examination and can be difficult to demonstrate in the brief testing typical of examinations at the bedside or in the consulting room. Such behavioral disorders can be most obvious in everyday life, such as setting the table, gardening, cooking, or washing the car. The clinician must pay careful attention to the observations of relatives and friends.

The core of frontal cognitive disorders is impairment in planning, sequencing, holding responses, and sustaining a steady behavioral output. Attention is focused only for short times and hence there is easy distractibility.

Many tests address particular aspects of these deficits, among which the authors find especially commendable the go/no-go paradigm and the alternating sequences test. In the go/no-go paradigm the patient

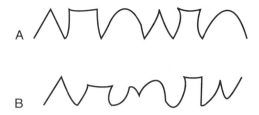

Figure 25-12. Alternating sequences test. **(A)** Normal; **(B)** patient with frontal tumor. Note perseverations.

is instructed to raise the index finger in response to one tap and not to raise it in response to two taps. The taps are produced with the examiner's pen, of course without the patient seeing the movement. In the alternating sequences test the patient is asked either to make serial movements of the hand (striking the table with palm, edge, and fist successively) or to draw a zigzag line consisting in alternately pointed, rectangular, and domed elements (Fig. 25-12). In the first test afflicted patients cannot withhold erroneous responses, and in the second they cannot follow the correct sequencing. Both tests show a great deal of perseverations.

Reduced Initiative

The whole demeanor of the patient with reduced initiative suggests a diminished motivation and an absence of the normal desire to enter into conversation with people or to pay attention to external events. Such patients are not hostile, but their cooperation is faulty because they lack the normal drive that makes people interested in events and tasks that come up with each moment of life. This kind of mood is called apathy (Greek *a*, lacking; *pathos*, emotion) and in severe cases abulia (Greek *a*, lacking; *boule*, will). Abulia is most impressive in patients with large bifrontal tumors or with degenerative frontal atrophies such as Pick's disease, in which the patient sits or lies immobile, indifferent to the surroundings, and answers questions after a long delay in a feeble, whispered voice. In a less severe form, this disorder, may make history taking slow and incomplete, with the patient speaking only in laconic sentences and falling silent, requiring frequent prompting and long waits before responding.

Disinhibition of Behavior

Some patients, most often those with lesions affecting the inferior surface of the frontal lobes, display a propensity to make jokes, often of a rather crude sort, puns inappropriate to the present situation, and comments most often contrasting with their previous social personality and upbringing. This pathologic jocu-

---

THE MAIN ELEMENTS OF THE
FRONTAL SYNDROME

1. Contralateral grasping, groping; bilateral so-called magnetic apraxia, imitation, utilization behavior, apraxia of the left hand, alien hand, neglect, impersistence
2. Disorders of micturition and defecation
3. Disorders of planning, sequencing, producing a steady behavioral output, holding responses
4. Apathy and abulia
5. Moria/Witzelsucht

---

lar behavior is termed Witzelsucht (German for compulsive joking) or moria (Greek for folly).

Traditionally, disorders that involve area 4 (contralateral paralysis) or 44 on the left side (Broca's aphasia) are not included in the frontal syndrome (summarized in the box above).

Vascular Supply

Arteries

The arteries supplying the frontal lobe derive from both the anterior and middle cerebral arteries. The entire medial surface of the frontal lobe (see Fig. 35-16) and almost all of the pole is from surface branches of the anterior cerebral artery. On the convex surface, the posterior half of the frontal lobe is supplied by surface branches of the middle cerebral artery, namely the prefrontal, prerolandic, and rolandic branches, in most cases arising from the upper division of the middle cerebral artery (see Fig. 35-15). On the inferior (orbital) surface of the frontal lobe, orbitofrontal branches of the middle cerebral artery anastomose with those of the anterior cerebral artery just lateral to the gyrus rectus (Figs. 35-16 and 35-18).

Veins

Most of the convex surface of the frontal lobe is supplied by veins that drain to the superior sagittal sinus. These veins vary somewhat in number, none of them being large enough or constant enough in position to have acquired an eponym such as those supplying the parietal and temporal lobes.

Disorders

Trauma

The frontal lobe, occupying two-thirds of the convexity and anterior in location, is especially subject to blunt injury and missile wounds. Closed head injury is common from vehicular accidents. Penetrating wounds in war may enter the frontal lobe from the convex surface, but they cause especial difficulties in management when the missile enters through a frontal sinus or from below via the orbit. Spinal fluid leaks and infection are especially prevalent in the latter two settings (see Ch. 6).

Tumors

The frontal lobe, being composed of so much of the cerebral white matter, is the most frequently recognized site of primary brain tumors (i.e., gliomas). Tumors arising in the frontal lobe are prone to grow across the corpus callosum (e.g., butterfly glioma, so-called because of its bilateral winglike appearance on brain imaging and at autopsy). The syndromes from these lesions may be bilateral or unilateral, depending on the relative size of the lesion in each hemisphere.

Like the other lobes, the frontal lobe is subject to metastases, which more often lodge in the regions of the border zones of the main cerebral arteries. In these regions blood flow may come to a standstill or even reverse direction momentarily, thus favoring the settling out of tumor microemboli.

Infections

Infectious particles can lodge in the arterial border zones for reasons similar to those of metastases (see above). Infection can spread from frontal, ethmoidal, or sphenoidal sinuses. Basal skull fractures can cause rhinorrhea with the attendant risk of meningitis (see Ch. 6).

Strokes

Infarction is far more frequently due to occlusion of the middle cerebral artery than to occlusion of the anterior cerebral artery (see Chs. 5 and 35). Most of the infarcts are explained by embolism. Hemorrhages are fairly common in the frontal lobe in hypertension and in a setting of congophilic angiopathy (see Ch. 36).

Degenerative Diseases

Alzheimer's disease commonly involves the frontal lobe to a lesser extent than the parietal and temporal regions. Pick's disease causes a severe atrophy of the frontal lobes. Frontal involvement tends to cause elements of the frontal lobe syndrome, most especially reduced initiation of activity.

PARIETAL LOBE

Anatomy and Implied Physiology

The parietal lobe (from the Latin for belonging to or bounded by a wall) is bounded anteriorly by the central (rolandic) fissure, anteroinferiorly by the lateral (sylvian) fissure, and superoposteriorly, along the superior margin of the hemisphere, by the short lateral segment of the parieto-occipital fissure. The parietal lobe, decreasing in size at its extends posteroinferiorly, has no other natural landmark to separate it from the temporal and occipital lobes (see Figs. 25-1, 25-2).

On the medial side of the hemisphere, the parietal lobe remains bounded anteriorly by the central fissure and posteriorly by the same parieto-occipital fissure, now deep and long. The rear part of the paracentral lobule and the precuneus are thus part of the parietal lobe.

On the convexity, the expanse of the lobe is subdivided first by the postcentral sulcus, which runs roughly parallel to the central fissure, making the posterior border of the postcentral gyrus. In the upper third of the parietal convexity (Fig. 25-1), the intraparietal sulcus, running posteriorly from the postcentral sulcus to the occipital lobe, separates the superior from the inferior parietal gyrus, traditionally and hereafter termed lobules. The location of the intraparietal sulcus high on the convexity accounts for most of the superior parietal lobule lying on the medial surface of the hemisphere.

In humans the inferior parietal lobule is strikingly well developed; hence the convolutions are very sinuous as they bend repeatedly, their sulci deeper than those in the frontal lobe. Moreover, the configuration of the inferior parietal lobule is quite variable, not only between individuals but even from one hemisphere to the other. Two gyri are of particular importance physiologically and clinically, namely, the supramarginal gyrus (area 40), which is formed like a cap over the termination of the sylvian fissure, and the angular gyrus (area 39), which caps the end of the first (superior) temporal sulcus. When examining postmortem specimens it can be difficult to distinguish one gyrus from the other. The authors recommend following Dejerine's advice, namely, to look first for Jensen's intermediate sulcus, a short furrow directly in line with the parieto-occipital fissure. The gyrus angularis is just behind Jensen's sulcus.

Histology

Three narrow strips of cortex labeled from anterior to posterior areas 3, 1, and 2 (Fig. 25-6) make up the primary somatosensory area (also known as S1). The histologic appearance is almost exclusively that of koniocortex. Area 3 is made up of thin koniocortex located mostly in the posterior bank of the central fissure. Just behind, in areas 1 and 2, koniocortex is admixed with numerous pyramidal cells. Although roughly 40 percent of the Betz cells are said to be found in the parietal lobe, virtually no Betz cells are found in the posterior half of the superior lobule and the whole of the inferior lobule. The secondary somesthetic unimodal area, separate from the primary in areas 3, 2, and 1, occupies the superior parietal lobule as area 5 (Fig. 25-6).

The multimodal association areas behind the primary somatosensory cortex in the superior and inferior parietal lobule have the histologic appearance of the homogeneous, homotypical cortex seen in other regions of the cerebrum (see introductory paragraph of this chapter).

Pathways, Cortical Areas, and Physiology

Primary Sensory Cortex. S1 receives thalamic projections from the ventral posterolateral and ventral posteromedial nuclei (Fig. 25-7). These nuclei process inputs from the median lemniscus, spinothalamic, secondary trigeminal tracts and from the gustatory pathways from the nucleus of the solitary fasciculus (Ch. 29). The majority of fibers from the primary sensory area project onto area 3, which serves as an association system for links to other brain regions.

In the postcentral gyrus, regions of the body are represented as a "sensory homunculus." As with its motor homunculus counterpart in the precentral gyrus (see the section Frontal Lobe above) this large-mouthed, large-tongued little man is head down, hand with big thumb in the upper third of the gyrus, foot over the margin of the hemisphere, in the paracentral lobule (Figs. 25-10 and 25-11).

Such localizations are useful for rough clinical topographic diagnosis (in such disorders as sensory jacksonian epilepsy, when the jacksonian march of tingling can successively involve foot, leg, hand, and face, or in those focal postrolandic lesions that produce the cheiro-oral syndromes (Greek: *cheiros,* hand; Latin *os, oris,* mouth), in which concomitant tingling or numbness of the ipsilateral lips and hand denote a lesion of the contralateral postcentral gyrus. (Similar cheiro-oral motor syndromes are thought to reflect a comparable lesion in the motor cortex but have also been documented from infarction in subcortical pathways.)

Sensory evoked responses of newborn primates indicate that homuncular organization is genetically programmed. However, in humans it has proved more difficult to obtain sharp localization data, in part because much of the recording is made over the intact calvarium, and only feeble signals are obtained after highly focal stimulation of, say, a digit. The site at which stimulation evokes sensation at a certain body site seems rather variable, although the somatotopic organization appears reliable (i.e., the hand is higher than the face and the leg higher than the hand). By evoked response mapping, the hand area has been found most frequently in the upper third of the postcentral gyrus, near the site of the largest bend (see also Ch. 23).

While there may be a highly organized homunculus in normal subjects, the exact location for each sensory receptor zone and the degree of organization do not appear to be the same for each type of stimulation. In primates, some postrolandic cells have been found that respond to any types of stimulus (plurimodal) while others respond only to touch or to pain. Furthermore, the specificity for the site of stimulation varies, some cells responding to contact anywhere on a limb while others appear to require extremely circumscribed sites and still others respond to movement of a joint irrespective of the load conditions (changes in muscle activity involved in producing the same movements under load).

The close interaction between vision and motor function also influences the threshold response for certain types of cells. Some cells dramatically lower their threshold as a noxious stimulus approaches under visual guidance, while at other times they make no anticipatory response when the target approaches unseen. PET studies have demonstrated activation of the postrolandic regions in response to voluntary movements as well as to passive or active somatosensory stimulation. Neurologists may have to revise traditional simplistic notions of a homunculus to provide closer overlap with the work of contemporary physiologists.

Posterior Parietal Region. The posterior parietal region, as studied in the monkey, has massive, generally reciprocal, connections with three main cerebral systems: sensory, limbic, and reticular. First, there are connections with S1 through the secondary areas and with the thalamus, chiefly the pulvinar (reciprocally linked with the visual areas and receiving from the lateral and medial geniculate bodies) and the lateroposterior nucleus (receiving from the ventral posterior nucleus). Second, there are links with the limbic system, mostly the cingulate and retrosplenia gyri (see the section Temporal Lobe, below), and, like the whole cortex, the posterior parietal region receives projections from the nucleus basalis. Third, there are connections with the reticular system (i.e., the thalamic intralaminar nuclei) the locus ceruleus (adrenergic), and perhaps the raphe nuclei of the brainstem (serotoninergic).

While it would be wrong to transpose pari passu anatomic features of monkeys to humans, in whom they are both much more elaborated and much less precisely studied, it is reasonable to take monkey data as a basic pattern in approaching human organization.

Inferior Parietal Region. In primates, neurons in the inferior parietal region fire in response to multimodal stimuli and appear to be the highest-level processors of all information used in preparing motor responses. Such neurons show a capacity of behavioral judgment (e.g., they fire maximally when the animal is thirsty and liquid provides the stimulus to look at or to reach). The activity of these cells is likely to subserve attention and motivation. Conversely, their destruction is likely to play a key role in asomatognosia (Ch. 19) and neglect (see the section Frontal Lobe, above and Ch. 20).

In humans, PET studies have shown activation in the superior parietal lobule along with the motor cortex, supplementary motor area, and ipsilateral cerebellum when the index finger tracks a moving target under visual guidance. Increasing the complexity of the task by providing a reference target in addition to the moving target increases the activity in the superior parietal region, corroborating the role of this area in integrating multimodal activities, as suggested by animal studies.

It has also long been known in animals that lesions of the parietal association cortex can cause an exaggerated withdrawal reaction after cutaneous contact. This was interpreted by D. Denny-Brown (New Zealand-born neurologist in the United Kingdom and United States, 1901–81) as loss of an essential function of the parietal lobe, namely to promote exploring, reaching, and manipulating in the extrapersonal space. Such withdrawal reaction or avoidance behavior has been described only in patients with very large parietal lesions.

In a broader view, while the role of the parietal lobe seems to be to prepare and launch action, that of the frontal lobe is for deliberating, delaying, and possibly canceling action. Loss of the normal balance between the two lobes would account for the withdrawal behavior associated with parietal lesions (frontal predominance) or to the forced grasping and groping reflexes produced by frontal lesions (parietal predominance) (see section Frontal Lobe, above).

The inferior parietal lobule is continuous with the multimodal temporal and occipital cortices. This vast region appears to be endowed with activities that subserve the highest cognitive functions in humans. Moreover, the left and right hemispheres are not equivalent, and their lesions cause clinically different disorders (e.g., aphasia and ideational apraxia on the left side, see below). The notion of dominance is thus inherent to the study of the physiology and pathophysiology of the posterior parietal cortex of the non-dominant hemisphere (see Ch. 20). The authors know of anatomic studies documenting a longer superior temporal plane on the left than on the right side, corroborating that language function is left-side dominant, but do not know of studies suggesting a larger development of areas 39 and 40 on the left side although the longer left sylvian fissure has often been assumed to reflect such development.

Deep Pathways. Two dense tracts run deep in the parietal lobe. The *superior longitudinal fasciculus* (or fronto-occipital tract of Onufrowicz) is the superior part of the arcuate fasciculus (Fig. 25-8). It leaves au passage collaterals to the parietal lobe. The clinical consequences of its lesions are not well known, but it is suspected that lesions in these tracts account for the syndromes of optic ataxia (see the section Occipital Lobe, below).

The *optic radiations* pass through the inferomedial portions of the parietal lobe en route to the occipital lobe, their course being close to the outer ventricular wall (see Ch. 26). Lesions of the superior part of the radiations (i.e., those coursing through the depths of the parietal lobe) should cause contralateral homonymous inferior quadrantanopia. However, hemianopia, not merely quadrantanopia, is as frequent. A disorder of optokinetic nystagmus is characteristic of parietal lesions. In this condition, when the targets are rotated toward the damaged side, the nystagmus is of diminished amplitude and frequency as compared with the normal nystagmus resulting from targets rotated toward the intact side (see Ch. 26). It is a good rule that in a patient with hemianopia, a normal optokinetic nystagmus makes a parietal lesion unlikely.

Both parietal lobes are linked by fibers of the corpus callosum. For the consequences of their disconnection, see section Corpus Callosum, below.

Arteries

The arteries supplying the lateral surface of the parietal lobe derive mainly from the middle cerebral artery. Usually the supply is limited to three branches—the rolandic, anterior parietal, and angular (to the angular gyrus). Virtually none of the parietal lobe receives supply from the deep lenticulostriate branches of the middle cerebral artery.

The anterior cerebral artery supplies the rear part of the paracentral lobule and the precuneus. Moreover, this artery supplies the higher third of the lobe on the convexity (Fig. 35-15). Along the border or watershed zone, distal branches of the anterior and middle cerebral arteries anastomose end to end. Posteriorly, branches of both arteries also anastomose with those of the posterior cerebral artery.

CLINICAL SYNDROMES FROM PARIETAL LESIONS

Unilateral lesions either side
  Cortical sensory syndrome
  Quadrantanopia or hemianopia
  Disorders of optokinetic nystagmus to the lesioned side
  Rarely, contralateral muscle wasting (Silverstein syndrome)
Lesions on the dominant side, include in addition
  Wernicke aphasia in which alexia can be predominant (see Ch. 18)
  Bilateral idomotor and ideational apraxia
  Gerstmann syndrome (see Ch. 19)
  Rarely, bilateral tactile agnosia (see Ch. 19)
Lesions on the nondominant side include (in addition to unilateral lesions, either side, listed above)
  Asomatognosia
  Anosognosia
  Constructional apraxia
  Dressing apraxia
  Prosopagnosia, loss of topographic memory, color agnosia (often bilateral lesions, but evidence that the right-sided ones are more significant (see Ch. 19)
Bilateral lesions
  Balint's syndrome (see Occipital Lobe)

Veins

The superior longitudinal sinus courses along the superior margin of both parietal lobes, so that bilateral parietal infarction is characteristic of occlusion of the sinus. The great anastomotic veins of Trolard and Labbé drape over the lobe (Fig. 35-23).

Clinical Syndromes

The clinical disorders due to parietal lesions are one of the mainstays of clinical neurology. Consequently, they have been considered individually in several chapters of this book and are summarized below. The schematic classification in the box calls for reservations, that is some disorders (e.g., asomatognosia) can result from lesions on either side but are more evident with right-sided lesions, while some other disorders imply generally bilateral lesions, those on one side being more significant (e.g., prosopagnosia and right-sided lesions). The text below considers circumscribed lesions in more detail.

Postrolandic Lesions

Too few instances of isolated focal lesions limited to the postrolandic convexity exist to permit exploration of the possible range of syndromes. A very few examples of isolated infarction have presented with pure sensory loss, sparing any disturbance in motor function. As with prerolandic motor lesions, rare cases of highly circumscribed losses in sensation have been described, some limited to the face, to the face and hand, to the thumb and index and middle fingers, or to the hand and foot. Likewise, instances have been described of patterns of numbness approximating those of a root or peripheral nerve distribution, known as pseudoradicular sensory loss. They have usually roughly approximated the ulnar or the median territory. While the tactile threshold is not blunted in the affected body parts, there is decreased sensitivity to alterations in stimulus strength, suggesting a narrowing of the range of response. Rarely, a postrolandic lesion produces hallucinations of touch or feeling the persistence of immediately preceding experiences.

Classically, postcentral lesions are said to feature loss of the ability to discriminate objects by the unique combination of size, weight, shape, density, and texture, a loss known as *astereognosia*. As mentioned above, some of the disturbance could be attributed to blunting of tactile sense or to impaired fine manipulation, but even by passive manipulation aided by the examiner in a hand that can detect touch, reports document the absolute inability of some patients to offer any description of the stimulus. Selective loss of detection of a single property of discrimination, such as size, texture, or weight, are so rare that neither author has an example in his experience. The usual finding has been that the patient performs well enough in any given single task having but one component such as size.

Hopes have dimmed that a single clinical test of higher sensory function could suffice to indicate a parietal lesion. Critchley's suggestion, dating from the 1950s, that impairment of the ability to estimate weights (barognosis) is an especially sensitive sign, has not been borne out in the authors' experience, nor has Luria's claim that minor lesions of the parietal system cause as their first sign the loss of Charpentier's illusion. (Charpentier's illusion is the imprinting of size asymmetry by the repeated squeezing of two objects of grossly different size, followed immediately thereafter by grasping two same-sized objects. The subject discovers that the object in the hand that previously squeezed the larger now feels as if it were now squeezing the smaller, and vice versa.) Likewise, the

time-honored test of naming numbers or letters written by the examiner on the patient's index fingerpad or palm and that of using the compass for "two-point" discrimination, which are two other popular tests taught to generations of students, have only occasionally shown value in predicting clinicoanatomic findings by brain imaging. A better correlation with lesion location appears to exist for impairment of the ability to name objects palpated actively (i.e., the patient manipulating the object) or passively (i.e., the object being moved by the examiner through the patient's dormant fingers and palm).

In the larger postrolandic lesions, the disturbances in sensorimotor function are often more striking. A distinctive observation is the patient's inability to find the site on the affected side being subjected to noxious stimuli. When the normal side is subjected to the same pinch, the site is found immediately and the stimulus removed. However, when a painful pinch is made unseen on the affected arm or leg, or sometimes even the face, the patient is promptly aroused to movements suggesting discomfort, even pain, and yet the normal contralateral limb fails to move to the site of the pinching and remove the noxious stimulus. The implicit lack of localization is commonly observed by the opposite hand reaching no further than the midline of the trunk, rubbing the abdomen or thorax as if seeking relief. This failure of topographic localization in the presence of preserved perception of a noxious stimulus suggests that the postrolandic region plays a vital role in localization of somatosensory stimuli but a less important role in detecting noxious stimuli per se. Often, the nature of the painful stimulus is not described by the patient, who may even say there is no pain, a finding suggesting that the arousal may not be the conscious awareness of pain so much as an activation of the reticular activating system from the ascending volley of noxious stimuli.

Complaints of pain following postrolandic lesions is also uncommon. Despite the common reports of numbness and sensory loss to testing of touch and pinprick, description of postlesion pain in the affected parts is far less common, although one instance of dental pain from a primary parietal lobe brain tumor (glioma) has been reported.

Other unusual and poorly understood syndromes include the loss of muscle mass (amyotrophy), known as *Silverstein's syndrome*, in the limbs contralateral to a parietal lesion. The arm is usually the limb most affected. Least understood has been the finding of loss of eye closure ipsilateral to the parietal lesion.

Posterior Parietal Lesions

Although no gross weakness occurs, impairments are commonly observed in the explorative finger movements, the precision of grip, and the skill, speed, and force of manipulation of objects in the contralateral hand. The resultant syndromes are easily labeled as dyspraxias, reflecting an impairment in the normally tight coordination between the sensory and motor cortices.

Posterior parietal lesions in humans all produce a degree of impairment in response to contralateral space. These disorders, described in more detail under the terms unilateral spatial neglect and various categories of dyspraxias, affect ocular motility and limb activities in varying degree. The disturbance most easily detected is impaired opticokinetic nystagmus for tracking of targets toward the midline from the affected visual field. In more advanced disturbances, the accuracy of reaching into space is impaired, with the patient failing to touch a visually displayed target, usually reaching medial to the site. Such disturbances have been reported even in the absence of clinically evident disturbance in response to pinprick, cold, or touch, or in the naming of palpated objects and with full visual fields to confrontation testing. In the most severe cases, organized whole body movements have been impaired and the patient has had difficulty even turning over in bed.

Posterior parietal lesions also impair exploratory ocular search for the same reasons that they affect limb and trunk movements. The lesion makes it difficult for the patient's eye movements to be used to outline the shapes and fine details of the thematically relevant portions of complex visual displays such as action pictures, while preserving the more practiced metronomic horizontal movements in reading. This syndrome of impaired ocular search with preserved ocular movements, noted by Balint (R. Balint, Hungarian neurologist, 1874–1934) in his famous 1909 report, were characterized by him by several terms, the first, the unusual "Seelenlähmung des 'Schauens'" translated by most reviewers as *psychic paresis of gaze*, a term Balint recognized as a neologism by his insertion of quotation marks around "Schauens" or gaze, immediately after which he cited in the title the second feature, optic ataxia. By the former term he seems to have meant what others have come to describe as an apraxia of ocular searching movements. By optic ataxia he meant an impairment in the use of vision to reach, touch, or grab objects under visual guidance, and a need to rely on touch. This is the reverse of the familiar "sensory ataxia," in which lesions of the posterior columns make it difficult for the patient to walk on the basis of proprioception and a need to rely on visual cues for balance. Balint's patient was also characterized by a third term, more easily translated as *disturbance in spatial attention*. This feature was characterized as difficulty in seeing into the periphery of the visual field. The combination of these disturbances impaired the ability of the patient to apprehend as a whole the meaning of complex visual displays and scenes. The lesions found at autopsy were extensive, bilateral, and high in the parietal regions and over the posterolateral occipital and inferior temporal regions (roughly in the border zones between the middle and the posterior cerebral arteries) (see Ch. 35). Balint himself attributed much of the disturbance to disruption of the links between the occipital and frontal systems. Since his time, rare cases have been reported of a unilateral disturbance in exploration of space resulting from a contralateral occipital or occipito-parietal lesion.

In the generation that followed Balint, terms such as *simultanognosia* were popularized to explain this syndrome and were used to suggest a disturbance in a putative capacity to integrate the meaning of elements of a picture. With the decline in emphasis of the once popular gestalt concepts of cerebral function as the basis for explanations of these findings have come other explanations: more modern interpretations of Balint's patient place greater weight on the impaired ocular movements in searching a display (see also the section Frontal Lobe and Ch. 19).

It was partly gestalt psychology that at its height as a field in the 1920s through the 1940s helped spawn the many eponymic syndromes popularized at the time, which were based on the notion that the parietal lobe served to integrate multimodal (i.e., visual, auditory, and somatosensory) sensory function. In this view, parietal lesions thus reflect several functions, which item by item would seem separate from one another. These syndromes include Balint's (see above), Gerstmann's (right-left confusion and finger agnosia, agraphia, and acalculia), Wolpert's 'simultanognosia' and many others. Although Balint's syndrome has a good record of predicting the clinical correlation with biparieto-occipital lesions, there has been less success with many of the others.

Medial Parietal Lesions

Little is known of the clinical effects of lesions in this region. One report of multilead stereotaxically placed electrode stimulation described illusions of visual motion from stimulation near the parieto-occipital fissure, which occurred despite the lack of eye movements.

Diseases

Infarction

Occlusion of the parietal branches of the middle cerebral artery is usually caused by embolism. Since the embolic material must pass by several more anterior branches en route, several branches are generally occluded. However, occasionally a small embolic particle can selectively occlude one branch, causing highly focal deficits that allow detailed studies of the parietal lobe functions.

In a setting of collapse or cardiac arrest or bilateral internal carotid artery occlusion, the upper parietal region is liable to suffer (bilaterally) from perfusion failure (see Ch. 35) because it is at the most distal end of the endangered vascular territory. In such cases, there can be a large band of infarction along the watershed zone between the three main cerebral arteries, hence across the parietal lobe. Various combinations of apraxias and agnosias are characteristic of such cases. In unilateral occlusions of the internal carotid artery with poor collateral supply, similar lesions can occur unilaterally.

Thrombosis of the superior longitudinal sinus, as mentioned above, often causes bilateral parietal infarction. Computed tomography (CT) or magnetic resonance imaging (MRI) easily pick up the hemorrhagic (venous) infarction and show the thrombosis of the sinus. The diagnosis could also include hemorrhage in unilateral infarcts. Hemorrhage, of course, would contraindicate anticoagulants, whereas venous infarction indicates anticoagulation as early as possible (see Ch. 35).

Hemorrhage

The parietal lobe is the most frequent site of hypertensive hemorrhage and a possible site of hemorrhage due to amyloid angiopathy (see Ch. 36).

Trauma

The parietal lobes are especially at risk from falling objects. Injuries from stabs, bullets, gunshot, and fragments are commonplace in war and currently in many cities in civilian practice. Concussion by a blow under the chin often causes contrecoup lesions of the parietal lobes. The transverse skull diameter is smaller in the parietal than the frontal region; survivors of through-and-through bullet or fragment wounds are more frequently found than for frontal wounds.

Infection

Bloodborne infectious particles can be preferentially deposited along the arterial border zones (see above). Like the other lobes, the parietal is a frequent target for infection. Progressive multifocal leukoencephalopathy, a viral disease in immunocompromised patients, is more frequent in the parieto-occipital region, and often begins clinically as dyspraxia and later as disorders suggestive of hemineglect.

Tumors

Seeding of metastatic cancers also can occur preferentially along the arterial border zone for the same reasons as that of infections, hence metastases are also frequent in the parietal lobe. Likewise, with its large volume of white matter the lobe is a favorite site for gliomas to develop.

Degenerative Diseases

Severe involvement of the association cortex of the parietal lobe occurs in Alzheimer's disease. Aphasia and apraxia are early and frequently encountered disorders. Parietal involvement is also a feature of Pick's and Creutzfeldt-Jakob diseases.

Several cases of slowly progressive apraxia with MRI and PET evidence of atrophy predominating in the parietal lobe have been reported during recent years. There was also, in most cases, constructional and dressing apraxia. Dementia has not been a feature, except in a few cases and late in the course of the disease. Involuntary movements have been frequent, suggesting the involvement of the basal ganglia, but slowly progressive apraxia is likely to be distinct from corticobasal degeneration in which there is also a constructional apraxia. The few pathologically documented cases have shown Alzheimer or Pick lesions or a dense gliosis with lesions of the white matter. The characteristic lesion of corticobasal degeneration involving extensively the basal ganglia with particular inclusions were absent. Obviously, slowly progressive apraxia is reminiscent of slowly progressive aphasia (see the section Temporal Lobe). Both currently share a similar lack of definite classification.

TEMPORAL LOBE

The temporal lobe is the most heterogeneous of all the cerebral lobes, since it harbors not only two primary sensory (auditory and olfactory) cortices and the uni- and multimodal cortices shared with other lobes, but also anatomic structures that rank among the phylogenetically oldest in the human brain.

Anatomy and Implied Physiology

The anatomy and anatomic nomenclature of the temporal lobe are complex but of special importance for the clinician, since many particular parts of the lobe are involved in many pathologic processes (e.g., epilepsy, behavioral disorders, and temporal herniation). Details of temporal anatomy have taxed the imagination and memory of generations of students, so the authors have intended here to provide a simplified refresher of the salient features of the lobe.

The temporal lobe has the shape of a triangular pyramid with superior, lateral, and inferior surfaces and an anterior tip, the temporal pole. The temporal lobe lies below the sylvian fissure (Fig. 25-1). Most of the lobe is connected with the rest of the cerebral hemisphere by a narrow band of white matter, the isthmus

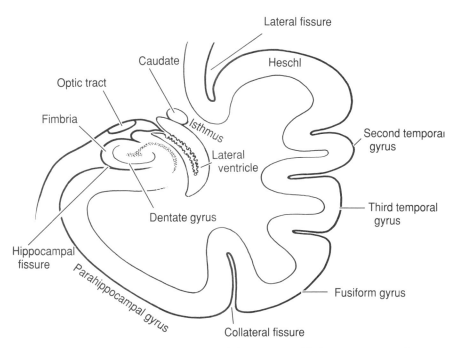

Figure 25-13. A schematic macroscopic view of the temporal lobe on a coronal section (see text).

(from the Greek for narrow part), through which all tracts that arrive or leave the lobe must pass (Fig. 25-13). Lesions of this strategic causeway obviously have considerable clinical consequences but remain imperfectly understood.

The medial part of the lobe lies in the middle fossa of the skull just atop the tentorium cerebelli and is subject to herniation when the pressure is high above the tentorium (see Ch. 17 and the section, Temporal Herniation, below). The temporal pole is lodged in the hollow of the greater wing of the sphenoid bone, just below the ridge of the lesser wing. This embedded location accounts for the pole being particularly liable to lesions in cerebral concussion (see below and Ch. 6).

The inferior surface of the lobe lies atop the middle ear, on the petrous bone, whence infection can spread directly through the tegmentum tympani to the substance of the lobe to cause a temporal abscess. Posteriorly its principal gyri, the lingual and fusiform, blend into the occipital lobe (see Occipital Lobe).

The superior surface (i.e., the first temporal gyrus) hardly appears on the convexity of the brain and mostly constitutes the inferior bank of the lateral fissure (Fig. 25-1). Anteriorly, it merges with the insula. Its midpart constitutes Heschl transverse gyri (Fig. 25-6, areas 41, 42), corresponding to the primary auditory cortex with a tonotopic arrangement of incoming auditory fibers (see eighth cranial nerve in Ch. 29). The Heschl gyri are surrounded by secondary areas

of unimodal cortex. Posterior to areas 41 and 42 is the vestibular area, its exact site still not well defined. Still more posterior lies the planum temporale, the cortical area between Heschl gyri and the posterior margin of the lateral fissure. Its rear limits are somewhat uncertain.

In most humans the planum temporale is longer and larger on the left side, providing an anatomic basis for the localization of right-handedness and language functions to the left hemisphere. Conversely, there is evidence that this asymmetry is lacking in developmental dyslexia. Such structural features can now be documented by special CT and MRI studies. In primates, evidence has accumulated that the planum temporale contains a multimodal cortex linked by bidirectional fibers to the unimodal sensory areas (auditory, somatosensory, visual) and other postrolandic association areas. There would be heavy projections to and through the pons to the cerebellum (temporopontine tract, see Ch. 22). These findings have encouraged speculation that the cerebellum plays some role in modulating nonmotor as well as motor functions and suggest that the planum temporale has functions that make its central role in the brain response to sensory input as important as its role inferred for language.

The first and second temporal gyri, on the lateral surface of the brain, are separated by the first temporal sulcus (Fig. 25-1 and 25-13), an anterior furrow capped posteriorly by the gyrus angularis, a typical multimodal cortex (Fig. 25-4A and Fig. 25-6, area 39), which belongs to the parietal lobe. However, multimodal cortex extends forwards along the sulcus. On the left side, the anterior part of the Wernicke area lies in the rear portion of the first temporal convolution (see Ch. 18).

Similarly, the second and third temporal sulci separate the second and third temporal gyri, mostly unimodal cortex. The fourth temporal gyrus, termed the fusiform or occipitotemporal gyrus, is bounded medially by the deep, anteroposterior collateral fissure (Fig. 25-14), which continues anteriorly as the rhinal fissure. Both fissures herald the transition with the old brain (paleocortex), which in most animals subserves olfaction, while in humans the so-called olfactory or parolfactory cortex is involved in emotional and motivational activities (see discussion of the limbic lobe below). Outside the collateral fissure (thus close to the old cortex) lies a band of multimodal cortex (Fig. 25-6, area 36).

Medial to the fusiform gyrus and medially bounded by the hippocampal fissure is the fifth temporal gyrus (Fig. 25-14), termed *parahippocampal* because it lies just beneath the hippocampus (see below). The more medial part of the gyrus is known as the *subiculum* (from the Latin for little step). The rostral part of the gyrus, with an enlarged fold, the uncus (from the Latin for

hook), and the lateral olfactory stria (see first cranial nerve in Ch. 29) constitute the pyriform lobe (from the Latin for pear-shaped), an old cortex belonging to the primary olfactory cortex.

Above the hippocampal fissure, the most medial part of the temporal lobe constitutes the hippocampus or hippocampal formation, so named because on coronal sections it resembles a seahorse (Greek *hippos*, horse, *kampen*, sinuous) (Fig. 25-14). From the subiculum, the hippocampus curves medially, dorsally, and inward, ending in a thin semilunar gyrus, the dentate (from the Latin for notched) gyrus or fascia (from the Latin for band) dentata.

The hippocampus makes a bulge on the floor of the inferior horn of the lateral ventricle, and the shape of this bulge resembles a ram's horn, hence its name 'Cornu Ammonis' (from the Latin for horn of Ammon, a God of ancient Egypt depicted as a ram). The superior surface of the hippocampus is covered by a layer of white matter, the alveus (from the Latin for hull) (Fig. 25-14), composed of axons of the pyramidal cells of the hippocampus (see below) that gather into the fimbria (from the Latin for fringe), which in turn courses posteriorly, being the origin of the posterior pillar of the fornix (Latin: arch) (Fig. 25-14). The choroidal plexus inserts on the free edge of the fimbria and invaginates into the ventricle. When the hippocampal fissure is opened, the gyrus dentatus can be seen. Anteriorly, this gyrus begins as a smooth band across the uncus (Giacomini's band) and then, taking its notched appearance, it accompanies the fimbria toward the splenium of the corpus callosum. There they separate, the gyrus dentatus passing over the callosum as a thin gray layer, the indusium griseum (from the Latin for gray tunic), a vestigial convolution that contains tiny strands of myelinated fibers, the medial and lateral striae. Beneath the genu of the corpus callosum, the indusium and striae connect with the paraterminal (or subcallosal) gyrus (Fig. 25-6, area 25) and Broca's diagonal band (see first cranial nerve in Ch. 29). The stria terminalis is part of the central autonomic network (see also Ch. 34).

As noted above, besides isocortex, the human brain contains phylogenetically older cortices, the paleocortex and the still older archeocortex. Both are present in the temporal lobe, but to better grasp their significance, it is convenient here to understand their situation in terms of the concept of the limbic lobe.

As a whole, the old cortex constitutes a belt around the interhemispheric commissures and upper brainstem known as the limbic lobe (Latin: *limbus*, border) (Fig. 25-3). This includes the subcallosal gyrus, pyriform lobe, hippocampus, retrosplenial gyrus, and cingulate gyrus. Some authors include in addition the anterior part of the insula and the temporal pole. It

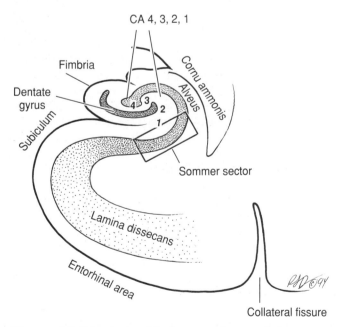

Figure 25-14. A simplified nomenclature of the microscopic features of the fifth temporal gyrus (see text). CA1, 2, 3, and 4 are fields individualized by Lorente de Nó with Golgi silver impregnation. Rose's fields, individualized with Nissl's stain, are not mentioned because they seem currently less in use. For Sommer's sector, see text.

can thus be seen that the temporal lobe is an essential part of the limbic lobe. A still more comprehensive concept is the limbic system, incorporating the subjacent nuclei, the septal nuclei (Fig. 25-6, area 25), and the amygdala and closely related regions such as the hypothalamus, medial forebrain bundle, and medial tegmental region of the midbrain (see below). The limbic system is believed to play a fundamental role in emotional, autonomic, and visceral activities, hence terms such as "visceral brain" or "circuit of emotions" can still be found in the literature.

Proceeding inward from the convexity, the first changes in the temporal cortex begin within the collateral fissure (Fig. 25-14) in the paleocortex of the entorhinal area, so named because it lies medial to the rhinal fissure (Greek: *ento*, inner). First there is a dropout of the fourth layer of the isocortex, which is replaced by a layer with rare cells, the lamina dissecans. Further simplification in the subiculum and hippocampus results in a cortex with three layers: polymorphic, pyramidal, and molecular. Similarly, the dentate gyrus has a three-layered cortex although without a pyramidal layer and with a prominent granular layer suggestive of a receptive function.

The thalamic connection of the temporal lobe is the projection of the medial geniculate body to the auditory primary area. It is a characteristic feature of the hippocampus and gyrus dentatus that, of all parts of the hemisphere, they do not receive direct projections from the thalamus.

Many transmitters have been located in the hippocampus: acetylcholine, norepinephrine with afferents from the locus ceruleus in the pons, leu- and met-enkephalin, among others. The terminals of the granule cells of the gyrus dentatus have a high concentration of zinc.

The arrangement of cells and fibers in the hippocampus is remarkable for its regularity, a feature reminiscent of the cerebellar cortex (Ch. 22). Pyramidal cells, among which are particularly arborized ones with biapical dendrites termed *double pyramidals,* receive afferents running transversely above and below them. Lorente de No (Spanish anatomist and physiologist, 1902–1990) characterized several hippocampal regions, chiefly by silver impregnation, termed CA1, 2, 3, and 4 (the end folium, in the hilus of the gyrus dentatus) (Fig. 25-14), CA standing for Cornu Ammonis.

In a much simplified view, the main afferents and efferents of this system are as follows. The entorhinal area receives information from the adjacent temporal multimodal cortex, from the so-called olfactory cortex, and from the septal area. Each pyramidal cell of the entorhinal area projects to a row of granule cells in the gyrus dentatus (via a complex bundle termed the *perforant path*). Each of the granule cells, in turn, projects to a row of pyramidal cells in CA3, whence projections are sent to CA1. Axons of CA3 and CA1 enter the alveus and fimbria, as already mentioned, and then the fornix. The latter is a quite large tract (it contains more fibers than the corticospinal tract or optic nerve), which links, mostly ipsilaterally, the hippocampus with the hypothalamus (mammillary bodies), the anterior and intralaminar nuclei of the thalamus, and the septal area. In addition, the fornix contributes rostrally to the medial forebrain bundle (to the basal forebrain) and caudally to the midbrain tegmentum.

Almost all pyramidal cells of CA3 are multimodal, viz., they respond to all sorts of combinations of sensory modalities. Moreover, they both display a capacity for habituation (i.e., they respond less and less to the same repeated stimulus) and have a strong capacity to be alerted by a new stimulus (novelty-conscious cells).

Finally, anatomy and physiology suggest that the hippocampus can be the final common path for signals that have been analyzed and integrated through the isocortex. Moreover, experimental and pathologic evidence shows that the arrival of these signals in the hippocampus marks their entry in the processes of memory (Ch. 21).

Most of the cells of the superior, lateral, and inferior surfaces of the temporal lobe belong to uni- or multimodal cortex. The former analyzes incoming signals from the primary olfactory and auditory areas. The latter further analyzes these signals and in addition makes an integrated synthesis of the elaborated information with cross-modality (somatosensory, visual, and linguistic) signals whose multimodal cortices lie either in the temporal lobe or in its confines.

No obvious clinical disorder results from destruction of the primary olfactory area (see first cranial nerve in Ch. 29) and yet this region still contains significant olfactory structures (see the section Temporal Epilepsy, below). Unilateral destruction of the primary auditory cortex does not cause deafness, although more subtle tests (dichotic listening, see eighth cranial nerve in Ch. 29) show that the ear contralateral to the damaged temporal lobe has defective discrimination. Destruction of both transverse gyri cause temporal (cortical) deafness (Chs. 18, 19, and eighth cranial nerve in Ch. 29).

Experimental data in the macaque monkey show that the multimodal cells are endowed with two chief characteristics. First, they are more and more stimulus-specific or, in other terms, more and more specialized (e.g., some have been claimed to respond preferentially to the arrival in the visual field of the animal's own hand). Face recognition has been especially well studied, showing cells specific for faces versus other objects and for various views of the face and head. Populations of cells rather than single cells seem involved in parallel processing, the so-called grandmother cells, which store face-specific engrams. These observations in animals have their human counterpart in the occurrence of prosopagnosia (Ch. 19).

The second chief characteristic of the multimodal cells is their ever more sophisticated capacity to integrate cross-modality stimuli. Electrical stimulation of the temporal cortex in humans (prior to surgery for epilepsy) has evoked full, vivid, recollections of fragments of the past in scenes in school, office, church, or family settings with the particular characters, sounds, music, weather, and mood of these experiences. Stereotactically implanted depth electrode recordings have, however, shown that such experiential responses are associated with seizure activity in the amygdala and hippocampus rather than in the temporal neocortex.

From similar evidence and from the distortions of perceptions that occur in temporal epilepsy (see below), it is currently thought that the temporal multimodal cortex is instrumental in such psychological achievements as perception of line orientation, edges, depth, distances, sizes, shapes, and hue saturation and the inner sense of time.

The main internal structures of the lobe are the amygdala, the inferior horn of the lateral ventricle, and part of the optic radiations. (For the various tracts that link the temporal lobe with other regions of the hemisphere, namely the uncinate fasciculus, arcuate fasciculus, cingulum, and superior longitudinal fasciculus, see the general discussion of lobar anatomy that precedes the descriptions of individual lobes.) The inferior fronto-occipital fasciculus connects the peri- and parastriate areas with the inferior and medial temporal lobe. In fact, this tract appear to consist of a series of contiguous short bundles, and its role is not settled.

The many afferents of the uncus, which is located near the temporal pole, are from unimodal and multimodal cortex (e.g., temporal isocortex, frontal association areas, and the limbic system). The uncus also has reciprocal connections with the dorsomedial thalamus, the reticular formation, and the locus ceruleus. The main efferent path is the ventral amygdalofugal projection to the hypothalamus; the amygdala has few if any olfactory functions. Its stimulation in humans causes fear, rage, aggressive behavior, and emotional reactions with a strong autonomic component. Some stimulations cause adversive turning of eyes and head, with movements of licking, chewing, and swallowing (see Temporal Epilepsy, below). Bilateral ablations cause a dramatic change in behavior, with normally aggressive animals becoming placid and tame. Lesions affecting the uncus and adjacent medial and inferior temporal regions in animals and humans may precipitate the Klüver-Bucy syndrome (named for the American neuroscientist and neurosurgeon H. Klüver and P. Bucy), featuring docility; loss of fear of dangerous objects (e.g., snakes or sharp instruments), propensity to carry all objects to the mouth and hypersexuality.

Last but not least, the tail of the caudate nucleus terminates on the central nucleus of the amygdala, a probably significant relationship but one for which no firm data are available. The amygdala and hippocampus have been implicated in a variety of autonomic, visceral, and endocrine functions. There is also evidence in animals that they could play a role in immunologic processes.

The lower part of the optic radiation, after leaving the lateral geniculate body, sweeps around the tip of the horn of the lateral ventricle (see Ch. 26). Hence the typical field defect is a contralateral superior quadrantanopia. However, there is such variation in the forward looping of the radiations that the defect also shows many variations, among which it can be congruous or incongruous and can extend into the inferior quadrant although remaining denser in the superior quadrant. In rare cases hemianopia is possible, in contradistinction to the classical rules of topical diagnosis.

The temporal lobe is also linked with the contralateral hemisphere through the corpus callosum (see Corpus Callosum, below) and the anterior commissure, which connects the anterior and lateral parts of both lobes.

Arteries

There are three distinct arterial territories. The middle cerebral artery supplies the superior and lateral surfaces. Its branches arise from the lower division (assuming that the stem of the artery divides into two main divisions), but often a branch for the temporal pole has arisen before the bifurcation, with the remainder of the superior and lateral surfaces supplied by the middle and posterior temporal branches. These two latter vessels drape over the lobe, coursing posteroinferiorly. Their distal segments anastomose end to end with branches of the posterior cerebral artery in a border zone or watershed area, which courses along the inferolateral margin of the hemisphere.

The posterior cerebral artery supplies the third and fourth temporal gyri and the adjacent parahippocampal gyrus. The anterior choroidal artery supplies the anterior two-thirds of the hippocampus, the amygdala, and the medial part of the parahippocampal gyrus. Isolated infarction of the hippocampus is probably very rare.

Veins

On the lateral surface of the lobe, superficial veins drain into the middle cerebral vein or into the lateral sinus. The inferior anastomotic vein of Labbé (L. Labbé, French surgeon, 1870–1939) courses caudally and inferiorly from the great anastomotic vein of Trolard (P. Trolard, French anatomist, 1842–1910) to the lateral sinus (Fig. 35-23). Labbé's vein was the classical most posterior limit for left temporal lobectomies (a boundary not exceeded for fear of causing language disorders), although its variable location and course calls for more sophisticated criteria (e.g., cortical stimulations) to achieve this goal. Veins of the inferior surface, including hippocampal veins, drain into Rosenthal's basal vein (F. C. Rosenthal, German anatomist, 1780–1829). As some veins of the middle ear drain into meningeal veins and the superior petrosal sinus, thrombophlebitis of these veins can play a role in the pathogenesis of temporal lobe abscesses due to otitis media. The veins of the temporal pole drain into the sphenoparietal sinus, and tearing of these veins as they cross the subdural space is likely to account in part for the high frequency of lesions of the pole in brain concussion (see below and Ch. 6).

Dysfunctions, Displacements, Diseases

Language disorders such as word deafness and Wernicke aphasia are described in Chapter 16 and memory disorders in Chapter 21.

Temporal Lobe Epilepsy

Some of the clinical disorders described below (also discussed in Ch. 79) can originate in any limbic structure and even in cortical areas projecting to the limbic system. However, they usually originate in the mesial part of one temporal lobe, and with others that originate on the convexity of the temporal neocortex, they are conveniently considered here under the traditional (if disputable) term of temporal lobe epilepsy (TLE), also currently known as partial complex epilepsy.

TLE is a major issue for clinicians for several reasons. It is one of the most frequent complex partial epilepsies (for a definition see Ch. 79) in neurologic practice. It has the richest symptomatology of all focal epilepsies, owing to the complex anatomy and physiology of the temporal lobe (see above). Since the early studies of Hughlings Jackson TLE has fascinated neurologists for the insight it provides into brain functions. Many cases can be well controlled by medical therapy, but a good number require surgery.

The symptoms of temporal seizures result from paroxysmal discharges in the primary or secondary olfactory or auditory cortices or in the secondary visual cortices. Consequently the spectrum of the epileptic phenomena varies from simple sensation-like events (e.g., a noise) to distortions of perception (e.g., changes in size, distance, shape, and depth of the visual field) and even to experiential recollections with cross-modal activations (e.g., scenery with characters, music and landscape). Such experiential fits, however, imply the participation of the limbic part of the lobe, which can, in addition, cause behavioral disorders with emotion-like and motivation-like components (see below). Dysmnestic disorders and disorientation in time are frequent. Consciousness is almost always disturbed.

During the fit, the gaze is vacant or the patient is absorbed by an epileptic activity (automatisms, see below). No contact with those around can be established. A period of amnesia covers the fit. Some of these partial seizures proceed to a generalized fit. Some TLE episodes only cause a temporary loss of contact with the surroundings. This is termed "temporal absence" or "temporal pseudo-absence" (to keep the word "absence" for petit mal [see Ch. 79]).

The many kinds of mesial TLE can only be outlined here. The most frequent olfactory seizure is the uncinate fit (named after the uncus), in which the patient is seized by a hallucination of smell and often of taste, usually of an unpleasant character. Auditory seizures are complex resurgences of fragments of melodies or songs or even words, sentences, bits of conservations when the seizure is left-sided. Vertiginous (vestibular) seizures are distinctly rare. Visual fits are elaborate hallucinations of persons or animals, often in a scene that brings back the ambience of this particular event. During such fits consciousness is disturbed ("dreamy state" is Hughlings Jackson's oft quoted expression). Some patients have special feelings of déjà vu (French: already seen), or jamais vu (French: never seen), which perhaps result from a mismatching of the abnormal neural activation with the templates of memory. Some fits called gelastic epilepsy (Greek: gelas, joy) begin by an outburst of laughing, while in others called procursive epilepsy, the patient runs forward.

Fits of fear or rage obviously imply the participation of the limbic lobe. An epigastric rising sensation at the beginning of a seizure is also characteristic. Disordered sexual drive is frequent. There are movements of the lips, tongue, and jaw as in chewing and tasting. Frequently also the patient displays a simple activity such as chafing the hands or buttoning a coat, searching in a pocket, or looking around on the floor or under a table, as if searching for something. Epileptic fugues are rare, and during them violence and assault are rare. They can result from TLE or from postictal confusion in generalized epilepsy. They can, of course, raise difficult medicolegal issues.

TLE is seen mostly in young people. The history of birth and early years must be elicited as precisely as possible (see below), seeking especially evidence of a long, difficult labor, circumstances that suggest anoxia, such as delay before the first breath and cry, febrile convulsions during infancy, and delayed motor "milestones." Other points in the life history include trauma, meningitis or encephalitis, or brain abscess. Arteriovenous malformations are also possible. Tumors are rare. In older patients, tumors, stroke, and trauma are the usual causes.

The evaluation of a patient with TLE begins with surface electroencephalography (EEG) and brain imaging. Whenever possible, MRI should be performed since it provides the best brain imaging, showing the fine anatomy and to a certain extent the pathology of the temporal lobe. In severe cases, which prove medically intractable, further investigations in specialized centers are warranted. These include long-duration wake and sleep EEG with video recordings, telemetry, EEG with stereotactically implanted depth electrodes (Ch. 11), SPECT (Ch. 15), PET (Ch. 14), all of which are studies aimed at localizing and identifying the core focus of the initial epileptic discharge. Such procedures are performed when surgery is considered a possible and valuable therapeutic alternative.

The complex pathology of TLE can be outlined as follows. First, the most common abnormality lies in the temporal lobe but is not specific for TLE since it can be found in nontemporal epileptics who have had frequent convulsions. This abnormality is a loss of neurons with consequent gliosis, so-called hippocampal sclerosis. The lesion predominates in Sommer sector (Wilhelm Sommer, German physician, 1852–1900), which corresponds to CA1 (Fig. 25-14). CA3 and CA4 (the end folium) also are vulnerable, while for unknown reasons, CA2 is more resistant. Lesions frequently extend into the amygdala, uncus, and parahippocampal gyrus. There is also loss of cells in the dentate gyrus. Such lesions result from ischemia-anoxia, and pathogenetic hypotheses have been proposed.

A tentorial herniation through the incisura of the tentorium cerebelli (see the section Tentorial Herniation, below) could happen at birth during labor, compressing the anterior choroidal artery and the posterior cerebral artery (hence the term incisural sclerosis sometimes used for hippocampal sclerosis). Alternatively, febrile convulsions in early life could cause anoxic damage to the especially vulnerable hippocampal cells (febrile convulsions indeed are found in a fair number of TLEs). In both situations, the early lesion would "ripen" to become epileptogenic in childhood,

adolescence, or adulthood. As can be seen, the significance of hippocampal sclerosis is ambiguous; whether it can be a cause or a consequence of TLE or both is not settled.

Second, in some cases, with or without hippocampal sclerosis, a focal lesion is found in the temporal lobe. It can be an extrinsic lesion, such as a scar of trauma, abscess, infarction, or hamartoma (e.g., cavernous angioma) or a tumor (generally low-grade glioma in the young). Alternatively, it can be an intrinsic lesion, consisting of islets of abnormal neurons and glial cells. This latter type of lesion is difficult to diagnose, and it is not easy to draw a firm line between normal and abnormal.

Third, in about 20 percent of cases, no pathology is found. It should also be kept in mind that a genetic factor is possible in TLE, a family history of epilepsy is found in 40 percent of patients with hippocampal sclerosis.

For medical treatment of TLE, many neurologists use carbamazepine as the first-choice drug (see Ch. 79). In medically intractable cases and those in which there is a well circumscribed unilateral temporal epileptic focus, either at the convexity or more frequently in the mesial temporal lobe, total or partial lobectomy can be considered.

Temporal Herniation

The skull is compartmentalized by thick sheaths of dura mater (Fig. 25-15). On the midline the sagittal falx cerebri separates the two hemispheres, from the calvarium to the superior surface of the corpus callosum. Posteriorly, the tentorium cerebelli inserts on the petrous ridges and along the lateral sinuses to separate the middle from the posterior fossa. A large semiovale vent, the tentorial notch or incisura, allows the midbrain to pass from one fossa to the other. With the midbrain is the top of the basilar artery, which divides into the diverging posterior cerebral arteries, each of which crosses the edge of the notch to gain access to the medial temporal and occipital lobes. The anterior choroidal artery courses backward between the midbrain and the temporal lobe. Between the origins of the posterior cerebral and superior cerebellar arteries, the oculomotor nerve emerges near the midline, coursing anteriorly and superiorly to the cavernous sinus. En route, the nerve crosses the superior surface of the petroclinoidal ligament, just medial to the uncus.

As stated above, the medial part of the temporal lobe hangs just atop the free edge of the incisura, even to the point that, in the normal subject, usually 3 to 4 mm of the uncus bulges into the notch.

The living brain is a semiliquid jelly (77 percent water), so that when there is a temporal or lateralized

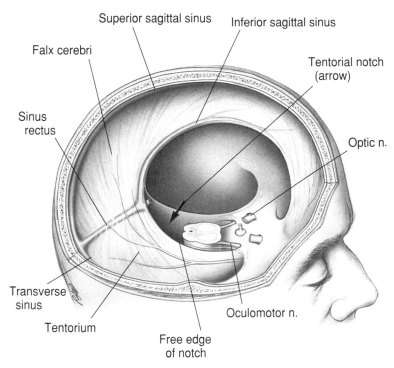

Falx cerebri

Superior sagittal sinus   Inferior sagittal sinus

Tentorial notch
(arrow)

Sinus
rectus

Optic n.

Transverse
sinus

Tentorium

Oculomotor n.

Free edge
of notch

Figure 25-15. The compartmentalization of the skull by dural sheaths. The arrow is in the tentorial notch or incisura.

lesion anywhere in the hemisphere causing supratentorial increased pressure, that pressure pushes down the medial temporal lobe into the slit between the edge of the notch and the midbrain (Fig. 25-16 (2) and Ch. 19). This is traditionally termed *uncal herniation,* although adjacent parts of the parahippocampal gyrus also can herniate and the subthalamic structures often are displaced as well. Several consequences ensue, knowledge of which is vital in clinical neurology. First, the evidence or even the suspicion of temporal herniation precludes lumbar puncture, which can raise the gradient of pressure across the notch, thereby causing more herniation and even death. Second, some of the causes of temporal herniation are amenable to treatment (see below), provided that irreversible brainstem lesions have not occurred.

In progressive, unchecked cases, the herniated tissue first compresses the oculomotor nerve against the petroclinoidal ligament or over the clivus. The outer, parasympathetic, fibers suffer first, resulting in a fixed mydriasis, called Hutchinson's pupil (see also Ch. 27). As a rule, this unilateral mydriasis is ipsilateral to the herniation. With more damage, ptosis and opthalmoplegia can occur.

Second, the herniated tissue can laterally push the midbrain against the opposite edge of the notch, and

the push can be so strong that at postmortem it is common to see a quite macroscopic indentation on the contralateral midbrain (Kernohan's notch (J. W. Kernohan, Irish-American pathologist 1896–1981). The clinical consequence of this lesion, contralateral to the primary hemispheric lesion, is a Babinski sign ipsilateral to the herniation.

Third, decreased alertness, drowsiness, stupor, and coma can appear, often in quick succession, due to dysfunction or lesions of the reticular formation. Also, diencephalic herniation due to rostrocaudal pressure can be associated, causing a caudal displacement of the brainstem.

Fourth, compression of the posterior cerebral artery as it crosses the edge of the notch can cause ischemia or infarction of the posterior hippocampus, optic radiations, and calcarine region. Visual field defects are hardly detectable in stuporous patients, but survivors can display hemi- or quadrantanopia. In large herniations, the flow in the anterior choroidal artery can be compromised, with resultant lesions of the anterior hippocampus (see Ch. 35, Fig. 35-17).

Fifth, while the brainstem can, to a certain extent, shun pressure, the basilar artery is anchored to the circle of Willis. Displacements of the brainstem and probably fluctuations in these displacements, with

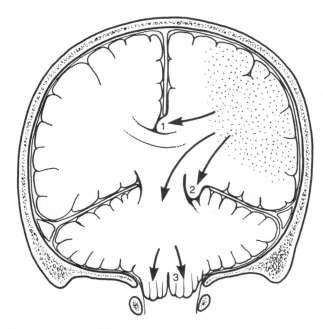

Figure 25-16. The main kinds of herniations. (1) Subfalcial: the cingulate gyrus is pushed across under the falx. The symptomatology is unknown. (2) Temporal-tentorial (see text). (3) Cerebellar-foramen magnum. The tonsils and paraflocculus are pushed down across the foramen, compressing the medulla oblongata and high cord and causing hydrocephalus, unilaterally or bilaterally, as shown here. Cerebellar-foramen herniation causes pain in the neck, stiff neck, head tilt, and paresthesias over the shoulders. Tonic extensor spasms are the classical sign (also termed "cerebellar fits"). Death by respiratory arrest can occur at any moment. (From Zülch, 1969, with permission.)

fixed penetrating arteries, account for hemorrhages in the tegmentum and hypothalamus known as Duret's hemorrhages. (H. Duret, French neurologist and surgeon, 1849–1921). Such lesions also account for stupor and coma, Cheyne-Stokes respiration and neurogenic hyperventilation, and disorders of oculocephalic and labyrinthine reflexes.

Finally, the lateral displacement and the hemorrhagic lesions of the brainstem occlude the aqueduct of sylvius, causing hydrocephalus (see Ch. 59), which can play a role in the disorders of consciousness and causes bradycardia and high blood pressure. Death is usually due to apnea, sometimes after apneustic breathing (see Ch. 17).

Temporal herniation obviously is a nonspecific syndrome. It can result from any supratentorial, lateralized, space-occupying lesion. By space-occupying lesion is meant not only the primary lesion (usually an expanding one) but, in addition, the surrounding edema and the consequences of the loss of autoregulation of the cerebral arteries and the blockage of cerebrospinal fluid (CSF) circulation.

The common causes are large infarctions or hemorrhages in the territory of the internal carotid artery, for which there is currently not much treatment, but also treatable lesions, namely, epidural (extradural) hematomas and cerebral abscesses. In such cases, temporal herniation usually occurs quickly—within minutes, hours, or a few days after the onset of the causal affection. In subdural hematomas the supratentorial pressure increases more slowly, so that temporal herniation can occur weeks or months after the causal cranial trauma. However, once the first symptom has appeared (mydriasis, drowsiness) the evolution to disaster can be quite rapid, so that emergency therapeutic measures are mandatory.

Infections

The medial temporal lobe is the predominant site for the most frequent of all virus encephalitides, namely that due to *herpes simplex* (see Ch. 48). The lesions are frequently bilateral, often beginning in the entorhinal region, but occasionally are somewhat more lateral. The suddenness of onset may mimic infarction, and instances of severe isolated residual amnestic disorders could suggest a misdiagnosis of Wernicke-Korsakoff encephalopathy. The hemorrhagic lesions are well appreciated on CT scan on a coronal view, although MRI offers better images without resorting to special angles.

Temporal lobe abscess (see also Ch. 39) was the feared complication of otitis media and mastoiditis in the days before antibiotic therapy. It could also complicate sphenoid infection. The spread of infection could be direct, through bone and dura, or could be due to thrombophlebitis (see above). The onset of focal clinical disorders is usually rapid; these may include amnestic dysnomia or Wernicke aphasia on the left side, epilepsy, and sometimes a contralateral upper quadrantanopia and lower face paresis in a patient with fever and headache. Abscesses resulting from otitis media are generally due to enteric organisms.

Tumors

Brain tumors are discussed in detail in Chapter 51 to 58. Primary and secondary tumors of course grow in the temporal lobe. Their focal symptoms are more or less quickly progressive according to their degree of malignancy. They are similar to those of any focal space-occupying lesion in the temporal structures (see above, abscess). Temporal lobe gliomas cause seizures, although in many patients these are antedated by changes in personality, mood, and behavior. Meningiomas of the sphenoidal ridge, one of the preferential sites of intracranial meningiomas, can cause uncinate fits (see below) and infiltrate the temporal bone.

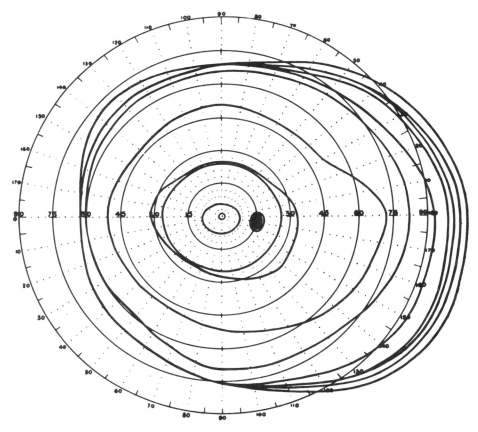

Figure 25-17. A rendering of the visual field plotted as a flat display. (From Traquair, 1949, with permission.)

Radiation therapy focused on the pituitary can cause delayed expanding lesions in the temporal lobe, often difficult to distinguish from malignancies.

Arachnoid Cysts

These uncommon lesions are often found fortuitously on a CT or MRI done for another reason. Rarely, they cause focal disorders or increased intracranial pressure. One of their preferential sites is in front of the temporal pole and very large ones can enlarge the middle fossa and elevate the lesser wing of the sphenoid. Most are asymptomatic and require no treatment. For symptomatic ones a neurosurgical opinion should be sought. The treatment of these otherwise benign lesions is difficult.

Trauma

Trauma is discussed in detail in Chapter 6. The temporal poles are at special risk in blunt trauma with concussion, owing to the configuration of the middle fossa and the course of the polar veins (see above). CT scan is not the best tool to show lacerations and contusions of the poles because the dense signal caused by the underlying bone obscures the brain im-

ages. MRI, being relatively insensitive to bone signal and exquisitely sensitive to blood signal, accurately displays the hemorrhagic lesions.

Immediate and often lasting disturbances in memory, mood, and sometimes behavior are common and likely to result from damage to the entorhinal-amygdala-hippocampus system. After a delay, epilepsy can appear. Later, the diagnostic problems are compounded by those of litigation and compensation (see postconcussion syndrome, Ch. 6).

Stab, bullet, shrapnel, or gunshot wounds are, of course, commonplace in war but by no means rare in civilian practice. A modern cause of casualty is the discharge of nails by air-powered drivers. In all cases, in addition to temporal lobe damage there may be damage to the cavernous sinus and internal carotid artery or even to the basilar artery. These vascular lesions in some cases may not produce catastrophic bleeding as long as the object remains in place. Under no circumstances should it be touched or pulled back on the spot. Craniotomy is needed to assess the situation, remove the object, ensure the arrest of whatever hemorrhage can be found, and obtain a watertight dural seal.

Stroke

Stroke is discussed in detail in Chapters 35 and 36. Occlusion of the lower division of the middle cerebral artery is ordinarily due to small emboli from the heart. The relatively straight course from the stem of the artery to its posterior temporal branch guides most emboli to the superior temporal plane, leading to Wernicke aphasia on the dominant side with or without contralateral homonymous hemianopia. Occlusion of the anterior and middle cerebral branches is far less common, and no specific syndrome of these arteries has yet been individualized. Infarction of these territories in the nondominant hemisphere can cause confusion and agitation.

Occlusion of the posterior cerebral artery usually causes contralateral homonymous hemianopia through infarction of the sides of the calcarine fissure or, where the infarct predominates on the lower optic radiations, causes contralateral superior quadrantanopia. The clinical consequences of damage to the inferior temporal cortex are mainly visual; agnosic disorders, and color dysnomia have been described from infarcts affecting the lingual gyri (see the section Occipital Lobe, below). In left-sided infarcts, a degree of anomia is a usual sequel. Infarction of the posterior hippocampus produces a severe amnestic state when bilateral or even when unilateral and left-sided in right-handed individuals (see Ch. 21).

The effects of occlusion of the anterior choroidal artery are often mitigated by the collateral supply of neighboring arteries, but in some cases the anterior hippocampus can be destroyed with severe amnesia. There is also a dense hemiplegia caused by destruction of the corticospinal tract in the lower internal capsule. In the dominant hemisphere the infarct may also affect the thalamus, in some instances causing a syndrome of aphasia. This syndrome can sometimes improve remarkably (see Ch. 18).

Hemorrhage in the temporal lobe is frequent. In the dominant temporal lobe hemorrhage can cause sudden Wernicke aphasia, which can sometimes remarkably improve (see also Ch. 18). With a large hematoma a hemiparesis, at least affecting the lower face, may occur.

Thrombosis of the Lateral Sinus

The rare thrombosis of the lateral sinus presents with the same features as infarction or hemorrhage although its onset can be progressive and the lesions more lateral. The hemorrhagic infarct, once known as a "red" infarct because of its grossly hemorrhagic appearance on gross anatomic specimens, is characteristic of venous infarction (see Chs. 5 and 35) is easily picked up by CT or MRI, which in addition shows the thrombosis of the sinus. Delays in diagnosis may result in greatly enlarged volume of infarcted tissue. The differential diagnosis is with a hematoma that would contraindicate anticoagulants, whereas anticoagulation should be indicated as early as possible in venous infarction (see also Chs. 5 and 35).

Dementias

In Alzheimer's disease (see Ch. 60), a progressive deficit of memory is usually the first clinical disorder to appear, at least the first to be noticed by the family. At about the same time, examination discloses anomia (i.e., lack of words in naming tests) (see Ch. 18) and disorientation in time, generally more severe than disorientation in space. Characteristic Alzheimer lesions (neuritic plaques, neurofibrillary changes, granulovacuolar degenerations) typically predominate in the hippocampus, particularly in the CA1 zone, entorhinal cortex, and subiculum (Figs. 25-13 and 25-14). A severe atrophy of the hippocampus can be shown by MRI.

In Pick's disease (lobar atrophy (see Ch. 61), the brunt of the lesions bear upon the insula, amygdala, and hippocampus. The temporal lobe as a whole is often involved, although characteristically and for unknown reasons, the first temporal gyrus is strikingly spared. In some patients symptoms and signs that are likely of temporal origin including anomia and jargon, can be prominent, but the most frequent language disorder is a reduction of language that is more probably of frontal origin. Alterations in sexual behavior are frequent.

In primary progressive aphasia lesions, due to Pick's or Alzheimer's disease, spongiform changes, or Creutzfeldt-Jakob disease (see Ch. 50) are found around the left lateral fissure in the inferior frontal gyrus and the temporal cortex.

Schizophrenia

Decreased volume of the hippocampus and amygdala is prominent among the pathologic changes found in schizophrenia. It can be demonstrated by MRI. Other temporal pathologic changes include lesions in the superior temporal gyrus, related to auditory hallucinations; reduced cell counts; heterotopias; and disruptions of cortical layers, which would be more frequent on the left side in association with schizophrenialike psychoses. After either left or right temporal lobectomy (for temporal epilepsy, see above), schizophrenialike psychosis can occur.

OCCIPITAL LOBE
Anatomy and Physiology

The smallest of the cerebral lobes, the occipital lobe, makes up about one-eighth of the cerebral volume and is the posterior pole of the cerebral hemisphere.

It is devoted to receiving and processing visual information. Barely visible on the lateral surface of the hemisphere, it is bounded superomedially by the short parieto-occipital fissure and inferiorly by the small preoccipital notch. In between, there are no gross anatomic distinctions separating the occipital from the temporal and parietal lobes (Fig. 25-1).

On the lateral cerebral convexity the lobe is sometimes divided by the lateral occipital sulcus (Fig. 25-1) and sometimes by two small anteroposterior sulci, so that superior, middle, and inferior occipital gyri can be described. However, the complexity of the gyri in the occipital convexity makes this the least well described and classified part of the whole human brain.

On the medial surface there is less variation. Anteriorly, the lobe is limited by the deep and long parieto-occipital fissure, which together with the calcarine fissure below, forms the boundaries of the *cuneus* (from the Latin for wedge). The calcarine fissure, very deep and about 5 cm long, makes a bulge into the occipital horn of the lateral ventricle. Because of its shape, this bulge is known as the *calcar avis* (from the Latin for bird claw), hence the name of the fissure. Below the calcarine fissure, the lingual gyrus belongs partly to the inferior surface of the lobe, which lies atop the tentorium cerebelli. It extends anteriorly to the rear part of the collateral fissure (see section Temporal Lobe, above). Beyond the collateral fissure, the posterior part of the fusiform gyrus is in the occipital lobe while its anterior part is in the temporal lobe (occipitotemporal gyrus).

The medial surfaces of the two occipital lobes are separated by the falx cerebri, which, behind the splenium of the corpus callosum, inserts on the ridge of the tentorium cerebelli along the sinus rectus, which drains blood to the confluens sinuum. In the substance of the occipital lobe the occipital horn of the lateral ventricle extends backward adjacent to the calcar avis. As can be seen on many CT and MRI scans, there is often considerable asymmetry in the size of the occipital horns, the larger usually being the left.

Histology

The banks of the calcarine fissure and a small part of the cuneus and lingual gyrus form the primary visual area (Fig. 25-6, area 17), a thin zone of small sensory receptor cells (koniocortex), remarkable by the high number of granule cells and by the greatly thickened external band or stripe of Baillarger that can be seen with the naked eye, hence the name of area striata for area 17. The band is also named for Francisco Gennari (1750–97), an Italian medical student when the band was described.

The termination of the optic radiations on the calcarine cortex (i.e., the geniculocalcarine tract) is considered in more detail in Chapter 26 (see Fig. 26-8). The large macular projection extends 1 to 2 cm over the posterolateral surface of the lobe. The rostral part of the calcarine cortex extends forward almost to the level of the splenium and is concerned with peripheral vision. The horizontal meridian of the visual field nearly coincides with the plane of the calcarine fissure.

Around area 17 are areas 18 (parastriate) and 19 (peristriate) (Fig. 26-5), unimodal areas that merge anteriorly and inferiorly with multimodal cortices in the parietal (areas 39, 40 and temporal areas 23, 36) lobes (Fig. 25-6). This is a simplified account of the visual cortex, convenient for clinical purposes. Physiologic studies have unraveled a much more complex organization, (e.g., several subfields have been individualized in area 17).

Pathways

There are at least two important thalamooccipital projections: (1) the optic radiations from the lateral geniculate body to area 17 and (2) reciprocal connections from the pulvinar to areas 18 and 19 and the inferior parietal lobule (see section Parietal Lobe and Fig. 25-7). In addition, the pulvinar receives from and projects to the superior colliculus, and there is a topographic representation of the contralateral hemifield in the pulvinar.

The great transverse bundles forming the corpus callosum are separable into several groups (Fig. 25-8). The *forceps major* links the cuneus, calcarine cortex, and parietal gyri on the convex surface, including the angular and anterior parietal gyri. Its fibers pass through the dorsal portion of the splenium of the corpus callosum, forming a bulge in the superomesial wall of the occipital horn of the lateral ventricle. Such fibers, which cross the splenium in the midline, link areas 18 and 19 on both sides. Just below the forceps major is the *calcar avis*. These two structures in the mesial ventricular wall show the close relationship between transcallosal fibers and the primary visual cortex. The *forceps minor* is a fiber band of the callosum, which passes below the calcar avis, linking the lingual and second and third occipital gyri. The lateral wall and floor of the occipital horn are made by the *tapetum* (from the Latin for rug), the fiber system connecting the temporal lobes, which passes through the body of the splenium of the corpus callosum. On the outer side of the tapetum and the lateral side of the horn, fibers from the occipital lobe to the superior colliculus and lateral geniculate body make up the *internal sagittal stratum*. On the outside edge of these pathways are the optic radiations, sometimes termed the *external sagittal stratum*.

Two major fiber systems run in an anteroposterior

direction (Fig. 25-8). The *occipitofrontal fasciculus* of Onufrowicz links the occipital and the frontal lobes, leaving *au passage* collaterals to the parietal lobe (see the section Parietal Lobe, above). A role in visual guidance of movement has been assumed for this tract. The *inferior longitudinal fasciculus* seems to spread anteroinferiorly, lateral to the optic radiations. It has been considered as linking the occipital and inferior temporal regions and possibly having a role in reading comprehension. However, recent data have shown it to be actually a series of subcortical U fibers rather than a bundle, casting doubt on its role in language function.

Some Physiologic Aspects

For diagnostic purposes, clinicians use gross symptoms and signs that result from lesions of the visual areas or optic radiations, namely the anopias (see Ch. 26) and the visual agnosias (see Ch. 19). Recent years have witnessed impressive advances in the physiology of the visual cortices. These must be known by clinicians and can well provide the basis of novel investigations in patients.

These advances have resulted from various sectors of research: single-cell recordings from the occipital cortex; histologic techniques using horseradish peroxidase transport (which maps the origin of fibers) or cytochrome oxidase (which stains particular fiber features as "blobs"; and autoradiographic techniques using ^{14}C-2-deoxyglucose uptake, which reflects cellular and synaptic activation following specific stimuli. Only a simplified and brief account of these physiologic data can be given here.

Several Visual Systems

It has been recognized that the population of ganglion cells in the retina (see Ch. 26) includes two kinds of cells, each of which triggers a specific chain of physiologic events extending down to the occipital cortex.

The vast majority of ganglion cells are small (formerly called midget cells), hence their name P cells (Latin: *parvus*, small). They are responsible for macular vision. In the lateral geniculate body, their axons synapse in the parvocellular portion (layers 3, 4, 5, and 6). After passing through the visual radiations, fibers from these cells terminate in the occipital cortex in subarea 4Cβ of area 17 (it is mentioned above that are 17 has been divided into subfields). From there they project into area 18 and farther into the multimodal cortices. This P system subserves color opponency, low contrast sensitivity, and high spatial resolution.

The other type of cell population contains the M cells (Latin: *magnus*, large), whose axons synapse in the magnocellular part of the lateral geniculate body (layers 1 and 2). These large geniculate neurons project onto the 4Cα subarea of area 17, whence another set of neurons projects onto the midtemporal cortex. These M cells subserve high contrast sensitivity, low spatial resolution, fast temporal resolution, and stereopsis; they are color-ignorant.

A third system, termed the blob system, probably receives from P and M cells. It may analyze colors and process brightness data.

During early maturation in the human, synaptogenesis is rapid between the second and fourth month after birth, stabilizing some time between 8 months and 11 years. Thereafter the synaptic number seem to remain stable until old age. In animals, the intact corpus callosum mediates the development of binocular responses and degree of visual acuity, which suggests that some features of the visual system are dynamically acquired, while others are preprogrammed.

Visual Field Representation

In the striate cortex, the vertical meridian seems neither over-represented nor duplicated. The magnification factor from the retina seems to be similar across species, reaching a maximum of 15 mm per degree of visual angle in the fovea, the angle spreading out broadly with increasing distance from the foveal region along the striate cortex. This confirms the different sizes and shapes of human visual fields as a function of differences in target size. Targets as small as about 1 mm can be detected by normal subjects only within the small macular area; targets 1 cm in size may be detected at several degrees of angle from the midline; and those as large as a moving pillow can be detected everywhere. The normal visual fields can be plotted as if displayed on a flat surface (Fig. 25-17) or they can be plotted like a geodesic survey map, forming a "hill" of steadily steepening sides to reach a shallow plateau atop which is a narrow pinnacle (Fig. 25-18).

Stimulus Specificity of the Visual Cortex

From retina to occipital cortex, each cell has a receptive field (i.e., the region of the visual field over which the firing of the cell can be influenced). Retinal ganglion cells and lateral geniculate body cells have circular receptive fields with either *on* or *off* centers and opposite surrounds. They fire best when a small circular spot of light is flashed on or put out in the right (adequate) place (i.e., the receptive field of one eye). Some processing of the retinal input takes place in the lateral geniculate body, whose cells, for instance, are more sensitive to differences in retinal illumination than to the illumination itself, but few if any geniculate cells are binocularly influenced.

The striate cortex has few cells with circular recep-

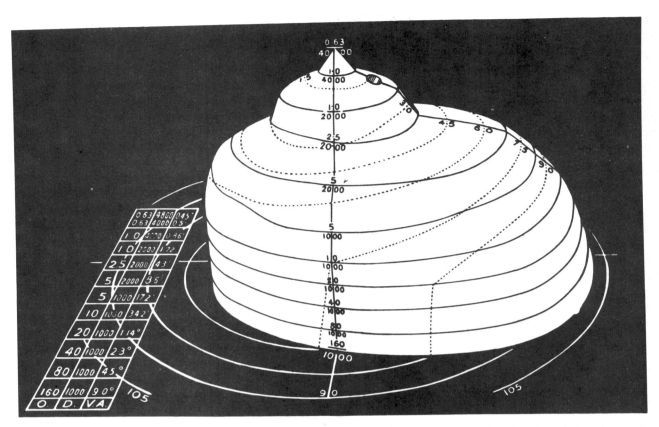

Figure 25-18. The "hill of vision" plotted as if it were a geodesic survey map showing the relative size of the fields as a function of target size. As the smaller targets have smaller fields and require more visual discrimination, they are shown higher on the hill. (From Traquair, 1949, with permission).

tive fields. The most effective stimuli are long, narrow rectangles of light terms *slits,* dark bar presented against a bright background, or straight line borders separating areas of different brightness termed *edges.* Moreover, cells fire only or maximally when such stimuli are presented with a specific orientation. All cells that respond to a given orientation are arranged in columns perpendicular to the surface and extending the whole cortical width. There are cells, termed *simple,* that respond only to one specific oriented stimulus (e.g., a slit), with still evidence of *on* and *off* cells. Orientation columns are narrow slabs arranged in such a fashion that a microelectrode penetrating the cortex tangentially records clockwise or counterclockwise changes in axis orientation corresponding to rotations through 180 degrees.

Besides the so-called simple cells, there are *complex* cells, which are receptive to the same stimuli but keep firing while the stimulus is moved across the retina provided that the axis of orientation remains adequate. Such cells often show opposite responses to movements in the opposite direction. Complex cells would receive inputs from several simple cells. Fur-

thermore, there are *hypercomplex* cells, which have the capacities of several complex ones and have particular connections with the lateral geniculate body. In summary, the vertical columnar organization of the striate cortex subserves the perception of retinal position, line orientation, ocular dominance (see below), and probably direction of movement. The plan for integrative function of the striate cortex itself has a feature in addition to those of single cell detectors: horizontally oriented connections found between cellular columns may permit the striate system to survey larger fields of vision than are detected by a given field of a single cell.

The farther from the striate cortex, the more specific the form of the stimulus required to activate cells. With increasing distance, the simple cells (those responding to stimuli having a simple feature such as width or straight edge) give way to complex and even hypercomplex cells, some of which respond to visual stimuli so specific as to encourage the view that some single cells might be activated only by a unique shape (e.g., that of a subject's hand).

A cortical patterning according to *ocular dominance*

is another characteristic of the visual cortex. In area 17, the bulk of the inputs from the lateral geniculate body is distributed to separate, parallel slabe perpendicular to the surface and extending the whole cortical width. These ocular dominance columns are alternately more sensitive to events from the left and the right retina. As with orientation columns, a set of ocular dominance columns corresponds to a field of 180-degree of rotational axes.

Corticofugal Projections

Apart from retinal projections via the lateral geniculate body to the striate cortex, retinal projections also find their way to the superior colliculus, where they appear to mediate detection of movement but not shape or size. This "second system" for vision has been thought to be the means by which moving stimuli are detected in the large, low-acuity portions of the visual fields outside the high-acuity foveal region. Once the stimuli are detected, the foveal discrimination system can be directed to the site of interest.

This view of visual function has extremely important functional significance in the many and far-flung anatomic linkages from the striate areas to the frontal, temporal, parietal, and even brainstem and cerebellar regions of the brain.

The clinical implications of this high degree of specificity suggests that patients could show extremely circumscribed functional disturbances if clinicians were able to set the stage for proper testing.

Arteries

The bulk of the occipital lobe is supplied by the posterior cerebral artery. The trunk of the artery gains the brain by passing over the free edge of the tentorium cerebelli (Fig. 35-16 and 35-17). There it fiburcates into an anterior division for the inferior surface of the temporal and occipital lobes and a posterior division giving rise to the occipito-parietal and the calcarine arteries. The latter runs backward to supply both sides of the calcarine fissure. Before that a branch to the splenium of the corpus callosum is given off.

The territory of the posterior cerebral artery over the occipital pole is variable—sometimes extended, sometimes small. Whatever the case, branches of the posterior cerebral artery anastomose end to end with those of the middle cerebral artery on the convexity and those of the anterior cerebral artery on the medial surface and over the splenium.

Veins

Veins of the convexity drain into either the superior longitudinal or the lateral sinuses. Veins of the medial surface drain into the ipsilateral internal cerebral vein or into the great vein of Galen (see Ch. 35 and Fig. 35-21).

Clinical Syndromes

Several syndromes due to occipital lesions are considered in other chapters of this book. For field defects see Chapter 26 and for visual agnosias see Chapter 19.

Occipital Blindness

The traditional term for occipital blindness is "cortical" blindness. However, lesions of the white matter are present in such cases, and so-called cortical blindness can result from purely subcortical lesions, as in bilateral (usually successive) lesions of the optic radiations.

There is a loss of vision with preservation of the pupillary light reflex, since the central part of the reflex arc is in the brainstem. Optokinetic nystagmus (see below) cannot be elicited. With rare exceptions, no cortical visually evoked potential can be obtained. In this clinical setting the patient may experience visual hallucinations (see below). Denial of blindness (anosognosia) by such patients, said to be "blind to their blindness," is a striking finding (see Ch. 19).

Among the many causes, the most frequent is stroke, especially bilateral infarction of the posterior cerebral artery territory. Occipital blindness can be a transient ischemic attack. Other causes include trauma (in concussion, occipital blindness can be transient), tumors (usually quite large), and Creutzfeldt-Jakob disease, mainly in its so-called posterior form, formerly termed *Heidenhain variant* (R. Heidenhain, German histologist, 1835–1897) (see Ch. 50).

Color dysnomia

Difficulties in naming or matching colors result from many causes, the most frequent being inherited color blindness. Color dysnomia may also simply be part of an aphasia, in which case there is no primary disorder of vision.

Color dysnomia of cerebral visual origin is termed dyschromatopsia or achromatopsia. Such patients report that colors are perceived as dull, pale, faded, and all are grayish. Lesions of the lingual gyrus probably have a key role, and some patients with double-sided lingual gyrus infarcts have had bilateral color dysnomia. Field defects in the upper quadrants and prosopagnosia (Ch. 19) are usually present in such cases.

Dysplexia Without Agraphia

There are two main kinds of alexia (see Ch. 18). First, alexia can be part of aphasia when agraphia and disorders of spoken speech are also present. The lesion is usually parietal in location, involving the posterior portion and usually including the left angular gyrus (see Fig. 18-8).

Second, alexia (or dyslexia) without agraphia is a striking syndrome, which results from purely occipital lesions. Patients cannot read printed or cursive text, including what they may have just written normally. Although patients typically say that the displays are letters and words, the attempts to read aloud or for comprehension show a striking lack of correlation between the semantic meaning of the visual display and the actual words spoken by the patient.

The syndrome is not frequent, but every seasoned neurologist knows of at least one case. Dejerine's (J. Dejerine, French neurologist, 1859–1917) case from 1892 is archetypal. The patient could read neither letters nor words, not even musical notes. The closest to an accurate naming of lexical stimuli was the patient's recognition of the masthead of a newspaper, which had a distinctive typeset. Language was otherwise normal as tested by conversation, and he could write normally, either spontaneously or under dictation. Only copying, which requires visual cues, was defective. There was also a right homonymous hemianopia with right hemiachromatopsia. Postmortem, an infarct was found that interrupted the left optic radiations, the callosal fibers that convey visual data from the right to the left visual area and also interrupted the fibers that link the left visual area to the left gyrus angularis (Fig. 25-19). The case was interpreted as showing that the left gyrus angularis (taken at the time as a reading center) was deprived of visual inputs owing to damage to the projecting fiber system, hence the alexia. The spared language areas in the parietal, temporal, and frontal lobes were taken to explain the normal language function in speaking and auditory comprehension.

Dejerine's famous diagram left unsettled how the lesion (marked by an "x") achieved the disruption that causes the alexia. In the years since, possibilities entertained by subsequent readers of this case have included the disruption of transcallosal fibers en route to the left calcarine cortex, where they join those of the left visual radiation; interruption of fibers passing beyond the left calcarine cortex to some mutual junction point near the occipital pole shared by transcallosal fibers and postcalcarine cortex projection fibers, which they jointly passed through in going from the inferior parietal white matter to the angular gyrus; and transcallosal fiber projections directly to the left angular gyrus, unjoined to those from the left calcarine region.

Dejerine's seminal case prompted many subsequent case reports of disturbances in reading, none of which have directly answered the question of the pathophysiologic effect of the lesion posed by Dejerine's diagram.

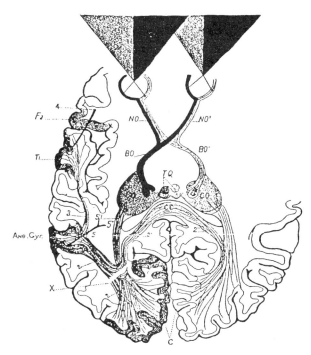

Figure 25-19. The lesion location found by Dejerine to explain alexia without agraphia (lesion location designated by "X"). Note that its position may allow it to have achieved effects on one or more pathways.

The exact pathway carrying the information necessary for reading comprehension from stimuli seen by the right hemisphere has never been fully clarified. Surgical section of the posterior half of the corpus callosum, occasionally necessary for surgical access to the third ventricle from above, has been shown to cause an alexia for the visual field served by the nondominant hemisphere. This has been explained by interruption of the fibers crossing the corpus callosum from right to left (hereafter assumed to be the left hemisphere). The alexia is limited to the left visual field. Visual forms are well discriminated, since no lesion has affected the radiations or calcarine cortex, but the lexical content of the material cannot be understood. This syndrome supports the simple disconnection hypothesis described above, which indicates that fully formed lexical information is transferred across the corpus callosum but does not indicate the fate of this information once it reaches the left hemisphere.

In naturally occurring lesions the callosum is but rarely affected alone, and at least some of the lesion lies in the posterior portion of the dominant hemisphere on the fiber systems that have already crossed through the callosum from the nondominant hemisphere. Unless the lesion causes complete destruction of all the crossing fibers, alexia rarely occurs, which suggests that naturally occurring diseases do not cause specific fiber destruction or that such a specific pathway does not exist within the left hemisphere. Instead, dyslexia occurs to differing degrees of severity, in some instances even taking different clinical forms depending on where and how these fibers are injured.

When infarction is limited to the left cortex, a contralateral (right) hemianopia occurs but with no alexia. The patient quickly adjusts to the initially surprising inability to see to the right. Words seen are easily named, the only hint of dyslexia occurring at times on the extreme right-hand end of very long and unfamiliar words, which is explained by the hemianopia. These observations suggest that information reaching the left hemisphere from the right does not pass through the left calcarine cortex, which argues against dyslexia from the first explanation (see above) of Dejerine's diagram.

Infarction of the mesial occipital region forward of the calcarine cortex and under the corpus callosum can cause right hemidyslexia of short duration but not permanent alexia. The lesion is presumed to destroy only some of the crossing fibers in the lower portion of the callosum.

Acute hemorrhage in the occipital pole may precipitate alexia for reasons still unclear. Usually, the alexia is not persistent. Trauma, even surgical removal of the occipital pole, also does not produce the permanent alexia that occurs from total infarction of the left posterior cerebral artery territory. These findings suggest that some lexical information must pass to or toward the pole from both sides but that other parallel pathways must exist or else the main pathway does not entirely pass through the pole. A few reports claim that the visual fields were full on both sides and yet the patient had an absolute alexia, the explanation having been found or inferred to be a lesion at the occipital pole.

The most severe form, absolute alexia, usually requires infarction affecting almost the whole of the posterior cerebral artery territory, causing the expected right-sided hemianopia from destruction of the visual radiations and calcarine cortex, but also destroying the transcallosal fiber systems after they have crossed into the dominant hemisphere also destroying whatever systems link these transcallosal pathways with the left parietal convexity. Recent work in which brain lesions were plotted on a computerized grid and the locations of those lesions causing hemianopia without alexia were subtracted from those of lesions causing alexia has suggested that a mainly dorsal pathway via the forceps major of the corpus callosum is the critical pathway, not the caudal or inferior pathways speculated by some workers. This region is not uniquely affected by disease, so the conundrum set forth by Dejerine's original diagram remains unsettled, but clinicians can rely on the observation that complete alexia is a sign of near total infarction of the left posterior cerebral artery territory.

Balint's Syndrome

Balint's syndrome has been discussed in the section, Parietal Lobe.

Palinopsia

Palinopsia (Greek: *palin*, again; *opsis*, sight) is visual perseveration. The patient continues to perceive the image after the object has disappeared. It is generally a brief, transient event. The palinopic image occupies either the whole field or part of it, sometimes the blind field of a hemianopia. Parieto-occipital lesions, more often on the right side, are the focal causes. Migraine and some drugs (e.g., mescaline) can cause palinopsia.

The limited case material reported leaves many features of palinopsia unsettled, but there seem to be two forms. One of these features persistence of reappearance of some or all of a visual image immediately after it has disappeared from the environment. In the other form, images reappear only some time later and persist for varying periods of time. The images that reappear are quite striking, given that the delay between the disappearance of the original stimulus and its reappearance may be hours, even days, and the image may persist into the following day. A peculiar feature of the palinopic images are their tendency to be incorporated in the appropriate position into current visual stimuli, such as extra limbs on a person. Frank hallucinations and illusions of visual movement are common accompaniments of both types. The disorder is usually temporary, giving way to more severe visual disturbances as the underlying tumor enlarges or fading away in weeks as the effects of the acute stroke subside. Whether the palinopic effect represents a form of seizure remains unknown, although it remains common practice to treat such patients with anticonvulsants.

Visual Deformations

Visual deformations are deformations of images (e.g., objects as seen as too small (micropsia) or too big (macropsia) or there are illusions of movement, of depth, or of orientation. These deformations occur with occipital or more often occipitoparietal or occipitotemporal lesions. They are frequent in temporal lobe epilepsy (see section, Temporal Lobe).

Visual Hallucinations

Many patients dare not to complain that they "see things" for fear of being considered crazy. Actually, visual hallucinations are quite frequent and clinicians must be prepared to deal with them.

In principle, visual hallucinations can result either from some cause that provokes a neuronal discharge (a focal lesion in epilepsy, or some drugs) or from visual deprivation viz., too few stimuli reaching the visual cortex (blindness, amblyopia, hemianopia). Admittedly, many cases do not fit simply into that very broad classification.

Visual hallucinations, which are visual perceptions without object, are either elementary or complex. When elementary, they are flashes of light, bright zigzags, snowflakes, or geometric shapes. Their origin is chiefly occipital. Complex hallucinations take the form of persons, animals, or landscapes. Their origin is occipitotemporal or temporal (see the section Temporal Lobe). Multimodal hallucinations (e.g., visual and olfactory) have a temporal origin.

The large range of pathophysiologic settings of visual hallucinations (see above) indicates that they can occur in many different circumstances. In peduncular hallucinosis (the term refers to the peduncles of the midbrain), the lesions usually are in the midbrain but not in the peduncles. The hallucinations are well formed characters, for instance animals that appear mostly in the evening and move around. As a rule the patient considers that these images have no objective support. Visual hallucinations are a feature of the hypnagogic state (i.e., the state between waking and sleep), and they are then prominent in narcolepsy or the narcolepsy-cataplexy syndrome (see Ch. 78). They are also a major feature of the onset of ophthalmic migraine (see Ch. 24). As previously mentioned, they are a typical symptom of some temporal lobe seizures.

Florid visual hallucinations occur in the ethanol and barbiturate withdrawal syndromes.

Abuse of drugs (e.g., LSD, mescaline, phencyclidine, cannabis, amphetamines, cocaine) can cause visual hallucinations, or the drugs may even be taken for that effect. Many therapeutic agents can also provoke visual hallucinations—antiparkinsonian drugs, antidepressants, and anticonvulsants, among others. This is more likely to occur in old patients with poor vision and in our experience in old Parkinson disease patients, perhaps because of the lesions in the midbrain. Visual hallucinations, resembling peduncular hallucinosis, in old people with poor vision is sometimes termed the *Charles Bonnet syndrome*.

Diseases

Trauma

Falls on the occiput can cause a flash of simple visual hallucinations. Occipital blindness can occur and can be transient.

Tumors

Gliomas are possible but relatively rare in this small lobe. On the other hand, metastases are frequent, probably because blood flow is at rest in the border zones of the three main cerebral arteries, which favors the settling out of tumor microemboli in these regions.

Strokes

Infarction is due to occlusion of the posterior cerebral artery (see Ch. 35), mostly caused by embolism. Total infarction is rare but can occur when the internal carotid artery is occluded and the posterior cerebral artery is mainly fed by this internal carotid. On the left side, total infarction causes, in addition to a right homonymous hemianopia, severe memory disorders (see Ch. 21), alexia, and a degree of dysnomia. Occlusion of the calcarine artery by a small embolic particle is frequent and is the usual cause of pure or isolated homonymous hemianopia.

Hemorrhages due either to hypertension, amyloid angiopathy, or vascular malformations are relatively rare. Some may affect the occipital pole, causing a short-term hemianopia from disturbance of the adjacent regions of macular representation.

Degenerative Diseases

Alzheimer's disease involves the parietal and temporooccipital regions, thus causing agnosias and disorders of visual exploration of the environment. Creutzfeldt-Jakob disease can severely involve the occipital cortex and even cause occipital blindness (see above).

Some cases of dementia termed *posterior cerebral atrophy* begin with posterior (i.e., occipital and parietal disorders): visual agnosia (Ch. 19), Balint's syndrome (see above), Gerstmann's syndrome (see the section Parietal Lobe) and transcortical sensory aphasia (Ch. 18). Such cases that have come to postmortem have shown either Alzheimer or Creutzfeldt-Jakob lesions or subcortical gliosis. Obviously, these example cases are close to progressive aphasia (see the section Temporal Lobe) and progressive apraxia (see Parietal Lobe), and they await clarification.

CORPUS CALLOSUM

Anatomy

The corpus callosum is a dense mass of white matter roughly 12 cm long, resembling a pulled-apart scroll in sagittal section, thicker in front and at the back, and thinner in the intervening parts, which connects the two cerebral hemispheres (Fig. 25-3). The extreme anterior end, known as the *rostrum,* is thin, and just posterior, the callosum thickens considerably, its bulbous shape known as the *genu* (Latin: knee). The middle portion of the callosum, which is quite thin, is known as the *isthmus* or body and the posterior end as the *splenium* (Latin: bandage).

Although the core of the corpus callosum is made up entirely of interhemispheric fiber pathways, its upper surface hosts parallel thin bands of gray and white matter passing from back to front. These thin bands, known as the *indusium griseum,* are considered to be a remnant of the hippocampal system in lower animals, shrunken to almost invisible threads in the human. On its undersurface, the callosum forms the roof for the third ventricle, and its sides abut the head, body, and tail of the caudate nucleus, forming the roof of the lateral ventricles. Near its midline on the undersurface, the callosum provides the upper attachment for the fornix along most of its course, and it also forms the roof support for the septum lucidum at its anterior end.

The size of the corpus callosum is related to brain weight. Its relative size varies along the course, reflecting the different populations of fibers that make up the structure. In strongly right-handed men, the midportion (isthmus) of the callosum is thinner than among ambidextrous people and among women. Some evidence suggests that callosal thickness increases in middle age in women while it declines in men. Some studies have found the callosum thicker in females, but others have not shown sex-based differences.

The estimated 300 million fibers passing through the callosum are arranged in three layers, rather like a bias-ply tire. The central layer is more or less arranged in the transverse plane, while the thinner layers above and below run at a bias at roughly right angles to each other.

Physiology

The directly transverse fiber systems are the most frequently described of the callosal components. These link homologous sites in the two hemispheres. Appreciation of the homologous site projections requires special stains after focal lesions. In whole-brain sections stained to demonstrate white matter, the pale, obvious staining reflecting the degeneration near the callosal lesion fades quickly into the bulk of the centrum semiovale. Anteriorly, fibers of the forceps anterior link the anterior regions of the two frontal lobes. Posteriorly, the transverse bundles forming the corpus callosum are separable into several groups (see also the section Occipital Lobe). The *forceps major* links the cuneus, calcarine cortex, and parietal gyri on the convex surface, including the angular and anterior parietal gyri (Fig. 25-8). Its fibers pass through the dorsal portion of the splenium, forming a bulge in the superomesial wall of the occipital horn of the lateral ventri-

cle. Just below the forceps major is another prominent bulge, the *calcar avis,* produced by the indentation from the calcarine fissure and cortex. These two structures in the mesial ventricular wall show the close relationship between transcallosal fibers and the primary visual cortex. The *forceps minor* is a fiber band of the callosum, which passes below the calcar avis, linking the lingual and second and third occipital gyri. Fibers of the corpus callosum that separate the ventricles from the optic radiation are known as the tapetum.

Of clinical importance is the fact that transcallosal links to homologous regions do *not* include the primary visual cortex (area 17), the hand and foot regions of the primary motor cortex, or the primary sensory cortex. These latter regions are linked indirectly through their associative cortex to transcallosal fibers, which project to homologous regions of association cortices.

Direct stimulation of the callosum during its exposure at operation has yielded evidence of regional functional localization within the structure. Considering it from front to back in equal tenths, stimulation in the anterior five tenths yields evoked potentials entirely within the frontal lobes; in the sixth to eighth tenth, the responses are still mainly frontal and occasionally in the temporal and parietal lobes; and stimulation in the ninth and tenth segment yields evoked responses only in the parietal and occipital lobes.

Arteries

The arterial supply is mainly from the anterior cerebral artery over the superior surface and via the posterior choroidal branches of the posterior cerebral arteries on the inferior surface. The rostrum and genu are also supplied by branches from the anterior communicating artery. Throughout the length of the callosum, the branches of the anterior cerebral and choroidal arteries are concentrated along its outer wall, differing in size and length, but all of them penetrate into the fiber network and are oriented among the transverse fibers.

Clinical Syndromes

The principle of the syndromes of callosal disorders is the lack of transfer of information from one hemisphere to the other. These disorders take different forms depending on the sites where lesions occur in the callosum.

Following section (sometimes performed for epilepsy or for surgical access to the third ventricle) or infarction of the anterior portions of the callosum, sparing the splenium, the failure of information transfer from the hemisphere dominant for speech and language prevents right-handed patients from performing skilled movements with the left hand to dictated command, since the right hemisphere depends on the auditory discrimination and language functions of the left hemisphere for the instructions to perform the motor movements demanded by the examiner. Likewise, objects placed unseen in the left hand are not named because the sensory discriminations made by the right hemisphere fail to cross the damaged callosum and inform the dominant hemisphere of the features of the palpated stimulus sufficiently for it to be named aloud. Similar disorders of interhemispheral transfer explain the failure to reproduce with the right hand those positions of the left hand created by an examiner manipulating the left hand. Callosum-damaged patients often state that their own hand, presented passively in the left visual field, is not their own (alien hand sign, see section Frontal Lobe). The finding that complex right-hand movements are difficult to learn following dictated instructions or visual examples suggests that the left hemisphere normally draws upon the greater spatial skills of the right hemisphere. When transection of the callosum produces clinical findings, the "disconnected' hemispheres appear to function independently in the judg-

ment of positions in space within each visual field (Fig. 25-20). It still remains unclear how the severity of the clinical disturbances fade over time.

Apart from disturbances in motor function, each of the sensory modalities may be affected. Minor noxious stimulation to the left side of the body is often poorly described by patients who have undergone complete callosal section, but more severe stimuli are well appreciated even if the exact site of the stimulus is not well described.

For hearing, a small hemorrhage in the posterior half of the callosum appears sufficient to suppress interhemispheric transfer of information heard by the right hemisphere in dichotic listening tests. These tasks reflect the attempt to understand the meaning of two competing words or strings of words that are presented simultaneously, one word or set in one ear, another word or set in the other. For example, "Seated at a football" could be presented to one ear and "He caught the table" could be presented to the other. Ordinarily, the normal brain should hear these as two meaningful sentences such as "Seated at a table" and "He caught the football." Typically, hemispherectom-

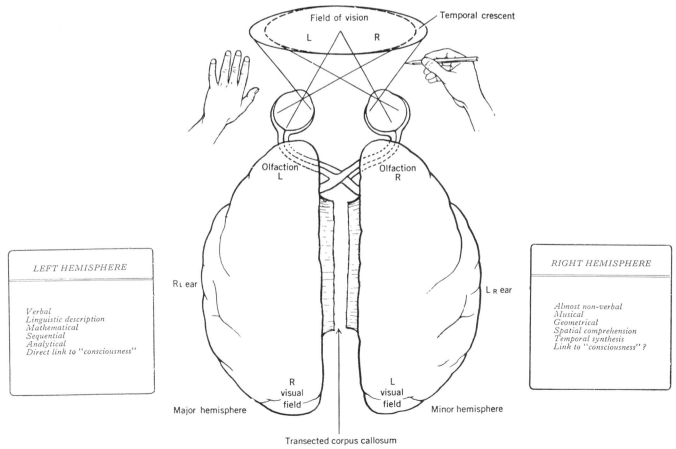

Figure 25-20. Schematic representation of functions considered limited to each hemisphere.

ized patients show extinction to sounds from contralateral space in dichotic listening tests as do callosum-sectioned patients when asked to report the words heard in the left ear (which sounds are preferentially projected to the right side of the brain).

When the callosal section from anterior to posterior leaves as much as one-third of the posterior callosum intact, there is only slight impairment of interhemispheric transfer of somatosensory and auditory (dichotic listening) information and no abnormality for visual tasks. If even small parts of the splenium remain, the interhemispheric transfer of visual information remains largely intact.

Lesions in the posterior end of the callosum involving the splenium interfere with naming or other ways of responding to visual displays for visual stimuli projected into the nondominant (right) hemisphere but produce no disturbances for those projected into the dominant hemisphere (see also the section Occipital Lobe). (For the purposes of discussion the left visual field is hereafter considered to be the source of visual stimulation to the hemisphere nondominant for speech and language.) Left-sided visual displays may arouse a pointing or reaching response with the left hand, but the patient is unable to name aloud or point to the object when hearing the name dictated or when shown the printed name of the object in the right visual field.

In the simplest form of absent naming, the patient either acts as if displays in the left visual field do not exist or acknowledging that they exist, cannot recall their names, or acts as if any printed letters, words, or even musical notes are unfamiliar shapes. Familiar logos, such as the script shapes characteristic of Coca-Cola, Gothic lettering, or typesets typical of certain newspapers and magazines may be used by the patient to name the display and thus express familiarity with the material. However, if the examiner deliberately uses the logo and replaces it with another word, such as "cacaza" for Coca-Cola, the name expected is the more likely to be uttered. Letter forms from alphabets unfamiliar to the patient are rejected, and misoriented letters can be manually reoriented properly by the patient.

Diseases

Naturally occurring lesions damaging fiber pathways of the corpus callosum are rare. Many of the syndromes attributed to lesions of the callosum are actually from injuries to the pathways well into one hemisphere, as is the usual case in dyslexia from left occipital lesions (see the section Occipital Lobe).

Trauma

During the sudden deceleration of the moving head as in striking the floor in a fall or the automobile dash-board during an accident, the sliding forward of the brain as a whole pushes the genu of the callosum against the falx cerebri and may result in laceration. After trauma, brain swelling on one side may displace the swollen hemisphere so much across the midline that the callosum is folded slightly or suffers partial infarction when the medial frontal region herniates under the inferior edge of the falx cerebri (see Ch. 6).

Tumors

Primary tumors arising in the frontal lobes commonly spread across the corpus callosum, the tumor in the diverging fibers on either side of the callosum giving a double-sided fanlike appearance on brain imaging or cut section of the brain at autopsy, which is often described as a butterfly glioma. Whether gliomas arise wholly within the callosum has been difficult to determine.

Stroke

Infarction, the best known of stroke lesions, typically occurs from occlusion of the anterior cerebral artery, which usually includes a large portion of the medial frontal region on one or the other side. Although such patients comprise the bulk of the source of studies on interhemispheric transfer, there remains concern that the contribution fo the medial hemispheric lesion could easily be overlooked. In the acute phase after infarction, mutism and long delays before any form of voluntary response are a common findings, lasting for days or weeks.

Multiple Sclerosis

Lesions of the corpus callosum are frequent in multiple sclerosis and characteristic of the disease. In advanced cases, atrophy of the callosum is common and correlates fairly well with the clinical severity of the disease but not with its mere duration or with the age or sex of the patient or with abnormality in visual evoked responses. Evidence of impairment of motor, auditory, and sensory transfer has been reported in multiple sclerosis.

Metabolic and Degenerative Disease

Disease that selectively affect the white matter also commonly affect the corpus callosum, but the clinical manifestations are often difficult to relate to callosal involvement. In some cases they resemble those of bihemispheric disconnection, but more often the frontal lobe syndrome (see section, Frontal Lobe) causes a picture resembling frontal brain tumor. Included in the list of diseases affecting the callosum are the nutritional disturbances that bring about necrosis of its central fiber systems known as the Marchiafava-Bignami disease (see Ch. 67) and multisystem atrophy (see Ch. 76).

Surgery

Surgical section of the corpus callosum is usually performed for treatment of epilepsy in the hope of blocking bihemispheric spread of seizure activity. The group of patients whose callosum is sectioned in part for access to the third ventricle for tumor removal make up a smaller data set. The smallest group of callosal sections are the rare cases in which section is performed for rupture of an anterior communicating artery aneurysm with discharge of blood into the anterior callosum. Awareness that section of the splenium may impair reading in the left visual field has long been heeded by surgeons.

Small surgical section of the isthmus of the callosum for access to the third ventricle typically causes no clinically obvious disturbance in function. Special testing of dichotic listening and complex interhemispheric transfer of somatosensory information is needed to demonstrate deficits. Patients undergoing callosal section for control of epilepsy have often shown a surprisingly intact capacity for interhemispheric transfer of information.

More worrisome is the risk that the callosum incision will transect the fornix lying just below. Severe disorders of recent memory have been described from bilateral fornix section and even from unilateral section if the fornix serves the hemisphere dominant for speech and language.

ANNOTATED BIBLIOGRAPHY

Adler A. Disintegration and restoration of optic recognition in visual agnosia. Arch Neurol Psychiatry 1944;51:243.

Detailed analysis of a survivor of Boston's Cocoanut Grove nightclub fire, whose gradual improvement in visual function passed through several stages.

Agostini E, Coletti A, Orlando G, Tredici G. Apraxia in deep cerebral lesions. J Neurol Neurosurg Psychiatry 1983;46:804.

Detailed description of the clinical findings.

Ajuriaguerra J, Hecaen H, Angelergues R. Les apraxies: variétés clinique et latéralisation lésionelle. Rev Neurol (Paris) 1960;102:494.

A classic clinical description.

Albert NL, Soffer D, Silverberg R, Raches A. The anatomic basis of visual agnosia. Neurology 1979;29:876.

Mostly posterior cerebral territory infarctions.

Alexander MP, Fischer RS, Friedman R. Lesion localization in apractic agraphia. Arch Neurol 1992;49:246–51.

Poor morphology from superior parietal lobule lesions despite adequate motor power, sensory function, and awareness of meaning of words and letters.

Alexander MP, Warren RL. Localization of callosal auditory pathways: a CT case study. Neurology 1988;38:802–4.

Case report of posterior callosal hemorrhage and dichotic listening tests.

Amarenco P, Cohen P, Roullet E et al. Syndrome amnèsique lors d'un infarctus du territoire de l'artère choroidienne antérieure gauche. Rev Neurol (Paris) 1988;144:36–9.

One of the few reported.

Andrew J, Nathan PW. Lesions of the anterior frontal lobes and disturbances of micturition and defaecation. Brain 1964;87:233–62.

Good evidence accounting for incontinence from frontal lobe lesions.

Arboix A, Junque C, Vendrell P, Marti-Vilalta JL. Auditory ear extinction in lacunar syndromes. Acta Neurol Scand 1990;81:507–11.

Studies of the transcallosal pathways from subcortical infarction.

Balint R. Seelenlähmung des "Schauens," optische Ataxia, und rämliche Störung der Aufmerksamkeit. Monatsschr Psychiatrie Neurol 1909;25:51.

Full description of the disordered motor and visual behavior that may follow bilateral parietooccipital lesions.

Banks G, Short P, Martinez J et al. The alien hand syndrome. Clinical and postmortem findings. Arch Neurol 1989;46:456–9.

Case report.

Barnes CL, Pandya DN. Efferent cortical connections of multimodal cortex of the superior temporal sulcus in the rhesus monkey. J Comp Neurol 1992;318:222–44.

Observations that the temporal lobe receives inputs from all primary modality cortical regions and transmits outputs to the pons and cerebellum.

Basso A, Luzzatti C, Spinnler H. Is ideomotor apraxia the outcome of damage to well defined regions of the left hemisphere? J Neurol Neurosrug Psychiatry 1980;43:118.

The answer is yes in some cases.

Berrebi AS, Fitch RH, Ralphe DL et al. Corpus callosum: region specific effects of sex, early experience and age. Brain Res 1988;438:216–24.

Changes with age in men and women.

Bizzi E. Discharge of frontal eye field neurons during eye movements in unanesthetized monkeys. Science 1967;157:1588.

Discharges only keep the eyes deviated but do not cause deviation.

Blythe IM, Kennard C, Ruddock KH. Residual vision in patients with retrogeniculate lesions of the visual pathways. Brain 1987;110:887–905.

Detection of movement sufficient for localization but no discrimi-

nation of size or shape in 25 patients with extensive occipital lesions when tested in the blind areas.

Bonhoeffer K. Klinischer und anatomischer Befund zur Lehre von der Apraxie und der "motorischen Sprachbahn." Monatsschr Psychiatrie Neurol 1914;35:113.

Clinical classic for mutism after bilateral deep frontal lesions.

Brodman K. Vergleichende Lokalisationslehre der Grosshirnrinde. 2nd Ed., JA Barth, Leipzig, 1925.

Buchsbaum MS. The frontal lobes, basal ganglia, and temporal lobes as sites for schizophrenia. Schizophr Bull 1990;16:379–89.

The behavior looks like schizophrenia.

Canaple S, Rosa A, Mizon JP. Maladie de Marchiafava-Bignami: disconnexion interhémisphérique, évolution favorable, aspect neuroradiologique. Rev Neurol (Paris) 1992;148:638–40.

Detailed neuroradiologic study of two survivors with some clinical details of the dyspraxias.

Carpenter MB, Sutin J. Human Neuroanatomy. 8th Ed. Williams & Wilkins, Baltimore, 1983.

Basic reference.

Carpenter RHS. Neurophysiology. 2nd Ed. E Arnold, London, 1993.

Clear and astute.

Carpenter WT Jr, Buchanan RW. Medical progress. Schizophrenia. N Eng J Med 1994;330:681–90.

Good review with elements of pathology.

Castaigne P, Lhermitte F, Gautier JC et al. Arterial occlusions in the vertebro-basilar system—a study of forty-four patients with post-mortem data. Brain 1973;96:133.

Most are embolic from the vertebral artery or from the heart.

Cavada C, Goldman Rakic PS. Posterior parietal cortex in rhesus monkey: II. Evidence for segregated corticocortical networks linking sensory and limbic areas with the frontal lobe. J Comp Neurol 1989;287:422–45.

The classical association cortex of the frontal lobe is parcelled into sectors with specific connections with posterior parietal subdivisions.

Chai SY, McKenzie JS, McKinley MJ, Mendelsohn FA. Angiotensin converting enzyme in the human basal forebrain and midbrain visualized by in vitro autoradiography. J Comp Neurol 1990;291:179–94.

Rather focal distribution.

Clark CR, Geffen GM. Corpus callosum surgery and recent memory. A review. Brain 1989;112:165–75.

Damage to the fornix, not to the callosum, explains memory loss.

Cobb S. Foundations of Neuropsychiatry. Williams & Wilkins, Baltimore, 1958.

Costello AL, Warrington EK. Dynamic aphasia: the selective impairment of verbal planning. Cortex 1989;25:103–14.

Description of the disorder task by task.

Cusick CG, Gould HJ 3d. Connections between area 3b of the somatosensory cortex and subdivisions of the ventroposterior nuclear complex and the anterior pulvinar nucleus in squirrel monkeys. J Comp Neurol 1990;292:83–102.

Area 3b has somatotopically organized connections with the ventroposterior thalamus and pulvinar nucleus, which contains a representation of all parts of the body, including the face. The authors believe that thalamus nuclei project to several cortical sites and cortical sites receive several different inputs.

Damasio A, Damasio H, Chang Chi H. Neglect following damage to frontal lobe or basal ganglia. Neuropsychologia 1980;18:123.

Large and small lesions may cause impaired responses to contralateral stimuli.

Damasio AR, Damasio H, Van Hoesen GW. Prosopagnosia: anatomic basis and behavioral mechanisms. Neurology 1982;32:332.

Usually posterior cerebral infarcts.

Dejerine J. Contribution a l'étude anatomo-pathologique et clinique des différentes variétés de cécite verbale. C R Soc Biol (Paris) 1892;4:61–90.

Magnificent seminal case.

Dejerine J. Sur un cas de cécite verbale avec agraphie, suivi d'autopsie. Mem Soc Biol 1891;3:197.

The first well described attempt to define alexia with agraphia.

Dejerine J, Regnard M. Monoplégie brachiale gauche limitée aux muscles des éminences thenar, hypothenar et aux interosseus. Astéreognosie, epilepsie jacksonienne. Rev Neurol (Paris) 1912;1:285.

Clinical classic of the pseudoneuropathic syndromes.

Denny-Brown D, Chambers RA. The parietal lobe and behavior. Res Publ Assoc Res Nerv Ment Dis 1958;36:35–117.

The early theory of frontal-parietal imbalance.

DeRenzi E, Colombo A, Faglioni P, Gilbertoni N. Conjugate gaze paresis in stroke patients with unilateral damage. Arch Neurol 1982;39:42.

More common in nondominant hemisphere lesions.

Doody RS, Jankovic J. The alien hand and related signs. J Neurol Neurosurg Psychiatry 1992;55:806–10.

Seven case histories and an overview.

Ebeling U, Reulen HJ. Neurosurgical topography of the optic radiation in the temporal lobe. Acta Neurochir (Wien) 1988;92:29–36.

A modern treatise on the course of the visual radiations in the temporal lobe.

Elberger AJ. Binocularity and single cell acuity are related in striate cortex of corpus callosum sectioned and normal cats. Exp Brain Res 1989;77:213–6.

The younger the age when the corpus callosum is sectioned, the worse the binocular representation and acuity.

Freund HJ. Premotor area and preparation of movement. Rev Neurol (Paris) 1990;146:543–7.

Clear, concise update.

Freund HJ. Abnormalities of motor behavior after cortical lesions in man. In Mountcastle VB, Plum F (eds). Handbook of Physiology. Sect. 1: The Nervous System. Vol 5, Part 2. American Physiological Society, Bethesda, MD, 1987, pp. 763–810.

Scholarly review.

Freund HJ. Abnormalities of motor behavior after cortical lesions in humans. In Brookhart JM, Mountcastle VB (eds). Handbook of Physiology. Sect. 1: Neurophysiology. Vol. 2: Motor control. Part 2. American Physiological Society, Bethesda, MD, 1981, pp. 763–810.

Detailed analysis of the effect of prerolandic and rolandic lesions on movements in humans.

Galaburda AM. Developmental dyslexia. Rev Neurol (Paris) 1993;149:1–3.

Asymmetry of the planum temporale lacking in developmental dyslexia.

Gestaut JL, Benaim LJ, L'amyotrophie d'origine pariétale: syndrome de Silverstein, Etude clinique et electrophysiologique. Rev Neurol (Paris) 1988;144:301–5.

Recent examples of amyotrophy from parietal lesions.

Gazzaniga M, Bogen J, Sperry R, Dyspraxia following division of the cerebral commissures. Arch Neurol 1967;16:606.

Brain functions if two separate systems were at work.

Gentilucci M, Fogassi L, Luppino G et al: Somatotopic representation in inferior area 6 of the macaque monkey. Brain Behav Evol 1989;33:118–21.

Details of monocellular recordings.

Georgopoulos AP, Taira M, Lukashin A. Cognitive neurophysiology of the motor cortex. Science 1993;260:47–52.

Computer model for organization of the control of neurons governing motor movements.

Gerstmann J. Syndrome of finger agnosia, disorientation for right and left, agraphia and acalculia. J Neurol Neurosurg Psychiatry 1940;44:398–408.

One of the better-known "parietal" syndromes.

Geschwind N. Disconnection syndromes in animals and man. Parts 1 and 2. Brain 1965;88:237.

Clinical classic drawing on the old literature.

Gibb WRG, Luthert PJ, Marsden CD. Corticobasal degeneration. Brain 1989;112:1171–92.

The seminal paper.

Gilbert CD, Wiesel TN, Columnar specificity of intrinsic horizontal and corticocortical connections in cat visual cortex. J Neurosci 1989;9:2432–42.

Horizontal connections linking striate cell columns may allow

single cells to collect information from far larger areas of the visual field than those of the specific receptive field of the cell.

Glaser JS. Neuro-ophthalmology. 2nd Ed. JB Lippincott, Philadelphia, 1990.

Knowledgeable and practical.

Godoy J, Luders H, Dinner DS et al. Versive eye movements elicited by cortical stimulation of the human brain. Neurology 1990;40:296–9.

Surprising range of sites can cause turning of the eyes.

Grafton ST, Mazziotta JC, Woods RP, Phelps ME. Human functional anatomy of visually guided finger movements. Brain 1992;115:565–87.

PET studies show a role for the superior parietal lobule.

Head H, Holmes G. Sensory disturbances from cerebral lesions. Brain 1912;34:102–213.

The clinical classic for cerebral dysfunction.

Herbaut AG, Cole JD, Sedgwick EM. A cerebral hemisphere influence on cutaneous vasomotor reflexes in humans. J Neurol Neurosurg Psychiatry 1990;53:118–20.

Premotor convexity lesions cause contralateral dysautonomic responses.

Huttenlocher PR, de Courten C. The development of synapses in striate cortex of man. Hum Neurobiol 1987;6:1–9.

Aging and synaptic density in human striate cortex.

Jones Gotman M, Zatorre RJ. Olfactory identification deficits in patients with focal cerebral excision. Neuropsychologia 1988 26:387–400.

Minor losses from lesions of either side.

Joseph JP. Role of the dorsolateral prefrontal cortex in organizing visually guided behavior. Brain Behav Evol 1989;33:132–5.

Dorsolateral prefrontal cortex guides responses to remembered or current events and objects in the behavioral surround that have not yet been fixed in the fovea of the eye.

Kalaska JF. The representation of arm movements in postcentral and parietal cortex. Can J Physiol Pharmacol 1988;66:455–63.

Populations of sensory cortex cells code patterns of joint movements.

Katayama S, Kito S, Miyoshi R, Yamamura Y. Mapping of somatostatin receptor localization in rat brain: forebrain and diencephalon. Brain Res Bull 1990;24:331–9.

Current maps.

Kennard A, Viets HR, Fulton JF. The syndrome of the premotor cortex in man: impairment of skilled movements, forced grasping, spasticity and vasomotor disturbances. Brain 1934;57:69–84.

Classical, disputed description.

Klekamp J, Riedel A, Harper C, Kretschmann HJ. A quantitative study of Australian aboriginal and Caucasian brains. J Anat 1987;150:191–210.

No differences found in the size of the striate cortex, but it projects farther onto the convex surface in the aborigines.

Klüver H, Bucy P. Am J Physiol 1937;119:352.

The first of a series of papers published through 1939 detailing animal experiments and humans with temporal lobe lesions displaying the elements eventually known as the Klüver-Bucy syndrome.

Krubitzer LA, Kaas JH. Responsiveness and somatotopic organization of anterior parietal field 3b and adjoining cortex in newborn and infant monkeys. Somatosens Mot Res 1988;6:179–205.

A homunculus for sensory functions is evident in newborns.

LaPlane D, Degos JD. Motor neglect. J Neurol Neurosrug Psychiatry 1983;46:152.

Clinical classic describing the syndromes.

Lazorthes G. Le Systeme Nerveux Central. Masson et cie, Paris, 1967.

Leger JM, Levasseur M, Benoit N et al. Apraxie d'aggravation lentement progressive. Etude par IRM et tomographie à positrons dans 4 cas. Rev Neurol (Paris) 1991;147:183–91.

Four cases and a nosologic review.

Lhermitte F. Human anatomy and the frontal lobes. Part II: Patient behavior in complex and social situations: the "environmental dependency syndrome." Ann Neurol 1986;19:335–43.

Motor behavior subjugated to the external world.

Lhermitte F, Pillon B, Serdaru M. Human autonomy and the frontal lobes. Part I: Imitation and utilization behavior: a neuropsychological study of 75 patients. Ann Neurol 1986;19:326–34.

Motor behavior subjugated to the external world.

Leiguarda R, Starkstein S, Berthier M. Anterior callosal haemorrhage. A partial interhemispheric disconnection syndrome. Brain 1989;112:1019–37.

Motor and somatosensory but not visual disturbances.

Lenz FA, Dostrovsky JO, Tasker RR et al. Single unit analysis of the human ventral thalamic nuclear group: somatosensory responses. J Neurophysiol 1988;59:299–315.

Details of studies showing frequency and topographic representation of response to mechanical stimulation.

Liepmann H. Das Krankheitsbild der Apraxia (motorischen Asymbolie). Monatschr Psychol 1900;8:15–44, 102–32, 182–97.

Full theses of dyspraxia, including ideomotor disorders.

Liepmann H, Maas O. Fall von linksseitiger Agraphie und Apraxie bei rechtsseitiger Lähmung. Z Psychol Neurol 1907;10:214.

An early example of ideomotor dyspraxia.

Luria AR. Higher Cortical Functions in Man. Basic Books, New York, 1966.

A clinical classic for those interested in the pavlovian view of neurology; full of references.

Magnusson M, Pyykko I, Jantti V. Effect of alertness and visual attention on optokinetic nystagmus in humans. Am J Otolaryngol 1985;6:419–25.

Not much optokinetic nystagmus when inattentive.

Martinot JL, Hardy P, Feline A et al. Left prefrontal glucose hypometabolism in the depressed state: a confirmation. Am J Psychiatry 1990;147:1313–7.

Evidence that depression is related to focal injuries.

Matelli M, Luppino G, Fogassi L, Rizzolatti G. Thalamic input to inferior area 6 and area 4 in the macaque monkey. J Comp Neurol 1989;280:468–88.

One region controlling distal movements receives input from one thalamic area, while regions controlling proximal movements receive their main inputs from another.

Mathews TJ, Marus G. Otogenic intradural complications: (a review of 37 patients). J Laryngol Otol 1988;102:121–4.

A recent review of an old problem.

Meldrum BS, Bruton CJ. Epilepsy. In Adams JH, Duchen LW (eds). Greenfield's Neuropathology. 5th ed. E Arnold, London, 1992.

First-class neuropathology text.

Mesulam MM. Principles of Behavioral Neurology. 3rd ed. FA Davis, Philadelphia, 1987.

Classical reference.

Mesulam MM. Frontal cortex and behavior. Ann Neurol 1986;19:326–34.

Clear review.

Mesulam MM. A cortical network for directed attention and unilateral neglect. Ann Neurol 1981;10:309.

Thesis was new at time of this publication.

Michel D, Laurent B, Convers P et al. Douleurs corticales. Etude clinique, electrophysiologique et topographique de 12 cas. Rev Neurol (Paris) 1990;146:405–14.

Twelve remarkable cases of pain from cortical lesions.

Mitz AR, Godschalk M. Eye movement representation in the frontal lobe of rhesus monkeys. Neurosci Lett 1989;106:157–62.

Eye movements are more broadly represented in the frontal lobes than previously described.

Mohr JP, Foulkes MA, Polis AT et al. Infarct topography and hemiparesis profiles with cerebral convexity infarction: the Stroke Data Bank. J Neurol Neurosurg Psychiatry 1993;56:344–51.

Wide range of syndromes, with a single lesion rolandic and vice versa.

Mohr JP, Leicester J, Stoddard LT, Sidman M. Right hemianopia with memory and colors defects in circumscribed left posterior cerebral artery territory infarction. Neurology 1971;21:1104.

The term agnosia would be misleading.

Mohr JP, Rubinstein LV, Kase CS et al. Gaze palsy in hemispheral stroke: the NINCDS Stroke Data Bank. Neurology 1984;34(suppl. 1):119.

Deep lesions cause more persistent distrubance than do superficial ones.

Neal JW, Pearson RC, Powell TP. The ipsilateral corticocortical connections of area 7 with the frontal lobe in the monkey. Brain Res 1990;509:31–40.

Description of a feedforward and feedback system.

Newman RP, Kinkel WR, Jacobs L. Altitudinal hemianopia caused by occipital infarctions. Arch Neurol 1984;41:413.

Upper altitudinal anopsia but no "agnosia."

Norback CR, Strominger NL, Demorest RJ. Thalamus. pp. 365–373. In: The Human Nervous System. 4th Ed. Lea & Febiger, Philadelphia, 1991.

Pakkenberg B. What happens in the leucotomised brain? A postmortem morphological study of brains from schizophrenic patients. J Neurol Neurosurg Psychiatry 1989;52:156–61.

Widespread degeneration.

Pause M, Freund HJ. Role of the parietal cortex for sensorimotor transformation. Evidence from clinical observations. Brain Behav Evol 1989;33:136–40.

Impaired manual skills from parietal lesions in humans.

Pelletier J, Habib M, Brouchon M et al. Etude du transfert interhémisphérique dans la sclérose en plaques. Rev Neurol 1992;148:672–9.

Impairment of motor, sensory, and auditory transfer.

Penfield W, Boldrey E. Somatic motor and sensory representation in the cerebral cortex of man as studied by electrical stimulation. Brain 1937;60:389–443.

Remarkable range of movements from a given site and sites giving rise to a given movement.

Penfield W, Rasmussen T. The Cerebral Cortex in Conscious Man. Blakiston, New York, 1959.

Penfield W, Rasmussen T. The Cerebral Cortex of Man. MacMillan, New York, 1952.

Clinical classic describing details of movements from surface stimulation.

Pierrot-Deseilligny C, Gray F, Brunet P. Infarcts of both inferior parietal lobules with impairment of visually guided eye movements, peripheral visual inattention and optic ataxia. Brain 1986;109:81–97.

Unusual bilateral lesions of the deep parietal white matter, which produced elements of Balint's syndrome.

Pierrot-Deseilligny C, Rivaud S, Gaymard B, Agid Y. Cortical control of reflexive visually guided saccades. Brain 1991;114:1473–85.

Impaired ocular saccades for movements contralateral to superior parietal lesions.

Pillon B, Signoret J-L, Lhermitte F. Agnosie visuelle associative. Role de l'hémisphere gauche dans la perception visuelle. Rev Neurol (Paris) 1981;137:831.

Attacks the traditional thesis.

Pötzl O. Die zweite Gruppe der optischen Agnosien. In Aschaffenburg G (ed). Handbuch der Psychiatrie. Die Aphasielehre: I. Optische-agnostischen Störungen. Franz Deuticke, Vienna, 1928, P. 80.

An underquoted classic. Thoughtful discussion of the implications of the terms.

Rakic P, Yakovlev PI. J Comp Neurol 1968;132:45–72.

Classic article on embryology.

Rao SM, Bernardin L, Leo GJ et al. Cerebral disconnection in multiple sclerosis. Relationship to atrophy of the corpus callosum. Arch Neurol 1989;46:918–20.

Callosal atrophy correlated with poor left ear performance on dichotic listening tests.

Richer F, Martinez M, Cohen H, Saint Hilaire JM. Visual motion perception from stimulation of the human medial parieto occipital cortex. Exp Brain Res 1991;87:649–52.

One of the few reports of medial parieto-occipital function.

Risse GL, Gates J, Lund G et al. Interhemispheric transfer in patients with incomplete section of the corpus callosum. Anatomic verification with magnetic resonance imaging. Arch Neurol 1989;46:437–43.

Considerable variation in the syndromes from anterior callosal section in chronic epileptics.

Rizzolatti G, Berti A. Neglect as a neural representation deficit. Rev Neurol (Paris) 1990;146:626–34.

Neglect is a representational deficit consequent to lesions of neural centers responsible for the organization of motor acts, in which space is coded in nonretinal coordinates.

Roberts GW, Bruton CJ. Notes from the graveyard: neuropathology and schizophrenia. Neuropathol Appl Neurobiol 1990;16:3–16.

Structural abnormalities may underlie schizophrenia.

Roland PE. Somatosensory detection of microgeometry, macrogeometry and kinesthesia after localized lesions of the cerebral hemispheres in man. Brain Res 1987;434:43–94.

Authoritative review.

Roland PE, Seitz RJ. Positron emission tomography studies of the somatosensory system in man. Ciba Found Symp 1991;163:113–20.

One of many excellent papers in this symposium.

Rosa A, Demiati M, Cartz L, Mizon JP. Marchiafava Bignami disease, syndrome of interhemispheric disconnection, and right handed agraphia in a left hander. Arch Neurol 1991;48:986–8.

Elements of disconnection syndrome with this disease.

Rubens AB, Benson DF. Associative visual agnosia. Arch Neurol 1971;24:305.

The disconnection model.

Sedat J, Duvernoy H. Anatomical study of the temporal lobe. Correlations with nuclear magnetic resonance. J Neuroradiol 1990;17:26–49.

Imaging of the gross anatomy of the temporal lobe.

Segraves MA, Goldberg ME, Deny SY et al. The role of striate cortex in the guidance of eye movements in the monkey. J Neurosci 1987;7:3040–58.

Striatal lesions in the monkey produce disturbance of saccades and smooth ocular tracking.

Sergent J. Processing of spatial relations within and between the disconnected cerebral hemispheres. Brain 1991;114:1025–53.

The two hemispheres can operate independently for spatial discrimination.

Squire LR, Zola Morgan S. The medial temporal lobe memory system. Science 1991;253:1380–6.

Thorough review of memory mechanisms.

Stanton GB, Deng SY, Goldberg ME, McMullen NT. Cytoarchitectural characteristic of the frontal eye fields in macaque monkeys. J Comp Neurol 1989;282:415–27.

The cells mediating eye movements seem to be large layer V pyramidal cells.

Stein BE, Price DD, Gazzaniga MS. Pain perception in a man with total corpus callosum transection. Pain 1989;38:51–6.

Tactile and low-intensity noxious stimuli were not well detected in the non-dominant hand but more intense stimuli were.

Steinmetz H, Volkmann J, Jancke L, Freund HJ. Anatomical left right asymmetry of language related temporal cortex is different in left and right handers. Ann Neurol 1991;29:315–9.

Asymmetries are evident in the newborn, with the planum temporale on the left longer than the right in right handers.

Tootell RB, Silverman MS, Hamilton SL et al. Functional anatomy of macaque striate cortex. J Neurosci 1988;8:1500–30, 1531–68, 1659–93, 1594–609, 1610–24.

Long series of articles covering in detail the macaque striate cortex, emphasizing ocular dominance, binocular interactions, retinotopic organization, color, contrast and magno-parvo-cellular streams, and spatial frequency.

Traquair HM, Introduction to Clinical Perimetry. 6th Ed. Mosby, St. Louis, 1949.

Tusa RJ, Ungerleider LG. Fiber pathways of crotical areas mediating smooth pursuit eye movements in monkeys. Ann Neurol 1988;23:174–83.

Wide projections from the striate cortex connect it to the ipsilateral occipitoparietal cortex, by an interhemispheric callosal pathway to the opposite side and by a corticosubcortical pathway to pontine nuclei. Fiber pathways link the superior parietal region with occipital, frontal and pontine systems subserving sensory, motor, and spatial systems.

Tusa RJ, Ungerleider LG. The inferior longitudinal fasciculus: a reexamination in humans and monkeys. Ann Neurol 1985;18:583–91.

Not a long band (fasciculus) but a series of short connections (U fibers) resembling a long band.

Victoroff J, Ross GW, Benson F et al. Posterior cortical atrophy: neuropathologic correlations. Arch Neurol 1994;51:269–74.

Clinical homogeneity, pathologic heterogeneity.

Von Monakow K: Die Lokalisation im Grosshirn und der Abbau der Funktion durch Kortikale Herde. JF Begman, Wiesbaden, 1914.

Full literature review to that time.

Walter A, Mai JK, Jimenez Hertel W. Mapping of neuropeptide Y like immunoreactivity in the human forebrain. Brain Res Bull 1990;24:297–311.

More maps.

Wilson FAW, Scalaidhe SPÓ, Goldman-Radic PS. Dissociation of object and spatial processing domains in primate prefrontal cortex. Science 1993;260:1995–8.

Different neurons code information for stimulus identify versus stimulus location.

Witelson SF, Goldsmith CH. The relationship of hand preference to anatomy of the corpus callosum in men. Brain Res 1991;545:175–82.

The less the preference, the thicker the central portion of the callosum.

Wolfram Gabel R, Maillot C, Koritke JG. Systematisation de l'angioarchitectonie du corps calleux chez l'homme. Acta Anat (Basel). 1991;141:46–50.

Blood supply studies in 20 brains.

Wolpert I. Die Simultanagnosie: Störung der Gesamtauffassung. Z Gesamte Neurol Psychiatrie 1924;93:397.

Early effort to account for the defective description of thematic pictures.

Wood CC, Spencer DD, Allison T et al. Localization of human sensorimotor cortex during surgery by cortical surface recording or somatosensory evoked potentials. J Neurosurg 1988;68:99–111.

Reliable hand areas can be found.

Zatorre RJ, Samson S. Role of the right temporal neocortex in retention of pitch in auditory short term memory. Brain 1991;114:2403–17.

Studies of patients with focal lesions.

Zülch K-J. Brain Tumors. Oxford University Press, Oxford 1969.

26

The Optic Nerve (Cranial Nerve II) and Vision

J. C. Gautier and J. P. Mohr

The retina and the optic pathways subserve vision, the most important sensory system in the human brain. Many diseases with many symptoms and signs can damage the visual system, and they constitute an essential part of clinical neurology. The optical part of the eye, in front of the retina, allows the physician a direct view of the retina, head of the optic nerve, and retinal vessels, which share many normal and pathologic features with intracerebral vessels of the same size. There is much truth in the aphorism, "he who knows neuro-ophthalmology knows neurology."

RETINA AND VISUAL PATHWAY

The visual pathways are basically organized as are other sensory systems with the exception that, like the olfactory nerve (see Ch. 29), the optic nerve, so-named originally because it hangs from the brain as do as the other nerve, is actually a part of the central nervous system itself. Its "peripheral" nerve components are entirely contained within the retina. The system is made up of receptors and three neurons: bipolar, ganglion, and thalamocortical.

Retina

The retina (Figs. 26-1 and 26-2) is a nervous membrane in which the pattern of receptors and neurons is inversed. It is very thin (100 to 350 μm) and transparent, allowing light rays to pass through it before they reach the receptors. These, the rods and cones, are just internal to the pigment epithelium and basal choroidal membrane (Bruch's or Henle's membrane) in a close relationship with the choroid, a pigmented membrane with a rich network of blood vessels. Rods are present throughout the retina and subserve vision in dim illumination. Cones subserve sharp and color

vision. At the posterior pole of the eye in the macula (from the Latin for small spot) and its central part, the fovea (from the Latin for small pit), about 100,000 cones are concentrated in the fovea. In normal photopic vision, objects are focused on the fovea, where central fixation or central vision is concentrated.

From the visual receptors, impulses are transmitted to bipolar cells and then to ganglion cells. Axons of the latter converge on the optic disc or papilla (from the Latin for nipple) located 3 to 4 mm on the nasal side of the fovea, thus forming the optic nerve. Fibers from the macula course straight to the disc; those from the superior and inferior temporal quadrants arch around the macular area. The macular area is devoid of blood vessels, making it optimal for macular stimulation by light rays.

The disc (Plate 26-1) itself is devoid of receptors, and when the visual fields are tested clinically, the area represented by the disc appears as the *blind spot*. When seen through an ophthalmoscope, it is normally well rounded and pale pink (more so on the nasal side), with clear-cut edges (more so on the temporal side). Its depressed center, the pit or cup, is normally symmetric in both eyes.

The central retinal artery emerges from the cup and divides into superior and inferior branches, which in turn give each a temporal and a nasal branch. Consequently, there is a retinal artery branch for each retinal quadrant. In about 15 percent of people, a cilioretinal artery from the posterior ciliary circulation emerges at the temporal side of the disc and supplies a cecocentral retinal area (Plate 26-1). Four retinal veins converge to the disc. They are crossed along their course at varying points by the arteries and then share with them a common adventitial sheath. Blood to the outer layers of the retina, particularly rods and cones, is supplied by

397

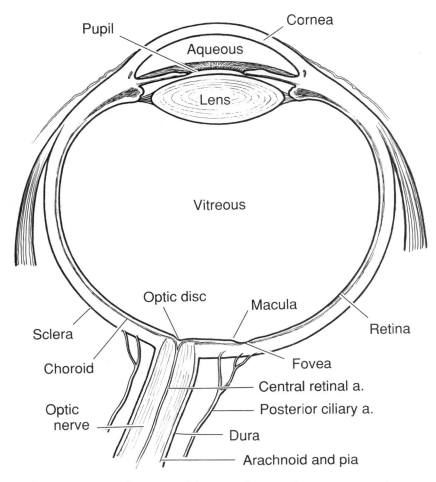

Figure 26-1. Horizontal section of the eye, showing the main anatomic structures.

diffusion from the choroid. Bipolar cells, ganglion cells, and their nerve fibers are supplied by the retinal arteries. Like the brain, the retina has no lymphatic vessels.

As a result of the cameralike optical apparatus of the eye, with a lens inverting and reversing the environmental image, the superior visual field is projected on the inferior retina and the temporal field on the nasal retina. This inversion is retained throughout the visual system: optic nerve, chiasm, optic radiations, and calcarine cortex. Besides, throughout the visual pathways, fibers from the superior retina remain superior and conversely. Lesions of the retina result in various defects of the ipsilateral monocular visual field from blindness to scotomas (from the Greek for obscuration) that reflect the location and shape of the damaged retinal part.

Optic Nerve

The disc is the beginning of the optic nerve. The axons of the ganglion cell leave the eyeball through the lamina cribrosa, which, as is suggested by its name, is a sieve made by holes in the sclera. There, they acquire a myelin sheath with oligodendrocytes. Thus, the optic nerve is not, like the other cranial nerves, covered with Schwann cells for the maintenance of myelin but is, instead, a tract of the central nervous system itself. It courses posteriorly to the optic foramen through which it enters the skull and in which it lies with the ophthalmic artery and branches of the carotid sympathetic plexus. Dura mater surrounds the nerve from the optic foramen to the lamina cribrosa, and the subarachnoid space also extends forward so that the nerve is surrounded by cerebrospinal fluid. Septa of connective tissue from the pia mater divide the nerve in columns. The optic nerve is 4 mm thick, which allows good visualization by computed tomography (CT) and magnetic resonance imaging (MRI). Its length is 25 to 30 mm; the distance from eyeball to optic foramen is 20 mm. Its gently curving, slightly sinuous appearance is, therefore, normal.

Each optic nerve contains 1.1 to 1.2 million fibers. Both optic nerves make up 42 percent of all cranial

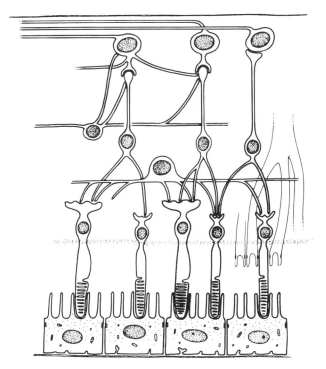

Figure 26-2. Schematic diagram of the neuronal connections and glial structures in the retina, showing the pigment layer below, and neuronal connections linking to the ganglia cell layer.

nerve fibers, a measure of the importance of vision in the human brain. All along the visual pathways, the macular representation (i.e., the number of fibers conveying impulses from the macula) greatly exceeds that of the peripheral retina. In the optic nerve, the macular fibers are central.

The blood supply of the optic nerve comes from the internal carotid artery through the ophthalmic artery. There are two distinct territories. The posterior part of the nerve is supplied by centripetal branches of pial arteries; the head of the nerve (the laminar and prelaminar parts) is supplied by the posterior ciliary arteries and also by the choroid and pial arteries. It was formerly thought that the supply came from an anastomotic circle (of Zinn-Haller), but this appears uncommon. When present, the "circle" is incomplete. Thus, the supply of the nerve head does not depend on the central retinal artery. Histologically, the ciliary and central retinal (after it has entered the optic nerve) arteries are also different. The former are elastic rich and the latter, elastic poor, which probably accounts for their different vulnerability to some pathologic processes (e.g., giant-cell arteritis) (see Ch. 38).

Lesions of the optic nerve result in defects in the monocular field from blindness to central scotomas (Fig. 26-3). The fovea-macular fibers are particularly vulnerable to many pathologic processes, which explains the decrease in visual acuity; central scotomas for color vision are characteristic of early disorders.

Optic Chiasm

The optic chiasm is a flat rectangular white tract (see Fig. 25-1). Optic nerves arrive at its anterior angles, and optic tracts leave at its posterior angles. It lies in the chiasmal cistern of the cerebrospinal fluid in association with important structures: below the sella turcica and pituitary gland, behind the anterior part of the third ventricle, and above the proximal parts of the anterior cerebral arteries and anterior communicating artery, on both sides of the internal carotid arteries as they emerge from the cavernous sinuses.

The chiasm (from the Greek for crossing) is a commissure in which 2.4 million fibers partially decussate. Fibers from the temporal retina pass into the ipsilateral optic tract (i.e., they do not cross). Fibers from the nasal retina cross to pass into the contralateral tract. Inferonasal fibers that course along the anterior notch of the chiasm (i.e., between the optic nerves) bend slightly in the contralateral optic nerve before passing into the optic tract. Nasal macular fibers cross, but temporal macular fibers do not. Fibers from the superior retina remain superior. Finally, the posterior notch of the chiasm (i.e., between the optic tracts) is occupied by superior nasal fibers and macular fibers. From this complex arrangement, it can be understood that the typical field defect of chiasmatic lesions is bitemporal hemianopia from damage to both crossing fibers from the nasal retinal (Fig. 26-3), although many other subtle field defects are possible.

Optic Tract and Lateral Geniculate Body

Each optic tract sweeps posteriorly around the cerebral peduncle along with the anterior choroidal artery and vein of Rosenthal. Just before reaching the lateral geniculate body, the tract gives off a medial arm containing fibers that mediate pupillary impulses and enters the brachium of the superior colliculus (Fig. 26-4). The lateral geniculate body is a separate part of the thalamus, in the roof of the collateral trigone or atrium. It has a conical shape with an inferomedial basis in which the tract fibers enter to synapse with the geniculocalcarine (thalamocortical) neurons. The lateral geniculate body contains six layers of cells numbered from below. Fibers from the ipsilateral eye are in layers two, three, and five, and those from the contralateral eye are in layers one, four, and six.

The optic tract and lateral geniculate body are supplied by the anterior choroidal artery from the internal carotid artery and branches of the posterior cerebral artery from the vertebrobasilar system.

Only one postmortem example of infarction of the

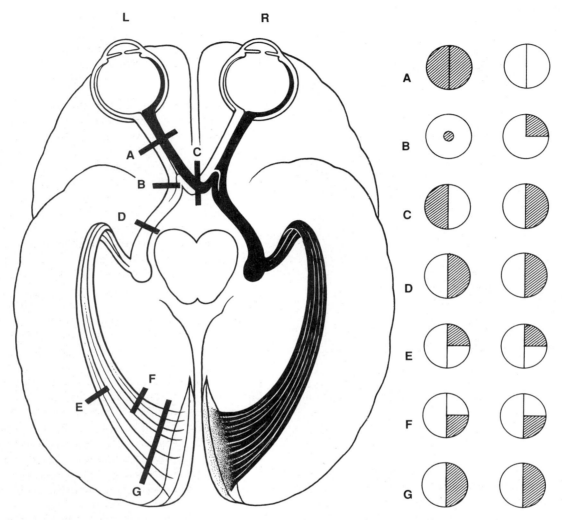

Figure 26-3. The course of the optic pathway depicting the optic nerves, chiasm, tracts, and visual radiations and, at right, the extremes of the visual field disturbances expected from a lesion at each site. Actual lesions rarely are as complete or discrete as shown and frequently yield less complete disturbances than are depicted.

lateral geniculate is known to the authors. In contrast to the usual claim that the fibers of the optic radiations are not well sorted at the level of the lateral geniculate, this patient's visual field defect was strikingly congruous (i.e., showed the same abnormality in the vision of each eye) and demonstrated a defect that was an upper quadrantanopia plus a portion below the horizontal meridian, from 12:00 o'clock to 4:00 o'clock.

Optic Radiations

Axons of cells of the lateral geniculate body leave its superior part to course posteriorly to the calcarine fissure in the occipital pole. Together, they form the optic or visual radiations. Fibers that convey impulses of the superior retina course straight to the occipital

cortex along the wall of the posterior horn of the lateral ventricle. Inferior fibers loop downward and laterally around the tip of the temporal horn of the lateral ventricle (Meyer's or Archambault's loop, named for Adolph Meyer [1866–1950, German-born American neurologist] and L. Archambault [1879–1940, American neurologist]) before coursing posteriorly to the calcarine fissure. Fibers pass above and under the occipital horn of the lateral ventricle to end in the medial aspect of the occipital lobe in the striate cortex of the calcarine fissure.

The optic radiations receive their blood supply from the internal carotid artery by way of the anterior choroidal artery (anterior part); the middle cerebral artery (middle part), from the vertebrobasilar system by way of the posterior cerebral artery (posterior part).

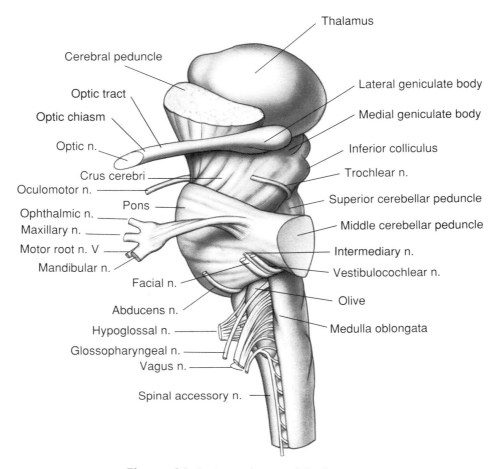

Figure 26-4. Lateral view of the brainstem.

The typical field defect of lesions of the radiations is homonymous hemianopia in which vision is impaired in the temporal and nasal fields of the same visual space (i.e., right or left) (Fig. 26-3).

Nongeniculate Visual Systems

Two visual systems that do not take the geniculo-occipital cortex route have been identified. The first, centered on the superior colliculus, deals with localization of of objects in space. In the superior colliculus and in the pulvinar, with which it is linked, there is a retinotopic representation. This system steers movements of the eyes that foveate an object entering into or moving across the visual field. Fibers from the superior colliculus inhibit pause cells in the paramedian prepontine reticular formation (see Ch. 28), which allows saccades to occur. On the other hand, cells of the superior colliculus are inhibited by fibers from the substantia nigra, which oppose incessant movements of the eyes. This system could account for some perception of movement in blind fields, particularly in occipital blindness (see Ch. 25), an occurrence known

as the Riddoch phenomenon (George Riddoch, British Neurologist, 1889–1947).

The second system, sometimes termed the accessory optic system, is made of retinal fibers that project to nuclei in the midbrain and pons. Inputs take part in feeding the cerebellum with data that permit computation of corrections of the position of the head according to movements of the eyes.

Occipital Cortex

The primary visual cortex (area 17) is termed the *striate cortex* because of the stria of Gennari, a thin myelinated tract that is a prominent feature of its fourth or granular layer. Optic radiations synapse in this fourth layer. Area 17 lies mainly in the depth of the fissure; only approximately one-third is on the surface of the brain (Fig. 26-5). Posteriorly, it extends 1–2 cm onto the lateral aspect of the occipital lobe. Anteroposteriorly, the striate cortex measures about 5 cm, and the macular representation occupies about the posterior 2.5 cm, including the most posterior part of the lateral surface of the occipital lobe. Fibers from the

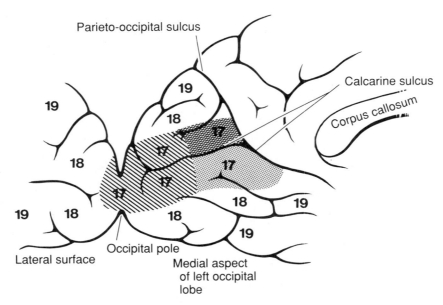

Figure 26-5. Mesial view of the occipital pole (right side of figure) demonstrating the topographic projection of the visual fields on the calcarine cortex and the extension of area 17 around the occipital pole to the lateral convexity (left side).

superior retina occupy the superior lip of the fissure and those from the lower, the lower.

The blood supply of area 17 depends mainly on the calcarine artery, a branch of the posterior cerebral artery. The middle cerebral artery supplies the part of the striate cortex on the lateral surface of the occipital lobe. There are individual variations in the territories of the posterior and middle cerebral arteries. In case of occlusion of one of them, a compensatory circulation may come from the other.

Area 17 is surrounded by area 18 (parastriate cortex), which is richly connected with area 18 of the other hemisphere but appears to have little connections in the ipsilateral hemisphere. The interhemispheric pathway crosses through the splenium of the corpus callosum. It would appear to integrate the two halves of the visual fields. It is also likely that, from the posterior parietal lobe (Brodmann's area 39), parietofrontal pathways play a role in horizontal fast eye movements (saccades) and parietomesencephalic pathways in horizontal smooth pursuit movements. Area 18 is surrounded by area 19 (peristriate cortex), which extends mainly onto the lateral aspect of the occipital lobe up to the posterior parts of the parietal and temporal lobes (Fig. 26-5). Its blood supply there depends on the middle cerebral artery. Area 19 plays a major role in the integration of visual messages.

The typical field defect of damage to the calcarine cortex is homonymous hemianopia (Fig. 26-3). Damage to the superior lip or inferior lip of the calcarine fissure results in inferior or superior altitudinal hemianopia. Destruction to both areas 17 or both radiations results in occipital (so-called cortical) blindness.

EXAMINATION OF VISION

Visual Acuity

Visual acuity is essentially the power of resolution of the eye. Different methods of evaluation are used in different countries. For example, the patient may face a Snellen's chart at a distance of 6 m (using the metric system), or the patient may stand at a distance of 20 feet (using the English-American system) and read down to the last legible line. The results are reported with two figures (e.g., 6/6 [metric] or 20/20 [English-American]). The figures compare the patient's vision with normal vision; a score of 6/20 would mean that, at 6 m, the patient could only read what a normal eye would have read at 20 m.

In neurologic practice, near cards are convenient. Each eye must be examined separately. The patient wears corrective glasses. Poor vision with glasses means either that glasses are inadequate or that there is another pathologic condition. This may be resolved by the stenopeic or pinhole test in which the patient looks at a distant object through a small hole in a cardboard. This ensures only parallel rays pass through the pinhole, eliminating the need for focus, and concentrates light onto the center of cornea and onto fovea. Poor vision that is improved by looking through a pinhole is due to a refractive error.

Examination of Fundus Oculi

Funduscopy is part of every clinical neurologic examination, whatever the patient's primary complaint. Skill and experience stem from practice. Beginners are encouraged to buy their own instrument and look at as many fundi as possible.

The examination is carried out in a dim room with the direct ophthalmoscope, which provides a ×15 magnification. The right eye must be examined with the right eye, with the ophthalmoscope in the right hand and the examiner on the right side of the patient. Neurologists with one poor eye either hold their breath or look at the fundus from behind the supine patient. The latter is instructed to look at a distant object, not at the light. Ophthalmoscopes are provided with beams of various sizes and colors. In neurologic practice, the larger round white beam is generally convenient. A smaller beam would be used for small pupils or strong glare from the iris. Many ophthalmoscopes are supplied with batteries. As soon as these begin to wear out, they should be changed. The pupil must not be dilated routinely for several reasons. First, it is usually unnecessary in neurologic practice. Second, in certain settings (e.g., head trauma), the changes in pupillary diameter are an essential part of neurologic monitoring. Third, it may be dangerous in people at risk for narrow-angle glaucoma; before dilation, patients must always be questioned on this point. Fourth, the pupil must not be dilated in patients with an artificial lens implant. When dilation is mandatory, short-acting drops must be used, and 2 percent pilocarpine is instilled at the end of the examination.

Transparency of the parts of the eye that are in front of the retina (Fig. 26-1) can be assessed by looking at the pupil from 15 to 30 cm with high plus lenses provided that the pupil has a diameter of at least 5 to 7 mm. To begin, one obtains the red reflex (i.e., the pupil appears red, although with the naked eye it is black). This red hue is due to the red-pink color of the choroidal background. With +10 to +2, vitreous opacities can be seen. Then, from −1 to +1, the retina comes into focus. The examination should first note the *disc*, which is reached by following a vessel as it gets broader and is examined from out to in, that is, the edge, color, vessels, and cup. Some frequent benign features are visibility of small pits of the lamina cribrosa, early myelination of the nerve fibers (i.e., in front of the lamina cribrosa), presence of drusen (i.e., colloid bodies, buried in the disc, with a bunch-of-grapes appearance), and a pigmented crescent on the temporal side of the disc. It is customary next to examine the *macula*, two disc diameters on the temporal

side, which appears as a pinhead point of bright light reflection. In older patients, it is often pigmented. Heavy pigmentation and hemorrhages point to macular degeneration. The rest of the *retina* is normally pink because of the choroid background. It is more or less pigmented, according to ethnic characteristics. Lastly, the *vessels* are followed up to two disc diameters from the disc. Arteries are bright red. Normally, their walls are not seen. What is seen indeed is the column of red cells, with often a central light streak caused by the reflection of light on the posterior wall of the vessel. Veins are bluish, larger than arteries, in a proportion of about 5:3. In many normal sitting subjects, the veins appear to pulsate, but an absence of pulsations is not necessarily pathologic. Arteries cross over the veins without a change in the caliber of the vein.

Myopia and hypermetropia are common conditions with particular fundus features with which one must be familiar. In myopia, the disc is larger and paler than normal, frequently with a *myopia crescent* (i.e., a whitish crescent on one side of the disc). The choroid may be thin, which gives a pale tinge to the fundus, with sometimes visible areas of white sclera. In hypermetropia, the disc is smaller and pinker.

Visual Fields

Confrontation

Each eye is assessed separately. The patient and examiner face each other at a distance of about 1 m, and the patient is instructed to look steadily into the corresponding examiner's eye (e.g., patient's right eye into examiner's left eye). For a quick assessment of the peripheral fields, index fingers are moved well above and then well below the horizontal meridian of the field. First one and then the other index finger is moved, then both are moved simultaneously since in some cases the patient perceives a single stimulus appropriately but only one of two simultaneous stimuli.

Then the inner and central field are examined using a small white target. With cooperating patients, it is easy to localize the blind spot, which may be enlarged in case of papilledema. Scotomas are found and outlined by bringing the white target from outward to the point of fixation along a number of radii in the field. Field defects that result from a lesion of the macular fibers may be evident with red targets only. This is especially true for lesions of the chiasm because macular fibers course in the anterior notch of the chiasm (see above). One must remember that sensitivity to red normally fades out beyond the central 20 degrees of the field.

In another method, the examiner presents simultaneously one hand in the temporal field and the other hand in the nasal field. In a depressed field, the hand appears darker or blurred. This is a simple and sensitive method that avoids the gross stimulus of movement.

When a field defect is only suspected or its characterization is insufficient, examination with Bjerrum's tangent screen or Amsler's charts should be performed. Field defects are reported on the charts as visual field data not as visual lesions (i.e., what the patient sees is outlined).

In the obtunded or uncooperative patient, visual fields may be roughly evaluated by bringing attractive objects in the peripheral field or by the presence or absence of a blink in response to a threatening quick movement of a finger toward the eye from the peripheral visual field.

Ophthalmodynamometry

By exertion of a graded pressure on the eyeball, intraocular pressure is increased. When it equates with the diastolic systemic arterial pressure the retinal arteries pulsate. With still increased pressure on the eye, intraocular pressure equates with systolic systemic pressure when blood flow in the retinal arteries ceases. This is the basis of ophthalmodynamometry, which measures the pressure in the ophthalmic artery and gives a fair idea of the pressure in the internal carotid artery. The main interest lies in the comparison of figures from both eyes. Formerly, ophthalmodynamometry was much valued in carotid artery disease, but its results are often open to question. It has been superseded by ultrasonic examinations.

Visual-Evoked Potentials

Intermittent visual stimuli determine transient electrical changes along the optic pathways. With temporally and spatially well-defined series of stimuli, electrical events are reproducible with specific characteristics. These may be recorded from the scalp with summation and computer-averaging techniques. The usual stimulus is a black-and-white checkerboard reversed at set intervals. The two most significant signals are N70, a negative wave that occurs at 70 ms, and the macular-derived P100, a positive wave that occurs at 100 ms. Transient visual-evoked potentials are useful in many pathologic conditions, especially optic nerve lesions (see Ch. 11).

Fluorescein Angiography

Fluorescein, injected intravenously, outlines vessels of the fundus when looked at with the ophthalmoscope or photographed with blue light. It does not leak through normal vessels. A main interest for the neurologist is the diagnosis of papilledema from pseudopapilledema. In the former only, the dye leaks out the vessels of the disc with a fluorescence that lasts several minutes. Drusen autofluoresce, but because there is no leakage of dye, fluorescein angiography is also useful in the diagnosis of papilledema, which some drusen may mimic closely. The patient must be told that the skin and urine will be yellow for 1 day.

VISUAL SYNDROMES

Retina

Degenerative retinal diseases may involve the pigment epithelium and photoreceptors layers in retinitis pigmentosa. The most important instances in adult neurology are Refsum's disease and Kearns-Sayre's syndrome. Treatment with some phenothiazine derivatives at high dosages may be a cause. Macular degeneration is a frequent and distressing cause of reduced vision in aging people.

Retinal arteries may undergo chronic changes or acute occlusions or ruptures. It is unlikely that true atherosclerosis develops on the central retinal artery and its branches because atherosclerosis is usually absent on vessels of such small size (diameters about 180 and 90 μm, respectively). In chronic hypertension, the media of the arterial wall undergoes hypertrophy, giving a broader than normal light reflex. Veins are compressed where they are crossed by arteries (nicking) because of the common adventitial sheath. With more severe atherosclerosis, retinal arteries assume a copper-wire and then a silver-wire appearance. In acute hypertension, arteries are narrowed, either diffusely or with focal constrictions. Soft exudates (cotton-wool patches) result from the interruption of orthograde and retrograde axonal flow with accumulation of organelles at the edges of infarcted areas. Deep hard glistening exudates are mostly seen in severe hypertension associated with diabetes mellitus. They predominate around the fovea and have a radiating disposition (macular star).

The shape of hemorrhages depends on the pattern of the fibers among which they develop. Splinter, flame-shaped, or linear hemorrhages are found in the superficial nerve fiber layer. They are present in hypertension and blood disorders. They may have a white or yellow center as a result of an accumulation of leukocytes (Roth's spot). These are observed in subacute bacterial endocarditis, blood diseases, or embolic retinopathy. Small circular, well-defined hemorrhages (*dot and blot*) develop in the outer plexiform layer. They are found in diabetes mellitus, occlusions of carotid arteries, and blood diseases with high viscosity. Hemorrhages with a horizontal top and curved inferior limit, resembling a boat, develop between the retina and the hyaloid membrane that surrounds the vitreous. These preretinal or subhyaloid hemorrhages result from a sudden increase in intracranial pressure (e.g., subarachnoid hemorrhage or trauma).

Infarction results from permanent or long enough transient occlusions of retinal arteries. Brief transient occlusions result in transient disorders.

Infarction as a result of occlusion of the central retinal artery causes a sudden painless loss of vision of the eye. Where there is a cilioretinal artery of good size, central vision may be spared. The arteries are pale and small, and the retina is pale and edematous with a cloudy appearance. By contrast, the macula in front of which there are no fibers (see above) stands out as a bright red area (cherry-red spot). With arterial flow being absent or slow, the venous flow is segmented (cattle trucking). After edema has subsided, the retina is pale, and the optic disc becomes pale because of the disappearance of the axons of the infarcted ganglion cells (optic atrophy). Infarcts caused by retinal branch occlusions are sectorial, with a corresponding sectorial visual defect. Permanent occlusions of the central retinal artery and its branches are mostly embolic (atherosclerosis or cardiac disease). In patients over 50 years of age, giant-cell arteritis must always be considered (see below).

Occlusions of brief duration of the central retinal artery and branches cause amaurosis fugax (i.e., transient monocular blindness), which is a sudden painless loss of the whole or part (frequently superior or inferior) of a monocular field. In many patients, blindness progresses and regresses as if a shade was pulled down or up or rarely from the side. Most attacks last less than 10 minutes and many less than 5. The main cause in people older than age 40 is atherosclerosis, with the most frequent lesion being a stenosis at the bifurcation of the common carotid artery. Examination of the retinal arteries may find yellow-orange cholesterol crystals, usually at bifurcations and more often on the temporal retina. They are flat small plaques that do not necessarily interrupt blood flow. They are debris of an upstream, usually carotid, atherosclerotic plaque. In a few instances, during an attack, long white-gray bodies have been seen progressing slowly or intermittently in the arteries. They are thought to be platelet aggregates, built on and detached from a similar atherosclerotic lesion. In amaurosis fugax, the risk of permanent visual loss is relatively low, but transient monocular blindness is a good marker of atherosclerosis and of an increased risk of stroke and myocardial infarction. Cardiac embolism, low-pressure retinopathy caused by multiple occlusions of extracranial cerebral arteries, high blood viscosity, giant-cell arteritis, glaucoma, migraine, and papilledema are other causes. In the young patient, amaurosis fugax is often idiopathic and benign; invasive investigations must be considered cautiously.

Occlusion of the central retinal vein occurs at the lamina cribrosa. The onset is a severe painless loss of monocular vision. Usually, light and hand movement perception are retained. In severe cases, the fundus shows massive hemorrhage. The veins, where they can be seen, are dark, dilated, and tortuous. Numerous exudates are present. Occlusion of branches, often the superior temporal, appears to occur at an arteriovenous nicking (see above). The usual basic condition is atherosclerosis, and the main cause is hypertension. Associated diabetes mellitus is common. Blood dyscrasias with increased viscosity are also causal factors.

Diabetic Retinopathy

Diabetic retinopathy is so common in diabetic patients and the neurologic complications of diabetes mellitus are so common that the neurologist must be acquainted with the features of the fundus. Most of the lesions tend to predominate at the posterior pole of the eye. Microaneurysms are the first to appear. They are discrete, minute (20 to 90 μm) red dots. Fluorescein angiography visualizes a good number that cannot be seen with the ophthalmoscope. Hemorrhages are of the dot-and-blot type or linear. There are soft and hard exudates. Neovascularization (i.e., new vessel formation) is characteristic. New vessels may grow into the vitreous, with a high risk of severe hemorrhage.

Optic Nerve

Optic Disc

Papilledema is important for the neurologist because it implies increased intracranial pressure, suspicion of a tumor, and immediate investigations. The mechanisms of papilledema are not entirely clear. A basic fact is elevated pressure of the cerebrospinal fluid around the intraorbital part of the nerve. This could theoretically hinder flow in the central retinal vein, but this does not explain satisfactorily the development and appearance of papilledema. It would rather seem that high pressure around the nerve hinders axoplasmic flow, with consequent swelling of the axons at the nerve head.

The usual clinical presentation is swelling of both discs with no visual impairment. In early papilledema, the disc is pinker than normal, and there is slight blurring and elevation of the nasal edge. Venous pulsations are absent, but they can be normal. Conversely, the presence of pulsations of veins makes papilledema very unlikely. With full-fledged papilledema, the "angry" papilla is elevated above the retinal surface, numerous small vessels run on its surface, and the cup may be filled. The margins are blurred with poor visibility of vessels. There are peripapillary hemorrhages and exudates. When necessary, fluorescein angiography could help in the diagnosis with pseudo-papilledema (see above). In malignant hypertension, there may be papilledema, but in addition, there are florid retinal lesions.

Unilateral papilledema is a feature of compression of the ipsilateral optic nerve by an intraorbital space-occupying lesion (e.g., a sheath meningioma). Optic atrophy on the side of a meningioma near the optic foramen may coexist with contralateral papilledema in the rare Foster-Kennedy's syndrome.

Papilledema must be relieved as soon as possible because vision is at stake. Blackouts of a few seconds, and thus somewhat distinct from the more protracted amaurosis fugax of carotid disease (see above), are classically ominous because secondary optic atrophy with loss of vision could develop rapidly. The disc becomes pale with grayish and slightly blurred edges as a result of gliosis. Papilledema may also be due to pseudotumor cerebri and drugs such as vitamin A, steroids, tetracyclines, and nalidixic acid.

Papillitis

The clinical presentation of papillitis is swollen discs similar to those of papilledema but with severe loss of vision and often deep eye pain (see below).

Optic Atrophy

In optic atrophy, the axons of the ganglion cells are damaged and eventually die. Secondary optic atrophy is due to unrelieved papilledema (see above). In primary optic atrophy, the fibers are damaged by various causes: inflammatory, metabolic (inherited or acquired), vascular, or compressive. With severe atrophy, the disc is chalk white with sharp edges and very few vessels on its surface. The pits of the lamina cribrosa are too clearly visible. Where the macular bundle is particularly damaged, pallor predominates on the temporal side of the disc. There may be blindness. In less severe cases, there is loss of visual acuity and color perception, and there is a sluggish pupillary light reflex. The typical field defect is a central scotoma. When optic atrophy is due to retinal or nerve infarction, the defects may be total, altitudinal, or sectorial. Cases of primary optic atrophy coming to the neurologist are usually monocular, although in some heredo-degenerative diseases of the nervous system (e.g., Charcot-Marie-Tooth disease or Friedreich's ataxia) bilateral optic atrophy may occur. Toxic, nutritional, and hereditary cases are bilateral.

Ischemic Optic Neuropathy

Usually, ischemic anterior optic neuropathy occurs, which means infarction of the laminar and prelaminar part of the nerve. The frequent cause is occlusion of posterior ciliary arteries, but occlusion of the central retinal artery or ophthalmic artery is possible. Visual loss and field defects depend on the extent and location of the lesion. Often, the sudden painless loss of vision is noticed on awakening. The disc is usually swollen with small linear hemorrhages. There is little recovery. After some weeks, optic atrophy develops.

In a patient over 50 years of age, giant-cell arteritis is the first diagnosis considered because of the high risk of involvement of the other eye and therapeutic implications. Prior to infarction, amaurosis fugax may have been neglected. Temporal and scalp arteries may be inflamed and tender, and there may be jaw claudication, pain in muscles and joints (polymyalgia rheumatica), fever, sweating, weight loss, malaise, and asthenia. The erythrocyte sedimentation rate is nearly always increased in the range of 80 to 100, but this may be lacking or moderate. High-dose corticosteroid therapy is an emergency treatment. The results of biopsy of a temporal artery must not be awaited before starting therapy. Besides, the arterial biopsy findings may be negative in this segmental arterial disease.

The most common type of anterior optic ischemic neuropathy, however, remains idiopathic, the so-called arteriosclerotic type. Its mechanisms are obscure. An absent or small cup on the disc is frequent, resulting in packing of the nerve fibers in the lamina cribrosa. This type of nerve infarction is rarely heralded by amaurosis fugax. It frequently involves the central part of the nerve with a severe visual loss. In one of two or three patients, the second eye is involved within months or years. Migraine and polycythemia are other causal factors of ischemic optic neuropathy.

Optic Neuritis or Retrobulbar Neuritis

This is a common syndrome at any age, particularly in young adults and children. Optic neuritis (or neuropathy) may be unilateral or bilateral. Unilateral optic neuritis begins by a visual haze, which progresses over a few days, sometimes to near blindness. There is discomfort or pain in and above the eye, particularly on eye movements. The fundus is normal, although in a number of cases, there may be some disc swelling. Later, the disc will be pale (more so on the temporal side). The field defect is a central scotoma and, in a few patients, a total monocular blindness. In moderately severe cases, exercise or a hot bath may transiently exacerbate the visual loss (Uhthoff's sign). After 1 to 2 weeks, some degree of recovery is usual to a good functional level. However, in patients with apparent full recovery, color vision may remain impaired. Visual-evoked potentials are a sensitive examination and characteristically show a delay in the P100 with a normal or abnormal waveform.

Unilateral optic neuritis in a young patient, in

northern countries at least, raises immediately the possible diagnosis of multiple sclerosis. Where the diagnosis has not been previously established, MRI has superseded the examination of the cerebrospinal fluid for slight lymphocytic pleocytosis and oligoclonal bands. In young patients with clinically isolated optic neuritis, MRI shows brain lesions in about 50 to 60 percent at first examination. In a young patient with no previous history, the risk of multiple sclerosis has been estimated from 35 to 75 percent. Among the risk factors, the presence of HLA-DR2 might be taken into account.

In neuromyelitis optica (Devic's disease), generally considered a variant of multiple sclerosis, severe visual loss is bilateral (successive or simultaneous) to be followed quickly by paraplegia.

In children, optic neuritis is often bilateral and presents as a papillitis (i.e., the disc is swollen with hemorrhages). The episode follows diseases such as measles, mumps, chicken pox, or infectious mononucleosis. The prognosis in regard to multiple sclerosis is far better than in adults.

In many cases of unilateral optic neuritis, no cause is found. Rare but important causes include orbital cellulitis, dysthyroid states, radiation, mucocele of the sphenoid sinus, and carcinomatous meningitis. In compression (meningiomas, pituitary tumors, or aneurysms and tumors of the optic nerve), the course is usually relentless. Exceptions can obviously occur, and whenever the slightest doubt might exist, CT or, preferrably, MRI must be performed. Bilateral optic neuritis may be successive in multiple sclerosis. True bilateral concomitant optic neuropathies are characterized by the often insidious and generally slowly but sometimes acute (methanol) or subacute loss of visual acuity with central scotomas. Vitamin B$_{12}$ deficiency is a classical cause. Tobacco (pipe) and alcohol are commonly invoked causes in which deficiencies in vitamins B$_1$ and B$_{12}$ and other nutritional disorders play a role. Many drugs may be toxic to the optic nerve, and a careful inquiry is mandatory. Halogenated hydroxyquinolines have caused subacute myelo-optic neuropathy in Japan and elsewhere. Jamaican optic neuropathy is peculiar to young blacks. Among relatively common drugs, chloramphenicol, isoniazid, digitalis, disulfiram, and streptomycin have been implicated. Finally, heredodegenerative diseases and ophthalmologic causes of bilateral progressive visual loss must be considered.

Chiasm

With the exceptions of pituitary apoplexy and some leaking aneurysms, interferences with chiasmal function result from slow-growing adjacent tumors: pituitary adenomas, meningiomas, craniopharyngiomas, aneurysms, and granulomas, as in sarcoidosis. Metastatic tumors are intermediate with a subacute course. The disc is pale in about 50 percent of the cases.

Visual fields should be clinically plotted eye by eye with a red and white target. The typical defect is bitemporal hemianopia. When the pressure from the lesion comes from above, the defect begins and predominates in the lower bitemporal quadrants and, when it comes from below, in the upper bitemporal quadrants. Commonly, one temporal field is severely affected while the other shows a small defect only. CT or, preferably, MRI is mandatory, and angiography is often required.

Optic Tract and Radiations

Because homonymous hemifield fibers, mainly superior ones, join in the tract fairly near to the chiasm, lesions of the tract tend to result in incongruous homonymous hemianopia (i.e., the defect is not similar in the two eyes). This is contrasted with congruous homonymous hemianopia, which suggests a lesion of the calcarine cortex. However, even with calcarine lesions, precise congruity may be lacking. To elicit Wernicke's hemipupillary defect, strict methodologic conditions are mandatory.

Lesions of the optic radiations are mostly vascular in origin. Tumors rank second and trauma, third. Anterior temporal lesions may involve Meyer's loop, resulting in a homonymous superior quadrantanopia or a homonymous hemianopia that predominates in the upper quadrants. Lesions of the superior part of the radiations in the inferior part of the parietal lobe result in a homonymous hemianopia more severe in the lower quadrants, and the reverse is true for lesions of the inferior radiations in the temporal lobe. Destruction of the calcarine cortex, usually by infarction, results in a homonymous hemianopia, which in principle, spares macular vision because macular projections extend well over the occipital tip on the lateral aspect of the brain and are supplied by the middle cerebral artery. On the other hand, patients with a profound lasting arterial hypotension, such as during cardiac arrest, may have large central scotomas caused by infarction of the macular cortical projection in the border zones between distal middle and posterior cerebral arteries. Only the superior or inferior bank of the calcarine fissure can be infarcted, resulting in altitudinal hemianopia. After destruction of both occipital poles, generally as a result of embolism, there is occipital blindness in which the patient often has anosognosia (i.e., the patient is not aware of the blindness probably because the very notion that vision exists has disappeared). In this setting, denial of blindness is frequent. The pupillary reactions are of course normal. Occipital blindness in a transient vertebrobasilar ischemic attack is not rare. In visual agnosias, the patients are able to tell the shapes, colors, and sizes of objects, but they do not know what they are (i.e., they cannot identify them). They can do this through another sensory channel (e.g., touch). Inability to recognize letters or words visually is alexia, a part of aphasia. These disorders result in broad terms from lesions of areas 18 and 19 (see above). Alexia results from lesions of the angular gyrus in the dominant hemisphere. There is an agnosia for faces, called prosopagnosia, and an inability to understand visually the meaning of an entire picture while details are well recognized. This is called simultanagnosia.

Deformations of images are usually of retinal origin. Bilateral macropsia or micropsia, however, is due to temporal lobe disease, often as part of an epileptic seizure. In lesions near the vestibular nuclei in the brainstem or with parietal lesions, objects may appear tilted.

Visual hallucinations (i.e., visual perceptions without an object in the exterior world) may be zigzags, fortifications, or spectra and are common in migraine. Elaborate hallucinations, with persons, or landscapes, suggest occipitotemporal lesions and are often part of an epileptic seizure or part of the withdrawal syndrome from ethanol or barbiturates. A visual image may persist after the object has disappeared. This persistence is called palinopsia, which occurs in depressed but not blind fields.

COMMON OCULAR DISEASES FOR THE NEUROLOGIST

Before reaching the retina, light rays must got through the tissues and refractile media of the eye (Fig. 26-1), diseases of which may hinder vision and also the examination of the fundus. Therefore, neurologists must be acquainted with the most common of them.

Conjunctivitis is usually of no neurologic significance.

Corneal opacities are mostly scars from infections and trauma and can result from a wide array of metabolic disorders. Corneal clouding is a feature of several hereditary metabolic diseases of infancy and childhood. A golden-brown corneal ring (Kayser-Fleischer ring) is diagnostic of hepatolenticular degeneration.

In the *anterior chamber* (Fig. 26-6), the main pathologic condition is glaucoma, which is elevated intraocular pressure caused by a bad flow of the aqueous fluid. The latter is secreted by the ciliary process, part of the ciliary body in the posterior chamber (Fig. 26-6), which then flows behind the iris and through the pupil into the anterior chamber. The fluid flows out from the anterior chamber by passing into Schlemm's

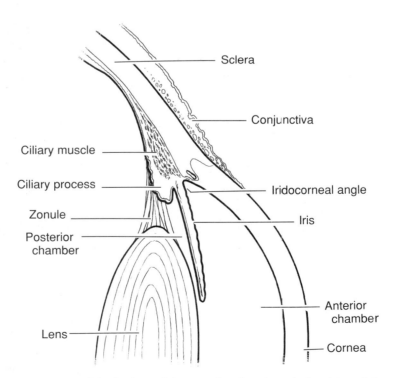

Figure 26-6. Cross section of the limbus of the eye showing the relationships of the canal of Schlemm, iridocorneal angle, iris, and ciliary process.

canal in the iridocorneal angle made by iris and cornea. Normal pressure is about 15 mmHg. When it exceeds 20 mmHg, the cup of the optic disc becomes excavated, and vision is greatly endangered.

Chronic glaucoma is a common condition, particularly over 40 years of age. Most cases have a normal iridocorneal angle (open-angle glaucoma). The outflow of the aqueous fluid is impaired for generally unknown reasons, although there is often a family history. A few patients have a narrow iridocorneal angle and also a narrow anterior chamber. This is narrow-angle glaucoma, which involves a risk of acute glaucoma because of acute closure of the angle. This acute closure may result from dilation of the pupil when the iris is tucked up in the narrow iridocorneal angle. There may be also an abnormal outflow of fluid between the iris and lens that builds up pressure in the posterior chamber and pushes forward the base of the iris, thus contributing to angle closure.

Acute narrow-angle glaucoma can thus be precipitated by mydriatic drops. In acute glaucoma, the eye is red, the pupil is dilated, the cornea is hazy, vision is reduced, and there is pain in and around the eye. Nausea and vomiting may be prominent. The eyeball is stone hard (pressure can be elevated to 60 mmHg or more). Acute glaucoma is an immediate and major threat to vision. Emergency measures are instillation of miotic drops: pilocarpine 4 percent, two drops every 5 minutes, acetazolamide or mannitol intravenously, and glycerol orally. An ophthalmologic opinion must be obtained without delay.

Neurologists must also keep in mind that many common neurologic drugs (e.g., those used in parkinsonism and the tricyclic antidepressants) are dangerous in patients with narrow iridocorneal glaucoma. When mandatory, their use implies careful ophthalmologic monitoring.

The *lens* is a transparent, elastic (allowing accommodation) tissue with highly specific structural and biochemical characteristics. Being avascular, its nutritional elements (e.g., glucose) come from the aqueous fluid. This accounts for its high vulnerability to metabolic disorders. Changes are mainly opacities (i.e., cataracts). The common causes of cataract are aging and diabetes mellitus. Cataract may be the cause of monocular diplopia. It is a feature of myotonic dystrophy (see Ch. 82).

The *vitreous* is a viscous gel closely packed against the retina, ciliary body, and lens. Tearing of retinal or ciliary vessels may cause vitreous hemorrhage. Vitreous hemorrhages are a main feature of Eales' disease in which stroke and white matter lesions have been reported. Floaters are a frequent source of anxiety. They are gray spots that move slowly when the head has just moved and are mainly noticed in bright light (mountains or seashore). They are small particles due to physicochemical changes in the vitreous and are benign. However, a sudden flurry with flashes of light would suggest retinal detachment.

The *uvea* is composed of the iris, ciliary body, and choroid. Iritis is a disease of the iris, cyclitis of the ciliary body, and iridocyclitis of both. Iridocyclitis is termed anterior uveitis. Disease of the choroid, often associated with retinal involvement (chorioretinitis), is termed posterior uveitis. Uveitis may be infectious, parasitic, dysimmune, or frequently of unknown origin. It may be associated with meningitis and encephalitis in Vogt-Koyanagi's syndrome, Harada's disease, and Behçet's disease.

ANNOTATED BIBLIOGRAPHY

Bernstein EF (ed). Amaurosis Fugax. Springer Verlag, New York, 1988.

All aspects and problems of amaurosis fugax with anatomic updates of optic nerve vasculature.

Brodal A. The Cranial Nerves. Anatomy and Anatomico-Clinical Correlations. 2nd Ed. Blackwell, Oxford, 1962.

A classic.

Carpenter MB, Sutin J. Human Neuroanatomy. 8th Ed. Williams & Wilkins, Baltimore, 1983.

Reference book.

Cogan DG. Neurology of the Visual System. CC Thomas, Sprinfield, IL, 1966.

A classic.

Fisher CM. Some neuroophthalmological observations. J Neurol Neurosurg Psychiatry 1967;30:383–92.

Clinical pearls.

Glaser JS. Neuro-Ophthalmology. 2nd Ed. JB Lippincott, Philadelphia, 1990.

A scholarly book that reflects also the best down-to-earth experience.

Jacobs L, Kinkel PR, Kinkel WR. Silent brain lesions in patients with isolated idiopathic optic neuritis. Arch Neurol 1986;43:452.

MRI showed CT missed multiple sclerosis lesions in one-half of the cases.

McDonald WI. Diseases of the Optic Nerve. In Asbury AK, McKhann GM, McDonald WI (eds). Diseases of the Nervous System Clinical Neurobiology. WB Saunders, Philadelphia, 1991.

A good update with much experience.

McLeod D. Reappraisal of the retinal cotton-wool spot: a discussion paper. J R Soc Med 1981;74:682.

Clear, concise, and convincing demonstration of the pathogenesis of soft retinal exudates.

Mohr JP, Sidman M, Stoddard LT, Leicester J. Right hemianopia with memory and color deficits in circumscribed left posterior cerebral artery territory infarction. Neurology 1971;21:1105–13.

Lateral geniculate infarct with quadrantanopia and sectoranopia.

Ormerod IEC, Miller DH, McDonald WI et al. The role of NMR imaging in the assessment of multiple sclerosis and isolated neurological lesions. A quantitative study. Brain 1987;110:1579–616.

A nice MRI study of multiple sclerosis, optic neuritis, and related problems.

Wilkinson IMS, Russell RWR. Arteries of the head and neck in giant-cell arteritis. Arch Neurol 1972;27:378.

An article on elastic-rich and elastic-poor arteries with seminal ideas on giant-cell arteritis.

27
The Pupil

J. C. Gautier and J. P. Mohr

The pupil (Latin: *pupa*, little doll, which is said to have been used to describe the human pupil because a tiny image of the beholder is reflected in it) is the name given to the hole in the iris (from the Greek for rainbow). It regulates the amount of light that enters the eye. The size of the pupil changes from moment to moment to adapt to changes in the level of illumination in the environment by the antagonistic balanced control of the parasympathetic and sympathetic systems on the muscles of the iris. The pupil size is reduced by the action of the circular pupilloconstrictor sphincter, controlled by parasympathetic innervation. Dilation is mediated by the sympathetic-dependent radial pupillodilator muscle fibers. These pupillary-controlling muscles are called *internal* or *intrinsic* as opposed to the *external* or *extrinsic* muscles that move the eyeball.

Pupillary tonus and movements are reflex activities with a reflex arc at the level of the brainstem and are also controlled by higher (hemispheric) structures. The documentation of the basic reflexes of the pupil are of such vital importance that a clinical examination might be said to be incomplete until the pupils have been examined.

NORMAL PUPILS

Normal pupils are central, circular, and symmetric in size. Inequalities are called anisocoria; those up to 1 mm are common and considered normal. The size of the pupil commonly undergoes slight variations, known as hippus. Constriction is called miosis, and dilation is mydriasis.

The examination is made in dim light, and each eye is examined separately. A hand-held magnifying lens is recommended. To diagnose an unreactive pupil, the light that illuminates the retina must be bright, but the light of the ophthalmoscope is not bright enough.

To assess a problem of pupillary size of unknown duration, old photographs may be useful.

Pupillary Light Reflex

Retinal illumination is the chief determinant factor of pupil size, and illuminating the retina with a flashlight allows the physician to study the pupillary light reflex (PLR). The reflex arc is made of four neurons. The first is in the retina (i.e., rods and cones) and bipolar and ganglion cells, which pass their response to the second, the intercalated neurons in the pretectal area of the high brainstem. From there, the pathways reach the third neuron, the Edinger-Westphal's nucleus, a parasympathetic large cluster of cells that is part of the dorsal nucleus of the oculomotor nerve. Finally, axons play on the cells the axons of which (the short ciliary nerves) arise from the ciliary ganglion, a small nervous corpuscle on the lateral aspect of the optic nerve, 7 to 8 mm in front of the optic foramen.

This simplified account of the reflex arc (Fig. 27-1) shows that the afferent arm of the reflex is the retina, optic nerve, optic chiasm (in which nasal pupillomotor fibers cross, but temporal do not), and optic tract and its medial branch that bypasses the lateral geniculate body and enters the brachium of the superior colliculus to end in the pretectal area beneath the superior colliculus. The intercalated neurons are crossed and uncrossed in the gray substance around the aqueduct. The efferent arm is the parasympathetic fibers that are part of the oculomotor nerve in which they lie superficially.

Normally bright light shone on the retina causes a brisk contraction of the ipsilateral pupil (direct reflex). Because the pupillary pathways are twice crossed (see above) a symmetric brisk contraction of the opposite pupil occurs (consensual reflex). The constriction holds on as long as the light stimulus is kept on, although a slight dilation after the initial constriction is

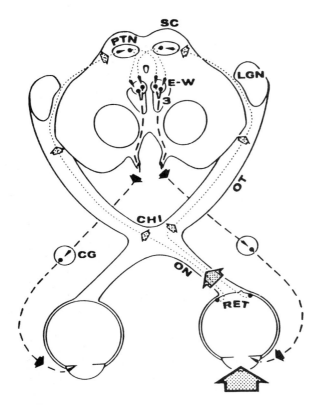

Figure 27-1. Pupillary light reflex. Light in left eye (dotted arrow) stimulates retina (RET), whose afferent axons (*fine dashed lines*) ascend optic nerve (ON), decussate at chiasm (CHI), and terminate in pretectal nuclear complex (PTN). Lateral geniculate nucleus (LGN) is bypassed by these pupillomotor fibers. The PTN is connected by *crossed and uncrossed* intercalated neurons to both Edinger-Westphal parasympathetic motor nuclei (E-W), which compose the dorsal aspect of the oculomotor nuclear complex (3). Preganglionic parasympathetic fibers (*heavy dashed lines*) leave ventral aspect of midbrain in the substance of the third cranial nerves. After synapsing in the ciliary ganglia (CG), the postganglionic fibers innervate the pupillary sphincter muscles. Note that uniocular light stimulus evokes bilateral and symmetric pupillary constriction. Brainstem diagram represents section through level rostral to superior colliculi (SC). (From Glaser, 1990, with permission.)

normal. An afferent pupillary defect is characterized by absent direct and consensual responses with consensual response on illumination of the opposite eye. An efferent pupillary defect is characterized by absent direct response with the presence of a consensual response. Pupillary responses are sluggish when there is loss of acuity from lesions of the retina, optic nerve, or chiasm.

Near Reflex and Accommodation

Near vision requires accommodation, which depends primarily on changes of shape of the lens. However, the pupil also plays a role, albeit minor, by increasing the depth of focus. Therefore, in near vision, there is pupillary constriction, sometimes called *near synkinesis*. The near reflex can be elicited by electrical stimulation of Brodmann's area 19. Pupillary constriction depends on initiation of convergence, which itself is dependent on the initiation of accommodation. The pathways of this reflex are not well known. The important clinical fact is that they are distinct from those of the PLR. The former may be present, although the latter is absent (see Argyll Robertson's pupil).

In some patients, near vision is difficult to obtain. A watch is a good target. Some people need their own finger brought by the examiner at short visual distance. In old people with small pupils and in all those with black irises, pupillary constriction may be difficult to assess. To bypass these difficulties, the eye is first brightly illuminated, which results in constriction, then under that bright light, near vision determines normally an additional constriction.

Spasm of the near reflex may be unilateral or bilateral, thus mimicking unilateral or bilateral paralysis of the abducens nerve. The presence of miosis in the adducted eye(s) is the telltale sign. Spasm of the near reflex is commonly of hysterical nature, but some cases are concomitant with lesions, usually in the posterior fossa.

Pupillary Sympathetic Pathways

The sympathetic pathway (Fig. 27-2) takes a long and complicated course to reach the eye. The cells of the first neuron lie in the posterior hypothalamus. Axons course caudally and ipsilaterally in the lateral tegmentum of midbrain, pons, and medulla. They course still more caudally in the intermediolateralis part of the cervical cord near the posterior angle of the anterior horn and synapse with the second neuron from C8 to T2 (Budge's ciliospinal center, named for J. L. Budge, 1811–1888, German physiologist). Axons of the second neuron exit from the spinal cord with the ventral roots, chiefly T1, accessorily C8 to T2. Sympathetic fibers then ramify as white rami and course dorsally to the cervical sympathetic chain, which lies behind the common carotid artery and jugular vein. This part of the sympathetic pathway passes over the pleura of the apex of the lung and under the subclavian artery. The fibers then course rostrally through the inferior (stellate) and middle cervical ganglion without synapsing. Finally, they synapse in the superior cervical ganglion. Thus the first and second neurons are called preganglionic. Axons of cells of the superior cervical sympathetic ganglion are postganglionic fibers. They make a plexus around the carotid artery. Fibers for sweat and hair erection course with the external carotid artery. Fibers for the eye are part of the sympathetic plexus around the internal carotid artery. They

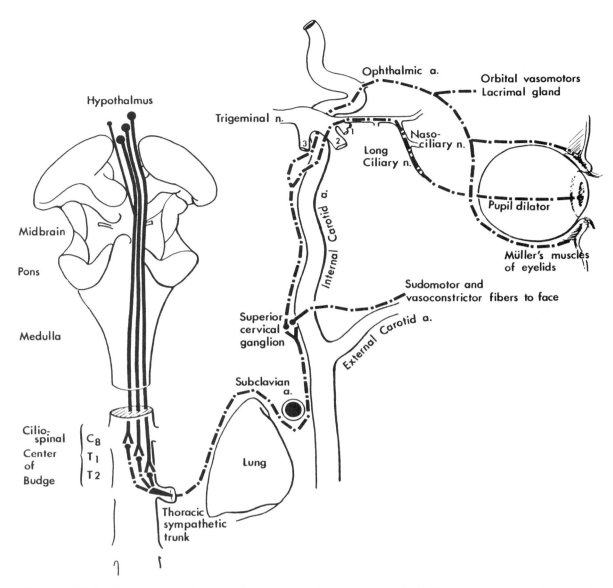

Figure 27-2. Ocular sympathetic pathways. Hypothalamic sympathetic fibers compose a polysynaptic (?) system as they descend to the ciliospinal center. This intra-axial tract is functionally considered the "first-order neuron." The second-order neuron takes a circuitous course through the posterosuperior aspect of the chest and ascends in the neck in relationship to the carotid system. Third-order neurons originate in the superior cervical ganglion and are distributed to the face with branches of the external carotid artery and to the orbit via the ophthalmic artery and ophthalmic division (*1*) of the trigeminal nerve. *2, 3:* maxillary and mandibular branches of the trigeminal nerve. (From Glaser, 1990, with permission.)

anastomose with the ophthalmic nerve, a branch of the trigeminal nerve, and leave it in the orbit as the nasociliary nerves that innervate the pupillodilator and Müller's muscle, a tiny smooth muscle in the upper and lower lids (J. P. Müller, 1801–1858, German anatomist). They also give trophic fibers for the melanin cells of the uvea. There is experimental and human evidence that frontal areas influence pupillary size because their stimulation determines contralateral, and sometimes ipsilateral, dilation of the pupil.

PUPILLARY SYNDROMES

Bernard-Horner or Horner Syndrome

This classic syndrome is named after C. Bernard (1813–1878, French physiologist) and J. F. Horner (1831–1886, a Swiss ophthalmologist). Bernard discovered the condition experimentally, and Horner reported the first human case in 1869. The main elements are ptosis (from the Greek for falling), miosis, and enophthalmos. Ptosis results from the paralysis of

Müller's muscle and, therefore, is slight. Both a drop of the upper and elevation of the inferior lids occur, accounting for the narrowing of the interpalpebral fissure. Miosis is usually well marked, with a pupillary diameter of 1.5 to 2 mm. Light and near reflexes are retained. The existence of enophthalmos has been denied. At least, it is more apparent than real. In the complete oculosympathetic syndrome, there is in addition absence of sweat on the ipsilateral side of the face, which is most evident on the forehead. The abnormality in sweating is usually either transient (caused perhaps by the action of circulating epinephrine) or absent (when sympathetic lesions are distal to the external carotid artery).

The long route of the sympathetic makes it vulnerable to many various lesions. Thus, Bernard-Horner syndrome can be a part or can reveal many various diseases. In its brainstem part, the usual cause is cerebrovascular disease (e.g., in the lateral medullary [Wallenberg's] syndrome, see Ch. 35). Trauma and syringomyelia account for most cases of cervical cord origin. The first thoracic segment (T1) can be damaged during delivery or in such occasions as motorbike accidents when the inferior brachial plexus is overstretched (Klumpke-Dejerine syndrome). Cancer of the apex of the lung can be revealed by Bernard-Horner syndrome (Pancoast's syndrome). In the neck, occlusions of the internal carotid artery, particularly dissections, either spontaneous or from trauma, are the chief cause, and Bernard-Horner syndrome may be the only sign of a carotid artery dissection. Malignancies are also a frequent cause. Bernard-Horner syndrome has been reported after neck manipulation, presumably as a result of carotid artery dissection. Transient Bernard-Horner syndrome is a chief feature of cluster headache.

In congenital Bernard-Horner syndrome, the ipsilateral iris is lighter (heterochromia). T1 injury at birth has been proposed as a mechanism. A few patients present with Bernard-Horner syndrome for which no cause is found. In such cases, pharmacologic tests could separate preganglionic from postganglionic lesions. Several tests are available. It would seem that failure of dilation by hydroxyamphetamine 1 percent is the clearest clue to postganglionic lesions.

Argyll Robertson's Pupil

The association of miosis and loss of light reflex with retention of near reflex described by Douglas Argyll Robertson (Scottish neurologist) in 1869 is one of the most celebrated signs in clinical neurology. Generations of students have learned the syndrome's features by believing a prostitute (who has neurosyphilis) can accommodate but not react (see Ch. 16). With few reservations, it is diagnostic of tertiary neurosyphilis

(tabes). The absence of light reflex is significant when there is no gross loss of acuity. The sign is bilateral, and the pupils are small, unequal, and irregular. There is a variable degree of iris atrophy. It has been often reasoned that the lesions should involve the region rostral to the oculomotor nucleus. The authors know of three cases that have undergone postmortem examination: one in a case of progressive hypertrophic neuropathy of Dejerine-Sottas disease, one in a case of malignant lymphoma infiltrating the orbit, and one in leprosy. In the three cases, the lesions involved the ciliary ganglion and/or the short ciliary nerves; the midbrain was normal.

In diabetes mellitus, a dissociation of light reflex and near-vision accommodation is occasionally found. The pupils, however, are usually mydriatic. Some authorities have stated that miosis is possible, in which case it would be a true Argyll Robertson's pupil. This must be very rare indeed. In pinealomas and tumors of that region, the light-near dissociation may be present, but here again, the pupils are usually not miotic.

Marcus Gunn's Pupil

This finding of delayed dilation of the pupil despite illumination is a good sign of unilateral optic neuritis, commonly caused by multiple sclerosis. To demonstrate the sign, the examiner swings alternatively the flashlight to each eye for periods of 2 to 3 seconds (swinging flashlight test). After a few switches, the pupil on the diseased side dilates in spite of illumination, with the contralateral dilation overcoming consensually the weaker direct response.

Tonic Pupil

The tonic or Adie's pupil (named after the Australian physician, W. J. Adie, 1886–1935) is enlarged and unilateral, the opposite of that in the Bernard-Horner syndrome. The disorder is noticed because, at the onset, troubles with accommodation are frequent. The tonic pupil contracts to light and near reflex but very slowly, over minutes or hours. After cessation of illumination or near vision, it dilates but again very slowly. There is denervation supersensitivity to the weak parasympathomimetic metacholine 2.5 percent. It may occur at all ages and in both sexes, but the typical case is a 30- to 50-year-old woman. Pathologically, there is a loss of cells in the ciliary ganglion. Usually, no cause is found. The tonic pupil is frequently associated with absent or weak deep reflexes (Holmes-Adie syndrome). We know of two reports of Holmes-Adie syndrome postmortem with examination of the spinal ganglia. In both, there was evidence of neuronal loss and, in one, evidence of lesions of the dorsal tracts likely to be consequences of the spinal ganglion damage. The unilateral tonic pupil is considered a benign condition. Bilateral tonic pupils would raise more suspicion of an associated nervous disease. Tonic pupils have been reported with postural hypotension, familial dysautonomia, the Riley-Day syndrome, and hereditary sensory neuropathy (see Ch. 80).

Pupil in Coma

Pupillary examination is particularly important when there are disorders of consciousness because the pathways of the pupillary reflexes lie in great part in the midbrain where those structures also lie on which consciousness depends. Because the pupillary pathways are relatively resistant to metabolic disorders, retention of pupillary reflexes in a comatose patient suggests metabolic coma (see Ch. 17).

From above down the neuraxis, causes of coma may involve or spare the pupil in different ways. Hypothalamic damage may cause an ipsilateral Bernard-Horner syndrome. Midbrain tectal and pretectal lesions may interrupt PLR while sparing the near reflex, in which case the pupils are 5 to 6 mm in diameter with a fluctuating size. Midbrain lesions may interrupt both parasympathetic and sympathetic pathways, leaving the pupils in midposition, 4 to 5 mm in diameter, often unequal and unresponsive to light. Both oculomotor nerves can be interrupted in the midbrain, leaving both pupils wide, unresponsive to light, and with paralyses of external muscles and ptosis. Bilateral pinpoint pupil with retained reaction to light suggest primarily pontine hemorrhage or massive infarction. A unilateral pinpoint pupil is either very rare or does not occur, which suggests that bilateral lesions of the descending sympathetic pathways must be present to reduce pupillary size to pinpoint.

Beyond the axis of the brainstem, injuries to the nerves that carry parasympathetic fibers can yield a widely dilated pupil from unopposed action of the intact sympathetic system. In uncal herniation, an ipsilateral mydriasis unresponsive to light is often present without paralysis of the external ocular muscles or ptosis. This is thought to be due to the superficial position of the parasympathetic fibers in the oculomotor nerve, as already mentioned. Farther distally, however (e.g., in the cavernous sinus), this particular vulnerability of parasympathetic fibers no longer obtains. Unilateral or bilateral oval pupils usually suggest progressive injury to the oculomotor nuclei complex, sometimes a phase in recovery. The causes are commonly cerebrovascular diseases.

Drugs: Therapeutic Use, Abuse, and Inadvertent Exposure

The common cause of small pupils is miotic drops for glaucoma (e.g., pilocarpine). Opiates, morphine, and heroin cause centrally small pupils. Amphetamines, cocaine, atropine, and scopolamine cause large pupils. People whose work involves such substances (e.g., nurses can inadvertently, by rubbing their eyes, instill a mydriatic or miotic). Nasal decongestants may contain ephedrine. Inadvertent instillation causes mydriasis. An isolated pupillary abnormality should always raise such possible diagnoses.

Episodic Pupillary Dysfunction

Some young healthy women experience periodic unilateral mydriasis that lasts minutes, hours, or days. There is usually some disorder of accommodation and discomfort in and around the eye. The cause and mechanisms are unknown.

ANNOTATED BIBLIOGRAPHY

Bartheson JD, Trautmann JC, Sundt TM Jr. Minimal oculomotor nerve paresis secondary to unruptured intracranial aneurysm. Arch Neurol 1986;43:1015–20.
Even partial cranial nerve III paresis with ipsilateral headache suggests berry aneurysms.

Brodal A. The Cranial Nerves. Anatomy and Anatomico-Clinical Correlations. 2nd Ed. Blackwell, Oxford, 1962.
A classic.

Cogan DG. Neurology of the Visual System. CC Thomas, Sprinfield, IL, 1966.
A classic.

Cogan DG. Neurology of the Ocular Muscles. CC Thomas, Springfield, IL, 1975.
A classic.

Collard M, Saint Val C, Mohr M, Kiesman M. Paralysie isolée du nerf moteur oculaire commun par infarctus des fibres fasciculaires. Rev Neurol (Paris) 1991;146:128–32.
A pathologically documented rare case.

Fisher CM. Some neuroophthalmological observations. J Neurol Neurosurg Psychiatry 1967;30:383–92.
Pearls.

Fisher CM. Oval pupils. Arch Neurol 1980;37:502–3.
A clinical curiosity but reliable sign of midbrain injury.

Garcin R, Gruner J, Man HX. Etude pathogénique du signe d'Argyll Robertson dans la névrite hypertrophique de Dejerine-Sottas. Document anatomo-clinique. Presse Med 1960;68:357–60.
A case with postmortem demonstration of the lesions responsible for Argyll Robertson's pupil.

Garcin R, Layani F, Lapresle J et al. Lèpre nerveuse a type de polynévrite sensitivo-motrice des quatre membres. Presse Med 1961;69:2597–600.
A case of leprosy with Argyll Robertson's pupil and postmortem evidence of ciliary ganglion lesions.

Gautier JC, Loron PH. Anévrismes disséquants de l'artére

carotide interne et syndrome de Claude Bernard-Horner. Rev Neurol (Paris) 1989;145:328–9.

Bernard-Horner syndrome may be the only sign of a dissection of the internal carotid artery.

Glaser JS. Neuro-Ophthalmology. 2nd Ed. JB Lippincott, Philadelphia, 1990.

A scholarly book that reflects also the best down-to-earth experience.

Grayson MF. Horner's syndrome after manipulation of the neck. BMJ 1987;295:1381–2.

Thought rare, possibly from carotid dissection.

Harriman DGF, Garland H. The pathology of Adie's syndrome. Brain 1968;91:401–18.

A pathologic document.

Lapresle J, Man HX. Signe d'Argyll Robertson dans un cas de lymphome malin avec lésions ciliaires. Rev Neurol (Paris) 1979;135:515–25.

A case with pathologic demonstration of the lesions responsible for Argyll Robertson's pupil.

Pierrot-Deseilligny C, Chain F, Gray F, et al. Parinaud's syndrome. Brain 1982;105:667–96.

Pathologic data and proposed mechanisms.

Plum F, Posner J. The Diagnosis of Stupor and Coma. 3rd Ed. FA Davis, Philadelphia, 1980.

The reference book on disorders of consciousness and the high brainstem.

Ruttner F. Die tonische Pupillenreaktion, Klinische und anatomische Untersuchungen. Mschr Psychiat Neurol 1947;114:265–330.

A thorough work.

Ulrich J. Morphological basis of Adie's syndrome. Eur Neurol 1980;19:300–95.

A case of Adie's syndrome with postmortem evidence of ciliary ganglion spinal ganglia and dorsal funiculi lesions.

28

Cranial Nerves III, IV, VI: The Oculomotor, Trochlear, and Abducens Nerves and Eye Movements

J. C. Gautier and J. P. Mohr

PRINCIPLES OF ANATOMY AND PHYSIOLOGY

As for other muscles, those of the eyes are controlled by upper central and lower peripheral neurons. The peripheral neuron cell bodies are contained in the nuclei of the oculomotor nerve (cranial nerve III), the trochlear nerve, (cranial nerve IV) and the abducens nerve (cranial nerve VI). The six muscles controlling each eye, known as the extrinsic or extraocular muscles (Fig. 28-1), are innervated by these nerves (see below). Frontal binocular human vision requires a special motor system because the objects perceived in normal vision must be projected on corresponding parts of each retina to allow fusion of the two retinal images, a process through which one sees one image only. Failure of such projection, when one object projects on noncorresponding parts of the retina, causes two objects to be seen, diplopia (from the Greek for double vision). Visual fusion thus requires that both eyes be yoked in all eye movements. This is accomplished by the six muscles of one eye being yoked in three pairs with their counterparts on the opposite side, namely lateral-medial rectus, superior rectus-inferior oblique, and inferior rectus-superior oblique (Fig. 28-2), with an anatomic organization for that yoking. Ocular movements are regulated by a system of complementary excitatory and inhibitory impulses. For instance, when one looks to the right, the right lateral rectus and the left medial rectus are activated while the right medial and the left lateral recti receive inhibitory impulses. In addition, postures and movements of the head, neck, and body influence eye positions and movements through informations of vestibular origin (vestibulo-ocular reflexes [VOR]).

The fundamental goal of the eye motor system is foveation or refoveation (i.e., either to catch up or maintain seen objects on the fovea or, more accurately, on both foveae). This goal is achieved by two types of ocular movements. In the first, the axes of both eyes remain parallel. These are the movements of the eyes known as versions, conjugate movements, or gaze. In the second, the axes of the two eyes temporarily lose their parallelism, with so-called vergence or disconjugate movements. Versions and vergence have two distinct anatomic and functional systems. The versional system can generate two kinds of eye movements: fast movements (also known as saccades) and slow movements.

The main types of saccades are either voluntary, such as when one scans a landscape visually or on command (e.g., look down or look up). Saccades of a reflexive type also can occur in response to the intrusion of a novel target in the peripheral visual field or to a sudden unexpected noise, in which case the head often turns with the eyes toward the stimulus. The rapid eye movements of paradoxic sleep and the quick phases of induced and pathologic nystagmus are also saccades.

Fast eye movements are quick, implying a high and short increase of innervation, which is provided by a *pulse generator* (i.e., a pool of burst neurons that fire with a short latency and a high frequency for a short time, ensuring quick foveation). The anatomic substrate of the pulse generator is the *paramedian pontine reticular formation* (PPRF) for horizontal saccades or the *rostral interstitial nucleus of the medial longitudinal fasciculus* (riMLF) for vertical ones (see below).

417

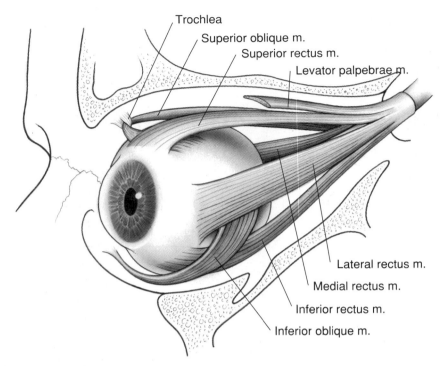

Figure 28-1. Origins and insertions on the globe of the extraocular muscles. The medial rectus is mostly hidden by the lateral rectus.

After movement, the eyes may be required to remain in the new position, which is not easily achieved given the viscous strength of the orbital content that tends to drag them back. A neuronal subsystem termed the *neural integrator* computes (integrates in the mathematic sense) the necessary energy that is dis-

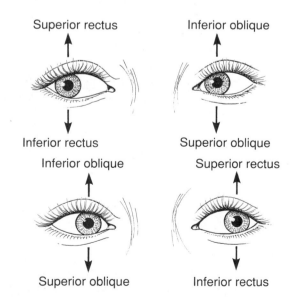

Figure 28-2. Muscles for vertical movements in abduction and adduction of the eyes.

pensed by tonic neurons. That momentum of energy is termed the *step*. Thus, the basic energy profile of saccades is a pulse-step mechanism. The anatomic substrate of the conceptual neural integrator is thought to include the flocculus, the nucleus prepositus hypoglossi, and the medial vestibular nucleus (Figs. 28-3 and 28-4). Between saccades, unwanted saccades are prevented by omnipause neurons that inhibit burst neurons.

Slow eye movements are either smooth pursuit (often abbreviated in pursuit) movements or VOR. Pursuit movements maintain foveation on a moving target, with the eye velocity normally matching target velocity. An immediate increase of innervation (step) followed by a linear increase (ramp) of neuronal firing is necessary to achieve this matching velocity. Pursuit movements are thus a step-ramp mechanism, differing from the pulse-step mechanism of the saccade.

VOR ensure compensatory eye movements to maintain foveation in response to new positions or movements of the body but mainly of the head. The inputs that control the eye movement responses are mainly from the semicircular canals, which send signals for acceleration. The semicircular canals and eye muscles are yoked to make the repositioning of the eyes caused by VOR occur in the plane of the activated semicircular canal. When head rotation is sustained, vestibular control fades out. The optokinetic system is then thought to prefer stabilization of the eyes. Inputs that control VOR also come from neck muscles.

For movements that require maintenance of foveation on targets that come to or recede from the observer along the axis that projects forward from the midline between the eyes, the vergence system is activated. Vergence movements are slow disconjugate movements in response to blur of near objects and asymmetric projection of the object on both retinas, maintaining fusion and avoiding diplopia.

The brainstem is the locus of both the version and vergence systems. It receives controlling inputs from the cerebral hemispheres, superior colliculi, and cerebellum.

The superior colliculi are two flat eminences in the rostral half of the tectum (Figs. 28-3 and 28-4) that show a rudimentary layer structure. Each superior colliculus can be divided in two parts: (1) superficial, which receives inputs mainly from retina and striate cortex, and (2) deep, which receives multimodal inputs among which are some from the frontal eye fields (Brodmann's area 8). Crossed and uncrossed tectopontine and tectobulbar fibers exit from the deep part. Some connect with the brainstem prenuclear structures of eye movements. Stimulation of the deep superior colliculi results in contralaterally directed saccades. In humans, the superior colliculi would act mainly on the position of the eyes and head, especially in reflexive saccades that respond to the arrival of a novel target in the peripheral visual field.

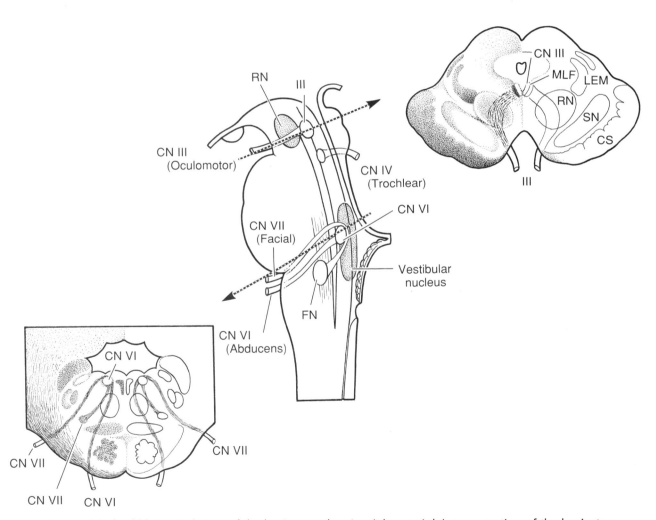

Figure 28-3. **(A)** Sagittal view of the brainstem showing (above, right) cross section of the brainstem at the level of the superior colliculus and (lower left) at the level of the abducens nucleus. The views include the oculomotor nerve (CN III), medial lemniscus (LEM), medial longitudinal fasciculus (MLF), red nucleus (RN), substantia nigra (SN), corticospinal tract (CS), abducens nerve (CN VI), vestibular nucleus, paramedian pontine reticular formation, facial nerve (N VII), spinal nucleus of the trigeminal, spinal tract of the trigeminal, and spinothalamic tract (see also Fig. 28-4). (*Figure continues.*)

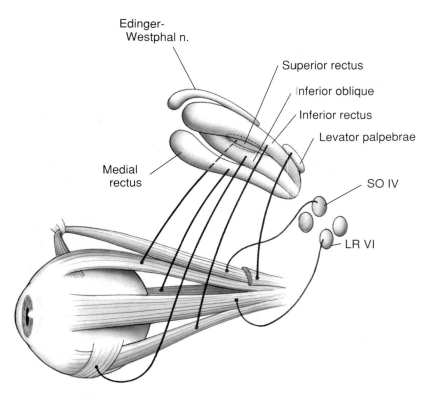

Figure 28-3 *(Continued).* **(B)** Lateral view of the oculomotor complex showing the Edinger-Westphal parasympathetic nucleus, inferior rectus, medial rectus, and superior oblique, which is crossed (i.e., one nucleus supplies the opposite eye); the trochlear nucleus supply to the superior oblique muscle (SO IV), which supplies the fibers to the superior oblique, also crossed; and the abducens nucleus (VI) for the lateral rectus (LR). The medial rectus neurons are clustered in three groups, each of which receives internuclear neurons from the contralateral abducens nucleus. Fibers to the lid levator are both crossed and uncrossed. (Modified from Buttner-Ennever, 1981, with permission.)

The cerebral hemispheres receive and process most of the retinal signals in the occipital lobes and neighboring regions of the parietal and temporal lobes (see Ch. 25). Visual signals are integrated with the extracorporeal and intracorporeal information that reaches the brain along other sensory modes and are integrated with those encoded in memory circuits. This inflow and background allow the parietal and frontal cortices to send commands to the prenuclear mechanisms (see below).

BRAINSTEM

Peripheral Neurons

Cranial Nerve III

The oculomotor nucleus lies ventral to the periaqueductal gray matter and superior colliculus (Figs. 28-3 and 28-4). It innervates the medial, superior, and inferior recti; the inferior oblique; and lid levators. Fibers to the superior rectus are totally crossed (i.e., elevation of the globe on one side is controlled by innervation from the opposite oculomotor nucleus). Innervation of the lid levators comes from a distinct single subnucleus, dorsal and caudal to the main nuclear complex, and is both crossed and uncrossed. There is evidence that a neural network that controls the lids lies rostral and dorsal to the oculomotor nucleus. The latter is made of large and small motor cells. Some of the latter innervate that layer of the extraocular muscles that lies against the bony walls of the socket (orbital layer), which histologically appears suited for tonic activity; hence they maintain the position of the eye. Large neurons would innervate the muscles of the inner layer (global layer) of the muscle and thus would be responsible for quick phasic activity. The parasympathetic Edinger-Westphal nucleus lies dorsal and rostral to the oculomotor nucleus complex (Fig. 28-3B) (see Ch. 34). The existence of Perlia's nucleus for convergence is not well established in humans.

Fascicular fibers that carry parasympathetic fibers course ventrally through the red nucleus (which is part of the reticular formation) and the medial part of the pes pedunculi to emerge in the interpeduncular space,

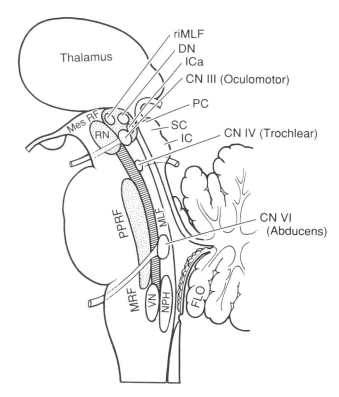

Figure 28-4. Important areas of the brain in regard ocular movements. Nucleus of oculomotor nerve (CN III); nucleus of trochlear nerve (CN IV); nucleus of abducens nerve (CN VI); Darkehewitsch nucleus (DN), inferior colliculus (IC); Cajal's interstitial nucleus (ICa); flocculus (FLO); medial longitudinal fasciculus (MLF); medullar reticular formation (MRF); mesencephalic reticular formation (Mes RF); nucleus prepositus hypoglossi (NPH); posterior commissure (PC); paramedian pontine reticular formation (PPRF); red nucleus (RN); rostral interstitial nucleus of MLF, (riMLF); superior colliculus (SC); vestibular nuclei (VN). (Modified from Pierrot-Deseilligny, 1985, with permission.)

close to the contralateral cranial nerve III (see Fig. 28-3). The nerve passes between posterior cerebral and anterior superior cerebellar arteries and then courses ventrally close to the posterior communicating artery. It enters the cavernous sinus between the free edge of the tentorium and the lateral aspect of the dorsum sellae. It courses ventrally in the superior part of the cavernous sinus, and as it passes in the superior orbital fissure, it divides into superior and inferior branches. The superior branch innervates the superior rectus and lid levator. The inferior branch innervates the other muscles mentioned above.

Cranial Nerve IV

The nucleus is continuous caudally with that of cranial nerve III (Figs. 28-3 and 28-4). Fascicular fibers run dorsally and medially and thus cross those of the contralateral cranial nerve IV on the midline in the ante-

rior medullary velum just caudal to the inferior colliculus. Cranial nerve IV is the one cranial nerve that exits dorsally from the central nervous system. This slender nerve turns forward around the cerebral peduncle and enters the cavernous sinus above the free edge of the tentorium. It leaves the cavernous sinus through the superior orbital fissure and innervates the superior oblique. This muscle slides in a tendinous pulley at the anteromedial angle of the socket, hence the name *trochlear* (from the Greek for pulley).

Cranial Nerve VI

The nucleus has a paramedian location just beneath the floor of the pontine part of the fourth ventricle (Figs. 28-3A and 28-4). Facial nerve fibers loop around the nucleus. Cranial nerve VI or abducens nucleus is made of two kinds of neurons: those that give off axons that enter cranial nerve VI and cells that give off internuclear axons (see below). Fascicular fibers course ventrally to exit in the pontomedullary sulcus about 1 cm from the midline (see Fig. 26-4). The nerve then ascends rostrally and laterally to enter the cavernous sinus about 2 cm below the posterior clinoid. This part of the nerve is in a close relationship with the tip of the petrous bone. It leaves the cavernous sinus through the superior orbital fissure and innervates the lateral rectus.

Brainstem Systems

In the brainstem, pools of neurons integrated into a circuitry provide the mechanism for versions and vergence. The following is a simplified account as a basis for clinical examination. For further information, the reader is referred to Glaser (1990), Leigh and Zee (1983), and Pierrot-Deseilligny (1985).

Horizontal Conjugate Gaze

As just mentioned, the abducens nucleus contains internuclear neurons (Fig. 28-4). The axons of these cross the midline and ascend in the medial longitudinal fasciculus (see below) to the medial rectus subnucleus of cranial nerve III. All horizontal versions originate in the nucleus abducens.

The *medial longitudinal fasciculus* (Figs. 28-3A, 28-4, and 28-5) is a paramedian myelinated bundle that extends from the midbrain to the caudal medulla where its fibers enter the sulcomarginal area of the anterior funiculus of the spinal cord. In addition to internuclear neurons from the nucleus abducens en route to the contralateral medial rectus subnucleus, it contains ascending fibers from the vestibular nuclei to the oculomotor nuclei; ascending and descending fibers to and from Cajal's interstitial nucleus; and a large group of tectobulbar, tectospinal, and pontine reticulospinal fibers.

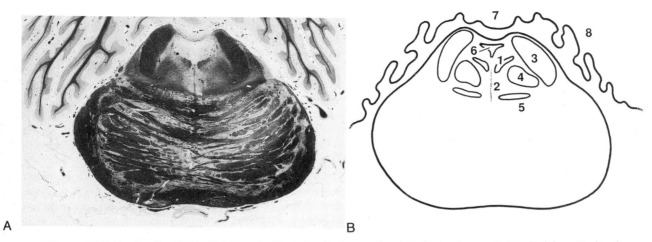

Figure 28-5. (A & B) Medial longitudinal fasciculus and related structures. *1,* Medial longitudinal fasciculus; *2,* paramedian pontine reticular formation (PPRF); *3,* superior cerebellar peduncle; *4,* central tegmental tract; *5,* medial lemniscus; *6,* fourth ventricle; *7,* vermis; *8,* cerebellar hemisphere.

The PPRF (Figs. 28-3A, 28-4, and 28-5) is a pool of neurons termed prenuclear or premotor because its cells fire just before and during horizontal versions. Excitatory and inhibitory impulses reach the PPRF from the vestibular nuclei, nucleus prepositus hypoglossi, posterior vermis, and flocculus of the cerebellum. Impulses also come from the contralateral superior colliculus through Meynert's decussation and the medial tectospinal tract and from the cerebral cortex.

At least three types of horizontal movements require separate consideration.

Horizontal Saccades. The PPRF is the neuronal pool in which all horizontal saccades are generated. The brainstem systems for horizontal saccades receive, in addition, controlling impulses from the cerebral cortex. From studies in the monkey, it appears that this control comes from both frontal and parietal areas. There are probably several parallel frontal pathways from the frontal eye field cortex, from the dorsomedial region in the supplementary motor area, and from the prefrontal cortex. They project contralaterally to the PPRF and ipsilaterally to the deep layers of the superior colliculus, either directly or by way of the caudate nucleus and pars reticulata of the substantia nigra. The parietal cortex, including probably an area in the ventral bank of the intraparietal sulcus, also projects onto the deep superior colliculus. There is now some evidence that parietal areas are devoted both to visual attention and to certain eye movements.

Horizontal Pursuit. The premotor cell pools and circuitry of horizontal smooth pursuit are still not well known. However, PPRF again plays a major role because lesions of this formation may result in an ipsilateral pursuit palsy. Cells in the dorsolateral pontine

nucleus, Purkinje cells in the cerebellar flocculus and posterior vermis, and cells close to the abducens nucleus all fire during pursuit. The medial vestibular nucleus and the nucleus prepositus hypoglossi are perhaps the premotor structures. Evidence of control from the cerebral cortex in humans is inferred by animal studies that show that cells in the MST area, which corresponds to Brodmann's area 39 in humans, fire during ocular pursuit movements. Furthermore, lesions of both areas 39 abolish pursuit movements. Pursuit-related fibers from area 39 may course in the posterior limb of the internal capsule to synapse in the ipsilateral dorsolateral pontine nuclei, providing a crossroad for inputs that come from parietal cortex and cerebellum.

Horizontal Vestibulo-Ocular Reflexes. The premotor cell pool is the rostral part of the medial vestibular nucleus, which sends inhibitory impulses to the ipsilateral nucleus abducens and excitatory impulses to the contralateral nucleus abducens.

Vertical Conjugate Gaze

The anatomic substrates of vertical versions are linked with, but rostral to, those of horizontal versions. They lie in the mesencephalon among the mesencephalic reticular formation (Fig. 28-4). The cells of the peripheral neurons are the subnuclei of cranial nerve III for the superior and inferior recti and the inferior oblique and the nucleus of cranial nerve IV for the superior oblique (Fig. 28-3B).

Vertical Saccades. The riMLF is located in the most rostral part of the medial longitudinal fasciculus, ventral and rostral to the accessory oculomotor nuclei, namely Darkschewitsch's and Cajal's nuclei and the nucleus of the posterior commissure (Fig. 28-4). The riMLF is the prenuclear cell pool for all vertical saccades. It contains burst and tonic neurons and receives inhibitory inputs from omnipause neurons.

There may be neurons for upward gaze and neurons for downward gaze. Bilateral lesions of the riMLF either suppress all vertical saccades or result in an impairment that is most evident on attempted downward saccades. The riMLF receives vestibular and cerebellar inputs and also inputs from the PPRF, although the latter may be less significant in humans than in animals. It receives, in addition, inputs from the superior colliculus and from the ipsilateral area 8. Efferent and/ or afferent fibers pass through the posterior commissure, a lesion of which results in paralysis of upward gaze. Lesions of fibers from Cajal's nucleus cause, in addition, bilateral eyelid retraction.

Vertical Pursuit. The anatomic substrate of vertical pursuit is still incompletely known. Cells in Cajal's nucleus and cells of some of the vestibular nuclei may act as premotor pools. The riMLF probably does not play here a prominent role.

Vertical Vestibulo-Ocular Reflexes. Vestibular nuclei are the prenuclear pools. The cerebellar control comes primarily from the flocculus.

Vergence

It can be assumed that cranial nerve III subnuclei for medial recti are the final pathway for vergence and that, simultaneously, the nucleus abducens receives inhibitory impulses. Furthermore, the medial longitudinal fasciculus is not essential for vergence because vergence is spared in lesions of this structure. The vergence mechanisms probably lie high in the brainstem because vergence paralysis is usually associated with paralysis of vertical versions. Neuronal pools lateral and dorsal to the cranial nerve III nucleus probably play a predominant role. Stimulation of areas 19 and 22 results in vergence as a part of the near triad.

CLINICAL EXAMINATION

Lids

The eyelids and interpalpebral fissure must first be assessed. Lids may be deformed by sties, chalazia, or basal cell carcinomas. In neurofibromatosis, the lid margin may take a characteristic horizontal S-shape. With eyes straight ahead, the upper lid covers 1 to 2 mm of the corneal limbus, and the lower lid is just at or on the corneal limbus. Exophthalmos (bulging eye) may be uni- or bilateral. Unilateral exophthalmos can be detected by looking from the rear over the head of the sitting patient. A benign form of hereditary exophthalmos, common in black people, features the

sclera covered by the lids on the vertical meridian of the iris. The two upper lids are yoked. Their synkinetic movements with the eyes are normally symmetric. Normally, the lids smoothly follow vertical versions. A lid lag, especially when unilateral, as the eyes follow a target from above downward, is highly suggestive of thyroid disease (von Graefe's sign). By the same mechanism of yoking, blinking is symmetric. In 1967, Fisher mentioned that asynchronous blinking is a sign of a very mild peripheral or nuclear seventh nerve palsy and that blinking is suspended on holding the breath, a useful maneuver in clinical practice to avoid interfering noises when the eyeball is auscultated for a possible bruit.

Retraction of the upper lid (stare) occurs in diverse conditions: hyperthyroidism, lesions of the posterior commissure (see above) or in its vicinity (Collier's tucked-lid sign) in progressive supranuclear palsy, and instillation of sympathomimetic drugs. Retraction of a ptotic lid occurs with jaw movements in Marcus Gunn's jaw-winking phenomenon, usually seen in young patients. It is usually unilateral. The ipsilateral pupil may be small.

Slight *ptosis,* or lid droop, is usually congenital. However, ptosis may result from lesions in the sympathetic pathway that causes paralysis of Müller's muscle. It is then of mild degree and associated with miosis (see Ch. 27). Ptosis may also be due to paralysis of the lid levator, when it is either mild, or the lid may hide the eye. A lesion of the oculomotor subnucleus on the same or opposite side may cause bilateral ptosis because fibers from the midline dorsal cranial nerve III subnucleus that supply the levator palpebrae are both being crossed and uncrossed (see above). The effort to overcome a unilateral ptosis may also determine contralateral lid elevation. In mild ptosis, there usually is a compensatory contraction of the frontalis with elevation of the brow. Unexplained ptosis requires an edrophonium test for a diagnosis of myasthenia gravis.

Bell's Phenomenon

In facial palsy caused by damage to the facial nerve itself (Bell's palsy) (see Ch. 29), on attempted eye closure, the globe on the paralyzed side can be seen deviating upward and outward. This normal synkinesis to lid closure, also known as Bell's phenomenon, can be tested by opposing forceful closure of the lids. Its occurrence implies pathways between cranial nerves VII and III nuclei. In patients who cannot elevate voluntarily, a normal Bell's phenomenon means that the neural network for upward gaze and the elevator muscles are functioning, and hence, that the disorder is supranuclear (e.g., in congenital elevator palsy). Although helpful when present, Bell's phenomenon is absent in some 15 percent of normal people.

Some patients with a unilateral cerebral lesion, on opposed forced lid closure, show a horizontal version instead of the normal response. This has been called spasticity of the conjugate motor mechanism, but it should be noted the version is in the direction opposite to the side of the lesion (i.e., contrary to that of a cerebral gaze palsy).

Positions of Eyes

In straight-ahead gaze, the axes of the eyes are parallel. Obvious deviations (known by the suffix, *tropia,* from the Greek for turning) cause no problems in diagnosis. Esotropia (Greek: *eso,* in) is eye deviation inward, and exotropia (Greek: *exo,* out) is deviation outward, in which case the light reflects, respectively, on the temporal and nasal sides of the center of the pupil in the deviated eye. Hypertropia is deviation upward, and hypotropia is deviation downward. Corresponding misplacements of the light reflex allow their diagnosis.

When slight, such deviations may require elicitation by a penlight held at the tip of the examiner's nose in the sagittal midplane of the patient's face. Normally, the pinpoint light reflex is right on the center of the patient's pupils or symmetric (i.e., either slightly lateral or nasal to these centers).

Testing Eye Movements

The cause of impaired visual acuity can be assessed by having the patient peep through a pinhole in paper or cardboard (see Ch 26). Visual fields are tested by confrontation (see Ch. 26). Saccadic movements are tested with alternate commands to gaze at two targets (e.g., pen and finger). Pursuit is assessed by having the patient follow a small slowly and smoothly moving target to ensure foveation. Convergence in old or inattentive patients is best tested by using the patient's forefinger tip as the target because this brings additional proprioceptive inputs to the eye movement.

During eccentric fixations and vergence testing, vestibular nystagmus may have been noticed (see below). In patients without spontaneous or gaze-evoked nystagmus, combining ophthalmoscopy with movements of the head can bring out disorders of the VOR.

Optokinetic Nystagmus

Passengers of a train gazing at the landscape or telegraph poles show an unwitting rhythmic characteristic eye movement with a slow phase directed contrary to the direction of the train and a quick reverse phase. The slow phase is a pursuit movement, and the quick one is a saccade. This can be reproduced by rotating a striped drum or a similar device and is termed optokinetic nystagmus, which is a highly complex reflex with several practical interests. First, it is lost or diminished in cases of deep parietal lesions when the drum is rotated toward the side of the lesion. Hemianopia per se does not suppress optokinetic nystagmus, suggesting that a positive (i.e., disturbed optokinetic nystagmus) is not due to a lesion of the geniculocalcarine tract; rather, it might be due to a lesion deep to the optic radiations damaging parietopontine fibers or the internal sagittal stratum, which conveys fibers from the occipital cortex to the superior colliculus and lateral geniculate body. Second, it may support the diagnosis of pure volitional (saccadic) gaze paresis with intact pursuit. Third, it demonstrates that hysterical patients or malingerers are not blind.

In the comatose patient, VOR can be tested by reflex deviations of the eyes. The oculocephalic reflex (doll's eyes) consists of reflex versions opposite to the direction of sudden, rapid passive head turning or extension flexions of the head. If the eyes deviate as expected, the pontine (horizontal) and mesencephalic (vertical) vestibular gaze mechanisms are still functioning. However, in comatose or severely ill patients or in patients suspected of increased intracranial pressure or brainstem lesions in cranial and cervical trauma, such maneuvers may be contraindicated for fear of adding to unknown injury of the neck. It is then better to resort to caloric stimulation (see below).

Testing Individual Extraocular Muscles in Strabismus and Diplopia

Among the six extrinsic muscles, only the medial and lateral recti have a single action, namely adduction and abduction, respectively. The four other muscles in the primary position have a mixed action of elevation or depression with torsion of the eye. However, when the eye is abducted, the superior rectus is an elevator, and the inferior rectus is a depressor. In adduction, in the adducted eye, the inferior oblique is an elevator, and the superior oblique is a depressor. This is the basis of testing individual extrinsic muscles (Fig. 28-2).

Strabismus or squint (Greek: *strabismos,* squinting) is a misalignment of the visual axes of the eyes. It may be paralytic or nonparalytic. Nonparalytic squint is concomitant (or comitant) because the angle of the axes remains unchanged in all directions of gaze. Paralytic squint is noncomitant because the angle widens when gaze is in the direction of the paralyzed muscle.

Nonparalytic strabismus is a disorder considered under the province of pediatric ophthalmology. The strabismus developed because the cause was unrecognized or neglected during infancy. Usually, one eye has amblyopia (i.e., the patient has monocular vision), and there is, of course, no diplopia. Divergent squint (walleyed) is also a feature of severe myopia. In some cases (alternating strabismus), the patient fixates alternatively with either eye, and both eyes have a good acuity.

Although nonparalytic tropias are now rare in adults, it is very common in the normal subject to find a tendency to squint, called a phoria. It is inapparent because it is overcome by fusional mechanisms that themselves depend on vergence (see above). Decompensation of phorias is a common cause of diplopia in adults, and neurologists must be acquainted with this condition.

Diplopia

In people with normal (binocular) vision, weakness of an extraocular muscle causes a deviation of the eye and, consequently, a misplacement of the fixation axis. The target projects on noncorresponding parts of the retinae, which causes double vision. Diplopia is a frequent complaint, and one with which the clinician must be prepared to cope with methodical step-by-step analysis. Not infrequently, a minimal degree of diplopia presents as a blur. The key to the diagnosis is covering one eye, which makes vision clear.

History taking is fundamental. Are the positions of the images side by side or under and over? Small vertical deviations in horizontal diplopias and small horizontal deviations in vertical ones should be disregarded as benign. Side-by-side diplopia is due to a defect in abduction or adduction. Over-and-under diplopias are due in most cases to a defect in vertically pulling muscles. Tilted images should suggest a weak superior or inferior oblique muscle. Double vision provoked or made worse by looking far away suggests a lesion of cranial nerve VI, that caused by downward gaze in reading or going downstairs, in cranial nerves III or IV. In many cases, adopting a tilt of the head to the side, up, down, or at an angle may cancel the diplopia by reducing the requirement for the paretic ocular movement in the affected eye.

In addition, in the diagnosis of the cause of diplopia, the duration of the complaint helps. Intermittent diplopia argues against a fixed structural lesion. Diplopia mainly in the afternoon or evening suggests myasthenia gravis. Pain in or around the eye at the onset of diplopia suggest infarction, with diabetes being a leading cause.

The examiner then records the position of the head. A tilt to the opposite shoulder is a good sign of cranial nerve IV paralysis. A turn of the head in the direction of a mildly weak lateral rectus is sometimes present. The position of the lids, drooping or retracted; the size of the pupils; and any sign of inflammatory disease of the eye and orbit are recorded. In many cases that come to the neurologist, diplopia results from paralysis of one of the motor nerves of the eye, and the examination is thus aimed at diagnosing which muscle

is weak. Conjugate gaze is tested on the cardinal position of the eyes with a linear object (e.g., a pencil held at least at 0.75 m in front of the patient). The pencil should be vertical in horizontal diplopia and horizontal in vertical ones. Whenever possible, the patient is asked to mimic with two fingers the position of the two images, according to the various directions of gaze. The position of the eyes should be recorded as soon as they are ascertained. Reasoning deductions and conclusions would come after the examination. In recent and complete paralyses (e.g., of cranial nerve VI), the eye is obviously deviated, and the eye does not move in the direction of action of the paralyzed muscle.

A very slight deviation of the visual axes, however, is sufficient to cause diplopia. In such cases, there is no tropia, and the weak muscle can be identified from characteristics of the false image. First, the false image that belongs to the paretic eye is less distinct because it does not project on the fovea. Second, diplopia occurs and increases (the gap between the images widens) when the target is moved farther in the field of action of the weak muscle. Failure of the palsied eye to turn in the direction of the target causes the image of the object to fall on the opposite retina farther and farther from the macula, resulting in a projection of the false image in the direction of action of the weak muscle.

Which eye sees the fainter image, projected off the center of vision, can be determined by covering each eye alternately and asking the patient which image disappears. It is often easier to use the red glass test. A red glass is put in front of the right eye. One image is red, and the other is white. It is easy for the patient to tell which of the two is peripheral. For example, in a paralysis of the right lateral rectus, the red image will be on the right. In a paralysis of the right medial rectus, the red image will be on the left. The same rules can be applied to vertical diplopias. In some diplopias, examination with the Maddox rod and the Lancaster green-red test may be necessary.

Myasthenia Gravis. At any age, any diplopia without a straightforward cause and a normal pupil should raise the suspicion of myasthenia gravis. Weakness of the extraocular muscles is transient, changing (i.e., involving successively different muscles), and often bilateral and involves muscles that cannot be accounted for by the dysfunction of one nerve. Ptosis is common. When necessary, it can be "facilitated" by sustained upward gaze or repeated eye closure. Quickly redirecting gaze from the downward position to the primary position makes the upper lid twitch before regaining its drooping position. Myasthenia can mimic all kinds of ocular nerve palsies, even internuclear ophthalmoplegia. Bilateral orbicularis oculi weakness is commonly present, which clinches the diagnosis. Throat and skeletal muscles may be involved to various degrees. Myasthenia gravis may be associated with thyroid disease or collagen disease. Edrophonium or neostigmine tests (see Ch. 81) are of fundamental diagnostic value.

Restrictive Ophthalmopathies. Lesions that restrict the contraction and stretch of eye muscles (e.g., fibrosis) can cause diplopia. In congenital diseases (e.g., Brown's congenital sheath syndrome of restricted movements of the superior oblique tendon) and in slowly developing diseases, such as chronic progressive external ophthalmoplegia (including all different subtypes of ophthalmoplegia plus), diplopia is rare, as it is also in myotonic dystrophy. The frequent condition and one that should not be missed by astute neurologists is dysthyroid ophthalmopathy. It can be part of Graves' or Hashimoto's disease. Typically, the restriction involves elevation because of retraction of the inferior rectus and is unilateral. The medial and superior recti are infrequently involved, and the lateral rectus is rarely involved. Clinical evidence of dysthyroidism is often absent or minimal (e.g., lid lag in downward movement of the eye). A forced duction test is positive. Computed tomography shows enlargement of the extraocular muscles. Biologic evidence of dysthyroidism must be sought by thyroid-stimulating hormone, triiodothyronine, and thyroxine tests. Orbital tumors, orbital pseudotumors, and the syndrome of Tolosa-Hunt can be causes of diplopia. Tumors can displace the eyeball and hinder the normal action of extraocular muscles. In orbital pseudotumors, there is an infiltration of the orbital tissues, including muscles, by inflammatory cells. It may occur at all ages but more often in young men. There is usually proptosis and sometimes pain. The Tolosa-Hunt syndrome is akin to orbital pseudotumor. The inflammatory granulomatous tissue and/or pachymeningitis are mainly located at the superior orbital fissure and anterior cavernous sinus. There is an aching pain in and about the eye, and there may be sensory deficit in the territory of the ophthalmic nerve. Spontaneous remissions and recurrences are possible. Symptoms and signs respond dramatically to large doses of corticosteroids.

Paralysis of convergence may be acute. It results in blur and diplopia in near vision. It may be due to trauma, encephalitis, or multiple sclerosis. Many cases have no recognizable organic basis.

Monocular diplopia may be due to astigmatism or corneal or mainly lens disease. Very rare cases have been ascribed to a cerebral pathologic disorder. (For decompensation of phorias into tropias, see above.)

NYSTAGMUS AND OTHER INVOLUNTARY MOVEMENTS

Nystagmus (from the Greek for drowsiness) refers to the slow drop of the head followed by a quick extension of the neck as so many have experienced on impending and indecent slumber. It is a to-and-fro involuntary movement of both eyes, rarely of one eye only. There are several kinds of nystagmus and a good number of involuntary eye movements are called nystagmus by tradition, although they are not true nystagmus. The mechanisms of the latter are not entirely known. In simple terms, (true) nystagmus results from disorders somewhere on the reflex arc that maintains the fovea in a steady position. Consequently, it is, in principle, due to visual defects or to defects in the mechanism that steady the eyes after a saccadic or pursuit movement (i.e., the neural integrator [see above]).

Nystagmus can be of the *pendular* type with roughly equal oscillations in both directions or the *jerk* type in which there is a slow displacement and a fast one. Although the slow movement is physiopathologically the meaningful one, the fast one, which is a saccade for refoveation, is the more conspicuous and, by convention, defines the nystagmus. Thus, nystagmus is said to "beat" to the left, to the right, upward, or downward. Frequently, a torsional movement of the eye is associated, usually referred to as rotary nystagmus. On lateral gaze, pendular nystagmus may convert to the jerk type. The examination begins with the patient's eyes in primary position and then in the cardinal positions, no more than 30 degrees away from the primary position. The patient is asked first to follow a target held at 50 cm at least to avoid the action of convergence mechanisms. To observe a torsional movement, the examiner should look at a conjuctival vessel. Then the patient is asked to look to the right, left, up, and down, which is a rough clinical means to suppress fixation. Suppression of fixation enhances vestibular nystagmus and is best achieved with the high plus lenses of Frenzel's glasses, which in addition, magnify the eyes and provide a good illumination. Ophthalmoscopy allows the physician to detect small degrees of nystagmus. With the ophthalmoscope, the disc, of course, beats in the direction opposite to that of the anterior segment of the eye.

In normal people, a few bilateral beats of nystagmus or "nystagmus jerks" can occur in extreme lateral gaze. They disappear when the eyes are back a few degrees to the primary position and have no pathologic significance.

Pendular Nystagmus

Pendular nystagmus is usually horizontal and rarely rotary. It increases with fixation attempts and damps on eye closure. It may be accompanied by head oscillations that indeed tend to counteract eye movements. There is no oscillopsia. The response to optokinetic nystagmus may be inversed.

In an adult, pendular nystagmus is either congenital or acquired. Congenital cases are most often associated with poor vision since childhood (e.g., as a result of albinism, congenital cataracts, or gross errors of refraction), although these visual defects do not account for the nystagmus. Acquired pendular nystagmus in adults is rare and results from demyelinating or arterial disease.

Miner's nystagmus was seen formerly in people who worked in poorly lit surroundings, with miners being the leading trade of workers in dark places. According to a proposed classic mechanism, vision in the dark was not foveated but rested on the peripheral retina without true fixation and, hence, constant eye movements that became established. Methane intoxication and nutritional defects have also been implicated.

Jerk Nystagmus

Jerk nystagmus is either horizontal, vertical, or both. A rotatory component is frequent. The fast movement is in the direction of gaze because it is a catchup saccade. The intensity of the jerks increases with gaze in the direction of the fast movement (Alexander's law). However, nystagmus may be unidirectional (i.e., the fast movement is always in the same direction, irrespective of the direction of gaze) or multidirectional, in which case the direction of the fast movement reverses with the direction of gaze. Jerk nystagmus may be either induced or spontaneous pathologic. Jerk nystagmus is induced by visual (optokinetic nystagmus) or vestibular (caloric, rotational, or positional) stimuli (see above).

Spontaneous pathologic nystagmus is a common neurologic sign of prime importance for the clinician. It is customary to distinguish vestibular and gaze-evoked forms.

Vestibular Nystagmus

Vestibular nystagmus results from an imbalance of inputs in or from the VOR subsystems. A simple way of understanding the disorders is to consider that, as it were, VOR on each side push eyes and body to the opposite side. Hence, physiologically, the eyes and body are stabilized on the midline. Impairment of VOR on one side results in displacement of the eyes and body on that side: the slow movement of nystagmus, Romberg's fall, and deviation of extended forefingers or past-pointing, all have this same fundamental significance. They have together been termed the vestibular syndrome. Vestibular nystagmus may be due to peripheral or central disorders.

Peripheral Vestibular Nystagmus

Peripheral vestibular nystagmus is usually unilateral and, of course, unidirectional, horizontal-rotatory, beating to the sound side, conjugate, and increased by loss of fixation. It is most often of short duration. The vestibular syndrome is "harmonious" (i.e., slow displacements of eyes and body are in the same direction because commonly vestibular dysfunction is one sided). Tinnitus and/or deafness, when present, are additional evidence of peripheral disease. There is no evidence of central nervous disease. Caloric and positional testing usually support the peripheral origin.

Central Vestibular Nystagmus

Central vestibular nystagmus is usually bilateral, with the direction changing, and may be disconjugate. It may be pure vertical or (rarely) pure rotatory, with both types being always central. Pure horizontal nystagmus suggests a central origin. Dizziness is common, but true vertigo is unusual. The vestibular syndrome is "dysharmonious" because of damage of crossed and uncrossed vestibular pathways by one or several lesions. The nystagmus is commonly of long duration (months or years). There is no tinnitus or deafness. There is often other evidence of central nervous system lesions. Table 28-1 summarizes the main clinical features of peripheral versus central vestibular nystagmus.

In clinical practice, distinguishing peripheral from central vestibular nystagmus is justified because the

Table 28-1. Peripheral and Central Vestibular Nystagmus[a]

	Peripheral	Central
Direction	Horizontal-rotatory	*Vertical*
	Rarely horizontal	*Pure rotatory*
	Unidirectional	*Multidirectional*
	Conjugate	*May be disconjugate*
Loss of fixation	Increased	Unchanged
Vertigo	Usually severe	Usually absent
		Dizziness frequent
Vestibular syndrome	Harmonious	Dysharmonious
Duration	Short: minutes, hours, days	Usually long: months, years
Tinnitus or deafness	Often present	Usually absent
Other evidence of central nervous system disease	Absent	Often present

[a] Italic features always belong to central nystagmus.

former is usually due to labyrinthine dysfunction, which allows the clinician to dismiss potentially severe intracranial disease. However, with the exceptions of acute end-organ (labyrinthine) disease and pure cerebellar infarction in the distal territory of the posterior cerebellar artery (see below), it must be realized that the peripheral-central distinction calls for several reservations. First, lesions of the vestibular nerve in the cerebellopontine angle can result in a mixed peripheral-central nystagmus (see Bruns' nystagmus), and lesions of the lateral medulla (see Wallenberg's Syndrome below) can involve peripheral neurons, that is, the distal part of the vestibular nerve and primary vestibular fibers en route to the cerebellum, the vestibular nuclei, and secondary neurons in the restiform and juxtarestiform bodies. Finally, it must be kept in mind that vestibular protoneurons (primary vestibular fibers) course to the vestibulocerebellum. Hence, a "peripheral vestibular syndrome" can be due to lesions of the central nervous system.

Wallenberg's Syndrome

In addition to motor, sensory, and autonomic components (see Chs. 30 and 35), the lateral medullary syndrome includes a severe peripheral vestibular syndrome: vertigo, nausea, and a horizontal-rotatory nystagmus beating away from the lesion. However, as a result probably of the mixed peripheral-central lesions mentioned above, more complex nystagmus patterns have been reported, such as monocular downbeat nystagmus, direction-changing nystagmus on closure of the eyes, and gaze-evoked eye and lid nystagmus inhibited by the near reflex. Saccadic lateropulsion has also been observed. Skew deviation may be present, which accounts probably for cases with diplopia. The clinical constellation of symptoms and signs is diagnostic of Wallenberg's syndrome, although the extent of the lesion may vary significantly. However, few of the above-mentioned reports of unusual types of nystagmus are substantiated by pathologic examinations. This casts doubts on their accuracy as it is now known that infarctions of the distal territory of the posterior/inferior cerebellar artery may be associated with lateral medullary infarction (see below).

Gaze-Evoked Nystagmus

By definition, this kind of nystagmus is not present in the primary position. It has also been called "gaze-paretic" nystagmus because it resembles gaze disorders seen in patients who are recovering from a contralateral gaze palsy after, for instance, a frontal infarction. Previous gaze palsy is, however, by no means a prerequisite to gaze-paretic or gaze-evoked nystagmus. Gaze-evoked nystagmus appears when the patient tries to assume eccentric gaze. The slow movement is toward the midline; therefore, the nystagmus is direction changing and beats in the direction of gaze. The amplitude of the slow and fast movements increases with the angle of gaze. The nystagmus may be disconjugate, despite the absence of structural lesion. Physiologically, a defective neural integrator has been held responsible for gaze-evoked nystagmus. Clinically, this type of nystagmus has no localizing value. It means dysfunction(s) at some point(s) in the systems that control conjugate gaze: the hemisphere, brainstem, and/or cerebellum. Symmetric (in horizontal versions) gaze-evoked nystagmus is commonly due to alcohol, phenobarbital, phenytoin, or some benzodiazepines. In such cases, an associated upbeating nystagmus is frequent; a downbeating nystagmus is uncommon. Multiple sclerosis, cerebellar lesions, and myasthenia gravis are possible causes. Asymmetric horizontal gaze-evoked nystagmus signifies a lesional, usually brainstem or cerebellar, cause.

In large schwannomas of the cerebellopontine angle and other extra-axial tumors of the posterior fossa, a coarse slow gaze-evoked nystagmus beating toward the side of the lesion can be associated (in the case of schwannomas) to a vestibular nystagmus (Bruns' nystagmus, named for L. Bruns, German neurologist, 1858–1916).

Other Types of Nystagmus
Upbeat

Primary position upbeat nystagmus is central in origin. It may result from drugs but is usually due to structural disease. Classically, it suggests damage to the brainstem tegmentum. However, it has been reported more precisely with lesions of the pontomedullary junction, of the anterior vermis, and of the inferior olives. Other causal conditions are Gayet-Wernicke encephalopathy, alcoholic cerebellar degeneration, and pontine myelinolysis.

Downbeat

In the primary position, the fast movement is downward. Here again it is central in origin. It is highly suggestive of a pathologic disorder near the foramen magnum, particularly of an Arnold-Chiari malformation. Other causal conditions are syringobulbia, basilar invagination, cerebellar degeneration, Gayet-Wernicke encephalopathy, and lithium toxicity. It may be associated with periodic alternating nystagmus, which too suggests pathologic findings around the craniocervical junction.

Periodic Alternating

In this striking disorder, a horizontal jerk nystagmus beats in one direction for about 1.5 minutes and then a pause (the null period) of 2 to 20 seconds, followed by beats in the opposite direction for about 1.5 minutes. It is central and suggests primarily caudal brainstem damage (see Downbeat, above). It should not be confused with rebound nystagmus (see below). It may be congenital or acquired. Baclofen has been reported to suppress this nystagmus in the acquired form.

Rebound

It is a gaze-evoked horizontal nystagmus that, on sustained eccentric gaze, fades and then, after a brief pause, reappears with a reversed direction. It would not be confused with periodic alternating nystagmus (see above). It is considered specific of cerebellar disease.

Rotatory

Pure rotatory nystagmus is always central in origin. It suggests medullary or thalamic lesions. It may be congenital. It is present in seesaw nystagmus.

Seesaw

This associates disconjugate vertical and torsional movements. One eye rises and intorts while the other falls and extorts. It can be present only in downward gaze or in the primary position. Most patients have a bitemporal hemianopia caused by a large parasellar tumor (e.g., a craniopharyngioma). Head trauma and arterial lesions can also be responsible, with the common physiopathologic denominator being likely damage to the upper brainstem.

Convergence-Retraction

On attempted upward gaze, there is no elevation of the eyes. Instead, the eyes converge and retract (nystagmus retractorius). The disorder is well induced with an optokinetic nystagmus drum rotating downward, thus challenging upward saccades. Convergence-retraction nystagmus is part of the dorsal midbrain or Parinaud's syndrome (see below).

Dissociated or Disconjugate

Dissociated nystagmus results from a lesion of the medial longitudinal fasciculus and is also called internuclear ophthalmoplegia (see below). The abducting eye contralateral to the lesion shows nystagmus beating in the direction of gaze, and there is a paresis of adduction of the ipsilateral eye. Myasthenia gravis may mimic this disorder. The least suspicion justifies a neostigmine or edrophonium chloride test.

Monocular

Nystagmus may be pendular and acquired in a patient with one seeing eye that becomes compromised. It can be of the jerk type, resulting from tumors, arterial lesions, or demyelinating disease of the posterior fossa.

Voluntary

Some people, sometimes several in the same family, have the ability to produce bursts of quick back-to-back horizontal saccadic versions for 20 to 30 seconds when they must "rest." Most, after about 10 seconds, grimace and close their eyes. This may be used as a party stunt or for malingering. This is not nystagmus.

Lid

Upward jerks of the lids frequently accompany upbeat nystagmus. Twitches of the lids on lateral gaze have been reported in the lateral medullary syndrome. Lid nystagmus induced by convergence has been found associated with rostral medullar or cerebellar lesions.

Tests for Nystagmus

Caloric Tests

Injecting cold or hot water in the external ear induces convection currents in the semicircular canals. This results in movements of the endolymph that mimic those that result from movements of the head. Contrary to what obtains in true head movements, only one set of semicircular canals is stimulated. Although caloric stimulation is a rather rough means to evaluate canal function, it is useful, especially in comatose patients.

After tympanic examination to ensure the ear is not clogged with wax or leaking blood and spinal fluid from a basal skull fracture, the head should, ideally, be elevated 30 degrees above the horizontal to provide the setting for a maximum stimulation of the horizontal canal. Irrigating one ear with cold water normally results within seconds in an initial eye deviation toward the stimulated ear followed by jerk nystagmus, the fast phase of which beats away from the stimulated ear. Hot water causes the initial deviation away from and then nystagmus beating toward the stimulated ear. There are two mnemonic tricks to remember this: (1) if one considers the direction of the nystagmus, COWS means cold opposite and warm same; or (2) if one considers the slow eye deviation, cold attracts and heat repels. A bilateral normal response means that the pontine VOR and horizontal gaze mechanisms are functioning. Bilateral simultaneous cold stimulation normally elicits a downward tonic deviation of both eyes followed by upward jerks. This means that the mesencephalic VOR and vertical gaze mechanisms are spared.

Canal paresis is an absent or decreased response to caloric stimulation. Directional preponderance is an imbalance in the nystagmus induced by testing of each ear. This can be of peripheral or central origin. Bithermal stimulation is an elaborate method in which each ear is irrigated in turn with 30°C and 44°C water that is 7°C below and above normal body temperature. Testing with 10 ml of ice water (0°C) yields rough information but is useful.

Positional Nystagmus

Although in caloric testing nystagmus is a normal response, it is an abnormal one in positional nystagmus. The sitting patient with the head rotated 45 degrees to one side is rapidly moved to a head-hanging position with the head 45 degrees below the horizontal (Fig. 28-6). This tests mainly the undermost utricle. The test is most often positive with peripheral, end-organ vestibular disease. In that case, a burst of vertical rotatory nystagmus appears after some 3 to 10 seconds, beating toward the undermost ear for some 10 to 15 seconds. There is concomitant dizziness and a sense of spinning. The test is positive for one ear only and, on repetition, elicits less and less nystagmus and vertigo. The test may, however, be positive with central lesions in the posterior fossa. In such cases, typically, the nystagmus is not delayed. It appears for both positions of the head, and responses do not wane with repetition.

Rotation-induced jerk nystagmus is a laboratory test in which the patient sits in a rotation chair. Both labyrinths are simultaneously stimulated, which corresponds to physiologic stimuli. During rotation, the fast movement is in the direction of rotation, and this is reversed when rotation is stopped.

Other Eye Involuntary Movements

Unwanted Saccades

Several pathologic eye oscillations are due to the intrusion of saccades. *Square-wave jerks* are small-amplitude conjugate saccades that briefly interrupt foveation. Then, after a pause, a reverse saccade restores central fixation. They may be normal with closed lids. Prominent square-wave jerks with open eyes have been reported in cerebellar disease, progressive supranuclear palsy, and Huntington's chorea. *Macrosquare wave jerks* are larger and have been observed in olivopontocerebellar atrophy and demyelinating disease.

Ocular flutter is characterized by bursts of horizontal conjugate saccades without intersaccadic interval.

Opsoclonus has the same features, but continuous saccadic bursts occur in all directions. During recovery, episodes of flutter appear and become predominant; opsoclonus may still be elicited by upward gaze. Flutter and opsoclonus may be due to viral encephalitis, neuroblastoma or other intracranial tumor or the paraneoplastic effects of a remote cancer, hydrocephalus, thalamic hemorrhage, lithium, thallium, and chlordecone.

Ocular Bobbing

Bobbing is a spontaneous quick downward jerk of both eyes followed by a slow return to midposition; it is usually seen in comatose patients. It suggests pri-

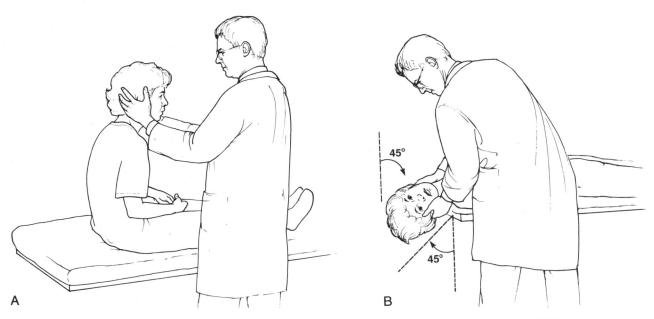

Figure 28-6. Performing passive head movement testing to determine ocular response. (**A**) The patient is started in the sitting position and then (**B**) rapidly placed in the head-hanging position with the head tilted 45 degrees below horizontal.

marily pontine dysfunction but has also been reported in obstructive hydrocephalus and metabolic encephalopathy. Inverse bobbing or dipping is a slow downward deviation with a quick return to midposition. Reverse bobbing is a quick upward deviation with a slow return to midposition. Reverse dipping is a slow upward conjugate movement, a short tonic phase, and a rapid return to midposition. Inverse and reverse bobbing and reverse dipping have no clear-cut topologic correlates.

Ping-Pong Gaze

In ping-pong gaze, every few seconds, the eyes deviate horizontally in alternate directions. Ping-pong gaze suggests bilateral cerebral lesions (bilateral cerebral infarction or posterior fossa hemorrhage).

Roving Eyes

Roving eyes are horizontal, sometimes vertical, random slow conjugate or disconjugate movements in comatose patients. They are similar or close to eye movements in light sleep and imply that brainstem mechanisms are functioning.

Oculogyric Crises

Oculogyric crises were peculiar to postencephalitic parkinsonism and can be seen as a side effect of phenothiazines. The eyes and lids are tonically elevated, and the neck is hyperextended for minutes or hours.

DISEASES THAT CAUSE NUCLEAR AND INFRANUCLEAR DISORDERS

Cranial Nerve III

The anatomic architecture of the cranial nerve III nucleus (see above) implies that cranial nerve III theoretical typical nuclear palsy would associate ipsilateral muscles weakness with paralysis of the contralateral superior rectus and partial bilateral ptosis. Cases with bilateral paralysis of elevation as a result of a unilateral lesion have been reported. Fascicular lesions cause ipsilateral eye muscle weakness with contralateral incoordination and tremor from lesions of the red nucleus and cerebellar pathways (Claude's syndrome), contralateral hemiplegia (Weber's syndrome), or contralateral hemiplegia and cerebellar incoordination (Benedikt's syndrome). There can be, in addition, a vertical gaze impairment (Nothnagel's syndrome). A few cases of pure cranial nerve III fascicular palsy have been reported. Mydriasis was not always present because probably of the fact that the parasympathetic fibers are lateral and can thus be spared. The trunk of the nerve may be compressed by a berry aneurysm, commonly located at the junction of the posterior communicating artery with the internal carotid artery.

The paralysis may be concomitant with a subarachnoid hemorrhage or present without clinical evidence of bleeding. However, there is usually orbital or facial pain. In most cases, there is paralytic mydriasis. Partial paralysis (i.e., without either ptosis, diplopia, or mydriasis) is possible. In tentorial herniation, an enlarged pupil is an early and common sign (see Chs. 17 and 25). On the other hand, in diabetes, cranial nerve III palsy is not rare. The infarction involves mainly the core of the nerve, thus typically sparing the pupil. There is also pain in and around the orbit. The prognosis in diabetic and in nontumor causes of cranial nerve III palsy is in most cases good in a few months. As already mentioned, sparing of the pupil is more frequent in nerve lesions in the cavernous sinus (aneurysms or tumors) than in lesions in the subarachnoid space. Aberrant regeneration of cranial nerve III fibers may be responsible for the synkinetic movements, such as retraction of the lid on attempted eye depression (pseudo-Graefe) or adduction. Cranial nerve III palsy has also been recorded in herpes zoster ophthalmicus, Fisher's syndrome, and ophthalmoplegic migraine. The latter begins usually in children, occasionally in an adult. In most cases, there is an extrinsic and intrinsic paralysis.

Cranial Nerve IV

Palsies are nearly always injuries to the peripheral nerve during its course outside the brainstem. They can result from head trauma and can then be bilateral. Blows on the head with pressure vectors directed to the tentorial notch impinge on the peduncle as cranial nerve IV turns around it. Cranial nerve IV palsy, however, can follow minimal head trauma. Tumors, diabetes, systemic inflammatory diseases, and even an aneurysm of the superior cerebellar artery adjacent to the nerve have been reported to cause cranial nerve IV palsy. There is a congenital fourth nerve palsy that is a phoria and may acutely decompensate into a severe tropia with diplopia.

Cranial Nerve VI

Because of the bilateral projections of the nucleus abducens, nuclear palsy of cranial nerve VI usually implies some difficulty in adducting the contralateral eye. Pure cranial nerve VI palsy, therefore, does not suggest nuclear palsy. Neither does it suggest fascicular lesions because the latter rarely involve cranial nerve VI alone but also cranial nerve VII (ipsilateral facial palsy) and/or the mesencephalic root of cranial nerve V (ipsilateral facial hypoesthesia) and the corticospinal tract (contralateral hemiplegia). These associated disorders are known as Foville's and Millard-Gubler syndromes. They are mostly due to demyelinating disease in young persons, arterial disease in elderly patients.

From its brainstem exit to its entry into the cavernous sinus, the sixth cranial nerve has a long course in the prepontine cistern where it can be damaged by expansions of nasopharyngeal carcinoma, meningitis, and tumors of the clivus (chordomas or meningiomas). The nerve crosses over the tip of the petrous bone where lesions from infections of the middle ear may cause cranial nerve VI and VII palsies with facial pain as a result of involvement of the trigeminal ganglion (Gradenigo's syndrome).

In the cavernous sinus, cranial nerve VI may be involved with cranial nerve III and IV and the ophthalmic branch of cranial nerve V by aneurysms of the carotid siphon, tumors such as meningiomas, pituitary apoplexy, or infections, but for some unknown reason, this nerve is especially vulnerable. An isolated cranial nerve VI palsy may result from cavernous sinus lesions. Cranial nerve VI paralysis is a rare complication of spinal tap. Diabetes mellitus and inflammatory systemic diseases (e.g., giant-cell arteritis) are possible causes.

Bilateral (or unilateral) cranial nerve VI palsy, sometimes associated with cranial nerve VII palsy, can result from head trauma when the examination must look for deafness, otorrhagia of blood or cerebrospinal fluid, and mastoid ecchymosis. Bilateral (or unilateral) cranial nerve VI paralysis is one of the most common false localizing signs of increased intracranial pressure.

SUPRANUCLEAR DISORDERS

Contralateral Gaze Palsy

With acute unilateral frontal lesions that interrupt the frontopontine pathways, there is a palsy of contralateral horizontal gaze. Hence, the eyes (and head) are deviated toward the lesioned side (i.e., "the patient looks at his or her lesion"). Caloric tests would elicit normal horizontal responses. When the opposite frontal lobe is normal, the paralysis is transient. During recovery, as already mentioned (see gaze-evoked nystagmus), gaze-paretic nystagmus can be elicited.

Ocluomotor Apraxia

With bilateral frontoparietal lesions, the eyes remain fixed on a target, a phenomenon that can perhaps be compared with a grasping reflex (see Ch. 25). Blinking interrupts fixation and allows foveation on another target. Thrusts of the head compensate to some degree the lack of eye movements. Oculomotor apraxia can be congenital. Males are more often affected. Familial cases have been reported. Bilateral posterior parietal and frontal lesions result in paralysis of pursuit

movements and of all types of saccades, except fast movements of vestibular nystagmus (see Ch. 25).

Parkinson's Disease

Blinking is strikingly rare, and together with the immobile facies, this gives the diagnostic "stare" of Parkinson's disease. Gaze paralysis is rare. Oculogyric crises (discussed earlier) occur in postencephalitic parkinsonism.

Progressive Supranuclear Palsy

The brunt of the pathologic condition in this degenerative disease bears on the high brainstem and subthalamic regions. Defects of vertical gaze are prominent, with downward paralysis as an often early sign. Upward and horizontal gaze are later compromised.

Parinaud's Syndromes

Parinaud's syndromes (H. Parinaud, 1844–1905, French ophthalmologist) are supranuclear palsies of vertical gaze that result from damage to the mesodiencephalic region. Saccadic and pursuit movements are usually involved. In many cases, the supranuclear nature can be demonstrated by the persistence of doll's head movements, Bell's phenomenon, and VOR. Besides, there is generally clear evidence that the nuclei and fibers of cranial nerves III and IV are spared. There are three subtypes of Parinaud's syndromes. Paralysis of downward gaze is the rarest. It results usually from bilateral infarction or hemorrhage in regions just caudal, medial, and dorsal to the rostral parts of the red nuclei. It has been proposed that such lesions damage the excitatory efferent tracts of the riMLF. Paralysis of upward gaze is the most common subtype. It results usually from unilateral arterial or tumor (mainly pinealomas and hydrocephalus) lesions in or near the posterior commissure. It has been proposed that such lesions damage excitatory efferent tracts from the riMLF that decussate through the posterior commissure en route to cranial nerve III and IV nuclei. The third subtype, paralysis of both upward and downward gaze, results from bilateral similar lesions or lesions that involve the whole riMLF as in the second subtypes. In all three subtypes, convergence may be altered or spared.

Internuclear Ophthalmoplegia

Unilateral interruption of the medial longitudinal fasciculus between the midpons and the medial rectus subnucleus results in failure of adduction of the ipsilateral eye during saccadic pursuit and vestibular horizontal versions. Adduction induced by convergence is usually spared. The abducting eye usually shows nystagmus, the mechanism of which is debated. When there is bilateral medial longitudinal fasciculi interruption there is often upbeating nystagmus. Skew deviation is frequent in uni- and bilateral types. In young adults, the common cause is multiple sclerosis, and the disorder is then commonly bilateral. In elderly patients, the common cause is infarction, with the disorder being commonly unilateral. Tumors, metabolic encephalopathies, Gayet-Wernicke's encephalopathy, and drug intoxication (phenothiazines and tricyclic antidepressants) are rare causes. Myasthenia gravis can mimic internuclear ophthalmoplegia, which would be proved by an edrophonium chloride test. The distinction between anterior and posterior internuclear ophthalmoplegia has very little, if any, practical value.

The One-and-a-Half Syndrome

A unilateral lesion involving the cranial nerve VI nucleus or the PPRF and medial longitudinal fasciculus results in an ipsilateral horizontal gaze palsy and a failure of adduction of the ipsilateral eye. The ipsilateral eye has no lateral movement, and the only horizontal movement of the contralateral eye is abduction, hence the colloquial term of "one-and-a-half syndrome." The contralateral eye is frequently exotropic and, on abduction, shows a nystagmus similar to that of internuclear ophthalmoplegia. The cause is usually infarction, rarely demyelinative disease or tumor.

Cerebellum

It has already been mentioned that some parts of the cerebellum are recognized pieces of the neural integrator. The vestibulocerebellum (flocculus, nodulus, ventral uvula, and ventral paraflocculus) plays a role in eye movements that respond to stimuli from the labyrinth and neck muscles in gaze-holding mechanisms. The flocculus plays a role in gaze velocity. Its lesions disturb smooth pursuit and can cause downbeat and rebound nystagmus. Downbeat and positional nystagmus have been related to lesions of the nodulus. The dorsal vermis and fastigial nuclei play a part in saccadic accuracy. Their failure results in dysmetria. Just as cerebellar modulation pervades all movements of all parts of the body, it pervades all eye movements to ensure stabilization of the eyes, quick adequate shifts of agonist-antagonist activity, and adequacy of amplitude.

Cerebellar disorders have been implicated in square-wave jerks, macrosquare-wave jerks, ocular flutter, and opsoclonus (described earlier). Cogwheel pursuit is slow pursuit with superimposed catchup saccades. Inaccurate saccades result from dysmetria, a basic expression of cerebellar dysfunction. A transient gaze palsy can result from an acute ipsilateral cerebellar lesion. Horizontal gaze-evoked nystagmus may be due to cerebellar dysfunction.

Skew Deviation

Skew deviation is a vertical, concomitant (or not), disconjugate deviation of the eyes. Although it is sometimes ascribed to cerebellar disease, it is likely to reflect a vestibulo-ocular disorder and thus is mainly observed in end-organ or brainstem from medullar to midbrain disease. When of cerebellar origin, it is likely to be due to a disorder of the vestibular pathways.

Infarcts in the Distal Territory of the Posterior Inferior Cerebellar Artery

Part of the primary vestibular fibers synapse in the flocculus, nodulus, uvula, and paraflocculus. Efferent fibers from flocculus, nodulus, and uvula project ipsilaterally on the vestibular nuclei. Acute destruction of these structures by infarction mimics acute labyrinthine dysfunction, with vertigo, nausea, gait disturbances, and nystagmus (see Chs. 30 and 35). The clinician's attention is called to direction-changing nystagmus, more prominent on the side of the lesion. This could help in the differential diagnosis. Similar clinical disorders have been reported with cerebellar hemorrhage. Cases reported with computed tomography do not allow precise correlations. The authors know of only three cases with a pathologic study (Duncan et al., Cases 1 and 2 and Amarenco et al., Case 6028). In Case 1, the flocculus was infarcted, but the nodulus was spared. In Case 2, the nodulus was infarcted. In Case 6028, the uvula and nodulus were infarcted. The infarcted territory in every case was that of the medial branch of posterior inferior cerebellar artery. The flocculus is in 97 percent of the cases supplied by the anterior inferior cerebellar artery and in 3 percent supplied by the posterior inferior cerebellar artery. The floccular lesion due to posterior inferior cerebellar artery occlusion in Case 1 suggests a very rare arterial supply. Again, it must be emphasized that the cerebellar lesion may be associated with a lateral medullary infarction. Symptoms and signs of the latter are liable to mask those of the cerebellar lesion. Hence, in Wallenberg's syndromes with no clear-cut acute labyrinthine dysfunction, whenever possible, magnetic resonance imaging is preferred to computed tomography for better definition of the lesion.

ANNOTATED BIBLIOGRAPHY

Amarenco P, Hauw JJ. Anatomie des arteres cerebelleuses. Rev Neurol 1989;145:267–76.

Update with pathologic correlations.

Amarenco P, Hauw JJ, Henin D et al. Les infarctus du territoire de l'artere cerebelleuse postero-inferieure. Etude clinico-pathologique de 28 cas. Rev Neurol 1989;145: 277–86.

There are no infarcts of the flocculonodular lobe. PICA does not supply the flocculus.

Baloh RW, Honrubia V. Clinical Neurophysiology of the Vestibular System. Contemporary Neurology Series. F A Davis, Philadelphia, 1979.

Clear, concise, clever vestibulology for the clinician.

Bartheson JD, Trautmann JC, Sundt TM Jr. Minimal oculomotor nerve paresis secondary to unruptured intracranial aneurysm. Arch Neurol 1986;43:1015–20.

Even partial cranial nerve III paresis with ipsilateral headache suggests berry aneurysms.

Blepharospasm. Leader. Lancet 1988;2:1059.

Good, concise account of neurophysiology and hypothetic pathology.

Brodal A. The Cranial Nerves Anatomy and Anatomico-Clinical Correlations. 2nd Ed. Blackwell, Oxford, 1962.

A classic.

Buttner-Ennever JA. Anatomy of the ocular motor nuclei. In Kennard C, Rose FC (eds). Physiological Aspects of Clinical Neuro-Ophthalmology. Chapman Hall Medical, London, 1989.

Fine functional anatomy of cranial nerve III nucleus complex.

Buttner-Ennever JA, Akert J. J Comp Neurol 1981;197:17–27.

Buttner-Ennever JA, et al. Ptosis and supranuclear downgaze paralysis. Neurology 1989;39:385–9.

Another premotor pool.

Carpenter MB, Sutin J. Human Neuroanatomy. 8th Ed. Williams & Wilkins, Baltimore, 1983.

Reference book.

Cogan DG. Neurology of the Ocular Muscles. CC Thomas, Springfield, IL, 1975.

A classic.

Collard M, Saint Val C, Mohr M, Kiesman M. Paralysie isolee du nerf moteur oculaire commun par infarctus des fibres fasciculaires. Rev Neurol (Paris) 1991;146:128–32.

A pathologically documented rare case.

Corbett JJ, Jacobson DM, Thompson HS et al. Downbeating nystagmus and other ocular motor defects caused by lithium toxicity. Neurology 1989;39:481–7.

One case with a postmortem examination showed cytotoxicity predominantly in the regions of the nucleus prepositus hypoglosssi and medial vestibular nucleus.

Dagi RL, Chrousos GA, Cogan DC. Spasm of the near reflex associated with organic disease. Am J Ophthalmol 1978;103:582–5.

Spasm of the near reflex is not always hysterical.

Daroff RD, Troost BT, Dell'Osso LF. Nystagmus and related ocular oscillations. In Glaser JS (ed). Neuro-Ophthalmology. Harper and Row, Hagerstown, MD, 1978.

A conceptualized clinical study with a glossary.

Duncan GW, Parker SW, Fisher CM. Acute cerebellar infarction in the PICA territory. Arch Neurol 1975;32:364–8.

The seminal paper on infarction of the vestibulocerebellum.

Fisher CM. Some neuroophthalmological observations. J Neurol Neurosurg Psychiatry 1967;30:383–92.

Pearls.

Gaze and Vision. Rev Neurol (special issue). Pierrot-Descalligay C, ed. 1988;145:499–664.

Twenty-two papers, eleven in English, eleven in French, giving an update of normal and pathologic eye movements.

Glaser JS. Neuro-Ophthalmology. 2nd Ed. JP Lippincott, Philadelphia, 1990.

A scholarly book that reflects also the best down-to-earth experience.

Grandas F, Elston J, Quinn N, Marsden CD. Blepharospasm: a review of 264 patients. J Neurol Neurosurg Psychiatry 1988;51:767–72.

Seventy-eight percent had Meige's syndrome.

Halmagyi GM, Rudge P, Gresty MA et al. Treatment of periodic alternating nystagmus. Ann Neurol 1980;8:609–11.

Baclofen was effective in two cases of acquired periodic alternating nystagmus and ineffective in one congenital case.

Huang CY, Yu YL. Small cerebellar strokes may mimic labyrinthine lesions. J Neurol Neurosurg Psychiatry 1985;48:263–5.

Cerebellar hemorrhage may mimic acute labyrinthine dysfunction.

Jankovic J. Etiology and differential diagnosis of blepharospasm and oromandibular dystonia. In Jankovic J, Tolosa E (eds). Facial Dyskinesias. Advances in Neurology. Vol. 49. Raven Press, New York, 1988.

An update with references and the diagnosis of eyelid closure.

Leigh RJ, Zee DS. The Neurology of Eye Movements. Contemporary Neurology Series. FA Davis, Philadelphia, 1983.

A must in the field.

Mays L. Neural control of vergence eye movements: convergence and divergence neurons in midbrain. J Neurophysiol 1984;31:1091–108.

Premotor pools for vergence.

Mehler MF. The clinical spectrum of ocular bobbing and ocular dipping. J Neurol Neurosurg Psychiatry 1988;51:725–7.

The fourth element of bobbing and dipping.

Najim Al-Dim A, Anderson M, Bickerstaff ER, Harvey I. Brainstem encephalitis and the syndrome of Miller Fisher. A clinical study. Brain 1982;105:481–95.

After ophthalmoplegia, facial weakness, often bilateral, is most common.

Oas J, Baloh RW. Vertigo and the anterior inferior cerebellar artery syndrome. Neurology 1992;42:2274–9.

Two patients with episodic isolated dizziness eventually developed stroke, which featured ataxia.

Pierrot-Deseilligny C. Circuits oculomoteurs centraux. Rev Neurol (Paris) 1985;141:349.

A fine review of experimental and human evidence.

Pierrot-Deseilligny C, Chain F, et al. The "one-and-a-half" syndrome. Brain 1981;104:665–99.

Fisher's basic findings expanded.

Pierrot-Deseilligny C, Chain F, et al. Parinaud's syndrome. Brain 1982;105:667–96.

Pathologic data and proposed mechanisms.

Pierrot-Deseilligny C, Gautier JC, Loron P. Acquired ocular motor apraxia due to bilateral frontoparietal infarcts. Ann Neurol 1988;23:199–202.

A study in failure of hemispheric commands of saccades and pursuit movements.

Pierrot-Deseilligny C, Schaison M, et al. Syndrome nucléaire du nerf moteur oculaire commun. À propos de deux observations cliniques. Rev Neurol (Paris) 1981;137:217–22.

Demonstration that the fibers to the superior rectus are crossed

Plum F, Posner J. The Diagnosis of Stupor and Coma. 3rd Ed. Contemporary Neurology Series. FA Davis, Philadelphia, 1980.

The reference book on disorders of consciousness and the high brainstem.

Spector RH, Troost BT. The ocular motor system. Ann Neurol 1981;9:517–25.

Brainstem control of eye movements and the clinical implications.

Symonds C. Vertigo. R Melbourne Hosp Clin Rep 1953;23:1–7.

Reflections of a great clinician.

Tatemichi TK, Duncan CM, Moser FG et al. Syndromes of paramedian thalamopeduncular arteries: clinical and MRI correlations in infarctions of the upper midbrain and thalamus. Ann Neurol 1987;22:159.

Magnetic resonance imaging used to image infarcts. Those above the midbrain produced impairment of upward gaze, some without oculomotor disturbances; some in the midbrain produced very circumscribed oculomotor dysfunction without involvement of the opposite side. None produced the pictures typical of midbrain compression in evolving mass

Troost BT. Nystagmus: a clinical review. Rev Neurol (Paris) 1989;145:417–28.

A practical update.

Tusa RJ. Cortical control of eye movements. In Kennard C, Rose FC (eds). Physiological Aspects of Clinical Neuro-Ophthalmology. Chapman Hall Medical, London, 1988.

Both saccades and pursuit movements are controlled by frontal and parietal areas.

29
Other Cranial Nerves

J. C. Gautier and J. P. Mohr

CRANIAL NERVE I (OLFACTORY NERVE)

The olfactory receptors are located in a restricted yellowish surface of the nasal mucosa on either side of the upper and rear part of the nasal cavity: the area olfactoria. There are about 20 million bipolar 5- to 15-μm receptor neurons with peripheral ciliated processes that undergo a constant renewal with a life span of about 1 month. The central processes are very thin (0.2 μm) unmyelinated axons that gather into bundles, passing upward through the cribriform plate where they are surrounded by meningeal sheaths and can be severed by sudden torquing movements of cerebral concussion. The neurons synapse with the dendrites of the mitral cells in the olfactory bulb (Fig. 29-1) that lie in the olfactory groove. Axons of these second-order mitral cells run caudally in the olfactory tract, which in turn, divides on either side of the anterior perforated substance into medial and lateral olfactory striae. Fibers in the medial olfactory stria cross the midline in the anterior commissure, providing the possibility of hemispatial localization of smell analogous to that for vision. Fibers in the lateral olfactory stria end in the amygdaloid complex and the piriform cortex in the anterior part of the temporal lobe. Olfactory stimuli thus reach the cortex through two neurons only and do not relay in the thalamus, an exception to the general organization of the sensory pathways. There is, however, some evidence that the medial temporal lobes and medial dorsal nuclei of the thalamus play a role in the recognition of smells. The trigeminal nerve also has a possible, but ill-defined, olfactory role.

The olfactory receptors in the area olfactoria are chemoreceptors that respond to stimuli representing odors, scents, and fragrances. Gustative receptors are also chemoreceptors to stimuli that convey the tastes of sweet, salty, sour, and bitter. Olfaction and gustation are closely linked physiologically and clinically. In a patient who complains of a loss of taste, olfaction should be first tested.

Clinical Assessment

In clinical testing, each side must be examined separately, with one nostril being occluded by the examiner because smell can be lost on one side only. Unilateral loss is the most significant clinically, but the patient may ignore it. The patient must sniff because, in quiet breathing, little air reaches the area olfactoria. Odors commonly used for testing include vanilla, coffee, lemon, and mint. It is a common annoyance when beginning the examination to find that odors from the little vials kept in wards and offices have faded away. Microencapsulated odors are now available. Asafetida has such a nasty scent that even subjects who feign a loss of smell can hardly avoid showing their disgust by facial expression or movement. Because ammonia testing stimulates the trigeminal receptors, it is not suitable for smell, but in a patient who claims a loss of smell (e.g., in litigation after head trauma), the claim of no sensation from ammonia makes malingering likely.

With each presented smell, patients are asked first whether they perceive an odor (detection) and second whether they recognize this odor. Many people are not good at identifying fragrances; so the sole perception of an odor has often been taken as meaning normal olfaction. However, this rather crude clinical rule is now open to question, and recent work distinguishes between detection and identification.

Anosmia (Greek: *a,* loss or absence, *nome,* smell) is a complete loss of smell. *Hyposmia* (Greek: *hypo,* deficient) is an incomplete loss and is rarely significant. Anosmia may be permanent or transitory.

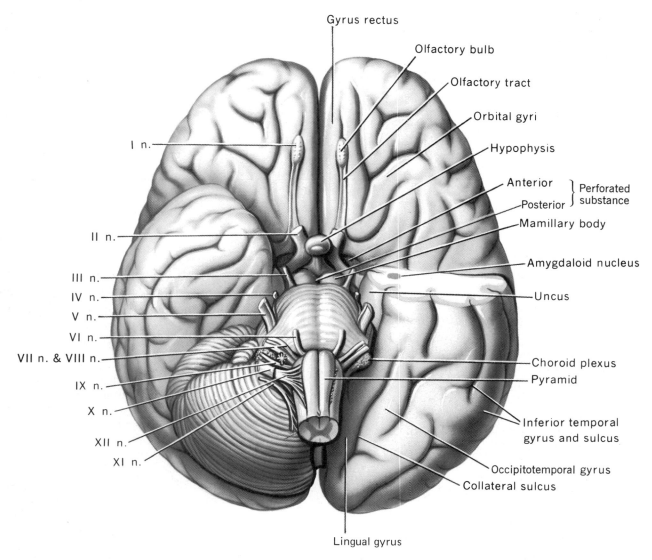

Figure 29-1. Inferior surface of the brain showing the cranial nerves. (From Noback et al., 1991, with permission.)

Disease States

The most common cause is disease of the nasal mucosa. Heavy smokers have a poor ability to smell. Anosmia commonly results from head trauma with or without fracture in the anterior fossa of the skull, neurosurgical procedures on the anterior fossa, subarachnoid hemorrhage, meningioma of the olfactory groove, frontal lobe tumors, radiations, and normal aging. Evidence from olfactory biopsy in post-traumatic anosmia suggests that receptor cells regenerate centrally directed axons that cannot get through fibrotic tissue in the cribriform plate. Many drugs can alter or suppress smell, as described by Schiffman in 1983. Anosmia can also be congenital as in albino pa-

tients and in Kallmann's syndrome when it is associated with hypogonadism. Anosmia may follow influenza.

Olfactory dysfunction has been reported in Alzheimer's, Huntington's, and Parkinson's diseases and Korsakoff's psychosis. In Alzheimer's disease, there are senile plaques and neurofibrillary tangles in the olfactory cortices; these may be found early in the course of the disease. Clinically, it has been reported that identification, not detection, of odors is disturbed early. Postmortem, it has been shown that the nasal epithelium shows unique lesions in Alzheimer's disease, which leads the clinician to consider a biopsy for pathologic examination and cell cultures. In Parkinson's disease, the defects in detection and identification have been found to be independent of cognitive, perceptual-motor, and memory deficits.

Olfactory hallucinations are due to disease of the central nervous system (see Chs. 25 and 79) or psychiatric disorders.

The olfactory nerve can be a pathway for infectious agents to reach the brain. Cases of rabies from inhalation of the virus have been reported.

CRANIAL NERVE V (TRIGEMINAL NERVE)

The largest of the cranial nerves, cranial nerve V is both a sensory and motor nerve. As a sensory nerve, it conveys sensory impulses from most of the skin and mucous membranes of the ipsilateral face and dura mater. As a motor nerve, it innervates the masticatory muscles, the temporalis, masseter, and pterygoids.

Sensory

Unipolar cells similar to those found in the spinal ganglia are found in the semilunar or Gasser's ganglion (see Figs. 29-1 and 26-4) (J. L. Gasser, Austrian anatomist, 1723–1765). The ganglion lies in a cleft of the dura mater atop the petrous bone known as Meckel's cave (J. F. Meckel, German anatomist, 1714–1774). The nucleus also has a few "peripheral" cells located in the mesencephalon, which form the rostral part of the nucleus of cranial nerve V (mesencephalic nucleus) and receive inputs from joint, muscle, and pressure receptors.

The peripheral processes of gasserian cells constitute the three main branches of cranial nerve V (see Fig. 26-4). These three branches each have a distinctive anatomy. The first is the *ophthalmic (V1)* branch, which passes forward to the orbit through the cavernous sinus and superior orbital fissure. The *maxillary (V2)* branch leaves the skull through the foramen rotundum and courses forward through the inferior orbital fissure and infraorbital canal. It reaches the face through the infraorbital foramen. The third, the *mandibular (V3)*, leaves the skull through the cranial foramen ovale and thus arrives into the infratemporal fossa. The skin territories of the three nerves are depicted in Figure 29-2. It should be noted that cranial nerve V1 innervates the cornea and cranial nerve V3 does *not* innervate the angle of the jaw. In addition, all three branches innervate the mucosa of the mouth, nose, paranasal sinuses, anterior two-thirds of the tongue, and the supratentorial dura mater. In the tongue, they convey general sensory but not taste impulses. Some trigeminal ganglion cells, mainly in V1, innervate supratentorial and caudal infratentorial vessels. As proposed by Moskowitz et al. this trigeminovascular system could play a key role in vascular headaches.

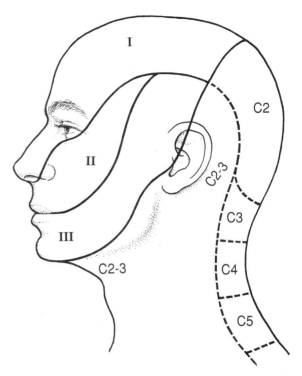

Figure 29-2. The fifth cranial nerve territory, with each major division: I, ophthalmic; II, maxillary; and III, mandibular.

The central processes of the gasserian cells form the sensory root (Fig. 26-4), which enters the tegmentum of the pons and divides into short ascending and long descending fibers. Ascending fibers convey tactile and pressure inputs and synapse in the principal sensory nucleus in the upper pons. Descending fibers convey thermal and pain inputs and run caudally well into the cervical cord at least down to C2. They synapse in the adjacent spinal trigeminal nucleus. From the principal sensory and spinal nucleus, postsynaptic (second-order or deutoneurons) form the ventral trigeminal tract and join the medial lemniscus to reach the thalamus. In the thalamus, cranial nerve V fibers synapse specifically in the ventroposteromedial nucleus. Uncrossed fibers from the principal sensory nucleus ascend to the ipsilateral ventroposteriomedial nucleus as the dorsal trigeminal tract.

Motor

The motor nucleus lies medial to the principal sensory nucleus. The efferent fibers exit medial to the sensory root (Fig. 29-1), pass under Gasser's ganglion, and together with the mandibular branch, exit through the cranial foramen ovale. They innervate the temporal, masseter, medial and lateral pterygoid muscles, the anterior bellies of the digastric and the mylohyoid muscles, the tensor tympani, and the tensor veli palatini. Some of the sensory branches carry also *autonomic* fibers that control lacrimal, salivary, and nasal secretions.

Clinical Examination

A time-honored test of the reflex arc mediated by the trigeminal nerve is the corneal reflex, a reflex closure of the lids (cranial nerve VII) in response to light touch of the cornea. The reflex is tested with a pointed wisp of cotton approaching laterally, with the patient looking toward the other side. This avoids defensive blinking. A decreased or absent response is an early sign of cranial nerve V sensory impairment but may also be diminished by a lesion in the contralateral hemisphere or even in the motor pathway from the hemisphere. This makes an abnormal response a general sign but not one that is specific for a monosynaptic reflex. Gently rolling a wisp of cotton in the nostril is also a good test of cranial nerve V1.

Motor disturbances cause muscle wasting and often striking hollowing of the temporalis. The bulk of the temporalis and masseter can be palpated by asking the patient to close the mouth forcefully. Pterygoids draw the jaw to the contralateral side (diduction). Their strength can be evaluated by opposing that movement, or patients can also be asked to open their mouth. When the pterygoids on one side are weak, the jaw is deviated to the weak side, and the open mouth is oval with the smaller part on the sound side (bouche oblique ovalaire of French neurologists).

The jaw reflex, the uppermost deep reflex, is a monosynaptic stretch reflex. The patient is asked to let the jaw sag open. The examiner taps with a forefinger, which is placed on the chin. A pathologically brisk response means that the lesion of the upper motor neurons is above the brainstem.

In the corneomandibular reflex, there is deviation of the jaw in response to corneal light touch. The response may be quick or slow. The latter is mainly seen in coma and has grave prognostic significance. This can be a normal response in infants. In elderly patients, it is generally evidence of corticobulbar bilateral lesions. The corneomandibular should not be confused with the corneomental reflex, which is a constriction of the ipsilateral mentalis, which responds to corneal stimulation, that can be seen in normal people. Other reflexes in which cranial nerve V is implied are tearing, sneezing, and vomiting.

Diseases of Cranial Nerve V

Trigeminal Neuralgia

Trigeminal neuralgia is the most common disorder of cranial nerve V. Although pathophysiologic theories have been proposed, it is correct at present to keep its full appellation: idiopathic or essential trigeminal neuralgia because it is a clear-cut entity that is separate from all other facial pains. In rare cases, the disease can be bilateral but very rarely simultaneous.

The typical patient with trigeminal neuralgia is older than 50 years and complains of short bouts (seconds) of sharp, severe, unilateral, stabbing, or shooting pain, often compared to an electric shock or lightning. Characteristically, the pain is provoked by contact (of the tongue, toothbrush, or food) on a precise small area, the trigger zone. After the pain, for a variable period, no pain can be elicited from the trigger area. In severe cases, patients make the best of this and eat quickly. Pain affects the fields of the maxillary or mandibular branches, rarely that of the ophthalmic. At the acme of the bout of pain, the patient often winces, hence the term "tic douloureux," which comes from a famous early description. However, trigeminal neuralgia is not a tic in the modern sense of the word. Apart from pain, the neurologic examination is altogether normal, and this is a prerequisite to the diagnosis. Although the diagnosis does not raise particular difficulties, it is not rare to see patients who have had many dental extractions or other misdirected procedures. Besides, trigeminal neuralgia can be heralded from hours to years by bouts of toothache or sinusitis-like pain, termed "pretrigeminal neuralgia."

The first treatment nowadays is carbamazepine, which involves medical monitoring for the low-frequency occurrence of rashes or agranulocytosis. The main disadvantage of carbamazepine is the common occurrence of dizziness and incoordination. In the authors' experience, these latter side effects happen most often when efficacious doses are given from the start. Their occurrence seems less frequent if the dose is started more slowly, at 50 mg twice a day, and increased slowly to the point of pain relief or intolerance. After some weeks of relief, doses are progressively and slowly decreased. As the natural course of the disorder is that of spontaneous remission, one can hope that there will be no pain at the end of a course of treatment. If pain recurs, the program can be resumed. Phenytoin, clonazepam, or baclofen are also worth trying, and in some patients, amitriptyline has been suggested. More recently, pimozide has been reported to be more effective than carbamazepine.

For patients who are intolerant or unresponsive to medical therapy, a variety of surgical procedures have been proposed. Surgical lesions must avoid cranial nerve V1 fibers to avoid corneal hypesthesia that could induce reflex tearing and a severe neuroparalytic keratitis. In addition, when the surgical lesion has caused facial hypesthesia, a severe, dull, aching pain (anesthesia dolorosa) may replace the original neuralgia. Section of the trigeminal root behind the gasserian ganglion, injection of alcohol of the ganglion, and tractotomy in the medulla are mainly of historical interest. Freeing the nerve root from vascular compressions has been performed in large series. All procedures that involve an intracranial approach must be considered with caution, particularly in elderly patients. Currently, thermocoagulation or compression of the gasserian ganglion, glycerol rhizotomy, and radiofrequency and cryotherapy lesions of the peripheral branches give a substantial number of good results at 1 year.

Infrequent "symptomatic" cases of trigeminal neuralgia may mimic at first the essential type. They are mostly due to multiple sclerosis (young patients, in which the pain can be bilateral) or syringobulbia, tumors of cranial nerve V, or a dolichoectatic basilar artery.

Sensory Defects

Sensory defects in the territories of cranial nerve V result commonly from trauma with or without fracture as the nerve branches and twigs exit from the skull. Paresthesiae are frequent. Sensory symptoms and/or signs can succeed dental procedures. Sinus tumors; tumors of the base of the skull (particularly of the nasopharynx); metastases, tumors, and aneurysms of the cavernous sinus; tumors of the trigeminal nerve; sarcoidosis; syphilis; aneurysms; and arachnoiditis are possible causes. Neurolemomas of cranial nerve V can originate anywhere on the course of the nerve and extend either proximally or distally. Apart from disorders of cranial nerve V (pain and sensory loss), they can cause palsies of other cranial nerves and present as tumors of the middle or posterior cranial fossa or both (dumbbell tumors). A small area of numbness on the chin suggests a metastasis to the base of the skull or mandible; numbness on the cheek suggests a tumor of the nasopharynx or inferior orbital fissure. The causes of "symptomatic" trigeminal neuralgia mentioned above can produce numbness and sensory deficits without pain. Some cases have been due to lupus erythematosus, Gougerot-Sjögren syndrome, scleroderma, or acquired immunodeficiency syndrome (AIDS). Trigeminal neuropathy is a term that should be applied to cases with no detectable cause. It should be kept in mind that the cause may be detected years after the clinical onset.

Inflammatory Diseases

The main and most common type is due to herpes zoster, which nearly always affects cranial nerve V1 (herpes zoster ophthalmicus) with vesiculation on the forehead. Lid swelling is common. The cornea may be involved, and ophthalmologic advice is required. Pain is severe in the early phase but usually quickly subsides. On the other hand, postherpetic neuralgia is both severe and chronic, mainly in old people. It is infrequently prevented by current treatments. Extrinsic and intrinsic ocular palsies are possible with a usually good outcome. Optic neuritis, either retrobulbar or with papillitis, is rare but usually has a poor outcome. Cases of stroke related to herpes zoster ophthalmicus are recorded.

Infections of the middle ear may involve the gasserian ganglion and adjacent parts of the nerve. Associated involvement of cranial nerve VI defines Gradenigo's syndrome.

THE CRANIAL NERVE VII (FACIAL NERVE)

The Intermediate Nerve, Cranial Nerve VII bis, Gustation

Cranial nerve VII is the motor nerve for the ipsilateral side of the face and plastysma of the neck. It is closely associated with the nervus intermedius, also known as the intermediate nerve, cranial nerve VII bis, and Wrisberg's nerve (H. A. Wrisberg, German anatomist, 1739–1808), which carries gustatory fibers and a few fibers for general sensation from the external ear (Fig. 29-3). Cranial nerve VII also carries parasympathetic fibers for the facial glands that serve lacrimation, salivation, and sweating.

The motor nucleus of the seventh cranial nerve lies ventrally in the tegmentum of the pons. Fascicular fibers make a dorsolaterocaudal loop that encircles the nucleus of cranial nerve VI and exit at the pontomedullary junction lateral to cranial nerve VI (see Figs. 26-4 and 29-1). The nerve then passes laterally in the cerebellopontine angle together with cranial nerve VII bis, cranial nerve VIII, and the internal auditory artery. With them, it enters the internal auditory meatus (see Fig. 26-4). In the temporal bone, it courses with the nervus intermedius in the facial canal, where it makes a first bend dorsalward (facial knee). In its intraosseous course, the nerve passes close by the tympanic cavity, and there, cranial nerve VII gives off the stapedial nerve for the stapedius muscle, which dampens the movements of the ossicles of the ear. The facial canal then makes a second bend and runs downward, and its course allows cranial nerve VII to exit from the skull at the stylomastoid foramen. The nerve in its extracranial course then proceeds forward in the parotid gland where it forms a plexus and gives off its terminal branches for all ipsilateral facial muscles. Among these, the most significant clinically are the orbicularis oculi and frontalis, innervated by the upper branches; and the orbicularis oris, buccinator, and platysma, innervated by the lower branches.

The ganglion containing the unipolar cells of cranial nerve VII bis lies at the sharp bend or knee of

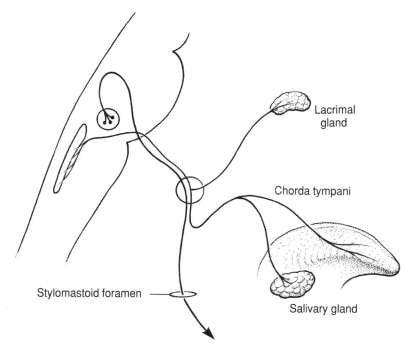

Lacrimal gland

Chorda tympani

Stylomastoid foramen

Salivary gland

Figure 29-3. Cranial nerves VII and VII bis. Autonomic fibers are not depicted (see text).

the facial nerve (see Fig. 25-4), hence its name "geniculate" from genu (from the latin for knee). Peripheral fibers carry taste impulses through fibers that have fused first with the lingual nerve (cranial nerve V3) and thence course through the chorda tympani in the tympanic cavity. These fibers join cranial nerve VII bis just distal to the stapedius nerve. From the ganglion, centripetal fibers run to the nucleus of the solitary tract in the medulla. A few peripheral cranial nerve VII bis fibers carry sensory cutaneous impulses from a small area of the concha. Physicians who place an otoscope in the external auditory canal often trigger a slight cough from the patient, an effect thought to be mediated by this small sensory cutaneous innervation.

Parasympathetic fibers from the superior salivary nucleus form two main outflow; the first is through the greater superficial petrosal nerve that leaves the intermediate near the geniculate ganglion to reach the sphenopalatine (synonym for pterygopalatine) ganglion. Postganglionic fibers innervate the lacrimal glands and glands in the nasal cavity. The second outflow consists of fibers running in the chorda tympani, which carry impulses to the submaxillary, sublingual, and other small salivary glands.

Clinical Syndromes

Facial Palsy. There are two main main kinds of facial palsy, one known as "peripheral" or "lower motor neuron" palsy, caused by an ipsilateral lesion of the lower motor neuron, and the other as "central" or "upper motor neuron" palsy, caused by a contralateral supranuclear upper motor neuron (i.e., corticopontine) lesion. Generally, peripheral palsies affect all cranial nerve VII-dependent muscles to more or less the same degree, whereas central palsies have more affect on the lower facial muscles. The frontalis and orbicularis oculi are often spared permanent weakness because of their bilateral supranuclear innervation.

In most cases of peripheral facial palsy, the clinical effects are obvious; in central palsies, the signs may be subtle ones that only seasoned neurologists would appreciate. The two main clinical tests rely on movements of the orbicularis oculi and orbicularis oris. Patients are first asked to close their eyes forcibly. Unexpectedly, a good number of normal people do not easily perform the order to close their eyes tightly and need explanations or the example of the examiner. In complete palsy, no closure is achieved, and Bell's phenomenon (see Ch. 28) is proof that the patient attempts to carry out the order. When there is only slight paresis, the interpalpebral fissure is often wider at rest, and blinking is rarer or weaker. On closure of the eyes, the eyelashes are incompletely buried on the paralyzed side.

Baring the teeth by grimacing tests the orbicularis oris. Some motor deficits of central origin do not appear during the carrying out of commands but can become suddenly obvious in smiling or in spontaneous facial mimicry during the interview. Humorous questions that elicit a spontaneous smile and efficacious quips are a part of good neurologic interviews. The authors have also noticed that a minimal unilateral drooling is often present, even in very mild facial palsies. Accessory tests are "wrinkle your forehead" (frontalis), "whistle" (orbicularis oris and buccinator), "pout" (orbicularis oris), "put your chin forward and draw your lips down" (platysma). In stuporous patients, pressing firmly on the angles of the jaw or on the eyebrows elicits an asymmetric wincing.

The sensory area of cranial nerve VII is too small and too overlapped by neighbor nerves to allow a clinical study. Absence of the cough on otoscopic examination is not a reliable sign. For taste examination, see below.

Lower Motor neurons Palsies (Bell's Palsy). Named after the Scottish neurologist Charles Bell (1774–1842), this common condition affects about 25 people of 100,000 per year, men and women alike. Positive serologic tests for herpes simplex virus have been reported in a high proportion of cases, but the condition is generally held to be idiopathic. At present, the traditional label of "paralysis a frigore" (i.e., caused by cold) is still commonly used. Diabetic patients are at a three to four times increased risk.

The onset is acute, with patients often becoming aware of their asymmetric face in the bathroom in the morning. Pain behind the ear in the preceding days is common. Facial paralysis is usually obvious but frequently incomplete; some degree of closure of the eyelids is often present. In severe paralyses, there is dysarthria, drooling, and difficulties in chewing and swallowing (the latter are an indirect consequence of paralysis of the cheek). Examination gives clues to the level of the lesions. Taste is often disturbed (for taste examination, see below), and normal taste suggests a lesion below the chorda tympani. Paralysis of the stapedius muscle results in harsh, painful sounds, and noises from jaw and facial muscles movements are no longer heard. Watering of the eye is common because of sagging to the lower lid, but in some cases, there is reduced lacrimation as a result of involvement of the great petrosal nerve fibers. This can be established by the Schirmer's test. Many patients complain of heaviness or numbness of the cheek, but there are no sensory signs. A possible concomitant involvement of the trigeminal nerve has, however, been reported but must be rare.

The full development of Bell's palsy may require a few days, but the diagnosis is usually straightforward at the first examination. However, four points must be given attention.

First, rare causes of acute facial palsy must be excluded, among which are ear disease (history of otitis media, defective hearing, vertigo, and dizziness), diffuse neuropathies such as Guillain-Barré and Miller Fisher syndrome (absent deep reflexes and involvement of other cranial nerves), and Ramsay Hunt's syndrome (vesicles in the external meatus, meaning geniculate herpes, see below).

Second, old patients commonly fear a stroke, and reassurance can be easily given. Younger and old people alike fear permanent disfigurement. Prognosis is then the foremost practical question. There are no certain predictive data, but the following are the usual guides. On the whole, 90 percent of the cases recover (i.e., all or nearly all of incomplete palsies and three-quarters of those with initial complete palsy). However, the patient should be warned that recovery may take from a few weeks to 3 to 4 months. Additional prognostic factors are early regression of taste disorders that would suggest recovery; paralysis of the stapedius muscle and reduced lacrimation would be of poor prognostic significance. Age older than 60, diabetes, and hypertension would also be unfavorable factors. Electromyographic evidence of denervation after 2 weeks indicates, at best, a long delayed recovery.

Third, therapy must be considered against a background of a good prognosis. Surgical decompression of the nerve trunk, proposed on the claim that the swollen nerve is compressed both in the bony canal and its perineurium, is no longer advised. For patients seen during the first week, a 10-day course of prednisone is used in descending doses (e.g., 40 mg daily for 4 to 7 days followed by tapering), with the usual precautions and monitoring of complications of steroid therapy. Some recommend such treatment only in severe cases because incomplete paralyses recover spontaneously. Electrical stimulation of facial muscles was formerly advocated but has been held responsible for spasm (see below).

In all patients, the eye must be protected from the consequences of absent or reduced blinking and/or reduced lacrimation by the use of eye drops (artificial tears) and an eye patch during sleep. When there is complete paralysis of the orbicularis oculi or there are signs of conjunctivitis, an ophthalmologic consultation is recommended.

Finally, only some 10 percent of patients are dissatisfied with their degree of recovery. Poor or mediocre outcomes are a result of contractures, synkinesias, and/or spasm. Synkinesias (i.e., involuntary ectopic concomitant muscular contractions, e.g., of the orbicularis oris when blinking and/or vice versa) are due to aberrant regeneration of nerve fibers. When severe, such movements are quite an inconvenience in some patients. On the other hand, a minor degree of synkinesia, of which the patient is unaware, is common in "good" recoveries. It is a telltale of antecedent lower motor neuron palsy and may clinch the diagnosis in patients who have long-standing facial paralysis (e.g., because of birth injury by forceps delivery) or who report a transient, undetermined (peripheral or central?) facial palsy and in the diagnosis of a slight hemifacial contracture. Facial synkinesias are elicited by asking patients to blink rapidly and smack their lips.

Another curious disorder caused by aberrant regeneration is the syndrome of crocodile tears in which the eye of the once-paralyzed side waters when the patient eats or thinks of good food. It is due to reinnervation of lacrimal glands by fibers originally pertaining to salivary glands.

Hemifacial spasm is characterized by bursts of involuntary facial movements with a permanent kind of contracture of the facial muscles, which reverses the facial deformation. The interpalpebral fissure is narrowed, and the corner of the mouth attracted toward the once-paralyzed side. It has been proposed that ephaptic excitations (Greek: *ephapse,* to touch), that is, pathologic stimulation of neighboring fibers by traveling impulses, could result from demyelination and account for these spasms. In such patients, there are also severe synkinesias. Mild form of postparalytic hemifacial spasm must be differentiated from facial myokymia, which is a continuous, fine, fibrillary, arrhythmic flickering of the muscles on one side of the face. It has been reported in multiple sclerosis, brainstem glioma, and Guillain-Barré syndrome. Short episodes of flickering of the eyelids are common and benign. They are said to be due to fatigue. Tics and epileptics clonus rarely raise diagnostic problems. For the treatment of hemifacial spasm, see below.

Other Causes of Lower Motor Neuron Facial Palsy. *Trauma,* most frequently fractures of the petrous bone can cause immediate cranial nerve VII paralysis with involvement of cranial nerve VIII, leading to deafness, vertigo, and transient nystagmus. A posttraumatic cranial nerve VII palsy can be delayed for some days and usually has a good prognosis. *Tumors* may cause progressive facial palsies. Cranial nerve VII neurinomas are rare. The authors have seen two cases with good results after microsurgery. Neighboring tumors include acoustic neuromas, tumors of the glomus jugulare, and cholesteatomas. Carcinomatous meningitis may be a cause of facial palsy. Paralysis of some facial muscles may herald malignancy of a parotid tumor. *Infections* are an uncommon cause of acute facial palsy. The best known is Ramsay Hunt's syndrome (J. Ramsay Hunt, English-born American neurologist, 1872–1937), which is due to infection of the geniculate ganglion by herpes zoster virus. There is

often involvement of cranial nerve VIII with tinnitus, loss of hearing, and vertigo. In addition to the vesicles in the external auditory meatus (see below), other vesicles may be present in the mouth, throat, retroauricular region, and neck, resulting from associated infection of cranial nerves IX and X and upper cervical ganglia. For the same reasons, for acute inflammatory peripheral neuropathies, facial paralysis is a common feature of Guillain-Barré and Miller Fisher syndromes. Peripheral facial palsy may be part of the AIDS and, in this setting, is likely to be due to metastatic lymphoma to the leptomeninges. Isolated facial palsy, closely resembling Bell's palsy, has been reported in human immunodeficiency virus-positive patients. Unilateral or bilateral facial palsy can occur in Lyme disease, when it can be associated with facial induration and erythema. Leprosy often involves cranial nerve VII.

Lesions of the fascicular fibers and/or nucleus of cranial nerve VII in the pons are mainly due to infarctions and hemorrhages. There is usually an associated cranial nerve VI paralysis and long tract symptoms and signs.

Peripheral facial palsy may be bilateral, concomitant, or successive. Bell's palsy may be successively bilateral. Acute bilateral concomitant facial palsy is common in the Guillain-Barré and Miller Fisher syndromes and may also be due to leukemia, Lyme disease, and infectious mononucleosis. Recurrent, usually successive, often bilateral facial palsy, facial edema predominant on the lips, and congenital fissures of the tongue make up the Melkersson-Rosenthal syndrome. The cause is unknown. Chronic unilateral or bilateral facial palsy is part of Heerfordt's syndrome, which is due to sarcoidosis (uveoparotid fever). In some instances, facial diplegias must be differentiated from myasthenia gravis and facial myopathies, facioscapular dystrophy, and dystrophia myotonica in which, among other signs, the eyelids and lips are easily prized apart against the patient's forced attempts at closure.

Upper Motor Neuron Palsies. Supranuclear lesions may lie from the upper brainstem to motor cortex and cause a contralateral facial paralysis. Central facial palsy, as already mentioned, affects the lower more than the upper part of the face. This, however, may not be obvious at the onset, even more so with brainstem lesions. In such cases, the usual association of central motor signs (e.g., brisk ipsilateral deep reflexes) is diagnostic. Infarctions, hemorrhages, and tumors are the common causes, but any kind of lesion can, of course, be responsible. In subacute and chronic cases, there may be a striking difference in facial movements that are normal or near normal on command ("voluntary movement"), although the palsy is obvious in "spontaneous" movements, mainly emotional ones (e.g., smiling).

Bilateral lesions result in severe bilateral facial paralysis that involve both the upper and lower parts of the face (facial diplegia). This can be part of a pseudobulbar palsy with dysarthria, dysphonia, dysphagia, and emotional incontinence. The cause is usually bilateral small infarcts (lacunae or small embolic infarcts) on the corticobulbar tracts. A resembling syndrome can occur in motor neuron disease in which case it is a true bulbar palsy with both lower and upper motor neuron involvement.

Facial diplegia can result from lesions of the frontal operculum on both sides. The clinical picture may be impressive with complete facial immobility, aphonia, profound dysphagia, and sagging of the mandible. Corticospinal signs can be minimal or absent. Previous history may or may not disclose a transient facial palsy. Facial central diplegia is usually of abrupt onset when the second lesion occurs. The common cause is opercular infarction as a result of cardiac embolism.

Hemifacial Spasm. Hemifacial spasm can be postparalytic (see above), but in most cases, it is "essential" (i.e., there is no evidence of previous facial palsy). It occurs mainly in middle age, more often in women. It begins usually as twitches of the inferior part of the orbicularis oculi that progressively become stronger as the contractions extend to the other ipsilateral facial muscles. Synkinesias are prominent. There may be facial weakness of the lower motor neuron type. Hemifacial spasm is readily distinguished from epilepsy, tic doloureux, and myokymia (see above). Blepharospasm, oromandibular tardive dyskinesias, and facial myoclonus, oculomasticatory movements with vertical ophthalmoplegia suggestive of Whipple's disease are bilateral; hemifacial spasm is rarely bilateral.

The mechanisms are still elusive. Current emphasis is on compression of the facial nerve as it emerges at the pontomedullary junction with resultant demyelination and ephaptic excitation (see above). There is also evidence of hyperexcitability of the facial nerve nucleus. The compression could be due to a loop of a cerebellar artery or to a dolichoectatic basilar or vertebral artery. Aneurysms, arteriovenous malformations, and cerebellopontine angle tumors with a possible predominance of epidermoids can also be responsible. Thus, such patients should undergo magnetic resonance imaging (MRI) or computed tomography (CT) with contrast.

In essential hemifacial spasm, medical treatment with phenytoin, baclofen, or clonazepam rarely brings sufficient relief. Alcohol injection of the facial nerve at the stylomastoid foramen usually interrupts the spasms for several months but results in residual paralysis. Using small doses of alcohol, the authors have had several good results at 1 year with minimal paralysis. Botulinus toxin blocks the release of acetylcholine from motor neurons. Injections of distal branches of the facial nerve can bring relief for 6 weeks to 6 months. Surgical exposure with decompression of the nerve has been reported to be successful in 75 to 90 percent of the cases. The complication rate is about 15 percent, and the complications include facial paralysis, hearing loss, and stroke. Recurrences are seen in less than 10 percent.

Blepharospasm. Blepharospasm is a focal dystonia characterized by involuntary, frequent, forceful, simultaneous closure of both eyes. It is often severe enough to hamper normal activities such as reading or driving. It is frequently associated with other facial or neck dystonias (Meige's syndrome). Blepharospasm is an organic disease with sometimes a suggestion of familial incidence. Electrophysiologic studies of the blink reflex show a state of hyperexcitability, which suggests a suprapontine disorder. Although the responsible lesions are not known, imaging evidence supports the concept that they probably lie in the diencephalic-brainstem region. Neurologic blepharospasm, of course, must be differentiated from reflex blepharospasm caused by ocular disease. Medical treatment is usually unrewarding. Crushing nerves to the orbicularis oculi has been superseded by botulinus toxin injections.

Taste

Receptors or taste buds lie mainly on the dorsal surface of the tongue and, in addition, in the palate, soft palate, cheeks, pharynx, larynx, and upper esophagus. A bud is made up of about 50 cells surrounding a pore and functions only in a fluid medium, which explains the loss of taste caused by dryness of the mouth. Taste buds are constantly renewed and have a life span of about 10 days.

From receptors, impulses are conveyed to the central nervous system by peripheral processes of the following cranial nerve ganglia: (1) *geniculate ganglion* (cranial nerve VII bis) from the anterior two-thirds of the tongue through the chorda tympani (fibers at first run with the lingual nerve, i.e., cranial nerve V3) and from palatal receptors through the greater superficial petrosal nerve; (2) *ganglion nodosum* (cranial nerve IX) from the posterior third of the tongue, soft palate, and pharynx; and (3) *ganglion nodosum* (cranial nerve X) from the epiglottis, larynx, and probably pharynx. In addition, some impulses may travel along fibers from the *semilunar* ganglion (cranial nerve V) as suggested by a possible preservation of taste after section of the chorda tympani and possible loss of taste after cranial nerve V root section. Centripetal fibers of the ganglia synapse in the nucleus of the solitary tract in the medulla.

Neurons of the second order have short projections to neighboring structures of the brainstem (e.g., trigeminal nucleus and nucleus salivarius) and long projections to the ventroposteromedial nucleus of the thalamus and to the lateral hypothalamus. There are cortical receptive areas in the parietal lobes.

The primary taste sensations are salty, sweet, bitter, and sour. In usual practice, salt and sugar are successively put on discrete parts of the tongue, and the patient is asked to identify the substance without drawing back the tongue. Quinine tests bitter, and a low voltage electric current could test sour.

Clinical Syndromes

Ageusia (Greek: *gueusis*, taste) and hypogueusia are loss and decrease in gustatory sensitivity, respectively. Taste acuity normally decreases in old age. Local disturbances, such as dryness of the tongue and mouth often with damage to taste buds, irradiation of mouth and neck, and many drugs (e.g., tricyclic antidepressants), are the usual causes. Anosmia and hyposmia should be suspected first in taste complaints (see cranial nerve I). Nutritional or hormonal disorders and malignancy may cause taste disorders. In idiopathic hypogueusia and foul taste (cacogueusia) and decreased smell with possible resulting loss of weight and depression, a deficiency of zinc in the saliva has been reported, with beneficial effects of therapy with oral zinc.

Ipsilateral agueusia in the anterior two-thirds of the tongue can result from cranial nerve VII palsy, with the main causes being Bell's palsy, trauma, and internal carotid artery dissection.

CRANIAL NERVE VIII (COCHLEAR-VESTIBULAR NERVE)

The traditional name of cranial nerve VIII is the "acoustic nerve," but the nerve subserves two distinct functions: hearing with cochlear fibers and the sense of position and motion with vestibular fibers. The union of fibers from labyrinth to brainstem is of great clinical significance because concomitant dysfunction of hearing and balance suggests labyrinth or nerve disease.

Cochlear Nerve

The receptors of sound are known as "hair" cells, which make up the organ of Corti, in the spiral-shaped structure of two and one-half turns of the cochlea in the inner ear (Fig. 29-4). Hair cells are in the fluid media known as endolymph that fills the membranous labyrinth. Endolymph has the chemical characteristics of an intracellular fluid with a high potassium and a low sodium concentration. The cells of origin of the first neuron are in the spiral ganglioN (Fig. 29-5). Their peripheral processes convey impulses from hair cells. Their central processes enter in cranial nerve VIII, which together with cranial nerve VII, cranial nerve VIII bis, the vestibular nerve, and the internal auditory artery run medially through the cerebellopontine angle to reach the brainstem at the pontomedullary junction, lateral to the companion nerve (see Figs. 26-4, 29-1, and 29-6). Fibers of the cochlear nerve bifurcate and synapse in the dorsal and ventral cochlear nuclei. The anatomy of second-order neurons that ascend in the brainstem is not fully known, but three principles of clinical relevance are established. First, the pathways are both crossed and uncrossed, and there are in addition commissural fibers so that a brainstem unilateral lesion does not result in simple deafness. Second, there are numerous relay nuclei (e.g., superior olivary nuclei, trapezoid nuclei, and nuclei of the lateral lemniscus), making auditory reflexes especially complex. Third, there is a strict tonotopic arrangement of fibers and cells from the cochlea throughout pathways and relays up to the cortex.

From the dorsal and ventral cochlear nuclei in the medulla, axons of second-order neurons ascend ipsilaterally and contralaterally by the intercalated relays just mentioned. The main bundle is the lateral lemniscus in the lateral tegmentum. Fibers give off collaterals to the reticular formulation. Most of the lemniscal fibers synapse in the laminated central nucleus of the inferior colliculus. Some may reach the contralateral inferior colliculus or the medial geniculate body directly. Fibers from the inferior colliculus reach the medial geniculate body through the brachium of the inferior colliculus. Geniculocortical fibers form the auditory radiation, which passes ipsilaterally through the sublenticular part of the internal capsule to end in the primary auditory cortex (area 41 and part of 42) on the dorsal surface of the temporal lobe, in Heschl's transverse gyri. The gyri are frequently larger and longer in the left hemisphere. Area 41 and part of 42 are surrounded by a belt of secondary auditory cortex: areas 42 and 22. Area 22 is connected with occipital, parietal, and insular areas. Some parts of the auditory cortex are connected with homologous contralateral areas through fibers of the corpus callosum.

Efferent auditory fibers carry regulating influences from higher levels (e.g., for sharpening the auditory discrimination by inhibiting certain frequencies or by controlling the activity of the stapedius and tensor tympani). Some of these fibers form the efferent co-

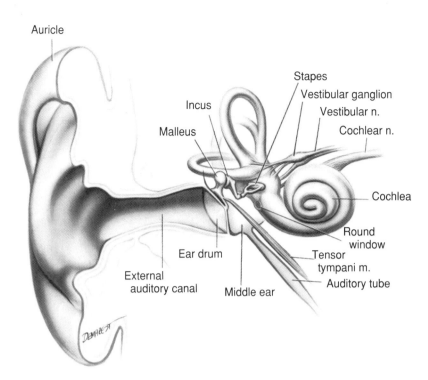

Figure 29-4. The semicircular canals of cranial nerve VIII.

chlear bundle, which leaves the brainstem with the vestibular nerve, joins the cochlear nerve in the labyrinth (Oort's anastomosis), and innervates the organ of Corti.

The cochlear nerve also contains autonomic neurons to the cochlea from the cervical sympathetic chain.

Clinical Examination

Tinnitus and Ear Noises. Tinnitus is frequent and rarely of neurologic significance, but it is a common cause of neurologic consultation because patients fear a disorder of the cerebral circulation. There is often an associated hearing loss. Tinnitus (from the Latin for jingling) is usually the term used to describe ringing or tingling, but it also refers to other ear noises: hissing, humming, buzzing, clicking, whistling, or cricket-like sounds. The main points to assess are whether the noise is uni- or bilateral. Bilateral noises are rarely of neurologic significance. A number of patients cannot answer this question, which usually means that they complain of noises "in the head" with no usual organic correlate. If the noise is rhythmical, a diagnosis is often possible. A quick click would raise the possibility of palatal myoclonus; a pulsatile noise (i.e., with a rhythm similar to that of the heart) suggests a cranial vascular lesion, either a dural or cavernous arteriovenous fistula, arteriovenous malforma-

tion, or rarely, a vessel-rich tumor. Auscultation of the skull, especially the mastoid and orbital regions, may transform the noise from subjective into objective. Caution is advised because some otherwise normal people may intermittently hear their pulsating blood flow on the pillow in the dependent ear. Nonrhythmical noises, by far the most frequent ear noises, are non-neurologic (i.e., result from ear disease). The exception is acoustic neuroma or other cerebellopontine space-occupying lesions that impinge on the cochlear nerve. Neurologic examination and contrast-enhanced CT or MRI, when necessary, should rule these out. After this, the neurologist can give reassurance and, when indicated, refer the patient to an otologist.

Deafness. Loss of hearing, a common complaint, occurs in about 6 percent of people. Deafness may result from two general mechanisms. Poor conduction of sounds in the middle ear (accessorily in the external ear) is known as *conductive* deafness and results from damping of the movements of the ossicles from otosclerosis or from adhesions in the ossicles. Dysfunction of the organ of Corti or acoustic nerve or central disorders are the cause of *sensorineural* deafness. Because central dysfunction is a rare cause of deafness and lesions of the auditory nerve are uncommon, most deaf patients are not seen by the neurologist. In clinical practice, however, the cochlear nerve must be rou-

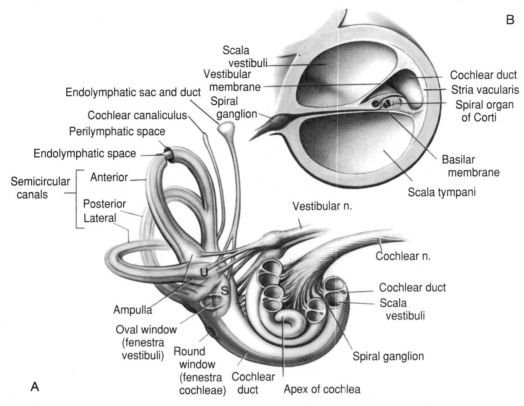

Figure 29-5. The labyrinth. **(A)** Right labyrinth, from the front. The perilymphatic space is between the bony labyrinth and the membanous labyrinth. The endolymphatic space is within the membranous labyrinth, which includes the three semicircular ducts, utricle (U), saccule (S) cochlear duct, and endolymphatic duct and sac. **(B)** Cross section through the cochlea.

tinely examined because unilateral progressive hearing loss may be unraveled in an unwitting patient.

A simple and reliable way to assess audition is to ask the patient to repeat numbers uttered from normal loudness to a whisper. Each ear is examined, with the other one being obturated by the vibrating tip of the examiner's forefinger. The patient's eyes are closed to avoid lip reading.

Time-honored clinical tests formerly thought to distinguish conductive from sensorineural deafness were proved to be unreliable. Their basis is that air conduction of sounds to the cochlea is more effective than bone (skull) conduction (i.e., air conduction greater than bone conduction). Sounds are produced by a 512-Hz tune fork set into vibration by a blow on the hand or knee not on wood or metal. In Rinne's test, the foot of the fork is placed on the mastoid and when the patient states that the noise is no longer heard, the fork is placed near the external meatus. Normally and in sensorineural loss, air conduction exceeds bone conduction; in conductive loss, bone conduction exceeds air conduction. In Weber's test, the foot of the

fork is placed on the midline high on the forehead. Normally, the noise is heard on the midline; in conductive loss, it is stronger on the diseased side and in sensorineural loss, on the normal side. For several reasons, disease of both ears, mixed deafness, and unreliable responses, these tests are not secure, and in a noninvestigated hearing loss, audiometry is required. Pure tone audiometry measures hearing loss from 250 to 8,000 Hz and allows a distinction between conductive and sensorineural disorders. Other investigations, sometimes of clinical interest for the neurologist, are acoustic impedance measurement, which checks the stapedius muscle and middle ear pressure; loudness recruitment (i.e., improvement of hearing with increasing intensities characteristic of hair cell dysfunction); and threshold tone decay (i.e., progressive decrease of a tone presented at threshold intensity, which is characteristic of nerve dysfunction).

Electrical studies of the auditory pathway and evoked auditory potentials (often, in practice, brainstem auditory-evoked potentials or brainstem auditory-evoked responses) are of great neurologic interest. With stimuli of well-defined intensity, tone, and

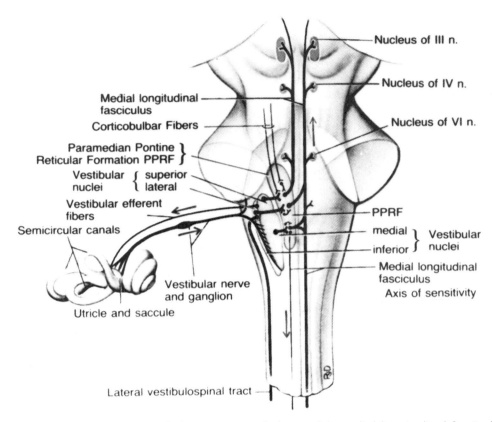

Figure 29-6. Pathways of the vestibular nerve, vestibular nuclei, medial longitudinal fasciculus, and lateral vestibulospinal tract.

interval, reproducible and specific electrical auditory events can be recorded on the scalp and computer averaged. Stimuli are usually clicks with monaural stimulation. The normal recording shows a series of waves that can be ascribed with reasonable probability to specified anatomic sites. Seven waves correspond to the cochlear nerve and the relay nuclei and pathways. The amplitude, shape, and intervals of the waves can be distorted by nerve or central nervous system lesions. Brainstem auditory-evoked potentials are of interest in all cranial nerve VIII lesions and in the brainstem lesions of multiple sclerosis and trauma. They may help in studies of nystagmus and in brain death. A very late wave (P300) on auditory tasks requiring attention and discrimination may have interest in the study of cognitive processes (see Ch. 11).

In dichotic listening tests, different auditory messages are simultaneously delivered to each ear, which allows the testing of the opposite cerebral hemisphere to some extent. Thus, the left hemisphere appears to manage linguistic material; the right hemisphere manages predominantly nonlinguistic messages (e.g., music, see Ch. 20).

Non-neurologic Causes of Deafness

Neurologists must be acquainted with the common otologic causes of hearing loss. These can be either of the conductive, sensorineural, or mixed types.

Hearing loss of mechanical origin can result from obstructive material in the external ear, including wax, external otitis, and foreign bodies, or actual damage to the conducting system from drum perforation or dysfunction of the ossicle chain from otitis media, acute or chronic, with the latter having its own late complications, including cholesteatoma. Other injuries may come from acoustic trauma from noise, barotrauma, quick descent from high altitude, or quick ascent from diving deep in the ocean. Otosclerosis is a genetic disease of the temporal bone that predominates in female patients. Stapedial fixation often results in asymmetric conductive hearing loss. Tinnitus is a frequent accompaniment. Cochlear invasion may cause associated sensorineural hearing loss, and vestibular invasion may cause dizziness. In van der Hoeve's syndrome, also known as osteogenesis imperfecta and blue sclerae, otosclerosis may be present. In Paget's disease (osteitis deformans), a mixed hearing loss is frequent. Neurologic disorders may be present. Hearing loss must also be due to dysfunction of the eustachian tube as a result of viral pharyngitis or barotrauma (common in passengers on alighting from airplanes). In the adult, it must raise the suspicion of a nasopharyngeal carcinoma. Aging is a common cause of otologic hearing loss (presbyacusis). Syphilis must be excluded. Ototoxic drugs can be anticancer chemical agents, quinine, furosemide, or ethacrynic acid but are mainly the aminoglycoside antibiotics. Among these kanamycin, tobramycin, and neomycin are the most offensive to cochlear hair cells; the brunt of streptomycin and gentamicin bears on vestibular hair cells. Hearing loss from salicylates usually regresses after arrest of therapy. Ménière's disease is due to a labyrinthine hydrops (i.e., enlargement of the endolymphatic space of unknown cause). A positive family history is present in one-half of the cases. The disease is characterized by a fluctuating progressive sensorineural hearing loss with typically low-pitched tinnitus and episodic, severe vertigo. The latter is often heralded by an increase in tinnitus and a sensation of ear fullness. It can be bilateral.

Neurologic Causes of Deafness

Trauma. Trauma concussion or fracture of the temporal bone may cause deafness. Longitudinal fractures usually result in the disruption of ossicles with conductive hearing loss. Transverse fractures usually also result in labyrinthine and nerve damage with deafness of mixed nature. In both types of fracture, there may be leakage of cerebrospinal fluid (CSF), which is through the ruptured drum (otorrhagia) in the former and through the eustachian tube in the latter. Hence, meningitis may be an early or later complication in both cases, and its late appearance should raise suspicion of sustained CSF leak. In transverse fractures, a peripheral cranial nerve VII paralysis is associated in about one-half of the cases.

Viral Meningitis. Particularly when viral meningitis follows mumps, it may cause deafness. In herpes zoster oticus, also known as Ramsay Hunt's syndrome (see cranial nerve VII), hearing loss is associated with vertigo, peripheral facial palsy, and a vesicular eruption in the concha and auditory meatus. Bacterial meningitis may damage the cochlear nerve. A severe sensorineural deafness is frequent in neurobrucellosis. Meningeal infiltrates in carcinomatous meningitis may also cause deafness.

Tumors. Tumors of the cerebellopontine angle compress the cochlear nerve. The most common is the acoustic neuroma, which nearly always arises from the vestibular nerve. Progressive, insidious, unilateral, sometimes unwitting, deafness is a hallmark of the clinical picture. Tinnitus is infrequent but, when present, is often of a high-pitched ringing type. Acoustic neuroma, hence deafness, may be bilateral. Before the age of 20 to 25, acoustic neurinomas are usually part of von Recklinghausen's neurofibromatosis with telltale café au lait spots and skin tumors. After age 25, skin features are often minimal or absent (central form of neurofibromatosis). In adults with von Recklinghausen's disease, the tumors may be in the temporal bone and not amenable to surgery. Other tumors of the cerebellopontine angle that can cause deafness are meningiomas, epidermoid cysts, and metastases. All glomus bodies beneath the base of the skull can give rise to enough local mass to cause deafness. The most frequent and that which most frequently compresses the cochlear nerve arises from the glomus jugulare.

Stroke. Whether ischemic or hemorrhagic, stroke is a rare cause of hearing loss. The labyrinth is supplied by the internal auditory artery, a branch of the anterior/inferior cerebellar artery, rarely a primary branch of the basilar artery. The internal auditory artery gives off cochlear and vestibular branches. Labyrinthine hemorrhage usually results from blood dyscrasia (e.g., leukemia) or sometimes from head trauma. Occlusion of the anterior/inferior cerebellar artery determines labyrinthine infarction with unilateral deafness, with or without tinnitus as a distinctive clinical feature. Rarely, unilateral or bilateral, labyrinthine infarction might be due to basilar artery occlusion. Isolated hearing loss or tinnitus are not reliable evidence of the so-called vertebrobasilar insufficiency. Patients with classic, common, or basilar artery migraine can complain of tinnitus. In Cogan's syndrome, presumed to be due to vasculitis, hearing loss, tinnitus, and vertigo are associated with antecedent, simultaneous, or subsequent interstitial keratitis. Some patients have also had panarteritis nodosa or sarcoidosis. Eventually, the second ear is involved.

Hearing loss from damage to the central nervous system is rare because, as already mentioned, auditory tracts and nuclei are both crossed and uncrossed. Lesions that damage both sides of the brainstem can result in deafness, but the whole clinical picture is then so severe as to preclude hearing examination. Deafness is rare in multiple sclerosis. Bilateral lesions that involve both Heschl's gyri in the temporal lobes are usually caused by cardiac embolism. They result in auditory agnosia (i.e., the patient is unable to identify spoken words, music, and nonlinguistic sounds). Some of these patients, however, can still distinguish pure sounds of different intensity and frequency, presumably as a result of the spared functioning of the medial geniculate bodies.

Pseudohearing loss may be due to hysteria or malingering. Additional clinical evidence and auditory-evoked potentials provide the diagnosis.

Sudden deafness is a clinical entity and an emergency that requires a full ear, nose, and throat and neurologic assessment. Many of the causes listed below as a checklist have been considered above. It may be due to head trauma, even a trivial injury, with or without perilymph leakage; a sudden burst of loud noise; viral neuritis and meningitis (e.g., mumps or zoster); labyrinthine hemorrhage; or labyrinthine infarction. If no such causes are present, syphilis and an exceptional form of acoustic neuroma must be excluded.

Despite the extensive list above, in most cases, however, the cause of sudden unilateral deafness remains elusive. Full or partial recovery is frequent. Some of these cases are Ménière's disease.

Vestibular Nerve

The role of the vestibular system is to stabilize the position of the body and the position of the eyes. For this, there are receptors to gravity, the position of the body, and changes in position of the head. Afferent messages are conveyed by vestibulospinal and vestibulo-ocular pathways. End-organ receptors are hair cells located in the rear part of the membranous labyrinth (Fig. 29-6). Receptors for gravity and the position of the head and body in response to linear forces are in two small globoid cavities: the utricle and the saccule. In each of these, hair cells are restricted to a small spot or macula. The cilia of hair cells are embedded in a gel topped by the otolithic membrane, which contains tiny crystals of calcium carbonate: the otoconia. The saccular macula is oriented in the sagittal plane and the utricular macula, in the horizontal plane. The weight of the otoconia acts as a permanent stimulus to counteract the force of gravity and linear forces. Behind the utricle, there are three semicircular canals: (1) anterior or superior, vertical; (2) lateral, horizontal; and (3) posterior, vertical. They correspond roughly to the three planes of space and are arranged in planes perpendicular to one another (Fig. 29-6). The canals are tubes with enlargements or ampullae where they join the bag-shaped utricle. There are two ampullae because the anterior and posterior canals join in their midpart. In each ampulla, there is a crest or crista, perpendicular to the long axis of the canal. This crista supports hair cells covered by a gel with an otolithic membrane but no otoconia. This fills the tube but can swing to-and-fro, acting like a valve. The utricle, saccule, and canals are filled with endolymph, a fluid of intracellular-like composition (see above, cochlea), while they are surrounded by perilymph, a fluid that resembles CSF.

The semicircular canals are receptors for changes in position or angular motions of the head and neck (i.e., rotations, flexions, and extensions). Such movements cause opposite movements of the endolymph in the canal that corresponds to the plane of the movement, with the flux of the fluid displacing the crista and consequently stimulating the hair cells. The resulting outputs to the vestibular nucleus allow adjustments of body and ocular positions. The canals are yoked on both sides (e.g., both horizontal canals or right anterior with left posterior. When the head is rotated to the right, the endolymph moves in the opposite direction in the horizontal canals, and consequently, the right horizontal canal is excited, with the left horizontal canal being inhibited. The canals are also yoked to pairs of ocular muscles that act in the plane of the particular canal (e.g., the left posterior canal is yoked to the right inferior rectus and left superior oblique). These connections explain some features of nystagmus caused by canal disease and also why labyrinthine, mainly utricular, dysfunction can cause elevation of one eye and depression of the other, resulting in skew deviation and diplopia.

Bipolar cells of the first neuron are in Scarpa's ganglion in the internal auditory meatus. Short processes synapse with hair cells. Long processes make up the vestibular nerve that runs together with the cochlear nerve through the cerebellopontine angle. Cranial nerve VIII enters the brainstem lateral to the intermediate nerve (Figs. 29-1 and 29-6). Primary vestibular fibers pass dorsally between the inferior cerebellar peduncle and the spinal trigeminal tract and bifurcate into short ascending and long descending branches that synapse with cells of the vestibular nuclei. As previously mentioned (see Ch. 22), some primary nerve fibers (i.e., protoneurons, running through the juxta-restiform body) pass directly to synapse in the ipsilateral nodulus, uvula, and flocculus of the cerebellum (vestibulocerebellum).

Four vestibular nuclei lie lateral beneath the floor of the fourth ventricle: superior (Bechterew's), lateral (Deiters'), medial (Schwalbe's), and inferior (Roller's). Mainly from the medial and lateral nuclei, largely uncrossed fibers of the vestibulospinal tract descend in the anterior and lateral funiculi of the spinal cord. Vestibulospinal fibers act mainly on extensor muscles. Crossed and uncrossed vestibulo-ocular fibers from all vestibular nuclei enter the medial longitudinal fasciculus (Fig. 29-6) and project chiefly to the nuclei of the oculomotor muscles. Other secondary fibers project to the cerebellum, mainly on the flocculus, nodulus, and uvula.

Two additional points must be stressed. First, projections on the vestibular nuclei are not limited to vestibular primary fibers. Various parts of the cerebellum, particularly the fastigial nuclei and vestibulocerebellum and the interstitial nucleus of Cajal, also project to the vestibular nuclei. Second, there are many commissural fibers between the two groups of vestibular nuclei, which account for the transient disturbances after unilateral vestibular lesions. Physiologic and pathologic evidence suggests vestibular projections to the thalamus (nucleus ventralis posterior lateralis pars oralis) and to the cortex close to the motor cortex and in the region of the intraparietal sulcus. There is evidence that, in humans, the vestibular cortex lies at least partly in the posterior insula. At present, no descending pathway from the cortex, corpus striatum, or colliculi has been firmly established.

Clinical Disorders

Vertigo, nystagmus, and imbalance are the three components of the vestibular syndrome. Vertigo is one of the most common complaints in neurologic practice. It is distressing and upsetting, and many patients fear a severe disease (e.g., tumors or cerebrovascular disorders). In reality, vertigo rarely heralds life-threatening disease, and in most cases, careful history taking and examination allow a reassuring diagnosis.

The first point is to be certain that one is dealing with vertigo for, quite often, patients with "vertigo" complain of fainting, swooning, lightheadedness, or anxiety, all troubles that can result from postural hypotension, anemia, cardiac dysrhythmias, or the frequent hyperventilation syndrome. The latter, commonly associated with anxiety is usually accompanied by pins and needles in the fingers and lips, findings that help separate it from vertigo. It is also useful to keep in mind that loss of consciousness is not characteristic of vertigo. Vertigo (Latin: *vertere*, to turn) implies an illusion of movement of the external world. Some patients maintain that the external world did not move and that "it turned in my head," an equivocal complaint at best. Most causes of vertigo are peripheral (labyrinthine), and in such cases, the movement of the surrounding space has been clearly experienced. Because canal disorders are the usual source of vertigo, spinning or whirling are characteristic complaints. It can help to ask the patient if the walls, windows, doors, ceiling, cars, buildings, and so forth really turned around. It is then rather surprising how many patients can add interesting precisions when properly asked. For clinical purposes, the three canals may be considered to lie in the three planes of space, allowing patients to be asked whether things turned like a wheel of fortune (frontal), around like a merry-go-round, like a dish on the table (horizontal), or like a mill wheel or a squirrel in its cage (sagittal). In the first two instances, the question is whether the world turned clockwise or counterclockwise; in sagittal cases, the patient is asked whether it turned head forward or backward. Rarely, patients complain of the sensation of being in an elevator that runs up or down too quickly. This would suggest utricular or saccular disease. Not all cases of vertigo result in an illusion of complete turning around of the external world. Such comparisons as being in a boat that rolls and pitches or remembrances of sea or travel sickness may help the diagnosis. In central nervous system disease, presumably caused by the wide dispersion of vestibular fibers, vertigo is rarely well defined in a plane. There can even be no movement of the external world, with the patient complaining only of giddiness and dizziness.

Vertigo is usually associated with autonomic disturbances: nausea, vomiting, pallor, and sweating. Again these can be severe in labyrinthine vertigo and are usually absent in central vertigo.

Nystagmus has been considered above (see Ch. 28). It is transient in peripheral vertigo and usually permanent in central vertigo. Nystagmus without vertigo is highly suggestive of central disease. Visual disorders are common in peripheral vestibular disease. In acute disorders, objects appear blurred and moving (in the direction of the fast phase of nystagmus). This is oscillopsia, which is usually transient. In acute lesions of the first and secondary neurons (e.g., in Wallenberg's syndrome), a few patients have been reported who experience a momentary tilt of space so that the patients see upside-down persons around their bed. In chronic vestibular disease (e.g., from ototoxic drugs), the eyes are not steady when the body moves. Typically, in airports or stations, the patients have to stop to read timetables and announcements.

Imbalance may be so sudden and severe it makes the patient fall down, which suggests canal disease. More often, the symptoms are milder. Sudden lurching or staggering while walking is common, and patients fear that people will think they are drunk. Among the many ways of demonstrating vestibular imbalance, Romberg's test, past-pointing, and deviation of the forefingers are usually mentioned. They are not clear-cut signs even in acute vestibular disease and can be compounded by proprioceptive disorders.

Doll's eye movements are normal compensatory movements of the eyes when the examiner turns the patient's head. They depend on vestibulo-ocular and pursuit reflexes. Their presence in a comatose patient means that vestibulo-ocular reflexes are functioning. For caloric tests, see Chapters 17 and 28.

The severity of vestibular symptoms varies largely according to whether the onset of the disorders is sudden or progressive and whether the end-organ and first neuron are involved compared with involvement of second neurons and nuclei in the brainstem. As previously stressed, infarction of the vestibulocerebellum (i.e., flocculus, nodulus, and uvula), caused by occlusion of the posterior inferior cerebellar artery or its branches, suddenly involves the vestibular protoneurons, which thus results in intense vertigo, nystagmus, dysequilibrium, vomiting, and malaise (see Ch. 22). This type of case apart, intense vestibular symptoms are highly suggestive of end-organ disease, and the more distressing the symptoms are, the more reassuring the diagnosis.

A carefully taken history is vital. If it is not the first bout of vertigo, it suggests peripheral disease. Special positions of the head or movements that elicit vertigo help suggest end-organ disease and warrant asking about and testing for triggering movements in an orderly way such as when having the patient turn over in bed, look up at a high shelf, or turn the head to the left and right before crossing the street. An associated disorder of hearing such as tinnitus or deafness and one-sided deafness suggest unilateral disease. A history of drugs such as aspirin, streptomycin, gentamicin, and other aminoglycosides may explain at least the tinnitus and, less often, the deafness.

A thorough neurologic examination is always requested. The main points are nystagmus, hearing, corneal reflexes, facial movements (facial palsy), and cerebellar and pyramidal signs (all these are used to exclude the rare acoustic neuroma that presents with vertigo). CT with contrast and MRI scanning are requested whenever there is any doubt about central or cerebellopontine angle lesions.

Main Causes of Vertigo

Ménière's Disease. (P. Ménière, French physician, 1801–1862) is a chronic disease with bouts of intense vertigo during several hours. The episode has often been preceded by a sensation of fullness in the ear and an increase in tinnitus. There is a chronic progressive fluctuating deafness. Some patients with Ménière's disease experience falling spells, the so-called otolithic catastrophe.

Acute Vestibular Failure. This has been dubbed vestibular neuronitis or neuritis, but proof of infection or inflammation is still lacking, hence the other appellations such as epidemic vertigo and vestibular neuropathy. It is a common disorder, chiefly in young adults, and is often preceded by a nonspecific, probably viral, upper respiratory infection. There is a distinctive absence of hearing disorder. The intense vertigo with severe vomiting, pallor, and sweating slowly subsides in a matter of days or a few weeks. Caloric stimulation shows canal paresis. Slow recovery is the rule. In older patients, acute vestibular failure has been assumed to result from vestibular artery occlusion.

Benign Positional or Paroxysmal Vertigo. This is probably the most common kind of vestibular dysfunction. Brief, vertiginous episodes, lasting a few seconds, occur when patients move their head. Such movements as lying back on the pillow, turning around, or sitting up in bed are particularly significant. The leading theory is that otoconia, broken off and loose in the endolymph, set down on the crista of the posterior/inferior canal, thus resulting in a denser receptor that sends false signals of angular movement when the head is moved (cupulolithiasis or canalolithiasis). Trauma or infection can be causal, but most cases remain idiopathic. Positional testing (see Fig. 28-6) to induce vertigo and nystagmus is diagnostic, although it must be kept in mind that many kinds of vertigo can be elicited or aggravated by positional changes of the head. Therapy by "liberatory maneuver" has been proposed.

Other Types. Vertigo is rare after damage to hair cells caused by *ototoxic drugs*. Imbalance that worsens at night and vestibulo-ocular unsteadiness are the main disorders (see above).

Vertigo is a feature of *basilar migraine*, mainly in young female patients. It is accompanied by other symptoms and signs, among which teichopsia and dimming of vision are diagnostic.

Occlusion of the basilar artery and, particularly, of its posterior/inferior and anterior/inferior cerebellar branches can cause vertigo. For years, it has been a sound clinical rule to consider *isolated* vertigo as nonsuggestive of a *transient ischemic attack*. Recent evidence has been presented, however, for a selective vulnerability of the vestibular labyrinth to ischemia. This could account for isolated bouts of vertigo caused by transient ischemic attacks in the vertebrobasilar system.

Despite anatomic and physiologic evidence that *neck muscles and joints* have a role in vestibular functioning, there is yet no firm evidence of vertigo as a result of neck lesions in humans.

CRANIAL NERVES IX (GLOSSOPHARYNGEAL NERVE) AND X (VAGUS NERVE)

The ninth cranial or glossopharyngeal nerve and the tenth cranial or vagus nerve, and a part of cranial nerve XI (the cranial roots of the accessory nerve) have much in common in their anatomic structure and physiologic significance.

Glossopharyngeal

Cranial nerve IX is predominantly a sensory nerve. The first sensory neurons are in two small ganglia located in the jugular foramen (foramen lacerum), namely the small superior (Andersch's) and petrosal

(Ehrenritter's) ganglia. Bipolar cells convey general sensation: tactile stimuli; pain; and thermal input from the posterior third of the tongue, middle and external ear, tonsil, posterior wall of the upper pharynx, and eustachian tube to the descending tract of cranial nerve V. Other bipolar cells convey taste sensation from the posterior third of the tongue to the tractus solitarius in the medulla. Efferent fibers from the inferior salivary nucleus run with cranial nerve IX and its branch, the lesser petrosal nerve, to the parasympathetic otic ganglion. Postganglionic fibers control saliva secretion, mainly from the parotid gland. From a motor cell group just rostral to the nucleus ambiguus in the medulla, fibers innervate the stylopharyngeus, an elevator of the pharynx.

Macroscopically, the nerve rootlets emerge from the lateral part of the medulla, rostral to cranial nerve X (Fig. 29-1). The nerve runs laterally to pass into the anterior compartment of the jugular foramen. Beneath the skull, on the side of the pharynx, the nerve arches forward between the internal carotid artery and the internal jugular vein and then between the internal and external carotid arteries. The carotid sinus nerve (Hering's), a branch of cranial nerve IX, is the afferent arm of the carotid sinus reflex. It conveys messages from the baroreceptors at the bifurcation of the common carotid artery to the nucleus of the solitary tract in the medulla through a negative feedback loop (an increased activity of baroreceptors causes a reduction in heart rate and arterial pressure), mediated by the efferent arm, which belongs to cranial nerve X.

The functional role of cranial nerve IX is closely linked with that of cranial nerve X. No specific signs of isolated cranial nerve IX function are known for certain. Testing taste on the posterior third of the tongue is beyond clinical feasibility. Touching the posterior wall of the pharynx with a stick normally elicits muscle contraction, with or without a gag reflex. These responses are shared by cranial nerves IX and X. Deficit of cranial nerve IX functions is part of the syndrome of the jugular foramen (Table 29-1).

Glossopharyngeal Neuralgia

Also called vagoglossopharyngeal neuralgia, this has many features similar to trigeminal neuralgia (see Cranial Nerve 5), that is, intense, short stabs of pain. The differences are in the location of the pain (the throat, ear, side of neck, and jaw angle) and in the triggering stimuli (swallowing and sometimes chewing or pressing the painful region). In some patients, there is a concomitant profound bradycardia with possible syncope. The diagnosis must exclude a nasopharyngeal or tonsillar tumor (so-called Schmincke tumor or lymphoepithelioma). Medical treatment is similar to that of trigeminal neuralgia.

Carotid Sinus Syncope

An over-response ("hypersensitivity") of the carotid sinus to stretch is a classic cause of brief loss of consciousness. The responsible stimuli are carried centrally by the carotid sinus nerve, with the response being bradycardia or transient arrest or even atrioventricular block with diffuse cerebral ischemia and syncope. A few convulsive jerks are common. The disorder can follow pressure on the bifurcation of the common carotid artery, classically by a tight collar or while shaving, but is more commonly found among those with severe bilateral carotid disease, in whom an atheroma presumably makes the carotid sinus response more easily evoked. Doppler studies are a good plan to exclude bilateral severe internal carotid artery disease in such cases. Simultaneous massage of both carotid sinuses is inadvisable. In patients suspected of having severe atherosclerosis, it is also unwise to undertake vigorous palpation, massage, or compression of the bifurcation of the common carotid artery. Carotid compression tests, if performed for studies of intracranial circulation, should be carried out well below the bifurcation to avoid the risk of breaking off a thrombus or atherosclerotic debris.

Vagus

Cranial nerve X contains sensory and motor fibers. Sensory bipolar cells of the jugular ganglion, located in the foramen jugulare, convey touch, pain, and thermal sensation from the back of the external ear to the trigeminal tract in the brainstem. Just beneath the jugular foramen, in the nodose ganglion, other bipolar cells convey sensations from the pharynx, larynx, and thoracic, and abdominal viscera to the tractus solitarius in the medulla.

Motor fibers arise from the nucleus ambiguus in the medulla and innervate the muscles of the soft palate (except tensor veli palatini, innervated by cranial nerve V), pharynx, and larynx (see below).

In addition, motor fibers from the caudal part of the nucleus ambiguus emerge as cranial rootlets of cranial nerve XI, join the cranial nerve XI trunk (cranial root of cranial nerve XI, see below) and soon leave it to join cranial nerve X above the nodose ganglion. They are aberrant cranial nerve X fibers and participate in the innervation of the pharynx and larynx. Motor autonomic fibers from the dorsal motor nucleus in the medulla synapse in peripheral parasympathetic ganglia. Postganglionic fibers innervate thoracic and abdominal viscera.

Macroscopically, cranial nerve X rootlets emerge caudal to those of cranial nerve IX, dorsal to the inferior olive (see Figs. 26-4 and 29-1). The nerve trunk passes laterally and then caudally in the foramen jugulare together with cranial nerve XI (see below). In the neck, the vagus lies behind the internal carotid artery and jugular vein in a common sheath. The nerve enters the thorax on the right over the subclavian artery and on the left over the aortic arch. Both enter the abdomen through the diaphragm, together with the esophagus.

Cranial nerve X gives off many branches to the pharyngolaryngeal muscles and to parasympathetic plexuses for the thoracic and abdominal viscera. Several points are of interest to the clinician. First, motor and sensory fibers to the soft palate branch off in the upper neck. Second, the pharynx and the larynx have distinct innervations, namely, (1) the nerves to the pharynx branch off in the upper neck and (2) branches to the larynx come from the recurrent laryngeal nerves with, however, the exception of the cricothyroid muscle, which is innervated by upper neck branch (see below). Both recurrent (Latin: *recurrens*, running or turning back) laryngeal nerves leave the main trunk at the thoracic level and must run back upward, although they have a different course. On the right, the nerve runs around the subclavian artery; on the left, it runs around the aortic arch. Ascending in the neck, both nerves pass between the trachea and thyroid gland. Diseases or surgery on the thorax and neck are thus the main causes of laryngeal paralysis.

Clinical Testing

Demonstration of the function of cranial nerve X is at present limited to an examination of the pharynx and larynx. Symptoms of pharyngeal dysfunction are reflux of air through the nose on phonation because the soft palate no longer occludes the opening of the nares to air coming from the larynx. Consequently, the voice takes up a nasal quality, most obvious on consonants. Other effects are a nasal reflux of food, chiefly liquids, as a result of the same deficit of the soft palate on swallowing. Dysphagia is the main symptom of paralysis of the constrictors of the pharynx. In unilateral lesions, it can be limited to intentional swallowing and frequent throat clearing or cough because froth tends to accumulate over the larynx. In bilateral lesions, the passage of solid foods (e.g., potatoes) can be hampered and often provokes coughing. Pulpy foods are easier to swallow.

Symptoms of laryngeal dysfunction include various degrees of weakness of the voice; hoarseness, which happens when a vocal cord is not tightly apposed with the opposite one; or stridor, which always means airway obstruction. It must be realized that, in unilateral or bilateral complete laryngeal paralysis, stridor can be absent. The patient may be voiceless, but the degree of weakness and hoarseness varies from case to case.

The main point for the neurologist is that stridor, which can herald acute asphyxiation, results chiefly from bilateral recurrent laryngeal nerve paralysis. In such cases, every laryngeal muscle is paralyzed except the cricothyroid muscles, which are innervated by upper neck branches of cranial nerve X (see above). As the cricothyroid muscles are tensors of the vocal cords, their unopposed action brings the cords in apposition, thus shutting the glottis (i.e., the chink between the cords) that serves as the entry of the larynx and trachea. Because a unilateral recurrent laryngeal nerve palsy can result in few symptoms and signs to the neurologist and bilateral palsy carries the high and urgent risk mentioned above, all planned neck surgery on both sides of the neck (e.g., bilateral carotid endarterectomy) requires preoperative laryngoscopy.

Signs of unilateral paralysis (e.g. in Wallenberg's syndrome, see Chs. 30 and 35) result in ipsilateral paralysis of soft palate, pharynx, and larynx. On the paralyzed side, the soft palate droops and does not elevate in phonation. When the patient says "Ah," the raphe (i.e., the uvula), instead of rising on the midline as it does normally, deviates to the sound side. The posterior wall of the pharynx is similarly deviated as if a theater curtain were pulled sideways to the sound side (curtain sign). The gag reflex can be lost. The voice is slightly hoarse and nasal. On laryngoscopy, the paralyzed vocal cord stands midway between adduction and abduction, in the so-called "cadaveric" position. In bilateral cranial nerve X paralysis, the soft palate also droops motionless on phonation, the gag reflex is abolished, and the voice is nasal.

Diseases

In its long course through the cranial cavity, the jugular foramen, neck, thorax, and abdomen, many kinds of lesions can damage cranial nerve X. In the medulla, motor neuron disease and infarction are the common lesions. Poliomyelitis is still a diagnosis in nonimmunized patients. Dysarthria and dysphonia raise consideration of the diagnoses of myasthenia gravis and polymyositis. In the meninges, tumors, carcinomatous meningitis, and infections are possible. At the jugular foramen, pharyngeal branches may be involved in diphtheria. In the neck, blunt or penetrating trauma and surgery are the main causes. Hoarseness is also an early sign of the Lambert-Eaton syndrome (see Ch. 81).

Because its deep thoracic course, the left recurrent laryngeal nerve can be involved by aortic aneurysms, dilation of the left auricle, carcinoma of the lung, and tumors of the mediastinum. Finally, either recurrent laryngeal nerve may be injured during thyroid, parathyroid, or carotid surgery.

CRANIAL NERVE XI (SPINAL ACCESSORY NERVE)

Cranial nerve XI is a purely motor nerve. Traditional anatomy includes a cranial root made of aberrant cranial nerve X fibers (see above, cranial nerve X). It is simpler to consider that cranial nerve XI has only a spinal root. Motor cells are in the anterior gray matter of the first five or six segments of the cervical cord. Rootlets emerging from the lateral aspect of the spinal cord (see Figs. 26-4 and 29-1) form a common trunk that ascends and enters the skull through the foramen magnum. The nerve trunk then descends, exiting from the skull through the jugular foramen. It runs down with the internal jugular vein and innervates the sternocleidomastoid and upper part of trapezius muscles. The lower part of the trapezius is innervated by the third and fourth cervical roots.

The sternocleidomastoid turns the head to the opposite side. The strength of the muscle may be tested and its bulk palpated when patients turn their head against the examiner's resistance or when the lying patient makes an effort to lift the head from the pillow. The trapezius is tested by asking the patient to shrug. The movement is weak on the affected side. In the patient standing at rest, the shoulder droops, and the scapula is slightly winged and rotated, with the lower end in.

The upper motor neuron innervation of cranial nerve XI is moot. With hemispheral lesions (e.g. stroke), the ipsilateral sternocleidomastoid (i.e. that which turns the head to the hemiparetic side) is weak, not the contralateral one. Therefore, an undecussated or a doubly decussated upper motor neuron pathway has been hypothesized.

The sternocleidomastoid and trapezius muscles may be weak and wasted in polymyositis and muscular dystrophy (e.g., myotonic dystrophy). Bilateral involvement is then suggestive of the diagnosis.

Diseases

Pathologic processes in the upper cervical cord, including syringomyelia, tumors, and amyotrophic lateral sclerosis, can damage cranial nerve XI. Tumors of the foramen magnum and the jugular foramen can impinge on the nerve. Cranial nerve XI is frequently involved in multiple cranial nerves palsies (Tables 29-1 and 29-2). In the neck, the nerve can be lesioned by trauma, surgery, and even by lymphadenopathies. Cases of painful paralysis with wasting have been reported, but most are idiopathic and recover.

CRANIAL NERVE XII (HYPOGLOSSAL NERVE)

Cranial nerve XII is a pure motor nerve for the ipsilateral part of the tongue. The motor cells of its nucleus lie near the midline under the medullary part of the fourth ventricle. In addition to motor corticobulbar fibers from both hemispheres, the nucleus receives afferent fibers from the reticular formation. Fascicular fibers pass ventrally and laterally. Rootlets emerge from the medulla between the inferior olive and the pyramid (see Figs. 26-4 and 29-1). The trunk of the nerve exits from the skull through the hypoglossal canal near the foramen magnum. In the neck, each

Table 29-1. Main Peripheral Syndromes of Multiple Cranial Nerve Paralyses

Site	Cranial Nerve	Main Causes
Superior orbital fissure, cavernous sinus	III, IV, V (V1), VI, ± proptosis	Tumors, aneurysms, thrombosis, granulomas (Tolosa-Hunt), infection, pituitary apoplexy, ischemic cranial nerve syndrome
Orbital apex	Same + loss of vision, papilledema, optic atrophy	Cranial nerve II glioma + same as above (often associated)
Apex petrous bone	V, VI	Tumors, infection
Cerebellopontine angle	VII, VII bis, VIII	Acoustic neuroma, dermoid, meningioma
Jugular foramen	IX, X, XI	Tumors (glomus jugulare), aneurysm
Laterocondylar space	IX, X, XI, XII	Tumors, lymph node lesions, granulomas, infectious mononucleosis, ischemic cranial nerve syndrome
Retroparotid space	IX, X, XI, XII, sympathetic	Dissecting aneurysm of the internal carotid artery + same as above
Meninges	Uni- or bilateral combinations	Nasopharyngeal carcinoma, carcinomatous meningitis, sarcoid, meningitides pachymeningitis, leukemia
"Diffuse" processes	Various combinations	Dysimmune neuropathies, e.g., Guillain-Barré and Fisher's syndromes, lymphomas, human immunodeficiency virus, bone disease of the base of the skull

Table 29-2. Main Classic Central Syndromes of Cranial Nerves[a]

Site	Cranial Nerve	Associated Lesions	Signs	Main Causes	Eponyme
Paramedian midbrain	III	Corticospinal tract	Oculomotor palsy + crossed hemiplegia	Infarction, aneurysm, tumor	Weber
Tegmentum of midbrain	III	Brachium conjunctivum + red nucleus	Oculomotor palsy, + crossed incoordination and tremor	Same as above	Claude
Same as above	III	Same as above + corticospinal tract	Same as above + crossed pyramidal syndrome	Same as above, tuberculoma	Benedikt
Tectum of midbrain	Uni- or bilateral III	Uni- or bilateral, brachium conjunctivum	Oculomotor palsies + incoordination + paralysis of gaze	Tumor	Nothnagel
Basis of the pons	VII, often VI	Corticospinal tract	VII + VI palsy + crossed hemiplegia	Infarction, tumor	Millard-Gubler Raymond-Foville
Tegmentum of medulla	X	Spinothalamic tract + sometimes descending sympathetic	Soft palate, vocal cord + Bernard-Horner pupil + crossed anesthesia	Same as above	Avellis
Same as above	X, XII	Corticospinal tract	Same as above + ipsilateral tongue paralysis	Same as above	Jackson
Retro-olivary medulla	V, VIII, IX, X sympathetic	Spinothalamic and spinocerebellar tracts	Same as above + corneal and face anesthesia, incoordination, nystagmus (crossed anesthesia spares the face)	Occlusion of vertebral or posterior inferior cerebellar arteries	Wallenberg
Dorsal medulla	X, XI	Spinothalamic tract + sometimes descending sympathetic	Same as Avellis + paralysis of sternocleidomastoid and trapezius muscles	Infarction, hemorrhage, tuberculoma	Schmidt
Hemimedulla	IX, X descending sympathetic	Corticospinal spinothalamic tract, restiform body	Same as Avellis + ipsilateral incoordination and crossed hemiplegia	Infarction	Babinski-Nageotte

[a] Parinaud's syndrome does not involve carnial nerves.

nerve crosses behind the ipsilateral carotid artery and then ascends to enter and innervate the tongue.

Cranial nerve XII is clinically tested by asking the patient to move the tongue quickly in and out and, to compare both sides, to push the tongue into either cheek while the examiner's finger opposes the movement on the cheek. In peripheral unilateral cranial nerve XII palsies, the protruded tongue deviates toward the affected side. At rest in the mouth, the tongue deviates toward the normal side. Wasting of the paralyzed half of the tongue is quick to appear with folding of the mucosa. Fasciculations are frequent. Unilateral paralysis does not impair speech.

Unilateral Paresis

The main causes of unilateral peripheral cranial nerve XII paralysis include tumors close to the foramen magnum, fractures of the skull base, syringobulbia, and carcinomatous meningitis and even isolated, transient palsy, in infectious mononucleosis. In the neck, the nerve may be injured by surgery or a dissecting aneurysm of the internal carotid artery. Hemiatrophy of the tongue is part of the syndrome of facial hemiatrophy. Unilateral lesions of the corticobulbar motor pathway from the opposite hemisphere usually produce a mild and transient paresis of the tongue, although a frank unilateral paralysis with an ipsilateral hemiparesis has been reported as a result of a small hematoma in the genu and anterior part of the internal capsule.

Bilateral Pareses

Bilateral lesions or the hypoglossal nucleus are a chief feature or motor neuron disease. Fasciculations of the tongue are an early sign. Eventually, the small, wasted tongue lies motionless, with still obvious fasciculations. Bilateral upper motor neuron (e.g., after bilateral strokes) results in pseudobulbar palsy (see Ch. 35). The tongue is small and spastic with slow, awkward movements. The gag reflexes and the jaw jerk are exaggerated.

Some patients complain of sharp pain and numbness of the tongue during head turning. This *neck-tongue syndrome* could be accounted for by sensory afferents of the tongue from the second cervical root, which could be compressed on rotation of an unstable upper cervical spine.

MULTIPLE CRANIAL NERVE PALSIES

Several cranial nerves can be involved by one pathologic process for two reasons: (1) the proximity of their nuclei or of their fascicular fibers, roots, and trunk as they run to and pass through the foramen of the skull (e.g., the syndrome of the jugular foramen or even beneath the skull as long as the nerves have not yet dispersed; and (2) the nature of the pathologic process, which either extends to large areas at the base of the brain (e.g., nasopharyngeal carcinoma) or selectively involves several particular cranial nerves for some still obscure (metabolic or immunologic?) affinity (e.g., Fisher's syndrome).

Involvement of several cranial nerves because of their close anatomic relationship can result from central lesions (i.e., in the brainstem) or peripheral lesions (i.e., outside the brainstem). The clinical diagnosis rests basically on the presence or absence of evidence of associated long tract dysfunction. Difficult cases are not infrequent. CSF examination, including the search for malignant cells, skull radiographs, CT, and MRI help to settle the diagnosis. Table 29-1 lists the main common peripheral syndromes. Table 29-2 lists classic central syndromes with their traditional eponymic designation, which can help the student to refer to historical papers. Except for Wallenberg's syndrome, these are extremely rare indeed and serve more to illustrate anatomy than to direct clinicians.

There is also evidence that concomitant paralysis of several cranial nerves could be due to a common arterial supply (i.e., a common origin of vasa nervorum). Three "associations" have been given as suggestive;

cranial nerves III, IV, VI, and V (V1), is so similar to the cavernous sinus syndrome (Table 29-1) and is caused by disease of a common supply from the internal carotid artery. "Associations" of cranial nerve V (V2 and V3) and cranial nerve VII or of cranial nerves IX, X, XI, and XII could result from disease or interventional embolization of common arterial supplies, respectively, from the middle meningeal artery and ascending pharyngeal arteries (i.e., branches of the external carotid artery).

Multiple cranial nerve palsies not accounted for by anatomic relationships are fairly frequent problems in clinical practice. Some are considered to be cranial forms of the Guillain-Barré syndrome with which they share elevated CSF protein levels (hyperproteinorrachia), absence of CSF pleocytosis, and a good prognosis. Others lack these diagnostic criteria, except for the usually good prognosis, although the disorders can recur. The nerve palsies are then often preceded by facial pain and headache from hours to months. Some can be due to a granulomatous infiltration of the meninges; other cases have been ascribed to Mycoplasma, infectious mononucleosis, varicella-zoster, aspergillosis, or Gougerot-Sjögren syndrome, and more recently also human immunodeficiency virus infection. However, many cases remain idiopathic. Invasion of the base of the brain by tumors or carcinomatous meningitis have a distinctive slower and relentless course. They can cause a paralysis of multiple cranial nerves on one side (Garcin's syndrome; R. Garcin, French neurologist, 1897–1971), in which the usual cause is a nasopharyngeal carcinoma.

ANNOTATED BIBLIOGRAPHY

Cranial Nerve I (Olfactory Nerve)

Brodal A. The Cranial Nerves. Anatomy and Anatomico-Clinical Correlations. 2nd Ed. Blackwell, Oxford, 1962.
A classic.

Conomy JP, Leibovitz A, McCombs W, Stinson J. Airborne rabies encephalitis: demonstration of rabies in the human nervous system. Neurology 1977;27:61–9.
A veterinarian inhaled the virus from a homogenate of rabid goat brain.

Doty RL, Deems DA, Stellar S. Olfactory dysfunction in parkinsonism: a general deficit unrelated to neurologic signs, disease stage or disease duration. Neurology 1988; 38:1237–44.
New symptoms and signs in Parkinson's disease.

Doty RL, Riklan M, Deems DA et al. The olfactory and cognitive deficits in Parkinson's disease: evidence for independence. Ann Neurol 1989;25:166–711
Further analysis in Parkinson's disease.

Esiri MM, Wilcock CK. The olfactory bulbs in Alzheimer's disease. J Neurol Neurosurg Psychiatry 1984;47:56–60.

Alzheimer-type lesions in the olfactory pathways.

Jafek BW, Eller PM, Esses BA, Moran DT. Post-traumatic anosmia. Ultrastructural correlates. Arch Neurol 1989; 46:300–4.

Biopsy of post-traumatic area olfactoria.

Koss E, Weiffenback JM, Haxby JV, Friedland RP. Olfactory detection and identification performance are dissociated in early Alzheimer's disease. Neurology 1988;38: 1228–32.

Olfactory disorders appear early in Alzheimer's disease.

Lancet D. Molecular view of olfactory reception. Trends Neurosci 1984;35–6.

Basic research in olfaction.

Moore-Gillon V. Testing the sense of smell. Br M J 1987; 294:793–4.

A good short account of practical details.

Noback LR, Strominger NL, Demarest RJ. Cranial nerves. In: The Human Nervous System: Introduction and Review. 4th Ed. Lea & Febiger, Philadelphia, 1991.

Ohm TG, Braak H. Olfactory bulb changes in Alzheimer's disease. Acta Neuropathol (Berl) 1987;73:365–9.

Alzheimer-type lesions in the olfactory pathways.

Cranial Nerve V (Trigeminal Nerve)

Brown JE, Preul MC. Percutaneous trigeminal ganglion compression for trigeminal neuralgia. J Neurosurg 1989; 70:900–4.

Experience in 22 patients.

Carpenter MB, Sutin J. Human Neuroanatomy. 8th Ed. Williams and Wilkins, Baltimore, 1983.

Reference book.

Fromm GH, Graff-Radford SB, Terrence CF, Sweet WH. Pretrigeminal neuralgia. Neurology 1990;40:1493–5.

Pain mimicking toothache or sinusitis can herald cranial nerve V neuralgia for hours or years.

Gautier JC, Hauw JJ, Awada A et al. Artères cérébrales dolichoectasiques. Association aux aneurysmes de l'artère abdominale. Rev Neurol (Paris) 1988;144:437–46.

Twenty-seven cases of trigeminal neuralgia among 204 cases of dolichoectatic arteries.

Gregg JM, Samle EW. Surgical management of trigeminal pain with radiofrequency lesions of peripheral nerves. J Oral Maxillofac Surg 1979;48:3–20.

Sixty-eight percent recurrences at 1 year but little sensory loss.

Guiot G. Valeur localisatrice et prognostique du réflex cornéo-ptérygoïdien. Le phénomène de la diduction lente maxillaire. Sem Hôp Paris 1946;22:1368–72.

The seminal article on the localizing significance of the reflex, the prognostic significance of the reflex, and the prognostic significance of the slow response.

Jannetta PJ. Microsurgical approach to the trigeminal nerve for tic douloureux. Prog Neurol Surg 1976;7:180–200.

Rationale of the operation by its main proponent.

Jolleys JV. Treatment of shingles and post-herpetic neuralgia. Br M J 1989;298:1537–8.

Relieves shingles but does not prevent neuralgia.

Lechin F, va de Digs B, Lechin M. Pimozide therapy for trigeminal neuralgia. Arch Neurol 1989;46:960–3.

Pimozide more effective than carbamezepine in a double-blind trial in 42 patients.

Lipkin WI, Parry G, Kiprov D, Abrams D. Inflammatory neuropathy in homosexual men with lymphadenopathy. Neurology 1985;35:1479–83.

Four of 12 cases had cranial nerve V involvement.

Lunsford LD, Bennett MH. Percutaneous retrogasserian glycerol rhizotomy for tic douloureux. Neurosurgery 1984;14:424–30.

Ninety percent excellent or good results.

Mittal B, Thomas DGT. Controlled thermocoagulation in trigeminal neuralgia. J Neurol Neurosurg Psychiatry 1986;49:932–6.

Eighty percent pain free at 1 year.

Moskowitz MA, Buzzi MG, Sakas DE, Linnik MD. Pain mechanisms underlying vascular headaches. Progress report 1989. Rev Neurol (Paris) 1989;145:181–93.

Review of evidence for a stimulating hypothesis.

Pollack IF, Jannetta PJ, Bissonette DJ. Bilateral trigeminal neuralgia: a 14 year experience with microvascular decompression. J Neurosurg 1988;68:559–65.

Good results reported in 89 percent of 22 procedures in 35 patients.

Pollack IF, Sekhar LN, Jannetta PJ, Janecka JP. Neurolemomas of the trigeminal nerve. J Neurosurg 1989;70: 737–45.

Clinical presentation, operative approach, and outcome in 16 cases.

Rushton JG, Olafson RA. Trigeminal neuralgia associated with multiple sclerosis: report of 35 cases. Arch Neurol 1986;13:383–9.

Facial pain frequently bilateral.

Schiffman SS. Taste and smell in disease. New Engl J Med 1983;308:1275–79, 1337–43.

Full review with many references.

Selby G. Diseases of the fifth cranial nerve in Dyck PJJ, Thomas PK, Lambert EH, Bunge R (eds). Peripheral Neuropathy. 2nd Ed. WB Saunders, Philadelphia, 1984.

Thorough review of cranial nerve V diseases.

Spillane JD, Urich H. Trigeminal neuropathy with nasal

ulcer. Report of two cases and one necropsy. J Neurol Neurosurg Psychiatry 1976;39:105–13.

Further data after the seminal article (Brain 82:391–416, 1959).

Trigeminal neuralgia (editorial). Lancet 1974;1:1326–7.

A good, short account.

Vincent D, Loron P, Awada A, Gautier JC. Paralysies multiples et recidivantes des nerfs craniens. Syndrome de Gougerot-Sjøgren. Rev Neurol (Paris) 1985;142:318–21.

Trigeminal sensory deficit is the most common among cranial nerve involvements.

Zakrzewska JM. Cryotherapy in the management of paroxysmal trigeminal neuralgia. J Neurol Neurosurg Psychiatry 1987;50:485–7.

Forty-one percent of 29 patients free of pain at 1 year with no sensory loss.

Cranial Nerve VII (Facial Nerve)

Adour KK, Wingerd J. Idiopathic facial paralysis (Bell's palsy): factors affecting severity and outcome in 446 patients. Neurology 1974;24:1112–6.

Hypertensives and diabetics patients older than 60 had a poorer prognosis; surgery was not beneficial.

Auger AD, Piedgras DG. Hemifacial spasm associated with epidermoid tumors of the cerebello-pontine angle. Neurology 1989;39:577–80.

High prevalence of epidermoids not confirmed.

Belec L, Georges AJ, Vuillecard E et al. Peripheral facial paralysis indicating HIV infection. Lancet 1988;2:1421–2.

Sixteen of 23 cases of acute isolated facial peripheral paralysis were seropositive for human immunodeficiency virus type 1 in Bangui, Africa.

Berlit P, Rakicky J. The Miller Fisher syndrome. Review of the literature. J Clin Neuro Ophthalmol 1992;12:57–63.

Full review of the 223 cases reported with ataxis, areflexia, and ophthalmoplegia.

Blepharospasm (editorial). Lancet 1988;2:1059.

Good, concise account of neurophysiology and hypothetical pathology.

Carpenter MB, Sutin J. Human Neuroanatomy. 8th Ed. Williams and Wilkins, Baltimore, 1982.

Reference book.

Digre K, Corbett JJ. Hemifacial spasm: differential diagnosis, mechanism and treatment, in Jankovic J, Tolosa E (eds). Facial Dyskinesias. Advances in Neurology. Vol. 49. Raven press, New York, 1988.

A review with references.

Dupuis MJM. Les multiples manifestations neurologiques des infections a Borrelia burgdorferi. Rev Neurol (Paris) 1988;144:745–75.

A clear and thorough review. Facial palsy, sometimes bilateral, is a feature in stage II of Lyme disease.

Fisher CM, Ojemann RG, Roberson GH. Spontaneous dissection of the cervico-cerebral arteries. Can J Neurol Sci 1978;5:9–19.

Two cases of dysgeusia among 16 cases.

Heukin RI, Schechter PJ, Hoye R. Mattern CFT. Idiopathic hypogeusia with dysgeusia, hyposmia and dysosmia. A new syndrome. JAMA 1971;217:434.

Disturbances of taste and smell caused by zinc deficiency.

Katusic SK, Beard CM, Wiederholt WC et al. Incidence, clinical features and prognosis in Bell's palsy, Rochester, Minnesota, 1968–1982. Ann Neurol 1986;20:629–7.

Population study.

Lapresle J, Fernandex Manchola I, Lasjaunias P. L'atteinte trigéminale sensitive au cours de la paralysie faciale périphérique essentielle. Presse Med 1980;9:291–3.

In 14 of 24 cases of Bell's palsies, there was facial pain or paresthesias with hypesthesia in 3. A vascular mechanism is proposed.

Najim Al-Dim A, Anderson M, Bickerstaff ER, Harvey I. Brainstem encephalitis and the syndrome of Miller Fisher. A clinical study. Brain 1982;105:481–95.

After ophthalmoplegia, facial weakness, often bilateral, is most common.

Schiffman SS. Taste and smell in disease. N Engl J Med 1983;308:1275–1343.

A good review with far-reaching consequences of smell disorders in medicine and many references.

Snider WD, Simpson DM, Nielsen et al. Neurological complications of acquired immune deficiency syndrome: analysis of 50 patients. Ann Neurol 1983;14:403–18.

Two cases of isolated cranial nerve VII palsy with CSF pleocytosis.

Stevens H. Melkersson's syndrome. Neurology 1965;15:263–6.

Two cases and a review of 184 articles.

Uldry PA, Regli F. Multinévrite des nerfs craniens et syndrome d'immunodéficience acquise (SIDA): 5 cas. Rev Neurol (Paris) 1988;144:586–9.

Two cases of peripheral facial palsy, one isolated in human immunodeficiency virus infection.

Wechsler AE, Ho DD. Bilateral Bell's palsy at the time of HIV seroconversion. Neurology 1988;39:747–8.

Neurologically isolated bilateral Bell's palsy in acute human immunodeficiency virus infection.

Cranial Nerve VIII (Cochlear-Vestibular Nerve)

Al-Deeb S, Yagub BA, Sharif HF, Phadke JG. Neurobrucellosis: clinical characteristics, diagnosis and outcome. Neurology 1989;39:498–501.

Seven of 13 patients (54 percent) with neurobrucellosis had a bilateral cochlear nerve palsy with profound or complete sensori-neural deafness.

Amarenco P, Hauw JJ. Cerebellar infarction in the territory of the anterior and inferior cerebellar artery. Brain 1990; 113:139–55.

A detailed report of 13 pure cases of this rather rare syndrome.

Amarenco P, Hauw JJ, Henin D et al. Les infarctus du territoire de l'artère cérébelleuse postero-inférieure. Étude clinicopathologique de 28 cas. Rev Neurol (Paris) 1989; 145:277–86.

A detailed pathologic study of infarcts of the vestibulocerebellum.

Baloh RW. Dizziness, Hearing Loss and Tinnitus. The Essentials of Neurootology. FA Davis, Philadelphia, 1984.

A clear anatomic and physiologic account with a survey of clinical issues.

Baloh RW, Honrubia V. Clinical Neurophysiology of the Vestibular System. Contemporary Neurology. FA Davis, Philadelphia, 1979.

Clear and thorough account of vestibular physiology and pathology.

Brandt T, Steddin S, Eng D, Daroff RD. Therapy for benign paroxysmal positioning vertigo, revisited. Neurology 1994;44:796–800.

Good reviews of the "maneuvers."

Carpenter MB, Sutin J. Human Neuroanatomy. 8th Ed. Williams and Wilkins, Baltimore, 1983.

Reference book.

Carpenter RHS. The vestibular apparatus, control of posture, in Hobsley M, Saunders KB, Fitzsimmons JT (eds). Neurophysiology. 2nd Ed. Physiological Principles of Medicine Series. E. Arnold, London, 1990.

A clear and up-to-date account of vestibular physiology.

Chiappa KH, Harrison JL, Brooks EB, Young RR. Brainstem auditory evoked responses in 200 patients with multiple sclerosis. Ann Neurol 1980;7:135–43.

Abnormalities detected electrophysiologically in clinically unsuspected lesions in 7.4 percent of patients.

Duncan GW, Parker SW, Fisher CM. Acute cerebellar infarction in the PICA territory. Arch Neurol 1975;32: 364–8.

The seminal article on infarction of the vestibulocerebellum.

Fisher C, Mauguiere F, Ibanez V, Courjon J. Potentiels évoques visuels, auditifs précoces et somesthésiques dans la sclérose en plaques (917 case). Rev Neurol (Paris) 1986; 142:517–23.

Brainstem-evoked auditory potentials detected clinically unsuspected lesions respectively in 13.7, 12.5, and 14.8 percent of definite, probable, and possible multiple sclerosis.

Konigsmark BW. Hereditary deafness in man. N Engl J Med 1969;281:713–827.

Thorough review of hereditary causes of deafness and associated syndromes.

Leigh RJ. Human vestibular cortex. Ann Neurol 1994;35: 383–4.

Review of a glimmering of evidence.

Nadol JB Jr. Hearing loss. N Engl J Med 1993;329: 1092–102.

Good update.

Noback LR, Strominger NL, Demarest RJ. The Human Nervous System. 4th Ed. Lea & Febiger, Philadelphia, 1991.

Ojemann RG. Acoustic Neuroma. In Contemporary Neurosurgery. Williams & Wilkins, Baltimore, 1979.

Thoughtful experience.

Pollack IF, Jannetta PJ, Bissonette DJ. Bilateral trigeminal neuralgia: a 14 year experience with microvascular decompression. J Neurosurg 1988;68:559–65.

Good results reported in 89 percent of 22 procedures in 35 patients.

Schuknecht H. Cupulolithiasis. Arch Otolaryngol 1969;90: 765–9.

The seminal article on detachment of the otoconia in benign positional vertigo.

Semont A, Freyss E, Vitte P. Curing the BPPV with a liberatory maneuver. Adv Otorhinolaryngol 1980;42:290–3.

Seminal article on this maneuver.

Starr A. Auditory brainstem responses in brain death. Brain 1975;99:543–54.

Responses were either absent or only wave 1 of normal amplitude, but prolonged latency was recorded.

Symonds C. Vertigo. R Melbourne Hosp Clin Rep 1953;23: 1–7.

Reflections of a great clinician.

Troost BT. Nystagmus: a clinical review. Rev Neurol (Paris) 1989;145:417–28.

Cranial Nerves IX (Glossopharyngeal Nerve) and 10 (Vagus Nerve)

Brain WR. Brain's Diseases of the Nervous System. 8th Ed. Oxford University Press, Oxford, 1977.

A good account of pharyngeal and laryngeal palsies.

Brodal A. The Cranial Nerves. Anatomy and Anatomico-Clinical Correlations. 2nd Ed. Blackwell, Oxford, 1962.

A classic.

Carpenter MB, Sutin J. Human Neuroanatomy. 8th Ed. Williams and Wilkins, Baltimore, 1983.

Reference book.

Cranial Nerve XI (Spinal Accessory Nerve)

Balagura S, Katz RG. Undecussated innervation of the sternomastoid muscle: a reinstatement. Ann Neurol 1980;7: 84–5.

Evidence for sternomastoid weakness ipsilateral to the hemi-

spheric lesions and review of the conflicting views on upper motor pathway.

Carpenter MB, Sutin J. Human Neuroanatomy. 8th Ed. Williams and Wilkins, Baltimore, 1983.

Reference book.

Eisen A, Bertrand G. Isolated accessory nerve palsy of spontaneous origin. A clinical and electromyographic study. Arch Neurol 1972;27:496–502.

Four cases of acute, idiopathic cranial nerve XI palsy, one with associated serratus anterior palsy. Diagnosis of winging of the scalpula.

Geschwind N. Nature of the decussated innervation of the sternomastoid muscle. Ann Neurol 1980;7:495–6.

Hypothesis of double decussation of the upper motor pathway.

Mastaglia FL, Knezenic W, Thompson PD. Weakness on head turning in hemiplegia: a quantitative study. J Neurol Neurosurg Psychiatry 1986;49:195–7.

Clinical evidence for a double decussation of the upper motor pathway to the sternomastoid muscle.

Cranial Nerve XII (Hypoglossal Nerve)

Bogousslavsky J, Regli F. Hémiparésie avec atteinte linguale. Hématome du genou de la capsule interne. Rev Neurol (Paris) 1984;140:587–90.

Discussion of an occasional case of unilateral tongue paralysis caused by a central lesion.

Bradac GB, Riva A, Stura G, Doriguzz C. Spontaneous ICA dissection presenting with 12th nerve palsy. J Neuroradiol 1989;16:197–202.

Dissection demonstrated by MRI.

Carpenter MB, Sutin J. Human Neuroanatomy. 8th Ed. Williams and Wilkins, Baltimore, 1983.

Reference book.

DeSimone PA, Snyder D. Hypoglossal nerve palsy in infectious mononucleosis. Neurology 1978;28:844–7.

A rare complication of infectious mononucleosis.

Lance JW, Anthony M. Neck-tongue syndrome on sudden turning of the head. J Neurol Neurosurg Psychiatry 1980;43:97–101.

Four cases in young people.

Multiple Cranial Nerve Palsies

DeSimone PA, Snyder D. Hypoglossal nerve palsy in infectious mononucleosis. Neurology 1978;28:844–7.

Isolated cranial nerve XII palsies and a review of multiple cranial nerve palsies in infectious mononucleosis.

Jorge L, Juncos JL, Beal MF. Idiopathic cranial polyneuropathy. A fifteen-year experience. Brain 1987;110:197–211.

Fourteen cases of Massachusetts General Hospital compared with six cases of Tolosa-Hunt syndrome.

Lapresle J, Lasjaunias P. Cranial nerves ischaemic arterial syndromes. Brain 1986;109:207–15.

Evidence for multiple nerves paralyses caused by a common origin of the vasa nervorum.

Masson C, Henin D, Decroix JHP et al. Pachyméningites crâniennes de cause indéterminée. Étude de 3 cas. Rev Neurol (Paris) 1989;145:16–23.

Idiopathic dural inflammatory lesions can cause multiple cranial nerves palsies.

Mayo DR, Boss J. Varicella-zoster associated neurologic disease without skin lesions. Arch Neurol 1989;46:313–5.

One case of multiple cranial nerves palsies with no skin lesions and serologic evidence for varicella-zoster virus infection.

Munsat TL, Barnes JE. Relation of multiple cranial nerve dysfunction to the Guillain-Barré syndrome. J Neurol Neurosurg Psychiatry 1965;28:115–20.

Five cases and a good review of the literature.

Panisset M, Eidelman BH. Multiple cranial neuropathy as a feature of internal carotid artery dissection. Stroke 1990;21:141–7.

Two cases and references.

Steele JC, Vasuvat A. Recurrent multiple cranial nerve palsies: a distinctive syndrome of cranial polyneuropathy. J Neurol Neurosurg Psychiatry 1970;33:828–32.

Palsies affected mainly the ocular and facial nerves. The sedimentation rate was frequently elevated. Prognosis is good, but palsies can recur.

Uldry PA, Regli F. Multinévrite des nerfs crâniens et syndrome d'immunodéficience acquise (SIDA): 5 cas. Rev Neurol (Paris) 1988;144:586–9.

One case with multiple ocular nerve palsies.

Vincent D, Loron P, Awada A, Gautier JC. Paralysies multiples et récidivantes des nerfs crâniens. Syndrome de Gougerot-Sjögren. Rev Neurol (Paris) 1985;141:318–21.

One case with five recurrences and a review of literature.

30
Brainstem

J. P. Mohr and J. C. Gautier

ANATOMY

The brainstem, a small structure made up of the medulla oblongata (usually shortened in common parlance to medulla), pons (from the Latin for bridge), and mesencephalon (from the Greek for midbrain), is roughly the size of the thumb and earned its name from its similarity to the stem of a plant for which the cerebrum would be the flower (see Fig. 26-2). Viewed as a transition structure, its design bears a resemblance to the spinal cord below it. Like in the cord, the major motor pathways have a ventral location. Similarly, the main thalamic-bound afferent somatosensory pathways are placed dorsally. Furthermore, the lower motor neurons that serve peripheral nerve functions for the tongue, oropharynx, face, and eye movements are ventral and ventrolateral. Finally, there is a dorsolateral location of the primary afferents that receive somatosensory input from the face and oropharynx and from the auditory and vestibular system. In contrast to the cord, the shape of the brainstem at its core is greatly distorted from the spinal cord design by the enormous enlargement of the central neuronal pool that serves alertness (sleep and wake functions) and by the enormous distortion that makes up the belly of the pons (the basis pontis) from the motor pathway that integrates the cerebrum with the cerebellum, which latter structure also changes the shape of the brainstem by its three major bridging pathways, the cerebellar peduncles, hanging off the back of the brainstem. Finally, the brainstem houses eye movements, vestibular reflexes, and major centers for autonomic function, including cardiorespiratory regulation.

The slender stalk that is the brainstem, which harbors so many vital functions, is in the confines of the posterior fossa of the skull, with its lower end passing through the foramen magnum, its upper end through the tentorium cerebelli, encased posteriorly and bilaterally by the cerebellum, and its ventral surface facing the clivus. These narrow confines subject the brainstem to compression and distortion in trauma and from mass effects in the cerebrum above and the cerebellum behind. Its position at the base of the skull makes its meninges collect much of the inflammatory material in meningitis. Diseases of the nearby sinuses and tumors of the skull base and nasopharynx also pose hazards.

SUBSECTIONS

The sheer number of structures makes many anatomy books display the brainstem as a sagittal view (see Fig. 28-3A) or as a series of cross-sectional levels like floors in a building (see Fig. 22-4.) Functional considerations show such divisions are arbitrary and a bit misleading. If the building metaphor is to be retained, it might be better to think of those structures in a large building that pass vertically through it, like the elevator shafts, stairwells, and plumbing and electrical systems, with less attention given to the individual floors. Looked at vertically, the brainstem links the spinal cord with the brain above by a large number of ascending and descending tracts, each of which, like the electrical cables or plumbing, play off onto each of the cross-sectional levels (see Fig. 29-3).

PATHWAYS

Afferent Pathways

The ascending or afferent systems from the spinal cord send the posterior columns and lateral spinothalamic tracts to the brainstem (see Figs. 22-6 and 22-7). These tracts synapse in the medullary region and pass their postsynaptic second-fiber systems rostralward toward the thalamus along pathways located in the same generally posterior and lateral locations. Those tracts that are already crossed at the level of the spinal cord, such as the spinothalamic, remain crossed; those that ascend ipsilaterally in the spinal cord, such as the posterior columns, cross after their synapse in the medulla, so that by midpontine levels, almost all of the afferent fiber systems from the cord are already crossed from their side of origin. The exceptions are those afferents that pass into the brainstem by way of the sensory cranial nerves, such as those that carry sensation from the oropharynx and face, via the glossopharyngeal and trigeminal nerves, respectively. These inputs enter the brainstem through the equivalent of the dorsal root entry zone (namely, main sensory nucleus of the trigeminal) and synapse in the equivalent of the zona gelatinosa (descending tract and nucleus of the trigeminal). After synapsing, they cross as the secondary trigeminothalamic tracts to join the pathways from the spinal cord.

In an ascending pattern analogous to that of the spinal cord, the brainstem portion of the posterior columns projects near the midline; those of the secondary spinothalamic tract lie more laterally. This rostralward projection of the sensory systems makes lesions of the brainstem mimic the sensory patterns of those of the spinal cord, with medially placed lesions disturbing position sense and vibration and lateral ones, pain and temperature.

As the ascending pathways pass toward their final destination in the thalamus, many of the fibers have other destinations in the brainstem. Only some 10 percent of the spinothalamic tract fibers present at the level of the foramen magnum actually reach the thalamus, with the remainder playing off onto some of the multimodal (plurimodal) neuronal pools, which run the length of the core of the brainstem.

An afferent system bound for the cerebellum also projects from the spinal cord, reaching the cerebellum by way of the inferior cerebellar peduncle, also known as the restiform body.

Efferent Pathways

The descending or efferent system has its own complexity (see Fig. 22-4). The pons is the synapse point for the descending fibers from the frontal lobe. These frontopontine fibers (Türck's tract, named for Ludwig Türck, Austrian neurologist, 1810–1868) project broadly across the basis pontis to the cerebellum via the middle cerebellar peduncle, also known as the brachium pontis. From the cerebellum projections pass out the superior cerebellar peduncle (brachium conjunctivum) bound toward the thalamus and eventually to the cortex (see Ch. 22).

The directly descending corticobulbospinal pathways pass through the central and ventral portions of the brainstem on the ventral surface of the midbrain. They are no longer distinguishable grossly in the pons because they pass among the frontopontocerebellar fibers so thoroughly that they cannot be recognized as distinct tracts. In studies of degeneration in humans using magnetic resonance imaging, the alteration in tissue density reflecting the atrophy has been best seen in the midbrain and medulla; that in the pons has been difficult to appreciate. In the medulla, the motor pathways emerge as distinct ventrally placed bundles (known as the medullary pyramids for their distinctive shape) and then cross through each other (decussation of the pyramids) over a short distance before descending into the spinal cord as the corticospinal tracts (see Fig. 22-4 and Ch. 31).

Other motor pathways, less easily distinguished anatomically, also pass downward from the thalamus and from the superior cerebellar peduncle and other brainstem structures, reaching the cord. They control aspects of motor tone, known by such names as the reticulospinal, vestibulospinal, and rubrospinal tracts (see Chs. 22, 25, and 27).

Special Structures

Unknown at the level of the spinal cord and approximating some of the functions usually thought to be reserved for the cerebrum, the brainstem is home to special centers for eye movements, a subject so complex as to have its own chapter in this text (see Ch. 28), as well as hearing and balance, two major sensory functions unique to the brainstem, which are mediated through the brainstem by the two major divisions of the eighth cranial nerve (see Ch. 29).

The brainstem also contains special motor systems for such activities as coordinated turning of the head and eyes, swallowing, cough, sneezing, hiccupping, yawning, and perhaps smiling. The former is mediated by the tectospinal tract. The second is by the nucleus ambiguus, which runs along the lateral portion of the lower medulla and is the source of the efferent projections that reach their end-organs via the glossopharyngeal and vagal nerves.

Less is known of the sites for the other functions and whether individual nuclear groups exist. Anencephalic infants have shown facial movements that look like smiling, which argues that the function may be generated in the brainstem and the cerebrum may not be necessary. Swallowing is thought to involve not only the medulla but inputs from the nucleus of the tractus solitarius. Hiccupping has been reported from medullary lesions after infarction, brainstem abscess, and pontomedullary tuberculomas, which indicates the effects may be from a highly focal lesion. The lesions that cause such symptoms usually affect the medulla, but whether the lesions achieve their effect by interruption of pathways, of nuclear groups, or of both is largely still unknown.

The brainstem also mediates the many autonomic functions and the special sensory functions of taste, hearing, and balance. For the former, in animals, chemoreceptor pathways from the carotid body have been traced by horseradish peroxidase into the caudal end of the nucleus and tractus solitarius, confirming its role in respiratory and blood pressure regulatory function. In its cephalad end in the pons, the nucleus mediates taste sensation brought to the brainstem by afferents from the trigeminal and glossopharyngeal nerves. The nucleus has been shown to have anatomic separation of general visceral nuclear inputs from the gustatory. This plan appears to exist throughout phylogeny, judging from the observation that horseradish peroxidase studies have shown such anatomic separation in species as remote from humans as fish. The two systems, although sharing an anatomic nucleus, also seem different in neurochemical transmitters, with the visceral system being reactive to calcitonin gene-related peptide and the gustatory, not. In animal studies, horseradish peroxidase degeneration pathways indicate that the nucleus of the tractus solitarius links its cardiovascular afferents with the noradrenergic cell group in the ventrolateral medulla, thus mediating reflex regulation of the circulation. Blood pressure has been found to increase greatly without changes in the cardiac rate during compression of the ventrolateral medulla in dogs, raising speculation that the two reactions are mediated at anatomically different sites. The anatomic sites that mediate respiration are less clear. Lesions of the medulla have long been known to modify respiratory and cardiovascular activity. For decades, the respiratory responsivity was believed to be mediated by specific receptors for pH and carbon dioxide located in the ventrolateral region of the medulla, although more recent work indicates the chemoreceptor functions occur in the carotid body itself, which sends its outputs to the nucleus of the tractus solitarius. Studies in humans have clearly indicated that the basic respiratory pattern can be altered by "mental" activity such as mental arithmetic and is subject to changes in cycles during the various phases of sleep.

The locus ceruleus, a thin structure that lies in the sagittal plane just below the cephalad end of the fourth ventricle and aqueduct, is a melanin-containing nuclear cluster the cells of which were understood from the early days of neurochemical investigations to be rich in norepinephrine. It has also been shown that the locus ceruleus has at least two major subsections, one noradrenergic and the other cholinergic, and that the locus ceruleus receives projections from a wide variety of neurons that carry an equally wide variety of neurotransmitters, among them norepinephrine, epinephrine, dopamine, acetylcholine, serotonin, histamine, and even neuropeptides like enkephalin and substance P. The neuronal projections of the norepinephrine cellular subsection of this structure are mainly to sensory nuclei, whereas the projection of norepinephrine-containing noncerulean neurons are mainly to motor nuclei within the brainstem, a finding in rats of poorly understood significance. Like the nucleus of the tractus solitarius, the locus ceruleus is one of the brainstem sites that receives afferent sensory projections that carry nocioceptive information, and stimulation of the locus ceruleus in animals has been shown to blunt the transmission of dorsal horn activity to noxious stimuli. The locus has also been implicated in sleep function. As one of the few sites that lack a blood-brain barrier, the locus may be subject to special effects of agents in the systemic circulation.

Running through the central regions of the brainstem is a plurisynaptic system of small neurons known as the reticular formation or reticular-activating system. This loose collection of neurons can be divided into ascending and descending pathways and is found along three caudocephalad zones in the median raphe and medial and lateral reticular regions. The formation follows a fairly compact course through the substance of the upper pons and midbrain and passes out of the brainstem through the medial thalamus. Major portions of the ascending sensory systems from the limbs, trunk, and head feed into the reticular formation, prompting arousal to afferent stimuli. A descending system, the reticulospinal tract, takes its origin from the reticular formation (see Chs. 25 and 27).

Not only grossly detectable anatomic pathways but also neurochemical pathways and regions have been mapped in the brainstem. In addition to the neurochemical transmitters found related to certain anatomic nuclei, neurochemical studies with immunoreactivity methods have shown regional localization for vasopressin in the dorsal pontine nuclei of animals and humans alike and for calcitonin gene-related peptide in the periaqueductal gray, locus ceruleus, nucleus solitarius, medial longitudinal fasciculi, lateral reticular nuclei, and area postrema. In animals, these regions receive projections from hypothalamic nuclei.

BLOOD SUPPLY

The whole brainstem receives its arterial supply from the two vertebral arteries, which fuse intracranially near the pontomedullary junction to form the basilar artery. From the basilar artery arise small penetrating branches and larger circumferential branches. The basilar ends in the circle of Willis, which often provides the major source of supply to the posterior cerebral arteries.

SYNDROMES

As in the spine, the cranial nerves may be interrupted in their course outside the substance of the brainstem. When such discrete injuries occur, there is generally no sign of disturbance of brainstem function itself. Such is the case in a lesion of a single nerve, examples of which are the acute facial (Bell's) palsy, oculomotor (third) or abducens (sixth) nerve palsies with selective disturbance of movement of one eye, acoustic nerve injury with unilateral deafness, disturbances in swallowing and speaking from interruption of the glossopharyngeal or vagal nerves, paralysis of the tongue from damage to the hypoglossal or lingual nerve, and loss of taste from a lesion of the nervus intermedius. (These syndromes are described in more detail in Ch. 29.)

To symptoms referrable to individual cranial nerves, a lesion of the brainstem occurs ipsilateral to cerebellar signs (because of the crossing and recrossing of the cerebellar pathways) and contralateral to "long tract" signs. Typically, the latter include weakness of the limbs on the opposite side of the body (as a result of damage to the corticospinal tract before it has crossed in the pyramids), impairment or loss of pain of the opposite side of the body (from injury to the spinothalamic tract already crossed in the cord below), occasionally an impairment of vibration and touch from involvement of the posterior columns whose thalamic-bound fibers cross in the medulla, and disorders of eye movements (see Ch. 28) and of autonomic function (see Chs. 16 and 34).

The more acute the cause is, the more likely brainstem lesions will present with dizziness and nausea and signs of rhythmic jerking of the eyes (nystagmus) at rest or on gaze in any direction. None of these signs are of great value in estimating the cause or the exact site or size of the disease within the brainstem. Weakness and incoordination, even confined to one or more limbs, are not easily localized and have been described from lesions in a number of sites, large and small, throughout the ventral brainstem. Weakness is an accompanying, not primary, sign that is not useful for precise lesion localization.

Despite these warnings, some symptoms or signs have considerable value in estimating the site of the lesion within the substance of the brainstem. Most of these have been made famous as eponyms, many caused by focal stroke (see below); some are based on a single case observation in the last century and inspired deductive reasoning without autopsy data. The best known and most reliable have come from a focal lesion that affects a cranial nerve nucleus or sensory tract, which makes the clinical syndrome easy to localize.

The most distinctive and best correlated with focal lesions of any of the brainstem syndromes is the lateral medullary syndrome described by Adolph Wallenberg (1862–1949, German physician) in 1895. The lesion, described here because it illustrates much of brainstem functional lesion anatomy, is usually caused by occlusion of the vertebral artery and results in an infarct some 7 to 10 mm in size that affects the posterolateral medulla. It may also extend to the olive and even affect the entire inferior surface of the cerebellum when the posterior inferior cerebellar artery branch of the vertebral artery is also involved, but most of the elements of the clinical syndrome seem adequately explained by the involvement of the lateral medulla.

The entire syndrome complex contains many features, most of which have been explained by a lesion that affects a pathway. The most common symptom, vertigo or dizziness, is not well explained but is usually attributed to a lesion that affects the vestibulocerebellar pathways. Vomiting, which is almost as frequent, is explained by a disturbance in the dorsal medullary tegmentum, said to be the vomiting center. Involvement of the adjacent descending sympathetic pathway causes a small pupil (miosis) from lack of sympathetic competition to the uninterrupted parasympathetic outflow from the midbrain; paralysis of ocular accommodation, which causes blurring of vision; and drooping of the eyelid from loss of sympathetic tone to the lid. This combination is known as Bernard-Horner syndrome (named for Claude Bernard, 1813–1878, French physiologist, and Johann Horner, 1831–1886, Swiss ophthalmologist). Injury to the descending sympathetic pathway also impairs sweating on the ipsilateral face and upper trunk. Injury to the adjoining descending nucleus and tract of the trigeminal nerve produces numbness of the face and the occasional complaints of sharp pain or stinging sensation and abolition of the corneal reflex. The nearby ascending spinothalamic tract is also usually affected, which causes contralateral numbness and lack of perception of pinprick, and often also of cold, on the neck, body, and limbs (spinothalamic tract) and ipsilateral face (ipsilateral descending nucleus and tract of cranial nerve V or contralateral from the crossed trigeminothalamic tract). Limb ataxia ipsilateral to the lesion is explained by involvement of the restiform body; a lesion of the vestibulo-ocular pathways explains the nystagmus and the ocular lateral pulsion (drift of the eyes conjugately to one side when fixation is prevented by covering the eyes) that is usually present. A few instances have been described in which the patient experiences sudden rotation (even upside down) of visual space for a few seconds, an experience so unique that both the patient and physician might not fully believe it has occurred. A hoarse cough and poor swallowing are accounted for by infarction of the lower portion of the nucleus ambiguus with paralysis of the ipsilateral velum and pharynx. Less easily explained is the common occurrence of hiccup, possibly explained by disturbance of nearby respiratory centers. In rare instances, severe respiratory failure has been described from unilateral lateral medullary infarcts that extend into the lower pons.

Other eponymic syndromes of focal brainstem disturbance are met far less frequently and are less well established to have such strictly localizing value. For medullary lesions, included among them are infarction of the medial medulla, causing ipsilateral weakness of the tongue and contralateral weakness of the limbs and trunk (Babinski-Nageotte syndrome, named for Joseph Babinski, 1857–1932, French neurologist, and Jean Nageotte, 1866–1948, French histologist). There are also a series of specific signs that relate to lesions of the medulla, without specific eponyms. In unilateral lesions of the medulla, severe respiratory insufficiency as a result of lack of spontaneous breathing while sleeping (Ondine's curse, from Greek mythology) or long periods without breathing have been described without most of the elements of Wallenberg's syndrome. Rare instances of sudden isolated severe hypertension have occurred. A few patients have been described in whom occlusion of the anterior spinal artery has caused infarction of the decussation of the medullary pyramids, resulting in bilateral severe (usually flaccid) paralysis of the limbs with no other signs. When the medulla suffers widespread damage, respirations are commonly entirely asynchronous, and in the agonal phases, episodic wide opening of the mouth occurs, so-called fishmouthing, with no movement of the chest wall.

In the pons, several distinctive syndromes have been described. A highly focal lesion of the facial nucleus, also involving the abducens nucleus, can yield isolated facial palsy and ipsilateral impairment of lateral gaze (Millard-Gubler or Raymond-Foville syndrome, four French 19th century neurologists). A focal lesion located in or near the medial longitudinal fasciculus may cause impairment of adduction on attempted lateral gaze to the opposite side (internuclear ophthalmoplegia), at times combined with an ipsilateral abducens palsy and nystagmus. At times, a lesion may lie across both medial longitudinal fasciculi and also cause abducens palsy, leaving preserved only lateral deviation of the eye in one direction (one-and-a-half syndrome) (see Chs. 23 and 24). In patients studied by magnetic resonance imaging, highly focal lesions

of the vestibular nucleus have been shown to cause selective loss of caloric responses; in animals, a highly circumscribed lesion of the cochlear nucleus causes selective loss of certain portions of the tone scale for hearing in one ear. A single small lesion in a variety of sites in the pons may occasion nystagmus, and a pontine location is especially likely when the nystagmus is seen in vertical gaze. Likewise, an asymmetric vertical position of the eyes, known as skew deviation, is commonly seen from a focal pontine or medullary lesion, usually in the upper reaches of the pons. A focal lesion at the posterolateral corner of the pons, usually explained by a small hemorrhage, and less often by infarction, may cause impaired lateral gaze of both eyes, accompanied by limb ataxia, and contralateral sensory loss is often observed. In large infarcts that affect both sides of the ventral pons, it is possible to destroy enough of the corticospinal motor pathways to cause bilateral paralysis of the trunk, limbs, face, and oropharynx, leaving the patient unable to make voluntary movements of these parts but still awake and able to hear, feel, see, and move the eyes vertically voluntarily. This state, known as the locked-in syndrome, is compatible with years of survival, given excellent nursing care, and illustrates the highly selective nature of brainstem pathways.

More extensive damage to the pons is required to cause intermittent conjugate sudden downward deviation of the eyes known as ocular bobbing. This sign is usually accompanied by other signs of major pontine injury, with the leading one being a state of coma and of tiny (so-called pinpoint) pupils caused by extensive disruption of the descending sympathetic projections. That the pupils are small from unopposed action of the parasympathetic system can be shown by further constriction in very bright light.

In the midbrain, occlusion of the small branches of the top of the basilar artery, which penetrate into the midbrain and thalamus, has been described (see Fig. 29-6). From unilateral focal infarction, ipsilateral oculomotor paralysis has been associated with a mild contralateral weakness or ataxia; bilateral medial infarction produces a bilateral oculomotor paralyses and limb weakness plus impairment of upward gaze from damage to supranuclear connections. More extensive infarction affects the mesencephalic reticular formation with stupor superimposed. In the syndromes of occlusion of penetrating arteries, which spare the midbrain but involve the thalamus, highly focal syndromes may occur such as the well-known effect of unilateral small lateral thalamic infarction (see Ch. 23).

Other well-defined focal lesions of the central and ventral pontine regions, usually from infarction, have been increasingly defined by brain imaging in recent years with a surprisingly narrow range of symptoms, most of them limited to weakness or ataxia of the contralateral limbs with few instances of diplopia, sensory changes, or impairment in consciousness. The degrees of severity have been difficult to predict from the size of the lesion, and a large number of them produce only minor forms of weakness, often with satisfactory clinical recovery; some may lead to severe paralysis of limbs and trunk on one but rarely both sides. Varying degrees of slurred speech (dysarthria) are often seen.

DISEASES

Stroke With Infarction

Symptoms of occlusion within the vertebrobasilar system (see Ch. 35) are related to focal dysfunction of the brainstem and adjacent cerebellum; when the posterior cerebral artery is supplied from the basilar artery, the temporal and occipital lobes may also be affected. Indeed, the presence of a homonymous hemianopia or quadrantanopsia can clinch the diagnosis of basilar artery disease when the motor or sensory features are not characteristic. Much of what was covered already (see above) has been derived from experience with focal brainstem infarction. The more limited the region involved is, the more local is the suspected microatheroma. The more widespread the signs are, the more likely it is that the basilar artery is affected. Dolichoectasia, an uncommon disease, has a predilection for involvement of the basilar artery, with the thickened and distorted walls blocking flow through side branches. Dolichoectasia is significantly associated with aneurysms of the abdominal aorta, and the latter must be looked for when the former has been demonstrated.

Some symptoms are suggestive of vertebrobasilar disease, included among these are diplopia, occipital blindness, paralysis of both legs, gait ataxia, whirling dizziness, or crossed symptoms (see above). Signs sufficient to diagnose vertebrobasilar disease include internuclear ophthalmoplegia, crossed motor of sensory loss, nystagmus, or bilateral simultaneously occurring paralysis.

Stroke With Hemorrhage

Hemorrhage into the pons (see Ch. 36) is the best known of the many causes of coma from stroke, with most hemorrhages being large enough to disrupt both sides of the pons and with it the reticular formation. Smaller hemorrhages, or those that are well away from the midline, cause symptoms indistinguishable from infarction, which makes it necessary to image the lesion before decisions are made about therapy and whether anticoagulants are considered. Primary hemorrhage in the medulla is virtually unknown; in the

midbrain, it is distinctly uncommon. Cavernous angiomas (see Ch. 37) have been reported in the pons. Some were so large that the brainstem was distorted, yet the individual syndromes reported and seen by the authors have been as highly focal as "peripheral" facial weakness, with facial and abducens palsy combined. Others were often benign. Severe hemorrhage is rare. The brainstem can be compressed from cerebellar hemorrhage with fatal results, often with the transition between an alert state and coma measured in minutes.

Trauma

The brainstem is usually spared the direct effects of trauma and is uncommonly affected even indirectly, but violent rotatory movements of the head may torque the upper brainstem enough to cause small shearing lesions. In a few famous instances, these lesions have affected the reticular activating system, plunging the patient into prolonged coma with few other signs (see Ch. 17). Gunshot and other penetrating wounds are poorly tolerated by the brainstem and are usually immediately fatal, a fact known to executioners and assassins who shoot forward from the base of the skull.

Tumors

Primary tumors (gliomas) that arise from the dense white matter of the brainstem often grow along the axis of the pathways for months, or even a few years, before they attain enough size or deactivate enough tissue to bring about focal symptoms. Those that arise along the floor of the fourth ventricle typically cause slowly evolving symptoms of nystagmus, internuclear ophthalmoplegia, and less often nausea and imbalance, which bring them to clinical attention. Primary tumors of the medulla are rare in adults. Even in children, they tend to arise from the structures around the fourth ventricle, such as the choroid plexus or cerebellum itself (medulloblstoma), often seeding into the cerebrospinal fluid down through the neuraxis. Metastases to the brainstem are exceedingly rare; most of the reported cases were curiosities found at autopsy. With increasing boldness, surgeons are attacking the brainstem itself not only for biopsy but also in attempts at gross or partial resection of tumors, a policy the wisdom of which has yet to be fully demonstrated.

Infections

Bacterial and granulomatous meningitis may invest the extraparenchymatous course of the cranial nerves, even clogging the subarachnoid space enough to cause hydrocephalus but rarely invading the brainstem itself. Brainstem abscess is rare enough to warrant case reports, many of which indicate the diagnosis was made only with difficulty because a brain tumor was considered more likely. The poliovirus can involve the motor brainstem nuclei. St. Louis encephalitis may affect nuclei in the brainstem, causing coma, but most encephalitides spare the brainstem. Acquired immunodeficiency syndrome is increasingly being reported, with instances of brainstem involvement early in the course of the disease.

Degenerative Diseases

The brainstem alone and in combination with the basal ganglia or cerebellum, is home to many so-called degenerative diseases (see Chs. 64 and 65). Suffice it to say that the "degenerative" process seems highly selective and, in some cases, seems attributable to loss of a particular neurotransmitter pathway. As a result, coma, internuclear ophthalmoplegia, dizziness, and other general manifestations of acute or widespread brainstem disease are usually absent.

Metabolic and Nutritional Diseases

Central pontine myelinolysis (see Ch. 71), a demyelinating disease seen in severe malnutrition, sometimes in systemic cancer, and following too rapid a correction of severe hyponatremia, usually presents at the end of life. The cases reported have included the evolution over several days of internuclear ophthalmoplegia, bilateral flaccid hemiparesis, dysarthria, and dysphagia, terminating in coma.

Demyelinating Disease

Multiple sclerosis commonly affects the brainstem; the syndromes are sometimes in isolation without hemispheral or spinal cord clinical elements (see Ch. 73). Vertical gaze nystagmus, ataxia, and dysarthria occurred so often in patients with the advanced form of the disease that this "Charcot triad" (Jean M. Charcot, French neurologist, 1825–1893, one of the founding fathers of neurology) was once considered a hallmark of the disease but is no longer. When the frequency with which spinal cord forms of the disease are considered that may produce striking unilateral or even bilateral paralysis from involvement of the corticospinal tracts, it is remarkable how uncommon such syndromes are from brainstem demyelination. Lesions that affect the spinal nucleus and tract of the trigeminal nerve are a common cause of tic douloureux in patients with multiple sclerosis. An instance of facial palsy inferred by magnetic resonance imaging to have been from multiple sclerosis has been reported. Lesions that affect the auditory pathway seem to be so rare that deafness as part of the syndrome argues against a diagnosis of multiple sclerosis. Autonomic dysfunction is common in patients with multiple sclerosis but is not correlated with the presence or location of brainstem lesions.

Migraine

Not usually affecting the brainstem, migraine in some instances can reproduce all of the symptoms of an evolving basilar occlusion over some minutes, followed by total reversal of the symptoms and signs to normal ("basilar migraine," see Ch. 24). The diagnosis can be entertained in younger patients, but thus far, no reliable methods have been created to give a clinician confidence in the acute stages of the syndrome.

ANNOTATED BIBLIOGRAPHY

Awerbuch G, Brown M, Levin JR. Magnetic resonance imaging correlates of internuclear ophthalmoplegia. Int J Neurosci 1990;52:39–43.

Many small lesions.

Babinski J, Nageotte J. Hémiasynergie, lateropulsion et myosis bulbaires avec hémianesthésie et hémiplégie croisées. Rev Neurol (Paris) 1902;10:358.

One of the classic brainstem syndromes.

Bickerstaff E. Basilar artery migraine. Lancet 1961;1:15.

Migraine can mimic the symptoms of acute brainstem ischemia.

Culebras A. Neuroanatomic and neurologic correlates of sleep disturbances. Neurology 1992;42:19–27.

The role of the brainstem in sleep.

Devereaux M, Keane JR, Davis R. Automatic respiratory failure associated with infarction of the medulla: report of two cases with pathologic study of one. Arch Neurol 1973;29:46–52.

Ondine's curse.

Fisher C. Some neuro-ophthalmological observations. J Neurol Neurosurg Psychiatry 1967;30:383–92.

Details of syndromes including those from brainstem lesions.

Francis DA, Bronstein AM, Rudge P, du Boulay EP. The site of brainstem lesions causing semicircular canal paresis: an MRI study. J Neurol Neurosurg Psychiatry 1992;55:446–9.

The magnetic resonance imaging-detected lesions seemed to affect the medial and lateral vestibular nucleus and proximal portion of the vestibular fascicle.

Gautier JC, Hauw JJ, Awada A et al. Artères cérébrales dolichoectasiques. Association aux anéurysms de l'arteria abdominal. Rev Neurol (Paris) 1988;144:437–66.

Not caused by atherosclerosis. Significant association with aneurysms of the abdominal aorta.

Hauw J, Der Agopian P, Trelles L, Escourolle R. Les infarctus bulbaires. J Neurol Sci 1976;28:83–102.

A clinical classic with some of the best-ever autopsy data.

Ho KL, Meyer KR. The medial medullary syndrome. Arch Neurol 1981;38:385–7.

Few examples.

Holmes G. The symptoms of acute cerebellar injuries due to gunshot wounds. Brain 1917;40:461.

World War I experience.

Ingvar D, Sourander P. Destruction of the reticular core of the brainstem. Arch Neurol 1970;23:1–8.

Profound coma.

Jones SL. Descending noradrenergic influences on pain. Prog Brain Res 1991;88:381–94.

Details of the function and projections of norepinephrine neurons in the locus ceruleus.

Kase C, Varakis J, Stafford J, Mohr JP. Medial medullary infarction from fibrocartilogenous embolism to the anterior spinal artery. Stroke 1983;14:413–18.

Clinical details of a bilateral pyramid lesion.

Kubik C, Adams R. Occlusion of the basilar artery: a clinical and pathologic study. Brain 1946;69:73.

A clinical classic.

Morruzzzi G, Magoun HW. Brain stem reticular formation and activation of the EEG. Electroencephalogr Clin Neurophysiol 1949;1:445.

The classic description of a brain region, stimulation of which produces arousal.

Sakai N, Yamada H, Tanigawara T et al. Surgical treatment of cavernous angioma involving the brainstem and review of the literature. Acta Neurochir (Wien) 1991;113:138–43.

Five new cases and a literature review indicating the remarkably discrete syndromes before surgery and the minor added effects of direct operation on the brainstem.

Tatemichi TK, Steinke W, Duncan C et al. Paramedian thalamopeduncular infarction: clinical syndromes and magnetic resonance imaging. Ann Neurol 1992;32:162–71.

Magnetic resonance imaging correlates of midbrain infarction delineated three syndromic clusters.

Wallenberg A. Acute Bulbäraffection (Embolie der Arteria cerebellaris inferior posterior sinistra). Arch Psychol (Frankf) 1895;27:504.

The original case report.

31

The Spinal Cord

J. C. Gautier and J. P. Mohr

The spinal cord (hereafter referred to as the cord) is a mere 2 percent of the volume of the central nervous system (CNS), but the frequent and varied diseases to which it is subject make up a fair part of a neurologist's activity. Although the cord is the least complex structure of the CNS, diagnosis of its disorders is not easy. All too often acute or chronic myelopathies remain insufficiently elucidated.

ANATOMY

The cord measures between 42 to 45 cm in length and fits inside the spinal canal, which, from the foramen magnum to the coccyx, measures some 60 cm in women and 70 cm in men. The greater rate of growth of the bony spine during fetal and immediate postpartum life explains the location of the cord's lower end at about the level of the L1–L2 intervertebral space (Fig. 31-1). It explains the relationship of cord segments and roots with the vertebral bodies, with the roots exiting at the intervertebral foramina above the cord levels in the cervical region and far below the termination of the cord in the lumbosacral segments. The termination site of the cord allows safe spinal puncture to be performed between the crest of L4–L5 or L5–S1 (see Ch. 9).

The width of the cord varies from 2 to 3 cm in the cervical enlargement and 3 to 4.5 cm in the lumbar, reflecting the large number of cells and radicular filaments that supply the limbs in these locations. Throughout its length, the cord occupies somewhat less than 50 percent of the cross-sectional area of the spinal canal, but particularly in the cervical region, the latter can be much narrowed by spondylosis. The cord is correspondingly small in the thoracic region.

A deep ventral and a shallow posterior dorsal midline fissure separates the two halves of the cord in the sagittal plane. Its center is occupied by a small canal lined with ependymal cells and filled with cerebrospinal fluid (CSF) and continuous rostrally with the fourth ventricle.

Movements of the spine have direct effects on the position and shape of the cord. The cross-sectional dimensions of the cord change with all movements. In extension, transverse folds appear on the cord surface, with the buckling of the posterior spinal ligament gently displacing the dural sac posteriorly and slightly compressing the cord dorsally while lengthening it ventrally. Neck flexion causes a change by several centimeters in the length of the cervical spine, and the cord and dura slide up by as much as 2 cm. Straight-leg flexion at the hip tugs the cord caudally. In all such movements, the nervous fibers undergo stretch.

Although the foramen magnum marks the anatomic boundary of the upper end of the cord, its structures closely resemble those of the medulla at this level, gradually changing shape and configuration as the cord descends through its length to end as the sharply tapered conus medullaris. Below this level, the remnant of the neuroectodermal bud is the filum terminale (Latin: *filum*, thread), which accompanies the arachnoidal sac to its termination in the second sacral segment. Still further below, a ligament runs down to its attachment point at the base of the coccyx. An abnormally short and thick filum terminale can be a source of clinical symptoms and signs (see below).

The cord is covered by the pia, a continuation of the pia of the brain. The CSF bathes the outside surface of the pia and is contained within the meshes of the arachnoid. The dura mater adheres firmly to the circumference of the foramen magnum, but below, it is separated from the spinal canal, so there is an extra- or epidural space, which contains venous plexi and fat but no lymph channels. The pattern of attachment of the spinal dura explains the technique of its removal at autopsy (see Ch. 7).

The cord does not simply hang by its weight in the spinal canal but is suspended by two rows of transverse denticulate ligaments (Latin: *denticulus*, small tooth), arising as pointed spicules between the anterior and posterior roots and inserting laterally on the dura. This arrangement makes the cord something like an accordion, capable of local bending and slight change in length but also limited in its capacity to tolerate displacement at any given length.

Throughout its length, the cord gives off paired filaments on both sides (Fig. 31-2) called roots: 8 cervical, 12 thoracic, 5 lumbar, 5 sacral, and 1 coccygeal. Ventral roots are motor, and dorsal ones are sensory (see Ch. 32). In humans, the first sensory cervical root is lacking, so that the occipital scalp, up to the line that runs from ear to ear, is innervated by C2 (see Ch. 23). Ventral (anterior) and dorsal (posterior) roots coalesce

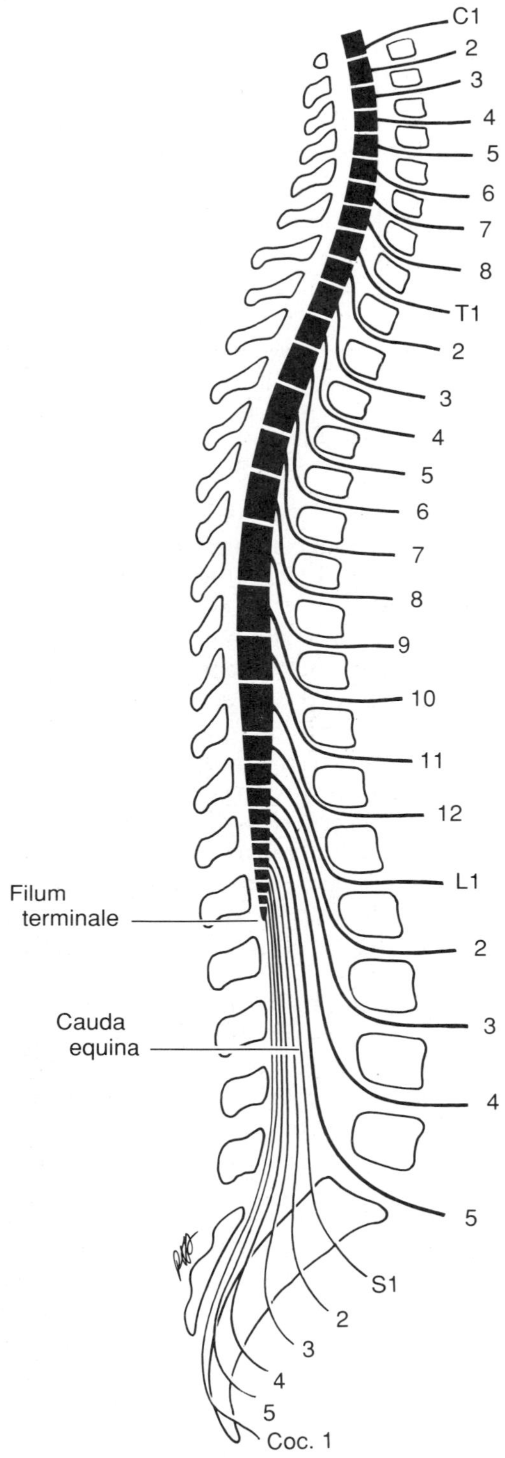

Figure 31-1. Spinal cord showing the exit points of the individual spinal nerves. Note the gradual separation of the shorter spinal cord from the longer spinal canal, resulting in longer vertical distances between the point of the origin of the spinal roots in the cords from their exit levels in the spinal column.

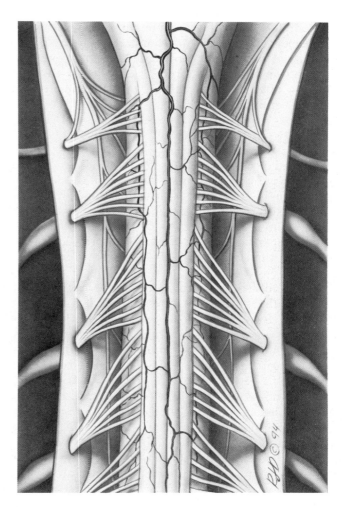

Figure 31-2. Spinal cord from a dorsal view, the arachnoid sectioned longitudinally and drawn away to each side, showing how the individual nerve rootlets arise continuously from the cord and form bundles that become the spinal nerves, passing through the dural sheaths.

to form the spinal nerve. The roots and spinal nerve in the spinal canal and intervertebral foramina are invested by an arachnoid-dural sheath, which extends to the intervertebral foramen. Consequently, they are bathed in CSF.

Below L1–L2, the spinal canal is occupied by a cluster of roots that resemble a horse's tail, hence the Latin name, cauda equina.

Blood Supply of the Cord

Just as there is an extracranial and an intracranial part of the arteries to the brain, there is an extraspinal and intraspinal arterial system for the cord.

Pial arteries (Fig. 31-3) on the surface of the cord make up three longitudinal systems of which the chief one is the midline anterior spinal artery, which sits astride the ventral cleft in the midline. The two smaller systems are the paired posterior spinal arteries that run dorsal to the root entry zones. Between these vessels, there is a coronal system, around the cord, that has no great anastomotic value. The penetrating or nutrient arteries arise from the pial arteries. Most of the parenchymatous branches at any level are end-arteries.

The anterior spinal artery originates from the union of an intracranial branch given off by each vertebral artery. Its runs caudally to the conus medullaris where it anastomoses with the posterior spinal arteries. The anterior spinal artery supplies blood to the anterior two-thirds to three-fifths of the cord, among which

is included the anterior horn and most of the lateral corticospinal tract (Fig. 31-3). Branches of the anterior spinal artery, known as sulcal arteries (Latin: *sulcus*, furrow), enter the anterior median fissure of the cord before penetrating it and turn alternatingly to the right and to the left, which explains the frequent asymmetry of infarctions. The posterior spinal arteries supply most of the posterior columns. The coronal system supplies a superficial rim of the cord and possibly the outer part of the lateral corticospinal tract.

The extraspinal arteries that supply the arteries on the cord arise from the aorta and course close to the spine, giving off branches that pass through the intervertebral foramina with the spinal nerves. These branches, in turn, divide in several vessels, among which is the neurospinal artery of Kadyi, which bifurcates into one anterior and one posterior branch, each of which divides into ascending and descending rami, which join to form the anterior and posterior spinal arteries.

Rostrocaudally, the arteries to the cord are derived from the vertebral arteries and branches of the subclavian, the intercostal and lumbar (branches of the aorta), the ileolumbar, and sacral arteries.

The feeding system of the anterior spinal artery shows many individual variations. In the 3-month-old fetus, there are as many radicular arteries as there are roots and cord segments. Eventually, few remain significant. In the adult, there are five to eight or even less vessels that supply the anterior spinal artery: usually, one at C6, one or two small ones in the superior thoracic region, and one to three in the lumbosacral region. One of the latter and often the only significant one is the great radicular artery of Adamkiewicz (A. Adamkiewicz, Polish pathologist, 1850–1921), which is found on one side only, more often on the left. Its origin varies widely from T8 to L2, more often from T11–L2. When its origin is high, and even when it is low, it has a large territory, spanning the lumbar and sacral territories (sometimes also the thoracic), which makes it an artery of great clinical significance.

The anterior spinal artery and its supplying arteries can be visualized by selective angiography, but this requires selective catheterizations of the vertebral, subclavian, intercostal, and lumbar arteries.

The arterial system of the cord has two "watershed" zones, which are reflected in the pathologic findings of cord infarction and hence have a high significance for clinical diagnosis (Fig. 31-4). The first watershed zone is intramedullary (i.e., in the spinal cord) and is located at the junction of the anterior and posterior spinal artery territories. In cases of critically low blood flow in the three systems (e.g., in collapse or occlusion of a major extraspinal feeding artery), there may occur a peculiar rounded site of infarction extending over

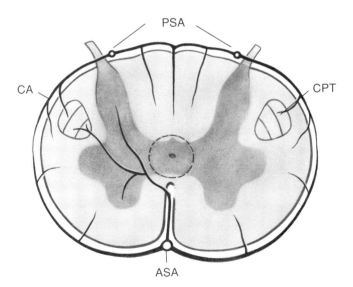

Figure 31-3. The arterial supply around and in the cord showing the anterior spinal artery (ASA), coronal arteries (CA), crossed pyramidal tract (CPT), and posterior spinal arteries (PSA). The dotted area represents the site of pencil infarcts (see text).

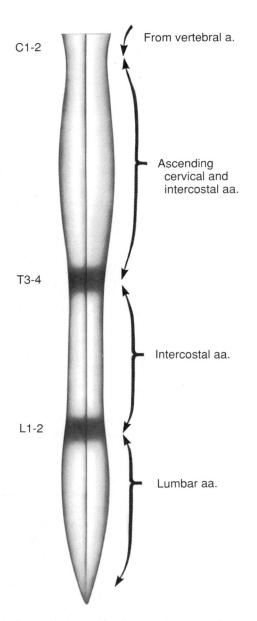

C1-2

From vertebral a.

Ascending cervical and intercostal aa.

T3-4

Intercostal aa.

L1-2

Lumbar aa.

Figure 31-4. Longitudinal view of the spinal cord showing the main sources of arterial supply to the cord. The darker zones represent the sites of the watershed zones between the main arterial territories.

several cord segments, known by its shape as a "pencil infarction." Pencil lesions, however, can also be seen in infarcts caused by thrombosis or embolism, not only from hypotension.

The second watershed zone results from the anterior spinal artery; in many individuals, it is poorly fed by supplying neurospinal arteries (see above). Ascending and descending branches of the latter can be of very small caliber or even fail to anastomose with neighboring vessels, in which cases the anterior spinal

artery runs an interrupted course. The most common sites of inadequate flow (watershed zones) are in the upper and lower thoracic cord (Fig. 31-4). Infarcts can also result from systemic circulatory failure (e.g., collapse or lesions extending along the aorta, i.e., dissection).

Spinal *veins* begin as radial veins draining into either sulcal veins and longitudinal venous channels or posterior longitudinal venous channels. Rostrally, these channels are in continuity with medullary veins and thus with cranial dural sinuses. The longitudinal channels (united by a coronal system) are drained by radicular veins that carry blood to the extradural venous plexus. These systems have no valves; so the blood can change direction, reflecting pressure in the neck, chest, or abdomen and can freely pass into the systemic venous system. Thus, the numerous anastomoses and multiple paths open to blood flow perhaps explain the rarity of venous infarction of the spinal cord. Also, the many anastomoses with pelvic plexi have been implicated in the vertebral metastases of prostatic carcinoma. Epidural venograms can display the venous system of the cord.

Gray Matter

The gray matter occupies roughly one-half of the cross section of the cord at each level. Like the brain and brainstem, its anterior or ventral portion is mainly motor in function; the posterior or dorsal portion is mainly sensory. As described in more detail in Chapter 22 on motor function, the anterior portion or horn of the spinal cord contains clusters of cell bodies that vary in size. The more numerous and large ones, known as the α neurons, individually control a single motor unit. The muscle groups supplied by these large neuronal cell bodies are organized in an orderly manner, in vertical columns extending over several anatomic segments. Those that supply the axial muscles of the trunk are the most medial in location; those that supply the extremities are more lateral; those that supply muscles for flexion are more ventral; and those involved in extension are more dorsal. Scattered among these large neurons are the smaller γ neurons the fiber outputs of which control the muscle spindles the response of which to muscle stretch contributes to muscle tone.

The tiny cell bodies that give rise to preganglionic sympathetic fibers are found in the intermediolateral portion of the gray matter. These fibers, which accompany the anterior roots exiting the cord, later separate from the spinal nerve to form the white communicating rami, which lead to the sympathetic trunk. A similar set of preganglionic fibers, this time parasympathetic in function, arise from these same areas in the sacral segments of the spinal cord.

Some cells in the central gray matter serve mainly a linking or feedback function. The afferent fibers that bear sensory inputs entering by way of the posterior or dorsal portions of the spinal cord, bearing information from the tendon organs, and are linked to the α and γ cell bodies by internuncial (Latin: *nuncius,* messenger) cells. Renshaw cells (named for the American neurophysiologist, B. Renshaw) playing on the α cells have a mainly inhibitory function.

The ventral roots also contain afferent fibers the functional significance of which is still not clear. Some enter the spinal cord directly through the ventral root; others may curve back to enter the dorsal root and horn.

CLINICAL SYNDROMES

General Principles of Clinical Diagnosis of Cord Lesions

Apart from diffuse or multifocal lesions of the cord (e.g., acute infectious myelitis or multiple sclerosis (see below), most lesions of the cord are focal. Consequently, first there are symptoms and signs at the level of the lesion, resulting from dysfunction of the anterior and posterior horns and roots. This first syndrome is termed the *local syndrome.* Second, symptoms and signs occur that result from dysfunction of the ascending and descending pathways of the cord, which are termed the *below-the-lesion* or *infralesional syndrome.* The task of the clinician is to recognize both syndromes to localize the site of the lesion. The upper limit of the symptoms and signs corresponds only roughly to the level of the lesion. To achieve this goal, the clinician must know the topography of the sensory dermatomes (see Ch. 23), the main sites in practice being T4 at the level of the nipple; T8, the lower rib; T10, the umbilicus; and L1, the groin.

When fibers of the spinothalamic tract are involved, there is a contralateral loss of pain and temperature below the level of the lesion (see Ch. 23). The upper limit of this part of the infralesional syndrome helps to localize the level of the lesion. However, the upper limit is often somewhat topographically indistinct because fibers of the spinothalamic tract decussate through several spinal levels or cross the cord obliquely. For the same reasons, the upper limit of anesthesia for pain and temperature can be more than one or two segments (dermatomes) below the actual level of the lesion. It is safer, when possible, to infer the level of the lesion from abolition of a reflex or local muscle wasting.

In recent years, progress in electrophysiology and imaging have considerably improved the diagnosis of cord disease. Somatosensory-evoked potentials can detect subtle defects in conduction of impulses in the pathways of the cord (see Ch. 11). Magnetic stimulation can also detect defects in conduction in the corticospinal tracts (see Ch. 11). Electromyography and nerve conduction velocities provide vital evidence in diseases of the motor cells of the anterior horn (see Ch. 12).

Computed tomography (CT) has provided definite progress in the diagnosis of lesions of the spinal cord, especially for tumors. The major advance, however, has come from magnetic resonance imaging (MRI), which allows an analysis of the cord, intra- and extradural spaces, and the spinal column. MRI with multiarray coils and fast spin-echo methods gives high-resolution images of the whole cord in about 5 minutes and allows measurements of the cross-sectional area of the cord. MRI has superseded myelography, which required injection of a liquid contrast medium into the intradural space and having the patient on a tilt table to make the contrast circulate by gravitational effect from the lower to the upper cord. Where MRI is not available, contrast myelography is still a useful tool, chiefly for compressive lesions and for some arteriovenous malformations. The latter, however, are best demonstrated by selective angiography (see above).

Pathways, Symptoms, and Signs

The anatomy of the motor, sensory, and cerebellar tracts of the cord; its gray substance; and the roots are described in Chapters 22, 23, and 32. It should be noted there are no symptoms and signs that can be attributed with certainty to lesions of the cerebellar pathways of the cord. The basic anatomy of the cord (Fig. 31-5) permits, in a simplified manner, an understanding of the clinical syndromes of cord lesions.

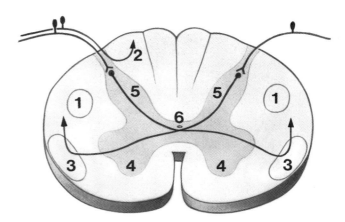

Figure 31-5. The main components of the spinal cord, including the corticospinal tracts (1); tracts of the posterior columns (2), which ascend ipsilateral to their point of entry into the posterior horn; spinothalamic tracts (3), whose fibers cross after entry into the cord (5); and the central canal (6).

Sensory Syndromes

The *dorsal (posterior) columns* are made up of the cephalad-bound axons of the large myelinated sensory fibers that supply responses to mechanical stimuli the cell bodies of which are in the dorsal root (spinal) ganglia. They do not synapse at their entry into the cord (Fig. 31-5). They could be considered parts of the peripheral nervous system and, indeed, degenerate as a consequence of lesions of the posterior roots (e.g., tabes dorsalis) (see Ch. 41). After entering the dorsal root entry zone, they remain ipsilateral and ascend in the posteromedial portions of the spinal cord (the posterior columns), sorting themselves to a medial location if they arise from the lower limbs and more laterally if from the upper limbs. They ascend to the caudal part of the medulla where they synapse in the nuclei cuneatus and gracilis. The dorsal (posterior) columns convey the clinically testable senses of joint position, vibration, and light touch.

The usual symptoms of dorsal (posterior) column dysfunction are ipsilateral paresthesias (see Ch. 23) (i.e., often described as "pins and needles," "ants," or "tingling"). They can also begin as sensations of numbness or deadness of part of the skin or a sensation of tight bands around the ankles. Paresthesias are not unique to dorsal column lesions but may also arise from lesions of the peripheral nerves, brainstem, and even sensory regions of the cerebral hemisphere. In severe lesions of the dorsal columns, there is a severe ataxia, predictably worsened by attempting to stand or walk in darkness or after closing the eyes (Romberg's sign) (M. H. Romberg, German physician, 1795–1873).

Lhermitte's sign (J. Lhermitte, French neurologist, 1877–1959) results from lesions of the dorsal columns in the cervical cord, rarely the thoracic. On flexing the neck, the patient experiences a sensation like an electric shock running in a few seconds from the cervical to the thoracic and lumbar spine and sometimes into the limbs. It is presumably due to the stretching tension of the demyelinated fibers (see Ch. 2). Most commonly, Lhermitte's sign means multiple sclerosis, although it can occur in a host of conditions.

The classic *spinothalamic tract* is made up of small, C-fibers, which enter the dorsal root entry zone and end in lamina II (substantia gelatinosa). The lamina of the substantia gelatinosa is complex, with lamina I receiving projections from peripheral nerves covering small receptive fields for noxious stimuli. Those in laminae IV to VI receive fibers with larger receptive fields and respond to innocuous and nocioceptive stimuli. None of those axons destined for the spinothalamic tract ascend in the posterior columns. Instead, the postsynaptic fibers decussate in front of the

---

CAUSES OF LHERMITTE'S SIGN

Multiple sclerosis
Cervical spondylosis
Cervical cord tumors
Radiation myelopathy
Pernicious anemia
Cisplatin toxicity
Pyridoxine toxicity
Nitrous oxide abuse
Cervical herpes zoster
Behcet's disease
Tumors of the thoracic cord
Tethered spinal cord

---

ependymal (central) canal (Fig. 31-5) in the anterior white commissure to form the spinothalamic tract that ascends to the ventroposterolateral nucleus of the thalamus, giving off, en route, many collaterals, particularly to the reticular substance of the brainstem.

The spinothalamic tract is laminated. Fibers from the lower limb are more lateral, and those from the upper limb are more medial within the tract. Within this general laminar arrangement is another system of projections. Fibers from laminae I to VI project mainly to the ventroposterolateral nuclei of the thalamus in topographic fashion, overlying those from the posterior columns. Those from laminae VII to X, the receptive fields of which respond to a wide variety of deep and superficial stimuli, project to the brainstem reticular formation on both sides and to the midbrain reticular formation, perhaps mediating arousal to noxious stimuli. They also project to the intralaminar and dorsomedial nuclei of the thalamus, which contain opiate receptors, perhaps subserving deep, poorly localized pain. Some of the dorsal horn fibers link ipsilaterally and contralaterally to internuncial or motor neurons to mediate nociceptive reflexes. A smaller number enter the cord at the ventral root.

Clinically, the spinothalamic tract conveys sensations of cold; warmth; both sharp, acute (epicritic) and diffuse, aching (protopathic) pain; and itch.

Symptoms of spinothalamic tract dysfunction include sensations of warmth, burning, cold, and itch, which when chronic, can be severe, diffuse, burning sensations analogous to thalamic pain (see Ch. 23). The chief signs of spinothalamic tract involvement are a contralateral hypoesthesia or anesthesia for cold, warmth, and pain.

The anatomy of the spinothalamic tract explains three distinctive spinal cord syndromes: the central cord syndrome and sacral-sparing and saddle anesthesia. The clinically distinctive *central cord syndrome* is explained by the anatomy of the second-order neurons of both spinothalamic tracts. These cross in the central cord just in front of the central canal. This unique anatomic setting allows lesions of that site (e.g., syringomyelia; see below) or spinal cord tumor to cause bilateral interruption of the spinothalamic tract, a feature of the central cord syndrome. When this syndrome occurs, as it does usually, in the cervical cord, there is a "suspended syndrome" (e.g., dissociated sensory deficit for pain and temperature) that affects the upper limbs and upper portion of the trunk, much like the shape of a sweater. In the lumbar region, a similar dissociation can result from infarction of the territory of the anterior spinal artery (Fig. 31-3).

Sacral sparing is explained by another feature of spinothalamic tract anatomy, its lamination. The sacral fibers are the first to enter the spinothalamic tract at the lowest end of the cord. As the tract enlarges as it ascends, fibers enter first from the lower limbs, then the trunk, and finally, from the upper limbs. After decussation, the sacral fibers are the most laterally located, with the trunk and upper limb fibers being more medially placed. This lateral location explains the sparing of sacral sensation in some instances of the central cord syndrome when the lesion is not large enough to affect the most laterally placed fibers. There is loss of pain and temperature on the lower limbs and trunk, but sensation to pinprick is spared in the perineum and adjacent buttocks.

Saddle anesthesia is a converse topographic pattern that occurs in lesions of the cauda equina. The hypoesthesia or anesthesia involves the perineum and genitalia but does not involve the legs or trunk because the lesion lies below the level(s) where these fibers enter the cord. Patients are said to "sit on their physical signs."

Motor Syndromes

As described in more detail in Chapter 22, the fibers of the *corticospinal tract* descending from the cerebrum undergo an incomplete decussation near the medullary-cervical cord junction, with roughly 70 to 90 percent of the fibers crossing the cord to form between three and four separate corticospinal tracts within the cord. The largest, the crossed lateral corticospinal tract, lies adjacent to the midportion of the gray matter and descends throughout the length of the cord to the lowest sacral segments, synapsing on cells in the ventral and dorsal horn of the gray matter and on cells of the intermediolateralis region. A smaller anterior (ventral) corticospinal tract contains uncrossed fibers, which descend in the medial and anterior portion of the cord white matter, with the fibers crossing through

the anterior commissure to synapse cells in the medial portion of the anterior horn, which are destined to control mainly trunk and proximal limb muscles. Two other smaller tracts, of unknown significance, include the uncrossed lateral corticospinal tract just ventral to the main corticospinal tract and a small tract containing crossed fibers descending in the posterolateral portion of the anterior columns in the cervical segments. Other descending motor tracts include two mainly uncrossed, the *reticulospinal tract*, related to sudden motor responses to startle stimuli, and the *vestibulospinal tract*, which mediates posture. Two others, mainly crossed, include the *rubrospinal tract*, ending in the cervical on upper thoracic cord and mediating flexor muscle movements, and the *tectospinal tract*, which terminates on internuncial neurons and mediates orienting responses to visual and auditory stimuli.

Dysfunction of the *descending motor pathways* is usually expressed as "the pyramidal syndrome" (i.e., fatigability, weakness, loss of dexterity, spasticity, exaggerated reflexes, and Babinski's sign). Despite the lamination of the corticospinal tracts, the motor equivalent of sensory sacral sparing is not clinically observed.

The symptoms and signs of lesions of the *anterior horn* are weakness, areflexia, fasciculations, and muscle atrophy (see Ch. 22).

Syndromes of Autonomic Dysfunction

Bladder dysfunction presents as urgency, frequency, and finally, incontinence or urinary retention with overflow incontinence. The former is common when there is a bilateral pyramidal syndrome (e.g., in pseudobulbar palsy). The latter is usually seen with lesions of the sacral cord, conus medullaris, or cauda equina. In acute cord dysfunction, such as that seen during spinal anesthesia, overflow incontinence may occur within hours.

Cord Hemisection

Disorders involving one-half of the cord (e.g., stab wounds, see Ch. 6) cause *Brown-Séquard syndrome* (Charles-Édouard Brown-Séquard, 1817–1896, a French neurologist who held posts in London, the Medical College of Virginia, Harvard, Geneva, and finally Paris, where he succeeded Claude Bernard at the College de France). This syndrome features ipsilateral weakness (descending corticospinal tract), loss of position and vibratory sense (dorsal column), and contralateral loss of pain and temperature (crossed spinothalamic tract) below the lesion (Fig. 31-5). If the lesion is truly a hemisection, there is often loss of lower motor function at the level of the lesion, ipsilateral autonomic dysfunction, and local hyperesthesia, as in

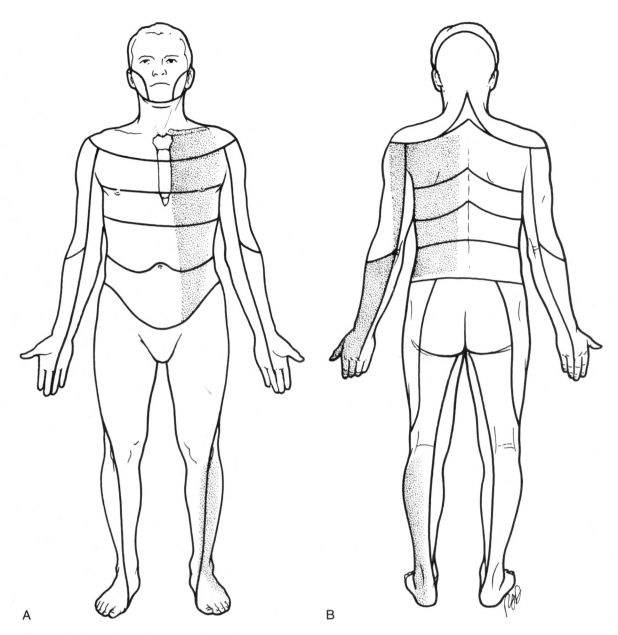

Figure 31-6. (A & B) Examples of incomplete hemisensory disturbances from lesions of the spinal cord, showing the syndromes may not be uniform.

complete cord transsection. Diseases causing true hemisections are rare, and incomplete syndromes are the rule (see Fig. 31-6).

Transsection of Cord

Transsection of the cord is an acute event, usually caused by trauma with fracture of the spine (see Ch. 6) and less often by infarction, hemorrhage, or myelitis. Motor, sensory, and autonomic function above the level of the lesion is retained and usually not even affected temporarily.

Immediately, at and below the level of the lesion, there is a flaccid paralysis because all function is lost, a state termed "spinal shock" and believed to be the result of the sudden disruption of descending excitatory impulses and an abolition of all somatic and visceral sensations below the level of the lesion. The bladder is areflexic with acute urinary retention. The bulbocavernosus reflex is usually the first to reappear, and when brisk and associated with evidence of severe cord damage, it is a predictor of poor recovery. Acutely, although many patients immediately experience illusions of movements of body parts below this level, the exact level for touch and vibration is less well delineated. For one or two segments above and below the lesion, touch and pinprick may show a permanent hyperpathia (from the Greek for exaggerated suffering) quality.

The state of spinal shock lasts some 6 to 8 weeks and sometimes longer. The first reflex to reappear is the inversed plantar response (Babinski's sign), which usually heralds the appearance of the triple flexion response to stimuli to the foot or leg (see Ch. 22). Also possible are flexor spasms, apparently separate from external stimuli, and after several months, alternating flexor and extensor spasms. Meanwhile, muscle tone reappears and evolves toward spasticity, and the tendon reflexes become hyperactive.

Incomplete lesions are more common. The sensory syndromes in such cases can be rather incomplete, often involving the trunk and only portions of the arm or leg, as illustrated by case material published long ago by von Monakow (Fig. 31-6).

Intramedullary Versus Extramedullary Lesion

When there is a cord syndrome, such as described earlier (transsections, hemisection, or central cord syndrome), the diagnostic problem is straightforward as to whether the lesion is intramedullary (within the spinal cord itself) or extramedullary (outside the cord) and if extramedullary whether intradural (inside the dura) or extradural (outside the dura).

Extramedullary lesions usually give less clear-cut symptoms and signs. All extramedullary lesions cause disturbance in cord function, first by means of distortion or compression of the cord. The ventral and lateral ligamentous attachment of the pia to the dura at every level prevents the cord from experiencing much distribution of stretch and compression, and compliance of the nervous tissue itself is rather limited. A mass outside the cord substance has little effect on cord function for more than a few segments above or below because of the lateral and ventral ligaments. It is believed that stretch of these ligaments by a mass at that site pulls on the attachment point at the pia and distorts and demyelinates the adjacent white matter pathways, with the most clinically sensitive being the corticospinal tract. The lamination of this tract with sacral and lumbar segments situated externally may explain the early appearance of "long tract signs" of stiff gait and easy fatigability in extra-axial compressive lesions, such as tumors, herniated discs, and arthritic spurs and bars. Reflex changes and signs of spasticity are surprisingly uncommon. Sensory loss may feature elements of the Brown-Séquard's hemicord syndrome but are not present often.

Whether the causative lesions is *intradural extramed-*

ullary versus *extradural* is an important distinction for reasons of diagnosing the likely cause and whether, if it is a tumor, it is benign (usually intradural) or malignant (usually extradural). Unhappily, clinical features that differentiate these two are almost completely lacking. Differentiation from purely intramedullary tumors can often be predicted with more confidence by the higher frequency of pain from the extramedullary lesions, which displace and place tension on pain-sensitive dura and roots; less often, there is loss of vibration and touch before loss of pain and temperature (the reverse of the central cord syndrome). Extramedullary intradural lesions are prone to produce radicular pains; extradural lesions more often produce local pain of the bony and ligamentous structures of the spine.

Some extramedullary disorders may mimic cord disease. Included among them are ganglionopathies (see Ch. 32), due to cisplatin or pyridoxine (vitamin B_6,) intoxication, which cause symptoms of dorsal column dysfunction. Pathophysiologically, they are similar (see dorsal columns, discussed earlier).

Cord Syndromes by Level

Cervical Cord

Acute *high* cervical injuries are often fatal because of the control of the diaphragm by the phrenic nerve (C3, C4, and C5) and of autonomic control from the lower medullary systems, which projects down into the upper cervical regions. For the survivors, transsection of the cord causes quadriplegia. *Midcervical* lesions cause weakness in the upper portions of the arms; those that affect roots C6–C8 involve the forearm and hand. Although most of the innervation of the hand comes from T1, motor findings and absence of reflexes (biceps; C5–C6; brachioradialis, C6; triceps, C7; pronator, C8–T1; and finger flexion, C8, see Ch. 22) are more helpful than sensory levels for the analysis of mid- and low cervical lesions. Autonomic disturbances may arise from injuries anywhere along the cervical cord, easily recognized by Bernard-Horner syndrome ipsilateral to the side of the lesion and by vasodilation, impaired sweating, and later trophic changes below the level of major cord injuries. Such disturbances are often absent or only slight with incomplete compressive lesions.

Thoracic Cord Syndromes

It is difficult to detect weakness of individual intercostal muscles on the thoracic wall. Nevertheless, paradoxic movements of the intercostal muscles in a slim patient occasionally give a clue to the level of the thoracic cord lesion. The T9-12 segments supply the muscles of the abdominal wall. Beevor's sign (C. E. Beevor,

1854–1908, British neurologist) (i.e., shift of the navel as the patient tries to sit up from a supine position), points to weakness of the upper abdominal muscles, suggesting a lesion near T9. The loss of autonomic function is similar to that from cervical lesions.

Lumbar Cord Syndromes

This segment of cord mediates movements of the legs through local lower motor neurons and provides passage for innervation of the genitalia, bowel, and bladder. The cremasteric reflex is an ipsilateral ascent of the testicle on scratching of the medial thigh and is mediated by L1–L2.

Weakness of individual muscles of the hips and legs, absence of cremasteric reflexes and knee and ankle jerks (see Ch. 22), and sensory deficits (see Ch. 23 and earlier discussion) suggest the level of the lesion. Upper lumbar cord lesions impair ejaculation. Sympathetic autonomic dysfunction does not occur from cord lesions below the L3 level (see Chs. 16 and 34).

Conus Medullaris Syndromes

This tiny sacrococcygeal and conus part of the cord contains sensory fibers to the perineum (saddle area) and important reflex arcs for sphincters and sexual function. Loss of erection and an autonomous bladder result from cord lesions from S2–S4. The bulbocavernosus and anal reflexes are also disturbed. Usually, there is associated loss of ankle jerks (S1). The bulbocavernosus reflex causes contraction of the bulbocavernosus muscle and of the external anal sphincter from scratch or stroking of the glans penis and is mediated by the S2–S4 roots. The anal reflex is shown as a contraction of the external sphincter on noxious stimulation—mild scratching the skin suffices—of the perineum or mucous membrane of the anus. It is mediated by the S4–S5 roots, damage to which can also interrupt the reflex.

Cauda Equina Syndromes

Lesions, usually tumors, of the cauda equina are properly considered lesions of nerve roots, the disturbance of which cause flaccid paralysis with areflexia (ankle jerks lost) and wasting of the legs and feet, saddle anesthesia, and sphincteric and sexual disturbances. The disorders can be unilateral. Pains in the sacroperineal region or radicular pain are frequent and early symptoms.

DISEASES

Spondylosis

From the age of 40 to 50 years and on, cervical spondylosis (Greek: *spondylos*, vertebra; *osis*, conditions affecting) is almost universal in the population. The ar-

thritic spurs, knobs, and bars that develop posteriorly from the margins of the vertebral bodies, together with degenerated, protruding discs narrow the intraspinal space and can impinge on the spinal cord and roots. Additional pathogenic factors are at play in flexion-extension of the neck; ischemia could occur because of transient repeated occlusions of the spinal arteries; folds of the ligamentum flavum in extension; and movements of the spinal cord and dura that slide up and down with flexion-extension while the cord is attached by the denticular ligaments. The anteroposterior diameter of the cervical spinal cord is normally 17 to 18 mm. In sturdy people and those with achondroplasias, it can be congenitally stenotic, making them more susceptible to cord compression with minor trauma (e.g., falls) (see Ch. 6).

In chronic spondylotic myelopathy, there is pain in the posterior neck with stiffness and limitation of passive movement of the neck, particularly that of lateral flexion. There is generally pain in at least one arm as a result of compression of a root. The most common lesions are at C5–C6, causing a C6 radicular syndrome with pain and numbness in the thumb and index finger, with diminished or absent biceps or brachioradialis jerks. With C7 involvement (C6–C7 vertebrae), paresthesiae are chiefly in the middle finger with diminished or absent triceps reflex. With C8 involvement (C7–T1 vertebrae), pins and needles and numbness affect the ring and small finger, and the pronator reflex is absent. Wasting of the hand rarely occurs because most of the hand muscles are innervated by T1.

Spasticity with hyper-reflexia is the main clinical token of cord dysfunction. It is usually obvious in one leg, but the Babinski sign is as a rule bilateral. It has been said that the presence of a Babinski sign in people older than age 50 years with no complaints is generally due to spondylitic myelopathy. Paresthesiae in the feet and sensations of tight bands around the ankles result from involvement of the posterior columns with diminished or abolished sense of position of the toes and of vibratory sense. A Lhermitte's sign is possible (see above). MRI is the best method of investigation. Where it is not available, lateral radiographs and myelography are useful.

Treatment decisions must be approached with caution. The mere (and common) presence of spondylosis is not reason enough to advise surgery; instead, it is the evidence of myelopathy. As a first step, it is common to advise a soft collar to immobilize neck movement. If this fails to alleviate symptoms, a few weeks of cervical traction can be attempted, hoping the separation of the compressed parts will be helpful. Patients often resort to chiropractic manipulations, hoping for relief, but no reliable means has been devised to determine which patients are at risk that such drastic movement of stiff parts may compress or dissect segments of the vertebral arteries with resultant stroke. Surgery for spondylotic myelopathy consists either of laminectomy or immobilization of the cervical spine by a graft. Despite traction or surgery, it is common for symptoms to persist. No controlled clinical trial has yet been undertaken to determine the benefits or surgery or to establish the setting under which it can most usefully be employed.

Lumbar Stenosis

Lumbar stenosis syndrome is that of the cauda equina (see above). It results from a congenitally shallow canal, spondylosis, or both. The clinical features are often characteristic. After long periods of standing (e.g., at cocktail parties or ceremonies) or on walking, especially downhill, painful paresthesias appear in both legs, often asymmetrically, ascending up to the buttocks. Weakness can force the patient to stop and sit. The ankle and knee jerks can disappear and reappear. Some of these complaints are easily misdiagnosed as claudication. In contrast to claudication, those with lumbar stenosis typically lack the acute pain, and stopping does not bring about a relief of symptoms. Relief is, instead, obtained by flexing the spine (e.g., flexing at the waist or lying on the side curled in the fetal position). Electromyography may show lumbosacral radiculopathies. Imaging, best achieved with MRI, shows the shallow canal. Laminectomy may be effective but often has to be extensive.

Trauma

See Chapter 6.

Tumors

Neoplasms may arise either within the cord (intramedullary) or outside the cord (extramedullary), the latter classified according to their intradural or extradural location. In all cases, the clinical syndrome features a progressive evolution, more or less reflecting the degree of malignancy. There are exceptions to these general rules in the astrocytoma, which in the cord is often a more indolent process than in the cerebrum.

Extradural tumors are the most frequent of the intraspinal tumors. Most of them are metastatic, usually an extension of nearby neoplasms and most often malignant. The spine is a favorite site for metastasis from primary tumors of the lung, breast, thyroid, and prostate and from local extension from lymphomas, less often from the bladder and bowel. The involvement of the vertebral body or pedicle often causes backache before evidence of disturbance in cord function. Weeks and months may pass between the emergence of the back pain and the more obvious signs of compressive myelopathy. A complaint of developing and unremitting isolated back pain warrants at least radiographs of the spine to seek evidence of bony erosion. MRI is a more definitive test.

Intradural tumors usually arise from supporting structures, most often meninges (meningiomas) or nerve sheath (neurofibromas), and are most often benign. They are common, accounting for 10 to 20 percent of all central nervous system neoplasms. Meningiomas most often arise in middle age, with neurofibromas somewhat earlier. Meningiomas are more common in aged women and are often in the thoracic region. Neurofibromas arise most often from posterior roots and can grow out through the intervertebral foramina, with their less-impeded foci of growth on either side of the foramen causing them to be thicker at either end (dumbbell tumors). In von Recklinghausen's disease, they are often multiple. Whatever their origin, these tumors cause inconstant local pain, with root pain being the more frequent.

When they have grown large, intradural tumors may displace the cord with a pyramidal syndrome, featuring spasticity; heightened reflexes; Babinski's signs, often asymmetric; and sensory disorders, which can be more or less clear-cut examples of Brown-Séquard's syndrome when there is lateral compression of the cord.

Uncommon causes of extramedullary tumors include epidermoids, chordomas (see below) and sarcomas. During the investigation of the tumor, the rare happy outcome (for reason of the better outlook with therapy) is the discovery of an arachnoid cyst or an arteriovenous malformation. The former is composed of partially sequestered arachnoidal diverticula. They occur most often in the thoracic region. Arteriovenous malformations may cause the same syndromes as any extramedullary mass and occur anywhere along in the surface of the cord (see below).

Intramedullary tumors are mainly ependymomas (often from the filum terminale) and astrocytomas. The high-grade malignant glial tumors so common in the cerebrum are more often histologically of lower grade in the cord. In middle-aged patients, tumors of the ependyma (ependymomas) of the central canal actually outnumber astrocytomas. Both occur more often in the cervical region. The characteristic clinical syndrome of intramedullary tumors is the central cord syndrome (see above), with less pain initially than the extramedullary tumors because the disease process may disrupt the crossing spinothalamic tract fibers before it enlarges enough to stretch pain-sensitive dural and vascular structures. A common retrospective history is an awareness that the legs and perineum do not appreciate the water temperature in the bathtub as readily as the hands and arms.

Other intramedullary tumors may be epidermoids, dermoids, teratomas, and hemangioblastomas; these last are rare and sporadic save for the congenital form associated with von Hippel-Lindau syndrome. Intramedullary metastases are not as rare as might be believed, but the diagnosis is difficult. All intramedullary tumors can be associated with syringomyelia (see Ch. 65).

Foramen Magnum Tumors

Tumors of the foramen magnum are rare but important because they are often benign (meningiomas or neurofibromas) and make for a difficult clinical diagnosis. Misdiagnosed, they can eventually be fatal. Pain is usually an early symptom, generally in the nape of the neck but sometimes in one arm. Weakness and sensory symptoms (mostly from the dorsal columns) characteristically progress in "square" fashion (i.e., one upper limb, the ipsilateral lower limb, the contralateral lower limb, and then the remaining upper limb). The lower cranial nerves can be involved. MRI and CT have greatly improved the ease of diagnosis. Where they are not available, myelography should be considered.

Lumbosacrococcygeal Tumors

Chordomas are malignant tumors that develop from remnants of the notochord and are almost always situated in the sacro-coccygeal region. Ependymomas of the filum terminale can reach a considerable size and cause papillary edema. Some can bleed, causing considerable siderosis (see Ch. 37). Uncommonly, there are cases of thoracolumbar extramedullary tumors with communicating hydrocephalus and dementia. A differential diagnosis of cauda equina tumors is the progressive cauda equina syndrome of acquired immunodeficiency syndrome (AIDS) (see Ch. 49).

Inflammatory Diseases

Acute dysfunction of the cord can result from trauma (see Ch. 6), infarction, or hemorrhage (see below) or from lesions related to infection or inflammation. By "acute" is meant disorders that develop within minutes to days and, by "subacute," those that take days or weeks to reach their full clinical picture.

Infection can damage the cord by direct access of viruses (e.g., poliomyelitis or herpes) or, rarely, of bacteria (e.g., abscess of the cord or epidural infections). Severe forms of myelitis can occur from Coxsackievirus and echovirus and from the virus in AIDS. Tropical spastic paraparesis occurs from human T-cell lymphotropic virus type I. Granulomatous fungal, mycobacteria, spirochetal, and parasitic diseases may involve the cord directly or affect it through meningitis or extradural mass lesions.

In another pathophysiologic group, the noxious process appears to be an autoimmune disorder resulting from a previous infection or immunization (e.g., postmeasles or postvaccinial myelitides). In many cases, the precise cause cannot be deduced.

Except for some viruses that have a special affinity for a particular part of the cord (e.g., polioviruses for the anterior horn cells), the various causes of acute myelitis (from the Greek for inflammation of the cord) are usually reflected clinically as transverse myelitis with distinctive clinical features. First, the lesions usually involve the thoracic cord, and hence, typically, a flaccid sensorimotor paraplegia occurs with bladder paralysis. Involvement of the cervical cord with acute quadriplegia is much less frequent. Second, the onset features paresthesiae that ascend from the perineum to the feet, legs, and trunk and stop at a sensory level. This level is clinically important because it means cord disease as contrasted to the rapidly evolving polyradiculoneuropathy (e.g., Guillain-Barré syndrome), in which there is no clear-cut upper sensory level. Third, the CSF usually shows a lymphocytic reaction (although an early polymorphonuclear reaction is possible), elevated total protein, and sometimes a reduction in the glucose level. In autoimmune processes, the lymphocytes can react with myelin basic protein. Finally, the diagnosis of lesions of the cord has been considerably improved by MRI, which shows high signals in T_2-weighted segments on several segments of the cord.

Except for cases that have a demonstrable cause (e.g., poliomyelitis in anterior horn cells or herpes in segmental cutaneous lesions), all cases that have an uncertain cause raise the possibility that the event may be the first clinical episode of multiple sclerosis (see Ch. 73).

For details of infectious disease, see Chapters 39 to 50. The main clinical features of the most frequent myelitides are outlined here.

Poliomyelitis (see Ch. 48) has become exceedingly rare in countries with high immunization rates. In other countries where the virus is common, the disease is usually a short-lived benign infection, leaving most children naturally immunized. The virus selectively invades the large cells of the anterior horn and the brainstem motor nuclei, causing flaccid paralysis of the muscles served by the roots the cell bodies of which are invaded. Areflexia and paralysis occur with a seemingly haphazard, asymmetric distribution. There are no sensory signs. In the days before the paralysis begins, there is usually a slight fever, malaise, and diffuse muscle pains in those limbs destined to become affected. Respiratory distress mandates admission to an intensive care unit. Recovery is variable, from near total to severe sequelae.

Herpesviruses (see Ch. 48) occur in the cord in two forms. Herpes simplex virus type 1 (oral herpes) more commonly causes an acute limbic encephalitis, rarely a myelitis. Similarly, herpes simplex type 2 (genital herpes) causes an acute lumbosacral radiculopathy, rarely a myelitis. The varicella-zoster virus causes a primarily ganglionic infection with pain and a vesicular eruption in a corresponding distribution (shingles). Sometimes, this can be followed by an acute myelitis when the eruption is thoracic. Immunocompromised patients are at special risk. Segmental pain heralds the cutaneous lesions as early as 7 to 10 days.

The cytomegalovirus, another herpesvirus, has been implicated in the myelitides in patients with AIDS. Monkey B virus can cause myelitis in laboratory workers.

Bacterial diseases (see Ch. 39) may cause myelitides as part of a systemic disease. They sometimes occur after trauma or neurosurgery. Only rarely does the process involve the cord, such as spinal cord abscess from *Mycoplasma pneumoniae* or *Listeria monocytogenes*. Usually, the infection develops in the epidural space as an abscess or granuloma, and the cord lesion results from vessel damage with infarction. Osteomyelitis, whether acute (*Staphylococcus aureus,* gram-negative organisms, or anaerobes) or subacute (tuberculosis or Pott's disease or brucellosis), can similarly cause cord infarction but also may compress the cord from the mass of the abscess itself. Focal or regional back pain and CT or MRI scans point to the diagnosis; the history, other systemic lesions, and CSF studies should detect the organism.

Chronic or subacute myelitides, such as syphilis or tuberculosis, can cause inflammation and occlusion of spinal arteries with infarction (meningovascular syphilis). In syphilitic meningomyelitis, there is a bilateral pyramidal syndrome with spasticity, enhanced reflexes, and Babinski's signs (Erb's spastic paraplegia). Tuberculomas and gummas of the cord are rare.

Parasitic myelitis may occur with many types of Schistosoma: *S. haematobium, S. mansoni,* or rarely *S. japonicum* (see Chs. 43 to 45). Myelitis is fairly frequent in Africa, South America, and the Far East. Granulomata form around the lumbosacral roots and conus, and the lumbar cord is usually involved. Rectal biopsy can provide a diagnosis. *Toxoplasma gondii* is a frequent cause of encephalitis in patients with AIDS and can also rarely cause myelitis.

Fungal infections are a cause of epidural lesions from hematogenous dissemination or to neighboring vertebral lesions; among the causes are Actinomyces, Coccidioides, Blastomyces, and Aspergillus (see Ch. 40).

Postinfectious, Postvaccinal (Autoimmune) Myelitides

These disorders are basically leukomyelitides (inflammations of the white matter of the cord), but the clinical picture is that of an acute transverse myelitis. The onset is within 1 to 2 weeks of a viral illness with exanthemata: measles, varicella, rubeola, or smallpox and more rarely after an immunization against cowpox or rabies. In all these cases, there often is an associated encephalitis and, particularly, involvement of the optic nerves. Pathologically, demyelinating lesions predominate around venules.

In principle, the clinical evolution is monophasic over a few weeks, but some cases, clinically indistinguishable from the others, will relapse as typical cases of multiple sclerosis (see Ch. 73). Particularly in those cases in which there is no apparent relationship with a viral illness or immunization, acute multiple sclerosis must be suspected. Cases caused by rabies vaccination should become much less frequent as the new vaccine from tissue cultures is used in place of the early vaccine made from spinal cord tissue.

Some cases, usually without a detectable cause, run a particularly rapid and severe course. They are termed *acute transverse necrotizing myelitides* because, pathologically, necrosis with hemorrhages is associated or predominates over demyelination. Some of these cases are associated with unilateral or bilateral involvement of the optic nerves (Devic's neuromyelitis optica, see Ch. 74). A *subacute necrotizing myelitis* occurs as a progressive myelopathy over several months, affecting mostly the lumbosacral cord. Many now believe the basic lesion is an arteriovenous malformation, although this explanation does not apply in other cases, especially those later shown to have an occult cancer (see below).

Retroviruses

In many patients with AIDS, a *vacuolar myelopathy* develops during the months prior to death. Symptoms and signs, usually thoracic in location, appear subacutely: weakness and sensory and sphincteric disorders. Pathologically, the lateral and posterior columns show vacuolations of the white matter. Myelin sheaths bear the brunt of the lesion.

Tropical spastic paraparesis is caused by human T-lymphotropic virus type I, an endemic disease in the French Antilles, the West Indies, Jamaica, Columbia, South America, Southern Japan, and Africa. Many sporadic instances are known. The clinical onset is in adults, mainly females. The retrovirus is transmitted either from mother to child, by transfusion, by intravenous injections, or by the sexual route. Clinically, tropical spastic paraparesis is a slowly progressive spastic paraparesis with sphincteric disorders and variable disturbance in sensation. Polyneuropathy is associated in some cases. Pathologically, the lesions fall most heavily on the corticospinal tracts and posterior columns with inflammatory demyelination or necrosis. Structurally similar to human T-lymphotropic virus but molecularly distinct, the human T-lymphotropic virus type II has also been reported in tropical spastic paraparesis associated with human T-lymphotropic virus type I, human immunodeficiency virus, or, recently, alone. The presence of antibodies in the serum and CSF can be detected by enzyme-linked immunosorbent assay techniques.

Multiple Sclerosis

Multiple sclerosis begins, in some cases, as an acute transverse myelopathy indistinguishable on clinical grounds from acute postinfectious myelopathies (discussed earlier), except that there is no history of skin rash or immunization (see Ch. 73). In most cases of chronic multiple sclerosis, the cord is involved, and there are infrequent cases in which the cord is the only part of the central nervous system involved by the disease.

The usual presentation is that of a paraparesis with fatigability and weakness on exercise, tingling and numbness of the legs, and urgency in micturition. The saying that "in multiple sclerosis, the patient complains of one leg and has signs in both" is commonly supported by clinical findings of brisk reflexes, Babinski's responses, and disorders of position and vibration on both sides. Abdominal cutaneous reflexes are often absent. MRI with multiarray coils and fast spin-echo methods confirms that the cord in involved in most patients. For further details, see Chapter 73.

Systemic Lupus Erythematosus

Acute transverse myelitis in patients with systemic lupus erythematosus is a well-known possibility. The onset is usually acute and evolves over a matter of hours. The basis would appear to be cord infarction (see Ch. 38). There is, however, a subacute myelopathy in patients with this disease that raises diagnostic problems with multiple sclerosis ("lupoid sclerosis").

Gougerot-Sjögren Syndrome

This is a fairly frequent immune disorder, occurring mostly in women. It is characterized by the sicca (from the Latin for dry) syndrome due to infiltration of the salivary and lachrymal glands by lymphocytes and plasma cells. Gougerot-Sjögren syndrome can be primary or secondary to various immune diseases (e.g., rheumatoid arthritis or systemic lupus erythematous). In primary Gougerot-Sjögren syndrome, an acute or chronic myelopathy is possible, often associated with involvement of the peripheral nervous system. Some

cases of myelopathy have a recurrent course, oligoclonal bands on CSF electrophoresis, and high signals in the white matter on T_2-weighted MRI. The differential diagnosis with multiple sclerosis is thus raised.

The diagnosis of primary Gougerot-Sjögren syndrome is supported by biopsy of accessory salivary glands and the presence of particular antinuclear antibodies: SSA and SSB (the SS stands for Sjögren's syndrome).

Subacute Paraneoplastic Necrotizing Myelopathy

This unusual disorder can be associated with lung carcinoma, solid lymphomas, and rarely colonic carcinoma. There is also a paraneoplastic affection in which anterior horn cells selectively disappear. Patients with ovarian carcinoma, Hodgkin's disease, or rarely, other carcinomas can have a subacute or chronic degeneration of the posterior and lateral columns together with loss of Purkinje cells of the cerebellum.

Myelopathies Caused by Toxic Substances

Clioquinol was at one time a drug used worldwide against acute (traveler's) diarrhea or chronic enteritis. In the 1970s, it was recognized that many long-term users, particularly in Japan, developed a subacute myelo-opticoneuropathy. The onset was acute or subacute with spastic paraplegia, sphincteric disturbances, and later amblyopia. Both optic and cord lesions usually produced lasting sequelae.

Several intrathecally injected chemotherapeutic agents, among them methotrexate and cytarabine, can cause an acute myelopathy.

A transverse myelopathy has also been reported with chemonucleolysis by chymopapain, as have fatal allergic reactions.

Myelopathies Caused by Physical Agents

Electric currents are well conducted by the nervous system, with the cord being specifically vulnerable to electric shocks. The injuries happen at work and at home; infants are frequent victims. The significant factors are the amperage (not voltage), duration of contact, resistance of the skin (which, if covered with water, is much less resistant), and path of the current (the cord is particularly at risk with arm-to-arm and arm-to-leg paths).

After an electric shock or a lightning strike, an immediate flaccid paraplegia with sensory symptoms may occur. It usually clears off within 12 to 24 hours. Delayed (weeks to months) myelopathy may occur, sometimes resembling amyotrophic lateral sclerosis (see Ch. 63).

Radiation myelopathy can occur early or late after radiation therapy of cervical and thoracic lesions. The early type appears after a few months, with distal paresthesiae and, frequently, a Lhermitte's sign. It wears off again in a few months and does not herald the delayed syndrome. The onset of the latter is delayed 1 to 5 years and is characterized by symptoms of posterior column dysfunction, which persists as spasticity of the legs, exaggerated reflexes, Babinski's signs, and disorders of pain and temperature, and are progressively added. At some time, a Brown-Séquard syndrome may develop. MRI shows an enlarged cord with high signals on T_2-weighted pulse sequences. Most pathologists believe a vascular process is responsible, although occlusions of arteries do not readily account for the slow progression of the disease. A case examined by the authors suggested a disorder of the permeability of the vessel walls with passage of plasma into the surrounding tissue, a pathologic picture also reported by others. Steroids have been beneficial in some cases. Fractionation of the radiation and a correct dose usually avoid this complication.

Another form of radiation myelopathy with weakness, atrophy of muscles, and areflexia has been reported. In such cases, it would appear that the anterior horn cells have been selectively damaged.

Caisson Disease

This condition and its name is an example of a disease state that resulted from advances in technology. In this case, it was the development in the last century of methods of building long-span bridges, which required the sinking of the wooden boxes (French, *caisson*) destined to be filled with concrete to support the piers to carry the cables for the roadway. The caissons had to be filled with pressurized air to prevent their walls from collapsing under the weight of the outside water while men dug down to the firm bedrock where the caissons finally rested.

Clinical consequences were first recognized in men who worked many hours under the high air pressures required inside the caisson. The nitrogen gas dissolved in the compressed air circulated harmlessly in the blood while the worker was in the high-pressure environment, but if he was returned too quickly to normal atmospheric pressure, the dissolved nitrogen trapped in the circulation was restored to gas form, causing widely disseminated hematogenous bubbles (decompression sickness), which occluded blood vessels, with the cervical and thoracic cord regions being especially susceptible to such effects. The clinical effects were extreme pain and involuntary flexion of the trunk ("the bends"). Ischemic lesions predominated in the posterior columns.

Rapidly acquired knowledge of these risks led to a schedule of limited-time exposures and the substitution of compressed air with oxygen mixed with gases better soluble than nitrogen. Caisson disease is now rare for workers in deep tunnels (sandhogs) and commercial deep-sea divers who are immersed in pressurized diving suits with attached helmets. Amateur and recreational divers still use compressed air in tanks but are warned to avoid excessive depths and not to emerge from them too quickly. However, those tempted to explore great depths in search of beautiful reef fish run the risk of wandering too deep, staying too long, and undergoing unwitting rapid decompression.

Patients with decompression sickness should be placed immediately in a hyperbaric chamber, if available, to redissolve the nitrogen and decompress the patient only slowly, a process that can take many hours.

Nutritional, Metabolic, and Endocrine Myelopathies

Several vitamin deficiencies can cause a myelopathy (see Ch. 71). *Subacute combined system disease,* from vitamin B_{12} deficiency, is now infrequent in Western countries because of the correct treatment of pernicious anemia, but it is still frequent in some parts of the world. Demyelination is most common in the posterior and lateral columns, especially in the heavily myelinated portions of the thoracic and cervical cord, leading to sensations of pins and needles in the legs with loss of vibration, sometimes high in the trunk, and proprioceptive sensation. Similar changes in the corticospinal tracts cause weakness and spasticity in the legs. The spasticity, weakness, and sensory changes cause an unsteady gait. If the accompanying polyneuropathy is advanced, deep tendon reflexes may be absent or diminished. The blood may not show the changes typical of pernicious anemia, and bone marrow specimens must be sought. Low levels of serum cobalamin support the diagnosis. Immediate and lifelong treatment with injected vitamin B_{12} is necessary. Recovery is possible with the early lesions.

Folate, given alone, can cure the anemia but not the myelopathy and may even make it worse. However, a few instances of myelopathy caused by folate deficiency have been reported.

Myelopathies also featuring combined system disease, but with lesions predominating in the posterior columns, have been reported from vitamin PP deficiency (*pellagra*) in malnourished persons, including prisoners and alcoholic persons.

A specific paraplegia, mainly observed in some parts of India and Africa, is due to *lathyrism* (i.e., a neuroexcitatory amino acid present in *Lathyrus sativus,* a pea grass the flour of which can be consumed during periods of starvation).

In *adrenoleukodystrophy,* there is a degeneration (i.e., a sudanophilic demyelination of the white matter of the brain together with atrophy of the adrenal glands). Typically, the skin takes on a bronzed tone. The histologic markers of this disease are the presence in brain and adrenal glands (and serum) of large quantities of very long chain fatty acids. A variant is *adrenomyeloneuropathy,* which can be a cause of spastic paraplegia in young adult men and a less severe paraparesis in heterozygous female patients. The diagnosis is supported by tests of adrenal insufficiency and the documentation of very-long-chain fatty acids in the serum.

Portocaval myelopathy presents clinically as a spastic paraparesis in patients with portal hypertension in whom surgical portosystemic anastomosis has been undertaken. More rarely, the disorder may be seen in patients with severe portal hypertension and, presumably, many spontaneous portosystemic shunts. Pathologic studies suggest that the primary lesion involves Betz cells in the precentral gyrus; hence, the term encephalomyelopathy may be more appropriate.

Arachnoiditis

In patients with multiple surgical interventions, chronic meningitis (e.g., tuberculous), contrast myelography with certain agents performed in the presence of blood in the spinal fluid, or multiple therapeutic subarachnoid injections, connective tissue can develop within the arachnoid, causing entrapment of the cauda equina and cord and may block the circulation of CSF. In earlier times, spinal anesthetic contaminated with a detergent was a cause. In some cases, no cause can be found.

There is usually an early onset of pain and paralysis when the pathologic process is launched by the introduction of an offending agent into the subarachnoid space. Otherwise, the picture is that of a progressive paraplegia with signs of cauda equina involvement (discussed earlier) and cord dysfunction. The CSF contains a few white cells and usually a high to very high protein concentration. Myelography shows a complete or incomplete block with irregularities in flow and pocketing of contrast, reflecting the adhesions and irregular masses of connective tissue. Surgical attempts at freeing up the adhered tissue are usually disappointing, and no real cure is available.

Syringomyelia

Syringomyelia (Greek: *syrinx,* tube) (see Ch. 65) involves a cystic degeneration of the central or paracentral spinal cord of unknown cause. The most common presentation is with a central cord syndrome, but partial Brown-Séquard forms are also common. The cervical region is most often affected, resulting in distinctive sensory loss and motor wasting in segments affected by the syrinx. The syrinx commonly extends into the medulla and, in rare cases, for the length of the spinal cord.

System Degenerations

These include pure motor, sensorimotor, and rare pure sensory syndromes. The *pure motor syndromes* include amyotrophic lateral sclerosis and primary sclerosis. Amyotrophic lateral sclerosis begins with cramps, and fasciculations appear, usually in the hands, in muscles that initially have their normal bulk and function. Atrophy of the small muscles of the hand appears within months, with, in one-third of cases, asymmetry in the affected muscles. The muscles involved first remain the most severely involved and continue to atrophy as fasciculations and weakness appear in shoulder, hips, and tongue. Weakness of the trunk occurs late. The rare but distinctive syndrome of primary lateral sclerosis features spastic weakness affecting the legs, and less often the arms, with hyperactive deep tendon reflexes and extensor plantar responses but no accompanying evidence of atrophy of the muscles or fasciculations and with no sensory disturbances. Of the *sensorimotor degenerative diseases,* the syndrome complex of Friedreich's ataxia is the best known. The spinal cord syndrome component features gradually developing spasticity, ataxia of the limbs and trunk, dysarthria, areflexia, and loss of position sense. Other spinocerebellar syndromes usually spare either sensory loss or show no spasticity (see Ch. 64).

Vascular Diseases

The blood supply of the cord has been summarized earlier in this chapter.

Infarction

Common in the brain, *infarction of the cord* is something of a rarity. Several reasons for the difference in frequency have been proposed, including a greater adequacy of collateral circulation or a higher resistance to infarction of cord tissue. The authors think that the basic fact is that the cord arteries are a rare target for cardiac embolism or atherosclerosis.

From Figure 31-3, it is easy to predict the main components of the syndrome of *anterior spinal artery occlusion,* the most common of cord infarcts: paraplegia or quadriplegia (central cord and corticospinal tracts), at first flaccid and later spastic; sensory disorders for pain and temperature (spinothalamic tracts lateral and crossing); sphincteric paralysis (central cord); and a characteristic sparing of dorsal (posterior) column function (i.e., preserved position and vibratory sense). The onset is usually sudden, or at the least rapidly evolving, typically hours ahead of the time table for the myelitides.

Rarely, it has been demonstrated that the anterior spinal artery or its branches were blocked by atherosclerotic, myxomatous, endocarditic, or malarial materials. Schistosomiasis is a possible cause, although the venous route is more likely in this condition (see Ch. 44). Among the better known are *fibrocartilaginous emboli*, rare elsewhere but reported several times in cord infarction. They can plug the spinal artery after trauma, but the trauma can be mild (the inferred source was horseback riding in a young woman whose case is known to the authors). Frequently, there is no clear history of a precipitating cause. The material is obviously fragments of intervertebral disc, but why and how it reaches the spinal vessels is a mystery. It is possible that the embolism is more widespread but that the spinal vessels are especially susceptible to clinical syndromes when occluded by such small material.

The bubbling nitrogen gas in caisson disease (see above) occludes the cervical and thoracic cord by obstructing vessels.

Inflammatory disease may occlude cord vessels from such causes as syphilis, other forms of chronic meningitis (tuberculous or neoplastic), and *metastatic malignancies,* which may so weaken the spine as to crimp the vascular supply to the cord. Even *spinal anesthesia* has been implicated.

Most of the causes of cord infarction lie outside the spine, as most causes of stroke in the brain lie outside the skull. Aortic disease ranks first with dissection, aortic aneurysms, and surgery following, all of which can block one or more segmental arteries that supply the cord. Aortography and catheterization through the aorta can dislodge atherosclerotic plaque or cause dissections. At one time, it was thought that a *spinal cord claudication* occurred from atherosclerosis of the aorta, obstructing many segmental arteries to the cord and causing weakness of the legs on walking, without pain, and relieved by rest, which was analogous to coronary insufficiency. The authors doubt such an entity exists.

There are no more than a dozen or so reported examples on record of *posterior spinal artery infarction.* Immediately after the sudden onset, the clinical picture is that of an acute transverse myelopathy. Much improvement occurs, amounting to near recovery. Syphilitic arteritis, trauma, atherosclerotic emboli, and intrathecal injection of phenol are among the causes.

Hypotension with vascular collapse may cause cord infarction, lesions thought to be explained by the watershed effect. They are located at the junctional areas of the anterior spinal artery (i.e., cervico- or lumbothoracic area) (Fig. 31-4). They may selectively involve the gray matter over several segments of the cord (pencil infarcts, Fig. 31-3), which can also be caused by aortic dissections with circulatory collapse.

Occlusion of *spinal veins* has been reported postmortem in a few cases. Infarction predominated in the gray matter, was extensive, and very hemorrhagic. Tumor, septicemia, and carcinoma of the pancreas have been associated.

Hemorrhage

Hematomyelia, literally meaning hemorrhage into the cord, is also rare compared with hemorrhage into the brain. It may be due to trauma or a bleeding diathesis and is a well-known complication of anticoagulant therapy. It causes an acute transverse myelopathy the clinical features of which are the same as those from other causes. Pain is not common enough to use this point in differential diagnosis. There has not yet developed a useful surgical therapy because evacuation of the clot is unlikely for fear of surgery resulting in even more damage to the cord.

Epidural or subdural spinal hemorrhage causes an acute compression of the cord, and the causes are similar to those of hematomyelia. Because of its potential reversibility, it is a neurosurgical emergency. No clinical features allow a differential diagnosis from hematomyelia; so the diagnosis rests mainly on clinical suspicion and imaging. MRI is the best available technique, with CT or contrast myelography used where MRI is not available.

Vascular Malformations

Two kinds of malformations occur: dural fistulae and arteriovenous malformations (see Ch. 37). In *dural fistulae,* the site of the abnormal arterial-to-venous communications (fistulae) lie in the dura, near a nerve root sleeve. They are usually recognized in late adult life. Enlargement of the vessels involved in the fistula can cause a progressive myelopathy, with exacerbations (sometimes occurring after exercise) and remissions, raising the differential diagnosis of multiple sclerosis. Hemorrhage is rare. MRI can show the enlarged vessels. Selective angiography shows the usually tortuous arterial feeders and the abnormally dilated draining veins. Selective embolization with quick-setting glues is the current therapy.

Arteriovenous malformations lie on the surface of the cord with a more or less extensive part within the cord. As a rule, there is a greatly enlarged tortuous vessel running along the posterior aspect of the cord. Aneurysms of feeding vessels are commonly encountered in these lesions of the brain but less so in arteriovenous malformations that involve the cord. Subarachnoid hemorrhage or acute transverse myelopathy may occur, but the usual problem is a progressive myelopathy, which may develop smoothly (from mass effect of distended vessels) or episodically (recurrent hemorrhage), raising the usual concern of multiple sclerosis. A bruit is only rarely heard over the spine, but auscultation is so simply performed and distinctly diagnostic when positive that it is a mandatory clinical step in the approach to patients with progressive myelopathy. Selective angiography shows the malformation. MRI may make the diagnosis with the serpentiginous appearance to the feeding vessels (MRI may be negative in small lesions that affect the lumbosacral cord and conus.) Occasionally, evidence of earlier hemorrhages can been seen from the presence of methemoglobin (seen as high-signal defects on T_1-weighted images) or hemosiderin (seen as low-signal defects on T_2-weighted images).

Developmental or Acquired Abnormalities of the Spine

Here briefly detailed are the main anomalies that involve the spinal cords and permit survival to adolescence or adult life when they reveal themselves clinically.

Spinal Defects

Skull base anomalies are most frequently a form of fusion, partial or total, of the axis with the foramen magnum. The size of the foramen magnum may be reduced (critical minimal diameter, 19 mm) with evidence of cord compression. The base of the skull may also be flattened (platybasia) from congenital or acquired causes of bone weakness (e.g., Paget's disease). There may also be an ascension of the bony structures that constitute the edges of the foramen magnum. The neck is often short with a low hairline. The clinical syndrome may feature cerebellar or cord syndromes from local compression, and closure of the foramen magnum may cause hydrocephalus (see Ch. 59). On lateral radiographs of the skull, the tip of the odontoid process is above Chamberlain's line (a line drawn between the posterior border of the hard palate and the posterior border of the foramen magnum).

Dislocation of the atlas from the axis with a forward slide, which can occur congenitally, results from trauma or from inflammatory lesions of the ligaments that hold these vertebrae together; rheumatoid arthritis is the most common such cause.

Diseases that enlarge the vertebrae (e.g., Paget's disease and achondroplasia) can cause cord compression. Ankylosing spondylitis can cause lumbosacral or cervical root dysfunction. Arachnoidal cysts that compress the thoracic cord may cause all the features of focal cord compression; they have been reported in Marfan's syndrome.

Dysraphic States

The general term of dysraphism (Greek: *dys,* bad; *raphe,* seam) refers to the imperfect closure of the neural tube. Rachischisis means split spine (Greek: *schisis,*

cleft) and connotes the frequently associated defects in the closure of the spine. Such abnormalities are usually found at either end of the cord, where the remnants of the embryologic notochord lie.

Arnold-Chiari malformation, named for the German pathologists J. Arnold (1835–1890) and J. B. Chiari (1851–1916), has two major forms. In *type I,* the medulla, fourth ventricle, and cord are in a low position in the cervical canal together with a tongue of cerebellar tissue (usually the tonsils). The cord, pushed caudalward by the medulla and fourth ventricle, is kinked. The foramens of Luschka and Magendie open in the cervical canal. The foramen magnum is occluded and the cerebellar tissue occupies the cisterna magna. Hydrocephalus is usually present from the obstruction of CSF at the foramen magnum.

In *Arnold-Chiari type II malformation,* there is an associated myelomeningocele (Greek: *myelo,* cord; *meninges,* membranes; *kele,* hernia), that is, parts of the cord and meninges extrude through a dehiscence of the vertebral laminae to form an exterior pouch.

Arnold-Chiari type I can produce symptoms and signs in adolescence or adult life. The onset can be abrupt with cord dysfunction caused by the commonly associated syringomyelia (see Ch. 65) or signs of high intracranial pressure or cerebellar ataxia. Concomitant defects in the caudal cord are frequent.

In the caudal part of the cord, several abnormalities can cause clinical disorders in the teens or early adult life. *Spina bifida* (from the Latin for spine divided in two) is frequent. The grossly obvious *spina bifida aperta,* that is, open, with extrusion of meninges (meningocele) and/or cord (myelomeningocoele) is recognized at birth. *Spina bifida occulta,* that is, concealed, can be, in some cases, suspected clinically, and examination of the lumbosacral region is part of a thorough neurologic examination. Spina bifida occulta is suggested by a tuft of hair on a dimple or palpable soft subcutaneous mass in the lumbosacral region. Many cases of spina bifida occulta are asymptomatic and diagnosed only by the gap in the bony spinal arch seen on radiographs. It can be associated with lipomas, dermoids, or sinus tracts. The latter should be suspected in recurrent meningeal infections.

In diastematomyelia (Greek: *diastema,* chink), there is a bony or fibrous protrusion in the lower thoracic or upper lumbar canal. The cord is split in two halves (diplomyelia) with two dural sacs. In adolescence or adult life, this can cause a traction myelopathy.

Tethered cord is an important cause of traction myelopathy, many cases of which make their clinical appearance in the early teens (age of growth) or in young adults. The cord it tethered (i.e., the conus lies below the L1–L2 level and is firmly attached by a short and thick filum terminale). A lipoma can be associated with this anomaly. Symptoms and signs can set in insidiously or be precipitated by trauma (e.g., fall on the buttocks or exercises that stretch the spine and normally would make the cord ascend in the spinal canal (see above), such as flexion at the hip, high kicks in ballet training, or rowing. Clinical features are rather different in children and adults and can be mixed in adolescents; foot drop, leg weakness, poor bladder control, and a Lhermitte's sign (see above) are all rather frequent. Cutaneous signs of dysraphism (see above) are common in children but are lacking in 50 percent of adults. In adults, diffuse pain, particularly in the perineum and anus is frequent. MRI is the best way to image the malpositioned cord and associated lipoma. It can sometimes show diastematomyelia (discussed previously). The basic principle of the treatment is section of the filum terminale to relieve the traction on the cord.

Syringomyelia (see Ch. 65) is significantly associated with all the congenital abnormalities of the rostral end of the cord.

Cordotomy

Used for relief of pain, cordotomy is intended to interrupt the spinothalamic tract in the hope of blunting the afferent signals reaching the brain. Its greatest use is for patients with asymmetric pain unresponsive to medical therapy. Although pain relief is usually achieved, the risks include persistent ipsilateral weakness, hypotension, and ipsilateral dysautonomia and permanent bladder paresis at rates from 10 to 30 percent, which are higher if bilateral cordotomies are undertaken. Indwelling (intrathecal) catheters for opioid infusions are becoming more common.

ANNOTATED BIBLIOGRAPHY

Abdel-Azim M, Sullivan M, Yalla SV. Disorders of bladder function in spinal cord disease. Neurol Clin 1991;9: 727–40.

Advice from an experienced team.

Alajouanine TH, Lhermitte F, Cambier J, Gautier JC. Les lésions post-radiothérapiques tardives du système nerveux central. Rev Neurol (Paris) 1961;105:9–21.

A pathologic study and review.

Barros TE, Oliveira RP, Rosemberg LA, Magalhaes AC. Hemisection of the cervical spinal cord caused by a stab wound: MR findings [letter]. AJR Am J Roentgenol 1992;158:1413.

A rare case.

Breig A. Overstretching of and circumscribed pathological tension in the spinal cord: a basic cause of symptoms in cord disorders. J Biomech 1970;3:7–9.

In neck flexion, the cord ascends by as much as 2 cm.

Critchley McD. Neurological effects of lightning and electricity. Lancet 1936;1:68–70.

A clinical classic.

DiTunno JF, Formal CS. Current concepts: chronic spinal cord injury. N Engl J Med 1994;330:550–6.

Thorough review.

Grundy D, Russell J, Swain A. ABC of Spinal Cord Injury. Tavistock Square, London, 1990.

A comprehensive series from emergency to late management.

Gutrecht JA, Zamani AA, Salgado ED. Anatomic-radiologic basis of Lhermitte's sign in multiple sclerosis. Arch Neurol 1993;50:849–51.

The sign is due to cervical dorsal column lesions and has many causes.

Hackney DB. Magnetic resonance imaging of the spine. Normal anatomy. Top Magn Reson Imaging 1992;4: 1–6.

Useful details of normal anatomy.

Hall S, Bartleson JD, Burton M, et al. Lumbar spine stenosis. Ann Intern Med 1985;103:273–5.

A pre-MRI review of 68 patients with good clinical and management data.

Heller JG. The syndromes of degenerative cervical disease. Orthrop Clin North Am 1992;23:381–94.

The spectrum of syndromes from different causes.

Jacobson S, Lehky T, Nishimura M. Isolation of HTLV-II from a patient with chronic progressive neurological disease clinically indistinguishable from HTLV-I-associated myelopathy/tropical spastic paraparesis. Ann Neurol 1993;33:392–6.

Human T-lymphotropic viruses types I and II.

Kidd D, Thorpe JW, Thompson AJ. Spinal cord MRI using multi-array coils and fast spin echo. II. Findings in multiple sclerosis. Neurology 1993;43:2632–7.

A rapid and sensitive method that shows the cord is involved in most patients.

Krol G, Heier L, Becker R et al. Value of magnetic resonance imaging in the evaluation of patients with complete and high degree block due to intracanal neoplasm. Acta Radiol Suppl (Stockh) 1986;369:741–3.

MRI findings are false negative in only 11 percent.

Maroon JC, Abla AA, Wilberger JI et al. Central cord syndrome. Clin Neurosurg 1991;37:612–21.

Authoritative modern review.

Mawson AR, Snelling L, Winchester Y, Biundo JJ Jr. 526 spinal cord injuries: experience of the Louisiana Rehabilitation Institute, 1965–1984. J La State Med Soc 1991; 143:31–7.

Most injuries cause incomplete syndromes.

McCormick PC, Stein BM (eds). Intradural spinal surgery. Neurosurg Clin North Am 1990;1(3).

Practical and timely thorough review.

Mirich DR, Kucharczyk W, Keller MA, Deck J. Subacute necrotizing myelopathy: MR imaging in four pathologically proved cases. AJNR Am J Neuroradiol 1991;12: 1077–83.

Differential diagnosis from acute transverse myelitis and arteriovenous malformation.

Miyasaka K, Akino M, Abe S et al. Computed tomography and magnetic resonance imaging of intramedullary spinal cord tumors. Acta Radiol Suppl (Stockh) 1986; 369:738–40.

MR superior to CT, even in 1986. (It has further improved.)

Pant SS, Rebeiz JJ, Richardson EP Jr. Spastic paraparesis following porto-caval shunts. Neurology 1968;18: 134–41.

The primary lesions were in the precentral gyrus.

Sliwa JA, Maclean IC. Ischemic myelopathy: a review of spinal vasculature and related clinical syndromes. Arch Phys Med Rehabil 1992;73:365–72.

Exhaustive review with much modern detail.

Smith KJ, McDonald WI. Spontaneous and mechanically evoked activity due to central demyelinating lesions. Nature 1980;286:154–5.

Observation in cats accounting for paresthesiae in Lhermitte's sign.

Thorpe JW, Kidd D, Kendall BE. Spinal cord MRI using multi-array coils and fast spin echo. I. Technical aspects and findings in healthy adults. Neurology 1993;43: 2625–31.

A new technique that quickly provides images of the whole cord with high resolution and allows measurement of the cross-sectional area of the cord.

Woolsey RM, Young RR. Disorders of the Spinal Cord. Neurological Clinics. 9. WB Saunders, Philadelphia, 1991.

An update on anatomic, physiologic, clinical, and pathologic findings; imaging; and bladder and sexual disturbances of normal and abnormal cord. Several distinguished contributors.

32
Peripheral Nervous System

J. C. Gautier and J. P. Mohr

A common mistake of beginners is to believe that the peripheral nervous system (PNS) is relatively simple so that the diagnosis of its diseases is relatively simple too. This error stems from two misconceptions, for both the gross anatomy and the fine anatomy and functions of the PNS are quite complex indeed.

The PNS is made of those parts of the nervous system that lie outside the central nervous system (CNS), (i.e., the ventral, dorsal, and lateral horns of the spinal cord, the ventral and dorsal roots, spinal ganglia, spinal nerves, plexuses, nerves, autonomic fibers, and ganglia). Except for the fibers in the posterior columns of the cord, all these cells and fibers are related to Schwann cells (T. Schwann, German histologist, 1810–82). The cranial nerves from C3 to C12 are parts of the PNS and share much of its pathology, but owing to their highly particular semiology, they are considered separately (see Chs. 28 and 29). For practical purposes, the term PNS applies to the motor, sensory, and autonomic cells and fibers that originate in or enter the spinal cord. Despite the need for a sound knowledge of the gross anatomy of the PNS for those engaged in the practice of neurology, the details are easily forgotten and must be refreshed as often as necessary. Even so, it is not always easy to locate clinically a lesion on a plexus or a nerve.

The fine anatomy of the PNS reflects complex functions. There are motor fibers of two types, A and γ (see Ch. 22); sensory fibers of various sizes (see Ch. 23) myelinated and unmyelinated of various thickness with various conduction velocities for each sensory modality; and fibers and ganglia of the autonomic system (see also Ch. 34). This complexity probably accounts for different degrees of vulnerability to metabolic disorders and to compression, reflected in the kaleidoscope of clinical disorders: pure motor, pure sensory, pure autonomic, and mixed disorders with numerous variants (e.g., of sensory-modality dissocia-

tions). This complexity is illustrated by the disappointing observation that no cause is found in about half of the patients who come to good neurologists with a polyneuropathy. Despite these problems, the PNS is a field of active research, which gives hope that the number of unsolved riddles will dwindle progressively. The aim of the present chapter is to set forth general principles of diagnosis and approach of the patients.

For the clinician, the complex conglomerate that makes up the PNS has two main characteristics, namely the length and the poor protection of its fibers. The amazing length of many PNS cells processes (e.g., 1.50 to 1.70 m for a cell in a lumbar spinal ganglion) implies an intense metabolic activity in the perikaryon with far distant axonal transport. The metabolic demands of such great lengths probably accounts for the vulnerability of these cells to many acquired or inherited metabolic derangements. On the other hand, the poor protection of PNS fibers that course along bones, joints, and ligaments from distal limbs to girdles and spine accounts for the frequency of traumatic, compressive, and entrapment disorders.

Nerve fascicles and individual fibers are surrounded by collagen with fibrocytes that form three concentric sheaths, the epineurium, perineurium, and endoneurium. The perineurium with its junctional cells may have a role of selective filtration analogous to that of the blood-brain barrier. Mast cells are present in the endoneurium. The blood supply depends on tiny vessels, the vasa nervorum. They are collateralized, but their occlusion can cause nerve infarction. In collagen diseases and the vasculitides, PNS involvement is frequent and often prominent. Nervi nervorum innervate the nervous sheaths. Their physiology and possible pathologic role are poorly known. Roots have several features of their own. They bathe in the cerebrospinal fluid, and hence disturbances of the latter are suggestive of root damage. Roots, in addition, have no epineurium and little perineurium, which is consistent with particular biologic characteristics and could account for the susceptibility of the roots to autoimmune disorders (Guillain-Barré syndrome), tabetic neurosyphilis, and diphtheritic toxins. The arachnoid ensheathes the roots as they pass through the intervertebral foramina, and this arachnoid sleeve can be torn off in traumatic avulsions of the roots. This lesion appears as meningoceles on myelography. Besides, in the intervertebral foramina the roots are liable to be compressed by a herniated intervertebral disk, annulus fibrosus, or ligamentum flavum.

DEFINITIONS OF TERMS

The term *neuropathy* conveys the general meaning of disease of the PNS. *Neuritis* is somewhat obsolete and should be reserved for cases with proven inflammation. *Polyneuropathy* has similarly replaced polyneuritis. It means a diffuse disease of nerves, usually involving at onset the distal ends of the limbs (the feet, then the hands), with a pattern of sensory and motor loss known as "stocking-glove." Polyneuropathy implies a systemic metabolic disorder, exogenous as when due to toxins, endogenous as when due to diabetes, or inherited as in Friedreich's ataxia or the ataxia of Charcot-Marie-Tooth disease (see Ch. 80). *Radiculopathy* means an affection of one or several roots as in herpes zoster or a herniated disk. *Polyradiculoneuropathy* means an association of polyneuropathy and radiculopathy. The deficit can affect nerves in their proximal as well as distal distribution, and there are abnormalities of the cerebrospinal fluid (CSF). *Mononeuropathy* is an affection of an individual nerve (e.g., the median or common peroneal nerve). It implies a local noxious agent, usually trauma, compression, or entrapment. A mononeuropathy can be the first event of a multiple mononeuropathy (also called mononeuropathy multiplex) in which two or more noncontiguous nerves are involved. It implies plurifocal causal lesions (e.g., occlusion of several vasa nervorum in polyarteritis nodosa).

BASIC PATHOLOGIC REACTIONS OF PERIPHERAL NEURONS

There are three fundamental reactions based on the site of the apparently primary insult: wallerian degeneration, which is the response to axonal transection, axonal degeneration (the dying-back phenomenon), and demyelination. Although this classification is useful, many neuropathies show lesions of both axons and myelin sheaths, this being due to the fundamental symbiosis between axons and their sheaths.

In *wallerian degeneration* (A. V. Waller, British physiologist, 1816–70), the distal parts of both axon and myelin sheath, severed from the proximal part, disintegrate. Wallerian degeneration can result from trauma, compression, entrapment, infarction, or tumor infiltration. Conduction is abolished distal to the interruption. Muscles supplied by the severed motor nerves undergo denervation atrophy. Regeneration can occur if the severed ends are close enough and not separated by interstitial tissue, but it is slow and often incomplete. If neighboring normal muscle fibers are available, sprouting of the proximal nerve end occurs, with enlargement of motor units. When the sprouting fibers are misdirected by interstitial tissue and fibrocytes, the axonal transport material accumulates at the severed end and forms a mass (neuroma). Regenerating fibers and those in neuromas are pathologically sensitive to mechanical stimuli. This sensitivity is the basis of Tinel's sign (J. Tinel, French neurologist, 1879–1952), which helps to locate lesions on peripheral nerves: percussion of the nerve elicits tingling sensations on the area of normal distal innervation.

In *demyelination* (often referred to as Gombault's segmental demyelination after F. Gombault, French neurologist, 1844–1904) the noxious agent affects primarily the myelin or Schwann cell, and the primary lesion is a complete or incomplete degeneration of the myelin sheath. The axon is relatively spared. Demyelination can result from compression, entrapment, immunologic disorders (e.g. Guillain-Barré syndrome), toxins (e.g., diphtheritic), inherited metabolic abnormalities (e.g., Refsum's disease). Conduction is slowed and there can be a conduction block. There is no muscle denervation. The lack of axon disruption allows a rapid and complete recovery when or if remyelination occurs.

Axonal degeneration (so-called dying-back neuropathy) results from a dysfunction of the whole neuron. Functional failure affects predominantly the longer and larger fibers, appearing first distally and then progresses proximad. Conduction disorders appear late in the course of the disease. Muscles, mostly distal ones, undergo denervation atrophy. There can be a slow (2 to 3 mm/day) reinnervation of distal structures with an often incomplete recovery. Among axonal degenerations some appear to result from a primary dysfunction of the perikaryon and others primarily from dysfunction of the axon, perhaps some disorder of the form of axonal transport. Primary diseases of the perikaryon are termed neuronopathies or ganglionopathies in the cases of cells of the spinal ganglia. Neuronopathies are exemplified by amyotrophic lateral sclerosis or organic mercury intoxication, ganglionopathies by the paraneoplastic pure sensory polyneuropathy. Primary diseases of the axons are termed ax-

Table 32-1. Pathologic Classification of Peripheral Neuropathies

Polyneuropathies
    Axonopathies
        Toxins: drugs, industrial
        Metabolic: diabetes mellitus, uremia, porphyria,
            endocrine diseases
        Vitamin deficiencies, alcohol
        Genetic: Charcot-Marie-Tooth disease
        Paraneoplastic: associated with myeloma or dys-
            proteinemia
    Myelinopathies
        Toxins: diphtheria
        Autoimmune: Guillain-Barré syndrome, chronic
            inflammatory neuropathy
        Genetic: Refsum's disease, Charcot-Marie-Tooth
            disease, metachromatic leukodystrophy
    Neuronopathies
        Motor: amyotrophic lateral sclerosis, hereditary
            forms, organic mercury intoxication
        Sensory (ganglionopathies): herpes zoster, para-
            neoplastic: pure sensory neuropathy
        Autonomic: Shy-Drager syndrome (acquired);
            Riley-Day syndrome (genetic)
Mononeuropathies and multiple mononeuronopathies
    Wallerian degeneration
        Trauma: compressions, entrapment, infarctions
        Diabetes mellitus, collagen diseases, vasculitides,
            leukemia, lymphomas, granulomas (leprosy),
            amyloid infiltration
    Myelinopathies
        Acute compressions, entrapment[a]
        Immune disorders (plexopathies)
        Genetic: tomaculous neuropathies

[a] Compression and entrapment can cause either demyelination or wallerian degeneration according to the degree of severity of the nervous insult.

onopathies and are the most common types of dying-back polyneuropathies (e.g., those due to alcohol or certain drugs). The pathological reactions of the peripheral neurons are at present the most convenient basis for a classification of diseases of the PNS (Table 32-1).

SYMPTOMS, SIGNS, AND POINTS OF EXAMINATION

Weakness of the lower motor neuron type (i.e., with flaccidity and wasting and reduced or absent reflexes) is the main motor complaint of neuropathies. The distribution of weakness depends on the type of neuropathy: mononeuropathy, plexopathy, radiculopathy, multiple neuropathy, polyneuropathy, or polyradiculoneuropathy (see above). The corresponding roots of the main deep reflexes are mentioned in Chapter 22.

Fasciculations and cramps are frequent in neuronopathies but uncommon in polyneuropathies. They can be a sequela of root disease (e.g., L5 compression by a herniated disc). There is a syndrome (Foley and Denny-Brown) of benign fasciculations and cramps, and it is a wise rule that fasciculations without atrophy or changes in reflexes are of no significance in young anxious patients. A disorder of the PNS is likely in Isaac's syndrome, in which myokymias are a prominent feature, and in the syndrome of painful legs and moving toes.

Sensory symptoms include dysesthesias, paresthesias, and pain. Dysesthesias and paresthesias are abnormal sensations felt either spontaneously or when the parts involved come into contact with some external object. They can be simple sensations or hypesthesias (e.g., as if the hand were in a silk glove), but more often there are "positive" symptoms (see Ch. 22), such as feelings of dead toes or fingers compared with dental anesthesia or as tingling, formication, and "pins and needles." Chafing the involved parts usually elicits or awakens the pins and needles with an "electric" sensation.

Spontaneous pain is frequent, and can be either dull or stabbing, or crushing. It may be permanent with exacerbations, often at night, or may come in brief, often repetitive bouts, as in the lightning pains of tabes dorsalis. Some pains are clearly position-dependent (e.g., L5 or S1 compression radiculopathy due to a herniated disk). Pain can have a burning quality, as in diabetic (burning feet) or alcoholic polyneuropathy or in herpes zoster or causalgia. Hyperesthesia means an increased sensitivity to stimulation. In hyperpathia the threshold to noxious stimuli is elevated (i.e., there is a degree of hypesthesia). However, if the noxious stimulus (e.g., a pinprick) is repeatedly applied, after a delay an exaggerated burning or stinging sensation is felt, which radiates from the stimulated point. Hyperpathia is a feature of various PNS lesions and is a cardinal feature of thalamic pain.

Sensory examination is considered in Chapter 23. Suffice it to mention here that light touch, pain, and temperature are tested from the insensitive area toward the sensitive area, except when hyperesthesia or hyperpathia is present, when the direction is reversed. All sensory modalities are usually affected, although sensory modality dissociations can occur (e.g., thermal and pain sensitivity can be affected while light touch, vibration, and joint position sense are spared in early leprous neuropathy, hereditary sensory polyneuropathy, and primary amyloid neuropathy). This dissociation reflects the predominance of lesions on small myelinated and unmyelinated fibers. The opposite dissociation (i.e., preservation of pain and temperature sensations with impairment of joint position and light touch senses) can be found in conditions involving loss of large myelinated fibers (e.g., Friedreich's ataxia or uremic polyneuropathy). In disorders involving severe proprioceptive deficit there can be a prominent ataxia, as in tabes dorsalis or diabetic pseudotabes.

In various neuropathies a postural or action tremor can be present and can, during action, mimic cerebellar incoordination. Its mechanisms are still obscure but may possibly involve selective deafferentation from muscle spindles or enhancement of physiologic tremor by minimal weakness.

Trophic changes affect feet, hands, and spine mostly in chronic polyneuropathies of early onset and long duration, such as claw feet and hands or kyphoscoliosis due to a chronic imbalance between paralyzed and less paralyzed muscular groups. Plantar ulcers and bone resorption are possible (e.g., in hereditary sensory polyneuropathy). Joints chronically pain-deafferented can be largely destroyed with little impairment of function in tabes dorsalis (Charcot arthropathy). In many chronic polyneuropathies the so-called trophic disorders are less severe, causing shiny, scaly, cold skin and irregular, brittle nails. Neuropathies with autonomic disorders (e.g., diabetes mellitus or amyloid neuropathies), feature postural arterial hypotension with dizziness and fainting on standing up (Ch. 34). When blood pressure is measured with the patient lying and standing, a drop of at least 30 mmHg is significant. Invariance of the R-R interval on the ECG on standing up or during the Valsalva maneuver also reflects a failure of cardiovascular reflexes. Pupillary abnormalities are frequent, with a light near-dissociation, but in contrast with the Argyll-Robertson pupil (see Chs. 27 and 34), there is usually mydriasis. Anhydrosis or excessive facial sweating during meals, bladder dysfunction, sexual impotence in the male, and bouts of nocturnal diarrhea followed by constipation are other signs of dysautonomia.

Points of Examination

As usual in neurology, the clinical examination is directed first to an anatomic (localizing) diagnosis and second to a causal diagnosis. To locate the pathologic process broadly means to identify a mononeuropathy, plexopathy, radiculopathy, multiple mononeuropathy, polyneuropathy, or polyradiculoneuropathy. When associated, cranial nerves and central nervous system disorders are of course valuable clues to the causal diagnosis. In PNS diseases electrophysiologic studies, whenever available and reliable, are indispensable for a sure anatomic diagnosis. By identifying the type of neuropathy, the field of search for a cause is greatly narrowed. However, when considered at large, the causes of PNS diseases embrace all the provinces of medicine (see the nonexhaustive Table 32-2. No branch of neurology other than PNS affections has such close and varied relationships to internal medicine. Therefore, the neurologist must be prepared to

perform a thorough clinical examination and to launch investigations in the various required directions (see also Chs. 7 to 16). As usual, taking the history is vital. The following are among many items, useful in practice: symptoms of unknown diabetes mellitus, concealed alcoholism, unusual hobbies (entrapment neuropathies), sojourns in areas endemic for leprosy, unmentioned use of drugs, especially new ones, family history of similar nervous disability, and when needed, examination of relatives.

Because nerves can be enlarged, palpation of the ulnar nerve above the elbow, the common peroneal nerve on the neck of the fibula, the great auricular nerve behind and below the ear, the supraclavicular nerves as they run over the clavicles, the superficial peroneal nerve on the dorsum of the foot, and the infrapatellar branch of the saphenous nerve can give causal clues to some neuropathies. Nerves can be thickened by various processes: granulomas and fibrosis in leprosy; concentric proliferation of Schwann cells ("onion bulbs") in hereditary hypertrophic neuropathy (Dejerine-Sottas syndrome); Refsum's disease; the hypertrophic form of Charcot-Marie-Tooth disease; chronic inflammatory polyradiculoneuropathy; amyloid deposits in amyloid neuropathy; neurofibromas, schwannomas, or sarcomas in von Recklinghausen's neurofibromatosis; and neuromas in traumatic lesions. In acromegaly the nerves can be thickened by connective tissue hyperplasia. In thin subjects, normal nerves are easily palpated, particularly on the neck and the instep of the foot, a reminder for caution in the diagnosis of enlarged nerves.

Electromyography can differentiate muscular atrophy due to lower motor neuron disease from that due to muscle disease and determine precisely which muscles are or are not denervated, thus contributing to the localizing diagnosis. Measurement of motor and sensory velocities allow distinction between axonal degenerations and demyelinating neuropathies (for details, see Ch. 12). Somatosensory evoked potentials also measure conduction velocities and help to localize lesions in proximal peripheral pathways (e.g., brachial and lumbosacral plexus neuropathies) (see Ch. 11).

In selected patients, muscle and nerve biopsy separates neurogenic from myogenic muscular atrophy and can give a clue to the cause (e.g., amyloidosis or vasculitis). Biopsy with teasing of nerve fibers has proven very valuable (see Ch. 8). CSF examination is mandatory for the diagnosis of polyradiculoneuropathy (see Ch. 9). Magnetic resonance imaging (MRI) of neuropathy can give detailed images of the peripheral nerves and could greatly improve diagnostic capacities in the forthcoming years. In polyneuropathies with no routinely detected cause, dysproteinemias, occult

Table 32-2. Causes of Peripheral Nervous System Lesions

Traumatic
    Direct injuries
    Compressions
    Entrapment
Infections
    Leprosy
    Herpes zoster
    Lyme disease
    AIDS
    HTLV-1
    Diphtheria
Ischemic
    Vasculitides
    Diabetes mellitus
    Direct injuries
    Compressions
    Peripheral atherosclerosis
Metabolic
    Vitamin deficiencies: B1/alcoholism, B6, B12 nicotinic
      acid, pantothenic acid
    Nutritional: malabsorption, postgastrectomy
    Uremia
    Porphyria
    Dysproteinemias: macroglobulinemias, myeloma, cryo-
      globulinemia
    Hypoglycemia
    Hypothyroidism
Toxic
    Drugs: amiodarone, cisplatin, chloroquine, dapsone,
      2′3′-dideoxynosine, disulfiram, hydralazine, isoniazid,
      metronidazole, nitrofurantoin, perhexilene, pheny-
      toin, stilbamidine, thalidomide, vinca alkaloids
    Heavy metals: arsenic, gold, lead, mercury, thallium
    Organic compounds: acrylamide, aldrin and dieldrin,
      carbon disulfide, hexacarbons, trichlorethylène, trior-
      thocresylphosphate

Immune
    Autoimmune polyradiculoneuropathy (Guillain-Barré
      syndrome)
    Chronic inflammatory demyelinating neuropathy
    Serum sickness neuropathy
    Infectious mononucleosis
    Sarcoidosis
Neoplastic, direct or remote effects
    Carcinoma, sarcoma
    Lymphoma
    Myeloma
    Primary tumors of PNS
Genetic
    Dominant
      Charcot-Marie-Tooth, hypertrophic and neuronal
        forms
      Amyloidosis
      Hereditary sensory neuropathy
      Tomaculous neuropathy
    Recessive
      Hereditary sensory neuropathy
      Hypertrophic neuropathy (Dejerine-Sottas)
      Refsum's disease
      Metachromatic leukodystrophy
      Globoid cell leukodystrophy (Krabbe)
      Abetalipoproteinemia (Bassen-Kornzweig)
      Analphalipoproteinemia (Tangier)

Abbreviations: HTLV-1, human T-cell leukemia virus 1; AIDS, acquired immunodeficiency syndrome; PNS, peripheral nervous system.

malignancy, and amyloidosis are the most likely etiologies.

THE ANATOMIC DIAGNOSIS OF ROOT, PLEXUS, AND NERVE LESIONS

Ideally, at the end of a clinical examination, the neurologist has collected a constellation of weak muscles, decreased or lost reflexes and sensory disturbances that betoken a root, a plexus, or a nerve lesion. Of course its analysis requires a knowledge of basic anatomy. The myotomes (i.e., the group of muscles innervated by roots, plexus, and nerves) are listed in Table 32-3 (see also Fig. 22-4). Testing individual muscles is depicted in Figures 32-1 to 32-26. Table 32-3 shows the roots corresponding to the deep reflexes usually elicited in practice (see also Ch. 22). The dermatomes (i.e., the skin areas innervated by sensory roots and their ganglia are shown in Figure 23-3.

Radiculopathies are first identified by their motor, reflex, and sensory distribution. Radicular pain is experienced not only in the dermatome (i.e., the area innervated by the sensory root) but also in the myotome (i.e., the group of muscles innervated by the anterior root). As they are often due to vertebral or intervertebral disk lesions, they are position-dependent and accompanied by low-back or cervical pain. Sneezing, coughing, or straining causes a brisk surge of CSF pressure in the arachnoid sleeve around the root and thus characteristically increases radicular pain. In herpes zoster, the skin eruption maps the involved dermatome.

Plexopathies

Brachial Plexus

The brachial plexus (BP) (see Fig. 22-3A) mixes motor and sensory fibers from C5 to T1 for the upper limb and the ipsilateral ventral (pectoral) and dorsal parts

Table 32-3. Nerve and Main Root Supply of Muscles

Nerve/Muscles	Spinal Roots	Nerve/Muscles	Spinal Roots
Upper Limb		Flexor digitorum	
Spinal accessory nerve		profundus III & IV	C7, **C8**
Trapezius	C3, C4	Hypothenar muscles	C8, **T1**
Brachial plexus		Adductor pollicis	C8, **T1**
Rhomboids	C4, C5	Flexor pollicis brevis[a]	C8, **T1**
Serratus anterior	C5, C6, C7	Palmar interossei	C8, **T1**
Pectoralis major		Dorsal interossei	C8, **T1**
Clavicular	**C5**, C6	Lumbricals III & IV	C8, **T1**
Sternal	C6,**C7**, C8	Lower limb	
Supraspinatus	**C5**, C6	Femoral nerve	
Infraspinatus	**C5**, C6	Iliopsoas	**L1, L2**, L3
Latissimus dorsi	C6, **C7**, C8	Rectus femoris	
Teres major	C5, 6, 7	Vastus lateralis Quadriceps	L2, **L3, L4**
Axillary nerve		Vastus intermedius femoris	
Deltoid	**C5**, C6	Vastus medialis	
Musculocutaneous nerve			
Biceps	C5, C6	Obturator nerve	
Brachialis	C5, C6		
Radial Nerve		Adductor longus	**L2, L3**, L4
Triceps Long head		Adductor magnus	
Lateral head	C6, **C7**, C8		
Medial head		Superior gluteal nerve	
Brachioradialis	C5, **C6**	Gluteus medius and	**L4, L5**, S1
Extensor carpi radialis	C5, **C6**	minimus	
longus		Tensor fasciae latae	
Posterior interosseous nerve		Inferior gluteal nerve	
Supinator	C6, C7	Gluteus maximus	**L5, S1**, S2
Extensor carpi ulnaris	**C7**, C8	Sciatic and tibial nerves	
Extensor digitorum	**C7**, C8	Semitendinosus	L5, **S1**, S2
Abductor pollicis longus	**C7**, C8	Biceps	L5, **S1**, S2
Extensor pollicis longus	**C7**, C8	Semimembranosus	L5, **S1**, S2
Extensor pollicis brevis	**C7**, C8	Gastrocnemius and	S1, S2
Extensor indicis	**C7**, C8	soleus	
Median nerve		Tibialis posterior	L4, L5
Pronator teres	C6, C7	Flexor digitorum longus	L5, **S1, S2**
Flexor carpi radialis,	C6, C7	Flexor hallucis longus	L5, **S1, S2**
Flexor digitorum			S1, S2
superficialis	C7, **C8**, T1	Abductor hallucis Small	
Abductor pollicis brevis	C8, **T1**	Abductor digiti minimi muscles	
Flexor pollicis brevis[a]	C8, **T1**	Interossei of foot	
Opponens pollicis	C8, **T1**		
Lumbricals I & II	C8, **T1**	Sciatic and common	
Anterior interosseous nerve		peroneal nerves	
Flexor digitorum		Tibialis anterior	**L4**, L5
profundus I & II	C7, **C8**	Extensor digitorum	**L5**, S1
Flexor pollicis longus	C7, **C8**	longus	
Pronator quadratus	C8–T1	Extensor hallucis longus	**L5**, S1
Ulnar nerve		Extensor digitorum	L5, S1
Flexor carpi ulnaris	C7, **C8**, T1	brevis	
		Peroneus longus	L5, S1
		Peroneus brevis	L5, S1

[a] The flexor pollicis brevis is often supplied wholly or partially by the ulnar nerve. (Modified from Medical Research Council, 1976, with permission.)

of the chest. Behind the clavicle the upper (C5 to C6), middle (C7), and lower (C8 to T1) trunks each split in anterior and posterior divisions. At the lateral border of the first rib, the anterior divisions form the lateral and medial cords while the posterior divisions form the posterior cord. The medial and lateral cords supply the volar, flexor muscles of arm, forearm, and hand (musculocutaneous, median, and ulnar nerves), while the posterior cord supplies the dorsal, extensor muscles of arm, forearm, and hand (axillary and radial nerves). The sympathetic fibers leave the cord mainly through the T1 ventral root.

A total lesion of the BP results in complete flaccid paralysis of arm and shoulder with anesthesia from midarm to hand, trophic changes, and a Claude Bernard-Horner oculosympathetic syndrome (see Ch. 27).

Damage to the upper trunk (C5 to C6) (Duchenne-Erb paralysis) is characterized by loss or weakness of arm abduction and forearm flexion. The brachioradialis muscle, which, as a flexor, is innervated by C6, is also paralyzed. Sensory loss is variable, often restricted to the lateral aspect of shoulder and arm. The biceps and brachioradialis reflexes are lost or decreased.

Isolated damage to the middle trunk (C7) is rare, although C7 radiculalgia due to cervical spondylosis is not. It is characterized by weakness of forearm extension with a lost or diminished triceps reflex.

Paralysis of the lower trunk (C8 to T1) results in paralysis and wasting of the muscles of the hand, the long extensors of the fingers being spared. The fingers are extended at the metacarpophalangeal joints and flexed at the interphalangeal joints, a characteristic position of the hand. There is sensory loss along the ulnar border of the hand and forearm, and there can be an oculosympathetic paralysis.

There are three cords to the BP, hence three types of cord paralysis (see Fig. 22-3A). Paralysis of the *lateral* cord involves fibers that make up the musculocutaneous nerve and the lateral part of the median nerve (i.e., C5, C6, and C7 fibers). There is paralysis of flexion of the forearm, wrist, and fingers and paralysis of pronation. Strikingly, the hand is normal. Abduction of the arm is also normal. The biceps and brachioradialis reflexes are lost or diminished. Sensory loss is restricted to a small area on the lateral aspect of the forearm. Paralysis of the *posterior* cord involves fibers that make up the axillary and radial nerves (i.e., C5, C6, C7, C8, and T1 fibers). There is paralysis or paresis of arm abduction and of extension of forearm, wrist, and fingers. The triceps reflex is lost or diminished. Sensory loss is restricted to the lateral aspect of shoulder and arm. Paralysis of the *medial* cord involves fibers that make up the ulnar nerve and the medial part of the median nerve (i.e., C8 and T1 fibers).

There is paralysis or paresis of the hand muscles, reflexes are normal, and sensory loss affects the medial aspect of arm and forearm.

The BP courses obliquely from the cervical spine to the shoulder girdle, gaining access to the axilla through a passage known as the *thoracic outlet.* Both cervical spine and shoulder girdle are mobile structures, so that in trauma to either or both, pathologic tractions with elongations or ruptures of nervous fibers can occur. From the cervical spine to the level of the clavicle, the plexus is covered only by skin, subcutaneous tissue, and fasciae, and hence is in an exposed position to stab or missile wounds. Fractures of the clavicle, first rib, or head of the humerus can cause plexus damage. The lower roots and trunk course first over the apex of the lung and then over the first rib, where they are behind the subclavian artery. The latter is behind the scalenus anterior (or anticus) muscle, in front of which courses the subclavian vein. Disorders of the artery and vein cause vascular syndromes that are to be distinguished from BP neuropathies. Diseases of the BP can be traumatic, compressive, tumoral, postradiotherapy, or due to some immune or allergic peculiar reaction of the plexical fibers. Not infrequently, the etiology remains undertermined. Trauma can occur during delivery with paralysis predominant on the lower plexus (Dejerine-Klumpke paralysis). Stabs, gunshot, bullets, and shrapnel cause lacerations, sections, or crush injuries. By far the most common cause of BP lesions in civilian practice is traffic accidents, especially motorcycle accidents, in which both driver and passenger can be involved as they hit the ground on a shoulder with the neck flexed laterally and away. In addition, at the very moment of being thrown off, the driver forcibly grips the handlebar, thus imparting a violent traction to the shoulder girdle. Upper plexus paralysis is the most frequent type of resulting paralysis. Total BP paralysis is common.

In *traction injuries* of the BP it is vital to know whether lesions result from root avulsions, which at present are irreversible, or from distal damage in the plexus. A spared serratus anterior means that the lesions are distal to the long thoracic nerve (see below). The presence of Tinel's sign also suggests a lesion distal to the spinal ganglia. Conversely, an oculosympathetic syndrome means a T1 root lesion. Electrophysiologic studies, somatosensory evoked potentials, and myelography help to sort out patients in whom surgical repair could be indicated. The prognosis is often poor. Compression injuries can cause BP deficits in two quite different conditions, entrapment and an inherited susceptibility of myelin to compression.

Cervical rib. Wasting of the hand may be associated with a cervical rib. In this case the C8 and T1 roots and the lower trunk are entrapped, stretched, and angulated under a sharp fibrous band extending from the tip of the C7 transverse process or a rudimentary C7 rib to the first rib. A similar band and syndrome in the absence of a bony abnormality is exceptional. Wasting of the hand with the above-mentioned fibro-osseous abnormalities is a rare condition, mainly seen in frail, middle-aged women. Wasting is generally obvious. Although it can predominate on the abductor pollicis brevis and opponens pollicis (see Figs. 32-13 and 32-14), and thus could at first glance suggest a carpal tunnel syndrome, wasting characteristically also involves the adductor pollicis, interosseous muscles, and hypothenar muscles (i.e., the territories of both median and ulnar nerves) (see Figs. 32-14 to 32-17). There can be some wasting on the ulnar side of the forearm. There is commonly sensory loss on the ulnar side of the forearm, sometimes extending to the ulnar border of the hand. Radiographs show a long, down-curving C7 transverse process or a rudimentary rib.

A fully developed cervical rib is exceptional and can well be on the side opposite to the wasted hand. Electrophysiologic studies suggest motor and sensory wallerian degeneration. Surgical excision of the fibrous band and bony abnormalities brings relief and usually stops the progression of wasting.

Wasting of the hand associated with a cervical rib is a clear-cut neurologic syndrome. It must be distinguished from a variety of neurovascular, thoracic outlet, and scalenus anticus syndromes, common to which are pain of non-neurologic location in the arm and vascular disorders. Compression and stenosis of the subclavian artery can be responsible for digital embolization (Raynaud phenomenon) or retrograde embolism into the vertebral artery. Compression of the subclavian vein can cause edema and a bluish hue of the hand. After sports or work that involve strenuous movements of the shoulder girdle, the vein can be thrombosed (effort-thrombotic syndrome). A vexing problem arises in patients who complain of acute or chronic pain in the arm, who have no wasting, and who have a cervical rib or large C7 transverse process and often have cervical spondylosis with degeneration of intervertebral disks. It should be remembered that 0.5 percent of the population have cervical ribs, and among those 90 percent are asymptomatic. This means that isolated pain in the arm and the presence of a cervical rib can be a concomitant, not a causally related, finding.

Heredofamilial Brachial Plexus Neuropathy. Heredofamilial BP neuropathy is an autosomal dominant disease in which peripheral nerve fibers have abnormal myelin sheaths. Morphologically the sheath is irregularly thickened, which gives the fiber a sausagelike appearance, hence the term *tomaculous* neuropathy (Latin: *tomaculum*, sausage). Pathologically the fiber is unduly sensitive to compression, possibly because the latter causes ischemia. Clinically, BP paralysis may result from trivial compressions or even occur when no significant compression can be found. Such patients are liable to suffer from similar paralyses of nerves in the limbs. The prognosis of each bout of paralysis is usually good.

Tumors. Tumors of the BP are generally benign schwannomas. Metastases from breast carcinoma, lymphosarcoma, or Hodgkin's disease can involve the BP. The most frequent source of metastases is carcinoma of the apex of the lung (Pancoast tumor), in which pain along the ulnar border of the forearm and hand can be an early symptom. The lower plexus is first infiltrated, with wasting of the hand and an oculosympathetic syndrome. After radiotherapy for breast carcinoma, when the dose may have exceeded 6,000 cGy, a progressive fibrosis can develop around the BP. The clinical onset (i.e., weakness and wasting of the hand) is delayed by about 1 year or sometimes by 5 to 10 years. The diagnosis is with tumor infiltration that is painful. Postradiotherapy BP neuropathy is a distressing condition that often progresses relentlessly for years, although it can unpredictably remain stationary for long periods of time and finally burn out. In the authors' experience, little if any benefit is to be expected from surgery.

Brachial Neuritis (Neuralgic Amyotrophy). Brachial neuritis is a not infrequent condition affecting males slightly more often than females at any age. It can follow a viral infection, cytomegalovirus, coxsackie virus, and parvovirus having been incriminated (see Ch. 48), or an immunization, or an injection of heroin or appear without any previous discernible cause. Formerly, it could follow an injection of serum as part of a serum sickness. The onset may be rapid enough to raise a suspicion of myelitis. Excruciating pain in the neck and around the shoulder is accompanied or followed after 1 to 3 days by muscular weakness and reflex and sensory impairment. The deltoid, serratus anterior, biceps, or triceps can be paralyzed or severely paretic. Rarely, all the muscles of the arm are paretic. Biceps and triceps reflexes can be reduced or abolished. Sensory loss is restricted to the outer aspect of the shoulder (over the deltoid) or the radial aspect of the forearm. Both sides can be affected. Pain abates in a few days to 2 to 3 weeks. The prognosis for motor function is good: improvement begins after 1 to 2 months, but full recovery can be achieved only after 2 to 3 years. Recurrences are rare.

Branches of the Branchial Plexus

Long Thoracic Nerve. The slender long thoracic nerve conveys motor fibers from C5, C6, and C7 to the serratus anterior muscle, which maintains the scapula on the thorax. Paralysis results in winging of the scapula (Fig. 32-1). There is some inability to raise the hand above the head. Causes include the carrying of heavy weights on the shoulder and use of tight straps, as when a patient is strapped on an operating table. Neuralgic amyotrophy, serum sickness, and injection of vaccines have been mentioned above. In some cases no cause is found, which is commonly the case in young girls.

Axillary Nerve. The axillary nerve leaves the posterior cord of the brachial plexus carrying motor and sensory fibers from C5 with a small supply from C6. It innervates the deltoid and teres minor muscles. When testing the deltoid (Fig. 32-2) care must be taken that the arm is in frank abduction since the first 15 degrees of abduction depend on the supraspinatus muscle (C5, C6, suprascapular nerve). Wasting of the deltoid is often striking. Sensory loss is restricted to a small area over the deltoid. Causes of axillary nerve paralysis include dislocation of the shoulder joint and fractures of the head of the humerus. The deltoid can, of course, be paralyzed in BP paralyses (see discussion of neuralgic amyotrophy, above).

Musculocutaneous Nerve. The musculocutaneous nerve conveys motor and sensory fibers from C5 to C6 and arises from the lateral cord of the BP. It innervates the biceps, brachialis, and coracobrachialis muscles (Table 32-3 and Fig. 32-3). Paralysis results in weakness or inability to flex the supinated forearm. The biceps reflex is abolished or diminished. Sensory loss involves the area of the lateral cutaneous nerve (i.e., the radial and volar aspects of the forearm). Fractures of the humerus are the main cause of isolated paralysis of the musculocutaneous nerve, but sometimes, compression, stabs, or missile wounds may be responsible. The authors know of one case precipitated by the sudden shifting of the weight of a heavy window air conditioner to the arm of one of two men carrying the unit.

Radial Nerve. The radial nerve terminates the posterior cord of the BP conveying fibers from C7 and C6 and additionally from C5 and C8. It is the nerve

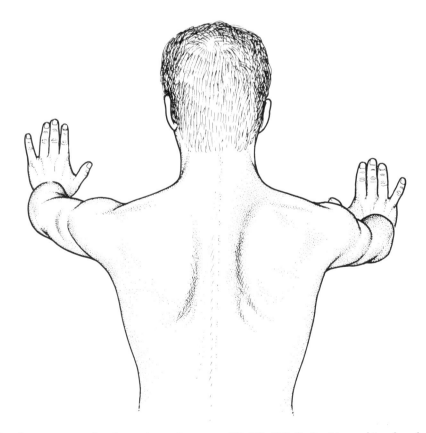

Figure 32-1. Serratus anterior (long thoracic nerve: C5, C6, C7). Patient is pushing hard against a wall. Right serratus anterior paralyzed; winging of the scapula.

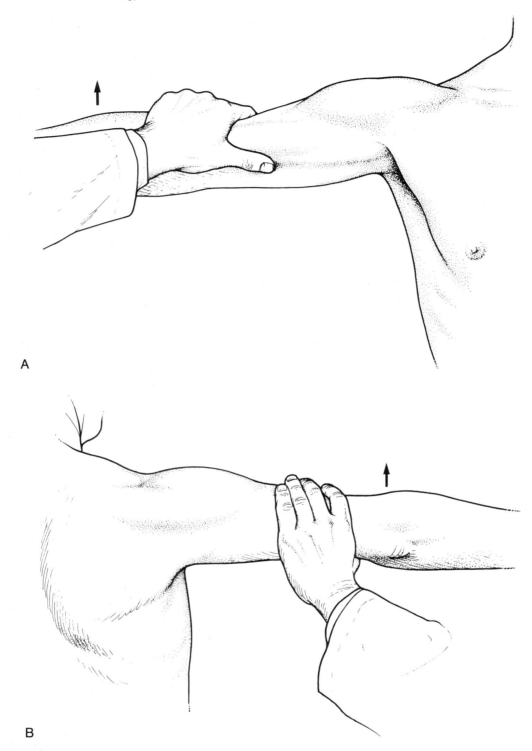

A

B

Figure 32-2. **(A)** Deltoid (axillary nerve: **C5,** C6). Patient is abducting upper arm against resistance. **(B)** Retracting abducted upper arm against resistance.

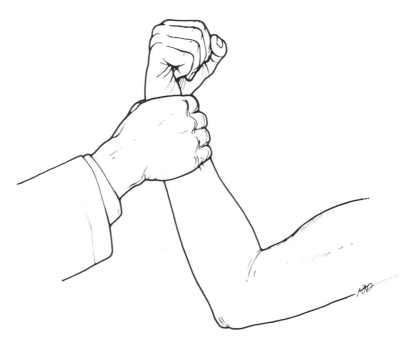

Figure 32-3. Biceps (musculocutaneous nerve: **C5,** C6). Flexion of the elbow and forearm, supinated against resistance.

of extension of the forearm (Fig. 32-4), wrist (Fig. 32-5), proximal phalanges (Fig. 32-6), and supination, extension, and abduction of the thumb (Figs. 32-7 to 32-9 and Table 32-3).

Lesions high in the arm cause paralysis of the triceps

with diminished or abolished triceps and brachioradialis reflexes, wrist drop, and fingers drop (flail hand). Fingers drop is due to the paralysis of the long extensors of the fingers (i.e., those that extend the proximal phalanges). Consequently when the examiner pas-

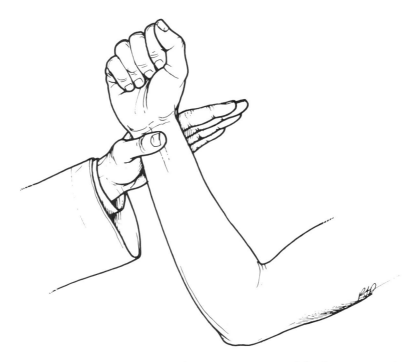

Figure 32-4. Triceps (radial nerve: C6, **C7,** C8). Extension of the forearm against resistance.

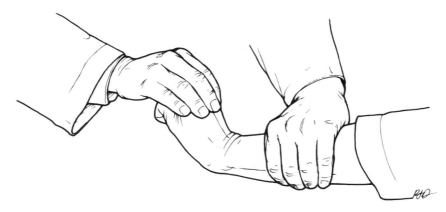

Figure 32-5. Forearm extensor muscles. Posterior interosseous nerve of the radial nerve (C7). Extension of the wrist against resistance.

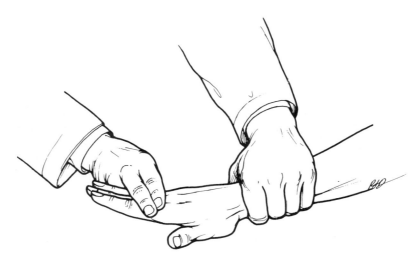

Figure 32-6. Extensor of the fingers. Posterior interosseous nerve of the radial nerve (**C7,** C8). Patient's wrist is firmly maintained while fingers are extended against resistance.

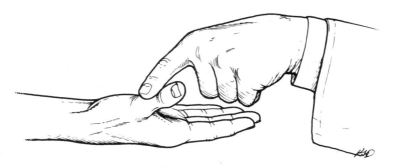

Figure 32-7. Abductor pollicis longus (posterior interosseous nerve: (**C7,** C8). Abduction of the thumb at the carpometacarpal joint in a plane at a right angle to the palm against resistance.

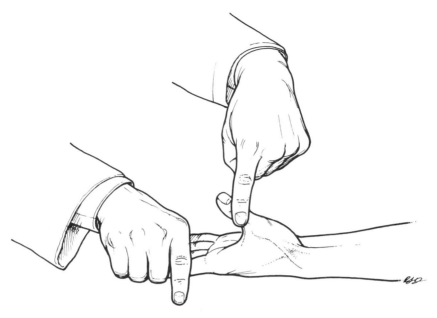

Figure 32-8. Extensor pollicis longus (posterior interosseous nerve of the radial nerve: **C7,** C8). Extension of the thumb at the interphalangeal joint against resistance.

sively extends the proximal phalanges (by supporting their volar aspect), the middle and distal phalanges extend normally under the normal action of the interosseous and lumbrical muscles (ulnar and median nerves). The triceps and brachioradialis reflexes are abolished or diminished. Sensory loss is usually limited to a small area on the dorsal base of the thumb and the anatomic snuff box.

High isolated lesions of the radial nerve, formerly mainly due to pressures (e.g., on crutches) are now rare. Lesions in the spiral groove are due to fractures of the humerus or to pressure during heavy sleep, such as might occur under anesthesia, after alcoholic intoxication (Saturday night paralysis), and after following sexual activity when one mate's head rests on the other's arm (known at one time as honeymoon

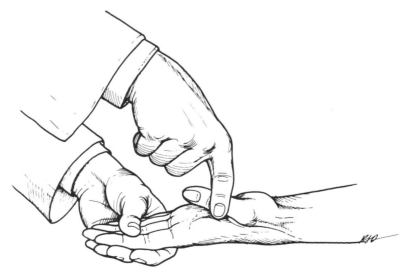

Figure 32-9. Extensor pollicis brevis (posterior interosseous nerve of the radial nerve: **C7,** C8). Extension of thumb at the metacarpophalangeal joint against resistance. The tendon of the muscle juts out as the lateral ridge of the snuffbox.

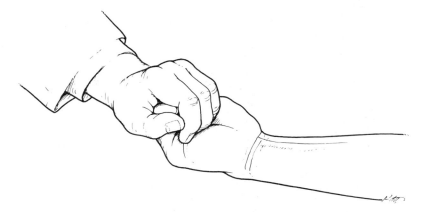

Figure 32-10. Flexor carpi radialis (median nerve: C6, **C7**). Flexion and abduction of the hand at the wrist against resistance.

paralysis). The triceps is not paralyzed and the triceps reflex is normal. Lesions below the elbow spare the brachioradialis and the brachioradialis reflex. The purely motor branch of the radial nerve (posterior interosseous nerve) may be paralyzed by entrapment as it passes through the supinator. Sensory loss is, of course, absent.

Paralysis of the radial nerve must be differentiated from C7 paralysis. In the former the brachioradialis is weak, and the brachioradialis reflex is abolished owing to involvement of C6. In the latter they are spared, and paresthesiae and sensory loss involve the middle finger. Small infarcts or small injuries of the precentral gyrus can cause wrist and fingers drop that could at first glance suggest radial nerve paralysis. In such cases, however, the interosseous and lumbrical muscles are weak, there is usually some weakness of the deltoid, and the reflexes of the affected muscles are brisk. The radial nerves has a particular vulnerability to lead intoxication.

Median Nerve. The median nerve conveys fibers from C6, C7, C8, and T1 and is formed by the union of the medial and lateral cords of the BP. It innervates

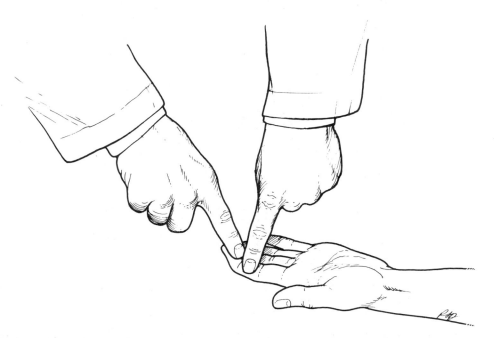

Figure 32-11. Flexor digitorum profundus I and II (anterior interosseous nerve of the median nerve, C7, **C8**). Flexion of the distal phalanx of the index finger against resistance with the middle phalanx fixed.

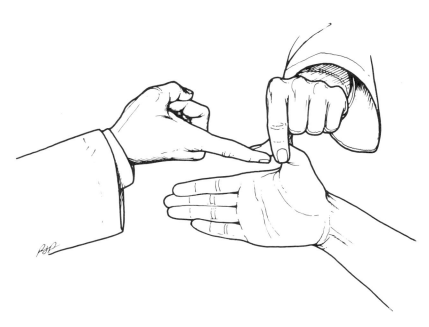

Figure 32-12. Flexor pollicis longus (anterior interosseous nerve of the median nerve: C7, **C8**). Flexion of the distal phalanx of the thumb against resistance. The proximal phalanx is fixed.

the pronators, the outer (radial) flexors of the wrist (Fig. 32-10), the flexors of the fingers (Fig. 32-11), particularly those of thumb (Fig. 32-12) and index finger, and the opponens (Fig. 32-13) and abductor brevis (Fig. 32-14) of the thumb (Table 32-3). Paralysis results in inability or weakness of these movements with wasting. The sensory area is distal to the wrist (see Fig. 32-27).

The median can be injured by stab or missile wounds. Partial injuries can result in causalgia (Ch. 23). Occasionally the nerve can be injured by dislocation of the shoulder. Around the elbow it can be damaged by fractures, catheterization of the brachial artery, or venipuncture in the antecubital fossa, or it can

be entrapped either by a fibrous band that passes from a spur of the humerus a few centimeters above the elbow to the epicondyle or as it passes through the two heads of the pronator teres (pronator syndrome). The purely motor anterior osseous nerve, which branches below the elbow, can also be entrapped by the pronator teres. As it innervates the flexors of the distal phalanges (Table 32-3), the patient characteristically cannot make an "O" between the tips of thumb and index.

Carpal Tunnel Syndrome. Carpal tunnel syndrome is the most common of all entrapment syndromes and a quite frequent issue in practice. Patients,

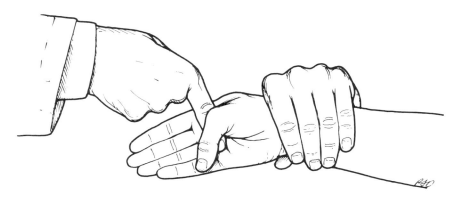

Figure 32-13. Opponens pollicis (median nerve: C8, **T1**). Pressing the base of the little finger with the thumb against resistance.

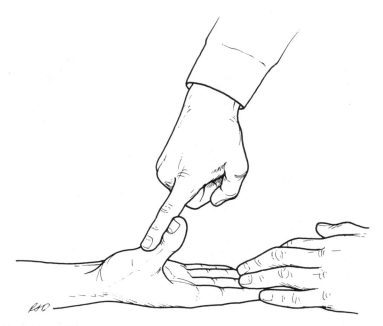

Figure 32-14. Abductor pollicis brevis (median nerve: C8, **T1**). Abduction of the thumb at a right angle to the palm against resistance.

mostly women, whose tunnel is narrower, complain of pins and needles in the fingers, especially at night. Shaking the hand or letting it dangle out of the bed brings relief. Besides numbness there can be trying pain, not only in hand and wrist but also in forearm and high in the arm, which should not be misdiagnosed as due to a root lesion. Also, patients commonly first assert that they feel tingling in all fingers, only to recognize on close scrutiny that the little finger is spared. In incipient cases, motor examination can be normal. Usually, however, there is weakness of op-

position and abduction of the thumb and a characteristic wasting of the lateral thenar pad, predominantly on the abductor pollicis brevis (Fig. 32-19). Sensory testing can show hypesthesia in the median nerve area. The index finger is the one with the most clear-cut involvement. There may be only slight deficit of two-point discrimination of the pulp of the index finger. Tingling can sometimes be provoked by forced flexion or extension of the wrist, and Tinel's sign can be present on tapping the carpal ligament. Electrophysiologic tests are needed even in clinically obvious cases to con-

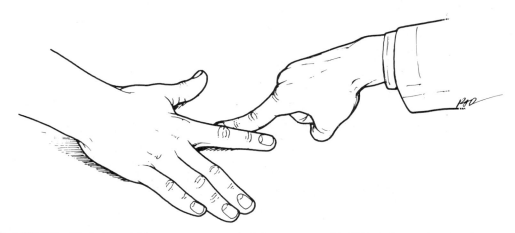

Figure 32-15. First dorsal interosseous muscle (ulnar nerve: C8, **T1**). Palm and index fingers flat on table. Abduction of the index finger against resistance.

firm the lesion at the wrist and to evaluate treatments. Bilateral cases are not exceptional nor are electrical abnormalities on the clinically normal side. Causes include past fractures of the wrist, rheumatoid arthritis, myxedema, acromegaly, and amyloid deposits as in multiple myeloma. Carpal tunnel syndrome can occur during pregnancy.

A local vulnerability of the median nerve can be due to a diffuse neuropathy (e.g., diabetic). Occupations that involve repeated flexion-extension of the wrist can play a causal role (e.g., painting). Rest brings relief, and together with splinting of the wrist may be sufficient in such conditions as pregnancy or myxedema, in which delivery or treatment should suppress the main cause of entrapment. Local steroid injections often have a temporary effect. In severe cases surgical decompression is required after the site of compression has been located as precisely as possible by electrical studies. A large decompression is needed.

Ulnar Nerve. Practically, the ulnar nerve carries fibers from C8 and T1 (Table 32-3) and arises from the medial cord of the BP. It innervates mainly muscles in the hand: all hypothenar muscles, all interossei (adduction-abduction of fingers) (Fig. 32-15), the two medial lumbricales, the flexor digiti minimi (Fig. 32-16), the adductor pollicis (Fig. 32-17), and part of the flexor pollicis brevis.

A complete paralysis results in a characteristic claw hand due to hyperextension at the metacarpophalangeal joints associated with flexion at the interphalangeal joints. Clawing is mainly due to the paralysis of the interossei, but it predominates on the ring and little fingers because the lumbricales of the index and middle finger, being innervated by the median nerve, counteract the flexion of the phalanges. Adduction-abduction of the fingers is abolished or very weak. Wasting is usually rapid and obvious, particularly in the web space between thumb and index finger (Fig. 32-18). Adduction of the thumb is paralyzed, as is well demonstrated by Froment's maneuver (Fig. 32-19). Sensory loss involves all or part of the ulnar area in the hand. The nerve can be palpated behind the medial epicondyle.

Stab or missile injuries can damage the ulnar, and partial injury can result in causalgia (Ch. 23). The usual lesions are around the elbow. Fractures, dislocations, or osteoarthritis of the joint can injure the nerve. Many years after incurring such elbow lesions or after a distal fracture of the humerus, an ulnar palsy can develop as a result of chronic strain of the nerve against a malpositioned medial epicondyle. Recurrent dislocation of the nerve from the posterior aspect of the epicondyle can cause dysfunction. Pressure palsy can also occur during heavy sleep or anesthesia. At the elbow, the ulnar passes into the cubital tunnel, (i.e., the aponeurosis of the flexor carpi, arching from the olecranon to the medial epicondyle). This can be

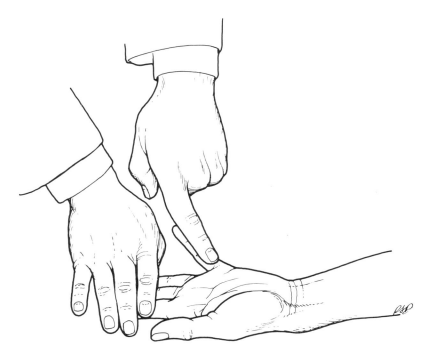

Figure 32-16. Flexor digiti minimi (ulnar nerve: C8, **T1**). Flexion of the extended little finger at the metacarpophalangeal joint against resistance.

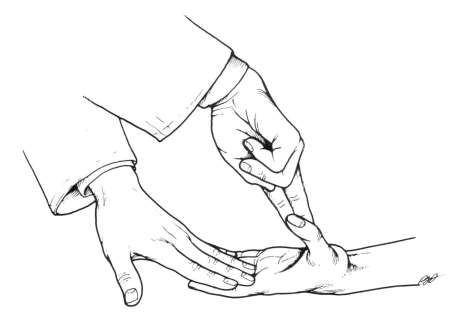

Figure 32-17. Adductor pollicis (ulnar nerve: C8, **T1**). Adduction of the thumb at right angle to the palm against resistance.

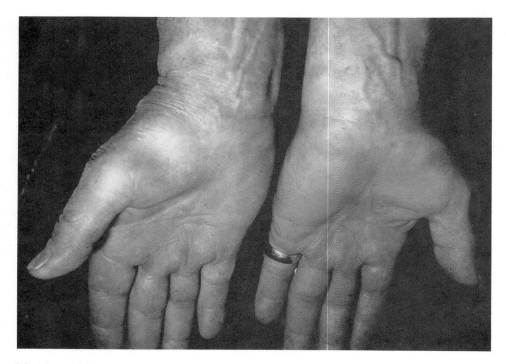

Figure 32-18. Left ulnar paralysis. The flexor pollicis longus (median nerve) substitutes for the paralyzed adductor pollicis.

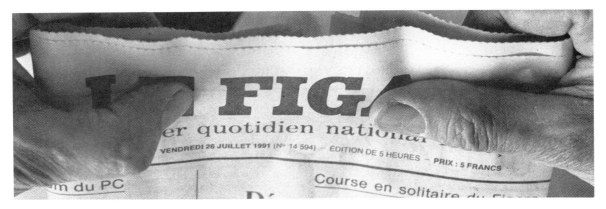

Figure 32-19. Right carpal tunnel syndrome. Lateral wasting of the thenar pad.

a site of entrapment. At the wrist, in Guyon's canal between the pisiform and the hook of hamate, the purely motor branch to the muscles of the hand can be compressed (e.g., during long cycling or long sessions of tree pruning). Compression here can also be due to rheumatoid arthritis, rarely to a ganglion.

Lumbosacral Plexus

The lumbosacral plexus (LSP) mixes motor and sensory fibers from T12 to S4 for the lower limb, perineum, and genitalia (see Fig. 22-3C). Testing of the muscles usually included in the neurologic examinations is depicted in Figures 32-20 to 32-26. The sen-

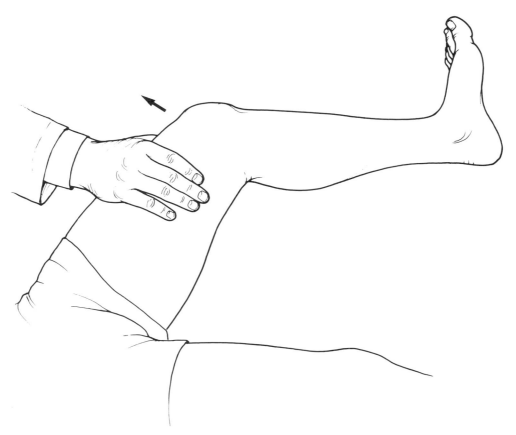

Figure 32-20. Iliopsoas (femoral nerve: **L1, L2,** L3). Flexion of the thigh against resistance, leg flexed at the knee.

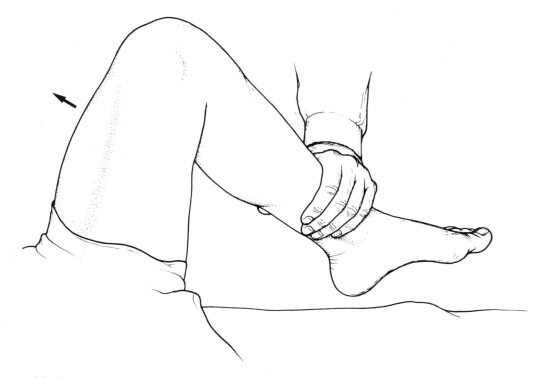

Figure 32-21. Quadriceps femoris (femoral nerve: L2, L3, L4). Extension of the leg against resistance with the limb flexed at the hip and knee.

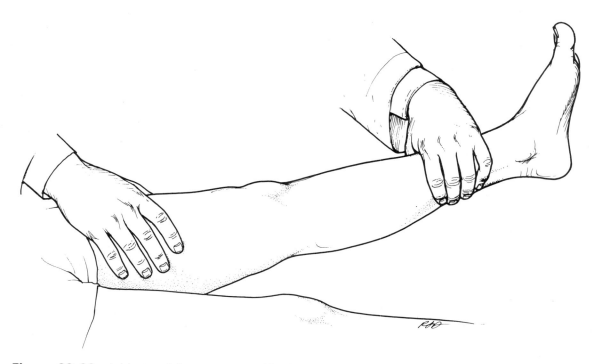

Figure 32-22. Adductors (obturator nerve: L2, L3, L4). Leg extended at the knee. Adduction of the limb against resistance.

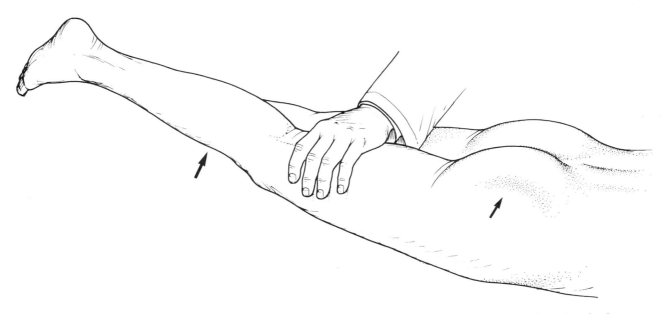

Figure 32-23. Gluteus maximus (inferios gluteal nerve: **L5, S1,** S2). Patient prone, elevating the leg against resistance.

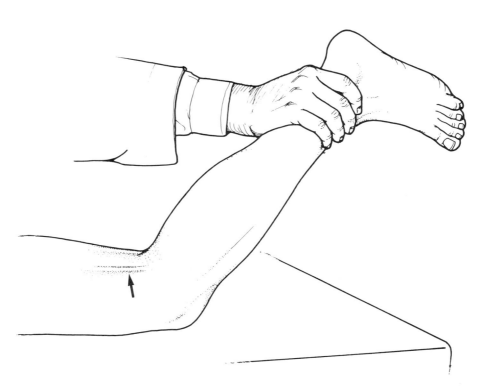

Figure 32-24. Hamstring muscles: semitendinosus, semimembranosus, and biceps (sciatic nerve: L5, **S1,** S2). Patient supine. Flexion of the leg at the knee against resistance. This maneuver provokes cramps in many normal people.

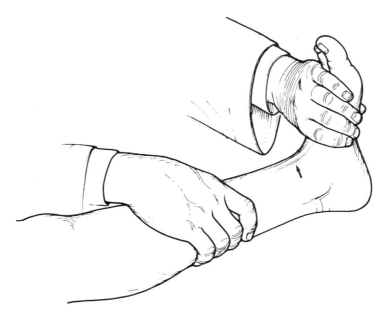

Figure 32-25. Tibialis anterior (deep peroneal nerve from the common peroneal nerve from the deep sciatic nerve: **L4,** L5). Dorsiflexion of the foot against resistance.

sory dermatomes and areas of individual nerves are shown in Chapter 23. LSP lesions result in ipsilateral weakness and wasting due to sensory and reflex losses that do not match root or nerve distribution. Pain is not increased by coughing or straining. Autonomic

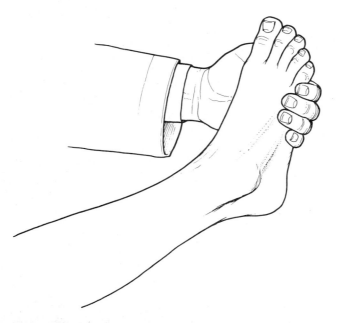

Figure 32-26. Peroneus longus and brevis (superficial peroneal nerve from the common peroneal nerve from the sciatic nerve: L5, S1). Eversion of the foot against resistance.

disturbances are an important clue, as they are absent in root lesions and present in plexus and nerve lesions.

Paralysis of the entire plexus causes paralysis and wasting of all muscles of the lower limbs and perineum, areflexia of knee and ankle jerks, anesthesia, including in the perineal region, autonomic disturbances, and usually, edema of the leg. In upper plexus lesions there is weakness of flexion and adduction of the thigh and extension of the leg, with sensory loss over the anterior thigh and leg. Lower plexus lesions result in weakness of the posterior thigh, leg, and foot muscles. Sensory loss extends to lower dermatomes, L5–S1 and sometimes the sacral dermatomes (saddle anesthesia) as well. Such cases must be differentiated from a syndrome of the cauda equina. Sphincter and genital disorders are the presenting symptoms. Ankle jerks are absent, and sensory loss is confined or predominates in the perineal area. CSF studies, myelography, computed tomography (CT) and MRI usually demonstrate the lesion.

When compared with the BP, the pathology of the LSP offers similarities and differences. The LSP exits from the strong lumbar spine and sacrum and courses behind the abdominal and pelvic viscera, with the outer thick shield of the iliac bone with iliac and buttock muscles. Thus, in contrast to the BP, the LSP is rather well protected against trauma but close to many viscera. Severe traffic accidents severe wounds in wartime or otherwise (e.g., shotgun and bullet wounds) can, however, cause avulsions, lacerations, and transections of roots and trunks. Injuries have occurred

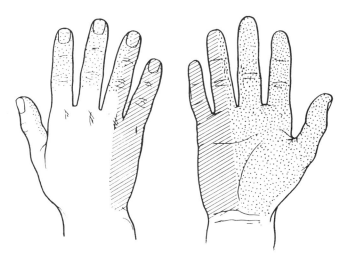

Figure 32-27. Sensory territories of the hand. The dotted area represents the region innervated by the median nerve; the stippled area represents the region innervated by the ulnar nerve; and the blank area, including the extreme lateral edge of the base of the thumb on the palmar view, represents the region innervated by the radial nerve.

during abdominal and pelvic surgery, at birth, and during parturition. Infiltration by adjacent tumors (kidney, colon, ovaries, uterus, prostate) or metastatic deposits compose a large part of LSP lesions. Postradiotherapy fibrosis can develop around the LSP. Compression of LSP can result from an abdominal aortic aneurysm, and the neurologic symptoms can be the early warning. A hematoma in the psoas muscle can occur in blood dyscrasies and particularly in patients treated with anticoagulants. Because of the close anatomic relationships between the LSP and psoas, there can sometimes be a transient LSP paralysis. The patient presents with a suggestive flexion and internal rotation of the thigh. An immune disorder analogous to neuralgic amyotrophy (see the section, Brachial Plexus) can involve the LSP. Vasculitides (e.g., polyarteritis nodosa) can cause various mononeuropathies or multiple neuropathies. Diabetic amyotrophy appears as a sudden painful paralysis of the quadriceps. The sensory loss involves the anterior aspect of the thigh and the medial aspect of the leg. It is difficult to be sure whether this is a plexopathy or a femoral nerve mononeuropathy (see below). Electrical investigations can help. The condition can be bilateral.

Lower Roots of the LSP. The L5 and S1 roots must be singled out, as they assume a considerable importance in practice because they are involved in sciatica, the traditional term applied to a common painful neuropathy of the lower limb. The L5 and S1 roots are in close anatomic relationship with the lateral part of the L4-L5 and L5-S1 intervertebral disks, respectively.

In a high proportion of middle-aged and aged people, these disks present degenerative lesions so that lifting a weight (e.g., a trunk or a piece of furniture) in a bent forward position, as well as a fall or lurch can rupture or rend the annulus fibrosus, particularly in its lateral part, which is not reinforced by the posterior longitudinal ligament.

In young people and adults, similar lesions can occur when strong pressures are imparted to the disk, as in accidents or some sports of feats of strength. Through the rent annulus the disk protrudes and the nucleus pulposus and other disk fragments can be expelled. Sometimes a detached piece of disc lies free in the spinal canal. Thus, the disc fragments impinge on either L5 or S1, or very rarely on both, causing the painful episode.

The pain of sciatica generally subsides in a few days or a few weeks, so that it is common to see patients who have had many episodes and who seek advice because of a recent long-lasting or a more severe attack. In such chronic cases the trigger effort can be trivial (e.g., sneezing or picking up a towel on the floor), or no particular circumstance can be found.

In the first episode(s) a sudden, severe, incapacitating low back pain or lumbago is usual. After a few hours or days pain appears in one inferior limb, for the condition is generally unilateral. Both L5 and S1 pains are felt in the buttock and descend along the posterior aspect of the thigh. L5 pain then proceeds along the outer aspect of the leg, while S1 pain proceeds on the posterior aspect. Usually pain is not felt beyond the malleoli. Distal paresthesiae are quite common however. In L5 disease they are located on the inner instep and first three toes, in S1 disease on the sole and fourth and fifth toes. In practice patients recognize that either the big or the little toe is numb and tingling. There is hypesthesia to light touch and pinprick in the same areas. In S1 disease the ankle jerk is depressed or lost. Years after, on a neurologic examination for another cause, a depressed ankle jerk frequently reminds the patient of a half-forgotten bout of sciatica.

L5 or S1 pain is typically increased by coughing, sneezing, straining (see the section Radiculopathies, above). Straight-leg raising (Lasègue maneuver) elongates the nerve and provokes pain. The angle at which pain stops leg raising should be noted, as it can help in evaluating progress. The same maneuver with the contralateral leg can provoke pain on the painful side.

Motor weakness is rare. L5 weakness predominates on the extensors of the big toe, and there can be difficulty in marching on the heel because of weakness of the foot eversors on the affected side. With S1 lesions tiptoeing can be difficult owing to ipsilateral weakness of the plantar flexors. Even with undelayed surgery, motor weakness frequently does not improve or after some improvement, the patient is left with fasciculations and frequent cramps in the paretic muscles.

Concomitant bilateral sciatica is rare. There is, however, a syndrome due to large median disk protrusions in which there is pain in both legs and disturbances of bladder and bowel control. Surgical decompression is performed only in an emergency. A safe clinical rule is to ask every patient with a sciatica (even unilateral) about possible sphincter troubles. Investigations of sciatica include radiographs of the spine and pelvis. When possible, myelography is replaced by CT or preferably MRI.

Prolapse of the L3-L4 disk with compression of L4 is much rarer. Pain radiates over the anterior aspect of the thigh and medial aspect of the leg. There is sensory loss over the same area. Weakness, when present, involves the quadriceps, with an impression of buckling on walking, and the flexors of the hip. The tibialis anterior muscle, which depends mostly on L4, is clinically weak or shows disturbances on electrophysiologic testing. The knee jerk is depressed or absent.

Branches of the LSP

Lateral Cutaneous Nerve of the Thigh. The lateral cutaneous nerve, a sensory nerve, conveys L2 and L3 fibers from the upper lateral aspect of the thigh. It can be entrapped as it passes through the inguinal ligament close to the anterior superior iliac spine. This causes meralgia paresthetica (Greek: *meros,* thigh), a sensation of numbness with often a disagreeable burning, icy quality over an area the size of the patient's hand on the lateral upper third of the thigh. The main causal conditions are obesity, pregnancy, diabetes mellitus, tight belts or pants, and surgical scars. Reassurance is often sufficient, and losing weight when necessary can bring relief. Corticoid injections can help. In a few cases surgery has been necessary. Neuromas are possible.

Obturator Nerve. The obturator nerve conveys motor and sensory fibers from L2, L3, and L4 and innervates mainly the adductors of the thigh (which are also flexors of the hip). Paresthesiae and sensory loss involve the inner side of the thigh. Damage to the nerve can be due to fractures, pelvic tumors and surgery, obturator hernia, diabetes mellitus, or polyarteritis nodosa.

Femoral Nerve. The femoral nerve conveys motor and sensory fibers from L2, L3, and L4. It innervates the psoas and iliacus, enters the thigh lateral to the femoral artery, and then innervates the quadriceps, pectineus, and sartorius. Depending on the level of the lesion, there is paralysis of extension of the leg with or without paralysis of flexion of the thigh. The knee jerk is abolished. The sensory area includes the anteromedial aspect of the thigh and the medial aspect of the leg. The main cause of femoral nerve lesion is diabetes mellitus. Polyarteritis nodosa or hematoma in the psoas can also be a cause (see above).

Sciatic Nerve. The sciatic nerve, a large nerve, conveys L4, L5, S1, and S2 motor and sensory fibers. It innervates the hamstring muscles and all the muscles below the knee. Complete paralysis results in inability to flex the leg and a flail foot. The ankle jerk is abolished. Sensory loss extends on the lateral aspect of the leg and the dorsum and sole of the foot. Nerve conduction studies exclude roots lesions. The nerve enters the thigh through the greater sciatic foramen and can be involved in fractures or tumors of the iliac bone and sacrum or can be compressed during delivery. It runs close to the posterior aspect of the hip and can be damaged by trauma or surgery of this joint. It can also be damaged by an injection placed too medially in the buttock. Comatose patients, particularly thin, emaciated ones, lying on a hard floor can develop a unilateral or bilateral paralysis. Partial injuries of the nerve can occasion causalgia (Ch. 23). Diabetes mellitus or polyarteritis nodosa can cause a sciatic mononeuropathy. At the upper end of the popliteal fossa the nerve divides into the tibial (medial popliteal) and common peroneal (lateral peroneal) nerves (see Table 22-3 and Table 32-3). Indeed, from the LSP to the popliteal fossa, the two branches of the sciatic nerve (i.e., the tibial, carrying fibers from the ventral divisions of the plexus and the common peroneal, carrying dorsal divisions) are juxtaposed, not mixed. Therefore stab or missile injuries in the buttock or thigh can result in isolated paralysis of one of the two terminal branches.

Common Peroneal Nerve. Motor fibers innervate the tibialis anterior, the peronei, and the extensors (dorsiflexors) of the toes. Paralysis results in a painless foot drop with steppage gait (see also Ch. 22). The ankle jerk is normal. The sensory area extends over the dorsum of the foot and lateral aspect of the leg, but as the lesion is often distal to the departure of the main cutaneous branches, sensory loss is often limited to the web space between the first and second toes. As it leaves the popliteal fossa, the nerve makes a turn around the head and neck of the fibula. It can be damaged in fractures and trauma. However, compression is by far the commonest cause, as the nerve lies on the bone, covered only by skin and subcutaneous tissue. Paralysis of the common peroneal nerve is also the most frequent of compression paralyses: prolonged cross-legged sitting, prolonged squatting, work that involves being on one's knees as slaters, and wearing of high boots are among the usual causal circumstances, especially in thin patients. Electrophysiologic studies show a conduction block at the level of the head of the fibula. Diabetes mellitus and polyarteritis nodosa can also cause a mononeuropathic paralysis.

Posterior Tibial Nerve (Tarsal Tunnel Syndrome). To enter the foot, the posterior tibial nerve passes behind and below the external malleolus in a passage limited outward by a ligament. There is much in common between carpal and tarsal tunnel syndromes. Both, indeed, can occur in one patient. Complaints are of disagreeable, burning numbness or tingling on the sole and toes. This is worse at night, and relief can come from letting the leg dangle out of the bed. There can be weakness of the abductor hallicis, sensory loss on the sole and plantar aspect of the toes, and a Tinel's sign on tapping the nerve below the ankle. Electrical studies can help. Venous engorgement can play a role in patients with varicose veins and edema. Diabetes mellitus can be an underlying condition. Surgical decompression is sometimes necessary.

ANNOTATED BIBLIOGRAPHY

Asbury AK, Johnson PC. Pathology of Peripheral Nerves. In Major Problems in Pathology. Vol. 9. WB Saunders, Philadelphia, 1978.

A clear introduction to clinical issues.

Bradley WC. Diseases of the spinal roots. In Dyck PJ, Thomas PK, Lambert EH, Bunge R (eds). Peripheral Neuropathy. 2nd Ed. Vol. 2. WB Saunders, Philadelphia, 1984.

A good, concise account.

Dawson DM. Entrapment neuropathies of the upper extremities. N Engl J Med 1993;329:2013–8.

Modern overview.

Dawson DM, Karup C. Perioperative nerve lesions. Arch Neurol 1989;46:1355–60.

A useful memorandum.

Filler AG, Howe FA, Hayes CE, et al. Magnetic resonance neuropathy. Lancet 1993;341:659–61.

Promising new technique.

Gilliatt RW. Thoracic outlet syndromes. In Dyck PJ, Thomas PK, Lambert EH, Bunge R (eds). Peripheral Neuropathy. 2nd Ed. WB Saunders, Philadelphia, 1984.

Written from top experience.

Gilliatt RW, Harrison MJG. Nerve compression and entrapment. In Dyck PJ, Thomas PK, Lambert EH, Bunge R (eds). Peripheral Neuropathy. 2nd Ed. WB Saunders, Philadelphia, 1984.

Written from top experience.

Hoffman M, Sacco RL, Mohr JP, Buda J: Cerebroappendicular embolism: simultaneous cerebral infarction and brachial plexopathy. Neurology 1993;43:620–1.

Rarely documented instances of brachial plaeuxs palsy from local infarction.

Medical Research Council. Aids to the Examination of the Peripheral Nervous System. Medical Research Council Memorandum No. 45. Her Majesty's Stationery Office, London, 1976.

The classical motor and sensory maps and charts.

Rowland LP. Cramps, spasms and muscle stiffness. Rev Neurol 1985;141:261–73.

Authoritative review.

Said G, Bathien N, Cesaro P. Peripheral neuropathies and tremor. Neurology 1982;32:480–5.

Fourteen cases and a review of hypotheses.

Tsairis P, Dyck PJ, Mulder DW. Natural history of brachial plexus neuropathy. Report on 99 patients. Arch Neurol 1972;27:109–17.

Basic paper.

33
Muscles

J. C. Gautier and J. P. Mohr

Muscle dysfunction can be the result of either lesions of the motor neurons (see Chs. 22 and 63) or primary diseases of the muscles. The latter make up a large and heterogeneous group with a wide variety of clinical features, too diverse to characterize easily. Chapter 82 is specifically devoted to the primary muscular diseases, to which the reader is referred. The aim of the present chapter is to provide some basic principles of clinical myology—that is, the clinical approach to primary muscular diseases. Table 33-1 lists the main forms of muscle disease, including the disorders of the neuromuscular junction. This classification is but one of many made in the hope of bringing some useful order to the range of individual conditions.

Despite the varying etiologies and names, diseases of muscle share some basic clinical features. First, the main symptom is weakness. Second, the axial muscles, (i.e., those of the head, neck, and trunk) and the proximal muscles of the limbs (those of the shoulder and pelvic girdle), are the most often affected. Third, deep reflexes are present and not exaggerated, but in the more advanced stages of muscle disease they can be depressed and even absent when there is extreme muscle wasting. Fourth, wasting is a cardinal feature although it is not universal. For some unknown reason(s), some muscles are affected and others are spared in regular patterns that are characteristic of particular diseases. In some syndromes the bulk of some muscles is actually increased, a condition known as *pseudohypertrophy*, usually explained by fatty infiltration. There is very rarely a true muscular hypertrophy in muscle disease. Fifth, there are no disturbances of sensory, autonomic, visual, auditory, and higher cerebral functions, which are the hallmark of diseases of the central nervous system. Their presence rules out primary muscle disease, except, of course, when both the central nervous system and muscles are involved. Indeed, the weakness-only separateness of myology

has made it something of a field apart from clinical neurology for many neurologists. Finally, in many primary muscular diseases there is an associated dysfunction of the cardiac muscle. Clinically it results in arrhythmias, conduction disorders, and cardiomyopathy. Every patient suspected of having a myopathy should have a thorough cardiac investigation.

These features distinguish most primary muscular disorders from lower motor neuron disease (see Ch. 22). Associated upper and lower motor neuron or sensory disorders are the chief clues to nonprimary muscle diseases.

SYMPTOMS AND SIGNS

Weakness (i.e., lack of strength) (see Ch. 22) is the principal symptom. Because the proximal muscles are the ones mainly affected, patients complain of increasing difficulties in combing their hair, reaching on high shelves, putting packs in racks, climbing stairs, and getting out of a low seat, car, or tub. Involvement of other muscles results in frequent complaints of ptosis, diplopia, difficulties in kissing, smiling, pouting, speaking, swallowing, holding up the head, and releasing grip on doorknobs or tools, according to the location and nature of the muscular disorder.

Fatigability is a prominent symptom of myasthenia gravis (see Ch. 81) but is also a common feature of most muscular diseases. The symptom is reflected in the appearance of weakness sooner than expected from repetitive efforts. In certain diseases with defects of energy metabolism, stiffness and tiredness can appear following an amount of physical exertion that would be without untoward consequences in normal people (exercise intolerance), or cold can precipitate the symptoms. There can be spontaneous pain (myalgia) or tenderness on muscle palpation (polymyositis).

517

Table 33-1. Synopsis of the Main Muscle Diseases

Genetic Myopathies	Acquired Myopathies
Muscular dystrophies	*Inflammatory*
X-Linked recessive	Infective
Duchenne, Becker, Emery-Dreifuss, scapuloperoneal	Viral, bacterial, parasitic
Autosomal recessive	Drug-induced (see below)
Limb-girdle (scapulohumeral, pelvifemoral), congenital	Idiopathic
Autosomal dominant	Polymyositis, dermatomyositis, inclusion body, granulomatous, eosinophilic
Facioscapulohumeral, scapuloperoneal, distal (Welander) oculopharyngeal	Neuromyositis
Myotonic disorders	*Endocrine and metabolic*
Myotonic dystrophy (Steinert)	Hyperthyroidism, hypothyroidism, Cushing's disease, Addison's disease, acromegaly, hyperthyroidism, osteomalacia
Autosomal dominant myotonia congenita (Thomsen)	*Other*
Paramyotonia congenita (Eulenburg)	Sarcoidosis, amyloidosis, remote cancer
Cytosolic and lysosomal deficiencies	*Toxic and drug-induced*
Acid maltase, Debrancher enzyme, myophosphorylase, phosphofructokinase, phosphoglycerate kinase, phosphoglycerate mutase, lactate dehydrogenase, myoadenylate deaminase	Acute
Mitochondrial myopathies	Alcohol, amphetamine, amphotericin B, barbiturates, carbenoxolone, diazepam, heroin, methadone, phencyclidine
Carnitine, carnitine palmityl transferase, pyruvate dehydrogenase deficiencies, chronic progressive external ophthalmoplegia, Kearns-Sayre syndrome, MERRF, MELAS.	Subacute
Myopathies with distinctive histologic abnormalities	Alcohol, emetine, heroin, ϵ-aminocaproic acid, clofibrate, simvastatine
Central core disease, multicore disease, nemaline myopathy, centronuclear myopathy, congenital fiber type disproportion	Hypokalemic
Familial periodic paralyses	Diuretics, laxatives, amphotericin B, carbenoxolone, licorice
Hypokalcemic, hypercacemic, normokalemic	Painless proximal
Uncertain origin	Corticosteroids, perhexiline, chloroquine
Malignant hyperthermia, idiopathic paroxysmal myoglobinuria	Painful with myokymia
	Lithium, cimetidine, clofibrate, salbutamol, isoetharine
	Myotonic: 20, 23-diazocholesterol
	Diseases of the neuromuscular junction
	Myasthenia gravis, congenital myasthenia, Lambert-Eaton myasthenic syndrome, botulism

Fatigue, a more persistent state not simply provoked by repetitive exertion, is another problem and a rare complaint in primary muscular diseases. In practice fatigue is mainly an attribute of systemic illness such as hepatitis or cancer and also of chronic depression. An ill-defined syndrome beginning with myalgia, headache, and occasionally low-grade fever, can last for months or more, with fatigue, poor mental concentration, and insomnia. Causal hypotheses have been proposed (e.g., Epstein-Barr virus and brucellosis) without convincing support. *Chronic fatigue syndrome* is the best label for this (possible) syndrome and must be preferred to such labels as postviral, chronic mononucleosis, or myalgic encephalomyelitis, for there is usually no evidence of encephalomyelitis. In the authors' experience there is almost always a strong depressive component in the syndrome, and the patients, often women, clearly benefit from antidepressant therapy.

Other important points of the clinical examination are the age of the patient, the tempo of the disease, and familial history with or without similar or related diseases. The search for consanguinity and a careful genealogic tree are essential for diagnosis and genetic counseling. Complaints of endocrine dysfunction and an exhaustive list of drugs recently and currently used are other main points of the clinical examination.

EXAMINATION

In every patient all chief muscles from head to foot must be tested. With experience this takes a few minutes. (For testing muscles that depend on cranial nerves see Chs. 28 and 29; for limb muscle testing see Ch. 22.) Frequently weakness is found in other muscles than those implied in the patient's complaints.

Patterns of Muscular Involvement

Several well-defined patterns of muscular involvement are frequently met with in clinical practice and, consequently, they have good pragmatic value for diagnostic orientation. Most of them can be due either to a primary muscular or to a nervous system disease—hence they imply a differential diagnosis.

In the following not all differential diagnoses have been considered but only those common diseases that should come first to the clinician's mind. Bilateral weakness of the orbicularis oculi with or without ptosis raises the suspicion of myasthenia gravis or facioscapulohumeral or oculopharyngeal myopathy. Diplopia is almost always present in myasthenia, absent in dystrophies. Bilateral facial weakness again suggests myasthenia gravis, myotonic dystrophy, facioscapulohumeral myopathy, and such congenital disorders as centronuclear nemaline myopathies or carnitine deficiency. Bilateral facial palsy is a common feature of Guillain-Barre and Fisher's syndromes. Patients presenting with bulbar palsy (dysarthria characterized by feeble and nasal speech, swallowing disorders, and sometimes a dropping jaw) have either motor neuron disease, myasthenia gravis, polymyositis, or a pseudobulbar palsy.

Those who cannot hold their head (floppy heads) owing to weakness of neck muscles suffer from either polymyositis, myasthenia gravis, or motor neuron disease. A few cases are due to myotonic dystrophy.

Where there is wasting in the upper limbs, selective involvement of the biceps and brachioradialis muscles with sparing of the deltoid is highly suggestive of dystrophy. Respiratory and trunk muscles can be chiefly involved in acute polymyositis, periodic paralyses, motor neuron disease, and the adult form of acid maltase deficiency (glycogenosis type II) (see Ch. 82). Occasionally the clinician may be faced with respiratory distress. Limb girdle weakness, expressed mainly by difficulties in getting up from squatting or from low seats, first suggests dystrophy in the young and polymyositis or thyrotoxic or steroid myopathy in adults.

LABORATORY

As a rule, laboratory investigations are needed. Among the main ones is the creatine kinase blood level, which reflects the amount of muscle breakdown and thus mirrors the severity and tempo of the disease. Modern investigations increasingly hinge on the electromyogram, which shows characteristically small polyphasic potentials (see Ch. 12), to test for hyper- or hypothyroidism. Muscle biopsy is often indicated (see Ch. 8).

ANNOTATED BIBLIOGRAPHY

Lombes A, Bonilla E, Dimauro S. Mitochondrial encephalomyopathies. Rev Neurol 1989;145:671–89.

A good update.

Mitochondria and nervous system diseases. Rev Neurol (Special issue) 1991;147:413–548.

Twenty-two papers (13 in English, 9 in French) covering many aspects of the topic.

Morgan-Hughes JA. Diseases of striated muscles. In Asbury AK, McKhann GM, McDonald WI (eds). In Diseases of the Nervous System. WB Saunders, Philadelphia, 1992.

Highly commendable review.

Swartz MN. The chronic fatigue syndrome. One entity or many? N Engl J Med 1988;319:1726–8.

Good review.

34
Autonomic Nervous System

E. Oribe and O. Appenzeller

The autonomic nervous system (ANS), largely involuntary, constitutes the part of the nervous system responsible for maintenance of internal homeostasis. Through the ANS the nervous system regulates visceral, endocrine, immune, behavioral, and pain functions. This regulatory function is exerted through the actions of autonomic nervous system reflexes acting through direct efferent innervation, hormonal effects, or the release of neuroeffector substances.

Dysfunction (failure and overactivity) of the autonomic nervous system may result in illness. The functional integrity of autonomic neurons may be affected selectively as a result of localized illness or diffusely as a result of systemic illness. Depending on the site and degree of involvement, the clinical manifestations of autonomic dysfunction may range from a local derangement of function with minimal clinical significance to a generalized disorder of body function severe enough to be life-threatening.

ANATOMY

Overview

All visceral functions are regulated through the actions of autonomic reflexes. Autonomic reflex pathways include specialized sensory receptors and their afferents, which carry information from the viscera to the autonomic centers in the central nervous system (CNS), where integration and processing occurs, together with efferent pathways and neuroeffectors, which execute the autonomic response.

Afferent information is integrated and processed by the central autonomic network centers. These project on the hypothalamus, which in turn produces a coordinated autonomic response. The hypothalamus regulates the ANS directly through its projections upon preganglionic neurons in the brainstem nuclei and the spinal cord or indirectly through the action of hypothalamic and pituitary hormones. Axons from autonomic preganglionic brainstem and spinal cord neurons exit the CNS traveling via cranial nerves and spinal ventral roots and then synapse with autonomic motor neurons within specialized ganglia. From here postganglionic fibers supply the target organs.

Endocrine, metabolic, and immune functions are also regulated through ANS feedback loops, which include specialized areas of the brain that are devoid of a blood-brain barrier (the circumventricular organs) and the central and the peripheral ANS. Although normally under central autonomic influences, local autonomic networks such as those controlling peristalsis, heart rate, and bladder function are able to function autonomously.

The ANS has three divisions: (1) the craniosacral or parasympathetic, (2) the thoracolumbar or sympathetic, and (3) the enteric nervous system. The parasympathetic and the sympathetic divisions innervate the smooth and cardiac muscle and the glands. The enteric nervous system innervates the gut, controlling motility and secretions.

The parasympathetic response is more rapid, selective, and short-lived than that of the sympathetic division. For example, the parasympathetic response is well suited to induce the almost immediate changes in heart rate that occur normally with breathing. The more selective parasympathetic response is explained in part by a lower ratio of pre- to postganglionic innervation than that of sympathetic innervation.

The sympathetic response, which is diffuse and relatively longer-lasting, is more suited for "fight or flight" responses. These are triggered by aversive or threatening stimuli and result in massive sympathetic discharges and release of epinephrine from the adrenal glands. They increase blood pressure and heart rate, produce bronchial and pupillary dilation, and glycogenolysis and cause inhibition of gut secretions and motility. Sympathetic responses are of relatively long duration owing to a slower disappearance of the main sympathetic neurotransmitter (norepinephrine) through re-uptake and diffusion from the synaptic cleft rather than through a rapid enzymatic degradation, as occurs with the main parasympathetic neurotransmitter (acetylcholine).

Afferent Autonomic Pathways

Afferent autonomic information originates from mechano-, chemo-, and osmoreceptors in the walls, parenchyma, and serosa of the viscera and blood vessels. The receptors sense changes in the body's internal milieu and can also signal events in the viscera that can evoke pain (e.g., the pain of cardiac ischemia or a distended viscus). Autonomic sensory neuron afferent fibers, whose cell bodies are located in the cranial and dorsal root ganglia, travel with parasympathetic and sympathetic nerves. The fibers then synapse with lateral horn cells as part of a local autonomic spinal reflex path or with dorsal horn cells from which afferent information is carried to the nucleus tractus solitarius, and from there to higher autonomic centers (the central autonomic network).

Central Autonomic Network

The central autonomic network consists of various nuclei within the brainstem and forebrain (i.e., certain areas of the parabrachial nucleus, the central gray matter, hypothalamic nuclei, amygdala, and the stria terminalis). These function together, controlling autonomic, endocrine, and complex behavioral responses, which allow survival of the individual (and ultimately the species) in an ever-changing environment.

Although knowledge regarding the complex interactions among nuclei and with the afferent and efferent pathways is limited to that learned from anatomic study of experimental animals (mainly rodents), it appears that in the human the central autonomic network participates in behavioral and cognitive functions through its links to the cortex and limbic system. Through the central autonomic network the ANS provides responses that are appropriate to and coordinated with each behavioral pattern.

The nucleus tractus solitarius receives diverse visceral information (such as taste and unconscious visceral modalities including baroreflex inputs) and serves as a relay that links central autonomic network afferents and efferents. Brainstem projections, which are part of feedback loops that are connected with higher central autonomic network centers involved in feeding and other complex behaviors, control functions such as mastication, swallowing, and salivation.

Efferent Autonomic Pathways

Sympathetic Division

Descending sympathetic pathways that originate in the hypothalamus, midbrain, pons, and medulla synapse with sympathetic preganglionic neurons within the intermediolateral gray matter of the spinal cord from levels T1 through L2. Axons from these cell bodies exit the spinal cord via ventral roots and travel with spinal nerves to form myelinated white rami communicantes (Fig. 34-1). From there, preganglionic fibers synapse with postganglionic autonomic motor neurons located within the paravertebral or the prevertebral ganglia.

The paravertebral ganglia are arranged as two interconnected chains, which run parallel to the vertebral column. The ganglia, in addition to the postganglionic neuron cell bodies, contain other cells that may have a modulatory function (e.g., the small intensely fluorescent cells), Most preganglionic fibers synapse with autonomic motor neurons located in the ganglia at their level of exit.

Unmyelinated postganglionic fibers (gray rami) leave the ganglia within the spinal nerves to supply blood vessels, sweat glands, and hair follicles. Some fibers form plexuses, which then innervate the thoracic and abdominal viscera (Fig. 34-2 and 34-3). Alternatively, some preganglionic axons may pass through paravertebral ganglia without synapsing to form the splanchnic nerves.

Preganglionic axons synapse with postganglionic autonomic motor neurons within the prevertebral ganglia (i.e., celiac, superior, and inferior mesenteric ganglia) or with secretory cells in the adrenal medulla.

The fibers from the T1 and T2 segments supply the face and neck via postganglionic fibers in the superior cervical ganglia. The heart, trachea, bronchi, lungs, and esophagus are supplied by the upper thoracic segments via postganglionic fibers from the cervical ganglia and upper thoracic ganglia. The T2 to T8 segments innervate the upper extremities via the postganglionic fibers in the lower cervical ganglion. The T5 to T10 segments innervate the stomach, gallbladder, lung, and pancreas via the great splanchnic nerve and celiac ganglia.

Sympathetic innervation of the gut originates in preganglionic fibers from T8 to L3 and their synapses with postganglionic fibers in the celiac and superior and inferior mesenteric prevertebral ganglia.

The adrenal medulla, receiving direct preganglionic sympathetic innervation, behaves as if it were a specialized sympathetic ganglion by secreting neurotransmitters and hormones such as epinephrine, which have profound systemic effects.

Pelvic viscera are innervated by the lower thoracic

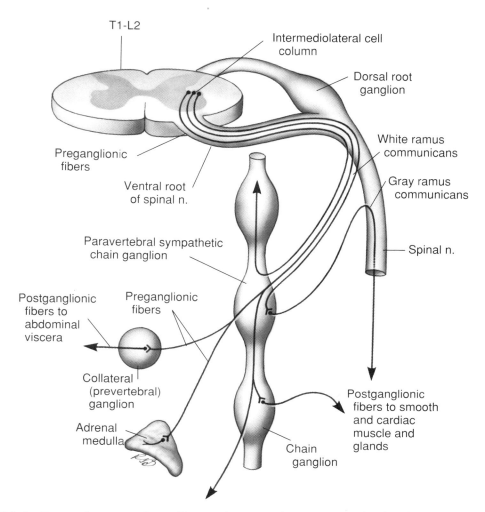

Figure 34-1. Pre- and postganglionic fibers in the sympathetic paravertebral and prevertebral ganglia. (Adapted from Appenzeller, 1990, with permission.)

and high lumbar segments via paravertebral ganglia and the hypogastric plexuses. The lower limbs are supplied by the lumbar and sacral segments via para-aortic ganglia.

Parasympathetic Division

The central connections of the parasympathetic division appear to originate from numerous sites in the brain, including the cortex, amygdala, hypothalamus, and mesencephalic central gray matter although the precise pathways are not known in the human. The preganglionic parasympathetic neurons are located in brainstem nuclei (Edinger-Westphal, superior and inferior salivary, dorsal vagus, and ambiguus nuclei) and in the interomediolateral cell columns of spinal segments S2–S4. Axons from preganglionic cells exit the CNS via cranial and sacral nerves to synapse in ganglia that are close to or within the organs they supply.

The Edinger-Westphal nucleus contains the oculomotor preganglionic neurons, which subserve the iris and ciliary muscles of the pupil. Efferent axons travel in the third cranial nerve and synapse with the ciliary ganglion cells in the orbit (see also Ch. 26).

The superior salivary nucleus contains cranial nerve preganglionic neurons, which innervate the cerebral vasculature and the lacrimal and mucous glands of the palate and nose via relays in the pterygopalatine ganglia.

Those neurons that innervate the sublingual and submandibular salivary and mucous glands of the mouth synapse in the submandibular ganglia. The inferior salivary nucleus contains the fifth cranial nerve neurons, which innervate the parotid and the mucous glands of the mouth after synapsing in the otic ganglia.

The smooth muscle and glands of the neck and of

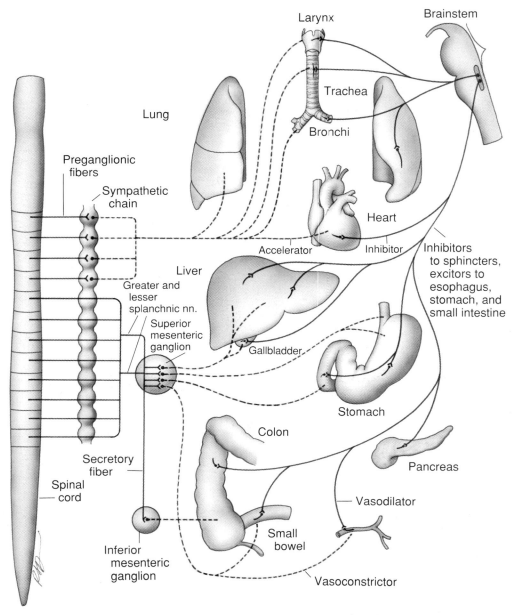

Figure 34-2. Pre- and postganglionic fibers of the autonomic innervation of the thoracic and abdominal viscera. Dotted lines represent postganglionic fibers of the sympathetic (thoracolumbar) division. Solid lines on viscera represent postganglionic fibers of the parasympathetic (craniosacral) division. (From Appenzeller, 1990, with permission.)

the thoracic and most abdominal viscera are supplied though the tenth cranial nerve (Fig. 34-2). The vagal nucleus contains preganglionic neurons regulating gut secretion, and the nucleus ambiguus contains neurons that control heart rate, bronchial tone, and other visceromotor functions. Neurons in the nodose ganglia relay visceral information to the nucleus tractus solitarius.

The parasympathetic efferent innervation of the gut originating from the brainstem travels with the vagus nerve, and that originating from S2 to S4 spinal segments travels through the pelvic splanchnic nerves. Efferent fibers then converge on enteric nervous system plexuses.

Sacral parasympathetic efferents travel via splanchnic nerves, synapse in the pelvic ganglia, and innervate the bladder and sexual organs. Afferent sensory fibers originate from the sacral dorsal root ganglia.

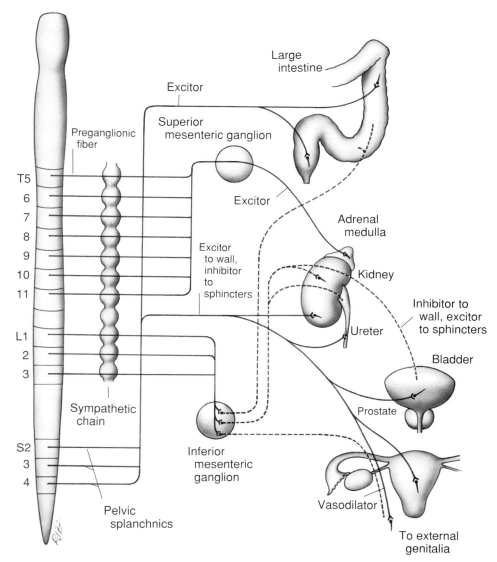

Figure 34-3. Pre- and postganglionic fibers of the autonomic innervation of the abdominal and pelvic viscera. Dotted lines represent postganglionic fibers of the sympathetic (thoracolumbar) division. Solid lines on viscera represent postganglionic fibers of the parasympathetic (craniosacral) division. (From Appenzeller, 1990, with permission.)

Enteric Nervous System

The enteric nervous system (ENS) participates in the regulation of the water and electrolyte milieu and motility of the gut. The ENS consists of afferent sensory neurons and networks of interneurons, which are capable of integrating and determining specific response patterns, which are then relayed via efferent neurons to the effector organs. As many as 80 to 100 million neurons are distributed as plexuses within the gut walls. In addition to Auerbach's myenteric plexus (L. Auerbach, German anatomist, 1828–97) between the two outer muscle coats and Meissner's submucous plexus (G. Meissner, German histologist, 1829–1905),

there are plexuses within the longitudinal and circular muscle layers and the mucosa. The myenteric plexus controls gut motility. The submucous plexus controls water and electrolyte transport across the epithelial membrane, provides gut secretions, and may provide a link with the myenteric plexus as part of what is thought to be a feedback loop regulating gut motility.

Although under the influence of the CNS through sympathetic and parasympathetic systems, the ENS is capable of functioning autonomously. Peristalsis and migrating motor complexes are examples of autonomous ENS functions. Prevertebral ganglia participate in spinal inhibitory reflexes and the enterocolic reflexes. The main sympathetic influence on the ENS is inhibitory through sympathetic nerves, and the parasympathetic influence is stimulatory through the vagus nerve.

Autonomic Neuroeffector Transmission

The autonomic neuroeffector transmission differs anatomically from that present in the striated muscle and the central and the peripheral nervous system. The autonomic synapse is a "nondirected" synapse lacking pre- and postsynaptic specialization. Autonomic terminals differ from somatic terminals by the presence of varicosities, which are distributed in series along axons (similar to beads on a necklace). The varicosities release neurotransmitters, which travel along the axons. Wide junctional clefts through which neurotransmitters diffuse, allow a "leakage" of neurotransmitter to adjacent areas and thus result in a greater spread of potentials. Smooth muscle fibers are organized into effector bundles of closely connected fibers, which are linked to each other through low-resistance gap junctions. The low-resistance junctions allow electrotonical coupling of adjacent cells, permitting a more rapid spread of potentials.

Acetylcholine (ACh) is the predominant neurotransmitter in the sympathetic and parasympathetic preganglionic as well as the postganglionic parasympathetic synapse. The main sympathetic postganglionic neurotransmitter is norepinephrine except for the sweat glands, adrenal medulla, and vasodilator fibers to muscle, in which the neurotransmitter is Ach.

ACh plays a fundamental role in ANS regulation at the level of the preganglionic and postganglionic parasympathetic and the postganglionic sympathetic sweat gland synapses and in the brain, where central autonomic pathways rely on cholinergic neurotransmission (i.e., pathways including the ventrolateral medulla, dorsal vagal nucleus, nucleus accumbens, and nucleus tractus solitarius).

Traditionally, cholinergic Ach receptors have been classified into muscarinic and nicotinic receptors, according to their response to muscarine and nicotine, respectively. Muscarinic receptors are present in postganglionic parasympathetic and postganglionic sympathetic synapses innervating the sweat glands as well as in the brain. Eight subtypes of muscarinic receptors have been identified so far, and it is expected that more will be found in the near future. Functionally, those that have been best categorized regulate gastric acid secretion (muscarinic receptors type M1), heart rate (muscarinic receptors type M2, cardiac), and contraction of gut smooth muscle (muscarinic receptors type M2, glandular). Their mechanism of action appears to involve a G-protein intermediate. Each subtype regulates different transduction pathways in

which cyclic guanosine monophosphate (cGMP), phosphatidylinositol, and C-kinases appear to participate.

There are three classic types of *nicotinic* receptors: those of the preganglionic parasympathetic and sympathetic synapse, those in the brain, and those innervating skeletal muscle. Nicotinic ACh receptors may function by opening cationconducting channels.

The pharmacology of adrenoceptors has allowed a convenient classification into α- and β-receptors. Norepinephrine stimulates mainly α-adrenoceptors, whereas epinephrine stimulates both α- and β-adrenoceptors. The α- and β-adrenoceptors are further divided into subtypes according to their response to different agonist and antagonist substances. Stimulation of α-adrenoceptors produces hydrolysis of phosphatidylinositol and leads to the formation of second messengers and ultimately, to release of calcium from intracellular stores. Release of calcium results in vesicle-mediated secretion, contraction of smooth muscle cells, and increase in turnover of cyclic nucleotides. α-Adrenoceptor stimulation decreases cyclic AMP synthesis. Stimulation of β-adrenoceptors results in the formation of cyclic AMP. Adrenoceptors mediate various vasomotor, secretomotor, metabolic, and hormonal effects (Table 34-1).

Table 34-1. Responses to Adrenoceptor Stimulation

Adrenoceptor	Response
α_1	Smooth muscle contraction (except gut where stimulation produces relaxation)
	Increased cardiac inotropism
	Sweat and salivary gland secretion
	Hepatic glycogenolysis; gluconeogenesis
	Renal sodium reabsorption
α_2	Vascular smooth muscle contraction
	Presynaptic inhibition of neuronal norepinephrine release
	Inhibition of insulin release
	Inhibition of lipolysis
	Platelet aggregation and degranulation
β_1	Increased cardiac inotropism and chronotropism
	Renal juxtaglomerular renin secretion
	Lipolysis
β_2	Smooth muscle relaxation
	Skeletal muscle glycogenolysis and potassium uptake
	Hepatic glycogenolysis; gluconeogenesis
	Salivary amylase secretion
β_3	Lipolysis

AUTONOMIC NEUROTRANSMITTER SUBSTANCES

Classic
  Acetylcholine
  Norepinephrine
  Dopamine
  Serotonin
Nonadrenergic-noncholinergic
  Purinergic
    Adenosine triphosphate
    γ-Aminobutyric acid
  Peptidergic
    Corticotropin
    Angiotensin
    Calcitonin gene-related peptide
    Cholecystokinin/gastrin
    Endothelin
    Enkephalin/endorphin
    Galanin
    Gastrin-releasing peptide/bombesin
    Luteinizing hormone-releasing hormone
    Neuropeptide Y/pancreatic polypeptide
    Neurotensin
    Peptide histidine isoleucine
    Somatostatin
    Substance P
    Vasoactive intestinal polypeptide
    Vasopressin
    Others
Diffusible
  Nitric oxide
  Carbon monoxide?

The knowledge that an individual neuron is able to synthesize, store, and release diverse neurotransmitter substances has made way for new fundamental physiologic concepts, which have replaced the classical one-nerve, one-transmitter paradigm. Early experiments in the 1960s leading to the discovery of the neurotransmitter role of adenosine triphosphate (ATP) were followed by confirmation that other purines, peptides, and gases act as autonomic neurotransmitters. Neurotransmitter functions have now been ascribed to numerous substances in addition to those already identified. These nonadrenergic, noncholinergic (NANC) neurotransmitters have been identified in most autonomic neurons. NANC substances participate, together with the classic monoaminergic (norepinephrine, 5-hydroxytryptamine, and dopa-mine) neurotransmitters and ACh in most, if not all autonomic synapses. Among the recently identified diffusible NANC transmitters are certain gases such as nitric oxide, which have been found to have major physiologic roles.

The effects of neurotransmitters on their target organs are complex and widespread. Not only does a neurotransmitter produce its effects directly, but it may also do so indirectly by modifying the effects (and the release) of other neurotransmitters. For example, NANC substances that are released in conjunction with other neurotransmitters act on postsynaptic receptors as cotransmitters or are able to modulate the effects of other neurotransmitters as neuromodulators. This occurs with the joint release of ACh and vasoactive intestinal polypeptide which together have an excitatory effect on gut motility, and the release of norepinephrine and adenosine triphosphate (ATP), which produce vasoconstriction.

Different autonomic nerve discharge frequencies can release different amounts of a transmitter, entirely different transmitters, or even different combinations of transmitters in a process appropriately termed *chemical coding*. The fact that the importance and function of each neurotransmitter also depends on its target tissue is further demonstration of the complexity of autonomic neurotransmission. For example, vasopressin, which has classically been known to promote antidiuresis and smooth muscle contraction, also produces vasodilation of cranial blood vessels.

The effects of transmitters are also influenced by circulating and locally released substances, either directly or through other local agents, thus providing further modulation of autonomic responses. For instance, vasopressin and atrial natriuretic peptide may regulate ANS responses not only when released locally but also by their systemic effects. The neuroeffector responses to autonomic transmitters have also been found to change with aging and disease.

Vascular Endothelium

Autonomic vasomotor control includes not only neural influences but also the release of paracrine endothelium-derived hormones and gaseous neurotransmitters. A major role of the vascular endothelium in regulating the diameter of blood vessels has become evident following the discovery that intact endothelium is necessary for ACh-induced vasodilation. Vascular diameter therefore reflects the sum of the vasomotor effects of perivascular autonomic nerves, the local release of endothelial substances, and also the effects of vasoactive substances released by blood constituents and circulating hormones (Fig. 34-4).

Several endothelial-derived factors have potent effects on vascular diameter. It now appears that nitric

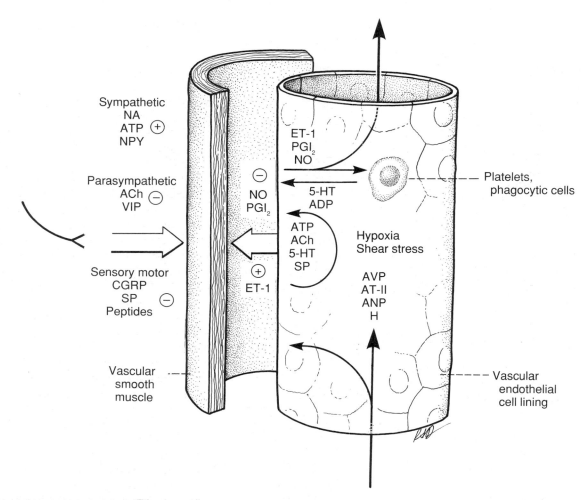

Figure 34-4. Autonomic neural, endothelial, and intravascular interactions regulating vascular tone. Perivascular nerves and sensorimotor nerves produce vasoconstriction and dilation through the release of NA, NPY, ATP, ACh, VIP, CGRP, SP, and other peptides. Endothelial cells release the powerful vasodilators NO and PGI_2 and vasoconstrictor substances such as ET-1 when stimulated by intraluminal shear stress, hypoxia, and various factors including those released by blood elements and those carried by the bloodstream. Local stimuli trigger release of NO and PGI_2 through the effects of ATP, ACh, 5-HT, and SP from endothelial cells. ACh, acetylcholine; AT, angiotensin II; ANP, atrial natriuretic peptide; ADP and ATP, adenosine di- and triphosphate; AVP, vasopressin; CGRP, calcitonin-gene related peptide; ET-1, endothelin-1; 5-HT, serotonin; H, histamine; NA, norepinephrine; NO, nitric oxide; NPY, neuropeptide Y; PGI_2, prostacyclin; SP, substance P; +, constriction; −, dilatation.

oxide identical with the endothelial-derived relaxing factor released by cholinergic stimulation of NANC terminals, is the major physiologic regulator of basal vasomotor tone. Nitric oxide produces smooth muscle relaxation through the formation of cGMP. In addition to being released by neural influences, nitric oxide and other endothelial vasoactive substances are released by hormones and also by increases in flow-shear stress. Endothelin-1, a vasoactive peptide (and neuropeptide) released from vascular endothelium (and perhaps from the neurohypophysis), has been

identified as the most potent vasoconstrictor (and also a potent vascular mitogenic factor) to date. It is possible that this peptide plays a fundamental role in determining vascular diameter by opposing the vasodilating effects of nitric oxide under certain conditions.

Endothelial substances can also act as neuromodulators by modifying the effects of the classic neurotransmitters (e.g., the vasoconstrictor effect of norepinephrine is amplified by endothelin-1. It is expected that the recent development of specific antagonists for nitric oxide and endothelin-1 and other neurotransmitter substances will allow significant discoveries in the field of autonomic physiology and pathology.

CLINICAL FEATURES OF AUTONOMIC DYSFUNCTION

History and Physical Examination

A basic knowledge of the anatomy and function of ANS reflex pathways is necessary to determine if autonomic dysfunction is present, to locate the site of dysfunction in the autonomic feedback loop, and to uncover the pathophysiologic mechanisms involved. Knowledge of the site of the ANS lesion is necessary for appropriate treatment.

The diagnosis of autonomic dysfunction relies on the presence of diagnostic clinical features, which sometimes require supporting evidence of abnormal autonomic testing results. On occasion, ANS dysfunction can be subclinical and detected through ANS testing.

The approach to the clinical evaluation of the ANS by history and physical examination should reflect its widespread regulatory role. Evaluation should be directed at revealing if autonomic dysfunction is focal, limited to a specific organ system, or if it is generalized, affecting multiple organ systems. Except as a result of trauma, ANS dysfunction is usually diffuse, but symptoms may remain relatively focal for long periods. As a rule, acute autonomic failure is usually symptomatic whereas chronic failure only becomes symptomatic when severe or additional stress (prolonged orthostasis, heat, cold, or altitude) is imposed on the system.

The history should not only focus on the presenting symptoms but should include an extensive review of ANS functions in search of evidence of widespread involvement. This includes investigating resistance to cold and altitude, heat tolerance, sleep patterns, skin color, sweating patterns, night vision, and orthostatic tolerance and searching for genitourinary and gastrointestinal symptoms.

Physical examination should include blood pressure and heart rate determinations after at least 5 minutes of supine rest and after 2 minutes of standing. In some cases, measuring blood pressure and heart rate under different conditions (e.g., after meals and exercise) may uncover ANS dysfunction. Skin and mucosal findings reveal temperature, sweating, and pilomotor, vasomotor, secretory, and dystrophic abnormalities (e.g., scaliness, smoothness, or hypertrophy). Their distribution may help to localize the site of an autonomic lesion. In some cases, neuroarthropathic (Charcot) joints may be a presenting feature of autonomic neuropathy. The pupils should be examined closely for differences in size and their response to light and the iris should be inspected for atrophy and color. Re-

---

AUTONOMIC SYMPTOMS

Orthostatic symptoms (lightheadedness, weakness, visual symptoms, syncope, neck pain, and pulsatile headache)

Sweating and thermoregulatory (decreased/increased sweating, heat/cold tolerance, piloerection)

Vasomotor (pallor, flushing, skin temperature changes)

Gastrointestinal (abdominal pain, diarrhea, constipation, bloating, vomiting)

Secretomotor (dry mouth/eyes, abnormal salivary production)

Urinary (incontinence/retention, loss of sensation of bladder function)

Sexual (erectile/ejaculatory impotence, loss of libido)

Visual (decreased accommodation, nocturnal vision impairment)

---

flex dartos muscle contraction (in response to scrotal and perineal stimuli—the scrotal reflex), internal anal sphincter contraction (in response to distension of the anus—the anal reflex) and bulbocavernosus contraction (in response to stimulation of the dorsum of the penis—the bulbocavernosus reflex) (see also Ch. 32) can help to localize some autonomic lesions.

Autonomic testing (see Ch. 16) helps confirm the presence and distribution of autonomic failure and may indicate the site in the autonomic feedback loop and the nature of lesions causing autonomic dysfunction. Other testing is aimed at determining the nature of the underlying illness causing autonomic dysfunction (e.g., searching for diabetes and other causes of autonomic neuropathies). Short corticotropin stimulation testing (e.g., time points at 0 and 60 minutes) to help exclude adrenal insufficiency and amyloid stains on subcutaneous fat, nerve, muscle, conjunctival, or rectal biopsy specimens should be considered in selected patients.

Autonomic Signs and Symptoms

Orthostatic Hypotension

Orthostatic hypotension is the most frequent and incapacitating sign of autonomic failure. The normal blood pressure and heart rate responses to standing are a fall in systolic blood pressure of 5 to 10 mmHg, an increase in diastolic blood pressure of 5 to 10 mmHg, and a rise in heart rate of 10 to 25 beats per minute. Different values have been used when defining orthostatic hypotension as symptomatic, but a fall in systolic pressure of more than 30 mmHg on standing, with symptoms, is a useful standard. It should be kept in mind however, that lesser decreases in blood pressure may be symptomatic, and conversely, greater falls in blood pressure may remain asymptomatic in some individuals.

When measuring blood pressure and heart rate responses to standing, supine values taken after at least 5 minutes (or ideally after 20 minutes) of supine rest should be compared with values after at least 2 minutes of quiet standing (the "early steady state"). Preferably, measurements should be made in the morning before the patient gets out of bed. Sitting blood pressure values are less reliable than standing values and sometimes are difficult to interpret. A significant increase in systolic pressure (>20 mmHg) on sitting may be a sign of ANS failure if the supine blood pressure is low, as this uncovers loss of blood pressure buffering capacity when compression of the splanchnic vascular bed by the sitting position increases venous return to the heart. In those patients who cannot tolerate the upright posture for enough time to permit blood pressure measurements, the maximum standing time can be used as an index of orthostatic tolerance. Normal blood pressure responses to standing up are different from those obtained by passive head-up tilting when activation of antigravity muscles is absent (see Ch. 16).

Symptoms of cerebral hypoperfusion are usually the initial complaints that bring the patient with autonomic dysfunction to medical attention. Orthostatic hypotension may manifest as generalized weakness, fatigability, headache, neck and upper back pains, visual disturbances such as blurring and dimming of vision, leg buckling, and on occasion focal neurologic deficits. Lightheadedness and presyncopal symptoms frequently occur in response to standing, sitting, and exercise. Loss of consciousness (syncope) occurs once the mean arterial pressure falls below a threshold of 70 mmHg (i.e., arterial pressures below 90/60 mmHg) when cerebral perfusion is compromised (age, training, sex, and altitude can alter the threshold pressure).

Syncope can be of either gradual or sudden onset. Clonic movements (so-called limb-shaking, often attributed to brain ischemia), incontinence, and rarely, seizures may be present. The role of orthostatic hypotension in the causation of disease such as transient ischemic attacks and ischemic stroke remains a subject of debate (see Ch. 35).

Orthostatic hypotension is due to a failure of the autonomic reflexes to adjust peripheral resistance adequately in response to the fall in venous return and cardiac output that occurs on assuming the upright posture (Fig. 34-5). The change in position from supine to upright produces a shift of blood on the order of 500 to 600 ml from the thoracic vessels into the legs and of 200 to 300 ml into the buttocks and pelvic veins. The increase of the transit time of blood though these venous capacitance beds (venous pooling) produces a decrease in venous return to the heart, which results in decreased cardiac output and blood pressure. The fall in blood pressure is detected by high-pressure arterial baroreceptors in the aorta and carotid sinus, which are continuously adjusting their afferent discharges in response to blood pressure changes. Blood pressure falls produce "unloading" of the arterial baroreceptors and a decrease in the inhibitory influence that they exert (via the ninth and tenth cranial nerves) upon the nucleus tractus solitarii and vasomotor centers in the medulla.

Disinhibition of the nucleus tractus solitarii and vasomotor centers results in increased sympathetic and decreased parasympathetic traffic, producing vasoconstriction, increased cardiac contractility, and acceleration of the heart rate. The efferent pathways from these centers include the tenth cranial nerve, sympathetic vasoconstrictor fibers are primarily to muscles, and sympathetic efferents to the kidney. In response to sympathetic activation there is also an increase in the release of renin from the kidney's juxtaglomerular apparatus, which activates the renin-angiotensin-aldosterone system.

Afferent baroreceptor information is also carried from the brainstem centers via norepinephrine pathways to the hypothalamus, from where the antidiuretic hormone vasopressin is released to the circulation from the neurohypophysis. Vasopressin produces vasoconstriction through its effect on vascular smooth muscle and water reabsorption through its effect on the distal and collecting kidney tubules. Neuropeptides such as endogenous opioids and endothelin-1 also play significant but as yet poorly defined roles in the baroreflex response.

In addition to baroreflex-controlled vasoconstriction, a local axon reflex causing constriction of arteriolar flow to limb, skin, muscle, and adipose tissue (the venoarteriolar reflex) further contributes to the increase in total peripheral resistance triggered by orthostasis. Decreases in circulating volume are detected by low-pressure cardiopulmonary receptors (cardiopulmonary baroreflex unloading), which also relay the information via the ninth and tenth cranial nerves to the vasomotor centers in the brainstem. The response is similar to that produced by arterial baroreflex unloading, with increased sympathetic outflow and release of neurohormonal substances. Decreased distension of the cardiac atria results in a diminished release of atrial natriuretic factor.

Together, both neuronal and hormonal responses

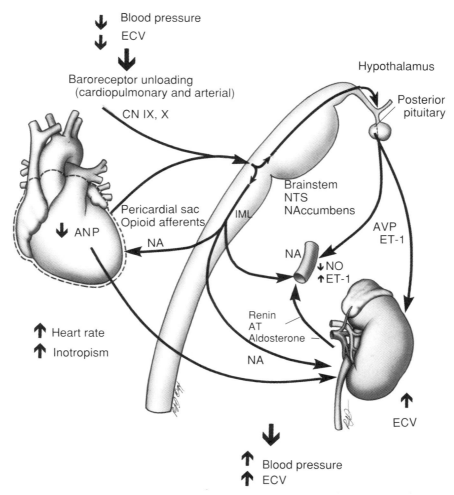

Figure 34-5. Neuronal pathways of the baroreflex response. Afferent information on blood pressure and blood volume from arterial and cardiopulmonary baroreceptors travels to the brainstem with cranial nerves IX and X. Brainstem neurons project to the preganglionic sympathetic neurons within the intermediolateral cell columns of the spinal cord and to the hypothalamus. Postganglionic sympathetic neurons innervate the heart, blood vessels, and kidneys. Falls in blood pressure (BP) or extracellular volume (ECV) produce "unloading" of the baroreceptors, which results in reflex parasympathetic withdrawal and sympathetic activation, increasing heart rate, inotropism, and vascular tone and promoting the release of renin from the kidney. The neural response is accompanied by increased release of AVP from the neurohypophysis and decreased release of ANP. The physiologic roles of hypophyseal and endothelial release of endothelin-1 (ET-1) and endothelial release of nitric oxide (NO) triggered by baroreflex activation are not yet fully defined. Opioid pathways appear to modulate baroreflex function. Together, complex neural (early) and neuroendocrine (later) responses result in increased peripheral resistance, extracellular volume, and cardiac output and blood pressure. AT, angiotensin II; ANP, atrial natriuretic peptide; AVP, vasopressin; IML, intermediolateral cell column; NA, norepinephrine; NAccumbens, nucleus accumbens; NTS, nucleus tractus solitarius.

promote increases in peripheral resistance and extracellular fluid volume, which tend to compensate for falls in blood pressure and circulating volume. The principle that neural responses are immediate and hormonal responses delayed and longer-lasting applies throughout the homeostatic control of the ANS.

If these mechanisms are intact but are unable to adjust sufficiently to changes in blood pressure or volume or are abnormal, abnormal blood pressure and heart rate changes will occur in response to orthostatic stress. Orthostatic hypotension may be present despite intact baroreflexes when there is severe intravascular volume depletion or excessive venous pooling or as an effect of vasodilator drugs. In these situations blood pressure falls are accompanied by increases in heart rate.

Table 34-2. Early Steady-State Blood Pressure and Heart Rate Responses to Standing (2 Minutes)

Response	Blood Pressure	Heart Rate	Cause
Normal	Systolic = Diastolic =, ↑	↑	
Hyperadrenergic	Systolic ↓, =, ↑ Diastolic ↓, =, ↑	↑↑	Hypovolemia Deconditioning/postural tachycardia Microgravity
Neurocardiogenic (Vasovagal)	Systolic ↓ Diastolic ↓	↓	↓ Sympathetic ↑ Parasympathetic due to exaggerated afferent discharge
Hypoadrenergic	Systolic ↓ Diastolic ↓	↑	Sympathetic failure with vagus intact
	Systolic ↓ Diastolic ↓	=	Sympathetic and vagus failure

In neurogenic orthostatic hypotension primary dysfunction of the afferent, central, or efferent baroreflex pathways results in insufficient sympathetic vasoconstriction to counteract the redistribution of blood to the dependent areas of the body. Usually, blood pressure falls rapidly on assuming the upright position, and the heart rate either is unchanged ("fixed") owing to both vagal and sympathetic dysfunction or does not rise above 110 beats/min when there is sympathetic damage but intact vagal function.

As opposed to patients with intact baroreflexes and orthostatic hypotension, patients with neurogenic orthostatic hypotension rarely have symptoms of autonomic activation such as sweating, pallor, tachycardia, nausea, and shortness of breath accompanying low pressures.

Typical patterns in blood pressure and heart rate in response to standing suggest different causes of ANS dysfunction (Table 34-2). Patients with neurogenic orthostatic hypotension may have falls in blood pressure during exercise and after meals (minimal and asymptomatic in normal individuals) related to muscle and splanchnic vasodilation, which is insufficiently opposed by the normal reflex sympathetic vasoconstriction of other vascular beds. Morning blood pressures tend to be lower, reflecting altered circadian blood pressure rhythms and overnight pooling of blood in the capacitance vasculature (veins). Supine hypertension, which is present in many patients with neurogenic orthostatic hypotension, reflects exaggerated sensitivity of postsynaptic adrenoceptors (denervation supersensitivity), which is thought to be due to an increase in the density of receptors. Centripetal volume shifts, deficient baroreflex function, and the hypertensive effects of medication used to treat orthostatic hypotension frequently aggravate supine hypertension. When severe, rises in blood pressure can cause retinal and cerebral hemorrhage. Even mildly elevated supine blood pressure may contribute to excessive nocturnal polyuria and sodium loss and aggravate orthostatic blood pressure falls present in the morning.

Denervation supersensitivity occurs more commonly with peripheral postganglionic than with central preganglionic disorders. The biochemical characteristic of neurogenic orthostatic hypotension is a failure to release norepinephrine appropriately upon assuming the upright posture (the normal increase is more than twofold). Patients with severe peripheral neuropathy may also have low resting plasma norepinephrine concentrations due to degeneration of postganglionic neurons. Hypovolemia may be present and be in part due to low plasma renin activity, which results from decreased β_1-adrenoceptor stimulation.

Mild and usually asymptomatic orthostatic hypotension is frequently encountered in the elderly. The causes are related to autonomic, cardiac, vascular, and volume homeostasis changes that occur with the aging process. A decline in baroreflex function and adrenoceptor sensitivity results in abnormal blood pressure and heart rate adjustments to posture. Altered cardiac pump function, often present in the elderly because of left ventricular hypertrophy and decreased early ventricular diastolic filling, reduces cardiac output and blood pressure. The decrease in cardiac output is aggravated by conditions that impair cardiac venous return, such as capacitance vessel blood pooling and hypovolemia. Hypovolemia may be present as a result of salt loss and extracellular volume contraction due to an age-associated decrease in renin and aldosterone production. Many elderly patients also have increased plasma levels of atrial natriuretic peptide, which promotes further salt loss.

Hypertension

Increased sympathetic activity producing hypertension and tachycardia can result from interruption of inhibitory baroreflex afferents to CNS cardiovascular centers. For instance, damage to the ninth and tenth cranial nerves found in autonomic neuropathies such as porphyria and Guillain-Barré syndrome result in hypertension through this mechanism.

Massive unbridled sympathetic outflow may occur when certain CNS autonomic pathways are interrupted. The result may be "autonomic storm," a dramatic syndrome including severe cardiovascular and respiratory manifestations such as neurogenic hypertension and pulmonary edema, myocardial ischemia and injury with contraction band necrosis, supraventricular and ventricular arrhythmias, and electrocardiographic abnormalities. During an autonomic storm there are clinical signs of sympathetic discharge such as dilated pupils, piloerection, pallor (see below).

Cardiac Arrhythmias

The sinus node pacemaker is influenced by both sympathetic and parasympathetic autonomic outflow. Sympathetic stimulation increases the heart rate by increasing the rate of sinus node diastolic depolarization while parasympathetic stimulation slows the heart rate by producing hyperpolarization of sinus pacemaker cells.

Afferent information from baro-, chemo-, and thoracic receptors is transmitted via the ninth and tenth cranial nerves to the brainstem, where it is integrated into the nucleus tractus solitarius nucleus tractus solitarii. Thermoreceptor, aortic, and cardiac receptor afferents also converge on the nucleus tractus solitarii, together with afferents from higher centers. Information is then relayed to the vasomotor center and the nucleus of the tenth cranial nerve, whence sympathetic and parasympathetic outflows are regulated. Preganglionic sympathetic nerves originating in the vasomotor center project onto cardiac sympathetic neurons in the intermediolateral gray of the upper thoracic spinal cord. From there preganglionic cardiac fibers converge mainly on the stellate ganglia and travel to join the parasympathetic fibers of the tenth cranial nerve, forming a plexus of mixed parasympathetic and sympathetic nerves that innervate the heart.

Sympathetic fibers innervate the sinus node, atria, atrioventricular node, ventricles, and coronary arteries. Preganglionic parasympathetic efferents from the nucleus ambiguus and the dorsal nucleus of the tenth cranial nerve travel with the tenth cranial nerve to the vicinity of the stellate ganglia, after which they course together with sympathetic fibers to innervate the heart. Parasympathetic fibers innervate mainly the sinus node, the atrioventricular node, and the atria. It appears that the sympathetic and parasympathetic nerves situated on the right side of the heart exert more effect on the sinus node than those on the left. Lesions affecting the heart rate feedback loop can

result in disorders of cardiac rate and rhythmicity. Tachycardia results from increased sympathetic discharge or from vagal dysfunction. Conversely, bradycardia results from sympathetic damage or excessive parasympathetic outflow.

The heart rate normally varies following inspiration and expiration. This is the respiratory sinus arrhythmia, which is mediated through the tenth cranial nerve and is dependent on the Bainbridge reflex (F. A. Bainbridge, British physiologist, 1874–1921). Lesions such as neuropathies that affect the integrity of the tenth cranial nerve result in decreased respiratory sinus arrhythmia and tachycardia at rest. The degree of denervation may vary from mild and subclinical as in early diabetic neuropathy to complete denervation in the transplanted heart. With complete denervation the heart rate responds mainly to the influence of circulating catecholamines and hormones. Heart rate responses to exercise and postural change are therefore slow (e.g., maximum heart rate rises occur after 5 minutes of standing). Physiologic aging is accompanied by a decrease in respiratory sinus arrhythmia and in other autonomic parameters.

Increased adrenoceptor stimulation does not usually induce arrhythmias in normal myocardium but may produce arrhythmias in the setting of cardiac ischemia. The main arrhythmogenic mechanisms include abnormal automaticity, after-depolarization, reentry, and triggered activity. Adrenergic stimulation reduces ventricular refractoriness (the arrhythmogenic shortening of the action potential may be opposed by endothelin-1 released during cardiac ischemia), lowers fibrillation thresholds, and promotes after-depolarizations, thus increasing the probability of cardiac arrhythmias. Conversely, enhanced parasympathetic tone may suppress arrhythmogenesis through direct effects on electrophysiologic mechanisms (but enhanced parasympathetic tone may also increase susceptibility to arrhythmias if it produces excessive bradycardia). Decreased heart rate variability is associated with an increased risk of sudden cardiac death (usually due to ventricular fibrillation) following myocardial infarction. In this circumstance vagal activation is thought to be protective.

Reflex Syncope

Diverse conditions such as carotid sinus sensitivity, glossopharyngeal neuralgia, aortic stenosis, hypertrophic cardiomyopathy, and inferior wall myocardial infarction can cause syncope by way of a common neural reflex that produces acute vasodilation in response to excessive afferent mechanoreceptor discharge. As opposed to neurogenic orthostatic hypotension, in which there is a defect in ANS pathways, the occurrence of reflex syncope implies the presence of functional ANS pathways.

The neurocardiogenic or vasovagal syncope (NCS), which has been studied extensively, is an example of a reflex mechanism that produces syncope. In patients with NCS and in normal individuals, the upright posture results in a progressive fall in venous return and cardiac output due to pooling of blood in the lower body. This combination triggers a reflex enhancement of sympathetic outflow, which increases cardiac contractility.

Current views on NCS propose that the increase in the force of myocardial contraction acting around a relatively empty heart chamber produces an exaggerated stimulation of ventricular mechanoreceptors. (Other hypotheses place the origin of exaggerated mechanoreceptor discharges in the atria and great veins.) Increased afferent mechanoreceptor discharges in turn trigger the von Bezold–Jarisch reflex (A. von Bezold, German physiologist, 1836–68, A. Jarisch, Austrian dermatologist, 1850–1902) producing vasodilation of resistance and capacitance vessels and bradycardia.

During syncope there may be an inappropriate heart rate response in the form of slowing (a vasovagal reaction), or there may be little change in heart rate (the vasodepressor reaction). During NCS microneurography recordings from peripheral sympathetic nerves show a sudden paradoxical reduction in sympathetic vasoconstrictor activity to muscle blood vessels, and plasma norepinephrine concentrations decrease, suggesting that vasodilation is due, at least in part, to sympathetic withdrawal. Because there is episodic, inappropriate slowing of the heart during NCS, it is believed that parasympathetic activity increases. It is not known however, whether disturbed autonomic cardiovascular regulation is present continuously in patients with NCS and if so, whether this predisposes to or causes syncope.

Although the trigger initiating this reflex autonomic response has not been identified, increased sympathetic cardiac stimulation before syncope may play an important role. However, recent reports of NCS in heart transplant patients (in whom afferent ventricular mechanoreceptor pathways are presumed to be interrupted) suggest that an alternate mechanism may be responsible for this syndrome in this setting. A possible role of CNS opiate mechanisms producing inhibition of sympathetic outflow during NCS has been proposed on the basis that indications that opiate receptor blockade reverses sympathetic withdrawal during hemorrhage in experimental animals. Syncope in response to emotional or pain stimuli may occur through a purely central mechanism that bypasses mechanoreceptor pathways.

Hyperthermia and Hypothermia

Thermoregulation, key to human survival, results in a body temperature that is maintained within narrow limits by the balance between heat production and heat loss. Thermoregulation is controlled mainly through convective and evaporative heat loss mechanisms. Changes in core temperature are sensed by thermosensitive neurons in the anterior hypothalamus, the brainstem, and the spinal cord. Afferent information is integrated in the hypothalamus, where core temperature is compared with the set point. Complex autonomic, endocrine and somatic responses are integrated by the ANS to match body temperature with the hypothalamic set point temperature.

A rise in core temperature leads to reflex vasodilation (convective heat loss) and increased sweat production (evaporative heat loss). Conversely, a decrease in core temperature produces a reflex increase in shivering by skeletal muscle (an involuntary thermogenic somatic function), cutaneous vasoconstriction, and decreased sweating. Complex thermoregulatory behaviors include seeking shelter, adjusting clothing, avoiding extreme environments, and other measures that assist in reaching thermoregulatory objectives.

Although thermoregulatory responses are generalized, cutaneous centrally mediated vasoconstriction and sweat production responses can be modified locally by the effect of temperature on effector organs. Of clinical significance, thermoregulation (together with other ANS homeostatic functions) is episodically depressed during sleep or by medications rendering the individual more susceptible to changes in ambient temperature.

Fever occurs when the hypothalamic set point is raised by pyrogenic substances and an intact thermoregulatory feedback loop raises body temperature to match the raised set point. In hyperthermia, the set point is normal (36° to 37.5°C) but thermoregulatory mechanisms are unable to eliminate enough heat. With hypothermia physiologic mechanisms involved in generating or conserving heat are dysfunctional or overwhelmed by low ambient temperatures. Hypothermia may occur with central (e.g., hypothalamic) or peripheral (e.g., spinal cord) lesions. Hypothermia with high spinal cord lesions results from the inability to prevent heat loss (vasoconstriction is deficient) and increase heat production (shivering is deficient).

Normal thermoregulatory sweating requires intact pre- and postganglionic efferent pathways. Sweating abnormalities (hyper- or hypohidrosis) may be focal or generalized. Focal abnormalities may have localizing value (e.g., a band of hyperhidrosis above a spinal cord lesion or the absence of facial sweating in Horner's syndrome). Areas of hypohidrosis may be present with peripheral nerve lesions (e.g., leprosy) or with peripheral neuropathies (e.g., distal "stocking" sweating deficits in diabetic or alcoholic neuropathies). More diffuse hypohidrosis may accompany primary autonomic failure. Generalized hyperhidrosis can result from situations in which there is increased sympathetic discharge and in tetanus.

Essential hyperhidrosis, a frequent condition of unknown etiology, usually involves hands, feet, and axillae. Excessive sweating without appropriate thermal stimuli is the hallmark of this condition. Definitive treatment usually involves sympathectomy.

Bladder Dysfunction

Normal urinary function relies on the integrity of autonomic mechanisms in the brain and the spinal cord. Afferent information from bladder mechanoreceptors travels through the parasympathetic pelvic nerves to the sacral spinal cord and through the sympathetic hypogastric and inferior splanchnic nerves to the lumbar spinal cord. Increases in bladder wall tension result in increased receptor discharge. Afferents from the striated sphincter and the urethra convey the sense of passage of urine through the pudendal nerve to the dorsal horns of the sacral spinal cord. Parasympathetic neurons with cell bodies in the S2–S4 intermediolateral gray send axons to ganglion cells in the pelvic plexus and the bladder wall via pelvic nerves.

Postganglionic neurons stimulate bladder smooth muscle contractions through release of ACh and NANC transmitters from their terminals. Sympathetic postganglionic neurons from lower thoracic and lumbar sympathetic chains travel to the bladder via hypogastric sympathetic nerves. β-Adrenoceptor stimulation inhibits the detrusor muscle, α-stimulation produces contraction of the bladder base and urethra, and α_2-stimulation inhibits, whereas α_1 enhances, parasympathetic activity of the ganglion cells. The somatic external muscle sphincter (and the anal sphincter) innervation originates in Onuf's nucleus in the sacral ventral horn and travels via the pudendal nerve. In addition, an extensive peptidergic neural network influences bladder function. The role of these nerves in human disease has not been elucidated.

Bladder filling occurs passively and depends on the properties of bladder smooth muscle and the ability to inhibit parasympathetic efferent pathways. Despite increasing volume during filling, bladder pressures remain low to permit continuous urine flow from the ureter. As filling progresses, there is increased sphincter constriction to prevent leakage of urine.

Voiding can be triggered either reflexly or voluntarily. Reflex voiding occurs when bladder volume exceeds a threshold (the micturition threshold). Increased bladder mechanoreceptor firing triggers sacral parasympathetic discharges, which produce detrusor muscle contraction and inhibit sympathetic and somatic efferents that relax the sphincters. Passage of urine through the urethra further enhances bladder contraction and ensures full emptying.

Voluntary voiding is controlled by the CNS and is dependent on the integrity of pathways involving the medial frontal gyrus and anterior cingulate lobes of the frontal lobe, the hypothalamus, the paracentral lobule, the brainstem, and spinal cord (lesions of the cortical areas disinhibit the excitatory hypothalamic effect on brainstem micturition centers). During voluntary voiding relaxation of the urethral sphincter and pelvic floor is accompanied by abdominal and diaphragmatic muscle contraction. Voiding commences once reflex detrusor contractions are triggered in response to increased bladder pressures. Voiding can be interrupted by voluntary contraction of the external sphincter.

Interruption of any of the reflex pathways results in urinary symptoms. Spinal shock produces complete loss of bladder function with initial retention of urine, excessive bladder filling, and overflow incontinence. With return of independent sacral parasympathetic function, bladder detrusor muscle contraction occurs, with lower volumes and pressures (neurogenic bladder). With destruction of the sacral cord pathways voluntary micturition is absent but reflex storage and voiding are still possible. With the denervated (or autonomous neurogenic) bladder, in which there is dysfunction of afferent and efferent parasympathetic innervation, both voluntary and reflex voiding are absent. Interruption of the posterior roots results in the atonic (or tabetic) neurogenic bladder, in which there is high residual bladder volume and inability to initiate micturition despite a sometimes intact sensation of bladder fullness.

Sexual Dysfunction

Normal sexual function relies on the integrity of the sexual response cycle, which is triggered by erotic stimuli and consists of four response phases (excitation, plateau, orgasm, and restoration). Despite anatomic differences, the physiologic responses (vascular, secretory, and smooth and skeletal muscle actions) involved are similar in both sexes.

With reflexogenic penile or clitoral erection, afferents travel from the perineal skin and soft tissue receptors to the sacral cord via the pudendal nerves. Interneurons within the cord integrate the parasympathetic response, which travels to the penis via preganglionic pelvic nerve fibers and then through postganglionic fibers to the trabecular muscle of the corpora cavernosa. Parasympathetic stimulation produces engorgement of the penis by releasing nitric oxide (a gaseous NANC transmitter), which relaxes the trabecular muscle and allows blood to fill the sinusoids. These compress the venules of the corpora against the tunica albuginea, resulting in outflow obstruction and thus engorgement. Psychogenic erections, which are initiated by a variety of complex stimuli, rely on intact supraspinal centers (hypothalamic and limbic) and lumbar sympathetic pathways. The sympathetic efferents travel with hypogastric, pelvic, and pudendal nerves. This anatomic distribution explains why sacral cord or cauda equina lesions abolish parasympathetic reflexogenic but still allow sympathetic psychogenic erections to occur.

The opposite occurs with lesions of the cord above the T12 segment. In men, during emission, sympathetic efferents produce closure of the internal urinary sphincter and contraction of the vas deferens, seminal vesicles, and prostate and propel semen and gland secretions into the posterior urethra. Ejaculation results from activation of thoracolumbar (T12–L2) sympathetic neurons, which travel through the pudendal nerves to produce contraction of the bulbocavernosus, ischiocavernosus, and periurethral muscles. In women these muscles produce rhythmic perineal contractions during orgasm.

With autonomic dysfunction erectile and ejaculatory impotence is frequent. In this situation erectile impotence responds to intracavernous injection of papaverine. If vascular pathology precludes erection, the response to papaverine is absent. Retrograde ejaculation (into the bladder) results from failure of the bladder neck to contract at the time of ejaculation. It is a common problem in diabetics with autonomic failure and as a sequela of prostate surgery.

Gastrointestinal Dysfunction

Normal gut motility, secretion, absorption, and blood flow rely on intact enteric (intrinsic) and sympathetic and parasympathetic (extrinsic) innervation. Lesions affecting the intrinsic innervation (e.g., amyloid infiltration of gut smooth muscle) cause constipation and intestinal pseudo-obstruction (symptoms and signs of intestinal obstruction in the absence of obstructive intestinal lesions). Lesions that interrupt the extrinsic innervation (such as neuropathies) affect coordinated peristalsis and result in hypo- or hypermotility states. In the absence of mechanical obstruction, dysphagia, regurgitation of food, bloating, and vomiting reflect esophageal and gastric autonomic involvement. Colic, abdominal distension, constipation, and diarrhea (which may be due in part to bacterial overgrowth) reflect small and large bowel autonomic dysfunction.

Diminished gastric motility causing gastroparesis,

PUPILLARY SYNDROMES

Sympathetic dysfunction
　　Horner's syndrome
　　　　Small irregular pupils, ptosis, decreased intraocular pressure, conjunctival vasodilation (acute), decreased accommodation, decreased facial sweating, increased facial temperature; intact facial sweating with postganglionic lesion
Parasympathetic dysfunction
　　Argyll-Robertson pupils
　　　　Small irregular pupils, poor response to light, respond to accommodation, constrict with physostigmine, and dilate poorly with atropine (central lesion)
　　Tonic pupil
　　　　Poor response to light and near accommodation, denervation supersensitivity (postganglionic lesion); accompanied by decreased deep tendon reflexes in Adie's syndrome

---

frequent in diabetes, presents as early satiety and postprandial nausea and vomiting, which when severe can lead to malnutrition. Diabetic gastroparesis has been attributed to vagal neuropathy and the effects of abnormal gut neuropeptide function. Numerous drugs (e.g., those with anticholinergic, adrenergic, or dopaminergic effects) can cause delayed gastric emptying. Diarrhea may result in part from the effects of bacterial overgrowth and decreased bile acid absorption (which promote steatorrhea and watery bowel movements).

Pupillary Syndromes

Interruption of sympathetic pathways from the hypothalamus to the superior cervical ganglia (central and preganglionic lesions) result in Horner's syndrome (miosis, ptosis, facial anhydrosis, decreased intraocular pressure, decreased accommodation, and iris depigmentation) (Fig. 34-6). Lesions between the hypothalamus and the ciliospinal center of Budge-Waller (J. L. Budge, German physiologist, 1811–88, A. V. Waller, British physiologist, 1816–70) in the spinal cord (caused by central lesions) usually result from cerebrovascular disease or tumor. Those occurring between the ciliospinal center and the superior cervical

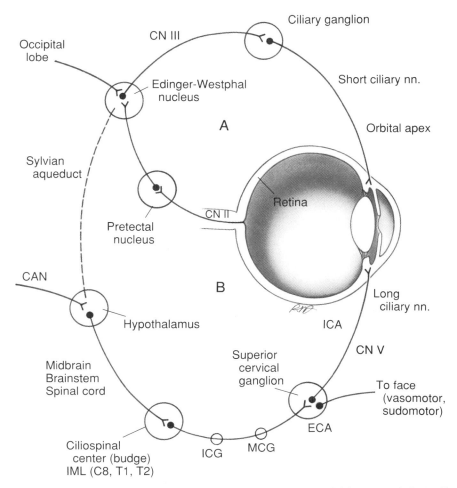

Figure 34-6. Neuronal pathways involved in pupillary constriction and dilation and clinically significant anatomic relations. **(A)** Pupillary constriction. Afferent fibers from the retina subserving the light reflex travel with the optic tract to synapse in the pretectal nuclei in the midbrain. Fibers from the pretectal nuclei, together with fibers originating in the occipital cortex subserving the accommodation reflex, project to both Edinger-Westphal parasympathetic nuclei in the anterior midbrain (bilateral projections allow a consensual pupillary response). Fibers leave the Edinger-Westphal nuclei, traveling uncrossed with the cranial nerve III, and synapse on cell bodies in the ciliary ganglia. Postganglionic fibers course with the short ciliary nerves to the ciliary and iris sphincter muscles, which produce accommodation and pupillary constriction. **(B)** Pupillary dilation. Sympathetic activation produces inhibition of the Edinger-Westphal nuclei via fibers from the posterior hypothalamus and contraction of the radial fibers of the dilator muscle of the pupil through a polysynaptic pathway. Fibers from the first-order neurons originating in the hypothalamus travel uncrossed through the brainstem to synapse in the ciliospinal center of Budge-Waller in the intermediolateral (IML) cell columns of the low cervical and high thoracic spinal cord. Fibers from second-order (preganglionic) neurons leave the spinal cord with the first two thoracic ventral roots, travel through the inferior (ICG) and middle cervical ganglia (MCG) to synapse in the superior cervical ganglia. Postganglionic fibers travel with the cranial nerve V through the superior orbital fissure and leave via the long ciliary nerves to innervate the dilator pupillae muscle, which dilates the pupil. ICA, internal carotid artery; ECA, external carotid artery; CAN, central autonomic network.

ganglia usually result from from low cervical and high thoracic region damage (trauma or tumors). Lesions distal to the superior cervical ganglia (postganglionic lesions) spare facial vaso- and sudomotor functions. These are produced by extra- and intracranial regional pathology (e.g., carotid artery, cavernous sinus).

The modern view is that disinhibition of the parasympathetic Edinger-Westphal nucleus by lesions situated in the ciliary ganglion results in Argyll-Robertson pupils (miotic irregular pupils, which respond poorly to light but accommodate well). Other central causes of parasympathetic disinhibition include the miotic pupils seen with sleep or narcolepsy, after exercise, and with use of drugs such as narcotics (where central disinhibition is accompanied by a local miotic effect). Postganglionic lesions (distal to the ciliary ganglion) causing parasympathetic dysfunction may result in tonic pupils (poor constriction in response to to light and near reflexes). Tonic pupils may occur in isolation or in association with loss of deep tendon reflexes, as in Adie's syndrome. (See also Ch. 27.)

Pain

Sympathetically maintained pain encompasses a variety of painful disorders that develop as result of trauma affecting the limbs, after visceral diseases or CNS lesions, or even spontaneously. The syndrome consists of pain and sensory abnormalities, abnormal blood flow, and sweating, and trophic changes are present in various combinations. Pain is usually burning (causalgic), and may be accompanied by hyperalgesias, which is frequently distributed beyond dermatomal, peripheral nerve, or plexus patterns. This syndrome is present with causalgia, reflex sympathetic dystrophy, shoulder-hand syndrome, and various other painful disorders.

Causalgia (Greek: *kausis,* burn) refers to burning pain, allodynia, and hyperpathia following injury of a peripheral nerve (see also Ch. 23). The clinical manifestations of reflex sympathetic dystrophy are similar to those present with causalgia, but there is no antecedent damage to a major peripheral nerve (usually nerve damage is minor). Involvement commences with a limb and can spread to other sites and be followed by trophic changes.

Sympathetically maintained pain is considered to be a primary autonomic disorder due to the presence of pain that improves following sympathetic blockade and to the prominent vasomotor, sudomotor, thermoregulatory, and trophic features that bespeak sympathetic dysfunction. The site of the sympathetic lesion (afferent or efferent pathways) has not yet been defined. A role of sympathetic dysfunction in sympathetically maintained pain has also been questioned on the grounds of a lack of rigorous scientific evidence implicating the sympathetic nervous system. To some investigators, autonomic abnormalities occur as epiphenomena and result from, among other causes underlying non-neurologic abnormalities, the effects of a locally mediated antidromic release of vasodilator substances, or immobility due to pain. The inconsistent response of pain to sympathetic blockade has also been cited as supportive evidence against a primary autonomic etiology in sympathetically mediated pain.

Treatment of sympathetically mediated pain involves sympathetic blockade. This can be done by regional block (usually intravenous phenoxybenzamine, bretylium, or guanethidine or steroids); by infiltration of sympathetic ganglia with local anesthetics, narcotics, and other agents such as phenol (chemical sympathectomy); or by surgical or radiofrequency ablation. The effects are not always predictable. Many patients require repeated blocks. Side effects include postsympathectomy pain in the sympathectomized area, in addition to autonomic symptoms expected from sympathectomy. Oral anticonvulsants and antidepressants may be of benefit in controlling postsympathectomy pain.

The role of the ANS in the genesis of migrainous and cluster headache attacks remains controversial. The abnormalities of pupils and other ANS function found during attacks and during interval (pain-free) periods in cluster headache may represent manifestations of the underlying process rather than the cause of attacks of pain. Similarly, in migraine the vasomotor and other sympathetic dysfunctions during headache-free periods are best regarded as epiphenomena until the pathogenesis of this disorder is elucidated.

EXERCISE, AGING AND THE AUTONOMIC NERVOUS SYSTEM

Autonomic Responses to Exercise

The autonomic responses to exercise are complex and require intact ANS pathways. Upon initiating a movement, the brainstem cardiovascular centers receive afferents from higher centers (the "central command") proportional to the muscle recruitment needed. A brief initial fall in blood pressure is followed by an increase in heart rate, blood pressure, and respiration, which allow adequate perfusion of active muscles. Increased sympathetic vasomotor outflow produces vasoconstriction, with redistribution of cardiac output to muscle and away from the splanchnic circulation. Accompanying this response there is a resetting of the baroreflex, which allows higher blood pressures to be achieved during exercise. Stimulation of muscle chemoreceptors (ergoreceptors) by local factors produced during muscle contraction promotes an increase in

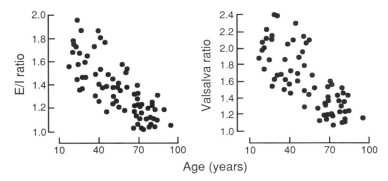

Figure 34-7. Heart rate variability in response to deep breathing and Valsalva's maneuver decline with advancing age in normal control subjects. E/I, expiration/inspiration ratio. Deep breathing, n = 76; Valsalva's ratio, n = 68. (See also Ch. 16.)

blood pressure, which further facilitates muscle perfusion. Also, metabolites produced by contracting muscle interfere with the release of norepinephrine at sympathetic nerve terminals and thus result in vasodilation, which permits increased muscle perfusion.

Chronic exercise that results in physical conditioning produces, among other effects, an increased vagal and a decreased sympathetic tone. Therefore, training may benefit patients with many conditions associated with enhanced sympathetic outflow such as hypertension, arrhythmias, myocardial infarction, patients at risk for sudden cardiac death, and also those with diabetes mellitus.

Age-Related Changes in Autonomic Function

Autonomic parameters used to measure autonomic function show a gradual decline with advancing age (Fig. 34-7). The decline in autonomic function with aging in part reflects age-related ANS cell loss. With aging, loss of axons in small, myelinated and unmyelinated fibers is accompanied by decreased effector organ response to neurotransmitters, resulting in declining autonomic function. Some neurotransmitters, notably norepinephrine, increase in the circulation with advancing age. An increase in this transmitter in perivascular nerves has also been found in the aged.

The decline in autonomic function with aging is not uniform: there is clear variation among individuals in the same age group. This variability may reflect the degree of physical conditioning, and cultural, dietary, and genetic factors. For example, physically conditioned elderly individuals have autonomic responses similar to those of far younger individuals. As compared with inactive individuals of similar age, those who are physically conditioned have a lower resting heart rate, increased stroke volume and cardiac output, and diminished total peripheral resistance. Thus, it is believed that physical training may delay the effects of aging on the ANS. Although it seems reasonable to assume that the salutory effects of physical conditioning may apply to other parts of the nervous system and other organs, this still remains to be established.

ANNOTATED BIBLIOGRAPHY

Abboud FM. Neurocardiogenic syncope. N Engl J Med 1993;328:1117–20.

Editorial.

Appenzeller O. The Autonomic Nervous System. An Introduction to Basic and Clinical Concepts. 4th Ed. Elsevier, Amsterdam, 1990.

Standard textbook.

Burnstock G, Milner P. Structural and chemical organization of the autonomic nervous system with special reference to non-adrenergic, non-cholinergic transmission. In Bannister R, Mathias CJ (eds). Autonomic Failure. A textbook of Clinical Disorders of the Autonomic Nervous System. 3rd Ed. Oxford University Press, Oxford, 1992, p. 107.

Neurochemical details.

Chapleau MW, Hajduckzok G, Abboud FM. Paracrine modulation of baroreceptor activity by vascular endothelium. News Physiol Sci 1991;6:210.

Vascular endothelium plays a role in baroreceptor responses.

Clerc N. Organisation fonctionelle du système nerveux autonome. In Serratrice G, Pellissier JF, Pouget J, Blin O (eds). Le Système Nerveux Autonome: Acquisitions Recentes. Expansion Scientifique Française, Paris, 1991, p. 5.

Review article.

Henry P, Brochet B, Tison F. Systeme nerveux autonome et maladie migraineuse. In Serratrice G, Pellissier JF, Pouget J, Blin O (eds). Le Système Nerveux Autonome:

Acquisitions Recentes. Expansion Scientifique Française, Paris, 1991, p. 218.

Details of ANS disorders in migraine.

Kaufmann H, Oribe E, Yahr MD. Differential effect of L-threo-3,4-dihydroxyphenylserine in pure autonomic failure and multiple system atrophy with autonomic failure. J Neural Trans 1991;3:143–8.

Benefits in patients with multisystem atrophy but not with pure autonomic failure.

Lance JW. The pathophysiology of migraine. In Dalessio D, Silberstein SD (eds): Wolff's Headache and Other Head Pain. 6th Ed. Oxford University Press, New York, 1993, p. 59.

Review article.

Loewy AD, Spyer KM (eds). Central Regulation of Autonomic Function. Oxford University Press, New York, 1990

Comprehensive review.

Ludbrook J, Evans R. Posthemorrhagic syncope. News Physiol Sci 1989;4:120.

Role of opioids

Ralevic V, Burnstock G. Neural-endothelial interactions in the control of local vascular tone. RG Landes, Austin, 1993.

Details of vasomotor control.

Robertson D. Orthostatic hypotension. In: Melmon KL, Morelli H (eds). Clinical Pharmacology. McGraw-Hill, New York, 1992, p. 84.

Comprehensive review.

Rowell LB. Human Cardiovascular Control. Oxford University Press, New York, 1993.

Comprehensive review.

Wallin BG. Intraneural recordings of normal and abnormal sympathetic activity in man. In Bannister R, Mathias CJ (eds): Autonomic Failure. A Textbook of Clinical Disorders of the Autonomic Nervous System. 3rd Ed. Oxford University Press, Oxford, 1992, p. 657.

Changes in age.

Section IV
Diseases of the
Nervous System

35

Ischemic Stroke

J. C. Gautier and J. P. Mohr

Ischemia (Greek: *iskhein*, to stop; *haima*, blood) is a critical decrease of the blood supply of a living tissue. Cerebral ischemia can be generalized (e.g., when due to cardiac arrest), or it can be focal, in the territory of a particular vessel. The clinical counterpart of focal cerebral ischemia is ischemic stroke as opposed to hemorrhagic stroke (see Ch. 5).

Ischemic infarctions make up 80 to 85 percent of all strokes (see also Ch. 5). The large majority of ischemic strokes result from disorders of the arterial circulation, a few from disorders of the venous circulation. Both as emergencies and as chronic disabling, distressing cases, they are the most frequent diseases seen by neurologists. Moreover, because the infarcts are sharply limited, often small, experimental-like lesions, they have been and are the main basis of neurologic semiology. C. Miller Fisher's words, "Neurology is learnt stroke by stroke," may be verified every day by juniors (and seniors).

ARTERIAL STROKES

Focal Cerebral Ischemia

To approach clinical issues, it is basic to have in mind an overview of the cerebral arterial supply, the development of thrombi in the arteries and heart, and the concept of perfusion failure. The following review provides a refresher in anatomy, emphasizing points of physiologic and pathophysiologic interest and leaving out most of the numerous anatomic variations that reflect the many changes of the cerebral arterial patterns during ontogeny.

Carotid and Vertebrobasilar Arterial Systems

The brain is supplied by two pairs of arteries, the carotids and the vertebrals. The right common carotid artery arises from the innominate, the left from the aortic arch (Figs. 35-1 and 35-2). At the level of the superior border of the thyroid cartilage, below and behind the angle of the jaw (there are variations of several centimeters above and below), the common carotid artery bifurcates into the internal carotid artery (ICA) and external carotid artery (ECA). The ICA ascends to the skull and brain with no important collaterals, while the ECA immediately divides into many branches for the neck and face. The ECA branches anastomose freely with their counterparts from the opposite side and with other neighboring arteries from the subclavian, including the vertebral artery near the base of the skull.

At its origin, the ICA is dilated to form a sinus or bulb, about 20 mm long, distal to which its caliber remains constant at about 5 mm. Close to the common carotid bifurcation are the carotid body, a chemoreceptor, and the nerve of the carotid sinus, which responds to stretching of the arterial wall by lowering blood pressure and slowing the heart.

The bifurcation is rather superficial, covered only by the sternocleidomastoid muscle and thus easily accessible to palpation (not to be done, see below), auscultation, insonation, trauma, and surgery. The ICA in the neck is usually straight, although in at least one-third of people it shows some tortuosity, kinking or coiling. During its extracranial course it is crossed by the lower cranial nerves, which accounts for their possible paralysis in ICA dissections. This condition also frequently causes a Claude Bernard-Horner syndrome due to involvement of the ascending sympathetic fibers traveling along the carotid from their origin in the superior cervical sympathetic ganglion (see Chs. 27 and 34). At the base of the skull, the ICA is just behind the transverse process of the atlas and can be bruised in sudden, forceful extension of the neck, a cause of ICA dissection. The ICA then enters the bony canal of the temporal bone, coursing dorsomedi-

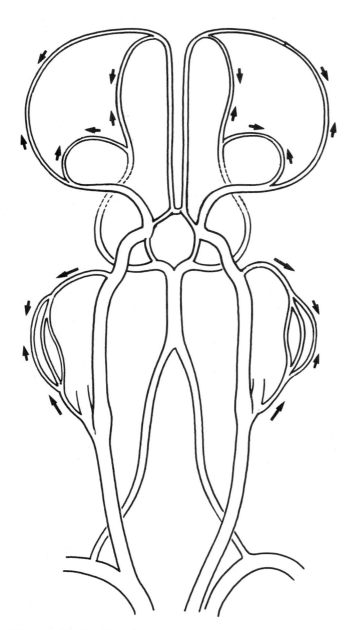

Figure 35-1. The cerebral arterial tree. Arrows indicate where, at each systole, blood flows meet at a dead point at middistance in the potential collateral channels. The external carotid artery—ophthalmic artery bypass is shown on both sides.

blood, and this site is classic for the development of arteriovenous fistula. The cavernous sinus is just behind the eye, so that the siphon can be auscultated and insonated through the ocular globe (see Ch. 13).

The ICA then becomes truly intracranial by piercing the dura, medial to the anterior clinoid process, passing upward and laterally below the optic nerve. This short stretch, usually less than 1 cm long, gives off in succession the ophthalmic artery, the posterior communication artery (Post Com A), and the anterior choroidal artery (AChA). The ophthalmic artery, the only collateral of significant size (others arising more proximally in the intracranial ICA are usually mere

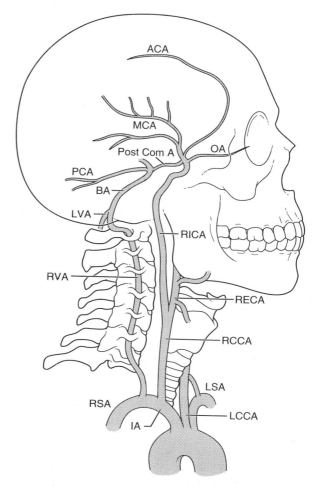

Figure 35-2. The cerebral arterial tree. A lateral view from the right. IA, innominate artery; RSA, right subclavian artery; RCCA, right common carotid artery; LCCA, left common carotid artery; LSA, left subclavian artery; RICA, right internal carotid artery; RECA, right external carotid artery; RVA, right vertebral artery; LVA, left vertebral artery; OA, ophthalmic artery; ACA, anterior cerebral artery; MCA, middle cerebral artery, PCA, posterior cerebral artery; Post Com A, posterior communicating artery. The anterior choroidal artery is not depicted.

ally to pass over the cartilage filling the foramen lacerum just beneath the gasserian ganglion, and then penetrates the cavernous sinus.

The cavernous portion of the ICA, 5 to 6 cm long, runs forward on the lateral aspect of the sella turcica, becoming more tortuous with age to form the S-shaped carotid siphon (Fig. 35-2). Within the cavernous sinus the artery is crossed by the third, fourth, fifth, and sixth cranial nerves. It is bathed in venous tiny twigs), enters the optic foramen with the optic nerve en route to the orbit to give rise to many branches, among which is the central retinal artery (see Ch. 26). The Post Com A runs dorsal to the posterior cerebral artery (PCA). Immediately after giving off these branches, the ICA bifurcates into the anterior (ACA) and middle cerebral (MCA) arteries (Figs. 35-1 and 35-2).

The *trigeminal artery,* a fairly frequent variant, results from the persistence of a fetal artery, which arises from the ICA as it enters the cavernous sinus and runs caudally to join the basilar artery, generally between the superior cerebellar (SCA) and anterior inferior cerebellar (AICA) arteries.

The *vertebral artery* is the first branch of the subclavian artery (Figs. 35-1, 35-2). Customarily, its course is divided into four segments. First, the artery runs dorsally and cephalad to enter the costotransverse foramen of the C6 (occasionally C5 or C7) vertebra to begin its intraosseous course cephalad. Here it is close to the stellate ganglion. Second, it courses in the transverse foramina from C6 to the axis. Third, the vertebral artery emerges from the transverse foramen of C2 and courses laterally to the transverse foramen of the atlas; after exiting, the artery makes a loop circling the posterior arch of C1 between the atlas and occiput. Fourth, it pierces the atlanto-occipital membrane and dura and becomes intracranial. At the pontomedullary junction both vertebral arteries unite to form the basilar artery. This fourth segment gives off the posterior inferior cerebellar artery (PICA). The basilar artery in turn gives branches to the brainstem and cerebellum (AICA and SCA), and at the pontopeduncular junction it bifurcates into the right and left PCAs. The vertebral artery provides the "roots" of the anterior spinal artery.

During its course in the neck, the vertebral artery is in close relationship with the cervical spine and craniospinal junction. This makes it vulnerable to trauma, especially forced movements of the spine and head. Inequalities of size between the two vertebral arteries are common, and one of these arteries can be so small as to be undetectable by ultrasound. Consequently, its nondetection makes it difficult to infer whether it is occluded. The artery can terminate in the PICA, in which case the distal segment that joins the BA is hypoplastic or absent. The artery can be auscultated and insonated in its first and third segments (see Ch. 13).

Pericerebral and Intracerebral Arteries

Unlike viscera that have a hilum and a centrifugal arterial supply (e.g., lung, liver, kidney), the brain, like the heart, has a centripetal arterial supply (i.e., the brain is enveloped by an arterial network from which

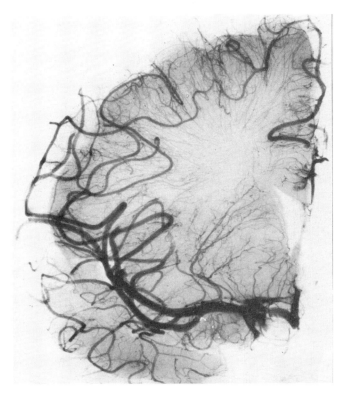

Figure 35-3. Pericerebral and perforator arteries. Author's specimen injected with lead carbonate. (From Russel, 1983, with permission.)

nutrient arteries perforate the tissue) (Fig. 35-3). Therefore these arteries, which penetrate the parenchyma, are also termed *perforators.* The brain vessels that make up the superficial network are the main branches of the ICA, the vertebral and basilar arteries, the PCA, and their ramifications.

Collateral Systems

When occluded at or beyond its origin, the extracranial ICA depends solely on the ophthalmic artery, whose orbital branches anastomose with those of the ECA around the rim of the orbit (ECA-ophthalmic bypass). This supply from the ECA is rarely sufficient to replace the normally robust flows from the ICA. By contrast, the extracranial vertebral artery has many anastomoses with branches of the subclavian and ECA that supply muscles and viscera in the neck, and occlusion of the vertebral artery below the skull base is often well compensated by collaterals.

Intracranially, the circle of Willis (Thomas Willis, 1621–1675, British physician and anatomist) is made by the anterior communicating artery (Ant Com A), which unites both ACAs, and the Post Com As, which unites the ICAs with the PCAs. It is a potentially major

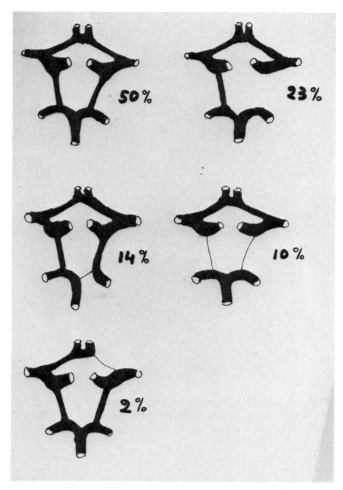

Figure 35-4. Main variants of the circle of Willis. (From Barnett et al., 1992, with permission.)

device for blood transfer from one ICA to the other and from the vertebrobasilar to the carotid circulation, or conversely. However, the circle is intact (i.e., has all its pieces of a significant size) in only 50 percent of people. In the remaining 50 percent, some defect impairs its functioning in one or several ways (Fig. 35-4). The functional value of the circle is essential in determining whether proximal ICA occlusion will cause cerebral infarction. Likewise, it is most important to know this value prior to carotid surgery, which implies temporary clamping of the artery.

Over the surface of the brain, meningeal anastomoses unite end to end the branches of the pericerebral and pericerebellar arteries in the border zones of their territories (Fig. 35-1) (see Ch. 5). There are many individual variations in number and size of these channels, but only rarely are the end-to-end anastomotic channels large enough to support instant retrograde flow

from one territory to another in the event of occlusion of a major cerebral artery or a branch thereof.

In the conditions of normal circulation, the anastomotic systems remain, in the main, potential. At each systole, blood flows meet and stop at a circulatory dead point around the orbit, roughly mid-distance in the Ant Com A and Post Com A and in the meningeal anastomoses (Fig. 35-1). Likewise, in the basilar artery, blood from both vertebral arteries flows side by side, usually without mixing.

Arrest of flow in one of these channels causes an instantaneous shift of the circulatory dead points (i.e., collateral circulation). However, to compensate efficiently for a suddenly occluded artery, the collateral channels must supply immediately an adequate volume of blood. This requires sufficient size (not always the case, see above) and sufficient blood pressure (a reason clinicians are reluctant to lower blood pressure much in ischemic strokes). Such propitious conditions obtain in some occlusions of the proximal ICA (clinically silent occlusions), or they may occur many times a day since vigorous rotation of the head is said to block the contralateral vertebral artery. In many cases, however, this immediate compensation is insufficient because of the small size or absence of the collateral vessels or because of unfavorable circulatory conditions (e.g., hypotension, increased blood viscosity). Another and major reason is that the material occluding the artery may be beyond the circle of Willis, which eliminates any role for it (see also below). Once occlusion is established, the size of functioning collateral channels increases with time, usually far too late to reduce the original risk of ischemia. This means that abundant ("superb") collateralizations seen on angiograms obtained long after strokes do not necessarily reveal the circulatory conditions at the time of the arterial occlusion. All too often, such rich collateralizations have developed only long after the stroke and perfuse only the old scars of infarction.

Last but not least is the question of how and when the collateral channels are set into action. Obviously, a gradient of pressure is necessary, which is expected to occur where there is arterial occlusion. With stenoses, however, the conditions favoring development of collateral flow are not so easily predicted. Mild to moderate stenoses reducing the arterial lumen by 40 to 70 percent have no such hemodynamic effect (i.e., they do not decrease flow or pressure). To become hemodynamically significant, a stenosis of average length must reduce the lumen by 75 percent and probably even more, 85 to 90 percent in many cases. For the often measured ICA in the neck, the critical cross-sectional area of the remaining lumen appears to be just about 2 mm². Any further reduction of the lumen diameter has dramatic effects on flow and pressure.

In practice, it is rare that angiograms demonstrate collateralization consequent to stenoses. Doppler ultrasound has been somewhat more sensitive in demonstrating such collaterals, but the available evidence shows that, with some exceptions, stenoses set collaterals into action only when extremely severe. The common belief that collaterals develop pari passu as stenosis increases is probably wishful thinking. As almost all thrombotic occlusions (see below) occur before or soon after stenoses have become hemodynamically significant, the collateral systems are usually caught unprepared by the sudden, profound circulatory change set up by arterial occlusion.

Parenchymatous Intracerebral Arteries

The vessels within the substance of the brain are end arteries. As soon as they leave the pericerebral network, penetrators behave as end arteries (Fig. 35-3) (see Ch. 5). Although there are microscopic anastomoses with neighboring penetrators, these provide no sources of collateral flow to compensate for the occlusion of a penetrator. The inevitable result for such occlusions is an infarct whose extent is the whole territory of the occluded penetrator.

Disease arising within the penetrator (e.g., lipohyalinosis, see below) confines the infarct to a single vessel. However, when the occluding material (anterograde thrombi, emboli) affects the origin of a major cerebral artery (e.g., the MCA), the material is usually long enough to occludes the ostia of those penetrators arising along the occluded arterial segment. At postmortem the extent of the infarct, gathering together the territories of several or many single penetrators is often strikingly proportional to the length of the occluding material along (Fig. 35-5), indicating the lack of collaterals for the penetrators and the adequate functioning of the collateral channels over the brain surface, sparing the cerebral surface branches. Failure of the cerebral surface collaterals gives rise to additional infarction over the brain surface distal to the occlusion (see also Ch. 5).

Thrombogenesis, Thrombi, Emboli

The vast majority of cerebral arterial occlusions are due either to local thrombus or to emboli broken off from arterial or cardiac thrombus.

First, and contrary to frequent improper terminology in some articles and books, the terms *thrombus* and *clot* are not synonyms. A thrombus is not a clot. A clot is blood solidified outside a vessel, (e.g., in a glass cup). Clotting results from the clotting process. At the microscopic level a clot consists of closely but randomly packed blood cells in a network of fibrin.

By contrast, a thrombus is blood solidified within a vessel (artery, vein, cardiac chamber). It results from

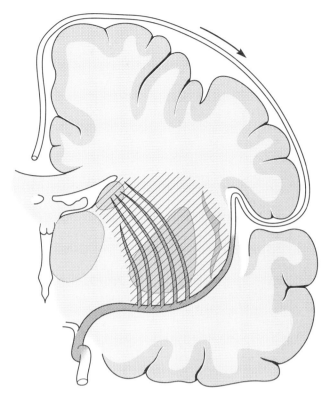

Figure 35-5. Occlusion of pericerebral arteries for more than a few moments inevitably causes infarction, as shown. Here the occluding material is an anterograde thrombus, originating from a proximal ICA primary occlusion, but it could as well be a long embolus. Hatched area: infarct (see Ch. 5). The extent of the infarct depends on the length of the occluding material and the capacity of the meningeal anastomoses *(arrow).*

thrombogenesis, not coagulation. Thrombi not only have a microscopic structure different from that of clots, but they have structures differing according to the vessel in which they have formed. Where blood flow is slow or stagnant, the structure of a thrombus resembles that of a clot, since it consists of closely packed red cells enmeshed in strands of fibrin. In arteries, where blood flow is rapid, thrombi cannot form simply through the process of stagnation. The triggering factor for thrombus formation is the loss of a fundamental property of the normal arterial endothelium namely active inhibition of the adhesion of circulating platelets. This loss of adhesion inhibition occurs in many diseases, detailed further below.

Thrombosis

Atherosclerosis serves as the paradigm of thrombogenic arterial lesions, but it can be assumed that the same principles hold true for other disorders (e.g., trauma, dissections, inflammation).

In atherosclerosis, occlusion due to progressive stricture is almost unknown. Occlusion is due to thrombus superimposed on a usually tight stenosis, with thrombogenesis probably developing as follows. When the plaque softens and pours debris in the bloodstream, platelets adhere to the exposed abnormal area, in the same fashion that they arrest hemorrhage when the vessel is ruptured. After the initial layering of platelets on the endothelium-denuded area, more platelets aggregate over the first that have adhered. The final result is a thrombus, snow white in appearance, termed the *white thrombus*. At this stage there is hardly any fibrin (the often used term "fibrin-platelet thrombus" is supported only by flimsy evidence), so that the white thrombus has little or no internal cohesion. It breaks off easily in tiny fragments, which may be carried distally, in some instances transiently plugging small arteries and then disintegrating rapidly. This can cause fleeting ischemia when the occluded vessels feed clinically sensitive regions of the retina or brain (transient ischemic attacks [TIAs], see below and Ch. 5), or it may perhaps have no clinical consequences when the vessels feed regions less subject to symptoms. Aspirin and other antiaggregant agents oppose this step of thrombogenesis.

It is likely that the process of thrombogenesis can terminate at that point in some cases. In others, for reasons not well understood but probably because in the vicinity of tight stenoses eddies and pools of sluggish flow are generated, a *red thrombus* becomes superimposed on the white one. The red thrombus means that fibrin has appeared, entrapping clumps of red cells. In large arteries (e.g., the aorta) with large thrombi, thrombi can show many successive layers in which platelets and red cells alternately predominate *(mixed thrombus)*. When such red or mixed thrombi embolize, the fragments are cohesive (fibrin is a coarse and adherent material) and thus liable to block arteries permanently or long enough to cause infarction. The presence of a red thrombus also means that the clotting process has played a part, which explains the fact that anticoagulants have a therapeutic influence on thromboembolic accidents.

Red or mixed thrombi are either mural (i.e. they adhere to the arterial wall) (Fig. 35-6), letting blood flow past (and carry off emboli), or occlusive, totally obliterating the arterial lumen. This is termed *primary atherosclerotic occlusive thrombosis*. For reasons not well understood, although the fact is most significant for clinicians, primary atherosclerotic occlusive thrombosis is very rare in the pericerebral arteries, with the exception of the basilar artery. This means that occlusions of large arteries beyond the circle of Willis are generally due to extracranial disease, either embolism or anterograde thrombus (see below).

Following the primary occlusive thrombus, *secondary*

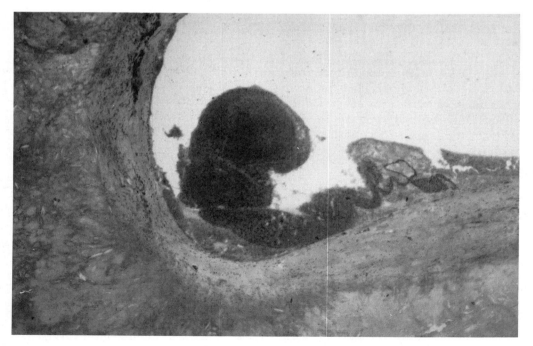

Figure 35-6. Mural thrombus in an atherosclerotic lesion at the origin of the ICA. It can obviously embolize or can grow upward to occlude the artery. (H&E.)

thrombi generally develop beyond and proximal to the primary occluded arterial segment. These anterograde and retrograde thrombi are mainly stagnation thrombi (i.e., they are made of packed red cells enveloped in a coat of platelets). This structure explains how, by gentle traction, surgeons can extirpate long segments of them in the hours or days following occlusion. The progression of these stagnation thrombi can be but is not always arrested at points where collateral flow is great enough to restore active blood flow in the occluded artery. For instance, an anterograde thrombus can be arrested by the reversed flow of the ophthalmic artery in occlusions of the ICA. Unfortunately, in a number of cases the anterograde thrombus may still progress, crossing the circle of Willis to enter the MCA or ACA. Thus occlusion of (often long segments of) pericerebral arteries can occur, with the inevitable consequence of cerebral infarction. This is the main mechanism of large infarctions due to ICA occlusion, with early death due to temporal herniation (see Chs. 17 and 25). Similarly, secondary thrombi can enter the basilar artery from vertebral artery primary occlusion or the PCA from basilar artery primary occlusion, with similar disastrous consequences. It is not well known whether secondary thrombi develop after occlusions due to cardiac emboli, nor is it well known whether secondary thrombi embolize and whether anticoagulants help to arrest their development.

Between veins and arteries, thrombi form quite often in the heart. As far as systemic emboli are concerned (see Embolism, below), they originate in the chambers on the left side of the heart, namely the left atrium, left appendage, or left ventricle. The exception comes with paradoxical emboli, in which the common defect is in the interatrial septum (see discussion of patent foramen ovale, below). Unfortunately, pathologic studies of intracardiac thrombi are scarce, and the authors do not know of one reference that could be cited on this subject. Presumably, since the circulatory conditions are quite different in the different parts of the heart and in different cardiac diseases, the structure of thrombi also differs in a fibrillating atrium, in a left appendage in atrial fibrillation (AF), in the left ventricle after myocardial infarction, or in dilated cardiomyopathies. A better knowledge of the presumably various structures of cardiac thrombi would allow a better understanding of the clinical features, prevention, and treatment of cardiogenic brain embolism.

Perfusion Failure

In the territory of patent arteries, ischemia may occur when blood pressure falls to critically low level. This perfusion failure is a mechanism obviously at play in generalized cerebral ischemia (see above and Ch. 17).

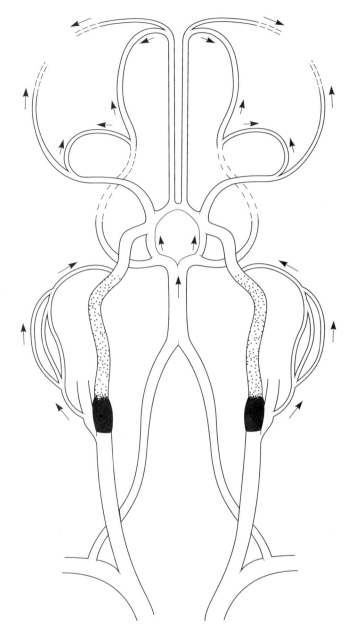

Figure 35-7. Occlusion of both ICAs, allowing the collateral channels to function *(arrows)*. Nevertheless, blood supply is wanting in the distal fields (perfusion failure) inasmuch as blood pressure is low.

Perfusion failure may also occur with multiple arterial occlusions (e.g., bilateral ICA occlusion [Fig. 35-7], because the meningeal anastomoses are insufficiently perfused for an adequate blood supply. As suggested by common sense, the most endangered brain regions are those farthest in the cerebral arterial tree (i.e., the distal fields, a term popularized by comparison made by German authors with the irrigation of meadows, *die letzten Wiesen,* the last meadows). As expected, the

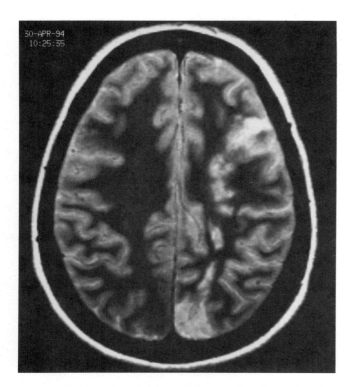

Figure 35-8. T₂-weighted MRI scan showing infarction scattered along the distal fields and border zones shared by the MCA and ACA, and also the MCA and PCA in a young woman with MCA stem stenosis and moyamoya disease.

brain lesions in such cases lie along the border zones of the major pericerebral arteries (Fig. 35-8) and spread varying distances in centripetal fashion into the adjoining vascular territories, the degree of spread away from the borderzones reflecting the degree of perfusion failure. In some cases the meningeal anastomoses are occluded, with the appearance of white threads to naked eye inspection. Such occlusions are likely the result of stasis, less probably the result of repeat embolism. That the lesions are essentially hypotensive in origin is shown by the fact that they also result from cardiac arrest and other sources of profound circulatory collapse. This process has often been termed *border zone infarction*. However, this term does not correctly convey the predilection for lesions to occur not only in the border zones but also in adjacent territories of the longest branches, overlying the upper and posterior convexity. The term also fails to explain the frequent sparing of the border zones formed by the shorter vessels in the frontal pole and anterolateral temporal lobe regions. *Watershed infarction*, another term often used, conveys the notion of a region of predilection for infarction but does not suggest the anatomic sites of the lesions.

Examples of perfusion failure in a setting of cerebral vascular disease are not often encountered currently in countries where surgical intervention for severe carotid stenosis is frequently undertaken, but they present fairly often in the small patient population with moyamoya (see below).

A few decades ago some clinicians held that many TIAs were due to ischemia in the distal fields, which overlie the upper part of the sensorimotor perirolandic strip, thus explaining TIAs mainly as examples of hypotensive episodes. Where hypotension is lacking, intermittent occlusion of tight ICA stenoses could be the triggering factor of transient distal perfusion failure. However, the current view among most clinicians is that the vast majority of TIAs happen without detectable hypotension and that the profound hypotension that occurs every night is well tolerated by most patients with tight stenoses or even silent ICA occlusions. The distal fields are also the regions where small emboli are expected to arrive. Since neither artery-to-artery embolism (ATAE) nor perfusion failure can really be ascertained in TIAs, it is reasonable to admit that we do not know the explanation in many cases. Instances have been documented in which pressure on a severely atherosclerotic common carotid bifurcation has caused a contralateral hemiplegia, one explanation being embolism, but others believe that such accidents are due to pressure on the carotid body and nerve of the sinus, with consequent lowering of blood pressure (see above).

While little doubt exists that perfusion failure explains some instances of hemispheric infarction, the process seems to account only for a minority of cases. Identification of patients with perfusion failure from high-grade large-artery stenosis or occlusion is now possible by using modern ultrasound and imaging techniques (see Chs. 10 and 13 to 15), so the role played by this mechanisms of ischemia is now more available for study than has been the case heretofore. Perfusion failure remains a subject of interest because this should be the setting in which an ischemic penumbra could most likely be expected to occur often enough to test theses of the benefits of neuroprotective agents (see Ch. 5). In some cases with a "low-flow" state, the clinical course seems remarkably stable despite near ischemic levels of cerebral blood flow, but in others this state seems to be a marker of future clinical events. Some clinicians have used metabolic or flow evidence of low-flow state to select patients for interventions such as prophylactic surgery. This subject continues to develop, and how important such findings will be in governing future patient management cannot be predicted.

SOURCES OF CEREBRAL EMBOLI

Heart
    Left atrium, left appendage, left ventri-
        cle, valves
Arteries
    Aortic arch, carotid and vertebral arter-
        ies, extra and intracranial
Pulmonary veins
Paradoxical embolism
    Right atrium, inferior and superior
        venae cavae

Embolism

Embolism is that process whereby fragments of thrombus or any other intracardiac or intra-arterial material are carried downstream and can plug vessels (Latin: *embolus*, a stopper). Since about the early 1970s, the frequency of the diagnosis of brain and retinal embolism has increased to the point that embolism, chiefly from the heart, is currently viewed as the most frequent cause of TIAs and cerebral infarction. Emboli originate from either cardiac or arterial thrombi (see below).

Emboli tend to lodge at bifurcations, branchings, and curvatures. The most common sites in the cerebral arteries are the bifurcations of the common and internal carotid and middle cerebral artery, in which case the embolus frequently occupies the stem of the artery. As the basilar artery is larger than is each vertebral artery, emboli entering the basilar artery are liable to be carried distally to the top, where the artery forks to form the PCAs. It is a sound clinical rule that sudden quadriplegia with oculomotor involvement ("top-of-the-basilar") suggests embolism, whereas quadriplegia with abducens paralysis, a sign of lower basilar disease, suggests thrombosis (see Ch. 30).

As opposed to in situ formed thrombi, emboli frequently drift along the occluded vessel. The time course of this movement cannot be predicted, so that the location of occlusions on angiograms does not necessarily shows the initial location of the embolus. Emboli frequently undergo spontaneous lysis and disappear or fragment into such small particles that they cannot be seen on angiograms. This explains the willingness of many clinicians, including the authors, to suggest a diagnosis of embolism in cases of stroke in which the angiogram shows no occlusion.

Emboli vary greatly in size, from microscopic to large enough to block the largest of the arteries supplying the brain. In the authors' experience, at least

20 percent of ICA occlusions result from cardiac embolism. Occlusions of large arteries beyond the circle of Willis commonly cause large, disastrous infarcts. At the other extreme, it is likely that some tiny emboli cause a small proportion of lacunes. As primary occlusive thrombi are rare in the cerebral surface arteries (see above), occlusions of small surface arteries are likely to be due to embolism. Thus, on clinical grounds embolism is the likely diagnosis in sudden-onset Wernicke aphasia or isolated homonymous hemianopia.

A number of occlusions, however, persist. Postmortem, the embolus is more or less recanalized and occludes a nonatherosclerotic artery, a criterion for the pathologic diagnosis of embolism. There are difficult cases in which the embolus has been incorporated into the vessel wall, thus resembling atherosclerosis.

Hemorrhagic Infarction. The drift and disappearance of emboli account for the possible leakage of blood through the damaged reperfused vessels (Fig. 35-9). Many embolic infarcts are pale (bland), but hemorrhagic infarcts are characteristic of embolism. From time to time hemorrhagic infarction is seen with a persistent arterial occlusion. Such mechanisms as a rich collateral circulation or episodes of hypertension have been suggested. As mentioned above, persistence of an occlusion at a site is no proof that this was the original site of occlusion—the embolus may have already drifted, so that the significance of its location remains debatable.

Cardiac Emboli and the Cerebral Circulation. The first large vessels branching off from the aorta are the innominate artery, the left common carotid

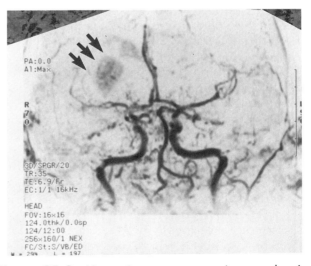

Figure 35-9. Magnetic resonance angiogram showing the recanalized MCA stem (left side of figure) and the hemorrhagic infarction in the territory of the lenticulostriates above *(arrows)*.

artery, and the left subclavian artery (Figs. 35-1 and 35-2). The large size of these vessels and the positions of their ostia, providing an almost straight line for particles leaving the heart, explain why at least 50 percent (and probably more) of systemic emboli reach the brain. Roughly 80 to 90 percent enter the carotid arteries. The course most frequent for emboli from the heart is into the MCA. This frequency still allows a substantial number of emboli to be carried into the vertebral arteries, so that the diagnosis of cardiac embolism is by no means rare in the posterior circulation. The chief cardiac conditions causing cerebral emboli have been listed in the box below.

Cardiac emboli that bypass the major branches of the aortic arch pass down the aorta and can occlude arteries to the kidney, spleen, gut, liver, and lower limbs. Such peripheral embolism occurring prior to, concomitant with, or following stroke of course suggests the embolic nature of the cerebral accident. In the authors' experience this is infrequently observed clinically. Postmortem evidence shows that many peripheral emboli, in fact the majority of renal and splenic emboli, are clinically silent.

Artery-to-Artery Embolism. The term artery-to-artery embolism refers to the origin of embolic particles from arteries supplying the brain. The authors prefer this term to "local embolism," because the latter is somewhat unclear. The concept of ATAE emerged around the early to middle 1960s for two chief reasons. First, it was found postmortem that the extracranial part of the cerebral arteries was often a nidus for silent thrombi and that the intracranial pericerebral arteries could be occluded by emboli from such thrombi. Second, fundoscopy during attacks of amaurosis fugax (see below) showed embolic material (i.e., fragments of white thrombi or cholesterol crystals) passing through the arteries.

Atherosclerosis is by far the main process generating ATAE from the aortic arch to the carotid, vertebral, and basilar arteries. Other lesions can also cause thromboembolism, including arterial trauma, dissecting aneurysms, and arteritides. Rarely, emboli from an aneurysmal sac plug the parent artery distally (see Ch. 37).

As mentioned above, arterial thrombi consist either of friable platelet clumps or of cohesive red or mixed cell aggregates. The former are liable to cause short-lived occlusions, hence TIAs. The latter are liable to block arteries permanently or long enough to cause infarction. It is uncertain whether such emboli tend to disappear as do platelet emboli and cardiac emboli (see above). ATAE generally follows the same course as do cardiac emboli and tends to stop, permanently or transiently, at the same points of the arterial tree

(see above). In a few cases, however, they can be carried along less expected routes. For instance, thrombus in the stump of an occluded ICA may occasionally be carried to the brain through collateral channels (i.e., by the ECA-ophthalmic bypass). Stenoses of the subclavian artery (e.g., due to a cervical rib) can generate thrombus, which in turn can embolize into the closely proximal vertebral artery.

In principle, the diagnosis of ATAE rests on criteria similar to those used for cardiogenic brain embolism: (1) a clinical cerebral episode of abrupt onset; (2) an arterial source (e.g., a stenosis of the ICA; and (3) the absence of a cardiac source. The diagnosis, however, is often compounded either by the coexistence of a cardiac source or by the presence of severe or multiple atherosclerotic lesions that raise the possibility that perfusion failure (see above) could have been operative in the cerebral episode. Cerebral and retinal ischemia can result from various mechanisms and causes, as listed below, and in individual cases it can be difficult to be sure that ischemia was due to ATAE. On balance, nevertheless, the authors believe that ATAE is the principal explanation for retinal transient ischemia (amaurosis fugax, see below) and also explains a good number of cerebral TIAs, but on the other hand they think that this diagnosis is probably too often accepted without due consideration of other possible mechanisms such as perfusion failure with severe stenosis (See Ch. 5).

Among questions that have been mooted, and this to some extent also pertains to cardiac emboli, is the

---

CARDIAC CONDITIONS CAUSING
CEREBRAL EMBOLISM

Atrial fibrillation, other dysrhythmias
Mural thrombus on recent or old myocardial
   infarction
Cardiomyopathies
Bacterial and nonbacterial endocarditides,
   nonrheumatic valvulitis
Prosthetic valves, catheterization, cardiac
   surgery
Mitral valve prolapse
Septal aneurysms
Patent foramen ovale
Other right-left shunts
Mitral or aortic valve calcification
Congenital heart disease
Left atrial myxoma, other tumors
Miscellaneous
Cerebral infarction of undetermined cause

mechanism of recurrent, stereotypical brief attacks (TIAs, see below) such as tingling in the hand in a patient with a tight ICA stenosis. For this symptom to result from emboli, the successive emboli would have to repeatedly take the same long and complex route to the same parietal arterial branch. Some clinicians accept this mechanism, whereas others doubt it and believe rather that the repeated TIAs result from repeated perfusion failures in the same regions farthest from the compromised source of supply, namely the proximal ICA (see Perfusion Failure, above).

A handful of instances suggestive of ATAE are known to the authors in which a contralateral hemiplegia immediately occurred in response to pressure on a tightly stenosed common carotid artery bifurcation. Precise information on the frequency of ATAE is, however, lacking. Relying on good circumstantial evidence, the authors believe that this mechanism is probably secondary to cardiac embolism when surface infarcts are considered.

No definite criteria have yet been developed that permit the assertion that a brain infarct was caused by ATAE. The mechanism is inferred when (1) the onset is sudden; (2) the clinical syndrome suggests a branch territory (on the whole ATAE infarcts are smaller than those due to cardiac emboli); (3) there is no cardiac source; and (4) the degree of stenosis, less than 80 to 90 percent, makes hemodynamic insufficiency (perfusion failure) unlikely.

Most ATAEs are elements of arterial thrombi broken free from the lesion. Cholesterol crystals alone are too small to cause infarction but can be seen as refractile bodies in the arteries. In some of the few cases of cerebral infarction attributed to cholesterol emboli, autopsies have shown some the arteries to be packed with atherosclerotic debris.

Ultrasound Monitoring of Cerebral Arteries

Ultrasound techniques now allow monitoring of the common carotid artery and the MCA for long periods of time (hours). Emboli generate high-intensity transient signals (HITS), easiest to detect as their density is lowest. Thus, air microbubbles are readily detected, but platelet clumps, thrombus fragments, atherosclerotic debris, and even fat are still detectable, although some are very tiny particles, as small as 200 to 400 μm or even less.

Monitoring the MCA in normal people yields no or very few HITS. However, in patients with a tight carotid stenosis, an amazingly high number of asymptomatic HITS has been recorded, and this number has been observed to drop sharply after endarterectomy. Recent data suggest that monitoring HITS could help in differentiating stable (asymptomatic) from unstable (symptomatic) ICA stenoses.

In patients with mechanical prosthetic heart valves, the number of HITS has been also high when compared with patients with bioprosthetic valves. Some of the HITS in this setting may be microcavitations caused by the mechanical prosthesis as blood passing through the aortic valve area swirls around the prosthesis. In some of the commonly used ventricular assist devices, HITS are recorded continually, suggesting continuous embolization of some sort. HITS have been shown to be correlated with large, acute, brain infarcts but not with lacunar strokes.

Advances are expected in the identification of the nature of HITS and the understanding of their biologic significance. It is hoped that ultrasound monitoring will provide markers of activity of potential arterial and cardiac sources of embolism, thus helping to define more accurately the increased stroke risk.

Arterial Diseases

Atherosclerosis

In most parts of the world, and particularly in countries with a Western style of life, atherosclerosis is among the leading cause of arterial strokes. The process of plaque growth is still debated. Suffice it here to repeat that occlusion almost never results from progressive stricture of the plaque but results rather from superimposed thrombus with its vital consequences on stroke pathogenesis (see Focal Cerebral Ischemia, above). At least as far as strokes are concerned, it could be said with much truth that without thrombosis, atherosclerosis would be a benign disease. The sites at which atherosclerosis selectively develops in the cerebral arterial tree are shown in Figure 35-10. In the ICA, roughly 8 of 10 primary occlusions occur at the origin and 2 of 10 in the siphon. Atherosclerotic primary occlusions are almost unknown from sinus to siphon, so that a lesion in that segment calls first for another diagnosis.

The process of atherosclerosis of the cerebral arteries is shared with arteries elsewhere in the body, namely the coronaries, aorta, and limb arteries. The same risk factors, with nuances, apply to all sites. These factors are age, arterial hypertension, cigarette smoking, diabetes mellitus, dyslipidemias, obesity, and high hematocrit.

Lacunar Infarcts, Fibrinoid Necrosis and Lipohyalinosis

Lacunes are small, deep infarcts, most often encountered in a setting of arterial hypertension. The name refers to the cavity or hole (Latin: *lacuna*, hole) that remains after macrophages have carried off the infarcted tissue. Lacunes are small lesions because they result from occlusion of small arteries, namely perfo-

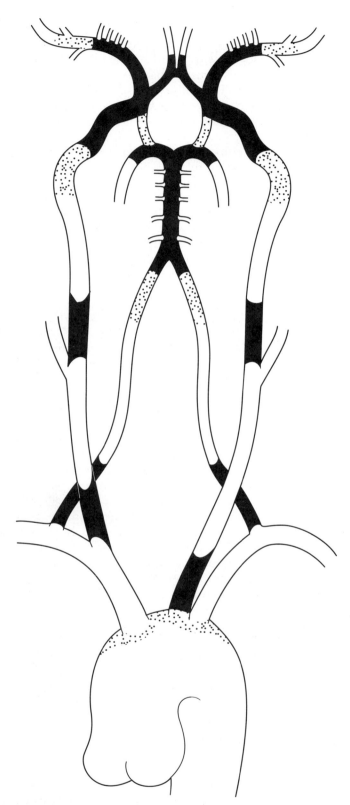

Figure 35-10. Distribution of lesions in the carotid artery territory. (Adapted from Barnett et al., 1992, with permission.)

rators (see Fig. 5-2). The majority of lacunes have a size in the order of 2 mm³, ranging from 0.2 mm³ to as large as 15 mm³ ("giant lacunes") in a few cases. The vast majority seem to be explained by lesions related to arterial hypertension and are also probably age-related, or it may be only the duration of hypertension that is significant.

In severe hypertension, the walls of arteries of the size of the penetrators (i.e., about 400 to 500 μm at their origin) undergo a lesion termed *fibrinoid necrosis* because the necrotic wall stains for fibrin. This may be the lesion initiating occlusion in some lacunes. Much more often, however, lacunes develop in a setting of moderately high hypertension with penetrators affected by a particular form of microatheroma termed *lipohyalinosis*. This means that the lesion combines hyalinosis (i.e., a loss of structure of the vessel wall, which takes a glassy look [Greek: *hyalos,* glass]) with conspicuous deposits of fat (Greek, *lipos,* fat). Lipohyalinosis is most probably the usual cause of penetrators artery occlusion, hence the usual cause of lacunes. Another cause of penetrators occlusion, at least in some cases, is atherosclerosis of the large, parent artery (branch occlusion). Clinically, separating occlusion of the ostium from that of the intracerebral perforator is rarely possible. In a few cases embolism can be the cause of occlusion.

Lipohyalinosis is uncommon in the surface gray matter, in large parts of the white matter (e.g., the optic radiations and the corpus callosum), and in the spinal cord, despite the presence of penetrators of similar small size. The lack of strict correlation of the topography of these small infarcts with small arteries means that from the neuropathologic standpoint, lacunes do not correspond to a uniform small vessel disease that could be considered as a cause of infarcts diffusely scattered through the brain. Rather, for reasons not well understood, lacunes are confined largely to certain neurovascular structures.

The vast majority of lacunes are found in the territory of the lenticulostriate branches of the MCA (Fig. 35-3), the thalamic perforants of the PCA (Fig. 35-11), and the paramedian branches of the basilar artery (Fig. 35-12). All these arteries share the same small size, are end arteries, and arise directly without branchings from large arteries. Perhaps they are particularly subjected to the strain of hypertension.

In general, the volume of the infarct matches the size of the occluded artery. As the penetrators vary very much in size and volume of supplied tissue, this explains the relatively wide variations in the size of lacunes (see above). Their distinctive locations occasion distinctive clinical syndromes (see below).

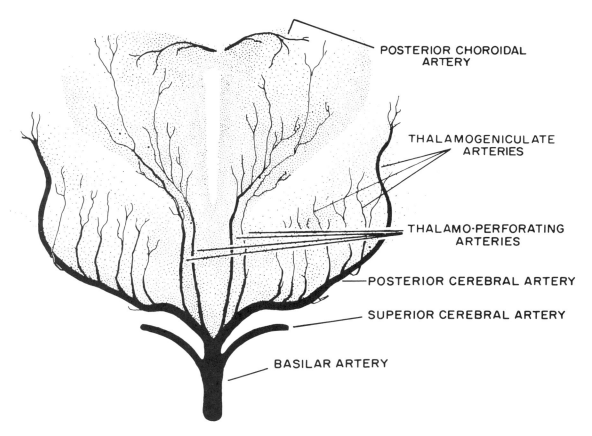

Figure 35-11. Thalamus with the usual arterial distribution. Note the multiple thalamogeniculate arteries. (Courtesy of Louis R. Caplan, M.D.) (From Barnett et al., 1992, with permission.)

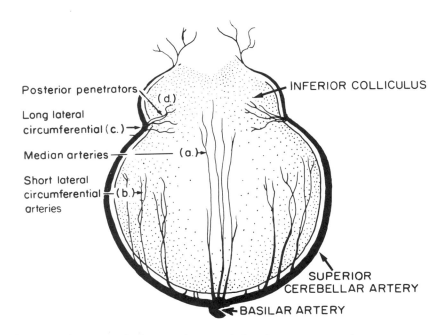

Figure 35-12. Rostral pons with the usual arterial distribution. *(a)* Median penetrating arteries; *(b)* short lateral circumferential arteries; *(c)* long lateral circumferential artery; *(d)* posterior penetrating arteries. (Courtesy of Louis R. Caplan, M.D.) (From Barnett et al., 1992, with permission.)

Dissecting Aneurysm

Currently often termed *dissections,* dissecting aneurysms result from the development of a hematoma in the arterial wall (where blood dissects the wall, hence the name), either in the outer layers of the media or subadventitia. ICA dissections are frequent, and vertebral artery dissections are not rare. The condition can be bilateral. In the ICA it is usual for the hematoma to ascend from just distal to the sinus to the base of the skull, where it stops at the entry of the bony canal. The hematoma compresses the arterial lumen and can cause intraluminal thrombosis with embolism. This explains the usual clinical picture, namely contralateral hemiplegia, ipsilateral oculosympathetic syndrome, and on angiograms, a long, irregular ICA stenosis from the sinus (not included) to the base of the skull (the string sign). In some cases the residual lumen is so small that only a flake of distal contrast agent can demonstrate that there is no occlusion indeed (pseudo-occlusion sign) (Fig. 35-13). If computed tomography (CT) or magnetic resonance imaging (MRI) of the neck is performed within a few days, the fresh wall hematoma can be displayed. Some ICA dissections cause only headache with an oculosympathetic syndrome, while others cause a paralysis of the vagus, spinal accessory, or hypoglossal nerves as they pass close by the dissected wall. Some ICA dissections lead to permanent occlusion, whereas others return to a normally patent lumen or leave an aneurysm or pseudoaneurysm, the future stroke risk of which remains unclear, posing difficult therapeutic problems.

Many dissections are spontaneous. In such cases it is customary to suggest that there is an underlying arterial disease, either focal (e.g., fibromuscular dysplasia, see below), or at the microscopic level, (cystic medial necrosis), but either diagnosis is usually difficult to prove. Search for systemic elastic tissue dysplasias (e.g., Marfan's disease, Ehlers-Danlos syndrome, or pseudoxanthoma elasticum) have been very rarely rewarding in our experience. Also, we have been impressed, over the years, by the number of dissections in women who were taking oral contraceptives. The authors know of two cases of basilar artery dissection in young women who took oral contraceptives.

Trauma to the ICA, either direct or indirect, can occur, for instance, in gymnastic exercises, in surfboarding, or at landing of parachutists, or in neck rotations, for instance chiropractic, where the vertebral artery is more often affected and is probably a more common site that formerly believed. Cases in which the evidence points to an ICA contusion against the transverse process of the atlas suggest that in such cases blood enters the artery wall and dissects it below the base of the skull. It is difficult to separate strictly traumatic cases from so-called spontaneous ones, for the trauma may be trivial and occur in the course of normal activities.

There are also dissections of intracranial arteries, which have not yet been well studied to our knowledge. Dissections of the *aortic arch* can progress along the extracranial neck arteries and cause TIAs or infarction. Dissections of the descending thoracic and abdominal aorta can cause transient ischemia or infarction of the spinal cord.

Fibromuscular Dysplasia

Fibromuscular dysplasia is a condition that usually also affects the renal arteries and is most frequent in women over 55. Pathologically, there are alternate segments of stenosis and ectasia, which account for the "string of beads" appearance on angiograms. This corresponds to alternate fibrotic and thinned segments (due to loss of elastic and sometimes muscular tissue). The lesions usually affect the cervical ICA beyond the sinus and can be bilateral. The vertebral arteries can be involved. Occlusion is most unusual. Dissection is possible (see above). In some 25 percent of cases there is an associated intracranial berry aneurysm. Fibromuscular dysplasia can be revealed by TIAs or subarachnoid hemorrhage or rarely in our experience by cerebral infarction. It is often a chance finding on Doppler ultrasound examination or angiograms for an unrelated condition.

Arterial Kinks

Arterial kinks are common (see above) and can be seen at any age, although their incidence rises with age. They can cause sharp bends in the artery, but these rarely achieve hemodynamic significance.

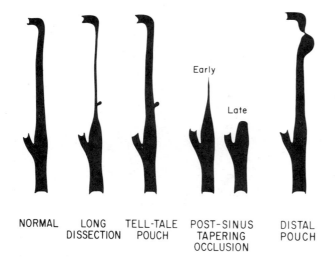

NORMAL LONG DISSECTION TELL-TALE POUCH POST-SINUS TAPERING OCCLUSION DISTAL POUCH

Figure 35-13. Arteriographic features of carotid dissection. (From Fisher et al., 1978, with permission.)

Dolichoectatic Arteries

As suggested by their name (Greek: *dolichos* long; *ek-tasis*, dilation), dolichoectatic arteries are too long and too wide. They are often calcified, which makes them easily detectable on CT. The basilar artery and the supraclinoid ICA are the arteries most often involved. Dolichoectatic arteries can cause ischemia but can also bleed or can compress brain, brainstem, or cranial nerves. There is a high percentage of associated aneurysms of the abdominal aorta.

Arteritides

Various kinds of vasculitides can affect intracranial arteries (see Ch. 38). The cerebral extracranial arteries also can be involved by several inflammatory processes, briefly described here.

The best known of these processes is *giant cell arteritis.* Arteries derived from the ECA and the vertebral arteries are the most frequently affected, probably because their walls are rich in elastic tissue. The cervical part of the ICA is infrequently involved, and the intracranial ICA and vertebral artery are usually spared, probably because they have only small amounts of elastic tissue. Cerebral involvement, on the whole, is rare and is due mainly to embolism from a thrombosed vertebral artery and occasionally from a thrombosed ICA. The main risk is blindness due to infarction of the retina or optic nerve. Any suggestion of giant cell arteritis in a patient over age 60 indicates the need for an immediate erythrocyte sedimentation rate test and corticosteroid treatment (see Ch. 38).

Another form of arteritis is the *aortic arch syndrome,* also termed pulseless disease or Takayashu disease. The aortic arch syndrome is the paradigm of disorders due to perfusion failure (see above). The pathologic process evolves slowly but is not well understood, and there are probably several diseases that can produce the syndrome. The early cases, in young Oriental women, showed an unspecific low-grade arteritis. In other cases, from India and Sri Lanka, there were inflammatory lesions of the elastic tissue of the aorta and its proximal branches with superimposed thrombus. Giant cell arteritis is a possible cause and one that should not be missed, since immediate treatment is mandatory (see above). Syphilis is a classical cause. Many of the cases seen in Europe and India have been due to a kind of hyperplastic atherosclerosis.

Congenital Abnormalities

Absence or hypoplasia of the ICA is rare. In adults the condition is usually brought to clinical attention by subarachnoid or cerebral hemorrhage due either to an associated berry aneurysm or to an abnormally developed collateral arterial supply. The absence or atresia of the carotid canal on skull x-rays is diagnostic.

Caution is warranted against making the diagnosis in error with magnetic resonance angiography (MRA). The authors have had cases mistakenly labeled "absence of ICA" in occlusion of the common carotid artery, and this occurred for the following reasons: (1) there was retrograde supply from the vertebral artery through the ECA with a feeble flow in the ICA; (2) the ECA flow was not printed out by the computer because, flowing caudad, it was interpreted as venous flow; (3) in addition, the anterograde flow in the ICA was too weak to reach the criteria for arterial flow in the computer program; and (4) the occluded common carotid artery was rightly absent on the angiogram. All these normal MRA data led to a gross misdiagnosis.

Tumors

Benign tumors such as chemodectomas or paragangliomas can develop immediately at the common carotid artery bifurcation (see above). Most are slow-growing masses that cause hoarseness and dysphagia and later, when larger, cause local pain and sometimes an oculosympathetic syndrome. Invasion of arteries by these tumors is uncommon, but metastatic laryngeal carcinoma is one cause.

Radiation Injury

Radiotherapy for neck tumors also irradiates the neck arteries. Years after the irradiation, TIAs or major stroke can result from postirradiation arterial lesions. These resemble atherosclerosis. The clue to the diagnosis is that some of these lesions involve the high cervical ICA or the common carotid artery, sites that usually are not severely involved by atherosclerosis. The history of irradiation is rarely missed, and in addition, many of these patients have on their neck telltale skin induration and telangiectasias. For the relationships with moyamoya, see below.

Moyamoya

Moyamoya (from the Japanese: for puff of smoke) is both a disease and a consequence of a disease. The name is derived from the haze in the basal brain seen on angiograms, which is explained by an enormous number of tiny arteries. In a setting of severe stenosis or occlusion of the distal ICA and its branches, these arteries are the greatly enlarged, normally tiny branches of the supraclinoid ICA and the circle of Willis, including the proximal MCA and ACA (Fig. 35-14).

Several disorders can cause the initial lesion of the parent arteries. In some cases there is a history of inflammation in the neck or head. Other cases are diagnosed several years after irradiation of a pituitary tumor. In still others, there is a poorly understood

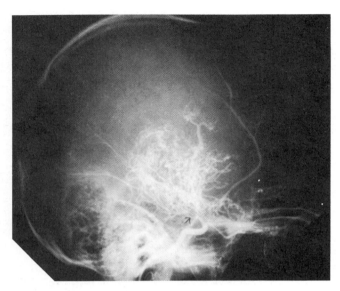

Figure 35-14. Typical angiographic findings of moya-moya disease. LICAG (lateral). (From Barnett et al., 1992, with permission.)

process of subintimal proliferation. The resemblance of this arterial hyperplasia with that of retinal arteries in low-pressure retinopathy (in patients with multiple extracranial occlusions) has led to the view that the striking collateral network could result from sustained hypotension in the distal ICA and branches. Interestingly, in a few cases of arteriovenous malformation of the origin of the MCA and ACA, moyamoya has developed in vessels just distal to the sites of ligation of vessels feeding the fistula. In such cases, the vessels showing the moyamoya effect appear to be serving as sources of anastomosis brought about by the low vascular resistance of the fistula.

In some cases, the enlarged, formerly tiny vessels participating in the moyamoya effect may be the source of cerebral hemorrhage (see Ch. 36).

CADASIL

CADASIL is an acronym for cerebral autosomal dominant arteriopathy with subcortical infarcts and leukoencephalopathy, formerly known is hereditary multi-infarct dementia. Recurrent subcortical infarctions begin in adulthood and can lead to pseudobulbar palsy and dementia. Migraine-like attacks and psychiatric disorders are possible. MRI shows small, deep infarcts and leukoencephalopathy. The penetrators of the white matter and basal ganglia are affected by a nonatherosclerotic, nonamyloid angiopathy. To date, eight unrelated European families have been reported. In two unrelated French families, genetic linkage analysis has shown the disease locus on chromosome 19q12.

Cardiac Diseases

Cardiac conditions causing cerebral embolism have been listed above.

Atrial Fibrillation

AF is by far the main cause of cardiac embolism. Flutter to a much lesser extent and rarely other dysrhythmias can also be emboligenic.

AF is a common disease, with an estimated prevalence of 0.4 percent in the population, rising steeply with age to reach 2 to 5 in those over 60. The sexes share equally. AF can complicate rheumatic endocarditis and valvulitis, myocardial infarction, coronary insufficiency, cardiomyopathy, the bradycardia-tachycardia syndrome (so-called sinus sick syndrome), mitral valve prolapse, and thyrotoxicosis. It can occur without evidence of cardiac disease, in which case it is known as idiopathic or lone AF.

In AF there is no effective atrial contraction, and hence there is stagnation of blood in the atrium and more in the appendage. Stagnation is considered the main factor inducing thrombosis. Atrial dilation increases the risk of thrombus formation and is maximal with mitral regurgitation. The risk of stroke in rheumatic valvular AF is increased 15-fold and in nonvalvular AF 5.7-fold. Patients under the age of 60 with lone AF are at lesser risk.

The classical teaching is that the sudden appearance of AF or of return to sinus rhythm, meaning return to normal atrial contraction (paroxysmal AF), carries particular risks of embolism. This is exemplified by the well-known risk of embolism with pharmacologic or electrical cardioversion, a risk estimated at 5.6 percent. This risk should be prevented to some extent by anticoagulation in the weeks preceding conversion. According to some studies, paroxysmal AF might carry a lesser risk than chronic AF, but the authors' experience does not support this contention. In chronic AF, the risk is always present but would be higher at the onset of AF (thus comparable with paroxysmal AF) and within about 2 weeks following an embolic episode.

The size of the emboli in AF vary widely. Thrombi large enough to fill the atrium (ball thrombi) are rare, but large emboli that can block a large artery (e.g., the ICA) are not rare. However, most emboli are small and are stopped in medium-size arteries (e.g., the MCA) or in distal branches.

Clinically, AF cause palpitations, and its onset may be concomitant with dyspnea and asthenia (due to decreased ventricular output), but such symptoms have little specificity and can well be absent or overlooked. A very rapid (higher than 120 beats/min) and irregular heart rate is almost always due to AF, whereas with a normal or slightly increased heart rate the diagnosis of AF is uneasy or impossible. Electrocardiography (ECG) readily shows AF, V_1 being usually the best lead to show the arrhythmia. In patients with a pacemaker, R-R intervals are, of course, equal, even though AF can be present. Long-duration ECG (Holter) monitoring may show paroxysmal AF. Positive results, however, are unlikely where there is no clinical or ECG abnormality.

Echocardiography is currently the preferred investigation to detect thrombi in the left atrium. *Transesophageal echocardiography* (TEE) is more sensitive than transthoracic echocardiography (TTE) and should be performed whenever possible. It shows thrombi in the left atrium body and the left appendage. TEE is also the most sensitive examination to detect spontaneous echo contrast ("atrial smoke") (i.e., reflectances in atrial blood) indicating a hypercoagulable state in addition to stasis.

Old, silent, brain infarcts are frequently detected by CT in patients with chronic AF after a recent stroke. Allowance must be made for patients in whom AF is first recorded after the stroke. In the authors' opinion, this reflects probably both the recent onset of AF and the well-known frequency with which patients with AF are unaware of their cardiac condition. However, the hypothesis has been suggested that infarcts involving the insula or brainstem could trigger AF.

Myocardial Infarction

Left ventricular thrombi develop mostly after large anterior, transmural, myocardial infarction because the wall and apex become akinetic, generating stasis, and the blood is in contact with the infarcted endocardium and myocardium, which induces thrombosis in about 30 percent of patients. The risk of cerebral embolism is more than 5 percent and can reach 15 percent in patients with a TEE-detected thrombus. It is highest in the first 10 days but persistent for the first 3 months. Since the risk of ventricular thrombus correlates with infarction size, strokes occur chiefly in patients with peak creatine kinase levels over 1,000. Anticoagulants, generally heparin followed by warfarin, decrease the risk by about 1 percent. Left ventricular thrombi can persist despite anticoagulation. In such conditions a thrombus forms in about 3 percent of patients.

Fibrinolysis, designed to minimize myocardial infarction, does not appear to reduce the incidence of left ventricular thrombi. Cases of cerebral embolism have been ascribed to disintegration of the ventricular thrombus after such therapy.

In chronic left ventricular aneurysms, thrombi are detected by TTE or TEE in almost half the patients.

The incidence of embolism, however, is much lower than that of thrombi in acute myocardial infarction. Protrusion and mobility of the thrombus into the left chamber carry a higher risk of detachment. Anticoagulation is generally recommended.

Akinetic segments of the left ventricular wall are a frequent TTE finding in stroke patients with a history of myocardial infarction. Their significance with respect to thrombosis and embolism is often uncertain.

Cardiomyopathies

Dilated cardiomyopathies cause blood flow stasis, and, additionally, there can be endocardial lesions inducing thrombosis. AF is also a frequent concomitant. The risk of cerebral embolism is 3 to 4 percent per year. Overall, however, cardiomyopathies are a very heterogeneous group and the risk in specific causes (listed in the accompanying box) has not been evaluated. Anticoagulation is recommended where a thrombus has been detected by TTE or TEE, where an embolic event has occurred, or where AF is present. Some recommend anticoagulation in all cases of dilated cardiomyopathy.

Hypertrophic cardiomyopathy, or idiopathic hypertrophic subaortic stenosis, can be a source of emboli, mostly where there is coexistent AF. A few conditions with left ventricular thrombi and embolism without evidence of cardiac disease has been reported.

Bacterial and Nonbacterial Endocarditides

Acute bacterial endocarditides and subacute bacterial endocarditides remain common in developing countries. In Western countries their incidence has sharply

---

CAUSES OF CARDIOMYOPATHIES

Ischemic
Idiopathic
Neuromuscular diseases
Amyloid alcoholism
Hypertrophic rheumatic myocarditis
Sarcoidosis
Catecholamine-induced
Viral
Peripartum
Hypereosinophilia
Chagas' disease
Adriamycin
Cocaine
Echinococcosis

Table 35-1. Main Types of Transient Ischemic Attacks

Carotid Territory	Vertebrobasilar Territory
Amaurosis fugax	Diplopia
Hemiparesis, monoparesis	Hemiparesis, monoparesis, paraparesis, quadriparesis
Numbness, tingling, affecting hand and/or foot	Numbness, tingling, affecting one or both sides of the body or perioral
Aphasia: anomia, paraphasias, jargon	Dysarthria
Homonymous hemianopia	Homonymous hemianopia
Shaking limbs	Gait disorders
	Vertigo
	Drop attacks
	Occipital blindness

declined, but the frequency is high enough that suspicion of the condition is well warranted. The diagnosis of subacute bacterial endocarditis can still be difficult. The traditional clinical adage that a hemiplegia with unexplained fever suggests subacute bacterial endocarditis is not obsolete, but it is well established that major cerebral embolism can occur with no systemic signs, prompting the recommendation that blood cultures be performed in any case in which the possibility of the diagnosis exists.

Embolism to the brain occurs in 15 to 20 percent of cases, mostly very early, within 48 hours of the diagnosis. However, after a few days of antibiotic therapy the risk decreases to 5 percent. This stresses that no delay in treatment is acceptable. The risk is highest with *Staphylococcus aureus* infection and mechanical prosthetic valves. Brain hemorrhage can occur either from rupture of a mycotic aneurysm or from pyogenic arteritis due to *S. aureus*.

In nonbacterial (marantic, verrucous) endocarditis, the valvular lesions vary from pinhead verrucae to large polyplike pedunculated growths shown by TTE or TEE. Marantic (from the Greek for wasting away) endocarditis can develop in cachectic, nonmalignant conditions, such as the acquired immunodeficiency syndrome (AIDS) (see Ch. 49). There can be a concomitant syndrome of diffuse intravascular coagulation so that at autopsy it can be difficult to distinguish lesions due to emboli from those due to in situ thrombosis. On balance, it is deemed that marantic endocarditis is complicated by brain emboli in about 30 percent of patients and accounts for about 25 to 30 percent of brain infarcts in patients with cancer.

Nonrheumatic valvulitides e.g., Libman-Sacks endocarditis, Behçet disease, syphilis) are rare causes of cerebral embolism.

Prosthetic Cardiac Valves

Prosthetic cardiac valves are either mechanical, requiring permanent anticoagulation, or bioprosthetic, having a lower risk of thromboembolism (but a higher rate of functional failure in 5 to 10 years).

Despite anticoagulation, the risk of embolism in patients with prosthetic mitral valves is 3 percent per year, and that in patients with prosthetic aortic valves is 1.5 percent per year. In anticoagulated patients many cerebral events are transient. Dipyridamole in addition to warfarin has been reported to lessen the risk. Antiplatelet agents alone as a treatment to prevent embolism with mechanical valves do not reduce the risk to acceptably low levels. The management of prosthetic valves during pregnancy is difficult and often not satisfactory.

Recently, Doppler monitoring of the MCA in patients with different kinds of mechanical cardiac valves has shown a higher number of microemboli signals likely to be microbubbles. The number of signals was variable according to the valve type. No clinical correlation has been identified (see discussion of HITS, above).

Cardiac Catheterization and Cardiac Surgery

In the early to middle 1980s, the cerebral risk of cardiac catheterization was evaluated at less than 0.1 percent of patients, and it is likely to be even lower nowadays. Embolism is the chief mechanism of the accidents. With the antecubital approach most complications occurred in the vertebrobasilar territory, probably because the catheter progressing in the subclavian artery was prone to roughen the origin of the vertebral artery. With the current catheters and the femoral approach, such danger has been greatly reduced.

All types of cardiac surgery can be complicated by systemic embolism. Of patients undergoing coronary bypass grafting, 5 percent suffer a stroke. Surgery with cardiopulmonary bypass, closed heart surgery, and heart transplantation carry a risk of cerebral embolism. The nature of the emboli is diverse: thrombus, atherosclerotic debris, fragments of valves, or particles of silicone or polyvinylchloride.

Mitral Valve Prolapse

Some years ago mitral valve prolapse was considered by some authorities to be a leading cause of stroke in the young. This estimate has been revised downward, and several studies have found mitral valve prolapse to be a possible cause of stroke in the young in about 4 percent of cases, which corresponds to the authors' experience. Mitral valve prolapse is present in 5 percent of the general population, mostly in young women. The majority have a normal variation of the mitral leaflet excursion and are at no special risk. A subgroup has a myxomatous structure of the leaflets, chords, and annulus and are at risk. This can be detected by echocardiography.

The authors have seen a fair number of patients with both mitral valve prolapse and patent foramen ovale (PFO) (see below). Contrast echocardiography should be performed whenever possible, and the diagnosis of mitral valve prolapse without other qualification as a cause of stroke should be accepted with caution.

Septal Aneurysms

Atrial septal aneurysms are a type of bulging of the interatrial septum in either atrium during the cardiac cycle. They are best detected by TEE and are present in 4 to 15 percent of patients with cerebral embolism but also in 0.2 to 4 percent of nonselected patients. A thrombus could form in such small pouches. A PFO is frequently associated (see below), and there can also be mitral valve prolapse and AF (see above).

Mitral Annulus Calcification

Mitral annulus calcification can rarely be a source of embolism; it is rather a marker of atherosclerosis. *Calcific aortic stenosis* can release small calcific emboli, which lodge in the retinal or cerebral arteries causing transient symptoms. Large emboli usually result from catheterization or balloon valvuloplasty.

Congenital Heart Diseases

Embolization can be due to cardiac dysrhythmias, paradoxical embolism (see below), or bacterial endocarditis. Most patients are cyanotic and prone to venous occlusion. Emboli have been chiefly reported in patients with the tetralogy of Fallot, ventricular or septal defects, or transposition of the great vessels.

Cardiac Tumors

Cardiac tumors are found in 0.05 percent of autopsies, 50 percent of such tumors being myxomas. Of the myxomas, 75 percent develop in the left atrium, attached to the interatrial septum in the region of the fossa ovale. Myxomas occur at all ages, most often in the 30 to 60 age group. Women are more affected than men in the proportion of 3 : 1. Familial cases have been reported. Emboli occur in 20 to 45 percent of patients and are composed of fragments of the soft, friable, tumor, sometimes of superimposed thrombus. AF is uncommon. Cardiac signs can be changing heart murmurs.

Cerebral embolism can be the presenting sign and is often recurrent. Other systemic emboli are frequent. Besides embolism, the tumor can obstruct the cardiac flow in the mitral ring, causing syncope, dyspnea, or congestive heart failure or causing systemic effects such as fever, weight loss, anemia, Raynaud's phenomenon, petechial rashes, or clubbing, thereby mimicking subacute bacterial endocarditis, collagen disease, and vasculitis. Such disorders disappear after removal of the myxoma. Any of these symptoms and signs, however, can be lacking, in which case stroke is the first manifestation. Cerebral embolism has been reported with a right atrial myxoma and a PFO (see below).

Rarely, myxomatous emboli can invade the arterial wall and produce multiple aneurysms, which rarely rupture. TTE or better, TEE readily shows left atrial myxomas as masses whose position changes from systole to diastole, sometimes protruding into the mitral ring. Cardiac CT or MRI can help in the diagnosis.

Other primary or secondary tumors can similarly embolize tumor tissue and superimposed thrombus.

Transcardiac Embolism

Emboli can enter the left cardiac chambers from the venous system (paradoxical embolism) or from the pulmonary veins (see below). Both of these sources are occasionally referred to as transcardiac embolism.

Paradoxical Embolism. A PFO (i.e., a nonclosure of the fossa ovale of the interatrial septum) is present in 25 to 30 percent of the population, providing a potential conduit to emboli from the right to the left atrium and thus to the systemic circulation. The process by which an embolus arising in the venous system reaches the arterial system is termed *paradoxical embolism* and is a time-honored concept in medicine. Until recently, however, it was considered a curiosity. With transcranial Doppler or echocardiography, whether TTE or TEE, it has become possible to screen large cohorts of patients, and it has been shown that in patients under age 55, a PFO is significantly more frequent in strokes with no cause found (cryptogenic strokes, see below) than in those of uncertain etiology and in a control group (54, 40, and 10 percent, respectively). The finding also holds true in older age groups, not merely in the young.

In a number of cases TTE, or TEE, or postmortem has shown the embolus astraddle the PFO. In vivo a PFO is demonstrated by injecting into a vein (usually the antecubital) a contrast material consisting of 10 ml of normal saline mixed with and agitated with 1.0 ml of sterile air. The arrival of the microbubbles in the left atrium crossing the PFO can be best detected by TEE (preferable to TTE) but the microbubbles implying the presence of a right-to-left shunt can also be detected in the MCA by transcranial Doppler ultrasound. A Valsalva maneuver or coughing during the test can "open" the conduit. As mentioned above, septal aneurysm and mitral valve prolapse can be associated. Rarely, the pulmonary angiomas of Weber-Rendu-Osler syndrome may be the cause of a right-to-left shunt in the absence of a PFO. The authors have encountered only one such example so far.

Clinically, the emboli enter the carotid circulation in 60 to 70 percent of cases, the same frequency for other cardiogenic emboli. When the history can be precisely taken, a Valsalva-like activity at the onset is frequently elicited. Studies using microbubbles have been able to calculate the frequency of particles reaching the various portions of the intracranial arterial tree, and the frequency data agree well with those of prior autopsy studies.

The source of embolism can be demonstrated by venography, and a high prevalence of occlusions of veins of the legs has been reported in patients with cryptogenic strokes. In some series, however, such occlusions were frequently lacking. This could be due to the delay between stroke and venography, to the difficulties in interpreting venograms, and perhaps to the transient character of some venous thrombi. Likewise, in cerebral infarcts due to AF, an atrial thrombus is not, by far, always found in the left atrium. On the other hand, there are large and small PFOs, a fact well documented postmortem. With biplanar TEE, patients with cryptogenic strokes have a larger PFO and more microbubbles in the left atrium than those with a stroke of known cause. It thus appears that both the size of the PFO and the degree of shunting can be and must be qualified.

There are yet no rules for therapy. Many patients receive aspirin or warfarin. A few have had transcatheter or surgical closure.

Paradoxical embolism can occur during puerperium. For fat and air emboli, see below.

Amniotic fluid emboli are characterized by sudden dyspnea, cyanosis, shock, and often death. Disseminated intravascular coagulopathy is frequent. Paradoxical cerebral embolism of amniotic fluid can occur and cause seizures. The latter could also be due to hypoxia resulting from pulmonary embolism.

It is the authors' impression that most stroke patients with PFO make a good recovery. Presumably, that could be due to the structure of venous thrombi, which are probably apt to disintegrate rapidly (see above).

Pulmonary Veins. In books and textbooks mention is made of systemic (and cerebral) emboli breaking off from thrombi in the pulmonary veins in patients with lung cancer or abscess or with bronchiectasis. While this is quite possible, the authors do not know of any definite case.

Miscellaneous

A number of cases of cerebral emboli have been recorded in patients with trichinosis, cysticercosis, or hydatidosis. Cerebral embolism of fibrocartilaginous fragments of the nucleus pulposus is also on record. It also occurs in the spinal cord (see Ch. 31) and is probably exceedingly rare in the brain. In both situations the pathophysiology is still a riddle.

Cerebral Infarcts of Undetermined Cause (Cryptogenic Infarcts)

In the current state of knowledge, 30 to 40 percent of brain infarcts that have been fully investigated remain of undetermined cause, either because there is more than one possible cause (e.g., cardiac embolism and atherosclerosis) or because no cause is found. In that large group (more than one-third of patients), many cases are clinically highly suggestive of cardiac emboli. It may be that the particle size sufficient to cause disabling stroke is small enough for the source not to be detected.

Improvements in technology have greatly improved recognition of causes for many otherwise unexplained ischemic strokes but nonetheless still leave many unexplained. Certainly no diagnosis will be forthcoming for those cases if there is failure to perform the appropriate tests, improper timing of otherwise appropriate tests, or normal findings or findings subject to ambiguity in interpretation on appropriate tests performed at the appropriate time. Testing is often deferred for patients of advanced age and those with coexisting severe disease and a poor prognosis, and in some cases it is deferred because of patient or physician unwillingness to undertake special tests or a casual confidence in a diagnosis based on clinical grounds alone.

Improper timing of the appropriate laboratory studies usually involves CT scans done too early and angiograms done too late. Angiograms for embolism that are obtained over 48 hours after the ictus have a yield as low as 15 percent for evidence of the responsible occlusion, even in those whose angiogram was initially positive. CT scans performed once only within a few hours of the onset of an ischemic stroke are normal in almost 50 percent of cases.

Test results without conclusive findings are obtained in a group that remains large enough to be worrisome. CT or MRI scanning may be positive and still leave the etiology of the infarction unclear. CT scans performed no matter how often may remain negative in some cases of small lacunar infarction when the lesion is below the limits of resolution of the CT scan technique, a problem especially applicable to the brainstem. Uncommon etiologies contribute to diagnostic problems, among them migraine, intracranial arteritis, and other entities not easily diagnosed. Of all the unproven mechanisms, embolism of indeterminable cause probably leads the list (see above).

Even when all known factors and modern imaging studies are taken into account, at least 15 to 20 percent of cases of stroke remain unsettled as to the mechanism of infarction.

SPECIAL PROBLEMS IN ISCHEMIC STROKE

Bilateral Ischemic Lesions

Bilateral infarction or transient ischemia of the occipital lobes causes occipital blindness. Bilateral infarction of the medial temporal lobes causes permanent amnesia (see above).

Bilateral lesions of the corticospinal tract, usually due to lacunes and more rarely to surface infarcts, cause a particular syndrome of *pseudobulbar palsy,* so named because it could at first sight suggest lesions of the medulla. Clinically, the limbs are mildly paretic with bilateral Babinski signs, brisk deep reflexes, and *marche à petits pas* (Dejerine). There is poor mimicry at rest and dysarthria with paralytic and dystonic components. Disorders of swallowing are common, and death can be due to choking. Usually, there is some urinary urgency. Loss of emotional control is characteristic, with outburst of *rire et pleurer spasmodiques* (spasmodic laughing and crying). Impairment of memory and some degree of dementia are possible but not invariably present, even in severe cases. The diagnosis is with occult or normal pressure hydrocephalus (see Ch. 59). A common clinical observation is pseudobulbar palsy appearing, sometimes for a limited period of time, after a mild stroke. Usually, it is a second stroke, the first one having been silent, or mild and forgotten. CT shows bilateral lesions.

Pseudobulbar palsy is not necessarily a stroke syndrome. Other diseases that can involve both corticospinal tracts can cause it, including trauma, multiple sclerosis, and motor neuron disease, although in the last case the disorders result from both pseudo- and true bulbar involvement.

Multi-infarct Dementia

The concept of multi-infarct dementia is complex and somewhat obscure in the opinion of the authors. There is, of course, no difficulty in agreeing that some patients with multiple surface infarcts causing aphasia, apraxia, agnosia, neglect, and memory and attention deficits have been labeled as demented. However, we have been impressed over the years by the normal or subnormal insight of such patients, a fact that does not easily accord with the diagnosis of dementia.

An important issue with multi-infarct dementia however, is that it could also be caused by subcortical lesions. Again, multiple, bilateral lacunes (see discussion of pseudobulbar palsy, above) can produce some degree of dementia, but this is not necessary, and there is clinicopathologic evidence that dozens of lacunes can exist without producing dementia.

The authors believe that the diagnosis of multi-infarct dementia is too often accepted and fully support the current studies attempting to segregate the dementias from the other disturbances of higher cerebral function in vascular disease.

Another point is that numerous lacunes often are concomitant with normal pressure hydrocephalus, the latter possibly accounting for part or all of the cognitive decline. Why some examples of *états lacunaires* (lacunar states) entail a degree of dementia is not clear. In some patients there has been evidence that some lacunes cause deafferentation of cortical areas or interrupt the interplay between cortex and basal ganglia.

A further issue has arisen with the word *leukoaraiosis* (Greek: *leuko,* white; *araiosis,* thin), meaning attenuation of the white matter on CT. It was assumed that this corresponds to lesions of the white matter that could account for the cognitive dysfunction. Leukoaraiosis has been shown to exist in some patients with multiple ischemic lesions but also occurs in other conditions, particularly in 19 to 35 percent of Alzheimer patients and in about 10 percent of normal people over age 60. Some have likened high-signal abnormalities on T_2-weighted MRI scans to leukoaraiosis. Both are mainly, but not only, seen in aging people with hypertension. Pathologically, the correlates of leukoaraiosis and high signals are not specific; they include thinning of myelin sheaths (myelin pallor), with a possible axonal loss and consequent gliosis. For the time being, it appears safe to think that the concept of leukoaraiosis has served mainly to direct attention to the problem without offering a definite solution.

Binswanger's Disease

Difficulties also arise with Binswanger's disease. In 1894 O. Binswanger (1852–1929, Swiss-born physician) reported from Jena, Germany, a chronic, progressive, subcortical encephalopathy in hypertensive patients. Whether it can be considered a single disease entity is uncertain, but reports are rare. To the knowledge of the authors, about 150 cases have been reported. Clinically, the onset is in the sixth or seventh decade, and pseudobulbar palsy with dementia develops in 3 to 5 years or more. Pathologically, the brunt of the lesions falls on the white matter, with sharply or ill defined areas of demyelination. The cortex, subarcuate fibers, and corpus callosum are spared. In most cases lesions predominate on the temporal and occipital lobes. Although Binswanger himself considered the disease separate from atherosclerosis or infarction, subsequent authors have not respected this distinction and currently include cases with large infarcts and lacunes under the term Binswanger's disease. Binswanger's patient had no microscopy at autopsy, but in subsequent cases intracerebral arteries have been reported to show extensive hyaline changes. On CT and MRI scans, leukoaraiosis is present, but this does not shed more light on the pathologic process (see Multi-infarct Dementia above).

The mechanism of the lesions is a riddle. No definite evidence has yet emerged for a metabolic disease of white matter that is separate from any vascular cause. Atherosclerosis is very unlikely since it can be absent or nonsignificant, and as a general rule, atherosclerosis does not selectively involve penetrators this far distal in the arterial tree. If the condition is a form of atherosclerosis, this would raise concern that it represents an unnatural form of the disease, possibly a form of edema. Recurrent ischemia that would selectively involve the penetrators of the distal centrum semiovale could be due, according to some authors, to repeated episodes of hypotension, but there is little support to that view. Finally, the concept of chronic ischemia, a revival of a 19th century hypothesis, has been suggested. If it exists, chronic ischemia would be analogous to an incandescent light bulb that can be dimmed by reducing the voltage (see Ch. 5). Such a process is at odds with the usual notion that ischemia first causes cell death when blood supply falls below a certain threshold, like the minimum voltage required to fire a fluorescent light. Some, finally, think that Binswanger's disease is a form of multi-infarct dementia (see above).

In recent years, there has been a trend to report Binswanger's disease with the diagnosis based mainly on the presence of leukoaraiosis on CT or MRI. This certainly cannot be taken as a specific support for the diagnosis (see Multi-infarct Dementia, above).

Hypertensive Encephalopathy

The term hypertensive encephalopathy does not mean the infarcts and hemorrhages with arterial changes that are common in chronic severe hypertension. Instead, it means acute cerebral disorders consequent to acute severe hypertension. Rather than a disorder featuring ischemic stroke, hypertensive encephalopathy is a hyperemic disorder (see below), but, for the sake of convenience it is dealt with here. It is a neurological emergency.

In this setting, animal experiments have shown that the cortical arteries take on a beaded appearance (i.e., there are alternating constricted and dilated segments). Evidence suggests that the constricted segments result from spasm while the dilated segments result from lesions of the vessel wall, likely due to spasm itself and to severe hypertension. This appears to be a breakthrough of autoregulation (see Ch. 5), and indeed, there is a pronounced increase in blood flow. In the dilated segments there is necrosis of medial muscles fibers and infiltration of plasma and fibrin, termed insudation or plasmatic vasculosis. Around the vessels and in the brain at large, there is evidence of plasma leakage and edema.

Hypertensive encephalopathy is probably common in developing countries. It has become rare in Western countries but could be present in the poorest ethnic groups. Moreover, the authors think that it is likely to be present in some or many of the cerebral accidents associated with drug abuse (see Ch. 68).

Characteristically, hypertensive encephalopathy occurs in young, previously normotensive patients with acute nephritis, toxemia of pregnancy, pheochromocytoma, lead poisoning, and rarely, porphyria. People with chronic hypertension are less liable to have hypertensive encephalopathy, probably because they have a hypertrophy of the arterial media (which can be likened to their left ventricular hypertrophy), which prevents the forced breakthrough of the vessel walls by severe hypertension.

Clinically, the episode of hypertensive encephalopathy is often heralded by headache, drowsiness, and vomiting concomitant with a severe rise in blood pressure, but there are exceptions. Convulsions occur, either generalized or focal. Acute visual failure is the second main feature and is due to occipital blindness. Various focal disturbances can occur, such as transient paralysis and aphasia. Drowsiness can lead to coma. Papilledema and hypertensive changes in the fundi are often lacking. Lumbar puncture must be avoided. CT shows areas of low density in the white matter.

Death is possible. With emergency antihypertensive therapy, the course is usually favorable. The cerebral disorders can regress in a matter of hours or even minutes. Sequelae are said to be rare when treatment has been prompt and efficient. However, occipital blindness, intellectual impairment, and epilepsy are possible.

The mainstay of treatment is immediate lowering of blood pressure. Several drugs are available. Sodium nitroprusside is given intravenously (0.5 to 0.8 μg/kg/min) under constant supervision. Diazoxide is given intravenously at a recommended dose of 150 mg in 15 to 30 seconds. It causes sodium retention. Hydralazine appears less effective and should be used cautiously in patients with coronary disease. There is an additional risk of occipital blindness if blood pressure is reduced excessively. To control seizures, intravenous phenytoin is recommended. To lessen cerebral edema, mannitol or glycerol (in the absence of renal failure) or dexamethasone can be used. Again, it is worth repeating that immediately lowering blood pressure is the key emergency measure. Where the above antihypertensives are not available, it should be remembered that venesection was formerly used with success.

Oral Contraceptives, Puerperium and Postpartum

Women of childbearing age who take oral contraceptives are at a higher risk of cerebral vascular accidents than those who do not. The risk is correlated with the dose of estrogens and is particularly increased for women over 35, those who are hypertensive, and those who smoke tobacco cigarettes. Infarctions can be of arterial or venous origin, the latter being due to sinus thrombosis (see Venous Strokes below). The cause of arterial strokes is less clear. Atherosclerosis appears to be unaffected by oral contraceptives. Cardiac embolism is not a likely cause. In some users, oral contraceptives induce an increase of low-density lipoprotein (LDL) cholesterol and a decrease of high-density lipoprotein (HDL) cholesterol, which perhaps play a part in inducing the accidents. Deficiency in antithrombin III and proteins C and S could induce a state of hypercoagulability, but obviously this could only apply to a small minority of cases. Estrogens per se can cause hypercoagulability, and leg phlebitis is another risk of oral contraceptives.

As stated above (see Dissecting Aneurysms), the authors have been impressed over the years by a number of dissecting aneurysms of the extracranial cerebral arteries in oral contraceptive users. We also have a number of cases in which the likely mechanism was transcardiac embolism from a leg thrombus through a PFO (see above). Oral contraceptives also increase the risk of cerebral infarction in migraine (see Ch. 24) and increase the risk of subarachnoid hemorrhage.

During pregnancy and the weeks following delivery, women are still at a higher risk of cerebral infarction, and in the experience of the authors, most of the strokes in young women (see below) are puerperium-related. Venous occlusion is possible, but contrary to classical teaching, arterial occlusions are more frequent.

Strokes in the Young

Estimates of strokes prior to age 40 vary widely from about 3 to 40 percent. What is certain is that every busy neurologist each year sees several of these particularly distressing cases. It is agreed that arterial ischemic strokes comprise the great majority of cases (there are also venous strokes and hemorrhages). As it is a subject of obvious interest, a good number of studies are available, but their value depends heavily on which investigations have been carried out and at what time with respect to the clinical onset. In several studies, only a few angiograms were obtained and with such delays (or unspecified delays) that lesions such as dissecting aneurysms were likely to have been missed, the angiograms showing either an occluded or a normal artery (see Dissecting Aneurysms, above). In other studies echocardiography was not available—or only TTE, not TEE—and contrast echocardiography was not done or rarely done. The question deserves further study.

With the available evidence, it appears that there is a host of possible causes, including, of course, rare diseases. However, there are leading causes such as dissecting aneurysms, trauma, and cardiac embolism. When venous infarctions are taken into account, oral contraceptives and puerperium are the main causes in women in the authors' experience. In that case, of course, an underlying abnormality may also be present (e.g., a defect in antithrombin III or protein C or S, or a cardiopathy), and extensive investigations are warranted.

Fat Embolism

Fat embolism has been evaluated as occurring in 90 percent of cases of major trauma and with TEE monitoring, in about 40 percent of patients undergoing major orthopedic procedures. Obviously, there are many subclinical or mild cases that go unrecognized. In severe, fulminant forms, the mortality rate is still 15 to 20 percent.

As the neurologic disorders of fat embolism mostly appear 1 to 5 days after trauma, the diagnosis in the presence of other cerebral consequences of the trauma can be difficult. Neurologic complications after fractures of the long bones should raise the possibility of fat embolism.

Rarely, fat embolism can occur in other settings such as acute pancreatitis, burns, joint reconstruction, diabetes mellitus, liposuction, cardiopulmonary bypass, caisson disease, and parenteral infusion of lipids. In sickle cell anemia, fat emboli can arise from foci of bone necrosis. Fat embolism also could occur in the puerperium, since fat from the vernix caseosa is a component of amniotic fluid.

There are two main views on the pathophysiology of fat embolism. According to the first one, called the mechanical theory, globules of fat pass from marrow into veins and then plug the lungs. The smaller droplets could pass through the capillaries, thus entering the systemic circulation. Another possible route is through a PFO (see above). In a recently reported case TEE monitoring showed the quantity of embolized fat to be closely correlated with the movements of the guide wire and nail in the femur shaft. In the second view, termed the biochemical theory, hydrolysis of fat particles in the lung releases toxic free fatty acids, which could disrupt lung capillaries. C-reactive protein, which is also elevated after trauma, could coalesce chylomicrons, thus forming fat globules. The two theories are not mutually exclusive.

Clinically, from 12 hours to 5 days or more after the fracture, the full-blown picture features a triad of respiratory distress (with hypoxemia), focal or diffuse (confusion, stupor) cerebral symptoms, and petechiae (mostly axillary and subconjunctival).

Diagnostic measures include chest x-ray, arterial blood gas analysis, and coagulation profile. Bronchoalveolar lavage or lung microcirculatory cytology, with stains for fat, has been proposed.

Prevention of fat embolism rests on minimal motion and early fixation of fractures. In the acute phase, the treatment is directed against respiratory distress. Corticoids, heparin, 5 percent ethyl alcohol, and low molecular weight dextran have been advised.

Air Embolism

Gases can appear in the blood in two settings. First, in decompression sickness nitrogen bubbles affect mainly the venous circulation of the spinal cord (see Ch. 31) but can also cause headache, visual scintillations, vertigo, nystagmus, and vomiting. Second, air can enter the blood through a vein injury, involving essentially veins above the level of the right atrium. Entry into an artery would require air under high pressure.

Venous air emboli in sufficient amount plug the branches of the pulmonary artery, causing sudden pulmonary hypertension. This could open a latent PFO, or if the foramen ovale is already patent, air passes from the right to the left atrium. However, air could enter the systemic circulation in the lung.

Clinically, where air is in large amount, chest pain with acute dyspnea is often the first symptom, soon followed by stupor or coma, seizures, blindness, and possibly other focal deficits. Bubbles can enter the retinal arteries and the heart (auscultation reveals churning, gurgling sounds due to frothy blood). Air readily visible on chest x-ray or echocardiograms would unequivocally confirm the diagnosis.

The setting of the accident is a major clue to the diagnosis. Air embolism may be due to trauma of the great vessels of the neck or to a host of medical maneuvers, which include insufflation (causing pneumoperitoneum or pneumorthorax), celioscopy, mechanical ventilation, extracorporeal circulation, surgery for a prosthesis of large joints, catheterization of large veins of the upper chest (e.g., the subclavian), lung biopsy, pleural puncture or lavage, and neurosurgery on a

sitting patient. Air embolism can also occur during pregnancy, in the puerperium, or during cesarean section, complicated vaginal delivery, or abortion. Air can enter an artery during arterial catheterization and cardiac surgery.

Where available, hyperbaric oxygen is probably the mainstay of emergency treatment. If not, the patient is turned on the left side to trap air in the right cardiac chambers, from which it can be aspirated.

ARTERIAL TERRITORIES AND CLINICAL SYNDROMES

Arterial Territories

Knowledge of the cerebral artery territories is the basis of the clinical diagnosis of ischemic lesions. It must, however, be used with two chief reservations. First, only a part of each territory is usually involved by ischemia because of either collateral supply or occlusion of only one or a few branches of a main artery. Second, the territories are subject to individual variations, one cause, for example being variations of the circle of Willis. A glance at Fig. 35-3, shows that in 14 percent of people the ICA territory is the whole ipsilateral hemisphere and in 2 percent it comprises the ACA territory of the contralateral hemisphere. Such constitutional differences explain why occlusion of an ICA can have widely differing consequences among individual patients. Furthermore, occlusions also modify the arterial territories along the same principles, so that additional occlusions can have far-reaching consequences (e.g., occlusion of an ICA contralateral to a silent occluded ICA can cause wide infarction of both hemispheres. Likewise, when one vertebral artery ends in the PICA (see above), occlusion of the contralateral vertebral artery can cause bilateral infarction of the brainstem, as would basilar artery occlusion. Knowledge of the average pericerebral arterial territories must be called on every day by the neurologist.

Middle Cerebral Artery

The MCA (Fig. 35-15) is the main branch of ICA bifurcation, both by its size and the course of its stem that continues the ICA. It supplies the lateral part of the orbital surface of the frontal lobe, the insula, and all of the convexity of the hemisphere except for the frontal pole and a 25-mm broad strip on the superior part of the convexity of the frontal and parietal lobes, which depends on the ACA, and most of the extreme end of the occipital lobe, which depends on the PCA. Through a dozen or so basal perforators, the MCA supplies the superior half of both limbs of the internal capsule; the caudate (except for the inferior portion of its head and its tail); the putamen, except for the inferior portion of its rostral pole; and the lateral part of the globus pallidus. It also supplies the optic radia-

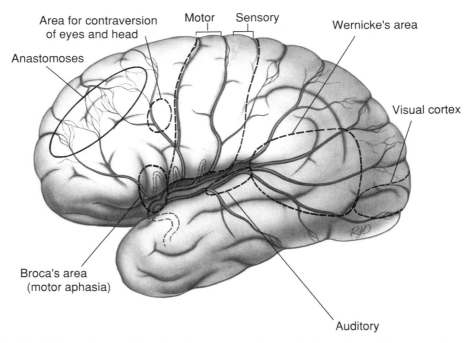

Figure 35-15. MCA territory, with major clinicoanatomic correlations shown. Examples of anastomoses that exist throughout border zones are shown in the superior frontal area.

tions, where it courses laterally to the occipital horn of the lateral ventricle.

Ischemia in the territory of the convexity branches causes a contralateral hemiparesis predominating on the arm and face, sensory disorders affecting the same body parts, contralateral homonymous hemianopia, and, when the dominant hemisphere is involved, global aphasia (see Ch. 18), apraxia (see Ch. 19), neglect, asomatognosia, or anosognosia (see Ch. 19), or sometimes delirium when the nondominant hemisphere is involved (see Ch. 20).

When ischemia is limited to the territory of the anterior surface branches of the MCA, the syndrome may feature contralateral motor and sensory deficit (see also Ch. 25) predominating on the arm and face, with motor aphasia when the dominant side is involved. When infarction occurs high over the convexity, there may be no strikingly obvious clinical disturbances. Rather, there is sometimes only mild weakness or slight impairment in skilled movements (dyspraxia) of the hand or forearm; slight weakness or faulty placement of the foot; impaired skilled movements of the leg; slowing in the promptness of spoken responses and laconic conversation; or rarely a dystonic leg placement, which appears as if the foot is adherent to the floor (so-called magnetic foot sign). Such signs might escape clinical attention in the early stages. Special clinical testing, including imitation of bicycling

movements of the legs and swimming movements of the arms, may reveal the disturbance in some cases.

With ischemia in the territory of the posterior branches, weakness is mild, sensory disorders can be prominent, and there is hemianopia and Wernicke aphasia with apraxia on the dominant side or hemineglect and anosognosia when the nondominant hemisphere is involved.

Where the territory of the basal perforators is involved, infarction of the internal capsular region causes a contralateral hemisparesis and sometimes a hemiplegia, whose form varies from one affecting equally face, arm, and leg (proportional hemiplegia) to one limited to one limb (see Lacunar Clinical Syndromes, below).

Anterior Cerebral Artery

The ACA territory (Fig. 35-16) is the frontal pole, cortex, and about 25 mm of underlying white matter of the internal part of the orbital surface of the frontal lobe and of the medial surface of the frontal and parietal lobes, including the corpus callosum except for the splenium. The parieto-occipital fissure usually is the posterior boundary of this territory. Soon after its origin, the ACA gives rise to a few basal perforators one of the larger of which, Heubner's artery (JOL Heubner, German physician, 1843–1926), supplies the inferior part of the head of the caudate, the ante-

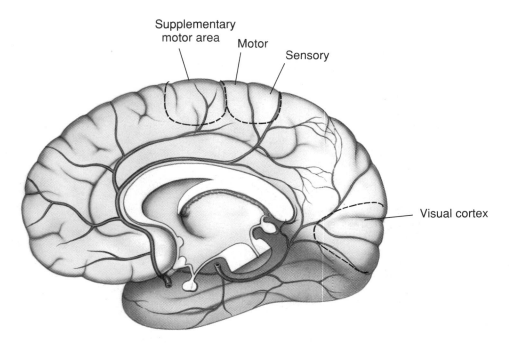

Supplementary
motor area   Motor   Sensory

Visual cortex

Figure 35-16. ACA/PCA territory, with major clinicoanatomic correlations shown. Note border zones between ACA and PCA.

rior part of the putamen, and the inferior half of the anterior limb of the internal capsule.

Ischemia in the distal ACA territory (the paracentral lobule) causes contralateral leg motor and sensory deficit (see Ch. 25), often with sphincteric disturbances. Recent evidence suggests various patterns of motor deficit with various prognoses in infarctions of the ACA territory. Lesions restricted to the paracentral lobule cause a severe, distally predominating leg weakness with little improvement. Lesions involving the medial part of the premotor cortex, the supplementary motor area, and the paracentral lobule cause a severe contralateral hemiplegia, predominant on the distal leg, and a less severe proximal weakness of the arm. The prognosis is good for the arm, poor for the leg. Lesions involving the medial part of the premotor cortex and the supplementary motor area but sparing the paracentral lobule cause a contralateral hemiparesis predominating on hip and shoulder, with a good recovery for both. Large frontal lesions cause abulia.

To the authors' knowledge, the clinical picture resulting from ischemia in Heubner's artery has not yet been clearly delineated. A few reports have mentioned memory disorders with infarction of the head of the caudate on the dominant side and weakness and slowness of movements on the contralateral side with infarction of the lower part of the anterior limb of the internal capsule.

Anterior Choroidal Artery

The AChA (Fig. 35-17) supplies the pyriform cortex; part of the amygdala and the uncus; part of the hippocampus with the fimbria; the medial part of the globus pallidus; the lateral part of the geniculate body and the initial segment of the optic radiations; the subthalamic region; the inferior half of the posterior limb of the internal capsule; part of the cerebral peduncle; and the choroid plexus.

The area is usually divided into many branches soon after it leaves the ICA to course dorsally between the temporal lobe and the cerebral peduncle. This is probably the reason why the clinical picture of ischemia in its territory is not frequent and has been recognized relatively recently. The AChA syndrome features contralateral hemiplegia (usually severe and proportional) because of the involvement of the lowest portion of the internal capsule, where the fibers are the most compact. There are varying degrees of visual and sensory impairment.

The infarct, being small, can escape detection by conventional CT scanning. Recent imaging techniques have shown it to involve the inferior part of the posterior limb of the internal capsule, often the medial pallidus, in about half the cases the cerebral peduncle, and in about one-third the medial temporal lobe and a thin rim of the posterior pole of the thalamus. In none of these cases has the upper, lateral wall

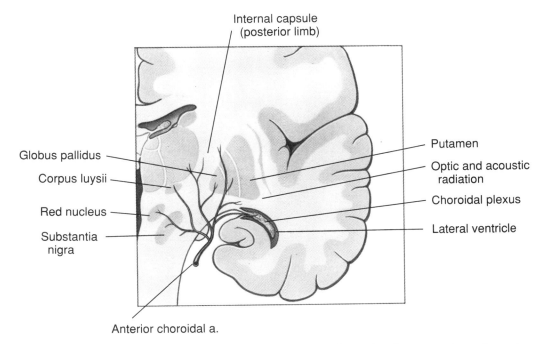

Figure 35-17. The anterior choroidal artery and the sites of supply of its main branches, shown in coronal section.

of the lateral ventricle been affected, a useful point to separate these infarcts from those due to ischemia in the lenticulostriate branches of the MCA territory.

Involvement of the AChA in temporal herniation is probably frequent. This mechanism, occurring in the fetus during labor, has been proposed to account for hippocampal sclerosis, a lesion common in epileptics (see Ch. 25).

Basilar Artery

The basilar artery (Fig. 35-18) is on the midline, ventral to the pons. It is formed by fusion of the two vertebral arteries. It gives rise to the AICA and the SCA, which loop dorsally around the pons to supply the cerebellum. Small branches arising from its posterior wall (paramedian penetrating arteries) penetrate the pons on each side of the midline, supplying the corticospinal tract, the medial lemniscus, and the nuclei and fascicular fibers of the third, fourth, and sixth cranial nerves, to which can be added the twelfth cranial nerve in the high medulla, supplied by the vertebral artery. More laterally, other branches (the short circumferential arteries) supply the corticospinal tract, the brachium conjunctivum, the spinothalamic tract, the central tegmental tract, the nuclei and fascicular fibers of the fifth, seventh, eighth cranial nerves, and the descending sympathetic pathway. At its bifurcation, it gives rise to perforators to both sides of the midbrain (Fig. 35-11).

Clinical and anatomic evidence suggests that here are many individual variants in the number and territories of the basilar artery perforators, so that the syndromes outlined below are subject to variations (Fig. 35-19). Finally, as mentioned, the basilar artery bifurcates into the PCAs, except in some 14 percent of people (Fig. 35-3).

As ischemia in the basilar artery involves both sides of the pons, the first tenet of the clinical diagnosis is the presence of bilateral disorders (for exceptions, see below). The second characteristic feature is involvement of cranial nerves whose nuclei lie in the pons or of other structures that lie in the pons (e.g., the medial longitudinal fasciculus). The characteristic clinical picture of basilar artery occlusion is quadriplegia with diplopia or gaze conjugate paralysis (see Chs. 28 and 29). Again there are many variants (see below). Frequently, there are associated symptoms or signs due to ischemia in the territory of the PCAs (hemianopia or occipital blindness), resulting either from propagated thrombus or from embolism.

Sudden occlusion of the top of the basilar artery, usually by embolism (see above), produces abrupt coma or stupor or an agitated delirium, visual hallucinations with quadriplegia, and a variety of ocular movement disorders, among which are paralysis of upward gaze, retraction nystagmus, retraction of upper lid, and skew deviation (see Ch. 28).

Occlusion of paramedian perforators results in con-

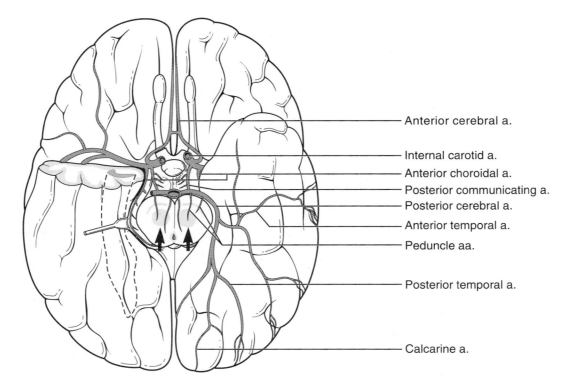

Figure 35-18. Basal view of the brain, showing the main branches of the circle of Willis. Note basilar penetrating arteries *(arrows).*

Labels for figure:
- Anterior cerebral a.
- Internal carotid a.
- Anterior choroidal a.
- Posterior communicating a.
- Posterior cerebral a.
- Anterior temporal a.
- Peduncle aa.
- Posterior temporal a.
- Calcarine a.

tralateral weakness with ipsilateral ataxia. Depending on how deep the band of infarction penetrates, a number of cranial nerves can be paralyzed. The most frequently involved is the abducens, followed by the oculomotor, while the trochlear, which lies dorsally, is off the paramedian territory. On the border of the paramedian territory, the facial nerve can be lesioned as it hooks around the abducens nucleus.

Further down, in the medulla, the hypoglossal nerve can be involved. Cranial nerve paralyses are ipsilateral to the lesion, while weakness due to corticospinal involvement and impairment of position sense and vibration perception are contralateral, hence the traditional term *crossed syndromes* applied to many syndromes of the brainstem (see Ch. 30). Ischemia in the territory of the short circumferential arteries causes contralateral weakness (corticospinal tract), sensory deficit for pain and temperature (spinothalamic tract), ipsilateral ataxia (brachium conjunctivum), paralysis of the seventh and eight cranial nerves, and an oculosympathetic syndrome (descending sympathetic), which again is a crossed syndrome. Palatal myoclonus can appear later as a result of involvement of the central tegmental tract, with consequent transsynaptic degeneration of the ipsilateral inferior olive.

In fact, occlusion of one or a few basilar artery per-

forators often occurs, owing to the fact that small basilar artery atherosclerotic lesions often occlude only the ostium of one or a few perforators (branch occlusion) (see Lacunar Clinical Syndromes, below). In such cases the infarct volume is very small and the clinical picture is monosympatomatic (e.g., pure motor stroke).

Posterior Inferior Cerebral Artery

The PICA is the collateral branch of the intracranial vertebral artery. It supplies a retro-olivary wedge of the medulla, part of the inferior surface of the cerebellum, and part of the dentate nucleus.

Infarction of the retro-olivary territory (Fig. 35-20) can result from PICA occlusion, but more often it is due to vertebral artery occlusion, blocking the ostium of the PICA. It causes Wallenberg's syndrome (A. Wallenberg, German neurologist, 1862–1949), one of the most reliable syndromes in clinical neurology. On the side of the lesion there is dysphagia and dysphonia (paralysis of soft palate, pharynx and vocal cord, and nucleus ambiguus); Claude Bernard-Horner syndrome with miosis, ptosis, and diminished sweating of the face and neck (descending sympathetic fibers); sensory disorders of the face, mainly of the responses to pain and temperature, with diminished or abolished corneal reflex (descending root and tract of the

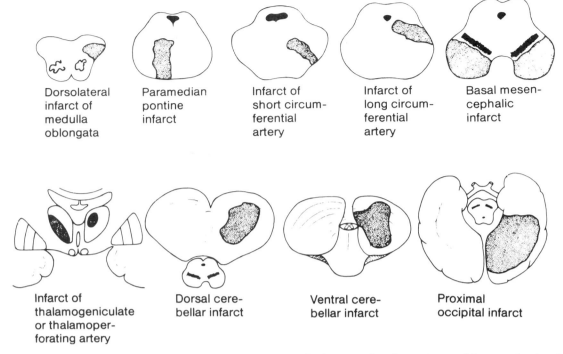

Dorsolateral infarct of medulla oblongata

Paramedian pontine infarct

Infarct of short circumferential artery

Infarct of long circumferential artery

Basal mesencephalic infarct

Infarct of thalamogeniculate or thalamoperforating artery

Dorsal cerebellar infarct

Ventral cerebellar infarct

Proximal occipital infarct

Figure 35-19. Schematic view of the principal types of infarcts within the territory of the vertebrobasilar system. (From Zülch, 1985, with permission.)

fifth cranial nerve); and cerebellar ataxia (restiform body). On the contralateral limbs and trunk there is impairment of pain and temperature sensation (spinothalamic tract). There is an acute, prominent peripheral vestibular syndrome with vertigo, nystagmus, and often vomiting (vestibular nuclei and protoneurones) see eighth cranial nerve in Ch. 29). In our experience, transient diplopia is frequent (skew deviation). Infrequent but quite distinctive for Wallenberg's syndrome are modifications of perception of the orientation of external objects (e.g., people are seen leaning on one side or even upside down). These also are due to acute vestibular disturbances. Hiccup is often present, but the site of the lesion is uncertain. Rarely, there is numbness of ipsilateral limbs due to involvement of the cuneatus and gracilis nuclei.

For isolated infarction of the lateral medulla, the prognosis is generally good, the usual sequelae being an oculosympathetic syndrome and some degree of hypesthesia on the ipsilateral face and contralateral body. The acute stage, however, can lead to sudden death, of poorly understood cause (although in a lesion of the medulla, disorders of cardiac and respiratory control are to be expected) or due to associated cerebellar infarction in the distal territory of the PICA. This can cause enough edema to produce potentially fatal brainstem compression, which could be treated by surgical removal of the infarcted cerebellar tissue, an option only occasionally required. Clinically, it is difficult or impossible to know whether a cerebellar infarct is associated with the medullary infarct (see below), so that whenever possible, CT or MRI is indicated. After the acute stage, apart the above-mentioned mild sequelae, a few elderly patients may complain of disagreeable, burning sensations over the contralateral body (spinothalamic tract, see Ch. 23). A few instances of Wallenberg's syndromes as a TIA have been reported.

Ischemia in the distal territory of the PICA, sparing the lateral medulla, causes sudden vertigo, vomiting, and nystagmus (an acute vestibular syndrome) because vestibular protoneurons are involved in the region of the flocculus (see eighth cranial nerve in Ch. 29). Ataxia can be minimal. Therefore, the differential diagnosis is with acute labyrinthine disorders. Imaging is diagnostic.

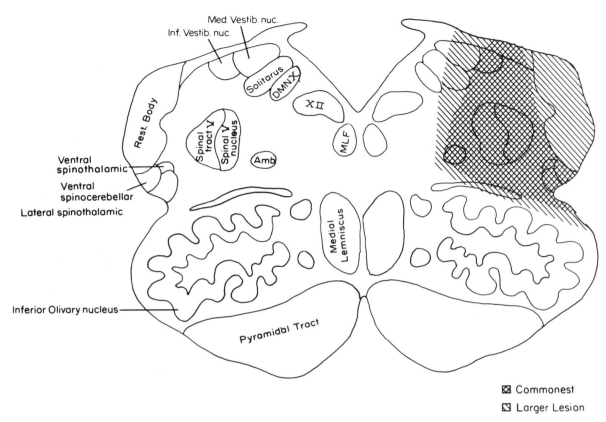

Figure 35-20. Lateral medullary infarction. The most common involvement and largest extent of the lesion are designated by checkerboard markings as described in the key. (Adapted from Currier et al., 1961, with permission.)

Anterior Inferior Cerebellar Artery

The AICA is a long circumferential artery, and, as such, supplies both the most lateral part of the pons and part of the cerebellum. Its size varies inversely with that of the PICA, hence its territory varies accordingly. It can supply the middle or inferior cerebellar peduncles, the spinothalamic tract, the fascicular fibers of the facial nerve, the descending sympathetic fibers, and part of the inferior surface of the cerebellum. Important from the clinical point of view is that it can give rise to the internal auditory artery.

Ischemia in the variable AICA territory causes variable clinical pictures, including vertigo, vomiting, deafness, ipsilateral ataxia and oculosympathetic syndrome, and crossed impairment of pain and temperature sensation. In practice, infarction in the AICA territory is a rare diagnosis, but sudden, unilateral deafness with any other evidence of brainstem or cerebellar involvement is highly suggestive.

Superior Cerebellar Artery

The SCA, another long circumferential artery supplies the most lateral part of the upper brainstem (i.e.,

the midbrain and rostral pons), the superior cerebellar peduncle, part of the dentate nucleus, and part of the superior surface of the cerebellum.

Ischemia in the SCA territory causes ipsilateral cerebellar ataxia, which can be mild or severe (superior cerebellar peduncle), postural tremor of the arm, oculosympathetic syndrome, and crossed impairment of pain and temperature sensation. Later, palatal myoclonus is possible, owing to crossed trans-synaptic degeneration of the contralateral inferior olive.

Posterior Cerebral Artery

The PCA (Fig. 35-18) arises from the basilar artery except in about 14 percent of people, a persistence of the fetal circulation (Fig. 35-3). From its origin to its junction with the Post Com A, it gives rise successively to perforators for the red nucleus, substantia nigra, medial part of the cerebral peduncle, nuclei and fascicles of the oculomotor and trochlear nerves, decussation of the superior cerebellar peduncles, rostral medial longitudinal fasciculus, medial lemniscus, and reticular substance of the brainstem. The PCA then gives rise to the thalamoperforant arteries, which supply the inferior, medial, and anterior parts of the thalamus. In some cases one PCA gives rise to these arteries for both thalami, and infarction in this territory has a characteristic butterfly shape in the high midbrain. Just before joining the Post Com A, the PCA gives rise to the thalamogeniculate arteries, which supply the central and posterior parts of the thalamus and parts of the lateral geniculate body.

As it loops around the midbrain, the PCA still also gives rise to perforators for the lateral part of the cerebral peduncle and corpora quadrigemina, and a branch, the posterior choroidal artery, gives rise to perforators for the pineal gland, posterosuperior thalamus, lateral geniculate body, and choroid plexus.

The artery then crosses the free edge of the tentorium cerebelli (where it can be squeezed in temporal herniation (see Chs. 17 and 25) and it supplies the inferior surface of the hemisphere rear of the temporal pole, with the posterior part of the hippocampal formation including the fimbria and initial fornix, as well as the occipital pole with the calcarine fissure and the distal part of the optic radiations. Usually, the PCA supplies a posterior part of the lateral surface of the hemisphere, and in some people this area can be extensive.

Ischemia in the PCA territory is rarely total because of the Post Com A. Ischemia in the proximal territory (i.e., prior to the junction with the Post Com A) causes various disturbances of ocular motility (see Ch. 28). Infarction of the posterolateral thalamus produces a contralateral pure sensory stroke with, less often, choreoathetoid movements, ataxia, or tremor. Thalamic infarction can give rise to delayed contralateral agonizing and burning pain, especially in older patients (Dejerine-Roussy syndrome, see Ch. 23).

More often, the infarction involves the hemispheric PCA territory. The most frequent site is a highly circumscribed region of the calcarine cortex, causing a pure contralateral homonymous hemianopia. When the upper bank of the calcarine fissure is spared, owing to collateral supply from the ACA across the cuneus, infarction limited to the lower bank yields a contralateral upper homonymous quadrantanopia. This diagnosis, however, is not always easily made, as the patient is usually anosognosic for the visual disturbance (see Chs. 19 and 25). When the lesion destroys both the left calcarine region and the splenium, there is alexia without agraphia (see Chs. 18 and 25). In some small infarcts anterior to the calcarine cortex and posterior to the splenium, isolated disturbances in spatial orientation are possible. Infarcts of the PCA hemispheric territory on the dominant side commonly cause a degree of anomia. Infarcts involving the fusiform and lingual gyrus cause disturbances in discrimination and naming of colors and can cause alexia in

the contralateral hemifield, a syndrome more obvious when the dominant hemisphere is involved. When the hippocampus is affected on the dominant side, an amnestic state also occurs (see Ch. 21).

Since the PCAs arise from a common arterial trunk, namely the basilar artery, bilateral simultaneous or successive ischemia, due to either propagated thrombus or embolism, occurs. The chief disorders are occipital blindness and a severe amnestic state, with various additional disturbances due to aphasia and agnosia.

Clinical Syndromes

Lacunar Clinical Syndromes

Because most occluding lacunar lesions are a form of mural disease, causing first stenosis and then thrombotic occlusion, TIAs are frequent, occurring in 20 percent of cases. In many cases the process of infarction evolves gradually, requiring hours or days to reach its peak. Lacunes being small lesions, they frequently involve one tract only, thus producing a monosymptomatic or "pure" syndrome.

Several distinct syndromes have been described from the small number of cases pathologically studied. *Pure motor stroke* is the most frequent syndrome, occurring in 60 percent of cases. The lacune may involve the corona radiata, internal capsule, pons, or rarely, the medullary pyramid. Although the syndrome is most easily diagnosed when the deficit equally affects the face, arm, and leg, sparing sensation and vision, language, and behavior, the diagnosis also applies when the weakness involves one part more than the other, and in a few cases the face is essentially spared. On the basis of CT scanning, three types of deep lesions have been recognized. Type 1 consists of capsuloputaminocaudate infarcts, which spread from the anterior to the posterior limb of the internal capsule, and into the adjacent striatum, and are large enough to qualify as giant lacunes. They cause profound hemiplegia and may disclose angiographic abnormalities of the MCA. Type 2 consists of capsulopallidal infarcts, located mainly in the posterior limb of the internal capsule. Type 3, anterior capsulocaudate infarcts, are also small, affecting the anterior limb. Although the posterior half of the posterior limb is considered to carry the motor fibers, the notion of homunculus whose face is anterior and whose leg is posterior in the plane of the internal capsule seems not to be a reliable chart for clinicopathologic correlation of lesions limited to the posterior limb of the internal capsule.

Syndromes featuring ataxia admixed with hemiparesis (*ataxic hemiparesis*) appear to be a clinical subset of pure motor strokes. Many have been documented from capsular infarction, especially when the lesions involved the genu and anterior limb. True dysphasia, dyspraxia, other disturbances of higher cerebral functions, and hemianopia have yet to be reported from lacunes.

Improvement in pure motor stroke occurs in a high percentage of cases. The incomplete, partial hemiparesis syndromes show the best prognosis, as do those with the smaller infarcts on CT scan, but cases of complete plegia with virtually total recovery have been encountered.

Pure sensory stroke has been documented from an infarct involving the ventroposterolateral nucleus of the thalamus, but in only a small number of cases has it been studied pathologically. A sensory component is part of Wallenberg's syndromes from lateral medullary infarction (see above), but whether such syndromes can arise from infarction of the upper brainstem or in pathways from the thalamus to the cortex has not been established. In one case small hemorrhage in the corona radiata was found to explain pure sensory stroke, and therefore infarction is not the unique cause.

Clinically, patients complain of striking alterations in spontaneous sensations. The parts may feel stretched, hot, sunburned, and tingling. Contacts of the skin with rings, watches, and sheets feel heavier on the affected side. The sensory complaints are sometimes greatly in excess of the deficits found on clinical examination. The diagnosis can be made most easily when the disturbance in sensation extends over the entire side of the body, involving the face and limbs, proximally as well as distally. Axial structures are often involved, including the scalp, neck, trunk, and genitalia right to the midline, even splitting the two sides of the nose, tongue, penis, and anus. This remarkable midline split is a clinical sign thought to be of value for separating thalamic from hemispheric sensory disturbances. Partial sensory syndromes occur more frequently in pure sensory stroke and may involve the face, arm, leg, or oral cavity, peribuccal area and hand (cheiro-oral syndromes), or peribuccal area and radial edge of forearm. The diagnosis of pure sensory stroke is certain on clinical grounds alone in such cases. How many permutations exist is a subject of some interest, since it could serve to further test current theories of the organization of the homunculus in the ventroposterolateral thalamus (see Ch. 23).

A few patients seen by the authors have experienced only TIAs.

Improvement usually occurs within weeks. The topography of the shrinking deficit may be rather unusual. Improvement in the trunk with persistence in the extremities, common in hemispheral disease, is only one of the patterns encountered. As already mentioned (see Posterior Cerebral Artery, above) in some patients agonizing, burning pain can appear (Dejerine-Roussy syndrome, see Ch. 23).

Sensorimotor lacunar stroke has been pathologically proved in only two cases. This contrasts sharply with the rising frequency of reported small, deep infarcts or of normal findings on CT or MRI in such patients, especially those with incomplete deficits. It is bad judgment to suspect a lacune when the clinical syndrome has both sensory and motor features, for the simple reason, already mentioned, that small, deep lesions tend to involve one tract. With sensorimotor syndromes, surface infarcts are the more likely.

Movement disorders, ranging from striking hemiballism through minor hemichorea to dystonia and action myoclonus and perhaps other movement disorders, have been attributed to small infarcts in the basal ganglia, thalamus, or subthalamic region. The movement disorder can be the first sign of the infarct or can appear as a more conventional sensory or motor syndrome fades, months after the initial stroke. The acute syndromes tend to be self-limiting, subsiding in days or weeks, but those that develop later can become increasingly severe and chronic.

Syndromes of pontine infarction are due to occlusions of basilar artery branches and, of course, comprise a heterogeneous group. They include the dysarthria–clumsy hand syndrome (usually with ipsilateral facial weakness and slight imbalance); crural paresis with ipsilateral ataxia (leg weakness, especially at the ankle), or arm and leg ataxia; pure dysarthria with no other focal signs; pure hemiparesis sparing the face; oculomotor paresis with cerebellar ataxia; and abducens palsy with pure motor paresis.

Technical limitations restrict CT imaging to only the larger lesions, with poor definition in the pons. MRI show lacunes as small as 1 mm^3. Owing to the small size of the involved arteries, angiography is not indicated.

Although lacunar syndromes prove to be amendable to a very reliable clinical diagnosis, from time to time they are mimicked by small surface infarcts, rarely even by a small hematoma. Therefore CT is indicated when a lacunar syndrome is diagnosed.

Arterial Syndromes from the Aorta to the Circle of Willis

Occlusion of a cerebral artery has variable consequences for the brain's blood supply. Beyond the circle, as stressed above, the area of ischemia or infarction can be minimized by the meningeal anastomoses, but ischemia (in short-lived occlusions) or infarction (in lasting occlusions) are inevitable. Here we briefly review the variable syndromes resulting from occlusion of the extracranial cerebral arteries.

Occlusion of the common carotid artery is rare and usually asymptomatic. The collateral supply comes from the ECA via an anastomosis from the vertebral artery. In some cases, however, blood can be diverted from the ICA to the ECA, thus stealing from the circle of Willis. This is an undesirable situation, which can be demonstrated by Doppler examination.

The consequences of occlusions of the ICA depend mostly on the configuration of the circle of Willis (Fig. 35-3), but also on the capacity of the contralateral ICA and of the vertebral arteries to supply blood to the circle. When there is no major defect in this arterial apparatus and the occluding material does not trespass on the circle (see above), ICA occlusion can even be totally silent clinically. Even cases of bilateral ICA occlusion can be clinically asymptomatic, and there are a handful of recorded cases in which the brain of asymptomatic patients was supplied only by one (usually greatly enlarged) vertebral artery. ICA occlusion, in other cases, features only TIAs, due either to transient failures of collateral circulation or to ATAE (see above). In unfavorable cases, owing to a poor circle of Willis or to propagating thrombus or embolism beyond the circle (see above), there is more or less extensive infarction. Often the infarct lies in the MCA territory because the ACA territory is still supplied by the Ant Com A. In a number of the author's cases, however, associated signs of dysfunction in the ACA, mostly sphincteric disturbances, were present (this finding is at the origin of the bedside adage "MCA + ACA = ICA." There are most unfavorable cases, however, occurring when the PCA arises from the ICA, in which most of the hemisphere can be infarcted, and cases in which one ICA supplies both ACAs, with the risk of bilateral infarction.

Occlusion of the innominate artery is rare and usually asymptomatic. It can cause a subclavian steal syndrome (see below) or cause a diversion of the common carotid artery blood into the right subclavian artery. This could be demonstrated by Doppler examination.

Occlusion of the subclavian artery, just proximal to the ostium of the vertebral artery, almost always occurs on the left side. It causes the subclavian steal, in which blood is diverted from the right vertebral artery into the left one, rarely from the basilar artery into the left vertebral artery. Very rarely, a similar abnormal hemodynamic situation exists on the right side. Patients are usually asymptomatic, and the diagnosis is suspected on the basis of a weak left radial pulse and a low blood pressure in the left arm. Doppler examination shows the steal (see Ch. 13). Rarely, patients complain of vertebrobasilar TIAs (see below), and vertebrobasilar infarctions have not been recorded. It is said that left arm exercise, by increasing the demand for blood, can provoke TIAs, but in the authors' expe-

rience, this view appears to be mostly theoretical. Surgery, formerly often advised, is currently exceptionally considered.

Occlusion of one vertebral artery at its origin is asymptomatic, provided that the other vertebral artery is of sufficient size. Occlusion of the intracranial segment is the usual cause of infarction in the PICA territory (see above). When the vertebral artery ends in the PICA, similar consequences may occur, and when one vertebral artery provides essentially the whole supply of the basilar artery, its occlusion leads to a full syndrome of basilar artery occlusion.

THE COURSE OF ISCHEMIC STROKES

The clinical hallmark of strokes is sudden onset. After this, however, quite differing courses are possible, according to the depth and duration of ischemia.

Completed Stroke

In many cases in which infarction has occurred, the deficit is maximal in a matter of minutes, follows a plateau for days or a few weeks, and thereafter some degree of improvement is usual. In such cases the clinician does not witness extension of the neurologic deficit. This course is traditionally termed *completed stroke* and is the most common course observed.

Worsening and Progressing Ischemic Stroke

In other cases, however, after the sudden clinical onset, the patient's status continues to deteriorate over days, either smoothly or in stepwise fashion. The frequency of this type of course is high, occurring in at least 25 percent of cases and perhaps even more frequently documented when the patient is studied closely. In former times such cases were called *stroke in progression,* a term that has largely been replaced by *worsening.*

The reasons for such worsening are poorly understood (see Ch. 5). Neurologic worsening is an unpredictable and decidedly nonuniform process for patients with ischemic stroke. The frequency varies somewhat according to the ischemic stroke subtype, being encountered least often in strokes of embolic mechanism and most often among those that appear due to thrombosis. In the latter group the frequency is the same regardless of whether the syndromes reflects occlusion of a large or small artery. The higher frequency in cases that seem to be thrombotic in nature raises the issue that the infarction may be due to perfusion failure (see above) and subject to waxing and waning of perfusion.

In trying to settle the issue of perfusion failure by studying the clinical features of progressing or worsening ischemic strokes, two types of worsening have been identified. In the first, the clinical syndrome of worsening adds new elements, involving parts not initially affected (e.g., the weakness involves the arm and leg when initially it involved only the leg). This type of worsening correlates in some cases with expansion of the lesion to contiguous areas of the brain, usually a reflection of perfusion failure or of extension of thrombosis. Worsening of this type may occur gradually or smoothly in the acute course of stroke or may take place in stepwise fashion over days or weeks. The pattern of delayed increments, separated by periods of stability, has been referred to as saltatory (Latin: *saltare,* to jump) progression, and while occurring uncommonly, it is distinctive and highly suggestive of perfusion failure from high-grade stenosis or thrombosis of large arteries or in other cases, from extension of thrombosis.

The second form of worsening represents intensification of the initial deficit with no change in the formula (e.g., arm weakness becoming arm paralysis), an effect that would suggest conversion of ischemia to infarction or edema surrounding the site of infarction (see Ch. 5). The intensification of the syndrome presumably explained by edema occurs in as many as 25 to 30 percent of patients with lacunar syndromes, who often revert back to their baseline syndrome within a week or so.

Transient Ischemic Attacks

In a third category, after the sudden onset the clinical disorders soon disappear because ischemia has been short-lived (transient arterial occlusions or transient perfusion failure) (see above). Such clinical episodes (TIAs) can herald brain infarction and therefore are of the utmost interest for stroke prevention. Their diagnosis and management are an important part of the everyday duties of most neurologists.

Traditionally, ischemic episodes that last less than 24 hours are considered to be TIAs. According to this definition, their annual incidence varies from roughly 2 to 8 per 1,000, with a prevalence from as low as 1 to as high as 77 per 1,000 persons, depending on the source of the study. TIAs are followed by stroke within 5 years in 25 to 51 percent of patients receiving no treatment, an outcome that, again, stresses the importance of their clinical diagnosis.

When the concept of TIAs was proposed around the early 1940s, it was believed that by segregating ischemic events lasting less than 24 hours, ischemic infarction would be separated from ischemia without infarction. Modern imaging and metabolic studies using SPECT and PET (see Chs. 14 and 15), however, have shown, in many instances of TIAs, alterations in brain structure (i.e., infarction) and perfusion deficits

persisting for hours or days despite complete clinical recovery.

There is a high correlation with tight stenoses in the affected territory for TIAS lasting a mere 5 to 10 minutes. However, when such attacks have been witnessed by physicians, it has been common for the patient's retrospective estimate to differ considerably from the observed duration of the attack. This suggests that the traditional description of TIAs, based on histories, is likely to underestimate their actual duration and to fail to appreciate the full picture of the spells.

The recent observations mentioned above, namely, that in many TIAs there is some structural damage, cast doubt on the usefulness of the concept of *reversible ischemic neurologic deficit,* a notion put forward as a bridge between TIA and infarction. Another practical consequence is that, however short their TIA, all patients should, whenever possible, undergo brain imaging to examine the possibility of clinically silent infarction. This point is of special importance when the patient is seen early, for with each passing hour, the probability of a normal outcome in the absence of medical or surgical intervention decreases steadily. In the largest trial to date for neuroprotective agents in acute ischemic stroke, the cohort of patients seen within 12 hours was large enough to permit analysis of their outcome at 4 days. Virtually none of those judged to have a neurologic deficit still present 12 hours after onset were normal by day 4, and the improvement toward normal occurred the least often in those who were most severely affected in their acute clinical syndrome. It is safer to assume persistence rather than to account on disappearance of an acute syndrome, especially when it is severe or moderately severe.

The clinical spectrum of TIA is the same as that of stroke. However, there are well recognized types that warrant being learned. It is customary to list them as pertaining either to the carotid or to the vertebrobasilar territory (Table 35-1), but the diagnosis of these territories is by no means always easy.

Amaurosis Fugax

The ophthalmic artery being a branch of the carotid artery, retinal ischemia is a marker of carotid disease, particularly atherosclerosis. Retinal infarction is rare in neurologic practice, and the common issue for the neurologist is transient monocular blindness or amaurosis fugax. This is a painless, brief (seconds, minutes) loss of sight of sudden onset involving all or part of the field of one eye. Characteristically, blindness develops as if a shade or curtain were drawn upward or downward, rarely sidewards. At the end of the episode, vision can recover, as if the shade were pulled in reverse fashion.

Attacks can be single or many, cases involving hundreds or even thousands of attacks having been recorded. In such repeated episodes, the pattern of blindness at onset and recovery is often stereotyped. In most cases there is full recovery, but in a few retinal infarction occurs. When patients have alternatively covered each eye during blindness, making sure the trouble was monocular, the diagnosis is straightforward. When this has not been done and in patients with one poor eye, the differential diagnosis must rule out transient hemianopia and migraine (see Ch. 24). Patients with amaurosis fugax can in addition have hemispheric TIAs, but very rarely simultaneously.

In a few patients fundoscopy during amaurosis fugax has shown white bodies, consisting of embolized white thrombi, slowly flowing down the retinal arteries. In others, after an episode or even with no amaurosis fugax fundoscopy has shown in the retinal arteries bright, yellow plaques of cholesterol (Hollenhorst's plaques). These tiny, flat crystals to not necessarily block blood flow. They originate mostly in atherosclerotic lesions at the origin of the ICA.

Amaurosis fugax thus should first raise the possibility of an ipsilateral (usually tight) ICA stenosis, all the more when the patient is a man over 40 with a bruit below the angle of the jaw. The bruit, however, can well be lacking, and as amaurosis fugax can herald a stroke at short notice, complete investigation, beginning with duplex Doppler ultrasound should not be delayed.

Fundoscopy during and after amaurosis fugax does not show abnormalities in many cases, and amaurosis fugax correlated with atherosclerosis accounts for probably less than 50 percent of the cases. The main mechanisms and causes of amaurosis fugax that must be considered when there is no ICA disease are listed in the accompanying box. The last item, No obvious cause, mostly covers cases in young patients with a benign outcome, suggesting that invasive procedures should be avoided in this setting.

Hemiparesis and Monoparesis

Table 35-1 shows that both hemiparesis and monoparesis can happen in the carotid and vertebrobasilar territories. When, as is frequent, they occur as pure motor strokes, the clinical diagnosis can be very difficult or impossible. The same remark applies to sensory disturbances.

Other Manifestations of Transient Ischemic Attacks

Aphasia is a reliable marker of left carotid artery territory disturbances. Quite often relatives or the family physician states that the patient was confused, which

---

CAUSES AND MECHANISMS OF AMAUROSIS FUGAX

Occlusive arterial disease
    Atherosclerosis or other lesions of the internal carotid artery (e.g., spontaneous dissection)
    Thromboemboli from the heart
    Arteritis
Low perfusion pressure
    Multiple occlusions of extracranial cerebral arteries
    Postural hypotension
    Arteriovenous fistula
    Intracranial hypertension
    Glaucoma
High resistance to retinal perfusion
    Migraine
    Malignant hypertension
    Increased blood viscosity
    Vasospasm
Miscellaneous causes
    Acute sharp pain
    Irrigation of the antrum
    Blowing the nose
    Sensitivity to cold
    Malaria
    Pregnancy
    Paraneoplastic retinopathy
    Interleukin-2 therapy
No obvious cause
    From Gautier, 1993, with permission.)

---

generally means aphasia. In the authors' opinion delirium is not a TIA.

Homonymous hemianopia pertains to both territories. In the authors' experience it is a rare TIA, and even rarer in the MCA territory. Occipital blindness is seen from time to time. Disorders of gait, dizziness, lightheadedness, and vertigo can be due to vertebrobasilar TIAs, but labyrinthine disease is a much more common cause and should be considered first. Drop attacks are most often cryptogenic. Shaking limbs must be clearly distinguished from that due to focal epilepsy. When TIAs are multiple, they most often remain of the same type in a given patient.

More TIA syndromes have been reported. Among the less common in the carotid territory is prosopagnosia (see Ch. 19). In the vertebrobasilar territory some distinctive attacks include deviation of one or both eyes, a feeling that the eyes are crossing or pulled medially or laterally, a sensation of falling asleep, hemiballismus, peduncular hallucinosis, or even a full

Wallenberg's syndrome. In the opinion of the authors, transient global amnesia is not a TIA.

Isolated symptoms such as diplopia, vertigo, or amnesia should not be accepted as TIAs unless proven otherwise, and nonfocal symptoms such as headache, dizziness, forgetfulness, or seizures are not TIAs.

Rarely, patients with severe perfusion failure can trigger their attacks by increasing the demand for blood supply in the compromised territory or by diverting blood from it. For instance, people with multiple extracranial arterial occlusions can trigger amaurosis fugax episodes by passing from dim light to sun or by bathing in a hot tub. Hyperventilation, causing reduction of carbon dioxide tension with vasoconstriction, can produce ischemia in a marginally perfused hemisphere and thus trigger contralateral involuntary, irregular limb-shaking movements. TIAs due to atherosclerosis are a good marker of coronary atherosclerosis, so that their diagnosis should lead to a cardiologic examination.

For long, TIAs were considered to be chiefly due to atherosclerosis in which case they could result from ATAE or perfusion failure (see above). Currently, where TIA patients can be submitted to full cardiologic investigation, cardiac embolism appears as probably the leading cause.

Differential Diagnosis

The differential diagnosis of TIAs is with epilepsy and migraine. In most cases the jacksonian march of clonic jerks or dysesthesias is diagnostic of epilepsy. A generalized seizure, either primary or following a focal fit, is not a TIA. Some particular types of epilepsy (e.g., ictal paralysis or inhibitory seizure paralysis) could be very difficult to prove or disprove. Migraine is a straightforward diagnosis when headache began in childhood or adolescence with a clear familial character (see Ch. 24). In *migraine accompagnée*, the visual symptoms and paresthesias have a slow buildup, which distinguishes them from TIAs and epilepsy. Late-life migraine accompaniments may occur without headaches and simulate TIAs or may actually be TIAs proper with a benign outlook.

POINTS OF CLINICAL EXAMINATION FOR ARTERIAL STROKES

Palpation of the bifurcation of the common carotid artery is contraindicated because it is not informative (it cannot distinguish the internal from the common and external carotids), it could dislodge a thrombus or plaque fragment, or it still could cause cardiac arrhythmia. When necessary (e.g., for Doppler studies), compression should be confined to the common carotid, as low in the neck as possible, and should be brief, limited to a few cardiac beats only.

Auscultation is best performed with the bell stethoscope. Tight stenoses may generate a systolic or systolodiastolic bruit, which has a harsh or high pitch when the stenosis is very tight. Stenoses that are not tight enough or too tight may generate no bruit, as of course is also the case with carotid occlusion, and thus the absence of bruit is of little significance.

Bruits arise from sources other than ICA stenosis. They may occur as radiated cardiac murmurs. Of course, auscultation of the heart is an important part of the examination. Cardiac murmurs are maximal over the precordium and typically peter out up the neck arteries. A systolic bruit below the angle of the jaw is very likely an indication of carotid stenosis.

The rare stenosis of the ECA cannot be distinguished from an ICA stenosis and requires Doppler evaluation (see Ch. 13). A carotid bruit may arise from augmented flow up a healthy ICA, which is compensating for contralateral occlusion or feeding an arteriovenous fistula (an arteriovenous malformation or a caroticocavernous fistula). In these latter cases the bruit may be of lower pitch than that of severe stenosis, but many exceptions are possible. Rarely, a neck bruit may represent augmented flow through a hypertrophied thyroid or a venous hum (the latter being interrupted by a Valsalva maneuver). Innocent bruits are frequent in children, in whom blood flow is rapid. Bruits are common over the subclavian arteries, but of little significance, except where the radial pulses are unequal (see discussion of subclavian steal, above).

The vertebral arteries should be auscultated at their origin and medial to the mastoid. On the mastoid, a bruit can signal an arteriovenous fistula or very rarely, a highly vascularized tumor. Such bruits are likely to be faint, and a quiet room is needed for auscultation.

Bruits over the eyeball may reflect a stenosis of the carotid siphon, may be radiated from flow to the siphon from the Post Com A, or may be due to an arteriovenous fistula (especially a caroticocavernous fistula) or malformation. To prevent eye movements that interfere with auscultation, the patient can be asked to stop breathing and to open the opposite eye and fix the gaze. Having the mouth hang loosely open usually prevents closing the eyes too tightly.

In the occasional patient ICA occlusion leads to extensive ECA collaterals, which can be seen on the brow or detected by palpating an increased pulse (as compared with the opposite side) in the ECA branches (facial, preaurcular, temporal), but this is rarely significant. Any anxiety to compromise collateral circulation by palpating these arteries is unwarranted, since their flow is trivial as compared with the greater volume carried by the faciomaxillary artery, which is not in the reach of palpation.

THERAPY

There are four major phases to the medical treatment of ischemic (as opposed to hemorrhagic) stroke: attempts to reverse the developing ischemia in the hyperacute stage; treatment of established infarction; prevention of recurrence; and prevention of the first-ever stroke (i.e., first stroke ever diagnosed, whether by symptoms or by discovery on brain scans).

Hyperacute Treatment

Thrombolysis

Thrombolysis seems a natural plan, given the assumption that it could clear away the occlusion, whether embolic or thrombotic in origin. Thrombolytic therapy, in principle, is the same as that used for evolving myocardial ischemia. For brain ischemia, much of the limited experience has been with tissue plasminogen activator but urokinase and streptokinase have also been used. A few examples of significant and sustained neurologic improvement have been documented when treatment was initiated within the first few hours. What remains uncertain is whether the timing of therapy is more important than specific dose and whether delays increase the risk of complications, negating any benefits. Ongoing clinical trials have yet to determine whether the selection of patients with actual occlusion can be made quickly and safely enough to use the agents in the brief time frame available before infarction develops and whether the dose required to achieve reliable recanalization will produce hemorrhage as often as it results in rescue of ischemic brain (i.e., if the benefits outweigh the hazards).

Neuronal Rescue

Neuronal rescue has become a major field of clinical investigation at present, the path having been opened by preclinical studies of brain ischemia in animal models. As cited in Chapter 5, the role of calcium in the process of brain ischemia has led to the development of many agents directed at blocking calcium entry into ischemic cells at one or many sites. Of the agents slowly working their way through clinical trials, promising findings have been generated by the first of them, the voltage-dependent, calcium channel antagonist nimodipine. In a large, multicenter trial of subarachnoid hemorrhage, as compared with placebo, the frequency of brain infarction was reduced by 34 percent and that of poor neurologic outcome by 40 percent with the use of oral nimodipine. For ischemic stroke, a recent meta-analysis of the nine double-blind trials showed a comparable reduction in clinical syndrome severity with 120 mg given as 30 mg every 6 hours for those treated within 12 hours of stroke onset. Those treated at 13 to 14 hours showed no benefits, and those treated after that time suffered a slightly worse outcome. Other agents are undergoing active trials. It remains unclear which agent will emerge as the most effective, but the findings with nimodipine establish the principle that neuroprotective therapy has a place, one that could alter the management of stroke in the direction of the hyperacute emergency approach given to myocardial ischemia.

Treatment for Hypertension

It is common for blood pressure to rise in the setting of hyperacute major stroke, especially from involvement of the brainstem, by as much as 5 to 30 mmHg, systolic and diastolic. Ample experience exists demonstrating that vigorous treatment of hypertension in the acute phase of the stroke may precipitate more clinical deficit. The authors caution against lowering the blood pressure by more than 20 to 30 mmHg systolic within the first 3 days after ischemic stroke.

Heparin

Heparin therapy, long a mainstay of treatment of the acute stroke, is an agent that forms a bridge between the principles of therapy to arrest stroke progression and those therapies hoping mainly to prevent recurrence. Unlike thrombolytic therapy, anticoagulation with intravenous heparin is not intended to dissolve thrombi but to impair thrombogenesis and prevent recurrent embolism. Whether heparin use can prevent worsening is the subject on an ongoing clinical trial, but there is general agreement, incompletely tested, that its use reduces the frequency of early recurrence. Furthermore, there is little argument that its use reduces the complications of immobilization, namely, venous thrombophlebitis and pulmonary embolism. Heparin is usually given intravenously, with no bolus, within hours of stroke onset by a maintenance infusion to keep the activated partial thromboplastin time at 1.5 to 2.5 times the control value. Arguments continue as to whether heparin could just as easily be given subcutaneously, whether a bolus is necessary to start the program, and whether the goal of an activated partial thromboplastin time of 1.5 to 2.5 times the control value is biologically necessary or merely a means for regulating the dose of the drug. Some clinicians hesitate to use heparin within the first 48 hours for fear it could encourage hemorrhagic conversion of an infarct, a concern that is appropriate for large infarcts but not a major concern for small ones. The authors advise erring on the side of caution and establishing on clinical and radiographic grounds that the infarct is small and that the stroke is not due to bleeding (e.g., a small hematoma misdiagnosed as infarct when brain imaging is not available) before planning heparin therapy. The risk of recurrence in the first 1 to 2 days is low, and the risk of hemorrhage from injudicious use of heparin could be high.

Treatment of Established Acute Stroke

Once established for many hours, brain infarction has proved remarkably resistant to any attempts at reversal. As indicated above, voltage-dependent calcium antagonists given later than 24 hours after onset may actually aggravate the effects of the infarct by increasing the collateral blood flow, which could increase brain edema. Treatments to halt brain edema have been remarkably unsuccessful, including among them use of steroids. Similar disappointments have been met in controlled clinical trials testing the possibility of increasing collateral flow by volume expansion, by potent vasodilation techniques such as carbon dioxide inhalation or nitroglycerin, and by plasmapheresis and phlebotomy to lower blood viscosity. Such programs are often resorted to for lack of suitable alternatives, but the results of clinical trials argue against their value.

Prevention of Recurrence and Prevention of First-Ever Stroke

Antiplatelet therapy is in well deserved widespread use in prevention of both primary (first ever) and secondary (recurrent) stroke. It is widely available, has a long history of safety, is inexpensive and easy to administer, and has recently been shown to have a beneficial effect in both settings. Upward of a dozen randomized placebo-controlled trials of aspirin in a setting of AF prior to first stroke or following TIA or minor stroke have shown significant risk reduction with aspirin as compared with placebo. Rates of reduction in stroke and vascular death of 20 to 50 percent have been documented, although some trials have shown less effect. The optimum dose of aspirin remains controversial, some European studies suggesting that as little as 30 mg/day may suffice, while others indicate that doses as high as 1,300 mg/day are needed. Side effects of nausea and gastrointestinal bleeding are somewhat higher in the high-dose group, but patients with arthritis have for generations consumed 10-fold higher daily doses, which makes the side effects issue less important than the higher likelihood of compliance with a single-dose 30- to 500-mg tablet. Some recent evidence suggests that more aspirin may be needed to achieve platelet suppression in patients with widespread atheroma than in healthy controls, a point prompting hesitation about the universal recommendation of ultra-low dose regimens of 30 mg/day until further testing is carried out.

Of the many other platelet antiaggregants, only ticlopidine has shown an effect only slightly superior to that of aspirin. When it is used in a dose of 250 mg twice a day, its effect peaks at 3 to 5 days (compared with aspirin, whose effects are immediate), and its use carries a small risk of neutropenia, rash, and disabling diarrhea, the occurrence of any of which prompts cessation of the drug. It can be used in patients said to be allergic to aspirin and is associated with none of the nausea that is not rare in aspirin users. In controlled clinical trials, its effects have been slightly superior to those obtained with aspirin. A derivative of ticlopidine, clopidogrel, is currently in clinical trials. It is more potent than ticlopidine in platelet antiaggregation and is said to have fewer side effects.

Anticoagulants are the main alternative to platelet antiaggregants. Until recently, the main basis for the use of anticoagulants had been the experience of many decades that anticoagulation seemed the most effective means of suppressing thromboembolic events in disorders associated with artificial (and diseased natural or native) cardiac valves, in which platelet antiaggregants seemed to be far less effective. This long-standing belief in the effectiveness of anticoagulants as compared with platelet antiaggregants has recently been confirmed in the only setting in which there have been modern clinical trials making direct comparison between the two classes of agents, namely in patients with AF who have not yet experienced an ischemic stroke. In five clinical trials, the anticoagulant warfarin has proved superior to the platelet antiaggregant aspirin by ratios of 2:1 and higher, depending on the study. At the doses of warfarin used, the dreaded complications of bleeding (systemic or intracranial, mild or fatal) have not occurred frequently enough to outweigh the benefits of warfarin.

Clearly, the ease of use and safety of platelet antiaggregants favors them in clinical settings in which patients have contraindications to anticoagulant use (e.g., unreliability, medical disorders likely to cause bleeding, greatly advanced age), but the recently completed trials have shown that it is possible to use warfarin safely under most conditions and achieve long-term benefits. A European trial reported in 1993 showed a similar superiority of warfarin in prevention of recurrent stroke in a setting of AF, indicating that the results do not apply only to previously asymptomatic patients.

What remains unclear is whether these differences would be equally evident in prevention of first or recurrent stroke when the cause of the stroke is not cardioembolic. Whether warfarin or aspirin offers better results in atherosclerosis, with complications of therapy taken into account, is the subject of a large trial currently underway, the Warfarin-Aspirin Recurrent Stroke study (WARSS), scheduled for completion in 1997.

Surgery for Hyperacute Stroke

In the carotid system the main efforts of surgery are directed at reestablishing the normal patency of the artery, removing a nidus of thromboembolism, and mitigating the effects of the perfusion failure. Surgical endarterectomy removes the offending plaque and thrombus, prevents embolism, and restores flow.

When acute stroke leads to the discovery of a totally occluded ICA, the management plan is unclear. The crucial angiographic finding that encourages an attempt to reopen the artery is the demonstration that the occluded portion extends for only a few centimeters from the origin and that the vessel is patent through its entire intracranial course. When dye is seen to enter the intracranial carotid retrograde through the ophthalmic artery and to fill back down the course of the artery to the base of the skull, this could indicate that the surgeon can attack the extracranial occlusion with less fear of dislodging an intracranial portion of the thrombus during the surgery. Such dislodgement might yield the very disastrous embolic stroke that the surgery is designed to prevent. Failure to demonstrate an operable carotid occlusion forces a decision to fall back on medical therapy, and here no uniform recommendations can be given from any clinical trial data. Aspirin once a day is recommended by many, while others resort to coumadin therapy.

In the immediate postoperative period, changes reflecting reactivation or loss of function of the nerve to the carotid sinus and of the carotid body may occur. These include a short-lived fall in blood pressure, sometimes striking, in the hours after surgery, which is thought by some to be due to reactivation of the function of the nerve to the carotid body, possibly long inactivated by having been embedded in a nondistensible wall. Operative section of the invisible tiny nerve may produce a short-lived dramatic rise in the blood pressure. The changes are usually self-correcting within a few days but may need medical treatment in the acute postoperative period. For patients with advanced pulmonary insufficiency, unintended removal of the carotid body may be followed by an increase in carbon dioxide tension and failure of response to hypoxia.

The demonstrated disease is often less severe than critical stenosis or occlusion. When dissection is found, most authorities recommend conservative management, since the lesion usually heals itself. Heparin is used for a few weeks, followed by platelet inhibitors, to minimize the risk of embolism during the healing phase.

Carotid endarterectomy under any conditions carries the small risks of intraoperative embolism from fragments of the plaque and of perfusion failure during the minutes when the carotid must be clamped below and above the operative field for removal of the plaque. When there is long-standing perfusion failure, rare instances occur in which the restoration of normal flow from successful endarterectomy reperfuses a vascular bed unable to tolerate the normal pressure, resulting in hemorrhagic infarction in the previously ischemic territory. Parenchymatous hematoma has even occurred, in some cases far removed from the vascular territory of the operation. Such outcomes usually occur within the first day or two after surgery or not at all. These observations have led to the recommendation that monitoring of blood pressure is needed, with a plan to prevent the dramatic rises in pressure that may follow unintended section of the nerve to the carotid sinus and to monitor the clinical effects of reperfusion.

Surgery for Prevention of Stroke After Transient Ischemic Attack or Stroke

The large North American Symptomatic Carotid Endarterectomy Trial (NASCET) and the European Cooperative Endarterectomy Trial (ECET) both demonstrated that endarterectomy strikingly reduced the frequency of ischemic stroke, ipsilateral to the operation and contralateral as well, as compared with aspirin therapy, for those patients whose stenosis was 70 percent or greater. Evidence of a benefit from surgery was apparent in the follow-up data within 3 months of surgery. This finding strongly suggests that once symptoms develop, further ischemia from ATAE, perfusion failure, or both is to be expected unless surgical intervention is undertaken. Compared with surgery, aspirin therapy had little benefit, but no formal trials have compared surgery with warfarin or with other (nonaspirin) platelet antiaggregants.

Prompt referral to experienced centers for surgical management has now become a widespread practice. In an effort to minimize untoward events, the authors recommend the approach to the patient be undertaken by noninvasive techniques wherever possible. Such techniques include duplex and transcranial Doppler ultrasound (see Ch. 13), the former to estimate the degree of extracranial stenosis and the latter to determine the extent of intracranial hemodynamic effects and assess the availability of collateral supply at the circle of Willis, as well as MRA to identify the anatomy of the lesion and thereby help guide the surgeon. Conventional cut-film angiography is still widely practiced at many centers, but its complication rate accounts for almost half of the untoward events associated with surgical management. In some centers balloon angioplasty is being undertaken in the same setting as conventional angiography, but this procedure carries the risk of dislodging plaque fragments, does not reliably rid the patient of the offending lesion, and may fail to suppress the risk of embolism from the same source thereafter. In coronary artery disease the procedure may spare the patient the great threat of open-heart surgery, while in carotid stenosis the disease process is literally right under the skin, easily accessible to the experienced surgeon.

When ulceration is shown without accompanying severe stenosis, opinions differ sharply as to the best management. Many are convinced that shallow ulcers and flat plaques are not a cause of stroke and represent at best an incidental lesion. Others strongly recommend surgery, since small ulcers with fibrin-platelet complexes have been found in microscopic studies of some such lesions. However, in postoperative specimens, ulcers have often been found with a smooth endothelium, without evidence of thrombus. Large, complex ulcerations are usually associated with severe stenosis, which makes the decision for surgery less difficult. Recent clinical trial data have not yet demonstrated the superiority of surgery over medical therapy in the absence of severe stenosis. Better insight into the best management still rests on the outcome of ongoing trials for the lesions with non-hemodynamically significant tight stenosis.

Surgery for Prevention of First-Ever Stroke

The risk of prophylactic carotid endarterectomy in experienced centers in asymptomatic patients was thought to be on the order of 1 percent, making some clinicians favor surgery while others have thought that the risks of stroke from surgery is far higher and can scarcely warrant the recommendation to have the operation. This issue has been settled to some degree by the results of a recently completed clinical trial, in which asymptomatic patients with more than 60 percent stenosis of the ICA agreed to randomization to a group for prophylactic carotid endarterectomy while the other group followed best medical therapy without planned surgery. Based on an analysis of 5-year event rates, the group having surgery experienced death or stroke ipsilateral to the side of the stenosis at a rate of 4.9 percent, as compared with a rate of just over 10.6 percent suffered by the nonsurgical group. These findings forced discontinuation of the study in late 1994 because of an outcome favoring surgery (P .006). The complication rate for surgery was 2.3 percent.

Prior to the release of these data, clinicians had difficulties in deciding which patients, if any, to refer for surgery. For some 20 percent of such patients with severe extracranial carotid stenosis, brain imaging discloses evidence of prior infarction, a finding that may also apply to those with carotid occlusion. Similarly, some patients showed blunted intracranial waveforms on transcranial Doppler (Ch. 13) and were thought by some clinicians to be at higher risk for stroke than those whose patterns of collateral flow showed normal intracranial velocities. Those with positive brain imaging results or blunted waveforms on transcranial Doppler were often referred for surgery, while those without such findings were withheld. This latter policy can be questioned given the current information.

Modification of Risk Factors

Cardiac disease is the largest risk factor for stroke. AF with rheumatic valvular disease increases stroke risk 17-fold and nonvalvular atrial fibrillation 5-fold. Increased risk also exists for patients with post-myocardial infarction thrombus or with cardiac ventricular aneurysm, PFO, mitral valve prolapse, or atrial septal aneurysm (see above).

Among the modifiable risk factors, hypertension overshadows the others, and its treatment is strongly advised. Hypertension increases stroke risk by a factor of 4.0 for men and 4.4 for women. So-called borderline hypertension confers a 2.0-fold higher relative risk. Even isolated systolic hypertension, once disregarded as benign, increase stroke risk 2.4-fold. Long-term effort to reduce blood pressure is an important adjunct to therapy, but the authors repeat their concern (see above) against too vigorous treatment of blood pressure in the hyperacute setting of ischemic stroke or where there are tight stenoses of cerebral arteries. Smoking (especially cigarettes) increases the risk of stroke to an extent depending on the smoking habit, ranging from a factor of 2 for light smokers to 5 for those smoking over a pack a day. Cessation of smoking lowers the risk, and 5 years after cessation the risk approaches that of the general population. Diabetes mellitus carries a 1.5- to 3.0-fold increased risk, probably secondary to microvascular disease and a greater tendency to atherosclerosis. Hypercholesterolemia, another modifiable risk factor, exerts its greatest threat to health through cardiac and peripheral vascular disease, with a surprisingly smaller impact on the outlook for ischemic vascular disease, but prudent physicians seek and treat hypercholesterolemia wherever found. Increased blood viscosity, associated with a hematocrit over 45, thrombocytosis, and leukocytosis are all known to be associated with increased risk of worsening in a setting of acute ischemic stroke and with increased risk of stroke. Normalization of these factors may favorably influence the course of acute ischemic stroke, but the matter has not yet been adequately tested in a therapeutic trial, and normalization has not been tested well for impact on prevention of first-ever stroke.

VENOUS STROKES

Venous strokes result from occlusion of cerebral veins due to thrombosis and are much rarer than arterial strokes. Their frequency is not precisely known, although in Western countries modern imaging, particularly MRI, shows that they are not as rare as suggested by autopsy series. They are likely to still be frequent in developing countries, all the more where infectious diseases and starvation prevail. The sexes are equally affected, except in the 20 to 35 age group, in which occlusion of cerebral veins predominates in women as a result of its causal relationship with oral contraceptives and the puerperium. Occlusion of cerebral veins is often a difficult clinical diagnosis but one not to be missed, since for many patients there is an efficient treatment, while the spontaneous course can be disastrous.

Anatomy

The blood of the brain is drained by cerebral veins into dural sinuses, which empty essentially in the internal jugular veins. Sinuses are channels within the dura. Their lumina are lined by an endothelium apparently similar to that of veins. Sinuses and cerebral veins have no valves, which allows blood to flow in either direc-

tion, providing an obviously advantageous opportunity for blood to divert from occluded vessels. Sinuses contain most of the arachnoid granulations through which much of but not all the cerebrospinal fluid is reabsorbed (see Ch. 59), which explains the Queckenstedt-Stookey maneuver (see Ch. 9) and the raised intracranial pressure that accompanies most occlusions of cerebral veins.

The more commonly occluded sinuses are the superior sagittal sinus, the lateral sinuses, and the cavernous sinuses (Figs. 35-21 and 35-22). The superior sagittal sinus runs in the superior border of the falx cerebri from the foramen caecum to the torcular herophili (Latin: *torcular*, press; Herophilus of Chalcedon, Greek physician and anatomist, born circa 325 B.C.). In some people the superior sagittal sinus is formed only to the rear of the coronal suture, and hence its poor or absent visualization in the frontal region on angiograms, CT, or MRI is not necessarily of pathologic significance. The superior sagittal sinus drains

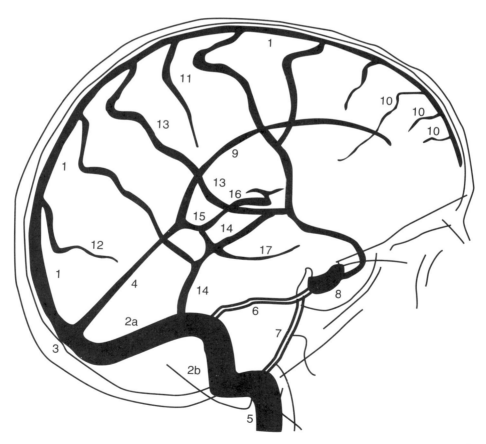

Figure 35-21. Superficial and deep cerebral veins and dural sinuses: *1*, superior sagittal sinus; *2a*, transverse and *2b*, sigmoid portion of lateral sinus; *3*, torcular herophili; *4*, straight sinus; *5*, internal jugular vein; *6*, superior petrosal sinus; *7*, inferior petrosal sinus; *8*, cavernous sinus; *9*, inferior sagittal sinus; *10*, frontal veins; *11*, parietal vein; *12*, occipital vein; *13*, Trolard's vein; *14*, Labbé's vein; *15*, great vein of Galen; *16*, internal cerebral vein; *17*, basal vein. (From Barnett et al., 1992, with permission.)

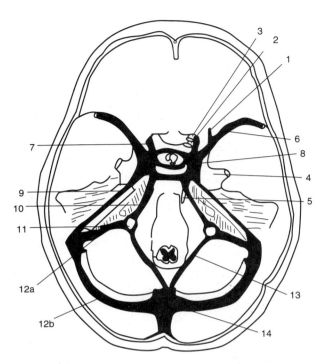

Figure 35-22. Cavernous sinus and dural sinuses: *1,* trochlear cranial nerve; *2,* carotid artery; *3,* optic nerve; *4,* trigeminal nerve; *5,* oculomotor nerve; *6,* sphenoparietal sinus; *7,* ophthalmic vein; *8,* cavernous sinus; *9,* superior petrosal sinus; *10,* inferior petrosal sinus; *11,* internal jugular vein; *12a,* sigmoid portion of lateral sinus; *12b,* transverse portion of lateral sinus; *13,* posterior occipital sinus; *14,* torcular herophili. (From Barnett et al., 1992, with permission.)

the major part of the cortex and centrum semiovale. Emissary veins connect it with scalp veins, which accounts for possible superior sagittal sinus thromboses after scalp injuries or infections.

The lateral sinuses join the torcular (where the superior sagittal sinus, the lateral sinuses, and the straight sinus meet) with the jugular bulb (Fig. 35-21). Its first or transverse portion runs within the insertion of the tentorium cerebelli on the occipital bone. Its second or sigmoid portion runs down medial to the mastoid and can be thrombosed in mastoiditis or otitis media. An emissary vein connects this part of the lateral sinus with the skin over the mastoid process, and it is said that this is why leeches applied to the mastoid region were in vogue as a treatment for strokes in the 19th and early 20th centuries. The lateral sinuses drain the posterior part of the cerebral hemispheres and parts of the cerebellum and brainstem. The right lateral sinus is often a direct continuation of the superior sagittal sinus and is frequently larger than the left lateral sinus. Therefore poor visualization or nonvisualization of the left lateral sinus is not necessarily of

pathologic significance. MRI allows the diagnosis of lateral sinus thrombosis with lateral sinus hypoplasia.

The cavernous sinuses (Fig. 35-22) are within the dura on each side of the sella turcica. They are divided by many fibrous septa (hence the name cavernous). The ICA siphon with the sympathetic plexus and the abducens nerve are within the sinus, while the oculomotor and trochlear nerves, together with the ophthalmic and maxillary nerves, run within its lateral wall. Both cavernous sinuses are largely anastomosed across the sella turcica by the coronary sinus, which explains why thrombophlebitis of the cavernous sinus can be bilateral. Posteriorly the cavernous sinus drains into the internal jugular vein via the superior and inferior petrosal sinuses (Fig. 35-21). Anteriorly, its main afferents are the ophthalmic veins, which accounts for the predominantly ocular symptoms and signs of cavernous sinus diseases (see below). Around the rim of the orbit, the ophthalmic veins anastomose freely with the veins of the middle third of the face. This accounts for cavernous sinus occlusions due to spreading infections from the face, the archetype of which is the furuncle on the upper lip or the nose. The cavernous sinuses are well visualized by CT and MRI.

The main superficial cerebral veins of the hemispheres are easily distinguished from arteries because they are larger and in contrast to the arteries, which wind over the convolutions and into the depths of fissures and sulci, they take a straight course over the cortex. Their walls are devoid of muscle fibers, which allows them to greatly dilate in response to occlusion. There is no precise correspondence with arterial territories. Superficial veins are either ascending, draining into the superior sagittal sinus, or descending, draining into the cavernous sinuses. Their number and location are very variable, which makes their absence on angiograms an unreliable sign of disease and in the authors' experience a cause of false-positive diagnoses. Two long veins run across the lateral aspect of the hemisphere, namely Trolard's great anastomotic vein (P. Trolard, French anatomist, 1842–1910) which extends from the superior sagittal sinus to the middle cerebral veins, and Labbé's vein (EM Labbé, French physician, 1870–1939), which connects the lateral sinus with Trolard's vein and sometimes with the superior sagittal sinus (Fig. 35-23).

Deep cerebral veins are formed on each side at the foramen of Monro, by the thalamostriate vein, the vein of the septum lucidum, and the vein of the choroid plexus. They run posteriorly side by side in the roof of the third ventricle and are sometimes termed internal cerebral vein (Fig. 35-21). Near its end, the internal cerebral vein receives the basal vein (of Rosenthal) (Fig. 35-21), which sweeps around the cerebral peduncles medial to the temporal lobe. Below the

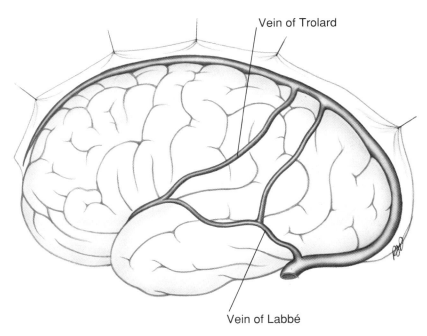

Figure 35-23. The two major cerebral surface veins.

splenium and above the dorsal midbrain the deep cerebral veins join to form the great vein of Galen (Galen of Pergamus, Greek physician, 131–201 A.D.), which drains into the straight sinus (Fig. 35-21).

Deep veins drain blood from the deep centrum semiovale, internal capsule, basal ganglia, and medial parts of the temporal lobe. In contrast to the superficial veins, the deep cerebral veins are remarkably constant. They are often beautifully shown on angiograms and during the heyday of angiography were quite useful for diagnosing displacements of deep structures.

Pathology

Opening the superior sagittal sinus is part of routine postmortems (see Ch. 7). Occlusion of sinuses and veins is due to red thrombi, sometimes infected. The authors do not know of detailed, recent microscopic studies of these thrombi. Thrombi in the superior sagittal sinus frequently extend into adjacent cerebral veins. Such data from autopsies characterize the most severe cases. Segmental occlusions are possible, and the authors know of an occlusion of a rolandic vein, about 2 cm long, which was responsible for focal seizures during a few days and was found at postmortem years afterward. Death was due to a colon cancer. Some segmental occlusions of this type can now be diagnosed during life with CT and even better with MRI.

The main characteristic of cerebral infarcts due to occlusion of cerebral veins is that they are hemorrhagic, the hemorrhagic lesions involving both the white and gray matter. This latter is a point of distinction from infarcts due to arterial occlusions, in which hemorrhages involve essentially the gray matter. The hemorrhagic changes can be prominent to the point that subarachnoid hemorrhages and subdural or intracerebral hematomas have been associated with venous infarction.

Blockage of the brain's supply of oxygen and glucose, which is typical of infarction from arterial occlusion, is not likely to have similar consequences in cerebral vein occlusion, in which it results from engorgement or clogging of the veins. However, the pathophysiology of brain infarction due to occlusion of cerebral veins has not, to the authors' knowledge, been addressed in recent studies.

Causes of Cerebral Vein Occlusion

The pathogenesis of occlusion of cerebral veins is imperfectly understood. Changes in the vessel wall, increased thrombogenic tendency, and venous stasis are more suspected than demonstrated in many individual cases. Septic thromboses are explained by the direct effect of microorganisms on thrombogenesis and clotting.

Infections either local (e.g., from head injuries), regional (e.g., sinusitis or otitis), or systemic (e.g., septicemia or viral diseases) are probably still the leading cause in developing countries. Their frequency has sharply declined in Western countries. Some occlusions are due to malaria (see Ch. 42) or to trichinosis. The puerperium is a leading setting for venous infarction in young women, and in Western life-style countries, oral contraceptives are another frequent cause. Occlusion of cerebral veins can be the only detectable finding or can be associated with an underlying disease (e.g., cancer), which implies an additional workup. Among systemic causes, the main ones are malignancies, connective tissue diseases, and inflammatory diseases such as Behçet disease (see Chs. 38 and 66). A few cases are related to a hereditary deficiency of antithrombin III or protein C or S.

This is not an exhaustive account of the causes, but even when the rarest ones have been considered, 25 to 35 percent of cases remain cryptogenic.

Clinical Features

Except for the cavernous sinus, which has a particular clinical picture (see below), extensive occlusion of cerebral sinuses and veins causes raised intracranial pressure (with symptoms of headache, papilledema, sometimes vomiting and obtundation, and abducens nerve palsy), generalized or focal seizures, and focal deficits. The classical clinical picture of superior sagittal sinus occlusion, namely bilateral deficit predominating on the lower limbs and alternating seizures, would be now rare. Recent series emphasize the frequency of isolated intracranial hypertension corresponding to the clinical features of pseudotumor cerebri, a diagnosis that should suggest cerebral vein occlusion. Seizures are present in 35 to 75 percent of the cases. Motor and sensory deficits and aphasia are possible, sometimes of brief duration as in TIAs. The onset can be acute, mimicking an arterial stroke, subacute, mimicking an abscess or encephalitis, or chronic, mimicking a tumor.

Examination of cerebrospinal fluid is crucial to rule out meningitis, inasmuch as many patients have fever and an elevated erythrocyte sedimentation rate. The examination shows elevated pressure, a raised protein content, red blood cells in most cases, and pleocytosis.

Imaging

Conventional angiography can show the absence of part or all of a sinus, signs to be interpreted with caution (see above). It can also show "corkscrew" veins, which are developed anastomoses between superficial veins.

In superior sagittal sinus occlusions, enhanced CT scan can show the empty delta sign, in which the nonopacified thrombus is surrounded by the opacified walls of the sinus. This is diagnostic but is present only in one third of patients because the empty delta sign can be lacking when CT is performed too early (in the first few days) or too late (after more than 2 months) in the course of the thrombus. It can also be lacking when the thrombus does not involve the posterior third of the sinus.

MRI detects blood flow and can visualize the thrombus with the process of conversion of oxyhemoglobin into methemoglobin. Early in the course of superior sagittal sinus thrombosis, the normal flow void is absent, so that the occluded sinus appears isointense on T_1-weighted images and hypointense on T_2-weighted images. After a few days, the thrombus is detected, appearing hyperintense on T_1-weighted and then on T_2-weighted images. Later, MRI can show the return of flow where there has been recanalization by the reappearance of flow void. The shortcomings of conventional MRI can be overcome by three-dimensional magnetic resonance flow imaging.

Cavernous Sinus Thrombosis

In acute cases cavernous sinus thrombosis with occlusion of the ophthalmic veins causes painful ophthalmoplegia, chemosis, proptosis, and sensory loss over the forehead. Bilateralization is possible (see above). There is high, fluctuating fever. High-dose, polyvalent antibiotic therapy is mandatory without delay. The differential diagnosis is with orbital cellulitis and mucormycosis, usually in ill-controlled diabetes mellitus. Caroticocavernous fistulas also present with chemosis, proptosis, and ophthalmoplegia. The loud systolic bruit heard over the eyeball and the angiograms are diagnostic. Besides the acute form of cavernous sinus thrombosis, there is a chronic, indolent form with mild proptosis and chemosis and an abducens nerve paralysis.

Treatment

In cerebral vein occlusion due to infection, high doses of broad-spectrum antibiotics are obviously needed immediately. Anticonvulsants are given to all patients by some clinicians but only to those who have convulsed by the majority. Measures that have been advised to reduce intracranial pressure include steroids, mannitol, acetazolamide, spinal taps, and various shuntings.

Anticoagulation is now widely recommended where there is no evidence of hemorrhagic infarction on CT. Even in cases with hemorrhagic infarction, anticoagulants appear beneficial. Provided that there are no contraindications to anticoagulation, heparin is first used, followed after a week or so by oral anticoagulants for a few months. Wherever possible, MRI allows monitoring the evolution of lesions. Use of fibrinolytics has not yet been fully assessed. A few surgical thrombectomies have been performed.

With early diagnosis and anticoagulants, the prognosis of nonseptic cerebral vein occlusions has undoubtedly improved. There are still fulminant forms and cases with sequelae (deficits, seizures, dural arteriovenous fistulas), but many patients make a total recovery. This confirms the long-known observation that for similar initial deficits, the prognosis is far better for venous strokes than for arterial strokes.

Septic occlusions of cerebral veins remain of poor prognosis with a high mortality, even where best care is available. Where emergency critical care is not available, it must be feared that the prognosis is disastrous.

ANNOTATED BIBLIOGRAPHY

Amarenco P, Hauw JJ, Duyckaerts C, Bousser MG. The prevalence of ulcerated plaques in the aortic arch in patients with stroke. N Engl J Med 1992;326:221–5.

Cerebral emboli from the aortic arch.

Amarenco P, Hauw JJ, Gautier JC. Arterial pathology in cerebellar infarctions. Stroke 1990;21:1299–1305.

Cardiac embolism the leading cause.

Amarenco P, Hauw JJ, Henin D et al. Les infarctus du territoire de l'artère cerebelleuse postero-inferieure. Etude clinico-pathologique de 28 cas. Rev Neurol (Paris) 1989; 145:277–86.

Cardiac embolism first cause of PICA infarctions.

Amaurosis Fugax Study Group. Current management of amaurosis fugax. Stroke 1990;21:201–8.

Current advice.

Ameri A, Bousser MG. Thromboses veineuses cérébrales. In Bogousslavsky J, Bousser MG, Mas JL (eds). Accidents Vasculaires Cerebraux. Doin, Paris, 1993.

110 personal cases and a review.

American-Canadian Cooperative Study Group. Persantine aspirin trial in cerebral ischemia: endpoint results. Stroke 1985;16:406–15.

No value for persantine alone or with aspirin.

Asymptomatic Carotid Atherosclerosis Study Group. Study design for randomized prospective trial of carotid endarterectomy for asymptomatic atherosclerosis. Stroke 1989; 20:844–9.

Background paper for ongoing study.

Baquis GD, Pessin MS, Scott RM. Limb Shaking. A Carotid TIA. Stroke 1985;16:444–8.

The event may mimic a seizure.

Barnett HJM, Mohr JP, Stein BM, Yatsu FM (eds). Stroke. 2nd Ed. Churchill Livingstone, New York, 1992.

Standard text.

Benomar A, Yahkiyaoui M, Birouk N et al. Middle cerebral artery occlusion due to hyatid cysts of myocardial and intraventricular cavity cardiac origin: two cases. Stroke 1994;25:886–8.

Should be considered in young patients in or from endemic areas.

Bernstein EF (ed). Amaurosis Fugax. Springer-Verlag, New York, 1987.

Dedicated volume.

Binswanger O. Die Abgrenzung der allgemeinen progressiven Paralyse. Berl Klin Wochenschr 1894;31: 1103–1105, 1137–1139, 1180–1186.

Details of the original case report.

Black IW, Hopkins AP, Lie CL, Walsh W. Evaluation of transesophageal echocardiography before cardioversion of atrial fibrillation and flutter in nonanticoagulated patients. Am Heart J 1993;126:375–81.

TEE improves the detection of thrombi in the left appendage. Even without detected thrombi, the risk of embolism with cardioversion is still present.

Bousser MG, Tournier-Lasserve E. Summary of the Proceedings of the First International Workshop on CADASIL. Stroke 1994;25:704–7.

Update on cerebral autosomal dominant arteriopathy with subcortical infarcts and leukoencephalopathy.

Buonanno FS, Moody DM, Ball RM. CT scan findings in cerebral sinovenous occlusion. Neurology 1982;32: 288–92.

The empty delta sign.

Butler MJ, Adams HP Jr, Hiratzka LF. Recurrent cerebral embolism from a right atrial myxoma. Ann Neurol 1986; 19:608.

Right atrial myxoma plus patent foramen ovale.

Caplan LR. Brain embolism revisited. Neurology 1993;43: 1281–7.

Inventory of current issues. Embolism, cardiac and artery-to-artery, frequent in the posterior circulation.

Caplan LR. Of birds and nests and brain emboli. Rev Neurol (Paris) 1991;147:265–73.

Embolism revisited. Meditation on the principles of brain embolism.

Caplan LR. "Top of the basilar" syndrome. Neurology 1980; 30:72.

Describes clinical features of lesions in the distal basilar artery territory.

Caplan LR. Occlusion of the vertebral or basilar artery. Follow-up analysis of some patients with benign outcome. Stroke 1979;10:277–82.

Emphasizes the time course and capabilities of collateral circulation.

Castaigne P, Lhermitte F, Buge A et al. Paramedian thalamic and midbrain infarcts. Clinical and neuropathological study. Ann Neurol 1981;10:127.

An approach to the complex clinical features of these small infarcts.

Castaigne P, Lhermitte F, Cambier J, Gautier JC. Obstruction bilatérale des carotids internes. Presse Med 1963;71: 757–60.

Long survival. Granular atrophy in distal fields.

Castaigne P, Lhermitte F, Gautier JC. Role des lésions artérielles dans les accidents ischémiques cérébraux de l'athérosclerose. Rev Neurol (Paris) 1965;113:1–32.

Infarcts correlated with thorough postmortem of cerebral arteries.

Castaigne P, Lhermitte F, Gautier JC et al. Arterial occlusions in the vertebro-basilar system. A study of forty-four patients with post-mortem data. Brain 1973;96:133–54.

Thrombi and emboli. The antero- and retrograde extension of thrombi. Most posterior cerebral artery occlusions are embolic.

Castaigne P, Lhermitte F, Gautier JC et al. Internal carotid artery occlusion. A study of 61 instances in 50 patients. Brain 1970;93:231–58.

Thrombi: their relationship with stenoses, their extension, and embolism.

Catron PW, Dutka AJ, Biondi DM et al. Cerebral air embolism treated by pressure and hyperbaric oxygen. Neurology 1991;41:314–16.

Two cases with good outcome.

Cerebral Embolism Task Force. Cardiogenic Brain Embolism. The second report of the Cerebral Brain Embolism Task Force. Arch Neurol 1989;46:727–43.

Update on the various causes.

Chamorro AM, Sacco RL, Mohr JP et al. Lacunar infarction: clinical–CT correlations in the Stroke Data Bank. Stroke 1991;22:175–82.

Difficult to predict the exact locus of the lesion in the internal capsule based on the clinical hemiparesis syndrome.

Cogan DG. Blackouts not obviously due to carotid occlusion. Arch Ophthalmol 1961;66:180–87.

Descriptions of amaurosis fugax and events of other origins.

Critchley M. The anterior cerebral artery and its syndromes. Brain 1930;53:120.

Review based on personal studies and the work done by C. Foix and Heubner. Autopsy data included.

Crystal HA, Dickson DW, Sliwinski MJ et al. Pathological markers associated with normal aging and dementia in the elderly. Ann Neurol 1993;34:566–73.

Currier R, Giles C, DeJong R. Some comments on Wallenberg's lateral medullary syndrome. Neurology 1961;11: 778.

Damasio H, Seabra-Gomes R, da Silva JP et al. Multiple cerebral aneurysms and cardiac Myxoma. Arch Neurol 1975;32:269–70.

Rare complications of myxomatous emboli.

David NJ, Klintworth GH, Friedberg SJ, Dillon M. Fatal atheromatous cerebral embolism associated with bright plaques in the retinal arterioles. Case report. Neurology 1963;13:708–13.

Report of a large discharge from a plaque. Cholesterol crystals in the retinal arteries was the clue to the diagnosis.

Delgado G, Urtasun F, Guridi J et al. Sindromes "lacunares" por hemorragías cerebrales espontaneas. Neurologia 1986;6:233–240.

A lacunar syndrome was found with 11 percent of cerebral hematomas.

Del Zoppo GHL, Poeck K, Pessin MS et al. Recombinant tissue plasminogen activator in acute thrombotic and embolic stroke. Ann Neurol 1992;32:78–86.

Recanalization occurs but is usually followed by infarction.

Donaldson JO. Neurology of Pregnancy. WB Saunders, Philadelphia, 1978.

Cerebral embolism during puerperium and postpartum.

Editorial. Left ventricular throbmosis and stroke following myocardial infarction. Lancet 1990;335:759–60.

Good, pithy, review.

Einhaupl KM, Villringer A, Meister W et al. Heparin treatment in sinus venous thrombosis. Lancet 1991;338: 597–600.

Heparin used even when the infarct is hemorrhagic.

El Koussa S, Chemaly R, Fabre-Bou Abboud V et al. Trichinose et occlusions sino-veineuses cérébrales. Rev Neurol (Paris) 1994;150:464–66.

Case report with a good, updated review.

Fabian TC. Unraveling the fat embolism syndrome. N Engl J Med 1993;329:951–63.

Fine editorial.

Falck RH, Podrid PJ. Atrial Fibrillation. Mechanisms and Management. Raven Press, New York, 1992.

Reviews of many cardiologic issues.

Fisher CM. Late-life migraine accompaniments. Further experience. Stroke 1986;17:1033–42.

Transient ischemic attack differentials.

Fisher CM. Lacunar strokes and infarcts: a review. Neurology 1982;32:871.

Summary of the over 20 syndromes attributed to lacunes.

Fisher CM. Reducing risks of cerebral embolism. Geriatrics 1979;34:59–66.

Risk of embolism was present in one-third of patients within 4 years after onset of atrial fibrillation.

Fisher CM. Transient paralytic attacks of obscure nature. The question of non-convulsive seizure paralysis. Can J Neurol Sci 1978;5:267–73.

Differential diagnosis of transient ischemic attacks.

Fisher CM. Some neuro-ophthalmological observations. J Neurol Neurosurg Psychiatry 1967;30:383–92.

How to auscultate the eyeball.

Fisher CM. Observations of the fundus oculi in transient monocula blindness. Neurology 1959;9:333–47.

The definitive initial observation of material moving through the retinal arteries during an attack of transient monocular blindness.

Fisher CM. Cerebral thromboangiitis obliterans (including a critical review of the literature). Medicine (Baltimore) 1957;36:160–209.

Cerebral thromboangiitis obliterans (Buerger's disease) probably does not exist.

Fisher CM, Adams RD. Observations on brain embolism with special reference to the mechanism of hemorrhagic infarction. J Neuropathol Exp Neurol 1951;10:92.

Seminal paper on the chief mechanism of hemorrhagic infarction.

Fisher CM, Karnes WE, Kubik CS. Lateral medullary infarction. The pattern of vascular occlusion. J Neuropathol Exp Neurol 1961;20:323–79.

Uusally the verebral artery is involved, not the posterior inferior cerebellar.

Fisher CM, Ojemann RG. A clinico-pathologic study of carotid endarterectomy plaques. Rev Neurol (Paris) 1986; 142:573–89.

Detailed study of 34 specimens. In only three was there embolism from ulceration in minor stenoses. No thrombus in many ulcers.

Fisher CM, Pearlman A. The non-sudden onset of cerebral embolism. Neurology 1967;17:1025–7.

Rare cases with prodromes or stepwise or fluctuating onset.

Foulkes MA, Wolf PA, Price TR et al. The Stroke Data Bank: design, methods, and baseline characteristics. Stroke 1988;19:547–54.

Large artery atheroma an infrequent cause of stroke.

Freund HJ. Abnormalities of motor behavior after cortical lesions in man. In Mountcastle VB, Plum F (eds). Handbook of Physiology. Section 1: The Nervous System. Vol 5, Part 2. 1987, pp. 763–810.

Scholarly review.

Gandolfo C, Moretti C, Dall'Agata D et al. Long-term prognosis of patients with lacunar syndromes. Acta Neurol Scand 1986;74:224.

Prognosis better than for some other forms of stroke; worse for those with severe hypertension, poor functional recovery, and pseudobulbar syndrome.

Gautier JC. Amaurosis fugax, editorial. N Engl J Med 1993; 329:426–8.

Updated review and advice in a brief editorial.

Gautier JC. L'angiopathie cérébrale moniliforme des toxicomanes. Signification physiopathologique. Rôle possible du spasme. Bull Mem Acad Natl Med 1988;172:87–93.

Beaded arteries similar in drug abuse and hypertensive encephalopathy.

Gautier JC. Clinical presentation and differential diagnosis of amaurosis fugax. In Bernstein EF (ed). Amaurosis Fugax. Springer-Verlag, New York, 1988.

Internal carotid artery stenosis found in 50 percent; many mechanisms and many diseases found in 50 percent.

Gautier JC. Stroke-in-progression. Stroke 1985;16:729–33.

Difficult theoretical and practical issues of a common situation.

Gautier JC. Cerebral ischemia in hypertension. In: Russell RWR (ed). Cerebral Arterial Disease. Churchill Livingstone, London, 1978, Pp. 181–209.

Neuropathology and pathophysiology of arterial lesions in chronic (lacunes) and acute (hypertensive encephalopathy) hypertension.

Gautier JC, Rosa A, Lhermitte F. Auscultation carotidienne. Correlations chez 200 patients avec 332 angiographies. Rev Neurol (Paris) 1975;131:175–84.

Bruit in 7 of 10 tight stenoses.

Gautier JC, Hauw JJ, Awada A et al. Artères cérébrales dolichoectasiques. Association aux anéyrismes de l'artería abdominal. Rev Neurol (Paris) 1988;144:437–66.

Not due to atherosclerosis. Significant association with aneurysms of the abdominal aorta.

Gautier JC, Dürr A, Koussa S et al. Paradoxical cerebral embolism with a patent foramen ovale. A report of 29 patients. Cerebrovasc Dis 1991;1:193–202.

Suggestive of diagnosis: Valsalva-like activity at onset, evidence of deep vein occlusion, concomitant pulmonary embolism, chronic pulmonary hypertension.

Gautier JC, Juilliard JB, Nauwelaers J. Les infarctus du territoire de l'artère cérébrale moyenne. Etude de 501 cas chez 484 patients. Bull Mem Acad Natl Med 1992;176: 43–55.

Cardiogenic embolism the leading cause of middle cerebral artery infarct.

Gautier JC, Pradat-Diehl, Loron P et al. Accidents vasculaires cérébraux des sujets jeunes. Une étude de 133 patients âgés de 9 à 45 ans. Rev Neurol (Paris) 1989;145: 437–42.

Arterial strokes found in 84 percent; main cause dissections. Venous strokes found in 7 percent, mainly caused by oral contraceptive use or puerperium. Hemorrhages in 9 percent; main cause hypertension.

Gautier JC, Durr A, Koussa S et al. Paradoxical cerebral embolism with a patent foramen ovale. A report of 29 patients. Cerebrovasc Dis 1991;1:193–202.

Suggestive of diagnosis: Valsalva-like activity at onset, evidence of deep vein occlusion, concomitant pulmonary embolism, chronic pulmonary hypertension.

Gent M, Blakeley JA, Easton JD et al: The Canadian American Ticlopidine Study (CATS) in thromboembolic stroke. Lancet 1989;1:1215–20.

Ticlopidine was superior to placebo.

Georgiadis D, Grosset DG, Kelman A. Prevalence and characteristics of intracranial microemboli signals in patients with different types of prosthetic valves. Stroke 1994;25:587–92.

Many high signals, likely due to bubbles. Number variable according to valve type. No clinical correlations.

Gray F, Dubas F, Roullet E, Escourolle R. Leukoencephalopathy in diffuse hemorrhagic cerebral amyloid angiopathy. Ann Neurol 1985;18:54–9.

Chronic ischemia insufficient to produce full thickness infarction may occur in Binswanger disease and in amyloid angiopathy from stenoses of the vessels supplying the deep white matter.

Grosset DG, Georgiadis D, Abdillah I. Doppler emboli signals vary according to stroke subtype. Stroke 1994;25:382–4.

High-intensity transcranial signals in large infarcts, not in lacunar strokes.

Hachinski VC, Lassen NA, Marshall J. Multi-infarct dementia. A cause of mental deterioration in the elderly. Lancet 1974;2:207–10.

Early concepts.

Hakim AM, Furlan AJ, Hart RG et al. Immediate anticoagulation of embolic stroke: a randomized trial. Stroke 1983;14:668–76.

Heparin better than placebo.

Hart RG. Cardiogenic embolism to the brain. Lancet 1992;339:589–94.

Recent review.

Hart RG, Foster JW, Luther MF, Canter MC. Stroke in ineffective endocarditis. Stroke 1990;21:695–700.

Good update.

Hartl WH, Janssen I, Fürst H. Effect of carotid endarterectomy on patterns of cerebrovascular reactivity in patients with unilateral carotid artery stenosis. Stroke 1994;24:1952–7.

Improved cerebral resistance as measured by transcranial Doppler was found in patients with severe preoperative impairments, and no changes were noted in those who were normal preoperatively.

Hinton RC, Kistler JP, Fallon JP et al. Influence of etiology of atrial fibrillation on incidence of systemic embolism. Am J Cardiol 1977;40:509–13.

High risk of embolism from fibrillation of any origin. Extracranial systemic emboli often silent.

Homma S, Di Tullio MR, Sacco RL. Patent cardiac foramen ovale associated characteristics of patient with cryptogenic stroke. A biplane transesophageal echocardiographic study. Stroke 1994;25:582–6.

Large patent foramina ovalia are significant, small ones probably not.

Hulqvist GT. Ueber Thrombose und Embolie der Arteria carotis und herbei vorkommende Gehirnveränderungen. Eine pathologish-anatomische Studie. Gustav Fischer Verlag, Stockholm, 1942.

The first and remarkable study of the carotid syndrome. Probably escaped wide acclaim because of World War II.

Hupperts RMM, Lodder J, Heuts-van Raak EPM, Kessels F. Infarcts in the anterior choroidal artery territory. Anatomical distribution, clinical syndromes, presumed pathogenesis and early outcome. Brain 1994;117:825–34.

Study of 77 cases (CT scan, not MRI) argues for inclusion of the paraventricular posterior corona radiata in the anterior choroidal artery territory, making this artery one of the territories capable of producing small, deep infarcts.

Jacobson JM, Terrence CF, Reinmuth OM. The neurologic manifestations of fat embolism. Neurology 1986;36:847–51.

Focal or diffuse cerebral lesions. Review of mechanisms.

Kase CS, Maulsby GO, deJuan E, Mohr JP. Hemichorea-hemiballismus and lacunar infarction in the basal ganglia. Neurology 1981;31:452–5.

One of many types of movement disorders from lacunes.

Kormorsky G, Hanson MR, Tomsak RL. Neuro-ophthalmologic complications of cardiac catheterization. Neurology 1985;38:483–5.

Artery-to-artery embolism possible but infrequent.

Kubick C, Adams RD. Occlusion of the basilar artery. Brain 1946;69:73–121.

The classical account of basilar artery occlusion, with excellent clinicopathologic correlation.

Lechat P, Lascault G, Thomas D et al. Patent foramen ovale and cerebral embolism. Circulation 1985;(suppl 3):134.

The seminal paper.

Lhermitte F, Gautier JC, Derouesne C. Nature of occlusions of the middle cerebral artery. Neurology 1970;20:82–8.

Most MCA occlusions are embolic, very few thrombotic.

Lhermitte F, Gautier JC, Derouesne C. Anatomie et physiopathologie des sténoses carotidiennes. Rev Neurol (Paris) 1966;115:641–72.

Causes and pathophysiology of thrombi in carotid stenosis.

Lhermitte F, Gautier JC, Derouesne C, Guiraud B. Ischemic accidents in the middle cerebral artery territory. A study in 122 cases. Arch Neurol 1968;19:248–56.

Among these accidents a group of infarcts whose cause was undetermined.

Lhermitte F, Gautier JC, Poirier J, Tyrer JH. Hypoplasia of the internal carotid artery. Neurology 1968;18:439–46.

A case with postmortem and review.

Leifer D, Buonanno FS, Richardson EP Jr. Clinicopathologic correlations of cranial magnetic resonance imaging of periventricular white matter. Neurology 1990;40: 911–8.

A variety of findings in patients with MRI findings in life showing periventricular white matter changes, some benign and others indicative of infarction.

Lindenberg R, Spatz F. Ueber die Thromboendarteritis obliterans der Hirngefässe. Virchows Arch [A] 1940;305: 531.

Now-defunct concept.

Lustgarten J, Solomon RA, Quest DW, Mohr JP. Endarterectomy based on Doppler and magnetic resonance angiogram without conventional angiogram. Neurosurgery 1994;34:612–19.

Possible to dispense with conventional angiography in some cases.

Marie P. Des foyers lacunaires de désintégration et de différents autres états cavitaires du cerveau. Rev Med 1901; 21:281.

The first major paper including histology on the subject.

Markus HS, Droste DW, Brown MM. Detection of asymptomatic cerebral embolism signals with ultrasound. Lancet 1994;343:1011–12.

Doppler high-intensity transcranial signals in carotid stenosis and mechanical heart valves.

Marshall RS, Mohr JP. Current management of ischaemic stroke. J Neurol Neurosurg Psychiatry 1993;56:6–16.

Current review.

Mast H, Thompson JLP, Völler H et al. Cardiac sources of embolism in patients with pial artery infarcts and lacunar lesions. Stroke 1994;25:776–81.

Left cardiac thrombi are significantly associated with pial (cerebral surface) infarcts, but other evidence for cardiogenic embolism did not separate pial from lacunar infarcts.

Meyer JS, McClintic KL, Rogers RL et al. Aetiological considerations and risk factors for multi-infarct dementia. J Neurol Neurosurg Psychiatry 1988;51:1489–97.

Attempts to relate infarcts to dementia.

Mohr JP. Cryptogenic stroke, editorial. N Engl J Med 1988; 318:1197–8.

Review of infarcts of undetermined cause.

Mohr JP. Neurological complications of cardiac valvular disease and cardiac surgery incliuding systemic hypotension. In Klawans HL (ed). Neurological Manifestations of Systemic Diseases. In Vinken PJ, Bruyn GW (eds). Handbook of Clinical Neurology. Vol. 38. North-Holland, Amsterdam, 1979, p. 143.

Older literature on syndromes of perfusion failure.

Mohr JP, Caplan LR, Melski JW et al. The Harvard Cooperative Stroke Registry: a prospective registry of cases hospitalized with stroke. Neurology 1978;28:754–62.

Embolism the most frequent cause of stroke.

Mohr JP, Kase CS, Meckler RJ, Fisher CM. Sensorimotor stroke due to thalamocapsular ischemia. Arch Neurol 1977;34:739–41.

One of the three autopsied cases reported.

Mohr JP, Orgogozo JM, Harrison MJG et al. Meta-analysis of oral nimodipine trials in acute ischemic stroke. Cerebrovasc Dis 1994;4:197–203.

Benefits if used within 12 hours.

Mokri B, Sundt TM Jr, Houser OW, Piepgras DG. Spontaneous dissection of the cervical internal carotid artery. Ann Neurol 1986;19:126.

Headache the most common early symptom. In 85 percent of patients the lesion resolved spontaneously.

Nogues M, Casas-Parera I, Starkstein S, Micheli F. Unusual manifestations of basilar artery ectasia. Eur Neurol 1988; 28:345–8.

Three patients reflecting the spectrum of basilar artery ectasia.

Patel A, Toole J. Subclavian steal syndrome. Medicine (Baltimore) 1965;44:289.

Few serious strokes.

Pell ACH, Hughes D, Keating J et al. Fulminating fat embolism syndrome caused by paradoxical embolism through a patent foramen ovale. N Engl J Med 1993;329:926–9.

Fat embolism monitored by transesophageal echocardiography during femur repair.

Pentschew A. Die granuläre Atrophie der Grosshirnrinde. Arch Psychiatrie Nervenkr 1934;101:80.

Older literature on autopsy material from perfusion failure.

Pessin MD, Duncan GW, Mohr JP, Poskanzer DC. Carotid artery territory transient ischemic attacks. N Engl J Med 1977;296:358–62.

High-grade carotid stenosis or occlusion found on angiogram in 50 percent of patients.

Pessin RS, Hinton RC, Davis KR et al. Mechanisms of acute carotid stroke: a clinicoangiographic study. Ann Neurol 1979;6:245–52.

Two-thirds are embolic, the rest from perfusion failure.

Petersen P, Boysen G, Godtfredsen J et al. Placebo controlled randomized trial of warfarin and aspirin for prevention of thromboembolic complications in chronic fibrillation. Lancet 1989;1:175–9.

Warfarin was superior to aspirin, 75 mg/day.

Petit H, Rousseaux M, Clarisse J, Delafosse A. Troubles oculo-céphalomoteurs et infarctus thalamo-sous thalamique bilateral. Rev Neurol (Paris) 1981;137:709.

Variety of top-of-the-basilar syndrome.

Petty GW, Lennihan L, Mohr JP et al. Complications of long-term anticoagulation. Ann Neurol 1988;23:570–4.

Safe if protimes are carefully monitored.

Petty GW, Tatemichi TK, Sacco RL et al. Fatal or severely

disabling cerebral infarction during hospitalization for stroke or transient ischemic attack. J Neurol 1990;237: 306–9.

Rare, but occurred when heparin was stopped for a planned procedure.

Poole JCF, French JE. Thrombosis. Atherosclerosis. 1961; 1:251–82.

A thrombus is not a clot.

Price TR, Gotshall RA, Poskanzer DC et al. Cooperative study of hospital frequency and character of transient ischemic attacks. VI. Patients examined during an attack. JAMA 1977;238:2512–15.

Large epidemiologic study.

Russell RWR. Observations on the retinal blood vessels in monocular blindness. Lancet 1961;2:1422–8.

Milestone observation on amaurosis fugax.

Sacco RL, Ellenberg JH, Mohr JP et al. Infarcts of undetermined cause: the NINCDS Stroke Data Bank. Ann Neurol 1989;25:382–90.

Many are unexplained.

Sacco RL, Freddo L, Bello JA et al. Wallenberg's lateral medullary syndrome. Arch Neurol 1993;50:609–14.

Modern review of 33 cases.

Schneider M. Durchblutung and Sauerstoffversorgung des Gehirns. Verh Dtsch Ges Kreisl Forsch 1953;19:3.

The first public promulgation of the perfusion failure concept.

Schneider R, Gautier JC. Leg weakness due to stroke. Sites of the lesions, weakness patterns, and causes. Brain 1994; 117:347–54.

The main patterns of leg weakness in anterior cerebral artery occlusion.

Sherman DG, Hart RG, Easton JD. The secondary prevention of stroke in patients with atrial fibrillation. Arch Neurol 1986;43:68–70.

Empirical guidelines.

Siebler M, Sitzer M, Rose G et al. Silent cerebral embolism caused by neurologically symptomatic high grade carotid stenosis. Event rates before and after carotid endarterectomy. Brain 1993;116:1005–15.

Before surgery many high-intensity transcardiac signals, after surgery few.

Stafford PJ, Strachan CJL, Vincent R, Chamberlain DA. Multiple microemboli after disintegration of clot during thrombolysis for acute myocardial infarction. Br Med J 1989;299:1310–12.

Cerebral embolism due to thrombolysis in coronary arteries.

Stollberger C, Slany J, Schuster I et al. The prevalence of deep vein thrombosis in patients wth suspected paradoxical embolism. Ann Intern Med 1993;119:461–5.

High prevalence.

Streifler JY, Furlan AJ, Barnett HJM. Cardiogenic Brain

embolism: incidence, varieties, treatment in stroke, pathophysiology, diagnosis and management. In Barnett HJM, Mohr JP, Stein BM, Yatsu FM (eds). Stroke. 2nd Ed. Churchill Livingstone, New York, 1992.

Review with many references.

Stroke Prevention in Atrial Fibrillation investigators. Stroke prevention in atrial fibrillation study. Final results. Circulation 1991;84:527–39.

Aspirin 325 mg/day compared with warfarin and placebo. Aspirin reduced the risk by 42 percent, warfarin did better.

Symonds C. Cervical rib: Thrombosis of the subclavian artery. Contralateral hemiplegia of sudden onset, probably embolic. In Studies in Neurology. Oxford University Press, London, 1970.

Retrograde artery-to-artery embolism.

Tatemichi TK, Chomorro A, Petty GW et al. Hemodynamic role of ophthalmic artery collateral in internal carotid artery occlusion. Neurology 1990;40:461–4.

When present, poor prognostic sign because other paths are absent.

Tatemichi TK, Foulkes MA, Mohr JP et al. Dementia in stroke survivors in the Stroke Data Bank cohort: prevalence, incidence, risk factors, and computed tomographic findings. Stroke 1990;21:858–66.

Difficult to see a clear relationship.

Tatemichi TK, Young WL, Prohovnik I et al. Perfusion insufficiency in limb shaking transient ischemic attacks. Stroke 1990;21:341–7.

Full study, indicating the factors precipitating the attacks.

Thompson PL, Robinson JL. Stroke after acute myocardial infarction: relation to infarct size. Br Med J 1978;2: 457–9.

Risk of cerebral embolism correlated with very high creatine kinase reflecting large infarct size.

Timsit S, Sacco RL, Mohr JP. Brain infarction severity differs according to cardiac or arterial embolic source. The NINDS Stroke Data Bank. Neurology 1990;40(suppl 1): 417.

Artery-to-artery embolisms smaller than cardiac emboli.

Timsit SG, Sacco RL, Mohr JP et al. Early clinical differentiation of cerebral infarction from severe atherosclerotic stenosis and cardioembolism. Stroke 1992;23:486–91.

Weakness limited to the hand and arm usually means carotid perfusion failure, and more severe syndromes mean embolism.

Venketasubramanian N, Sacco RL, DiTullio M et al. Vascular distribution of paradoxical emboli by transcranial Doppler. Neurology 1993;43:1533–5.

Basilar as well as middle cerebral locations.

Villringer A, Mehraein S, Einhaupl KM. Pathophysiological aspects of cerebral sinus venous thrombosis (SVT). J Neuroradiol 1994;21:72–80.

Experience with venous thrombosis cases suggests that arterial cerebral ischemia is usually a monophasic, abrupt, thrombotic process with only a small penumbra, while venous thrombosis is a continuing process of disequilibrium between prothrombotic and thrombolytic mechanisms. Heparin is believed to be effective because it blunts the prothrombotic state.

Vingerhoets F, Bogousslavsky J, Regli F, Van Melle G. Atrial fibrillation after acute stroke. Stroke 1993;24:26–30.

Hypothesis that some cases of atrial fibrillation could be due to stroke, particularly in infarcts involving the insula or brainstem.

Young SM, Fisher M, Sigsbee A, Errichetti A. Cardiogenic brain embolism and lupus anticoagulant. Ann Neurol 1989;26:390–2.

Intracardiac thrombi with circulating lupus anticoagulant.

Yufe R, Karpati G, Carpenter S. Cardiac myxoma: diagnostic challenge for the neurologist. Neurology 1976;26: 1060–5.

Three cases and a good review.

Zülch K-J. The Cerebral Infarct. Springer-Verlag, Berlin, 1985.

36
Parenchymatous Hemorrhages

J. P. Mohr and J. C. Gautier

Parenchymatous or intracerebral hemorrhage (ICH) accounts for approximately 10 to 15 percent of all strokes. It is 1.3 to 2.0 times as frequent as intracranial hemorrhage from aneurysm. Because some syndromes caused by hemorrhage mimic those of infarction, diagnosis of the cause of a stroke is not always reliable on clinical grounds alone (see below). A few forms of ICH are amenable to surgical therapy, while most are not.

ETIOLOGY

Normal cerebral arterial walls are remarkably resistant to rupture, but leakage or frank rupture may occur when these arteries within the brain are weakened by hypertension, infection, the poorly understood process known as *congophilic* or *amyloid angiopathy,* or anomalies in development.

Hypertension

The high incidence of an elevated admission blood pressure in patients with ICH, the presence of left ventricular hypertrophy on electrocardiography and in the autopsied cases, the higher incidence among blacks, and a slight familial tendency, have made clinicians consider hypertension so often when faced with a patient with ICH that the name *hypertensive hemorrhage* is still in common use.

Because hypertension has been traditionally identified as the greatest associated risk factor for ICH, numerous studies have sought to identify the underlying disease of the vessel that allows the hemorrhage. Working in the early days of microscopy, J. M. Charcot (French neurologist, 1825–93) and J. Bouchard (French neurologist, 1837–86) were the first to describe what they termed "miliary aneurysms" in brain specimens from ICH cases, which they believed represented true dilations of the arterial wall. The deep

location of these lesions suggested that the lesions explained ICH. R. W. Ross Russell found a higher frequency of miliary aneurysms in the brains of hypertensives, establishing a relationship between two. Subsequent workers, C. M. Fisher notable among them, found that the miliary aneurysms actually consisted of blood collected outside the vessel wall and were blood masses surrounded by either remains of the vessel wall or by fibrin. In Fisher's series, the rent in the arterial wall was at the site of the segmental disorganization now known as *lipohyalinosis*. These studies implied that ICH arose from a primary intimal lesion, distinct from miliary aneurysms, although tiny dissecting aneurysms could not be ruled out. Either form of vascular abnormality (simple weakening of the vessel wall by disease or dissecting aneurysm) could be responsible for rupture and hemorrhage. These studies also provided a link between the vascular pathology of hypertensive ischemic vascular disease and that of hemorrhage.

The involvement of the deep, small arteries cited above accounts for the frequency distribution of such hematomas: the putamen accounts for 35 to 50 percent of the cases, the thalamus for 10 to 15 percent, the pons for 5 to 12 percent, the cerebral lobes for 30 percent, and the cerebellum for the remainder (16 percent).

With rare exceptions, hypertensive ICH is a single event with rare instances of recurrence.

Cerebral Amyloid (Congophilic) Angiopathy

Cerebral amyloid angiopathy as a cause of hemorrhage is being increasingly recognized. The arterial disease it causes is characterized by amyloid deposits in the media and adventitia of medium-sized and small cortical and leptomeningeal arteries and is not associated with systemic vascular amyloidosis. Cases occur sporadically, save for a small number of familial instances with autosomal dominant inheritance. The usual sporadic case occurs in an elderly patient, about 30 percent of patients have progressive dementia, and hypertension is infrequent. The amyloid in the arterial walls can be seen on cerebral biopsy. The most common site is lobar, usually within the gray matter itself. Recurrence of hemorrhage is common, as compared with the great rarity of recurrence from hypertension, and is suggestive of the diagnosis.

Intracranial Tumors

Although well recognized as a cause of ICH, intracranial tumors are uncommon, accounting for some 1 to 2 percent in autopsy series. Most of them have been malignant, either primary (glioblastoma the most frequent) or metastatic (melanoma, choriocarcinoma, renal and bronchogenic carcinoma the leading examples), but rare instances of ICH have been found from meningiomas, oligodendrogliomas, or pituitary adenomas, the last-named occasionally a source of unexplained subarachnoid hemorrhage as well. These cases often feature large areas of low-density edema surrounding the hematoma, or in the presence of an area of post–contrast enhancement at the periphery of the hematoma, they frequently form a ring pattern on initial presentation with ICH.

Drugs and Other Factors

Repeated studies in recent decades seeking other explanations for TCH have found hypertension to be the leading single factor, even though others, including cigarette smoking, alcohol consumption, serum cholesterol levels, and coagulopathies from liver cirrhosis account for the remainder of cases.

Anticoagulants

Anticoagulants can easily be appreciated as a cause of ICH but are uncommon. ICH seems more common in anticoagulant-treated patients who are hypertensive. The locations of the ICHs that occur are usually the same as those of spontaneous hemorrhages, with a slightly greater incidence in the cerebellum. Brain hemorrhage need not be associated with signs of systemic bleeding. The slow leak of blood sometimes brings about a gradual or leisurely progression of the focal neurologic deficits, in some cases stretching out over days, making the diagnosis difficult on clinical ground alone. The prothrombin time or international normalized ratio (INR) is usually elevated well above the therapeutic range but need not be. ICH from an anticoagulant-type effect is also seen in some cases after use of fibrinolytic agents, including streptokinase, urokinase, and tissue-type plasminogen activator, which are increasingly being used in treatment of coronary, arterial, and venous thrombosis in the limbs

and pulmonary circulation and more recently also in the cerebral circulation. As with the ICH from anticoagulants, the exact mechanism of bleeding is unknown. Although excessively prolonged activated partial thromboplastin times are a common finding, some have been normal. Increased risk of ICH is associated with older age (>65 years), history of hypertension, and pre-tPA use of aspirin.

Coagulation status is also altered in patients with end-stage renal disease and those undergoing dialysis, and brain hemorrhage is not rare in either group.

Sympathomimetic Drugs

Sympathomimetic drugs are now a well-accepted cause of brain hemorrhage. The drugs implicated include amphetamines (most often methamphetamine, by either the intravenous or the intranasal route), oral pseudoephedrine, phenylpropanolamine (a component of many over-the-counter nasal decongestants and appetite supressants), and cocaine (especially in its precipitate form known as crack). The hemorrhage is usually associated with habitual use but in some cases occurs on first exposure. The cause has been attributed to transiently elevated blood pressure and drug-induced spasm or arteritis. The majority of the hematomas have been lobar in location.

A few instances of ICH have been reported among patients with granulomatous angiitis of the nervous system (see Ch. 38).

Unknown Causes

It must be admitted that many cases of parenchymatous hemorrhage remain unexplained, the frequency of such cases being perhaps as high as 30 percent. The most readily understood explanation is that the underlying lesion is too small to survive the effects of the arterial wall disruption, and histologic evidence of its presence is swept away amid the mass of the hematoma. The limitations of glass slide preparations used in traditional microscopy constitute another cause: in autopsy specimens, the dense clot of the hematoma makes it difficult to cut histologic sections when the material has been embedded in paraffin or celloidin, and the attempt frequently results in small tears of the tissue surrounding the hematoma, rendering serial section studies almost useless. Brain imaging is not yet sufficiently sensitive to detect the underlying cause of the hemorrhage in many cases. Finally, the pathophysiologic process (e.g., vasospasm induced by drugs) may be transient and thus not be detected at autopsy.

PATHOPHYSIOLOGY

How the rupture itself occurs is not known: a sudden increase in blood pressure coincident with exertion, emotional stress, and the like may serve to exceed the tolerance limits of vessel wall pressure, but many have bled with no history of predisposing activity (see also Ch. 5). Even pregnancy is no longer considered a risk of hemorrhage from arteriovenous malformations.

The leakage is thought to continue only for some minutes, as most spontaneous hemorrhages end before the patient reaches the hospital. In a few cases, the bleeding continues longer than the usual few minutes, with substantial increase in hematoma size accompanied by clinical deterioration. If bleeding does not arrest itself, the outcome is fatal. The usually self-arresting process does not then explain the commonly occurring clinical deterioration that continues for a day or more afterwards. It is generally believed that brain edema is the cause.

When the ICH involves the basal ganglia, it tends first to replace any gray matter nuclear group in which it arises (e.g., putamen, thalamus) and then tracks into white matter pathways nearby. The first stage produces an ovoid mass, the latter an irregular comma-shaped tail. Hematomas arising in the thalamus or the head of the caudate nucleus thus easily enter the ventricle, often with little displacement of brain parenchyma. This was sometimes misdiagnosed as due to a primary intraventricular hemorrhage in the days before good-quality brain imaging but is now recognized as quite rare. When the hematoma arises in the lobes, the dense fibers appear to inhibit the spread of lobar hemorrhage into the subarachnoid space, but the ventricular wall offers no such resistance for those hematomas that grow large enough to reach the ventricle. Cerebellar hemorrhage usually originates in the dentate nucleus and usually remains confined to one hemisphere. The bleeding sites in pontine hemorrhage are from the small paramedian basilar artery perforating branches. This produces a hematoma that extends symmetrically to involve the base of the pons bilaterally, with variable degrees of segmental extension, but the total volume of a pontine hematoma is quite small.

In the nonfatal cases, reduction in hematoma size occurs only slowly, over several months, frustrating rehabilitation efforts to alter the indolent, nonfluctuating clinical course that usually follows the hemorrhagic episode. Reduction in the hematoma mass is slow because the macrophages carrying off the hematoma must chisel down the mass only around its rim and do not penetrate all through it as in an ischemic infarction. Over many months the hematoma is reduced in size to a cavity whose orange-stained walls are filled with hemosiderin-laden macrophages, around which the surrounding tissue appears more or less normal. This is detectable on MRI, which helps in the differential diagnosis of old hemorrhage versus old infarction.

Throughout the entire spectrum of hematomas is the unresolvable issue of how much viable brain is displaced by the mass of the hematoma as compared with the volume of brain destroyed by the process of hemorrhage. Compared with the process of infarction, which tends to leave sharp borders between necrotic and healthy tissues, hematomas compress surrounding brain, rendering some of it immediately clinically inactive, but after some weeks to months, subsidence of the mass effect allows the surviving tissues to begin refunctioning.

CLINICAL FEATURES

Basal Ganglia Hemorrhage

The three sites most commonly affected are the putamen, thalamus, and caudate.

Putaminal Hemorrhage

The putamen is the most frequent site (40 percent of cases), with hemorrhage usually beginning in the posterior half of the nucleus. In large hemorrhages (i.e., those consuming the basal ganglia and extending into the ventricles or up into the centrum semiovale) the direction of hemorrhage spread varies: some enlarge in a roughly circular fashion, others track upward into the centrum semiovale, and some follow the arcuate fasciculus into the temporal lobe. The largest ones first displace and then destroy the adjacent internal capsule, next involve the thalamus, and extend laterally to bulge the insula outward. In fatal cases (up to 37 percent) the hematoma continues to accumulate, consuming in turn the putamen and adjacent internal and extreme capsules and then the thalamus; it enters the adjacent ventricle and spreads upward into the centrum semiovale and then both forward and backward to form an oval-shaped mass, which eventually herniates the hemisphere over the tentorium, with fatal results (Fig. 36-1). (See also Ch. 25 for discussion of the temporal lobe.)

These patients pose little problem in diagnosis. Their clinical features begin with a vague awareness of "something wrong," which is followed within minutes to hours by headache, vomiting, steadily evolving hemispheric deficit featuring contraversive eye deviation and sensorimotor syndrome, stupor, coma, and then the signs of herniation. The whole process is completed within a few hours of onset. Total unilateral motor deficit, coma, and clinical progression following admission all correlate with large hematoma size and poor functional and vital prognosis, as does ventricular extension of the hematoma shown by computed-tomography (CT) scan (see Ch. 10). Although careful history taking almost always establishes the smooth evolution of the syndrome, in some cases it is so rapid that the onset seems sudden to some observ-

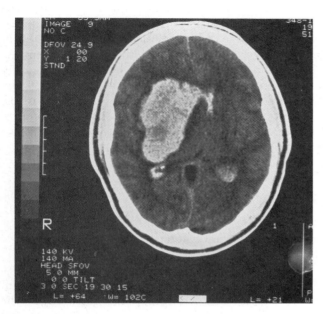

Figure 36-1. Huge, fatal putaminal hemorrhage entering the lateral ventricle through the caudate and destroying the ipsilateral basal ganglia and capsular structure.

ers, which may make it difficult to separate infarction from hemorrhage on clinical grounds alone.

The moderate-sized hemorrhage is more common than the massive hemorrhage. It begins in the same fashion but then ceases its syndromic development at varying degrees of hemiparesis, aphasia or nondominant hemisphere syndrome depending on the side involved, stupor (if the mass is large), and frequently, ipsilateral eye deviation, reflecting the involvement of the several pathways of hemispheric control over contraversive eye movements that pass via the capsular and basal ganglionic structures to the brainstem. Despite the location of the mass adjacent to the arcuate fasciculus, the syndrome of conduction aphasia is so rare that the authors know of only two examples. Repeating aloud is usually quite satisfactory even with moderate-sized hematomas. When dysphasia is present, it is usually severe and the lesion is large.

In moderate-size hematomas, the steadily progressing neurologic deficit at first seems destined to develop into an ever worsening clinical syndrome but then, after some minutes or an hour, fails to do so. Clinicians who have witnessed the evolving stages remain wary of continued worsening, but actual rebleeding is rare after the hemorrhage halts, and repeated brain imaging shows a stabilization of the volume of the hematoma. Although edema may follow, drastic worsening is rare.

At the far end of the size spectrum are the hemato-

mas that stop their development when still quite small (Fig. 36-2). The smallest mimic the highly circumscribed syndromes of lacunar infarcts (see Ch. 35). Features of the small hematomas are hemiparesis rather than hemiplegia, mild contralateral hemisensory deficits, and extraocular movements that are often normal. Almost all of these patients survive and leave the hospital with a mild functional disability. Signs portending a good functional and vital prognosis include partial motor deficit, alert mental status, normal extraocular movements, and full visual fields.

Thalamic Hemorrhage

Thalamic hemorrhage accounts for 10 to 15 percent of cases. It usually originates in the posterior half of the thalamus, entering the adjacent third and lateral ventricles when the mass is large. Large hematomas also extend laterally into the internal capsule, inferiorly into the subthalamus and dorsal midbrain, or upward into the centrum semiovale of the parietal lobe.

The basic clinical picture varies somewhat depending on the direction of spread of the hematoma. There is a rapidly evolving contralateral hemisensory syndrome accompanied by hemiparesis. Careful history taking may reveal that the sensory disturbance began before or seemed initially more prominent than the motor deficit, but an isolated hemisensory syndrome such as that produced by lacunar infarction (see Ch. 35) is rare. Vomiting occurs in half the cases, but head-

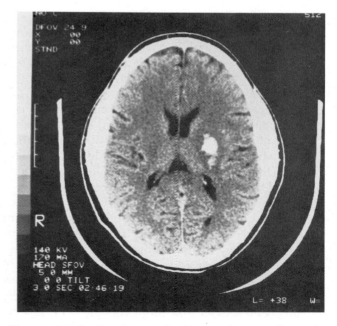

Figure 36-2. Small putaminal hemorrhage with a mass effect, causing a purely motor strokelike syndrome, mimicking a clinical diagnosis of lacunar infarction.

ache is uncommon, even in cases involving ventricular expansion of blood. This indicates that the headache in hematomas is due more to stretching of pain-sensitive structures than to the so-called irritating effects of blood. Although the lesion abuts the lateral geniculate body, hemianopia is uncommon.

When the mass spreads downward into the upper midbrain, Parinaud's syndrome (downward deviation of the eyes, impaired upward gaze, and miotic, unreactive pupils) is frequent. Other eye findings include skew deviation, eyelid ptosis, anisocoria with ipsilateral miosis, downward gaze palsy, and even transient opsoclonus. These signs suggest that the origin of the hemorrhage is in the subthalamus, although such origins are quite rare. In a few cases in which the main mass of the lesion lies superolateral to the thalamus, the contraversive eye deviation has been opposite to that expected ("wrong-way gaze"), for reasons incompletely understood. In the large hematomas involving the adjacent internal capsule, conjugate deviation of the eyes may occur.

When large, the hematoma causes a syndrome that so thoroughly mimics that of putaminal hemorrhage that no distinction can be made on clinical grounds alone (Fig. 36-3). Even interpretation of the brain images may make it difficult to decide where the hemorrhage began. When the lesion affects the dominant hemisphere, total aphasia is usually present. In such cases stupor or coma is also present, caused in part by the hydrocephalic and/or hemocephalic displacement of the midbrain.

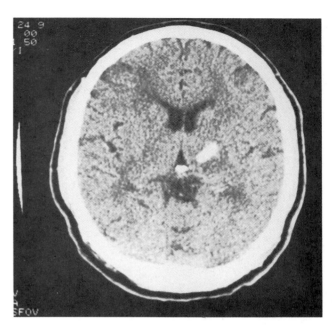

Figure 36-4. Small thalamic hemorrhage producing mainly sensory deficit.

Small hematomas may produce an incomplete hemisensory syndrome with only mild paresis and no eye movement disorders (Fig. 36-4). A small number of cases will suffer the Dejerine-Roussy thalamic pain syndrome (see Ch. 23). Smaller hematomas are also the source of the unusual aphasias distinctive for thalamic hemorrhage. There is typically a striking fluctuation in language function from virtually normal to paraphasic fluent speech (the state resembling delirium or the paraphasic disorders of speech in those sleep-deprived or in the process of falling asleep) and roughly parallels the striking variations in level of alertness and orientation of these patients. In the smaller lesions affecting the thalamus of the nondominant hemisphere, syndromes of hemineglect are common, mimicking those seen from damage to the parietal lobe.

Caudate Hemorrhage

Caudate hemorrhage has been increasingly recognized in recent years with improved brain imaging (Fig. 36-5). Usually lumped with putaminal hemorrhage as hemorrhage into the basal ganglia, caudate hemorrhage is worth separate consideration because the prognosis is usually benign. Approximately 5 to 7 percent of hematomas arise in the caudate, almost all of them in the head. As with hematomas in other sites, arterial hypertension is the usual cause, but caudate hemorrhage is occasionally caused by leakage from moyamoya disease changes in lenticulostriate

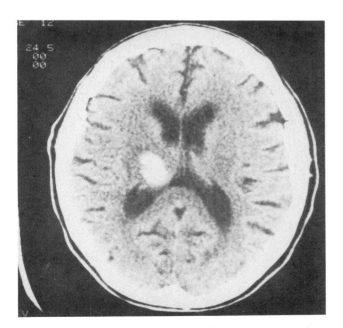

Figure 36-3. Moderately large thalamic hemorrhage spreading into the adjacent internal capsule.

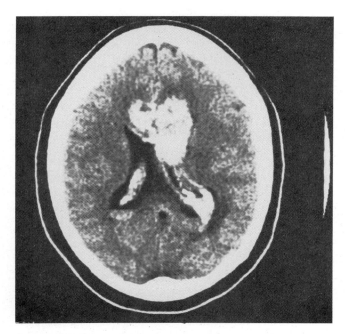

Figure 36-5. Large hemorrhage arising from the head of the caudate, extending into the lateral ventricle.

branches of the anterior and middle cerebral arteries (see Ch. 35).

The clinical picture features abrupt onset, headache, and vomiting, similar to that seen in putaminal hemorrhage. The hemiparesis may be mild and behavioral abnormalities, most often featuring disorientation, confusion, and severe short-term memory deficit (fornix), may be prominent features of the clinical picture. Much of the hemorrhage vents into the adjacent ventricle, where it mimics the CT or magnetic resonance imaging (MRI) picture of ventricular hemorrhage from ruptured anterior communicating artery aneurysm. The neurologic disturbance usually fades within weeks. Shunting for hydrocephalus and/or hemocephalus is rarely required.

Lobar Hemorrhages

Lobar hemorrhage has proved difficult to characterize with respect to both frequency and syndrome. If the many sites in the many cerebral lobes are grouped together, they are third in frequency behind the putamen and thalamus as a site, but if the cerebral lobes are considered individually, the lobe-by-lobe frequency is far lower. Hemorrhage in each individual cerebral lobe produces a different clinical picture, making generalizations as to syndrome difficult.

The clinical features of hypertensive hemorrhage and of hemorrhage from congophilic angiopathy are similar, since both arise from small arteries in the sub-

cortical white matter near the gray-white junction or in the gray matter itself. As the mass of the hematoma develops, its shape is limited somewhat by the tight mesh of the overlying gray matter and by the undulations of the gyri and sulci below. The resulting elliptical mass develops in a plane parallel to the overlying cortex, where pools of liquid blood may form, appearing on brain images as sedimented layers (Fig. 36-6). With time, reabsorption of blood leaves a shallow cavity, which led to the label "slit" hemorrhage formerly used by neuropathologists inspecting the brain at autopsy. The posterior half of the brain is the more frequent location for these hematomas, which roughly correlates with the distribution of small artery microaneurysms, known as markers for hypertension (Fig. 36-7). Lobar hemorrhages have a wider range of causes than do the hematomas in the deep nuclei, among them cerebral amyloid angiopathy, arteriovenous malformations, cavernous angiomas, metastatic and primary tumors, and arteritis.

The clinical picture varies with each lobar location, but lobar hemorrhages as a group are characterized by a higher frequency of seizures and headache and a lower frequency of coma as part of the initial clinical picture. Because of the great distance from the midbrain, a lobar hematoma of size comparable with that of one in the putamen or thalamus involves a lower risk for coma and brain herniation. Once the mass

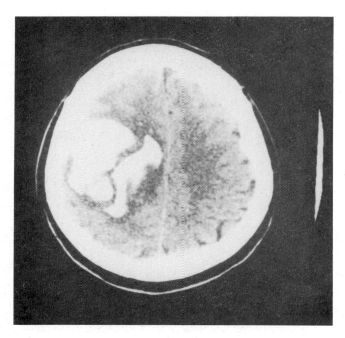

Figure 36-6. Large lobar hemorrhage showing involvement of adjacent gyri.

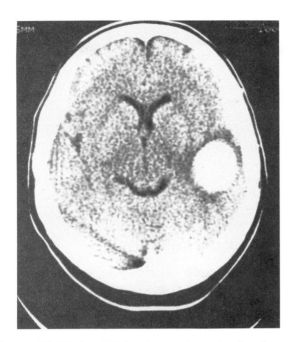

Figure 36-7. Small lobar hemorrhage having the acute globular appearance that later will shrink to an elliptical and finally to a slit shape.

subsides, a greater degree of clinical improvement can also be expected.

Brainstem Hemorrhage

Brainstem hemorrhage is a term broadly describing hemorrhage in any of the brainstem's major divisions (i.e., midbrain, pons, and medulla), but save for a few unusual examples, almost all cases occur in the pons, where the effects of hypertension on small perforating arteries is greatest.

Pontine Hemorrhage

Pontine hemorrhage (Fig. 36-8) occurs in several forms. When one of the small, paramedian pontine arteries gives way, blood pumped into the tightly compacted tracts and nucleus in the middle of the pons causes a syndrome that, in its fully developed form, is one of the most striking in clinical neurology. Disruption of the reticular activating system precipitates coma, usually within minutes, at the start of which occipital headache and vomiting may have occurred. Damage to the many descending motor pathways results in quadriparalysis, often with such violent decerebrate responses that the patient is thought to be having seizures. Ocular motility is disrupted in a variety of syndromes, ranging from paralysis of all gaze, including lack of response to ice-water caloric testing (see Chs. 28 and 29), to isolated sixth cranial nerve palsies and internuclear ophthalmoplegia, alone or in combination with sixth cranial nerve palsies. The pupils become so small that they have been called "pinpoint" but still react slightly to light (bright light and a hand lens are usually required to see the small amplitude of contraction), which shows that their small diameter is from loss of sympathetic tone from the damage to the descending pathways, not from parasympathetic excess. Dramatic changes occur in respiratory rhythm, from Cheyne-Stokes rhythm to inspiratory gasps and even apnea. Hyperthermia is common, with temperatures above 39°C and sometimes as high as 43°C. A fatal outcome is expected within a few hours, rarely days.

Smaller pontine hemorrhages offer at least a hope of survival, and those originating to one side of the midline or in the lateral tegmentum may mimic focal infarcts. Even examples of the syndromes of pure motor stroke and ataxic hemiparesis, (usually ascribed to a lacuna, see Ch. 35) have been reported. These smaller hematomas are often explained by cavernous malformations or by telangiectasias (see Ch. 37); the small amount of hemorrhage they cause may only slightly enlarge the lesion, with limited clinical effects.

Rarely, hemorrhage may develop in the midbrain. Cavernous angiomas or small arteriovenous malformations but not hypertension are the usual cause. The authors know of only one example of hemorrhage into the medulla, from a small cavernous angioma removed surgically.

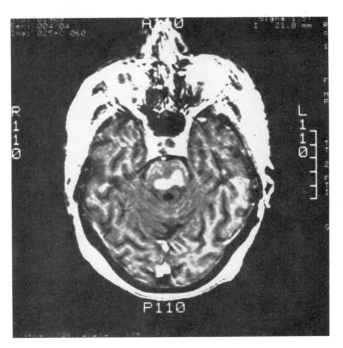

Figure 36-8. Small pontine hemorrhage on T₁-weighted MRI.

Cerebellar Hemorrhage

Cerebellar hemorrhage, described here last, is certainly not least in its clinical importance, as it is one of the few parenchymatous hematoma sites where surgical intervention may be life-saving and yield a remarkably mild long-term disability.

As with other sites, hypertension explains most cerebellar hematomas, which arise from distal branches of the posterior inferior cerebellar artery feeding the dentate nucleus. Save for the few caused by arteriovenous malformation or trauma, most hematomas arise in or near a dentate nucleus and remain mainly unilateral, often expanding into the fourth ventricle but rarely into the brainstem (Fig. 36-9).

Size plays a role in prognosis but is unrelated to the severity of the acute syndrome. The distinctive clinical features are a sudden inability to stand and walk, an absence of limb weakness, vomiting, which develops within a few minutes of onset of imbalance, headache, and dizziness. Examined supine, many patients pass almost for normal and vomit so readily from changes in head position that a diagnosis of labyrinthitis or viral gastroenteritis could easily be made. Yet when forced to stand up and attempt to walk, the patient amply reveals the ataxia and often has a horizontal gaze palsy to the same side as that of the hematoma shown on brain imaging. There are occasional examples of sixth nerve palsy, depressed corneal reflex, miosis, and, rarely, mild ipsilateral peripheral facial palsy. The ipsilateral gaze palsy is an important clinical finding since its presence stands in contrast to the absence of hemiparesis.

It is the unpredictability of cerebellar hemorrhage that makes its early clinical diagnosis important. Every case series contains instances of sudden deterioration leading to coma and death with little warning. No distinctive clinical picture has yet been determined that can safely predict a benign outcome. The cerebellar disturbance is maximal at onset and can get no worse, and no signs of impending brainstem compression occur until it is too late. Surgical management should be planned for each case as soon as possible (see below).

GENERAL LABORATORY FINDINGS

Fever, a rise in sedimentation rate, and a rise in the peripheral white blood cell count as high as 20,000/ mm³ have been observed frequently. Abnormalities in the electrocardiogram suggestive of subendocardial ischemia occur infrequently.

For those cases inaccesible to CT scanning, a lumbar puncture may be necessary in diagnosis. Many a pitfall exists in this effort. A hypertensive hemorrhage or one from cavernous angioma that is small or in the early phase of evolution may remain wholly within the parenchyma and not reach the ventricular wall or approach the subarachnoid space, leaving the cerebrospinal fluid (CSF) clear and colorless. When the CSF is clear, the protein is also usually normal. When the CSF is bloody, the fluid shows varying degrees of xanthochromia and protein values from normal to as high as 1,200 mg/100 ml.

The syndrome of cerebral herniation has followed lumbar puncture in some cases of large putaminal hemorrhage and may occur in thalamic or cerebellar hemorrhage, but it has not been at issue in pontine or "slit" hemorrhage. Lumbar puncture should be performed with patients lying on their sides, with as little CSF drawn off as is needed for the diagnosis.

IMAGING

The CT scan was the method of choice in the diagnosis of all hematomas prior to the advent of MRI. Both techniques (1) give a precise localization of the hemorrhage; (2) outline its size and configuration; (3) display the degree of hydrocephalus, ventricular shift, or compression; (4) show the presence of blood in the ventricular system; (5) give an indication of the degree of edema in the adjacent brain tissue; and (6) allow prediction of the residual clinical deficit following medical and surgical therapy. In the case of the CT scan, within the first week high densities are seen, but after 1 week isodensity or even low densities may be

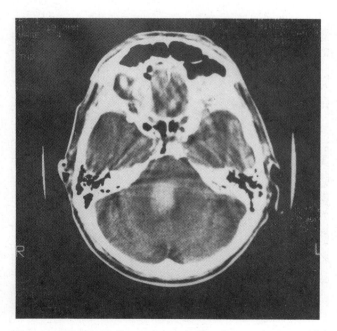

Figure 36-9. Unilateral cerebellar hemorrhage, which has entered the roof of the fourth ventricle.

Parenchymatous Hemorrhages

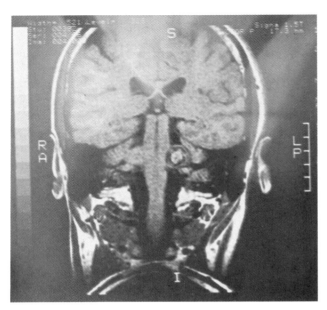

Figure 36-10. Cavernous angioma in the brachium pontis (right side of scan), showing the distinctive appearance of high- and low-intensity rings on T₁-weighted MRI.

present. The higher the density of the initial hematoma, the longer it will be seen on CT scan.

MRI has the advantage of remaining positive for years because of the paramagnetic properties of methemoglobin, a property that also helps to date the hemorrhage. It often shows a distinctive appearance for cavernous angiomas, with a contrasting high and low signal, one surrounding the other (Fig. 36-10) and some having the appearance of a tiger eye. At first this was thought to be a specific sign for cavernous angiomas, but enough examples have appeared involving small arteriovenous malformations that the sign can no longer be accepted as diagnostic for cavernous angiomas.

The only current value for arteriography is to exclude a vascular anomaly or neoplasm as the cause of the hemorrhage, these being diagnoses that come to mind most often in a hemorrhage affecting the cerebral lobes. Arteriographic findings in cases of hypertensive hemorrhage merely reflect the mass effect of the hematoma.

TREATMENT

Following confirmation of the hemorrhage, medical efforts alone cannot succeed in stopping the few cases of progressing hemorrhage. For those patients showing continued decline from the time of arrival at the hospital, whether to undertake emergency evacuation of the hematoma must be decided. Hematomas in the putamen, subcortical white matter, and cerebellum are amenable to surgical therapy, while those in the thalamus and pons are rarely operable because so many vital structures are likely to be damaged in the attempt.

The value of removing a putaminal or cerebral lobar hematoma has not yet been established for a patient who is showing signs of increasing neurologic deficit or decreasing state of consciousness. It has also not been established whether surgery improves the outlook for those with a stable moderate or severe neurologic deficit. Surgery has not proved useful for preventing a fatal outcome in massive hemorrhages with loss of pupillary reaction and brainstem function. It is particularly inadvisable to plunge ahead with surgery for lobar hemorrhages on the basis only of CT scanning, since some of these hemorrhages are from arteriovenous malformations, and the surgeon may face an insuperable task attempting to reduce the seemingly chaotic tangle of vessels for which the team is ill prepared. At the very least, transcranial Doppler ultrasonography, easily performed in emergency settings, may show the distinctive high-velocity, low-resistance profile typical of an arteriovenous malformation (see Ch. 13) and warn the surgical team of the underlying cause in time to undertake MRI or conventional angiography.

The situation is different with cerebellar hemorrhage, in which case the authors advise a plan for surgery. The difficulty of predicting the course of cerebellar hemorrhage prompts the suggestion that all such patients seen within 48 hours of onset be readied for surgery and all large hematomas (> 3 cm in diameter or seen on more than two levels on a CT scan) be evacuated as a prophylactic measure. The morbidity is slight and the functional outcome after some weeks is surprisingly good. No definite recommendations for management of the smaller hematomas can be made, but the authors' opinion leans toward surgery.

ANNOTATED BIBLIOGRAPHY

Berstein E, Diskant BM. Phenylpropanolamine: a potentially hazardous drug. Ann Emerg Med 1982;11:311–5.
Description of cases.

Biller J, Loftus CM, Moore SA et al. Isolated central nervous system angiitis first presenting as spontaneous intracranial hemorrhage. Neurosurgery 1987;20:310–15.
Case report.

Boudouresques G, Hauw JJ, Meininger V et al: Etude neuropathologique des hemorrhagies intracraniennes de l'adulte. Rev Neurol (Paris) 1979;135:197–210.
Details of neuropathology.

Brott T, Thalinger K, Hertzberg V. Hypertension as a risk factor for spontaneous intracerebral hemorrhage. Stroke 1986;17:1078–83.
Less the leading cause now than in former times.

Duret H. Etudes Experimentales et Cliniques sur les Traumatismes Cérébraux. Adrien Delhaye, Paris, 1873.

The classical report detailing hemorrhagic changes from herniation.

Fisher CM. The pathology and pathogenesis of intracerebral hemorrhage. In Fields (WS) (ed): Pathogenesis and Treatment of Cerebrovascular Disease. Charles C Thomas, Springfield, IL, 1961, p. 295.

A clinical classic.

Fisher CM. Pathological observations in hypertensive cerebral hemorrhage. J Neuropathol Exp Neurol 1971;30:536–50.

One of the few reports documenting the rent in the vessel.

Fisher CM, Picard EH, Polak A et al. Acute hypertensive cerebellar hemorrhage: diagnosis and surgical treatment. J Nerv Ment Dis 1965;140:38.

The article that defined the syndrome.

Franke CL, deJonge J, van Swieten JC et al. Intracerebral hematomas during anticoagulant treatment. Stroke 1990;21:726–30.

High prothrombin times.

Gautier JC. Segmental cerebral angiopathy of drug addicts. Physiopathological significance. Possible role of spasms. Bull Acad Nat Med (Paris) 1988;172:87–93.

Pathophysiologic hypothesis in French.

Gautier JC, Majdalani A, Juillard JB, Carmi AR. Hemorrhagies cérébrales au cours de la migraine. Rev Neurol (Paris) 1993;149:407–10.

Only six reported cases found. Recirculation in an infarct and dissecting aneurysm are among possible causes.

Gilbert JJ, Vinters HV. Cerebral amyloid angiopathy: incidence and complications in the aging brain. I. Cerebral hemorrhage. Stroke 1983;14:915–23.

Details of neuropathology.

Glick R, Hoying J, Cerullo L, Perlman S. Phenylpropanolamine: an over-the-counter drug causing central nervous system vasculitis and intracerebral hemorrhage. Neurosurgery 1987;20:969–74.

Drugs and hemorrhage.

Herbstein DJ, Schaumburg HH: Hypertensive intracerebral hematoma. An investigation of the initial hemorrhage and rebleeding using chromium Cr 51-labeled erythrocytes. Arch Neurol 1974;30:412–4.

Evidence that the hemorrhages bleed only for a short time.

Hier DB, Davis KR, Richardson EP, Mohr JP: Hypertensive putaminal hemorrhage. Ann Neurol 1977;1:152–9.

The first detailed study with CT scan.

Kase CS. Intracerebral hemorrhage: non-hypertensive causes. Stroke 1986;17:590–5.

Authoritative review.

Kase CS, Maulsby GO, Mohr JP. Partial pontine hematomas. Neurology 1980;30:652–5.

Evidence that small pontine hemorrhages may have a favorable prognosis.

Kase CS, Robinson RK, Stein RW et al. Anticoagulant-related intracerebral hemorrhage. Neurology 1985;35:943–8.

Cerebellar location seen more often than with spontaneous hemorrhages.

Kase CS, Williams JP, Mohr JP. Lobar intracerebral hematomas. Neurology 1982;32:1146–50.

Seizures occur in one third of patients.

Kelley RE, Berger JR, Scheinberg P, Stokes N: Active bleeding in hypertensive intracerebral hemorrhage: computed tomography. Neurology 1982;32:852–6.

Few examples.

Levine SR, Brust JCM, Futrell N et al. Cerebrovascular complications of the use of the "crack" form of alkaloid cocaine. N Engl J Med 1990;323:699–704.

A drug-induced hemorrhage.

Massaro AR, Sacco RL, Mohr JP et al. Clinical discriminators separate lobar and subcortical hemorrhage: the Stroke Data Bank. Neurology 1991;41:1881–5.

Useful clues.

Ott KH, Kase CS, Ojemann RG, Mohr JP: Cerebellar hemorrhage: diagnosis and treatment. Arch Neurol 1974;31:160–7.

No definitive syndrome predicts fatal outcome.

Regli F, Vonsattel J-P, Perentes E, Assal G: L'angiopathie amyloïde cérébrale. Une maladie cérébro-vasculaire peu connue. Etude d'une observation anatomo-clinique. Rev Neurol (Paris) 1981;137:181–94.

The first in a series.

Stein RW, Kase CS, Hier DB et al. Caudate hemorrhage. Neurology 1984;34:1549–54.

Definition of the syndrome.

Tapia JF, Kase CS, Sawyer RH, Mohr JP: Hypertensive putaminal hemorrhage presenting as pure motor hemiparesis. Stroke 1983;14:505–6.

Can occur when the lesion is small enough.

Tuhrim S, Dambrosia JM, Price TR et al. Intracerebral hemorrhage: external validation and extension of a model for prediction of 30 day survival. Ann Neurol 1991;29:658–63.

Useful algorithm.

Vonsattel JPG, Myers RH, Hedley-Whyte ET et al. Cerebral amyloid angiopathy without and with cerebral hemorrhages: a comparative histological study. Ann Neurol 1991;30:637–49.

Clinicopathologic study.

37

Subarachnoid Hemorrhage: Aneurysms and Vascular Malformations

J. P. Mohr and J. C. Gautier

It is not the existence of blood in the subarachnoid space but the disastrous effects of the usual cause, a ruptured intracranial aneurysm, that makes subarachnoid hemorrhage the major clinical problem it is. There are a number of other causes. Some degree of subarachnoid hemorrhage occurs during the molding of the head in the process of birth. Injuries to the head from falls may cause subarachnoid blood from contusions of the brain or tears of veins bridging the brain surface with the dura. Primary (parenchymatous) hemorrhages may leak blood into the ventricular space, from which it reaches the subarachnoid space following the cerebrospinal fluid (CSF) pathways. Finally, subarachnoid hemorrhage may follow the use of drugs that acutely raise blood pressure, leading among which are cocaine and phenylpropanolamine. However, these causes are so minor compared with the subarachnoid hemorrhage from aneurysms that it is this cause that occupies most of this chapter.

INTRACRANIAL ANEURYSMS

Aneurysms (their name derived from the Greek for dilation) account for 6 percent of strokes, leading the list for those that are fatal. The true prevalence of intracranial aneurysms remains difficult to ascertain. Autopsy studies have shown a prevalence of 17 percent for aneurysms as small as 2 mm while those than 3 mm or larger are present in less than 4 percent. The peak age for aneurysm rupture is between 55 and 60 years. Autopsy studies estimate that as much as 5 percent of the population may harbor aneurysms. The incidence of ruptured aneurysms has ranged from as low as 3.9 per 100,000 per year through a median

value of 11 per 100,000 per year to as high as 19.4 per 100,000 per year. These values have remained constant over the decades since statistics have been kept on causes of stroke, suggesting that little has been accomplished in the prevention of this disease.

A family prevalence is known, especially for the few patients with polycystic kidney disease, and the risk of aneurysmal bleeding is higher in those with connective tissue diseases (such as the Ehlers-Danlos and Marfan syndromes) and coarctation of the aorta, but otherwise there are few factors that predict the presence of a congenital aneurysm. A few other factors increase the risk of rupture, of which pregnancy is the leading one, with 12 percent to 25 percent of maternal deaths attributed to rupture. Size appears to be a factor, with increased risk of rupture associated with larger than 8 mm. Exertion and head injury are both suspected to be aggravating factors in rupture, but this has been difficult to prove. Exposure to drugs that drastically raise blood pressure may precipitate subarachnoid hemorrhage from aneurysms.

The issue of risk of rupture is important because of the high fatality rate for this disorder, estimated at just under 25 percent for the first rupture from data obtained from referral centers and as high as 50 percent for hospitals serving local populations. These findings suggest that many scarcely reach medical observation while alive, and fewer come into expert hands.

For the survivors major disability is common, with fully 64 percent of those discharged, even after successful surgery, never regaining the quality of life they had before the rupture.

Aneurysm Anatomy and Pathology

Aneurysms are thin-walled pouches distending the arterial wall (see Ch. 5). Congenital aneurysms, arising from defects in the media of the arterial wall, are named by their shape—*saccular* (arising from bifurcations, forming a berry-shaped bulge) or *fusiform* (Latin for spindle-shaped)—and comprise most of the circumference of the wall of an artery. A parallel classification is based on the cause: congenital for most of the saccular or fusiform aneurysms; mycotic (from the Greek for fungus) but used here for any infectious cause; traumatic or neoplastic for the remainder. Dissecting aneurysms, caused by spontaneous or trauma-induced fracture of a major artery, is classified under aneurysms for reasons of damage to and dilation of the arterial wall (see Ch. 5).

Congenital Aneurysms

Congenital aneurysms occur most often at the bifurcations of the large arteries at the base of the brain and the major branches of the circle of Willis (85 percent) and basilar artery (Fig. 37-1). This predilection makes the usual sites the junction of the anterior communicating artery with the anterior cerebral artery, the junction of the posterior communicating artery with the internal carotid, and the bifurcation of the middle

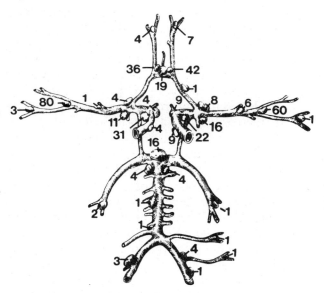

Figure 37-1. Drawing of the arteries at the base of the brain showing the location of 429 saccular aneurysms in 316 consecutive patients with aneurysms on an autopsy service. Approximately 90 percent of the aneurysms occur in the anterior cerebral circulation. Aneurysms are slightly more common on the right side of the intracranial vessels than on the left for reasons that are not apparent. (From McCormick, 1983, with permission.)

cerebral artery. In the basilar territory the most common sites are the top of the basilar artery, the junction of the basilar artery with the superior cerebellar artery or the anterior inferior cerebellar artery, and the junction of the vertebral artery and the posterior inferior cerebellar artery. Multiple sites occur in as many as 20 percent of cases. The intracranial internal carotid artery as it joins the circle of Willis may show an infundibulum (Latin, "funnel"), which is often a source of controversy when found on an angiogram; many consider it a harmless variant but others diagnose an aneurysm. The authors recommend the latter when the only image is an angiogram and suggest that such cases be further studied by magnetic resonance imaging (MRI) to determine if the "infundibulum" seen on the angiogram is actually the patent portion of an aneurysm whose larger, thrombosed component can be seen by MRI.

Three major theories of the development of congenital aneurysms remain popular. All three postulate a disorder of the arterial wall, which yields over years to the forces of systemic arterial pressure to balloon the vessel wall with a bulge containing an intimal lining and an adventitial surface devoid of media. The first explains aneurysm formation as a congenital defect in the muscular layer of the cerebral arteries. A second view theorizes that degenerative changes within the vessel wall eventually result in damage to the internal elastic membrane, creating a local weakness. The third is simply a combination of the other two. A role of systemic arterial hypertension is easy to envision but has not been clearly established.

Histologic studies show that aneurysms typically grow outward from a base on the arterial wall, most often at bifurcations, causing a bulge shaped roughly like a small balloon, sack (hence saccular aneurysms), or berry (hence berry aneurysms). The site of formation at the bifurcations of arteries has been related to small gaps in the musculature of the media at these points. Such media defects have been reported in 80 percent of the bifurcations of cerebral arteries in both aneurysmal and control cases.

The thickness and length of the base or neck and the size of the balloon or dome vary greatly from as small as 1 mm to as large as more than 2 cm. No internal elastic lamina is found in the neck. The normal vascular media is thin, the smooth muscle cells being replaced by collagenous connective tissue. The wall at the rupture site may be thinner than 0.3 mm. Although it is popular to envision the rupture site at the tip of the dome, rupture has been histologically documented in the base and in the neck, a finding that suggests that some aneurysms are not isolated from the circulation by the clip placed over the neck.

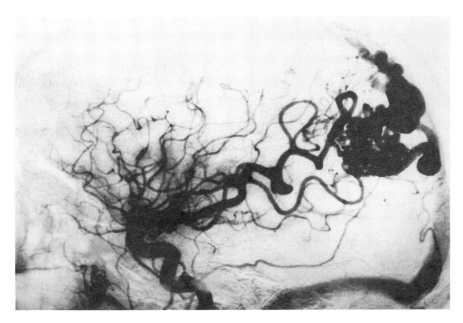

Figure 37-4. Lateral view of the brain showing a posterior hemispheric AVM supplied by branches of the middle cerebral artery draining to a large superficial vein.

are not as large as the usual AVM and they are less compact. Most of them occur adjacent to the walls of the lateral ventricle, making venous angioma a rare cause of ventricular hemorrhage. The prognosis is thought to be good. The rare *varix* is a single, anomalous, dilated vein, which is all but indistinguishable from a normal dilated vein.

CLINICAL FEATURES

Asymptomatic Unruptured Aneurysms

Before brain and vascular imaging became available, the diagnosis of unruptured aneurysm was difficult. Nowadays congenital and arteriosclerotic aneurysms are being increasingly discovered through the applica-

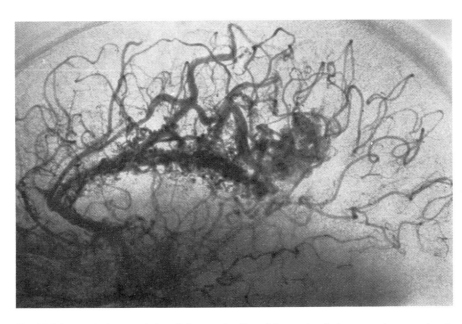

Figure 37-5. AVM consisting mainly of the pericallosal branch of the anterior cerebral artery along the corpus callosum.

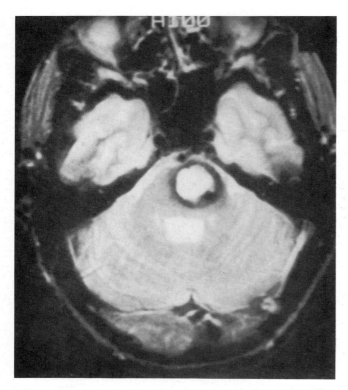

Figure 37-6. Large pontine cavernous angioma. This lesion produced only mild ipsilateral facial paresis.

tion of brain imaging (especially MRI) performed for another purpose. Their location in the subarachnoid space often prevents them from displacing nearby structures until they reach quite large size, and unless they rupture, the patient harboring the lesion has no idea that the aneurysm is present. Mycotic and neoplastic aneurysms affect the more distal vessels and can almost never be imaged by computed tomography (CT) or MRI.

Scant data exist on the risk of rupture for any type of aneurysm, making it difficult to formulate a fixed plan for management. Estimates that congenital or arteriosclerotic aneurysms over 8 mm in size are at higher risk for rupture in the succeeding decade have prompted some physicians to refer for surgery those patients whose aneurysms suitably placed for surgical reduction with minimum morbidity. For aneurysms more difficult to reach, no general recommendation can be made. Ideally, the risk of surgical reduction should be far less than that of hemorrhage, and prophylactic surgery is popular in many experienced centers, especially for the younger patients with a long life expectancy. The frequency of mycotic and neoplastic aneurysms is so low that no general plan has been formulated for their management prior to rupture.

Prior to rupture, many congenital and arterioscle-

rotic aneurysms enlarge to the point where they displaces adjacent brain structures. Of all the sites prone to cause symptoms, the posterior communicating artery aneurysm is best positioned to stretch a clinically sensitive structure, in this case the third cranial nerve in its extramedullary course between the brainstem and the orbit. The location of the pupillary constrictor fibers superficially on the third nerve causes pupillary dilation and loss of light reflex from stretch or injury to the nerve, a sign highly suggestive of an expanding (or recently ruptured) aneurysm at the junction of the posterior communicating artery and the distal internal carotid artery. It has been estimated that the aneurysm must be at least 7 mm in size. The motor palsy of the lid and extraocular muscles may precede pupillary dilation and loss of light and accommodation reflexes. If the third nerve palsy has been present for more than 10 days, the nerve's chances of recovering are not favorable.

When aneurysms of the top of the basilar artery, some congenital and some arteriosclerotic, enlarge, they displace the midbrain both posteriorly and by angulation, bringing about disorders of eye movements, weakness, and in some cases disorders of tone and posture. The dolichoectatic aneurysms are prone to such great enlargement as to dent the third ventricle from below, which in some cases causes symptomatic hydrocephalus on top of the other midbrain syndromes.

Giant aneurysm in the cavernous sinus may compress, even erode, the wall of the orbit, causing a sixth nerve palsy. An expanding supraclinoid carotid aneurysm may elevate the optic chiasm, nerve, or tract, causing a visual field defect that may be obvious only on clinical testing without the patient being aware of it.

For some aneurysms the only sign is pain, which may occur separately or in conjunction with the third nerve palsy and is typically located above the brow, radiating back to the ear. Pain in or behind the eye and in the low temple can occur with middle cerebral aneurysm expansion. Focal headache involving the occipital and posterior cervical region can occur with a posterior inferior cerebellar artery or anterior inferior cerebellar artery aneurysm. Mycotic and neoplastic aneurysms rarely enlarge to the point at which they can cause mass effects and are too distal in the arterial system to affect cranial nerves.

Prior to major rupture, as many as 50 percent of congenital aneurysms are subject to warning leaks, which may go unrecognized because of the minor syndromes they produce. These syndromes may include a variety of symptoms, including focal frontal or occipital headache and stiff neck, sudden headache with pain between the shoulder blades or at the back of the neck, sudden change in personality toward violent outbursts, and unexplained urinary or even fecal incontinence. None of these syndromes is distinct enough to make an easy diagnosis, but it is believed that if the diagnosis can be made before major rupture occurs, emergency management of the aneurysm can more easily be achieved. Warning leaks are almost unknown in mycotic and neoplastic aneurysms.

Syndromes of Vascular Malformations Prior to Rupture

Few symptoms or signs warn the patient of the existence of an underlying disease destined to cause hemorrhage. However, some patients with AVMs may have headaches or seizures. For decades it has been tempting to think that the large, tense arteries and veins involved in an AVM would be the source of headaches, but it has been difficult to show that such headaches occur more frequently than in the population of patients who do not have AVMs. The character of the headache, thought by earlier generations of neurologists to be distinctive for AVMs, is often indistinguishable from that of migraine (see Ch. 24). Despite a long-standing bias that repeated headache means an underlying AVM, especially when unilateral and always on the same side, the correlation has not proved reliable. Cranial bruits caused by arterial feeders to the AVM have a higher diagnostic value than does headache.

Seizures are a common form of presentation prior to hemorrhage for AVMs, occurring in as few as 28 percent to as many as 67 percent. They occur most often from lesions located more anteriorly in the brain and can take the classical focal or a generalized form, both of which occur in approximately equal proportions. Half of them are mild, and only about 15 percent are severe and poorly controlled by medication.

It is beyond doubt that a slowly progressive focal neurologic deficit may occur in patients with AVMs, affecting some 5 percent or so, but whether the progression can be attributed to a steal phenomenon (i.e., excessive shunting of oxygenated blood away from healthy brain into the fistula) is the subject of heated debate. The authors have encountered instances of progressive neurologic deficit, but in each case this has been best explained as a mass effect from a ballooned vein or artery displacing part of the brain or spinal cord, usually the latter. The concept of steal would be an important principle should it be established, but thus far it has not been.

Subarachnoid Hemorrhage

A rent in the wall of an aneurysm allows blood to escape under full arterial pressure, a fatal event unless the rupture is arrested. Increase of intracranial volume by as little as 100 ml is enough to cause coma, making even a short period of arterial bleeding sufficient to kill the patient from the mass effect alone. Mycotic and neoplastic aneurysms are more prone to uncontrolled bleeding, and the first hemorrhage is often fatal. For most patients with congenital and arteriosclerotic aneurysms, the rupture is self-limited, often causing transient coma from the initial high intracranial pressure. For a lucky few, the bleeding is so slight as to cause only a headache minor enough that no medical consultation is sought (see above).

It is believed that the sudden stretching of the pain-sensitive arachnoidal structures causes headache in all cases of subarachnoid hemorrhage, but for those suffering a sudden and large release of blood, the abrupt rise in intracranial pressure, which can approach that of systolic arterial pressure, causes loss of consciousness in half of the cases, in some before they can react to the pain. Headache is present for those who awaken. For those awake, vomiting is a symptom but does not correlate well with headache severity.

Aneurysms of any type whose rupture point is adjacent to brain structures may bleed directly into the brain or may fill a CSF cistern so completely as to cause a local mass effect, displacing the brain. The parenchymatous hematoma or cisternal mass may cause a variety of syndromes common to focal stroke, including hemiparesis, memory loss and abulia from frontal lobe involvement, aphasia when the dominant hemisphere is involved, and anosognosia and hemineglect with involvement of the nondominant hemisphere.

Distinctive syndromes of focal rupture are known. The middle cerebral artery aneurysm has several distinct variations. When an aneurysm in the bifurcation of the middle cerebral artery ruptures posteriorly into the sylvian fissure (Fig. 37-7), the fissure may be distended and the surrounding uninjured brain displaced, causing a clinical picture of brain herniation (see Chs. 17 and 25). Immediate evacuation of the mass and clipping of the aneurysm may not only be life-saving but may prompt a remarkable restoration of neurologic function. An aneurysm in the same location that ruptures into the adjacent temporal lobe may create a life-threatening mass that causes local uncal herniation, which was occasionally misdiagnosed as a primary temporal lobe hematoma in the days before adequate brain imaging. In rare instances the aneurysm may rupture inferolaterally, rending the arachnoid at the sphenoid ridge and causing a large subdural hemorrhage, which can threaten the brain with mass effect; the diagnosis of subdural hemorrhage is straightforward but the cause may not be obvious unless an angiogram is performed. In rare cases the middle cerebral aneurysm ruptures directly into the overlying brain, mimicking a putaminal hematoma.

Aneurysms of the anterior communicating artery typically cause a large hemorrhagic pocket between the two hemispheres, but some rupture upward into the rostrum of the corpus callosum, causing a striking syndrome of left-sided ideomotor dyspraxia. Other rupture directly posteriorly, damaging the septum, fornix, and anterior commissure, filling the third ventricle and causing a syndrome of hydrocephalus (see below), in this case hemocephalus. When the obtundation subsides as the hemocephalus clears, a severe, sometimes permanent, amnestic state remains. The third nerve palsy accompanying posterior communicating artery aneurysmal rupture has already been described (see above), but rupture directed laterally may cause a temporal lobe hemorrhage, mimicking that from the middle cerebral artery aneurysm.

Venous hemorrhage arising from the great vein of Galen or other veins posterior to the thalamus may cause a distinctive local subarachnoid hemorrhage that cuffs the midbrain (Fig. 37-7). The clinical course is usually benign, and this cause of subarachnoid hemorrhage yields no aneurysm on angiogram.

In the basilar territory, top-of-the-basilar aneurysms have distinctive clinical pictures (see above), but those arising from the cerebellar arteries where they branch from the basilar often cause such dramatic flooding of the prepontine cisterns as to cause some-

thing akin to tamponade of the posterior fossa. These patients frequently appear to have suffered cardiac arrest with temporary loss of all neurologic function, only to have it slowly reemerge after some minutes. During this time witnesses, including the authors, have found no evidence of neurologic function, which is slowly restored only minutes later, a clinical picture simulating that of cardiac arrest.

Syndromes of rupture of distally located mycotic aneurysms have all the features of lobar hematomas (see Ch. 37), and the mycotic origin of the hemorrhage is not often appreciated during life. Neoplastic aneurysms are often known to exist because of a tumor adjacent to the artery in question, and erosion of the artery, when large, is usually a fatal event.

In a few instances the initial neurologic deficits may have other explanations (see below) and usually improve over a matter of days.

Subarachnoid and Parenchymatous Hemorrhage

Hematomas arising within AVMs often expand initially within the confines of the AVM itself, tracking toward the ventricular wall and following deep venous drainage vessels where such veins exist. Hemorrhage in such cases may produce only slight additional damage to the adjacent healthy brain and vent mainly into the ventricle, causing acute hydro- or hemocephalus. Hematomas from AVMs with no deep venous drainage may expand into the adjacent brain. Many AVMs bleed from arterial or venous aneurysms embedded within the tangle of anomalous vessels and bleed with such violence as to mimic that of conventional arterial aneurysms.

Cavernous angiomas generally enlarge to only slightly more than their original size, causing neurologic disability but rarely a fatality.

For lobar hemorrhage from AVM, the clinical syndromes of hemorrhage contain few clinical clues to make AVM a leading diagnosis as compared with amyloid angiopathy, hypertensive hemorrhage, or aneurysm. Seizure occurring with clinical signs of hemorrhage (headache, vomiting, stiff neck, focal signs) may provide a clue but occurs in less than 2 percent of cases. An occipital lobe location, unusual for typical hypertensive hemorrhage, may be suggested by hemianopia without hemiparesis or sensory disturbance, but this also is infrequent. Rebleeding has been documented in AVMs but at widely varying intervals, sometimes of many years.

CLINICAL COURSE

For congenital and arteriosclerotic aneurysms, the initial hemorrhage is merely the first of a chain of events that often complicates the subsequent clinical course,

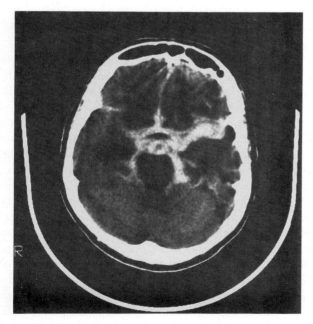

Figure 37-7. CT scan showing extensive subarachnoid hemorrhage with a large extension into the sylvian fissure (right side of scan) ipsilateral to the ruptured aneurysm.

which can be divided into the acute and chronic phases.

Leading among problems for survivors of the first rupture from aneurysm is *rebleeding*, which occurs in as many as 30 percent of all cases of congenital aneurysms, greatly increasing morbidity and mortality. The incidence of rebleeding is highest in the first 24 hours, often occurring during the early stages of transport to the hospital or during admission. Thereafter the rate is 1 to 2 percent per day, declining slightly day by day until 1 month. By 6 months the risk of rebleeding has fallen to 2 to 4 percent per year. Early surgical repair of the aneurysm has proved to be the only defense against this complication.

Hydrocephalus is a common complication from aneurysmal and AVM rupture at the base of the brain. It is evident on the first brain images from the blood flooded into the subarachnoid space. Ventricular size frequently increases between 4 days and 3 weeks following subarachnoid hemorrhage, after which it steadily regresses. Hydrocephalus may cause no detectable neurologic change, or it may be associated with profound stupor, appearing in a matter of hours. Mild drowsiness, urinary incontinence, and inability to move the eyes above the equator are associated with early mild to moderate hydrocephalus. Often hydrocephalus is transient and may not require specific surgical intervention.

Ventricular drains are a popular means of mitigating the hydrocephalus, but the authors have been impressed with the risk of infection, the risk of brain hemorrhage from the shunt tubing passed through the parenchyma, and the uncertainty that relief of the hydrocephalus has made a great difference in improving management or reducing morbidity. In some instances the obtundation has made the patient less subject to headache and in less obvious need of analgesics. However, shunting to prepare the patient for surgery is a useful practice.

Vasospasm, which is blamed for delayed neurologic deficits, remains a major problem in the setting of bleeding from aneurysms but is quite uncommon following rupture of AVMs. It is most commonly encountered in those congenital or arteriosclerotic aneurysms whose rupture discharges a large volume of blood into the subarachnoid space near the base of the brain; this is a common occurrence with aneurysms but uncommon with vascular malformatoins. The incidence varies widely (15 to 76 percent), but at least one-third of aneurysm patients suffer some form of spasm. Angiographic studies have documented a severe but short-lived spasm (minutes to 1 hour or more) when rupture has occurred during an angiogram. A few clinical series have documented some instances of transient acute focal deficit occurring within seconds or minutes of vessel rupture, mimicking transient ischemic attack. Its pathophsyiology remains a subject of considerable study (see Ch. 5).

In some cases, delayed focal deficits appear suddenly, suggesting some form of local embolism, from the aneurysm dome itself or from other sources not known. These sudden-onset syndromes typically persist unchanged, neither worsening nor responding to therapy. Apart from these unusual cases, the vast majority show an evolving syndrome that makes its first appearance on day 3 or 4 and that is correlated with arterial stenoses (spasm) on angiogram and with increase in intravascular velocities on transcranial Doppler studies (see below and Ch. 13).

Three major types of spasm have been described. *Diffuse spasm* is a nearly uniform narrowing over long distances of the major vessels, spreading out from their origins. *Segmental spasm* has the appearance of sausagelike bands of varying length. The most common form, *local spasm,* affects short segments of arteries in the vicinity of the aneurysm itself. The vessels most involved are those closest to the site of the aneurysm or where the densest subarachnoid clots are found. In cases in which serial angiograms have been performed for aneurysms affecting the circle of Willis, the spasm begins in one or more of its major cerebral arteries and spreads distally along the major CSF cylinders, passing over the convexity in the general direction of the superior sagittal sinus. Spasm affecting only the distal vessels is rare and when localized to a distal vessel suggests a diagnosis of arteritis (e.g., mycotic aneurysm).

The incidence, severity, and location of cerebral vasospasm in patients following subarachnoid hemorrhage can be predicted by early CT scan, which shows globular subarachnoid clots larger than 3×5 mm in the basal cisterns or layers of blood 1 mm thick or greater in the cerebral fissures (Fig. 37-6). CT scans that shows either no evidence of blood or its diffuse distribution are associated with a very low incidence of severe vasospasm. When severe, the syndrome of ischemia may prove resistant to all forms of therapy, and infarction large enough to be fatal is commonly recorded. Of all of the evolving complications of ruptured aneurysms, vasospasm is the worst.

Medical complications of subarachnoid hemorrhage include two that are specific to the hemorrhage: (1) electrocardiographic changes suggestive of coronary arterial ischemia, which may occur from overactive sympathetic nervous system discharge; and (2) hyponatremia and dehydration. For years the fall in serum sodium was considered a sign of inappropriate antidiuretic hormone secretion and subject to the usual treatment with fluid restriction. The risk of increasing vasospasm from dehydration and awareness that water as well as sodium are lost following subarachnoid hemorrhage have led to abandonment of this view. The effect is now thought of as cerebral salt wasting attributable to increased secretion of atrial naturetic hormone. Other complications for which the medical team must remain alert are those common in the bedridden state, such as bedsores, aspiration pneumonia, thrombophlebitis with pulmonary embolism, and perforated duodenal ulcer.

PROGNOSIS

In the aneurysm population overall, just under 10 percent die within the first 24 hours, roughly 50 percent survive 2 weeks, and the remainder survive with varying states of disability but half of these die within 5 years. The prognosis is worse for the 20 percent with multiple aneurysms. Rebleeding produces significant morbidity and mortality in the untreated patient. The risk of rebleeding within 1 month is approximately 33 percent, and the mortality rate from this second hemorrhage is 42 percent. Of long-term survivors approximately 3 percent can be expected annually to rebleed.

Grading systems have been devised to allow rapid assessment of the patient The Hunt and Hess scheme shown in Table 37-1 is the most widely used but is clearly not a unique means of appraisal. It is instead a simple means of conveying general status useful for telephone and conversational reporting. The scale has become a standard means of making a baseline assessment, which has often been used to estimate outcome. When the term "poor grade" is used, clinicians usually mean grades 4 or 5.

Table 37-1. Hunt and Hess Grading Scheme for Clinical Status

Grade	Clinicial Condition
0	Unruptured aneurysm
1	Asymptomatic or minimal headache and slight nuchal rigidity
1A	No acute meningeal or brain reaction, but with fixed neurologic deficit
2	Moderate to severe headache, nuchal rigidity; no neurologic deficit other than cranial nerve palsy
3	Drowsiness, confusion, or mild focal deficit
4	Stupor, moderate to severe hemiparesis, possible early decerebrate rigidity and vegetative disturbances
5	Deep coma, decerebrate rigidity, and moribund appearance

LABORATORY AND IMAGING STUDIES

White blood cell counts above 15,000 and low sodium values on admission are both poor prognostic signs, the former being related to vasospasm and the latter secondary to inappropriate antidiuretic hormone secretion or to an unknown factor. For reasons not yet understood, poor prognosis is also related to serum viscosity increases, with a hematocrit above 40 percent, high osmolality, and serum-fibrinogen level above 250 mg percent.

Lumbar puncture has been the time-honored test for subarachnoid hemorrhage. In true subarachnoid hemorrhage the CSF, drawn within 24 hours of onset, does not clot, and when centrifuged (to compact the cells in the bottom of the tube) has a a xanthochromic appearance (from the Greek for yellow-colored). Cell counts for red blood cells are expected to be in the thousands (mere dozens to hundreds are suspicious signs of a traumatic tap), and the counts should be approximately the same in the first and third tubes of CSF, showing the uniformity of the hemorrhagic fluid in the sample (CSF from traumatic taps usually has a far lower count in the later tubes) (see Ch. 9).

Brain imaging by CT scan using late-model equipment shows subarachnoid blood on the noncontrast scan in 75 percent of cases if the scan is obtained within the first 48 hours of aneurysmal rupture. The extent and location of subarachnoid blood are useful clues to the location of the aneurysm, but jet flow from the rupture site may occur across the base of the brain, providing a misleading localization in some cases. Localization of aneurysms down to 3 mm in size has been reported with use of high-resolution CT scan with contrast (see Ch. 10).

MRI has reliably detected aneurysms 0.5 mm or larger. More importantly, MRI can distinguish the thrombosed blood in the aneurysm dome, which is not adequately evaluated by angiogram (which images only the liquid blood), and can demonstrate old and new hemorrhages.

Transcranial Doppler ultrasonography has won a place for its ease of use at the bedside, as it offers an excellent means of demonstrating the presence and severity of vasospasm. An excellent correlation has been found between angiographic evidence of spasm and Doppler velocities above 100 cm/s to 120 mg/s. Flow velocities typically peak on the 11th and 18th days and normalize by the third to fourth week. The clinical importance is that these increases in velocities usually occur before the appearance of delayed ischemic defects and presage the increase in angiographically evident vasospasm. The sharp angle of the anterior cerebral artery with respect to the plane of insonation of the Doppler probe makes for poor signals from this vessel and a corresponding low incidence of detection of spasm.

Angiography, while losing favor, still remains the most commonly employed definitive method for aneurysm diagnosis. Where possible, selective angiography should be performed just prior to planned surgery, not only to localize the aneurysm but also to document its exact anatomy for approach. Because selective cerebral angiography can miss a subtle aneurysm, particularly of the anterior communicating artery or in the posterior circulation, repeat four-vessel angiography is still a common practice after about 1 week. If no aneurysm is found on the initial selective cerebral angiogram, the chance for repeat angiography to detect a subarachnoid hemorrhage is quite low (1 to 2 percent).

When no aneurysm is found, other explanations of subarachnoid hemorrhage include rupture of a small superficial cortical artery, a spinal cord AVM, an extramedullary aneurysm of the spinal cord (e.g., involving a cervical radicular artery or an anterior spinal artery aneurysm), an aneurysm of the artery of Adamkiewicz, or exposure to drugs. A toxic screen done within the first 24 hours of subarachnoid hemorrhage may reveal the cause.

When an angiogram has demonstrated an AVM, whether in a setting of acute hemorrhage or some time after the ictus, a decision must be made not only concerning the hematoma but the AVM itself (see below).

TREATMENT

In the immediate stages following rupture, clinical and brain imaging efforts are directed at assessing the clinical grade of the patient and discovering whether there is a reversible extracerebral mass effect from the released blood. The uncommon cases of acute subdural hemorrhage or large hemorrhagic mass trapped in the subarachnoid spaces of the sylvian fissure (see above) should prompt consideration of immediate operation, even in poor-grade patients, after angiography has clarified the location of the lesion.

Aneurysms

Where no extraparenchymatous mass lesion exists, the clinical grade of the patient and the size of the aneurysm dictate much of the plan. For all patients, oral nimodipine therapy at 60 mg qid is widely recommended, along with generous intravenous hydration to minimize the risk of vasospasm. The syndrome of salt (and water) loss is treated with fluid volume supplemented with crystalloid or colloid therapy as needed for a daily intake of 2 to 3 L of fluids. Use of 0.2 mg fludrocortisone assists in blunting the salt and water loss for those patients suffering the syndrome

of neurogenic hyponatremia. Anticonvulsants are a popular regimen, but no study has addressed their need or usefulness in prevention of seizures, an uncommon event in the early stages after aneurysm rupture. Electrocardiographic monitoring is also a common practice to detect treatable arrhythmias, which may occur in the first few days. Despite the availability of ϵ-aminocaproic acid to prevent rebleeding, its use has been discouraged by the higher frequency of delayed neurologic deficits attributed to spasm with this treatment.

In good-grade patients it has become commonplace in many centers to plan angiography to demonstrate the aneurysm and to undertake surgery within the first 24 hours. This offers the advantage of removing the aneurysm from the circulation, thereby eliminating the risk of early rerupture, and allows more aggressive management, with hypertension and volume expansion as needed for subsequent vasospasm. In experienced hands, there appears to be no advantage to delaying surgery.

Ventricular drains (see above) are used in some centers to reduce hydrocephalus (actually a mixture of hydro- and hemocephalus) in the hope that improvement of the neurologic syndromes attributable to the enlarged ventricles could allow better assessment of clinical disturbances attributable to the aneurysmal rupture and to any existing arterial spasm. Drainage also helps reduce intracranial pressure, which could reduce the severity of spasm and make planned surgery less technically difficult. The complications of infection and the small risk of provoking a brain hemorrhage by the insertion of the drain (through brain tissue to reach the ventricles) prompt caution in applying this procedure.

At the time of surgery, it was initially popular to flush the subarachnoid space in the hope of reducing the concentrations of blood products important in the genesis of vasospasm. This practice has largely been abandoned because the clots are difficult to dislodge and the benefit of flushing of CSF cisterns was not demonstrated. Use of tissue plasminogen activator, a thrombolytic agent, is under investigation, as is use of the 21-aminosteroid tirilazad mesylate, an inhibitor of iron-dependent peroxidation. When vasospasm does not respond to medical therapy, some centers have undertaken transluminal angioplasty to dilate the vessels in spasm, a technique not well enough developed as yet to be widely recommended outside specialized centers. Giant aneurysms, as well as those for which no neck can be found suitable for clip placement to isolate the aneurysm from the circulation, continue to pose difficult challenges for management. Intravascular procedures to place thrombotic coils within the dome of the aneurysm are being developed with the aim of thrombosing the aneurysm and nullifying its risk of rupture, but in some cases in which late follow-up angiograms have been obtained, the unclipped neck has continued to grow. The range of options for managing giant or unclippable aneurysms remains limited.

For mycotic aneurysms, angiography has been recommended for all patients with embolic symptoms in order to identify aneurysms prior to the occurrence of subarachnoid hemorrhage, but this policy has never been widely adopted. Those who harbor an aneurysm can be treated with high doses of the appropriate antibiotic and the aneurysm followed with repeat angiograms. If the aneurysm thromboses, no further treatment is necessary. However, if it enlarges, current recommendations are for resection of the diseased arterial segment or clipping of the aneurysm.

Surgical treatment is usually not an option for dolichoectatic aneurysms, and medical management is the rule. In these cases, focal infarcts may occur from occlusion of the tiny branches emerging through the thick wall of the artery. Anticoagulation is used in some centers to try to prevent occlusions in other arterial branches, but hemorrhage is also a natural risk for dolichoectatic arteries.

If the first angiogram does not demonstrate the aneurysm, it is no longer a widespread practice to repeat the study 1 to 6 weeks later, as was commonly done in the past. If the patient is of good grade and shows no sign of vasospasm within the first week, ambulation is allowed.

For some patients who remain in such poor grade as to contraindicate surgery or whose aneurysm is too large or unfavorable for surgery, medical management is all that is available. Treatment with nimodipine with adequate hydration (see above) for at least 3 weeks is the usual regimen, with cautious ambulation thereafter for those spared major focal deficits.

Arteriovenous Malformations

The large size of the lesion alone (sometimes a whole lobe) makes at least 30 percent of AVM patients untreatable. Those most favorable for treatment have an AVM smaller than half of a cerebral lobe; feeders easily identified on angiogram, with none feeding the malformation from the deep vascular territories; and drainage to the surface, not deep veins.

For therapy to succeed, total obliteration of the lesion is necessary. Anything less is almost as unsatisfactory as no therapy at all, as some of the smaller and more friable feeders left behind may enlarge within months to make an equally or more hazardous lesion as compared with that existing formerly.

Embolization of the lesion by means of microcatheters that deliver quick-acting glues, balloons, or fine metal or by means of thrombogenic coils may assist in reducing the size of the lesion to one manageable by direct surgical attack. In thoroughly experienced hands, surgical morbidity and mortality are low enough to favor the recommendation that all such lesions undergo operation, a recommendation that is inappropriate in inexperienced hands. In the current literature, fewer than a dozen teams can muster a series of as many as 100 operated cases, and for most of them the effort spans a decade or more. For AVMs and cavernous angiomas, successful surgery rids the patient of the risk of hemorrhage but does little to alter the course of seizures or even headaches.

ANNOTATED BIBLIOGRAPHY

Aminoff MJ. Treatment of unruptured cerebral arteriovenous malformations. Neurology 1987;37:815.

Argues against aggressive treatment.

Awad IA, Little JR. Perioperative management and outcome after surgical treatment of anterior cerebral artery aneurysms. Can J Neurol Sci 1991;18:120–5.

Details on hemodilution therapy as part of a large review.

Barnett HJM, Mohr JP, Stein BM, Yatsu F. Stroke. Churchill Livingstone, New York, 1992.

Standard textbook.

Brothers MF, Holgate RC. Intracranial angioplasty for treatment of vasospasm after subarachnoid hemorrhage: technique and modifications to improve branch access. AJNR 1990;11:237–47.

Early experiences.

Crawford JV, Russell DS. Cryptic arteriovenous and venous hamartomas of the brain. J Neurol Neurosurg Psychiatry 1956;19:1.

Details of neuropathology in a clinical classic.

Crompton MR. Cerebral infarction following the rupture of cerebral berry aneurysms. Brain 1964;87:263.

Pathology studies, some consistent with local embolism.

Disney L, Weir B, Grace M. Factors influencing the outcome of aneurysm rupture in poor grade patients: a prospective series. Neurosurgery 1988;23:1–9.

Poor outlook in patients with a poor initial clinical status can be predicted by whether they have had surgery, their clinical grade on admission, age, initial systolic blood pressure, and aneurysm size.

Fisher CM, Ojemann RG. Basal rupture of cerebral aneurysm—a pathological case report. J Neurosurg 1978;48:642.

Few reported but many may exist, adding to surgical burdens to place the clip proximal to the rupture site.

Fisher CM, Roberson GH, Ojemann RG. Cerebral vasospasm with ruptured saccular aneurysm—the clinical manifestations. Neurosurgery 1977;1:245.

Fine details.

Forbus WD. On the origin of miliary aneurysms of the superficial cerebral arteries. Johns Hopkins Med J H 1930; 47:237.

A classic article.

Freytag E. Fatal rupture of intracranial aneurysms: survey of 250 medicolegal cases. Arch Pathol 1966;81:418–24.

Evidence of a cause of sudden death.

Gautier JC, Hauw JJ, Awada A et al. Artères cérébrales dolichoectasiques. Association aux anevrysmes de l'aorte abdominale. Rev Neurol (Paris) 1988;144:437–46.

Abdominal aortic aneurysms in 50 percent.

Gilbert JW, Lee C, Young B. Repeat cerebral panangiography in subarachnoid hemorrhage of unknown etiology. Surg Neurol 1990;33:19–21.

Usually negative.

Hunt WE, Hess RM. Surgical risk as related to time of intervention in the repair of intracranial aneurysms. J Neurosurg 1968;28:14–20.

Description of the most popular rating scale for neurologic status.

Kistler JP, Crowell RM, Davis KR et al. The relation of cerebral vasospasm to the extent and location of subarachnoid blood as visualized by CT scan. Neurology 1983; 433:424.

The thicker the clots, the more the spasm.

Kondziolka D, Bernstein M, Spiegel SM, terBrugge K. Symptomatic arterial luminal narrowing presenting months after subarachnoid hemorrhage and aneurysm clipping. J Neurosurg 1988;69:494–9.

Some unexplained cases with very late spasm.

Kusske JA, Kelly WA. Embolization and reduction of the "steal" syndrome in cerebral AVMs. J Neurosurg 1974; 40:313.

Remarkable changes in neurologic deficit after correction of the AVM, the changes being attributed to better perfusion of the remainder of the brain. One of the few reported cases.

Lechevalier B, Houtteville JP. Cavernomes intracraniens. Rev Neurol (Paris) 1992;148:173–9.

Full pathologic and clinical details.

Lennihan L, Petty GW, Fink ME et al. Transcranial Doppler detection of anterior cerebral artery vasospasm. J Neurol Neurosurg Psychiatry 1993;56:906–9.

Transcranial Doppler ultrasound proved useful to detect and follow spasms in the middle cerebral artery but not the anterior cerebral artery because the anatomic course of the latter is at unfavorable angles for insonation by Doppler.

Locksley HB. Natural history of subarachnoid hemorrhage, intracranial aneurysm and arteriovenous malformation Based on 6368 cases in the cooperative study. Parts I and II. In Sahs, AL, Perret, GE, Locksley, HB Nishioka H (eds). Intracranial Aneurysms and Subarachnoid Hemorrhage. A Cooperative Study. JB Lippincott, Philadelphia, 1969, pp. 37–107.

Large cohort.

McCormick F. Vascular disease. In Rosenberg R. (ed). The Clinical Neurosciences. Vol. 3. Churchill Livingstone, New York, 1983, p. 38.

McCormick WF, Acosta-Rua GJ. The size of intracranial saccular aneurysms: an autopsy study. J Neurosurg 1970; 33:422.

The largest study of the range in size.

Mohr JP, Kase CS. Cerebral vasospasm. Rev Neurol (Paris) 1983;139:99–113.

Three syndromes defined.

Mohr JP, Stein BM, Hilal SK. Arteriovenous malformations. In Toole JF (ed). Vascular Diseases. Part II. in Vinken PJ, Bruyn GW, Klawans HL (eds): Handbook of Clinical Neurology. Vol. 10(54). 1989. pp 361–93.

Molinari GF, Smith L, Goldstein MN. Pathogenesis of cerebral mycotic aneurysms. Neurology 1973;23:325–32.

Experimental models.

New PFJ, Price DL, Carter B. Cerebral angiography in cardiac myxoma. Radiology 1970;96:335–45.

Neoplastic aneurysm.

Ohman J, Servo A, Heiskanen O. Risks factors for cerebral infarction in good grade patients after aneurysmal subarachnoid hemorrhage and surgery: a prospective study. J Neurosurg 1991;74:14–20.

Phillips LH, Whisnant JP, O'Fallon MW, Sundt TM. The unchanging pattern of subarachnoid hemorrhage in a community. Neurology 1980;30:1034–46.

Stable over the decades.

Pickard JD, Murray GD, Illingworth R et al. Effect of oral nimodipine on cerebral infarction and outcome after subarachnoid haemorrhage: British aneurysm nimodipine trial. Br Med J 1989;298:636–42.

This widely quoted trial randomized 554 patients with subarachnoid hemorrhage, comparing placebo with nimodipine 60 mg orally every 4 hours for 21 days. A 34 percent reduction of the incidence of cerebral infarction for those taking nimodipine and a 40 percent reduction in poor outcomes were achieved.

Raps EC, Rogers JD, Galetta SL et al. The clinical spectrum of unruptured intracranial aneurysms. Arch Neurol 1993;50:265–8.

Many occur with headache and as mass effect.

Rinkel GJ, Wijdicks EF, Vermeulen M et al. Outcome in perimesencephalic (nonaneurysmal) subarachnoid hemorrhage: a follow-up study in 37 patients. Neurology 1990;40:1130.

Mainly venous origins for the perimesencephalic cases.

Roberson GH, Kase CS, Wolpow ER. Telangiectases and cavernous angiomas of the brainstem: "cryptic" vascular malformations. Neuroradiology 1974;8:83

Schoerner W, Bradac GB, Treisch J et al. Magnetic resonance imaging (MRI) in the diagnosis of cerebral arteriovenous angiomas. Neuroradiology 1986;28:313.

MRI was far superior to CT.

Solomon RA, Smith CR, Raps EC et al. Deep hypothermic circulatory arrest for the management of complex anterior and posterior circulation aneurysms. Neurosurgery 1991;29:732–7.

Advanced techniques for large aneurysms.

Steinmeier R, Laumer R, Bondar I et al. Cerebral hemodynamics in subarachnoid hemorrhage evaluated by transcranial Doppler sonography. Part 2. Pulsatility indices: normal reference values and characteristics in subarachnoid hemorrhage. Neurosurgery 1993;33:10–18.

Transcranial Doppler imaging in a prospective study of 455 patients with subarachnoid hemorrhage showed elevated pulsatility indices initially, which normalized around day 10.

Taylor B, Harries P, Bullock R. Factors affecting outcome after surgery for intracranial aneurysm in Glasgow. Br J Neurosurg 1991;5:591–600.

Early surgery preferrable to delays.

Ter-Berg HW, Dippel DW, Limburg M et al. Familial intracranial aneurysms. A review. Stroke 1992;23:1024–30.

The frequency may be well below the 6.7 percent reported from retrospective reviews. Surgical treatment is recommended for those under age 70, and screening is suggested for those age 35 to 65.

Weber M, Vespignani H, Bracard S et al. Les angiomes caverneux intracérébraux. Rev Neurol (Paris) 1989;145:429.

Major series.

Weir B, Grace M, Hansen J, Rothberg C. Time course of vasospasm in man. J Neurosurg 1978;48:173–8.

Angiographic study.

Wiebers DO, Whisnant JP, O'Fallen WM. The natural history of unruptured intracranial aneurysms. N Engl J Med 1981;304:696–8.

Outcome predictable by size.

Wilkins RH. Aneurysm rupture during angiography: does acute vasospasm occur? Surg Neurol 1976;5:299–303.

Literature review showing acute spasm occurs.

Winn HR, Richardson AE, Jane JA. The long-term prognosis in untreated cerebral aneurysms: 1. The incidence of late hemorrhage in cerebral aneurysm: a 10-year evolution of 364 patients. Ann Neurol 1977;1:358.

Rupture rates as high as 2 percent per annum are reported.

38
Vasculitides

J. C. Gautier and J. P. Mohr

The central nervous system (CNS) vasculitides are a very heterogeneous group of diseases histologically characterized by inflammatory and often necrotizing lesions of the vessel wall. There is no satisfactory classification of this group of diseases. Table 38-1 enumerates the main disorders considered in this chapter.

Many of the arterial lesions are granulomatous. Veins are involved in many instances. With rare exceptions, the causes are generally elusive. Many are part of a systemic disease, but a few appear to be confined to the CNS. The diseases are important to neurologists because the inflammatory lesions of the vessels may cause thrombosis and occlusion with infarction or they may lead to rupture or aneurysm formation, resulting in hemorrhage.

It is widely believed that several CNS vasculitides are explained by one of three possible basic immune mechanisms. First, immune complexes may form at the arterial wall, activating complement components with accumulation of polymorphonuclear leukocytes, whose enzymes damage the vessel wall. Alternatively, circulating immune complexes may be deposited in vessel walls. Second, a direct attack on the vessel wall may occur from antibodies (e.g., in Kawasaki's disease), but this possibility is still unproved. Third, cell-mediated immune reactions may be present in many of the primary vasculitides, in which endothelial cells act as antigen-presenting cells with a response of T cells. Current hypotheses also include a possible role of perivascular microglial cells and smooth muscle cells in immune interactions bearing on the vessel wall. The histologic structure of granulomas also suggests a participation of monocytes and macrophages. Antiphospholipid antibodies, such as the lupus anticoagulant and anticardiolipin antibodies, although associated with a thrombotic tendency, may be markers for vasculitis.

Clinically, most vasculitides pose difficult diagnostic problems. As compared with atherosclerosis and cardiac embolism, the vasculitides are rare. Except when they are part of a florid systemic inflammatory disease, few of them have clear-cut clinical characteristics. The usual symptoms are mental confusion, delirium, and seizures rather than the more focal symptoms that usually characterize stroke due to infarction or hemorrhage. Arteriograms are often normal, since in many cases involved arteries are of less than 500-μm diameter, too small to be imaged by conventional angiography. When the vessels seen on angiogram are involved, the multiple successive stenoses ("beading") consistent with arteritis are not specific for the diagnosis (see below). In a fair number of cases there is an associated peripheral neuropathy, which is a clue to unusual CNS lesions and hence to vasculitis. In the end, brain biopsy to examine the meningeal and cortical vessels can be the key to the diagnosis.

VASCULITIDES ASSOCIATED WITH INFECTIONS

Pyogenic meningitides in the adult are mostly due to pneumococci, meningococci, *Haemophilus influenzae*, *Listeria monocytogenes*, staphylococci, and streptococci (see Ch. 39). Early in the course of the disease, the small and medium-size arteries, bathed in infected spinal fluid, are cuffed and invaded by neutrophils, lymphocytes, and hyperplastic endothelial cells bulge into the lumen. Veins are often involved and thrombosed. While such histopathologic changes are common, only in the more advanced cases does the process lead to occlusions with focal deficits, convulsions, and cranial nerve paralyses.

Arteries bathed by chronically inflammatory cerebrospinal fluid (CSF) of the chronic meningitides, such as tuberculous meningitis, meningovascular syphilis, or chronic pyogenic meningitis, can develop a particular obstructive reaction termed *endarteritis ob-*

Table 38-1. Causes of CNS Vasculitides

Associated with infections	Behçet's syndrome
Pyogenic meningitides	Associated with connective tissue disease
Tuberculous meningitis	Systemic lupus erythematosus
Syphilitic meningitis	Rheumatoid arthritis
Leptospiral meningitis	Scleroderma
Bacterial endocarditis	Gougerot-Sjögren's syndrome
Fungal meningitis	Relapsing polychondritis
Borrelia burgdorferi	Ulcerative colitis
Malaria	Celiac disease
Rickettsial diseases	Granulomatous conditions
Strongyloides stercoralis	Giant cell arteritis
Herpes zoster	Proximal
Cytomegalovirus	Cranial
Hepatitis B, streptoccocus	Intracranial
Acute serous otitis media	Sarcoidosis
Acquired immunodeficiency syndrome (AIDS)	Wegener's granulomatosis
Systemic necrotizing vasculitides	Lymphomatoid granulomatosis
Polyarteritis nodosa	Associated with malignancies
Allergic granulomatosis	Hodgkin's and non-Hodgkin's
and angiitis (Churg-Strauss)	lymphomas
Overlap syndrome	Lymphosarcoma
Kawasaki's disease	Hairy cell leukemia
Hypersensitivity vasculitides	Miscellaneous
Serum sickness	Cogan's syndrome
Cryoglobulinemia	Eales' syndrome
Henoch-Schönlein purpura	Irradiation
Associated with drugs	Cerebral thromboarteritis obliterans
	Idiopathic hypereosinophilia

literans, in which there is thickening of the intima first by a cellular infiltrate and later by fibrous tissue. Less marked alterations can occur in veins. When endarteritis is severe enough to stenose or occlude arteries, transient ischemic attacks or infarctions may occur. An especially severe basal meningitis with arteritis from *Leptospira* has been reported as a cause of moyamoya disease.

Other bacterial disorders include the endocardities, which can lead to emboli of infected vegetations; these emboli can result in arterial occlusions and infarction or in aneurysms that are often small, multiple, and distal on the branches of the middle cerebral artery. Such aneurysms can rupture. In addition, the source of infection can be in the lung, or a septicemia or cardiac surgery may be responsible.

Fungal arteritides and aneurysms develop mainly in immunosuppressed patients and can cause infarction or hemorrhage. The source is often an orbital or paranasal air sinus infection (*Aspergillus, Mucormycosis*) or lung infection (*Candida albicans, Nocardia asteroides*) (see Ch. 40).

Arteritis as part of other infectious disease have been reported, among them the ubiquitous Lyme disease (*Borrelia burgdorferi*), the diagnosis being supported by specific antibodies and an elevated specific antibody index in the CSF. An immune-mediated vasculopathy affecting arterioles and venules has been proposed as a key lesion in cerebral malaria (see Ch. 42). In typhus and scrub typhus an acute vasculitis of small brain vessels has also been reported, accompanied by perivascular typhus nodules. *Strongyloides stercoralis,* a nematode, can induce a so-called hyperinfection in immunosuppressed patients. It has been held responsible for cerebral vasculitis in a patient who had systemic lupus erythematosus. Delayed hemiplegia contralateral to herpes zoster ophthalmicus, causing a viral arteritis, is an infrequent but well-defined syndrome. It has also been reported following cervical *zoster* and herpes *oticus.* Inflammatory lesions of cerebral arteries and veins, probably due to cytomegalovirus, have been reported in an immunodepressed patient. A systemic necrotizing vasculitis has also been found associated with hepatitis B infection. Precedent hepatitis is rare. This association is not clearly delineated from polyarteritis nodosa, which it mimics closely and in which one-third of the patients have circulating immune complexes containing hepatitis B surface antigen. A less clearly causal relationship exists between systemic vasculitis and group A streptococcal infections and rheumatic fever. Vasculitis has also been reported after acute serous otitis media.

An isolated cerebral granulomatous arteritis occurred in a patient in whom human T-cell leukemia virus III (HTLV-III) (human immunodeficiency virus [HIV]) was isolated from brain tissue and CSF.

SYSTEMIC NECROTIZING VASCULITIDES

Polyarteritis nodosa (PAN) is an acute and subacute disease of small and medium-size arteries. The kidney, heart, and gastrointestinal tract are the organs most prominently affected. The involvement of the nervous system is often less obvious, but peripheral neuropathy occurs in over 50 percent of patients, while CNS involvement is found in approximately 30 percent, usually later in the course of the disease.

The arterial lesions in PAN are characterized by segmental fibrinoid or hyaline necrosis, with an inflammatory infiltrate predominating in the adventitia but involving all arterial coats. Thrombotic occlusion or rupture of the artery may occur, but aneurysm formation in the cerebral arteries is rare.

The manifestations of CNS involvement in PAN are headache, retinopathy, confusional states, often fluctuating with visual or other hallucinations, cranial neuropathies, seizures, and strokes due to infarction or hemorrhage. Cerebral angiography usually shows nonspecific occlusions or multiple stenoses of small and medium-size arteries. Celiac and renal angiography may reveal quasipathognomomic aneurysms. One-third of patients have circulating immune complexes containing hepatitis B surface antigens. Skin, muscle, or kidney biopsy can make the diagnosis. The prognosis, once poor, has been much improved by corticosteroids, usually employed with cyclophosphamide or azathioprine.

Allergic granulomatosis and angiitis, also termed the *Churg-Strauss syndrome*, closely resembles PAN, but lung involvement with asthma and high eosinophil counts are prominent features. Apart from frequent early brain involvement, the neurologic features are similar to those of PAN. The *overlap syndrome* is the term proposed for patients who have both PAN and Churg-Strauss features.

Kawasaki's disease occurs in infants. It is closely similar to PAN, although with prominent skin and lymph node involvement. Aseptic meningitis, seizures, and infarction due to occlusion of intracranial branch arteries have been reported.

Hypersensitivity vasculitides are the most frequent vasculitides in practice, but involvement of the CNS is infrequent. Serum sickness, now rare, includes as part of its syndrome a characteristic painful brachial plexopathy, a mononeuritis, or more rarely, an acute generalized polyneuropathy. Stroke due to middle cerebral artery occlusion has also been recorded, but its mechanism is obscure. Similar syndromes can occur after immunization, in drug-induced allergic vasculitis, or in the course of reticuloendothelial malignancies such as chronic lymphocytic leukemia, lymphoma, and multiple myeloma. Cases associated with cryoglobulinemia are also recorded. Henoch-Schönlein *purpura* is an affection of children, with possible seizures and hemiplegia due to a vasculitis. The differential diagnosis of brain disorders should also include hyponatremia.

VASCULITIDES ASSOCIATED WITH CONNECTIVE TISSUE DISEASES

Systemic lupus erythematosus (SLE) is a multisystem autoimmune disease with frequent CNS vasculitis. It is more common in women, with a peak age in the third and fourth decades. Despite the emphasis on vascular disease, many of the CNS disorders in SLE are not due to vasculitis, as there is evidence of the presence of antineural antibodies. Hypertension and renal failure are usually part of the clinical picture.

The basic arterial lesion in SLE is a fibrinoid or hyaline degeneration of small arteries without much inflammation. This lesion thus does not resemble the lesions of PAN. Deposits of immune complexes or immunoglobulins have not been demonstrated in the arteries. They have been found in the choroid plexuses, but they are not specific and have no clear clinical correlation. Occlusions of large arteries (e.g., internal carotid and middle cerebral) and occasionally of large cortical veins have been reported. Embolism from the noninfectious verrucous (Libman-Sacks) endocarditis is probably exceedingly rare.

Brain lesions usually occur as small foci of infarction in the hemispheres, basal ganglia, and brainstem or as multiple small hemorrhages, but large, often hemorrhagic, infarctions are part of the picture.

Since the lesions of SLE can affect any part of the CNS, they result in a wide spectrum of clinical syndromes. The common disorders are confusional states, headache, seizures, focal deficit, involuntary movements (e.g., chorea), athetosis, hemiballismus, cerebellar incoordination, retinal vasculitis, optic neuropathy, and paraparesis. Peripheral neuropathy is infrequent. The CSF is abnormal in one-third of patients: the protein is raised but usually less than 100 mg/L, and there is a moderate lymphocytic pleocytosis, usually less than 50 lymphocytes per mm^3. Electrophoresis shows an oligoclonal immunologic banding in many cases.

Such features, together with a frequent relapsing and remitting course of the clinical disorders, explain how an erroneous diagnosis of multiple sclerosis can be arrived at ("lupoid sclerosis"). However, cases that have been autopsied have shown vasculitic lesions, not demyelination, and isolated involvement of the CNS is rare. Skin, joint, kidney, or blood disorders are usually associated signs. Moreover, there can be evidence of an active immune disorder with false-positive venereal disease research laboratory (VDRL) test, lupus anticoagulant, and anticardiolipin antibody tests or increased DNA binding activity.

The prognosis, once very poor—over 80 percent of patients dying at 3 years, frequently as a result of CNS involvement—has been greatly improved with corticosteroids. High doses should be used with caution and for short periods, as side effects and complications can occur. Immunosuppressive agents such as cyclophosphamide or azathioprine are generally used along with the corticosteroids. Plasmapheresis can be considered in acute ("fulminant") SLE.

In rheumatoid arthritis, peripheral neuropathy is the commonest nervous complication. CNS vasculitis is rare, with lesions of small brain arteries similar to those of PAN leading to infarction or hemorrhages. Clinical disorders include confusional states, transient ischemic attacks, strokes, cranial neuropathies, chorea, sensorineural deafness, or paraparesis.

Scleroderma, or progressive systemic sclerosis is a systemic disease characterized by sclerosis of the collagen tissue in the skin, heart, lung, digestive tract, and kidneys. CNS involvement is extremely rare, and these very few cases could be due to arterial hypertension. CNS vasculitis is common where scleroderma is part of a mixed connective tissue disease (i.e., where there is concomitant evidence of SLE and polymyositis). Confusional states, headache, seizures, transient ischemic attacks, and strokes are possible. Occlusion of the terminal internal carotid artery has been reported.

Gougerot-Sjögren's syndrome is an autoimmune disease in which inflammatory cells damage the lachrymal and salivary glands, with resulting xerophthalmia and xerostomia (sicca syndrome). The Raynaud phenomenon and arthritis are frequent. Vasculitis has been documented in a few cases. GSS can occur in association with SLE, rheumatoid arthritis, and scleroderma. CNS involvement can determine ischemic optic neuropathy, strokes, myelopathy, and recurrent meningoencephalitis.

Relapsing polychondritis is a rare relapsing and remitting disease of cartilages, with rare CNS involvement. Peripheral neuropathy is still rarer. There is widespread necrotizing vasculitis. Confusional states, seizures, strokes, cranial neuropathies, ischemic optic neuropathy, and sensorineural deafness have been reported.

Cerebral vasculitis can also be associated with ulcerative colitis and celiac disease and with a necrotizing bowel disease (Köhlmeier-Degos) occurring most often in teenage boys.

GRANULOMATOUS CONDITIONS

Several diseases are discussed together in this section because their basic pathologic process is a granuloma. However, this grouping is mostly for the sake of convenience, as the causes and pathophysiology of these diseases are unknown and in all likelihood different.

Three of these diseases affect primarily the cerebral arteries either proximally (Takayasu's disease), cranially, or more truly extracranially (cranial arteritis) or intracranially (granulomatous angiitis of the CNS) (see Ch. 35). These different locations show that the brunt of the lesion involves arteries of different sizes. With slight (possibly significant) differences, the arterial lesion is characterized by a destruction of the inner media, with the presence of multinucleated giant cells and an inflammatory cellular infiltrate consisting of mononuclear cells, plasma cells, lymphocytes, and sometimes a few polymorphonuclear leukocytes.

In the proximal variety of Takayasu's disease (aortic arch syndrome), there is a gradual occlusion of the aortic arch and the innominate, common carotid, and subclavian arteries (see Ch. 35). Microscopically the lesions involve many other arteries, although the coronary and lower limb arteries are said to be spared. A less florid type of this disease is common in India, and a few cases of transient aortic arteritis are considered by some to constitute a distinct entity. Cerebral disorders include lightheadedness, giddiness, confusion, and seizures. Transient ischemic attacks, including drop attacks, are possible. Amaurosis fugax can be provoked by standing up or exercise or coming from shadow into bright light. The fundus examination can show low-pressure retinopathy. Bilateral or altitudinal transient blindness can be due to occipital ischemia. Pain in the arms on exercise is rare, but typically both radial pulses are abolished (pulseless disease). There is often claudication pain in the jaw on eating and sometimes ulceration of the scalp, palate, or nasal system. Insonation of the neck arteries and angiography show the proximal occlusion of the main branches of the aortic arch.

In approaching the diagnosis, atherosclerotic lesions and Behçet's syndrome (see below) must be excluded. Cranial arteritis (see below) can also result in proximal occlusions. Some cases of the aortic arch syndrome have had concomitant inflammatory evidence of fever, anemia, pleurisy, arthralgia, Raynaud phenomenon, erythema nodosum, and a high erythrocyte sedimentation rate (ESR). In such cases corticosteroids can be considered.

Cranial giant cell arteritis (formerly known as temporal arteritis) affects people of both sexes over the age of 60 (see Ch. 35). The large arteries (including the aorta, with possible dissection or aneurysmal dilation or occlusion of aortic arch branches) and medium-size arteries are involved. The disease could be rightly termed *extracranial,* as intracranial lesions are exceptional once the arteries have pierced the dura. Perhaps the paucity of elastic tissue in the intracranial arteries is the explanation. The extracranial internal carotid artery and the vertebral arteries may become thrombosed, with resulting transient ischemic attacks or infarcts (e.g., in the brainstem or occipital lobe). The most dreaded complication is blindness from acute ischemic anterior optic neuropathy, explained by involvement of the ophthalmic artery or of its ciliary branches. It may have been preceded by amaurosis fugax. Oculomotor palsies may also occur.

The lesions are usually severe on the branches of the external carotid artery, with inflamed, tender, pulseless scalp arteries. They are also responsible for headache and for pain in the jaw when eating or in the occipital region when lying down in bed. Muscle pains are common. There are often general symptoms such as fatigue, loss of appetite, weight loss, fever, sweating, and anemia. The ESR is over 50 mm/h in the majority of cases, although cases exist with a normal or slightly elevated ESR. Pain in the girdle muscles with a high ESR can be the foremost presenting disorder, known as polymyalgia rheumatica, a clinical variant of cranial arteritis. Biopsy of the temporal artery is the key examination, being positive in over 80 percent of the patients. The focal nature of the arteritic lesion accounts for the false-negative cases.

When the diagnosis is strongly suspected, corticosteroids must be started prior to biopsy, for they can prevent acute ischemic optic neuropathy. To ensure the best chances of positive results, biopsy should not be delayed, although in many cases lesions are still present during several weeks. High doses of corticosteroids (1 mg/kg every 24 hours) are recommended to begin. Typically, the patient feels well within 24 hours. For many clinicians, the diagnosis is strongly suggested by the speedy and dramatic improvement in constitutional symptoms. Headache and muscle pains must be controlled and the ESR kept below 30 mm/h. The patient must be weaned from corticosteroids very gradually, and where possible, they should be stopped altogether after approximately 2 years of treatment.

Intracranial giant cell arteritis (also called intracranial granulomatous arteritis, isolated angiitis, or angiopathy of the CNS) is a rare disease and a difficult diagnosis. Small vessels, both arteries and veins, of a diameter less than 200 μm are those mainly affected in the brain and spinal cord. The leptomeningeal vessels are generally severely involved, which is important when a brain biopsy is considered, but the disease may not be evident on the angiogram since the smaller vessels bear the brunt of the disorder. The pathologic changes include vessel infiltration with lymphocytes, polymorphonuclear leukocytes, monocytes, and multinucleated giant cells with granuloma formation. There may be fibrinoid necrosis of the vessel wall and even aneurysm formation. Ischemic or hemorrhagic nervous lesions involve the brain, brainstem, cerebellum, and spinal cord. In some cases clinically silent lesions have been found in thoracic and abdominal viscera. Direct attack on vessels by viruses, notably herpes zoster virus, and immune-mediated lesions have been reported. At present, there is no known etiology.

The disease affects both sexes at all ages, with a peak incidence in the 40 to 60-year range. Confusional states, drowsiness, stupor, seizures, focal deficits (e.g., hemiplegia, aphasia, hemianopia), elevated intracranial pressure with papilledema, and myelopathy are possible. The CSF usually shows increased protein content, which can be over 1,000 mg/dl, and a lymphocytic pleocytosis occurs, although rarely over 400/mm³. There can be a significant amount of red blood cells. Despite the frequent CSF findings, the examination can be normal. In principle, there are no systemic disorders that help to suggest the diagnosis.

Sarcoidosis is a systemic disease characterized pathologically by noncaseating (non-necrotizing) granulomas. The cause is unknown. Although infrequent, CNS disorders can be the presenting clinical features. Most are due to basal granulomatous meningitis with infiltration of the underlying nervous tissue and elevated intracranial pressure. A few cases of vasculitis involving arteries and veins have been reported, which resulted in headaches, seizures, confusion, or focal deficits due to infarction or hemorrhage. The spinal cord can be involved. In focal cerebral accidents, embolism from a sarcoid cardiomyopathy should be considered. The diagnosis rests on evidence of lesions in lungs, lymph nodes, liver, spleen, skin, eyes, phalangeal bones, heart, and muscles. Laboratory tests (e.g., the Kweim-Siltzbach reaction, anergy to tuberculin, increased CSF content of angiotensin-converting enzyme) are of poor sensitivity and specificity. Biopsy of a palpable lymph node or of the liver or muscle may show granulomas.

Wegener's granulomatosis involves small arteries and veins and causes necrotizing lesions of the respiratory tract, including the nose and paranasal sinuses. Glomerulonephritis is associated, but hypertension is rare. Myocardial infarction can occur. The ESR is elevated, with anemia and frequent thrombocytopenia. Granulomas can invade the CNS from contiguous lesions, or rarely, there can be a CNS vasculitis. Focal deficits due to infarction are rare, as are confusional states. Ophthalmologic disorders also result either from invasion of the orbit or from vasculitis that can involve the retina, optic nerve, uvea, cornea, or conjunctiva. Associated mononeuritis multiplex is frequent. The prognosis of the formerly rapidly fatal disease has been transformed by continued therapy with corticosteroids and cyclophosphamide.

Lymphomatoid granulomatosis is characterized by necrotizing granulomas that involve primarily the lungs. Some can progress to lymphomas. Skin lesions are frequent. A minority of patients have clinical CNS vasculitic involvement, with confusion, seizures, or hemiplegia. Mononeuritis multiplex and cranial neuropathies are also possible. The CSF shows an inflammatory reaction, frequently with abnormal cells. Prednisone, cyclophosphamide, and sometimes radiotherapy are the mainstays of therapy.

Behçet's syndrome is the eponym honoring the Turkish dermatologist who reported the first cases (see Ch. 66). The basic features are recurrent oral and genital aphthous ulcerations and hypopion iritis (i.e., pus in the anterior chamber of the eye) and in many instances a panophthalmitis. There are also skin disorders, ulcerations of the gut, synovitis, phlebitis of large and small veins, and aneurysms in the systemic and pulmonary circulation. Meningismus is the principal neurologic presentation. The cause is unknown. The pathergy test, a test of skin hypersensitivity, is positive in some patients during exacerbations: after 24 to 48 hours a sterile pustule develops at the site of a needle prick.

In Behçet's syndrome vasculitis is prominent and can involve large arteries (aortic arch, see above) and veins. Cerebral infarction (in about 25 percent of cases) and intracranial hypertension are frequent. Blindness usually results from occlusion of retinal vessels, but the optic nerve can be involved.

The disorder is most common in the eastern Mediterranean area, mostly in young men, and is associated with the HLA-B5 and HLA-B51 antigens. However, it is a worldwide disorder, well known in Turks living abroad. In Western countries most patients are women, and there is no association with HLA.

Therapy is based on corticoids for the acute exacerbations. Cyclosporine is the main therapy, with colchicine, chlorambucil and azathioprine among alternatives.

VASCULITIS ASSOCIATED WITH MALIGNANCIES

Cases of CNS granulomatous angiitis have been reported with Hodgkin's lymphoma, non-Hodgkin's lymphoma, lymphosarcoma, chronic myelogenous leukemia, and hairy cell leukemia. However, case reports of "vasculitis" associated with neoplastic angioendotheliosis and malignant histiocytosis do not, in the views of the authors, represent true vasculitides. In these cases the vessels are plugged with tumor cells, while any evidence of inflammation is most probably secondary to the endovascular malignant process.

VASCULITIS ASSOCIATED WITH DRUGS

Brain infarction or hemorrhage is frequent in drug abuse involving heroin, pentazocine (pyribenzamine in T's and Blues [common "street" names]), ephedrine, cocaine, free-base (crack) cocaine, amphetamine, metamphetamine (speed), methylphenidate, lysergic acid diethylamide (LSD), and phencyclidine (angel dust) (see Ch. 68). Drugs for use with oral diets or as decongestants, such as phenylpropanolamine, can result in similar accidents. The angiogram can be normal, probably depending on the timing of the examination. The usual appearance is that of multiple successive stenoses ("beading," "sausage-like," "moniliform") affecting the cerebral arteries (Fig. 38-1). This is generally taken as evidence of vasculitis. In cases in which postmortem examination or cerebral biopsy was performed inflammatory arterial lesions were found, involving all visceral arteries when a complete study was done. Their appearance has been likened to that of polyarteritis nodosa lesions.

The mechanisms of the arterial lesions are unknown. A direct toxic effect of the drug or an immune-mediated process has been suggested. However, the authors think that such lesions are also indistinguishable from those of experimental and human acute hypertension, in other words, of the lesions of acute hypertensive encephalopathy, in which necrosis of the vessel wall, due to prolonged vasospasm, induces a secondary inflammatory process. This hypertension could account for most of the reported cases, as most drugs have a known hypertensive effect, hypertension has been recorded in most patients, and clinical disorders included severe headache, nausea or vomiting, and seizures, as in cases of hypertensive encephalopathy. Moreover, second angiograms were usually normal (Fig. 38-1). Such a transient vasculopathy, termed *acute benign cerebral angiopathy* in mild cases, hardly corresponds to an immune-mediated vasculitis, and it could be that immune disorders, so common in drug abusers, have been a chance finding in those with so-called cerebral vasculitis.

As a caveat in the diagnosis of cerebral vasculopathies in drug abuse, many possible causes commonly exist for cerebral infarction or hemorrhage, including infectious endocarditis with emboli and aneurysms, opportunistic infections, bacterial and fungal meningitides, disorders of clotting, and chronic or subacute hy-

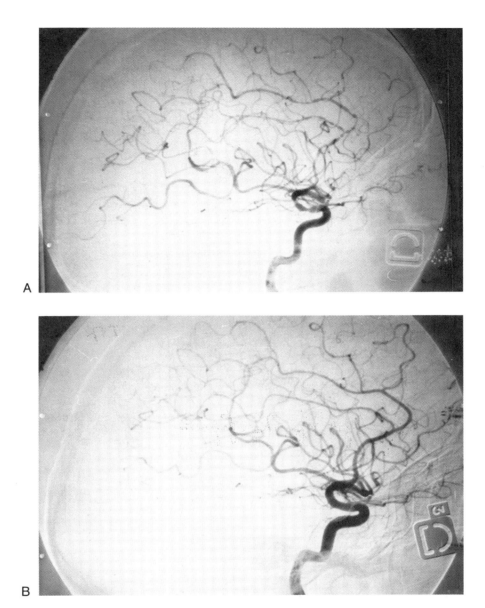

Figure 38-1. (A & B) A 36-year-old man suffered "bursting" headache with vomiting during intercourse prior to which he took cocaine. Twelve days after last intercourse, right (Fig. A) and left (Fig. B) carotid angiograms showed multiple beadings of carotid siphons, anterior and middle cerebral artery branches. Nine weeks later, carotid angiograms were normal.

pertension due to kidney disease. Hypotension, in cases of overdose, can cause border zone infarction. Finally, a given patient often takes several different drugs, and adulterants, contaminants, and foreign materials are frequently ingested or injected with the drug(s).

MISCELLANEOUS

Cogan's syndrome is defined by a nonsyphilitic interstitial keratitis associated with sensorineural deafness, often tinnitus, vertigo, and nystagmus. Headache, seizures, and focal deficits have been reported. The rare

pathologic data have shown a necrotizing arteritis close or similar to that of PAN. Eales' disease is characterized by recurrent retinal and vitreous hemorrhages related to retinal phlebitis or periphlebitis. Most patients are men. A few cases with CNS involvement have been reported, with a difficult differential diagnosis from multiple sclerosis. A postmortem case showed a vasculitis involving CNS small veins. CNS irradiation can cause delayed disorders due to vascular damage (see Ch. 58). An immune-mediated vasculitis has been hypothesized.

Cerebral thromboangitis obliterans (so-called von Winiwarter-Buerger's disease) was once a popular diagnosis, but the number of reported cases fell dramatically following the critical review of C. M. Fisher in 1957, and the authors do not know of a later demonstrating case. The white-gray solid leptomeningeal arteries that course over areas of border zone infarction are now generally believed to be thrombosed arteries, resulting from blood stagnation with possibly a prominent role of platelet stasis.

In the idiopathic hypereosinophilic syndrome, CNS disturbances, including behavioral changes, confusion, pyramidal disorders, and seizures, are possible. Peripheral neuropathy is more frequent. Some of these patients have evidence of vasculitis, but a eosinophil-derived neurotoxin may also play a role. Moreover, emboli from thrombi superimposed on endocardial fibrosis can cause transient ischemic attacks and strokes.

DIAGNOSING VASCULITIS ON ANGIOGRAMS

Pathologic-radiologic correlations strongly support the view that "beading," "sausage-shaped," and "moniliform" arteries on angiograms can correspond to focal or segmental lesions of arteritis (Fig. 38-2). However, from case reports based only on clinical information and angiographic images, it is obvious that these radiologic abnormalities have come to signify arteritis or vasculitis. As exemplified above, with the arterial changes due to drugs and sympathomimetic drugs,

Table 38-2. Possible Mechanisms of Arterial Beading

Conditions With Beading Arteries	Proposed Mechanism
Arteritis	
Hypertensive encephalopathy	Vasospasm
Subarachnoid hemorrhage	Vasospasm
Drugs	Possible vasospasm
Symphathomimetic agents	Possible vasospasm
Postpartum, eclampsia	Possible vasospasm
Migraine	Possible vasospasm
Pheochromocytoma	Hypertensive encephalothy
Acute benign cerebral angiopathy	Possible vasospasm
Chronic meningitides	Endarteritis obliterans
Multiple recanalizing emboli	
Radiation	

the authors believe that such a generalization is not warranted. Table 38-2 indicates conditions in which beading has been observed. It shows that several mechanism can play a role, although vasospasm in response to acute arterial hypertension appears to be the common denominator of most of these conditions.

ANNOTATED BIBLIOGRAPHY

Berlit P. Clinical and laboratory findings with giant cell arteritis. J Neurol Sci 1992;111:1–12.

An incidence of 3.4 per 100,000 per year for polymyalgia rheu-

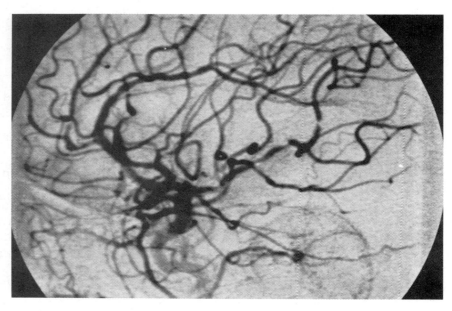

Figure 38-2. Lateral view of a middle cerebral artery angiogram showing multiple stenoses, consistent with arteritis.

matica or temporal arteritis was found for patients in Heidelberg. When the ESR was more than 90 mm/h, exacerbations of the illness (24) and complications were more frequent.

Biller J, Adams HP Jr. Non infectious granulomatous angiitis of the central nervous system. In Toole JF (ed.), Handbook of Clinical Neurology. Vol. 2, Part 3. Elsevier, Amsterdam, 1989.

A review with references.

Blackwood W. Pathological aspects of cerebral and spinal vascular disease. In Ross Russell RW (ed). Vascular Disease of the Central Nervous System. Churchill Livingstone, Edinburgh, 1983.

A clear and authoritative review.

Brown MM, Swash M. Polyarteritis nodosa and other systemic vasculitides. In Toole JF (ed). Handbook of Clinical Neurology, Vol 2, Part 3. Elsevier, Amsterdam, 1989.

A review with references.

Brust JCM. Stroke and drugs. In Toole JF (ed). Handbook of Clinical Neurology. Vol 2, Part III. Elsevier, Amsterdam, 1989.

A thorough, critical review, with references.

Fledelius HC, Nissen KR. Giant cell arteritis and visual loss. A 3-year retrospective hospital investigation in a Danish county. Acta Ophthalmol (Copenh) 1992;70:801–5.

Almost 20 percent of patients had significant visual loss in biopsy-proven giant cell arteritis.

Gautier JC. L'angiopathie cérébrale moniliforme des toxicomanes. Signification pathologique. Role possible du spasme. Bull Acad Natl Med (Paris) 1988;172:87–93.

Arterial lesions and mechanisms are probably similar to those in hypertensive encephalopathy.

Groothuis DR, Mikhael MA. Focal cerebral vasculitis associated with circulating immune complexes and brain irradiation. Ann Neurol 1986;19:590–2.

An irradiated patient with subacute bacterial endocarditis and circulating immune complexes.

Hankey GH. Isolated angiitis/angiopathy of the central nervous system. Cerebrovasc Dis 1991;1:2–15.

A review, with references.

Hatz HJ, Helmke K. Polymyalgia rheumatica und Riesenzellarteriitis; Diagnostik und Nebenwirkungsprofil bei niedrig dosierter Glukokortikoidlangzeittherapie. Z Rheumatol 1992;51:213–21.

Low-dose glucocorticoid therapy (< 10 mg of prednisolone) showed that osteoporosis was the main side effect.

Joy JL, Carlo J, Velez-Borras R. Cerebral infarction following herpes zoster: the enlarging clinical spectrum. Neurology 1989;39:1640.

A new case and references.

Koepper AH, Lansing LS, Peng S, Smith RS. Central nervous system vasculitis in cytomegalovirus infection. J Neurol Sci 1981;51:395–410.

A case and a review of cerebral herpes virus infection.

Laplane R, Fontaine JL, Escourolle R et al. Les manifestations neurologiques du purpura rhumatoide. A propos d'une observation anatomo-clinique. Ann Pediatr (Paris) 1973;20:525–8.

A case with cerebral vasculitis.

Levine SR, Deegan MJ, Futrell N, Welch KMA. Cerebrovascular and neurologic disease associated with antiphospholipid antibodies: 48 cases. Neurology 1991;40:1181–9.

A recent critical review of a still unclear field.

Lie JT. Primary (granulomatous) angiitis of the central nervous system: a clinicopathologic analysis of 15 new cases and a review of the literature. Hum Pathol 1992;23:164–71.

Clinical and pathologic features of 15 new cases are described.

Mas JL, Louarn F, Degos JD. Angéites non spécifiques du système nerveux central. Rev Neurol (Paris) 1983;139:467–84.

A review with references.

Moore PM, Harley JB, Fauci AS. Neurologic dysfunction in the idiopathic hypereosinophilic syndrome. Ann Intern Med 1985;102:109–14.

Vasculitis is possible, as is embolism too.

O'Duffy JD. Behçets syndrome. N Engl J Med 1990;322:326–7.

Succinct editorial.

Roman GC. Cerebral malaria: the unsolved riddle. J Neurol Sci 1991;101:1–6.

A critical review of the pathology of cerebral malaria and vessel lesions.

Yankner BA, Skolnik PR, Shoukimas GM et al. Cerebral angiitis associated with isolation of human T-lymphotropic virus type III from the central nervous system. Ann Neurol 1986;20:362–4.

Isolated cerebral granulomatous arteritis involving large, medium, and leptomeningeal arteries.

39
Bacterial Infections

John J. Halperin

Bacterial infections of the nervous system can cause a broad range of clinical syndromes, varying with the offending organism, the state of the host's defenses, and the route of bacterial introduction. At one end of the spectrum, cerebral abscesses can present as insidiously developing mass lesions in an afebrile patient; at the other, meningococcal meningitis can lead to septic shock and death within hours. Slowly reproducing and relatively less immunogenic organisms such as spirochetes can present such a diverse panoply of syndromes that they will be considered separately.

Clinical presentation will depend on the nature and location of the disease process. Brain abscesses present as mass lesions, often with seizures. Specific neurologic symptoms depend on abscess location. Epidural or subdural empyemas present as extradural masses, again with focal signs dependent on location. Bacterial dissemination within the subarachnoid space typically presents a more fulminant picture, with a very ill-appearing patient.

Unlike most viral infections of the nervous system, these syndromes are usually not self-limited, and so rapid diagnosis and therapeutic intervention is essential. It is unusual for meningitis and brain abscess to occur in the same patient as part of the same illness; only *Citrobacter diversus*, a cause of neonatal meningitis, will commonly result in postmeningitic abscesses. On the other hand, if a patient with a brain abscess appears to develop meningitis, this often reflects rupture of the abscess into the subarachnoid space.

MENINGITIS

Although under appropriate circumstances many different bacteria can invade the subarachnoid space, in the vast majority (80 percent) of cases bacterial meningitis is due to one of three organisms; *Haemophilus influenzae* (the cause of the majority of bacterial menin-

gitis cases, *Neisseria meningitidis* (less often the cause), or *Streptococcus pneumoniae* (least often the cause). Among the low-frequency causes are *Listeria monocytogenes*, *Escherichia coli*, and others too numerous and too infrequent to warrant mention. The cause varies with age (Fig. 39-1).

Epidemiology

Like all other nervous system infections, even these infections are relatively uncommon owing to the considerable difficulty that organisms have in invading the central nervous system (CNS).

Pathophysiology

As reviewed in detail by Martin et al. (1993), the three principal organisms cited above all invade through mucosal colonization. Each of these organisms has the ability to block mucosal immunoglobulin A and attack and neutralize mucosal defenses. *H. influenzae* and *N. meningitidis* can both colonize the nasal mucosa. As many as 20 to 40 percent of young adults may be asymptomatic nasopharyngeal carriers of meningococci, a state that, while noninvasive, does induce protective immunity.

Precisely what factors allow these organisms to become invasive in some circumstances but not others remain unclear. As many as 40 percent of patients with meningitis have had an antecedent upper respiratory infection, perhaps disrupting normal mechanical barriers, and thus permitting invasion. After colonizing the mucosa, invasive organisms disseminate hematogenously, this time avoiding intravascular defenses—blood cultures are positive in up to 80 to 90 percent of patients with *H. influenzae*, *N. meningitidis*, or *S. pneumoniae* meningitis. The organisms most commonly successful at this dissemination, namely these three and group B streptococci, all have thick polysaccharide capsules, which presumably protect them

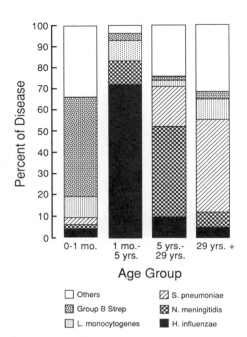

Figure 39-1. Causes of bacterial meningitis by age group. Strep, streptococci. (From Wenger et al. and the Bacterial Meningitis Study Group, 1990, with permission.)

against host defense mechanisms. Such organisms are particularly invasive in asplenic individuals, since the spleen normally plays a major role in eliminating encapsulated organisms from the bloodstream. The means by which the blood-brain barrier is ultimately crossed remains unclear, although a sustained bacteremia and adhesion to components of the blood-brain barrier appear to be necessary.

Once within the cerebrospinal fluid (CSF), the organisms can spread freely within the subarachnoid space along the length of the neuraxis, since resident immune defenses within the CNS are quite limited. As infection and the immune response to it evolve, a purulent exudate forms in the subarachnoid space, often particularly prominent at the base of the brain, where cranial nerves can be damaged in up to one-fifth of cases (particularly the third, sixth, and eighth cranial nerves). As many as 10 percent of children with bacterial meningitis will develop hearing impairment, particularly when meningitis is due to *S. pneumoniae*.

Initially the meningitis is accompanied by elevated intracranial pressure, presumably due to a combination of vasogenic edema related to cytokine production, obstruction to normal CSF pathways in the subarachnoid space or aqueduct of Sylvius, and obstruction of CSF resorption in the arachnoid villi. Unlike viral meningitis, bacterial meningitis usually leads to inflammation beyond the subarachnoid space. Left untreated, these infections usually rapidly evolve

to a meningoencephalitis. Cortical blood vessels (arteries and veins) passing through or adjacent to the inflamed subarachnoid space frequently become involved, which results in a vasculitis. This causes areas of cortical infarction (giving rise to cytotoxic edema), which in turn provides a more hospitable medium for bacteria to track into brain parenchyma.

Diagnosis by Bacterial Cause

With such a fulminant picture, rapid diagnosis is obviously essential. To some extent, the most likely organism in a given patient can be predicted by the clinical circumstances. *H. influenzae* is the most common cause of meningitis overall, but it affects children under age 5 predominantly (85 percent of invasive *H. influenzae* disease occurs in this age group). *H. influenzae* disease is also more common in asplenic individuals (either functionally asplenic, such as those with sickle cell disease, or anatomically asplenic). In children in the first few months of life, group B streptococcus is now the most common cause of meningitis, having replaced gram-negative organisms, the commonest cause until the past decade. In adults, *H. influenzae* generally only causes meningitis in the context of head trauma, in the presence of a contiguous ear, nose, or throat infection, or in the immunocompromised.

In young adults living in close quarters (military recruits, residential school or college students), epidemic meningococcal disease is the most likely cause of bacterial meningitis. *N. meningitidis* is also the second most common cause of bacterial meningitis in younger children. Fortunately, vaccination of at-risk groups against meningococcus and of children against *H. influenzae* B ("Hib") is making these two disorders less frequent.

In older adults, *S. pneumoniae* is the most common cause of meningitis, being responsible for up to 50 percent of adult cases. This can occur either as a primary infection or as a metastatic process, with primary infection in the lungs, ear, mastoid, or sinus, and a search for concomitant infection in these sites is important.

Finally, antecedent head trauma, including iatrogenic trauma such as neurosurgery, provides important bypass routes by which organisms can avoid the blood-brain barrier and cause infection. *Staphylococcus aureus* is a particularly common offender in trauma- and surgery-related bacterial meningitis and also occurs in the setting of endocarditis or other sources of bacteremia.

Gram-negative organisms can similarly cause meningitis in the setting of trauma, neurosurgery, or bacteremia, circumstances that can also lead to infection with obligate anaerobes, particularly if the bacteremia arises from an abdominal source or if otitis is present.

Quite distinct from meningitis due to the above organisms but worthy of mention because of its increasing incidence is meningitis due to *L. monocytogenes*. This disorder more typically occurs in newborns, in the elderly, or in patients with impaired cell-mediated immunity. Infection usually occurs by contact with dairy products, particularly in summer months. Meningitis can be typical of other bacterial meningitides but may be considerably more indolent. On occasion encephalitis may occur, particularly involving the brainstem, often with minimal evidence of meningeal involvement.

Clinical Features

The general clinical features of a patient with bacterial meningitis are of little help in differentiating among different organisms. Most patients complain of headache, malaise, and fever, and vomiting is common. The clinical search for meningism is essential. Stiffness of the neck is the chief sign. It is sought on passive flexion of the neck after the examiner's hand, placed under the occiput, has ascertained that the patient has relaxed as much as possible. The head is then slowly flexed; in young people the chin should reach the sternum. Stiffness only on rotational and lateral movements is not suggestive of meningeal origin. Painful inability of straight-leg raising (Kernig's sign) and flexion of the hip and knee on flexion of the head (Brudzinski's signs) are accessory signs. Neck stiffness is very common but not invariable, particularly in the very young and the elderly. In contrast to patients with viral meningitis, there is usually some degree of mental status change, with somnolence or mild confusion commonplace. On the other hand, photophobia is more common in viral meningitis. Patients are usually febrile and appear ill. The illness typically evolves rapidly.

Early focal CNS signs are most common with *S. pneumoniae*, which is particularly likely to cause arteritis and phlebitis. Recurrent bacterial meningitis is usually indicative of a CSF fistula (see Ch. 6). Polymicrobial infection, particularly including anaerobes, may occur with gastrointestinal neoplasms eroding into the sacral spinal canal.

As the meningitis process continues, neurologic impairment rapidly develops; seizures are frequent, occurring in approximately 40 percent of patients, as a result of cortical involvement. Overall, adult mortality from appropriately treated bacterial meningitis is about 20 percent, ranging from 6 percent with *H. influenzae* to 26 percent with *S. pneumoniae*.

Other clinical clues can provide presumptive support for a specific diagnosis. A disseminated petechial or purpuric rash should bring meningococcus to mind immediately, since it is present in about 50 percent of patients with meningococcal meningitis. Occasionally the closely related *Neisseria* organism, the gonococcus, can cause a strikingly similar picture.

Diagnosis

In addition to the diagnostic assistance provided by what is known about the epidemiology of these disorders and the associated signs and symptoms, the basic diagnostic procedure remains CSF examination (see Ch. 9). When there are concerns about raised intracranial pressure, an imaging study may be appropriate before performing a lumbar puncture. In the absence of a cerebral mass lesion or obstructive hydrocephalus, the risk of a lumbar puncture is relatively small and is significantly exceeded by the risk of failure to identify the causative organism. However, prudence would dictate that if the opening pressure is markedly elevated, only the minimum amount of fluid necessary be removed and treatment of intracranial hypertension then be instituted with mannitol.

Once fluid is obtained, it should be both Gram-stained and cultured. The commonest organisms can now be identified by antigen assays. Counterimmunoelectrophoresis, the technique originally introduced for this purpose, although still in use was always controversial because of the occurrence of significant numbers of both false-positives and false-negatives. More recently introduced assays appear to have significantly improved specificity and sensitivity, although none can be considered absolutely definitive. The CSF usually demonstrates a significant polymorphonuclear pleocytosis (up to tens of thousand per cubic millimeter, although with *Listeria* the count may be much more modest). Protein is usually significantly increased while glucose is generally depressed, although comparison with serum glucose is essential.

Blood cultures are also mandatory, since invasion of the neuraxis usually occurs in the setting of sustained bacteremia. Aspiration of skin lesions for Gram staining can be informative. Nasopharyngeal culture results can be confusing because of the high incidence of asymptomatic carriers of many of the responsible organisms.

Treatment

Therapy must be instituted as rapidly as possible, whenever bacterial meningitis is suspected. Although the blood-brain barrier impairs CNS penetration by many antimicrobials, in the presence of meningeal inflammation CNS penetration is somewhat improved. Even under these circumstances penicillin's entry into the CNS is quite limited, but several of the third-generation cephalosporins (ceftriaxone and cefotaxime but not cefuroxime) penetrate quite well and are effective against *H. influenzae*, *S. pneumoniae*, *N. meningitidis*, and Enterobacteriaceae. Unfortunately, these agents do not control *Listeria,* and if this is a real possibility, penicillin or ampicillin becomes necessary. With appropriate antimicrobials patients generally improve within a few days. Failure to do so should raise the possibility of an abscess, another source of infection, or a resistant organism.

The role of corticosteroids remains controversial. However, there is evidence in childhood meningitis that these are helpful in decreasing risk of complications, specifically damage to the eighth cranial nerve. Whether use of these agents is truly justified in circumstances other than efforts to control severely elevated intracranial pressure remains to be established. In emergency situations hyperventilation can be used to lower intracranial pressure. However, this technique also lowers cerebral perfusion and there are increasing data to suggest that this may be counterproductive, particularly when some degree of cerebral ischemia already exists.

BRAIN ABSCESS

Like other forms of CNS infection, brain abscesses are quite uncommon. The normal brain is an inhospitable environment for bacterial growth. Abscesses become established most easily when the brain is already damaged (e.g., by trauma or infarction).

Bacteriology

In the immunologically intact host, whether infection causes meningitis or an abscess seems to depend primarily on the specific infecting organism. While *N. meningitidis, H. influenzae,* and *S. pneumoniae* generally cause meningitis, most other streptococci, staphylococci, and gram-negative bacteria cause abscesses, even if their access to the CNS appears to be by the same route as the initial group of organisms. Only two bacteria, *Citrobacter diversus* in neonates or *L. monocytogenes* in any age group, commonly cause both meningitis and abscesses. Neonatal *Citrobacter* meningitis may result in abscess in up to 60 percent of cases. A smaller proportion of cases of *Listeria* infection can result in a cerebritis or actual abscess. When any of the other organisms commonly associated with abscesses are isolated from patients with meningitis, it can generally be inferred that an abscess has leaked into the CSF.

Most abscesses, particularly those occurring by contiguous spread, are polymicrobial. Approximately one-third of all isolated organisms are anaerobic, the remainder being aerobic or microaerobic. Streptococci are isolated from up to 70 percent of abscesses, *Bacteroides* spp. from up to 40 percent, and *Enterobacter* or *Pseudomonas* from up to 30 to 40 percent. The particu-

lar organism can provide a clue to the likely etiology of the abscess. *Staphylococcus* generally occurs in trauma or in hematogenous spread (e.g., endocarditis). *Fusobacterium* is often associated with dental disease. *E. coli* and *Proteus,* the commonest organisms responsible for gram-negative sepsis, typically follow bacteremic spread. *Pseudomonas* or *Proteus* are common with chronic otitis.

Pathophysiology

In those instances in which abscesses are able to form, it may well be that the nidus of infection becomes established after the local vasculature, either venous or arterial, is damaged, whether by a bacterial embolism or by local septic phlebitis and thrombosis. Infection reaches the CNS in much the same fashion as it does in meningitis—by local contiguous spread from chronic infection in the paranasal sinuses or the ear or hematogenous spread from the heart, lungs, or occasionally other sources. Hematogenous spread is particularly likely to occur when the normal filtration provided by the lungs is bypassed, as may occur in patients with right-to-left shunts, either in the heart itself or in the lung. As many as 1 percent of patients with the multiple-organ arteriovenous fistulas that characterize the Osler-Weber-Rendu syndrome suffer brain abscesses. Another example is provided by those in whom the primary infection occurs in the lung (e.g., pulmonary *Nocardia,* pulmonary abscess, or empyema).

Brain abscesses are more common in men than women. Most occur in young adults, and 25 percent occur in children. The age prevalence essentially parallels that of sinus and ear infections. About half of all brain abscesses arise from contiguous sources of primary infection, one-fourth are from hematogenous spread, and about 10 percent are from dental sources. In the remainder no source can be identified. Since abscesses associated with sinus or ear disease generally occur immediately adjacent to the site of extracranial infection, it must be assumed that bacterial spread occurs by direct extension. However, the mechanism by which bacteria cross the dura and invade the brain under these circumstances remains to be elucidated.

As might be expected from a localized lesion such as an abscess, much can be inferred about their pathogenesis from their location. Frontal abscesses typically occur in association with chronic frontal sinusitis or less commonly, with dental abscesses, particularly periapical abscesses of the molars. Typically, these infections are polymicrobial, including *Streptococcus* spp. (aerobic, anaerobic, and microaerobic), *Bacteroides, Fusobacterium,* and other gram-negative organisms. Temporal lobe abscesses are typically associated with chronic ear infections, as are cerebellar abscesses. In children, chronic otitis most commonly results in cerebellar abscesses; in adults the same source more often produces temporal lobe infection. Like abscesses associated with sinus infections, these are typically polymicrobial, sometimes including anaerobes but more typically aerobic organisms. Typical organisms in these abscesses are *Streptococcus, Bacteroides fragilis, E. coli, Proteus, Klebsiella, Pseudomonas* and *Enterobacter*. In trauma, surgical or other, the site of infection is obviously associated with the site of local disruption of brain, and *Staphylococcus* is particularly common. Brain abscess following surgery is actually extremely infrequent; infection of the incision itself, bone flap osteomyelitis, subdural empyema, and meningitis all occur more frequently.

In contrast, patients with hematogenously disseminated infection often have multiple smaller abscesses, except when the infection is due to *Staphylococcus*, which can rapidly form fairly large lesions with only a single organism responsible. As with other metastatic processes, the septic microemboli tend to lodge in watershed zones (i.e., at the gray-white junction and in the border zone between the distribution of the middle cerebral artery and the anterior and posterior cerebral arteries), which makes these the most common sites of these abscesses. Since the middle cerebral artery supplies all supratentorial watershed zones and since the supratentorial brain is so much larger than the infratentorial brain, most hematogenously originated abscesses are within the confines of the middle cerebral artery territory.

Clinical Features

The clinical picture of brain abscesses can be quite insidious. They typically present as a mass lesion, with headache in most patients, focal signs in the majority, lethargy in about half, seizures in about one-fourth, and fever in the minority. In general, if a patient presents with headache with or without focal signs and with evidence of extracerebral infection with an organism capable of causing brain abscesses, the index of suspicion should be quite high. The clinical course is typically subacute. Clinical and laboratory studies indicate a fairly typical sequence of events, which varies primarily in its time course but on average evolves over about 2 weeks. Following initial bacterial seeding, patients develop early cerebritis. Pathologic study demonstrates a central region of necrosis surrounded by an inflammatory response, with perivascular inflammatory infiltrates and vasogenic edema. This is followed by a stage of late cerebritis, in which the central necrotic zone becomes surrounded by a zone of fibroblast proliferation, with neovascularization. Early abscess formation is considered to occur when this surrounding zone consolidates into a distinct capsule. Finally, when this zone is fully condensed, a late abscess is considered to be present. Generally the capsule is thicker on the side of the abscess closer to the cortex—the reason for this is unknown.

Diagnosis

Modern imaging techniques (magnetic resonance imaging, [MRI] and computed tomography [CT] scanning) have greatly facilitated diagnosis, but the radiologic appearances of cerebritis and abscess often cannot be definitely differentiated from those of malignancies or some vascular events. Scans of cerebritis generally demonstrate a homogeneous area of contrast enhancement. Abscesses generally demonstrate thick enhancing capsules surrounding central necrotic cores.

Lumbar punctures in these disorders are high-risk and low-yield. Gram stains and cultures are negative in the vast majority of cases, since the infection is generally not in continuity with the subarachnoid space. Cell count is typically in the tens to hundreds, predominantly lymphocytes, with mild to moderate elevation of protein and usually normal glucose. A polymorphonuclear-predominant pleocytosis, particularly with a positive Gram stain, is typically present only if the abscess ruptures into the ventricles or subarachnoid space, a phenomenon that typically has disastrous consequences. On the other hand, as many as one-third of patients with brain abscess deteriorate significantly as a consequence of lumbar punctures.

Blood cultures are positive in about 10 percent of patients, presumably those in whom the abscess was due to hematogenous spread. Other laboratory assessment is rarely helpful. Early on, imaging studies demonstrate an area of cerebritis. Infections are most easily treated at this point, although diagnosis may be more elusive. Because of the neovascularity that occurs as part of the early response to infection, biopsy is associated with a significant risk of hemorrhage.

Treatment

Once an abscess cavity has formed, surgery is generally considered an essential component of management. Although medical management of abscesses may be possible, the presence of a large, infected, necrotic mass into which antibiotics must diffuse from the periphery makes such treatment quite problematic, and fairly prolonged courses of antibiotics are necessary. In contrast, with surgical drainage (stereotactically if necessary) or excision, 4 to 6 weeks of parenteral antibiotics is generally sufficient to sterilize the abscess. At this point it remains controversial whether abscesses should be just drained or actually removed; both techniques provide equivalent diagnostic information in terms of culture and histology, and studies indicate that the improvement in mortality is comparable with both techniques. However post-treatment sequelae, particularly seizures, which occur as a later sequela of abscesses in as many as 90 percent of patients, may be more common if the capsule is left in place. Further study of this issue is needed.

The use of steroids in brain abscess is also an area of some controversy. Although it is certainly clear that steroids are needed if a patient is in imminent danger of herniation because of cerebral edema, these agents do entail more than the usual complications in this patient population. In addition to impairing host immune defenses, steroids may impair blood-brain barrier penetration by antibiotics, particularly those, such as penicillin, that do not normally cross the blood-brain barrier easily. Steroids may also impede the walling off of the abscess, thereby impairing the patient's ability to contain the infection. The effects on vascular and blood-brain barrier permeability and on abscess wall formation also change the radiologic ring enhancement pattern that is diagnostic of abscesses and thereby may confuse diagnosis. Since seizures occur early on in up to half of patients with abscesses and later on in even a larger proportion, it is reasonable to treat these patients prophylactically with anticonvulsants.

Antimicrobial therapy is tailored to the specific organism. Even before cultures from a biopsy return, it is generally possible to pick appropriate agents based on the clinical circumstances. Penicillin in meningeal doses (20 million units/day IV) is generally included in all regimens. With a contiguous source, anaerobic coverage is generally essential. This is best provided with metronidazole (15 mg/kg loading dose, followed by 7.5 mg/kg every 6 hours), which penetrates the blood-brain barrier and abscess cavities easily and is extremely effective against the anaerobes likely to be present. When a gram-negative bacillus is likely, particularly with ear infections, a third-generation cephalosporin such as cefotaxime (2 g every 4 hours) or ceftizoxime is generally given in addition to metronidazole, either in addition to penicillin or with it. Aminoglycosides work poorly at the acid pH typical of the depths of an abscess. When the abscess is due to trauma or surgery, antistaphylococcal agents are essential; typically this is nafcillin (given as 1.0 to 1.5 g IV every 4 hours).

Treatment response is often followed with serial CT scans. Typically, by 4 weeks the cerebritis or abscess cavity will have diminished dramatically. If not, treatment may be extended another 2 weeks. Although it is commonplace to follow parenteral treatment with several months of oral therapy, few studies have been reported indicating that this improves outcome.

EXTRAPARENCHYMAL INFECTIONS

In addition to their occurrence within the brain parenchyma, abscesses can form in the potential space between the dura and the surrounding bone (epidural abscess) and between the dura and the pia-arachnoid (subdural empyema).

Within the skull subdural infections are more common than epidural ones, but in the spinal canal the opposite is true. The onset of an intracranial subdural empyema, like that of a brain abscess, may be insidious or fulminant, although fever is a far more common concomitant in subdural empyema. Patients usually present with headache, systemic symptoms, and focal neurologic signs dependent on the site of the infection. Like brain abscess, these infections are most frequently associated with contiguous disease—in half to three-quarters of patients this develops as a consequence of paranasal sinusitis, while in about one-fifth infection spreads from the ear. In subdural empyemas, unlike brain abscesses, usually a single organism is responsible for the infection, with streptococci causing about half of the cases and staphylococci about 20 percent. Therapy is with surgical drainage and appropriate antimicrobials. Since this requires coverage for both staphylococci and anaerobes, a common regimen is metronidazole and nafcillin or oxacillin. A third-generation cephalosporin such as cefuraxime may be substituted for nafcillin.

Epidural abscesses occur in the intracranial and intraspinal spaces. Intracranially, they are in many ways similar to subdural empyemas except that they are more insidious in their onset, presumably because the intracranial epidural space is more difficult to dissect. Within the spinal canal, however, epidural abscesses are the most common form of suppurative infection. These infections typically arise from hematogenous or contiguous spread. Hematogenous spread may occur in the usual fashion or via Batson's plexus, which is an interconnecting network of valveless venous channels extending through the spinal canal from the pelvis to the cranium, through which bacteria can spread, bypassing the heart and lungs. Direct spread may also occur from a vertebral osteomyelitis or from cutaneous furunculosis.

The intracranial syndrome mimics that of brain abscess. With intraspinal epidural abscesses, patients present with fever and initially minor local back pain, which becomes severe over days and is sometimes associated with radicular pain. When the abscess becomes large enough to compress the spinal cord, the progressive myelopathy may develop quite rapidly, presenting similarly to transverse myelitis and evolving rapidly to a syndrome of complete transection. The most common responsible organism is *Staphylo-*

coccus aureus, but other organisms, including gram-negatives, have been reported as well. Treatment usually requires decompressive surgery, often under emergency conditions, and at least 4 weeks of parenteral antimicrobials, typically nafcillin and a third-generation cephalosporin, targeted at the responsible organisms. If it seems likely that gastrointestinal anaerobes were contributory, metronidazole can be added.

ANNOTATED BIBLIOGRAPHY

Ashwal S, Tomasi L, Schneider S et al. Bacterial meningitis in children: pathophysiology and treatment. Neurology 1992;42:739–48.

Detailed discussion of pediatric meningitis.

Cunha B. The diagnosis and therapy of acute bacterial meningitis. In Schlossberg D (ed). Infections of the Nervous System, Springer-Verlag, New York. 1990, pp. 3–24.

Excellent review of bacterial meningitis.

Hristeva L, Booy R, Bowler I et al. Prospective surveillance of neonatal meningitis. Arch Dis Child 1993;69:14–18.

Good prospective study of neonatal meningitis.

Kaplan K. Brain abscess. Med Clin North Am 1985;69:345–60.

Review of clinical features, diagnosis and treatment.

Klein O, Neu HC. Use of antimicrobial agents to treat central nervous system infection. Neurosurg Clin North Am 1992;3:323–42.

Excellent discussion of therapeutic pharmacology.

Lebel MH et al. Dexamethasone therapy for bacterial meningitis: results of two double-blind, placebo-controlled trials. N Engl J Med 1988;319:964–71.

Martin JB, Tyler KL, Scheld WM. Bacterial meningitis. In Tyler KL, Martin JB (eds). Infectious Diseases of the Central Nervous System. F. A. Davis, Philadelphia. 1993, pp. 176–87.

Excellent overview of bacterial meningitis.

Osenbach RK, Loftus CM. Diagnosis and management of brain abscess. Neurosurg Clin North Am 1992;3:403–20.

Surgical versus nonsurgical considerations.

Roos KL. Management of bacterial meningitis in children and adults. Semin Neurol 1992;12:155–64

Good treatment overview.

Seydoux C, Francioli P. Bacterial brain abscesses: factors influencing mortality and sequelae. Clin Infect Dis 1992;15:394–401.

Review of 39 patients.

Sokolov RT, Meyer RD. Brain abscess and related focal intracranial suppuration. In Schlossberg D (ed). Infections of the Nervous System. Springer-Verlag, New York, 1990, pp. 93–104.

Good review of CNS abscesses.

Tunkel AR, Scheld WM. Pathogenesis and pathophysiology of bacterial meningitis. Clin Microbiol Rev 1993;6:118–36.

Excellent, detailed review of microbiologic pathophysiology.

Tyler KL, Martin JB, Scheld WM. Focal suppurative infections of the central nervous system. In Tyler KL, Martin JB (eds.). Infectious Diseases of the Central Nervous System. FA Davis, Philadelphia, 1993, pp. 157–75.

Good overview of CNS abscesses.

Wenger JD, Hightower AW, Broome CV and the Bacterial Meningitis Study Group. Bacterial meningitis in the United States: report of a multistate surveillance group. J Infect Dis 1990;162:1316–23.

Yang S-Y, Zhao C-S. Review of 140 patients with brain abscess. Surg Neurol 1993;39:290–6.

Review of clinical manifestations and treatment response in large cohort of patients.

40

Fungal Infections

John J. Halperin

Fungal infections of the nervous system occur primarily in the setting of the immunocompromised host. In the pre-AIDS (acquired immunodeficiency syndrome)/pretransplant era, these disorders were quite rare, but they now are becoming all too frequent.

Fungi normally are saprophytes (from the Greek for rotten plants), living on decaying organic material. They may colonize healthy hosts or even cause superficial infections, as occurs in oral thrush or cutaneous yeast infections. However, they only cause major illness when they become invasive. To differentiate superficial colonization from tissue invasion generally requires tissue sampling. Of course, the tissue sampled may be a body fluid not normally colonized by these agents, as when cryptococcal antigen is detected in blood or cerebrospinal fluid (CSF).

BASIC BIOLOGY

Fungi are more complex organisms than bacteria and are considerably more difficult to eradicate. They are typically an order of magnitude larger in size than bacteria and, unlike bacteria, are eukaryotic (i.e., they have a nucleus separated from the cytoplasm by a distinct membrane) rather than prokaryotic. Like bacteria, fungi can exist as unicellular organisms, referred to as *yeast* forms. Typically they are 3 to 5 μm in diameter, spherical, and often encapsulated, or they can form networks (mycelia) of branching tubules 2 to 10 μm in diameter, which are usually subdivided into separate cells by septae. Occasionally yeast and their progeny will adhere to each other in similar-appearing but less adherent structures referred to as *pseudohyphae* (Greek: *hyphe*, web). Like bacteria, they generally reproduce asexually, but their eukaryotic nature gives rise to a more complex reproductive process. While bacteria reproduce by dividing into two essentially equal daughter cells, yeasts bud, producing a large mother cell and a smaller daughter cell, which then matures. Mycelia reproduce by branching and by proliferating at their terminals. As a result of such differences in biology, it has been much more difficult to design therapeutic agents that kill fungi effectively while remaining relatively nontoxic to other eukaryotic cells, including those of the host.

Fungi can invade the nervous system either by hematogenous spread or directly. In general, those fungi that remain in yeast form are less tissue-invasive than are those that form hyphae. Large branching fungi such as *Aspergillus,* and *Nocardia,* the bacteria that can behave like a fungus, most commonly infect the host as inspired aerosols. The branching hyphae lodge in the airways, invade the lung parenchyma and blood vessels, and then, having bypassed the filtration usually provided by the pulmonary vasculature, metastasize directly to other organs, particularly the brain, where they lodge in blood vessels. The obstructed vessels thrombose, and the hyphae extend directly into the surrounding brain parenchyma. This typical sequence of events results in two common corollaries of cerebral infection with *Aspergillus* or similar organisms. First, many such patients have obvious cavitary pulmonary disease. Second, the distribution of cerebral lesions often follows the same watershed distribution (see Ch. 35) typically seen in metastatic neoplastic disease and other types of microemboli in the brain.

In contrast, yeast forms are less tissue-destructive. Hematogenously disseminated organisms invade the central nervous system (CNS), either through the choroid plexus or the cerebral vasculature itself, but are less likely to either obstruct vessels or form large contiguous lesions. Consequently, although *Candida* or *Cryptococcus* can cause parenchymal lesions, the predominant form of CNS involvement is a meningitis.

SPECIFIC ORGANISMS

Coccidioides immitis

C. immitis is one of the few fungi that commonly infect nonimmunosuppressed hosts, although the more severe forms of this infection do tend to occur in the immunocompromised. This soil saprophyte is widespread in dry, hot regions, being particularly endemic in the Americas (South, Central, and North) including Mexico. In the United States, the most affected regions are Arizona, California, particularly the San Joaquin Valley, New Mexico, and parts of Texas. Infection occurs after inhalation of spores.

Most infections are asymptomatic. About 40 percent of infected individuals have a transient flu-like illness, about 5 percent develop self-limited pulmonary disease, and less than 1 percent, many of whom are immunocompromised by human immunodeficiency virus (HIV), lymphoproliferative disorders, or medications, develop disseminated infection.

Diagnosis of this infection is typically made by culture, but this is quite slow—and hazardous to laboratory personnel. Detection of antibody in CSF can be useful, as can detection of antibody in serum or demonstration of skin test reactivity to either coccidioidin or spherulin, since such immunoreactivity generally only occurs in individuals with invasive disease.

In tissue, *Coccidioides immitis* normally grows as large, 20 to 100-μm diameter spherules. These can disseminate hematogenously, seed target tissues, proliferate, and incite local chronic inflammatory reactions. This process generally evolves over time, so that meningitis typically occurs several months after initial infection. In the CNS, infection causes a chronic meningitis, which, like many similar processes, tends to involve the basilar meninges primarily. As with other basilar meningitides, this results in chronic severe headache and frequently leads to cranial nerve palsies by local entrapment and raised intracranial pressure, with resultant changes in mental status, papilledema with altered vision, and progressive deterioration.

Untreated, this disease is invariably fatal, typically over the course of 1 to 2 years. Treatment is problematic, amphotericin B being the only useful agent. Blood-brain barrier penetration by this agent is inadequate in this infection, and intrathecal administration is generally necessary. The recommended dose is 0.6 mg/kg/day IV for 7 days, then 0.8 mg/kg every other day, to a total dose of 2.5 g or until toxicity requires cessation. At the same time 0.1 to 0.3 mg is given daily intrathecally via a reservoir. Fluconazole 400 mg PO daily is usually given in addition. Even with this modality, true cures are rare.

Candida

Candida spp. particularly *C. albicans,* are normal human commensals and are frequent causes of superficial disease. On occasion *Candida* may become invasive, again primarily among the immunocompromised. In tissue this organism assumes a yeast-like form, which is able to spread hematogenously. While the budding yeast may form pseudohyphae, the cells of these structures are less mutually adherent than are the cells of hyphae, so that tissue invasion is less prominent than with other fungi.

Dissemination incites an acute febrile illness, and multiorgan seeding with formation of microabscesses is possible, often evidenced by the presence of cottony infiltrates (*Candida* abscesses) in the retina on funduscopy. Such dissemination involves the CNS in about half of cases. This may be manifest as meningeal seeding, with a chronic meningitis or occasionally with parenchymal microabscess formation. Diagnosis generally requires culture of CSF or histologic demonstration.

Treatment of CNS infection requires amphotericin B, dosing as above, usually to a total of 0.5 to 1 g, which can be combined with fluconazole 200 to 400 mg/day, for up to 6 to 12 months or flucytosine 200 mg/kg/day, in four divided doses, for 3 days and then 100 mg/kg/day, in four divided doses, adjusting dose to maintain peak level at 70 to 80 and trough at 30 to 40 mg/L. Amphotericin B binds to ergosterol, the principal steroid of fungal walls, making the cell more permeable and leading eventually to cell death. Flucytosine is converted to 5-fluorouracil within fungal cells, where it then interferes with fungal DNA. This drug combination appears to be synergistic, since the amphotericin B-induced cell permeability increases flucytosine entry into the cells. Even though 50 percent of *Candida* infections are intrinsically resistant to flucytosine, this combination appears useful.

Cryptococcus neoformans

C. neoformans is an organism that is particularly widespread geographically. It is present primarily in avian feces, in which it may remain viable for up to 2 years. In tissue, the organism is a budding yeast, 4 to 8 μm in diameter, and it has a characteristic appearance in negative stains such as India ink preparations because of its thick polysaccharide capsule. The organism is classified into four distinct serotypes based on the polysaccharide composition of the capsule. Type A represents 95 percent of all isolates in the United States, where it is found primarily in pigeon droppings, D is the most common type in Europe, and B and C are rare. Polysaccharide structure plays an important role in determining virulence, perhaps by inducing immune tolerance to the organism or by impairing phagocytosis.

Aerosolized particles spread the disease. Often patients cannot recall a specific exposure. Initial infection involves the lungs and is often asymptomatic. The organism may then spread hematogenously to other organ systems and appears to have a predilection for involvement of the brain, where it initially is found in a perivascular distribution.

Prior to the onset of the AIDS epidemic, between 200 and 400 cases of cryptococcal meningitis usually occurred each year in the United States. About three-fourths of these patients had defective cell-mediated immunity, from either sarcoidosis, a lymphoproliferative disorder, or pharmacologic immunosuppression. Now, 5 to 10 percent of AIDS patients develop cryptococcal meningitis as well. Infection may also occur in immunocompetent individuals, particularly if the inoculum is especially large. Although the course is typically very chronic, in severely immunocompromised hosts it may be much more acute. Onset is usually rather indolent, however, and a majority of patients may be afebrile. As in other chronic fungal meningitides, meningism is not invariable and may be absent in 50 percent of patients. Also, as in other fungal meningitides, the CSF usually demonstrates a mononuclear pleocytosis, with decreased glucose concentration and modestly elevated protein content. The CSF may even be completely normal except for the presence of cryptococcal antigen.

Like other yeasts, *Cryptococcus* most typically causes a chronic meningitis. The basilar meninges are the most common site of involvement, with typical consequences, namely headache, cranial nerve compromise, obstruction to normal CSF flow with secondary raised intracranial pressure, altered consciousness and behavior, and chronic deterioration. Parenchymal involvement occurs as well, typically with multiple relatively small lesions involving the cerebellum and periventricular/periaqueductal structures.

Diagnosis can be confirmed by culture but can be made more expeditiously about half the time by negatively staining the sediment remaining after centrifuging up to 5 ml of CSF and looking for thickly encapsulated yeast forms. Cryptococcal antigen can be detected in CSF and serum in over 90 percent of patients. The titer of antigen in both fluids can be used to follow disease progression and response to therapy.

Untreated, cryptococcal meningitis is invariably fatal. Even with aggressive therapy, long-term neurologic sequelae are commonplace, although microbiologic cure can be obtained in the majority of immunocompetent individuals. Treatment is primarily with amphotericin B, aiming for a total dose of about 2.5 g. Intravenous administration is adequate in some pa-

tients, but blood-brain barrier penetration may be inadequate in others. Whether intrathecal administration improves morbidity or mortality significantly remains undetermined. Amphotericin B toxicity may be attenuated by using less of this highly toxic agent and adding flucytosine or fluconazole, these being the only three readily available antifungal agents that cross the blood-brain barrier. Fluconazole inhibits ergosterol production. Therefore it has been suggested that it might be counterproductive to use this agent in combination with amphotericin, which acts by binding to ergosterol. However, fluconazole, which is primarily suppressive and not curative, has the lowest toxicity of these three agents. As a result it is now being used for chronic suppression after initial amphotericin treatment, particularly in HIV-infected individuals in whom it is used on a lifelong suppressive basis after cryptococcal meningitis is diagnosed.

The end point for treatment remains difficult to define. Typically in non-HIV-infected individuals, treatment is stopped after 4 to 6 weeks, and a follow-up lumbar puncture is performed several months later, looking for either budding yeast forms, positive cultures, or a significant rise in antigen titer. However, even among immunocompetent individuals one-quarter will relapse with this regimen.

Aspergillus

A. fumigatus and other related *Aspergillus* spp. are similarly ubiquitous, being present primarily in decaying vegetable matter. The organism grows as a mold with septate hyphae, 2 to 4 μm in diameter. Despite the widespread prevalence of these organisms, systemic disease occurs rarely, and then almost exclusively in the immunocompromised, particularly in patients who are granulocytopenic.

Infection can occur by one of two routes. Most commonly inhalation of the organism results in a primary pulmonary infection, which may take the form of a disseminated pneumonitis or of a cavitating lesion. From this nidus the organism then invades the bloodstream and disseminates hematogenously. In a manner similar to behavior of neoplastic microemboli that are the presumed cause of brain metastases, the embolizing hyphae lodge in vessels in watershed areas in the brain. Once there, the vessels thrombose and the fungus grows through the vessel wall into the adjoining necrotic brain, forming a fungal abscess (Fig. 40-1).

In other patients, *Aspergillus* may invade the paranasal sinuses. As it directly invades local blood vessels, it causes necrosis. It can then invade through necrotic bone and soft tissue, penetrating directly into the cranial vault. Once intracranial, it frequently involves the cavernous sinuses or the vessels of the circle of Willis, where local invasion and thrombosis have obvious and disastrous consequences.

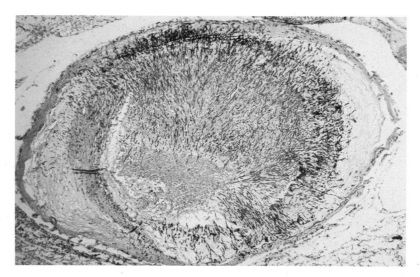

Figure 40-1. Light micrograph showing *Aspergillus* involving the walls of an artery.

Diagnosis is usually by tissue biopsy, preferably of involved pulmonary tissue or paranasal sinuses. Demonstration of *Aspergillus* in sputum of a patient with appropriate brain lesions should be considered highly suspicious for this disorder.

Treatment is primarily with amphotericin B, at doses of 1 mg/kg/day to a total dose of 2 to 2.5 g. This may be combined with flucytosine. Both drugs have been used for non-CNS disease. Their role in CNS infection is unclear. Results are mixed, particularly in the severely immunocompromised.

Mucormycosis

Mucormycosis (also known as *zygomycosis*, from the name of the genera containing the several related molds causing the condition) features infection with nonseptate hyphae, sharply branching at close to right angles, ranging from 6 to 50 μm in diameter. Responsible organisms are most commonly rhizopus and rhizomucor, ubiquitous molds found on decaying vegetable matter, animal feces, and substances high in sugar.

Despite the ubiquitous nature of these agents, infection is rare. It was initially described primarily in very poorly controlled diabetic patients but now is also known to occur in immunocompromised hosts. Typically infection begins as local black ulcerations in the nose or paranasal sinuses, followed by invasion of local blood vessels, leading to thrombosis and hemorrhagic infarction, followed by further local invasion. The infection readily proceeds through soft tissue and bone, invading the orbits or the base of the skull, followed by involvement of anything else in its path. If the infection invades the orbits, patients develop proptosis and difficulty in moving the eyes. Neurologic symp-

toms depend on the specific structures involved. Diagnosis is generally by tissue biopsy.

The infection is often fatal and requires aggressive surgical debridement, tight control of the underlying diabetes, or if possible, removal of causes of immunosuppression, and administration of amphotericin B, in doses of 0.8 mg/kg every other day, to a total of 2.5 to 3 g. In optimal circumstances cure is achieved in about half the cases of craniofacial mucormycosis.

ANNOTATED BIBLIOGRAPHY

Galgiani JN, Catanzaro A, Cloud GA et al. Fluconazole therapy for coccidioidal meningitis. Ann Intern Med 1993; 119:28–35.

Recent update on coccidioidal meningitis and tolerable long-term suppressive therapy.

Hoeprich PD. Cryptococcal and other fungal infections of the central nervous system. pp. 220–33. In Schlossberg D. (ed). Infections of the Nervous System, Springer-Verlag, New York, 1990.

Good review of fungal infections of CNS.

Lyman CA, Walsh TJ. Systemically administered antifungal agents. Drugs 1992;44:9–35.

Excellent and detailed overview of antifungal pharmacotherapeutics.

Saag MS, Powderly WG, Cloud GA et al. Comparison of amphotericin B with fluconazole in the treatment of acute AIDS-associated cryptococcal meningitis. N Engl J Med 1992;326:83–89.

Discussion of cryptococcal meningitis and its treatment.

Vincent T, Galgani JN, Huppert M et al. The natural history of coccidioidal meningitis: VA–Armed Forces Cooperative studies. Clin Infect Dis 1993;16:247–254.

Large series of coccidioides-infected individuals.

41
Spirochetal Diseases

John J. Halperin

SPIROCHETES

For reasons both sociologic and biologic, spirochetal infections of the nervous system have long been considered in a class by themselves. The two major neurotropic spirochetoses, syphilis and Lyme disease, share a number of important characteristics. Each has essentially one mode of transmission, which in each case makes a sociologic statement about the victim. Each starts as a fairly simple localized cutaneous infection, then disseminates, seeding various organ systems early on, and then enters a potentially long-lasting latent period, only to later cause significant symptoms in a subset of patients. Each organism reproduces slowly in vivo, even after the host has produced specific antibody against it, and may well attain a chronic symbiotic state in which, on the one hand, it causes the host no obvious problems but on the other, host defenses are able to keep it in check but not eradicate it. In neither disease is there an animal model that mimics all the neurologic effects of infection, making studies of pathophysiology difficult. Most importantly, both organisms are highly susceptible to widely available antibiotics, and at any stage of infection appropriate antimicrobial therapy will usually arrest further disease progression, although obviously such treatment cannot reverse nervous system damage that has already occurred. Finally, each of the two has been described as a great imitator, which probably largely reflects our ignorance about other disorders.

NEUROSYPHILIS

Syphilis is an infection of considerable historic interest. The responsible organism, *Treponema pallidum*, is a spirochete 6 to 15 μm long and 0.2 μm in diameter. Its external membrane consists primarily of lipid, with few exposed integral proteins, which is presumably the reason that host immune responses are so ineffec-

tive in controlling it. Although occasional cases have been transmitted by blood transfusion or other means, virtually all transmission is either by sexual contact or, far less frequently, transplacental. The organism is present in and shed from skin lesions and readily penetrates mucous membranes or nonintact skin. Once in a new host, it rapidly reaches local lymph nodes and from there can disseminate.

The host immune response includes production of antitreponemal antibodies, which can be measured by a fluorescent treponemal antibody-absorbed (FTA-ABS) test or similar tests and of anticardiolipin antibodies, such as those detected with the Venereal Disease Research Laboratory (VDRL) test or the rapid plasma reagin (RPR) assay. Whether the anticardiolipin antibodies are produced in direct response to the lipid coat of the spirochetes or to some interaction of the spirochete with the host is not clear. Neither of these types of antibody is useful either in eliminating the organism or in preventing reinfection. However, they do provide a ready means of diagnosis. The anticardiolipin antibody assays are inexpensive, easy to perform, and very sensitive but not entirely specific, which makes them screening assays. The antitreponemal assays are less sensitive but are highly specific, with false-positives occurring almost exclusively from infections with other antigenically closely related spirochetal diseases, which makes them most useful as confirmatory tests. Patients with Lyme disease and syphilis often cannot be differentiated on the basis of standard organism-specific antibody assays. However, the presence of sufficient anticardiolipin antibody to be detectable in a VDRL or RPR assay occurs almost exclusively in syphilis. Following adequate antimicrobial therapy, the RPR titer generally drops significantly or becomes negative; the FTA test usually remains positive indefinitely.

Clinical Course

Immediately following a patient's inoculation with the organism, there is a brief latent period lasting up to several weeks, during which the organism spreads to local lymph nodes, reproduces, and may even cause a spirochetemia. The patient then develops a local cutaneous lesion, known as a *chancre*, at the site of inoculation. This is an indurated, usually painless, ulcerating lesion in which spirochetes can be readily demonstrated. Even untreated, the chancre will slowly heal, but recurrent rashes are common, as is more widespread dissemination of the organism.

Within 1 to 2 months of the initial chancre's healing, the patient may develop secondary syphilis (i.e., symptomatic dissemination of the organism). This is usually marked by a widespread, multicentric mucocutaneous eruption, unusual in that it involves the palms and soles. While only 1 to 2 percent of patients with secondary syphilis will have symptomatic meningitis at this stage, as many as 40 percent may have a cerebrospinal fluid (CSF) pleocytosis, increased CSF protein, and/or detectable spirochetes in the CSF. This syphilitic meningitis can occur at any time during the first 2 years of infection, in 90 percent of cases independently of cutaneous dissemination. Syphilitic meningitis most commonly presents with headache and meningism and most typically affects the basilar meninges predominantly, with cranial neuropathies being commonplace. Alternatively, it may cause communicating hydrocephalus.

Once again, even without treatment, the infection may become latent, by which is meant that there is no evidence of active disease. During the first year after infection, defined as early latent disease, patients may develop relapsing disease or become reinfected. After 1 year these events both become quite unlikely, and patients enter the *late latent* period. Overall, about one-third of untreated patients progress to some form of latent disease and may ultimately develop long-term sequelae. In two-thirds, no further disease progression occurs.

Ultimately only 7 percent of untreated individuals will develop some form of symptomatic late neurosyphilis. Only patients who develop secondary disease are at risk for developing *tertiary* neurosyphilis. In particular, individuals who do not develop a CSF pleocytosis during the first year rarely if ever progress to develop late nervous system syphilis. Similarly, the 10 percent of patients who will develop syphilitic aortitis first develop lesions in the vasa vasorum of the ascending aorta at the secondary stage, leading ultimately to the obliterative endarteritis that damages the aorta in tertiary disease.

Late neurosyphilis is classically divided into three different types, although some degree of overlap is common: meningovascular syphilis, tabes dorsalis, and so-called generalized paresis of the insane. In all three, CSF examination usually demonstrates inflammatory changes (white blood cell counts in the low hundreds), mild to moderate increases in protein, and a positive CSF VDRL. Although the older literature describes patients with neurosyphilis without these positive findings, such cases must be viewed as potentially suspect, since most were reported at a time when our understanding of other pathophysiologic processes (e.g., atherosclerotic cerebrovascular disease) in the nervous system was at best rudimentary. The chronic inflammation leads to increased intrathecal immunoglobulin synthesis and not uncommonly to the presence of oligoclonal bands, which are probably organism-specific. The quantitative VDRL is a very useful marker of central nervous system (CNS) disease activity. The FTA is less helpful. Since a small proportion of peripheral blood immunoglobulin normally crosses the blood-brain barrier, the CSF FTA may well be positive simply as a reflection of passive transfer of peripheral blood antibody into the CSF, particularly when there is any blood-brain barrier disruption (see the section, Lyme Disease). Presumably this problem could be overcome by demonstrating intrathecal production of these antibodies, but since the CSF VDRL has always provided a simple and inexpensive marker of CNS disease, this more complex approach has never become popular.

Meningovascular syphilis is the result of chronic meningeal infection and inflammation and is the earliest of the three forms to appear (Fig. 41-1). On average this develops 7 years after primary infection, although there is considerable variability. The process results

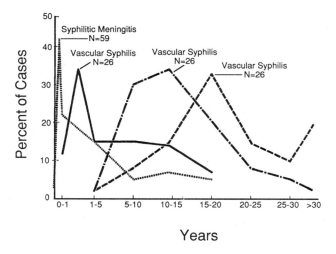

Figure 41-1. Interval between primary syphilitic infection and symptomatic neurosyphilis. (From Simon, 1985, with permission.)

in subacute occlusion of arteries, the middle cerebral artery territory being the most commonly involved, often with prominent involvement of deep penetrators, the lenticulostriate arteries, and resultant deep hemisphere infarcts. Unlike the typical abrupt onset of embolic strokes, these infarcts generally evolve over hours to days, often with a prodrome of headaches and psychiatric changes, including emotional lability. This disorder should be suspected in young adults who develop strokes without other obvious causes.

Tabes dorsalis similarly occurs in patients who have had meningeal involvement. For reasons that are unclear, men are affected far more often than women. This syndrome develops up to 20 to 30 years after initial infection and presents with prominent positive and negative signs of sensory system damage. Virtually all patients develop lightning-like lancinating pains, most commonly in the lower extremities, and at the same time develop predominantly large-fiber sensory loss. As a result of the latter they initially develop a sensory ataxia of gait and areflexia. Later on they develop difficulty with bladder function, which is thought to be primarily on a sensory basis. Eventually they lose the lancinating pains and also lose small-fiber sensory function. This, coupled with the chronic proprioceptive loss, leads to dramatic large joint destruction in the lower extremities (Charcot joints) from repeated injury. Pathologic abnormalities are seen in the dorsal roots, the dorsal ganglia, and the posterior columns. Which site is primary remains unclear. These same patients also commonly develop pupillary abnormalities, presumably on the basis of damage to the dorsal midbrain. The most commonly described form is the Argyll Robertson pupil—in these patients pupils are small and irregular and do not respond to light but do respond to accommodation (see Ch. 27).

Finally, general paresis of the insane also typically occurs one to two decades after initial infection. Like tabes, this syndrome is far more common in infected men than in women. These patients have widespread parenchymal disease, and clinical presentation tends not to be well localized. An old acronym merely demonstrates how widespread and nonspecific the syndrome may be—PARESIS: Personality, Affect, Reflexes (increased), Eye, Sensorium (hallucinations etc.), Intellect, Speech. The older literature is replete with colorful descriptions of grandiose personality changes in patients some of whom might have had other dementing diseases not as well recognized at the time.

Treatment

For early syphilis the treatment is straightforward. The organism is exquisitely penicillin-sensitive. Benzathine penicillin, 2.4 million units IM, cures 95 per-cent of patients with primary syphilis. Repeating this dose after 1 week is effective in secondary disease, and repeating it a third time is effective in patients with late latent disease if the CSF is normal.

Unfortunately these regimens do not produce highly effective concentrations of penicillin within the CSF, so that CNS syphilis is probably best treated with 10 to 14 days of intravenous aqueous penicillin, 12 to 24 million units/day. Although a variety of other regimens have been recommended for penicillin-allergic patients, none has ever been proved efficacious, or ineffective for that matter, in clinical trials. Therefore these patients must either be desensitized to penicillin or a more empiric approach must be tried, with treatment followed several months later with a follow-up lumbar puncture to see if the CSF pleocytosis has improved and if there has been a fourfold or greater drop in the CSF VDRL. Eradication of the organism apparently requires active participation by the host immune system.

In patients with the acquired immunodeficiency syndrome (AIDS), neurosyphilis may recur despite the above regimens, and even more aggressive courses have been recommended: up to 3 weeks of intravenous penicillin or penicillin followed by an oral agent. Neurosyphilis is considered to have responded when the CSF becomes inactive and the CSF VDRL has dropped at least fourfold.

LYME DISEASE

The term *Lyme arthritis* was first coined in the mid 1970s to describe a local epidemic of what initially was thought to be juvenile rheumatoid arthritis, occurring in the vicinity of the town of Lyme, Connecticut. Subsequent studies revealed that this was in fact a multisystem disorder, with frequent involvement of the heart, nervous system, and skin. As a result, the name of the disorder was broadened to the less restrictive *Lyme disease.* As the spectrum of clinical problems associated with this infection was more fully characterized, it became apparent that what had been thought to be a novel disorder was in fact very similar to one described in Europe shortly after the turn of the century. In 1910 European dermatologists first described the pathognomic skin rash, erythema chronicum migrans, now referred to just as erythema migrans, and two French neurologists, Garin and Bujadoux, described the most common neurologic concomitants of this tick bite-associated disorder in 1922.

Although this disease was originally defined in terms of its clinical phenomena, in particular its pathognomonic skin rash, in 1982 Willy Burgdorfer and colleagues succeeded in identifying the responsible bacterial pathogen, a tick-borne spirochete, which was subsequently named *Borrelia burgdorferi*. The following year, Eva Asbrink and colleagues identified a virtually identical organism as the agent responsible for European erythema migrans, as well for the disorder described by Garin and Bujadoux. More recent studies have demonstrated that this disorder in fact occurs virtually throughout the world, wherever humans and hard-shelled *Ixodes* ticks cohabit. Most recently sophisticated studies have suggested that slightly different *Borrelia* species may be responsible for this disease in different parts of the world—*B. burgdorferi* in North America, *B. garinii* and *B. afzelii* in Europe, and possibly other species elsewhere. This may in part explain the somewhat different clinical presentations described in different parts of the world, although these differences may also reflect bias of ascertainment, since this disorder was first defined as a dermatologic/neurologic disease in Europe but a rheumatologic/dermatologic one in North America.

The infection begins with the bite of the very small *Ixodes* tick, which has a three-stage life cycle. In its immature larval form, when its size is frequently likened to that of a period on a printed page, the tick takes one blood meal, typically from a small animal such as a mouse. If this blood donor is infected with *B. burgdorferi*, the tick will ingest spirochetes, which will then infect it and proliferate in its gastrointestinal tract. The tick then waits until its next life cycle stage, the nymph, for its next blood meal. Feeding is accompanied by injection of a variety of anticoagulants, local anesthetics, and enzymes. If the tick was previously infected, it may inject spirochetes into its new host along with these other compounds. If it was not already infected but the new host is, the tick will again have the opportunity to become infected. The tick will finally settle on a large animal to pass the winter and breed and it is this large animal that typically gives the tick its common name, the sheep tick (*Ixodes ricinus*) in Europe, the deer tick (*Ixodes dammini*) in northern North America. Humans become involved in this life cycle inadvertently, when they work (lumbermen, foresters, game keepers), play (hunters, campers), or stray into the wooded areas where field mice and ticks proliferate.

If an infected tick feeds long enough, typically at least 24 to 48 hours, its unwilling host may well be inoculated with spirochetes. It has been estimated that in endemic areas, no more than 1 to 2 percent of *Ixodes* tick bites result in infection. Conversely, at least one-third of patients infected with Lyme disease have no recollection of ever having been bitten by a tick or developing the acute rash. Although the tick bite itself is usually asymptomatic, within days about two-thirds of infected patients develop an enlarging, target-shaped rash at the site of the bite, representing the advancing front of invading spirochetes. Whether the other third do not develop the rash or develop it in an unobserved location such as the back remains unclear. In some individuals hematogenous spread will occur, occasionally leading to a similar but multifocal rash, typically with accompanying systemic symptoms. Untreated, the rash will continue to enlarge over days to weeks, often attaining diameters of more than 20 cm. Treated with appropriate antibiotics, the rash will disappear rapidly. Surprisingly, in most individuals this rash is also asymptomatic and may disappear unnoticed and untreated. However, at this early stage the infection disseminates and may set the stage for future multiorgan involvement. Recent studies using polymerase chain reaction techniques suggest that even the CNS may be seeded at this time. It is not yet known what proportion of patients with such seeding will go on to develop clinically significant problems from this, however.

Clinical Features

If the initial infection is not treated, about 10 to 15 percent of patients will develop acute nervous system involvement. The typical triad, first defined by Garin and Bujadoux, consists of lymphocytic meningitis, painful radiculoneuritis, and cranial neuritis, particularly facial palsy. Patients may develop all or some of this triad. In many individuals these symptoms may subside spontaneously, but resolution of the meningitis and radicular pain typically is accelerated by treatment with meningeal doses of appropriate antimicrobials. The meningitis is often surprisingly asymptomatic; lumbar puncture in a patient with Lyme facial palsy, for example, may demonstrate a significant pleocytosis, even in the absence of a headache.

A smaller number of patients may develop cardiac abnormalities, most commonly conduction abnormalities but occasionally myocarditis. Chemical evidence of hepatic involvement or myositis is also not uncommon, and some patients will develop arthralgias or frank arthritis.

Generally subsequent to this acute disseminated phase of the illness, a small subset of patients may develop what are considered late sequelae. In North America, Lyme arthritis figures prominently in this category and is typically a large-joint oligoarthritis (i.e., it typically affects large joints such as the knee, elbow, hip, or shoulder and tends to involve one joint at a time). In most instances this disorder responds to appropriate antimicrobials, but a subset of patients may continue to have recurring arthritis, a group that may be predisposed to this disorder by human leukocyte antigen (HLA) type, usually DR2 or DR4.

Diagnosis

Accurate diagnosis of Lyme disease has been challenging. The organism is somewhat fastidious and rather slow-growing, although with appropriate medium and growing conditions culture is possible. However the number of organisms present in involved tissues, with the exception of erythema migrans, is quite low, making culture quite insensitive. In the best of hands culture of CSF is positive in no more than 10 percent of patients with Lyme meningitis. As a result, most diagnosis has been based on serologic testing. This has been problematic, not only because of considerable technical variability in how this testing is performed but also because of a tendency to conclude that active infection is present when a single serologic test is positive, rather than using the more conventional method of observing a rise in titer.

Because of such problems, a vast literature has been produced consisting of anecdotes of patients with a single positive serologic test and disorder X, with causality implied. More recently several laboratories have been attempting to identify bacterial antigens in urine as well as other fluids. These techniques appear to be capable of reasonable specificity, but sensitivity is probably fairly low, and the relationship of test results to clinical phenomena remains to be established.

Perhaps more promising is the use of polymerase chain reaction techniques. This method has now been shown to be useful by multiple groups and appears to correlate well with what happens to patients. Although many problems remain with this procedure, it may be the best hope of diagnosis based on detection of the organism itself.

Diagnosis of CNS infection has actually been somewhat easier. As in many other infections, it is feasible to determine whether organism-specific antibodies are being produced within the CNS. Once the obvious cross-reactive bacteria are removed from consideration (e.g., those causing syphilis or relapsing fever), this technique is not susceptible to false-positives. If specific antibody is being produced within the neuraxis, the responsible organism must have invaded the CNS at some point, and therefore treatment based on the assumption of CNS infection is reasonable. The biggest drawback of this procedure is that intrathecal antibody production may appear to persist for years following successful treatment.

In measurement of intrathecal antibody, technical factors are key. It is impossible to define a normal range for concentration of specific antibodies in the CSF, since for any given individual the amount present will depend on the amount filtering in from peripheral blood, which in turn will be a reflection both of the concentration of those antibodies in peripheral blood and the permeability of the blood-brain barrier. The best way to allow for this is to perform each patient's assay with correction for CSF immunoglobulin concentration, something that can be done technically by measurement and appropriate dilution or by a capture assay. In either event, it is essential to know that the laboratory performing the CSF assay is performing it in an appropriate fashion.

Nervous System Involvement

Although the neurologic literature contains literally hundreds of reports of different manifestations of Lyme disease, the disorders clearly attributable to this infection can be simplified as described below.

Peripheral Nervous System

The peripheral nervous system is quite frequently involved. Although clinical manifestations may vary widely, it appears likely that virtually all are related to a mononeuropathy multiplex, the particular presentation depending on the severity and location of maximal disease involvement. A considerable body of evidence suggests that peripheral nerves are most likely to be involved in the part of the body that was the site of the tick bite—facial palsy with bites on the head, radicular symptoms in the bitten limb. This has been interpreted as suggesting that the spirochetes might be preferentially transported in peripheral nerves. While they are clearly too large ($20 +$ μm long) to be transported within axons, it remains possible that they might enter the nerve peripherally, where the blood-nerve barrier is incomplete, and then travel centrally within the perineurium.

The spirochete has been demonstrated to bind to endothelial cells. The pathology in nerve, as in the rest of the body, consists of perivascular inflammatory infiltrates, in nerve involving epineurial vessels partic-

---

PERIPHERAL NERVOUS SYSTEM
SYNDROMES WITH LYME DISEASE

Pathophysiologic mechanism
    Mononeuropathy multiplex
Clinical syndrome
    Mononeuropathy multiplex
    Radiculoneuritis
    Cranial neuritis
    Diffuse neuropathy
    Brachial plexopathy
    Lumbosacral plexopathy
    Guillain-Barré-like syndrome

ularly, without vessel wall necrosis (i.e., not a true vasculitis). Numerous studies have failed to demonstrate spirochetes, immune complexes, complement deposition, or other pathophysiologic clues to the mechanism by which this infection causes the nerve damage it does. However, it appears likely that a common pathologic process occurs in peripheral nerves of patients with facial palsy, painful radiculoneuritis, mild peripheral neuropathy, or plexopathies. In all, neurophysiologic studies demonstrate a disseminated axonal radiculoneuropathy, most consistent with a mononeuropathy multiplex. Although occasional patients have been described with a clinical course resembling the Guillain-Barré syndrome most of these have had a significant CSF pleocytosis and most have lacked clear evidence of peripheral nerve demyelination. Although rare cases of truly Guillain-Barré like presentations have been described, this certainly is not the typical presentation of Lyme neuropathy.

Without treatment the disease can range from an acute painful mononeuritis with weakness to a milder disseminated sensorimotor disorder, to a fulminating disorder with widespread weakness. Typically, the neuropathy improves following antimicrobial treatment, which indicates that the presence of organisms is required for persistence of the syndrome. In many patients, particularly those with more severe or painful presentations, a CSF pleocytosis occurs along with the neuropathy. This led to the early conclusion that such patients' disorders were due primarily to nerve root involvement. However, the near universal observation of significant abnormalities in sensory nerves, studied either neurophysiologically or pathologically, indicates that this process is much more disseminated in nature.

Cranial nerves are involved frequently. The facial nerve is the most frequently affected and Lyme disease is one of the few disorders associated with bilateral facial palsies, sarcoidosis and Guillain-Barré syndrome being the principal other causes. The eighth cranial nerve is also frequently involved, as are the nerves to the extraocular muscles. Other nerves are affected less frequently. Whether true optic neuritis occurs in Lyme disease remains to be established.

Central Nervous System

CNS involvement includes lymphocytic meningitis, which occurs in 10 to 15 percent of patients with Lyme disease. This may be asymptomatic or may have typical signs and symptoms of photophobia, headache, and meningism. *B. burgdorferi* can be cultured from CSF in about 10 percent of such patients. The polymerase chain reaction may be positive in a higher proportion. Several studies using the polymerase chain reaction have indicated that *B. burgdorferi* may pene-

---

CENTRAL NERVOUS SYSTEM SYNDROMES WITH LYME DISEASE

Extra-axial
    Lymphocytic meningitis
    Cranial neuritis
    Radiculoneuritis
Parenchymal
    Encephalomyelitis (acute and chronic)
Noninfectious (?)
    Parenchymal noninfectious (?)

---

trate the blood-brain barrier early in infection, even in the absence of an inflammatory response. What the implications of this are for future disease development and for optimal therapy remain to be determined.

Parenchymal CNS involvement is far less common. In areas highly endemic for Lyme disease, about five patients per million population at risk each year develop an acute or chronic inflammatory encephalomyelitis. White matter is involved more frequently than gray. As a result, long tract signs are frequent and seizures very rare. Although any part of the CNS may be involved, a myelopathic picture seems to be the most common one, particularly in more chronic cases. In most such patients, intrathecal production of anti-*Borrelia* antibody can be readily demonstrated. In most cases antimicrobial therapy is effective in arresting disease progression. As in other brain-damaging infections, residua may remain after treatment. Also as in other brain infections, longer courses of antimicrobial therapy (4 to 6 weeks) may be necessary to eliminate microorganisms. Finally, a chronic encephalopathy may occur. Many patients with symptomatic systemic Lyme disease have demonstrable difficulties with memory and complex cognitive functioning. Although in some instances this may reflect a milder form of encephalomyelitis, in most there is little to suggest the presence of brain infection. In these patients this disorder may be an effect of a soluble immunoneuromodulator produced in the periphery and affecting the CNS or of some other as yet to be defined mechanism. Some patients have had similar problems after treatment, and it has been postulated that this is a postinfectious disorder. It is hoped that additional studies using the polymerase chain reaction and measuring lymphokines and other immunomodulators will shed further light on this subject.

Regardless of the clinical presentation, most cases of true *B. burgdorferi* nervous system involvement re-

Table 41-1. Treatment of Lyme Disease

Type of Disease	Drug Regimen
Acute localized disease	Amoxicillin, 500–1,000 mg tid × 14–21 days, with or without probenecid, 500 mg tid or Doxycycline, 100 mg PO bid × 14–21 days (not in pregnant women or in children < 9 years old)
Acute disseminated, involving CNS (abnormal CSF)	Ceftriaxone, 2 g/day IV × 14–21 days or Cefotaxime, 2 g IV q8h × 14–21 days or Penicillin, 20 million U/day × 14 days
Late disseminated	Ceftriaxone, 2 g/day IV × 14–28 days or Cefotaxime, 2 g IV q8h × 14–28 days

spond readily to antimicrobial therapy (Table 41-1). Response may not be immediate and in severe cases recovery may be incomplete, but in the vast majority of cases treatment response is gratifying.

ANNOTATED BIBLIOGRAPHY

Ackermann R, Rehse KB, Gollmer E, Schmidt R. Chronic neurologic manifestations of erythema migrans borreliosis. Ann N Y Acad Sci 1988;539:16–23.

Description of late CNS disease in Europe.

Courevitch MN et al. Effects of HIV infection on the serologic manifestations and response to treatment of syphilis in intravenous drug users. Ann Intern Med 1993;118:350–5.

Evidence of persistence of T. pallidun after curative antibiotic therapy.

Davis LE, Schmitt JW. Clinical significance of cerebrospinal fluid tests for neurosyphilis. Ann Neurol 1989;25:50–5.

Good discussion of syphilis testing.

Fiumara NJ. Neurosyphilis. In Schlossberg D (ed). Infections of the Nervous System. Springer-Verlag, New York. 1990, pp. 262–7.

Good review of CNS abscesses.

Garin C, Bujadoux C. Paralysie par les tiques. J Med Lyon 1922;71:765–7.

First description of nervous system Lyme disease.

Gjestland T. The Oslo study of untreated syphilis. Acta Derm Venereol Suppl (Stockh) 1955;35(suppl. 34):1–368.

The natural history of untreated syphilis.

Halperin JJ, Luft BJ, Volkman DJ, Dattwyler RJ. Lyme neuroborreliosis—peripheral nervous system manifestations. Brain 1990;113:1207–21.

Overview of peripheral nervous system manifestations.

Halperin JJ, Volkman DJ, Wu P. Central nervous system abnormalities in Lyme neuroborreliosis. Neurology 1991;41:1571–82.

Overview of central nervous system manifestations.

Hansen K, Lebech A-M. The clinical and epidemiological profile of Lyme neuroborreliosis in Denmark 1985–1990. Brain 1992;115:399–423.

Overview of all nervous system manifestations in a well characterized population.

Johns DR, Tierney M, Felsenstein D. Alteration in the natural history of neurosyphilis by concurrent infection with the human immunodeficiency virus. N Engl J Med 1987;316:1569–72.

Worse outcome.

Keller TJ, Halperin JJ, Whitman M. PCR detection of Borrelia burgdorferi DNA in cerebrospinal fluid of Lyme neuroborreliosis patients. Neurology 1992;42:32.

Use of the polymerase chain reaction to diagnose Lyme disease.

Luger SW, Krauss E. Serologic tests for Lyme disease. Arch Intern Med 1990;150:761–8.

The problems with diagnostic tests.

Pfister HW, Preac MV, Wilske B, Einhaupl KM. Cefotaxime vs penicillin G for acute neurologic manifestations in Lyme borreliosis. A prospective randomized study. Arch Neurol 1989;46:1190–4.

Different treatment regimens for nervous system disease.

Reik L, Steere AC, Bartenhagen NH et al. Neurologic abnormalities of Lyme disease. Medicine (Baltimore) 1979;58:281–94.

Description of classic nervous system manifestations.

Simon R. Neurosyphilis. Arch Neurol 1985;42:606–13.

Excellent review of neurosyphilis.

Simon R, Bayne L. Neurosyphilis. In Tyler KL, Martin JB (eds). Infectious Diseases of the Central Nervous System. FA Davis, Philadelphia, 1993, pp. 237–58.

Textbook overview of CNS syphilis.

Steere AC, Malawista SE, Hardin JA et al. Erythema chronicum migrans and Lyme arthritis. The enlarging clinical spectrum. Ann Intern Med 1977;86:685–98.

Recognition of Lyme as a systemic disease.

Stiernstedt GT, Granstrom M, Hederstedt B, Skoldenberg B. Diagnosis of spirochetal meningitis by enzyme linked immunosorbent assay and indirect immunofluorescence assay in serum and cerebrospinal fluid. J Clin Microbiol 1985;21:819–25.

Establishes measurement of intrathecal antibody production as the method of choice for diagnosis of nervous system infection.

42
Malaria

Gustavo C. Román

Malaria is currently the most important human parasitic disease. Almost half of the population of the world is at risk, and more than 300 million individuals are thought to be infected. In Africa alone, over 1 million children die each year as a result of complicated malaria, including most prominently cerebral malaria. Resistance of the parasite to antimalarial drugs, insecticide-resistant mosquitoes, population migration, irrigation, deforestation, and also violence and warfare have prevented effective malarial control. A malaria vaccine appears promising, but its development may take at least another decade. Malaria can involve many organs and systems. However, the neurologic manifestations are usually life-threatening and require prompt action.

Cerebral malaria is an acute and severe encephalopathy produced exclusively by *Plasmodium falciparum* infection in humans. Cerebral malaria may complicate up to 16 percent of malaria infections. It occurs most commonly in children, young adults, and pregnant women in hyperendemic areas and also among nonimmune adults traveling from nonendemic areas.

PATHOLOGY AND PATHOPHYSIOLOGY

Changes in the brain found on postmortem examination include moderate cerebral edema, diffuse petechial hemorrhages, preferentially involving the white matter of brain, and slate gray discoloration from malarial pigment. Microscopically, ring hemorrhages occur predominantly around white matter arterioles. These are most likely the result of an immune-mediated vasculopathy leading to alterations of endothelial permeability, perivascular edema, diapedesis of leukocytes and erythrocytes, necrosis of the vessel wall, and intravascular microthrombosis. Despite intensive research and development of murine models, the pathogenesis of cerebral malaria remains unsolved. Plugging of cerebral capillaries and venules by clumped, parasitized red blood cells has been considered the main lesion. This cytoadherence is mediated by knobs that protrude from the surface of parasitized red cells. In addition, however, nonspecific, immune-mediated inflammatory responses, with release of vasoactive substances capable of producing endothelial damage and alterations of permeability, probably also occur. Serum concentrations of tumor necrosis factor (TNF) are significantly increased in children dying of cerebral malaria. TNF is one of the cytokines that can induce nitric oxide synthase, resulting in low nitric oxide within central nervous system (CNS) neurons and may help explain the reversible neurologic deficits of cerebral malaria.

CLINICAL MANIFESTATIONS

The onset of cerebral malaria is usually abrupt, but it may also develop as a late complication of falciparum malaria with multisystem involvement. Typically, the patient presents with fever, severe headache, and delirium progressing to stupor, commonly with hyperthermia reaching 40 to 42°C. There is rapid worsening from stupor to coma with fluctuations. Decerebrate and decorticate rigidity may occur. Funduscopic examination may show retinal hemorrhages. Generalized seizures occur in about 40 percent of adult patients and in most children. Partial seizures may occur, and transient focal neurologic signs are occasionally seen. Tendon reflexes and muscle tone are variable; brisk reflexes, extensor plantar responses, and ankle clonus may be elicited in half the patients and areflexia is a poor prognostic sign. Neck rigidity and Kernig's sign may be present. Cerebral malaria may also present with a clinical picture of psychomotor agitation and delirium resembling that of acute alcohol intoxication or an acute psychotic episode.

DIAGNOSIS

Infectious and metabolic causes of stupor and coma in the tropics should be excluded before a diagnosis of cerebral malaria is entertained. Hypoglycemia may mimic cerebral malaria and so must be included in the differential diagnosis. Heat stroke and exogenous intoxications should also be considered. A lumbar puncture is mandatory to exclude meningitis and encephalitis. In half the patients with cerebral malaria, the cerebrospinal fluid (CSF) is generally under normal pressure, with a few lymphocytes and a slight increase in protein content. A presumptive diagnosis of cerebral malaria can be made by exclusion of other diseases and by the demonstration of malarial parasites in peripheral blood. The degree of parasitemia cannot always be correlated with the severity of the cerebral involvement. It is important to treat the patient on clinical suspicion alone, since delay in treatment is accompanied by higher mortality.

TREATMENT

In patients from non-chloroquine-resistant areas, the recommended treatment is chloroquine, 10 mg/kg (of base) diluted in 10 ml/kg of isotonic fluid, by intravenous infusion over 8 hours, followed by 15 mg/kg/24 hours (5 mg/kg by intravenous infusion over 8 hours) to a total dose of 25 mg/kg. In chloroquine-resistant areas, treatment should be started with quinine dihydrochloride, with a loading dose of 20 mg/kg of salt diluted in 10 ml/kg isotonic fluid by intravenous infusion over 4 hours, then 10 mg/kg over 2 hours at 8-hour intervals until patients can swallow. Then quinine tablets, approximately 8.4 mg/kg q8h, are given to complete 7 days of treatment. Deep intramuscular injections may be given if intravenous treatment is impossible. The patient must be in bed to avoid postural hypotension. Hypoglycemia should be corrected and monitored frequently. Corticosteroids cannot be recommended because their use is accompanied by increased mortality. Lowering intracranial pressure by osmotic agents such as urea or mannitol may be beneficial. Fever should be controlled with acetaminophen and physical means. Aspirin should not be used because of its antiplatelet effects. Anemia should be corrected with packed red cells. Appropriate fluid and electrolyte balance is mandatory. Metabolic acidosis due to hypotension and shock should be corrected. A single intramuscular injection of phenobarbitone (3.5 mg/kg) is effective in preventing recurrence of seizures in cerebral malaria. Gram-negative sepsis is common in patients with severe malaria, and appropriate antibiotic therapy should be considered. Treatment with qinghaosu (artemisin), extracted from the leaves of *Artemisia annua,* appears promising, resulting in rapid parasite clearance. Artemisin suppositories (total dose 2800 mg over 8 days) are a major advance for the treatment of cerebral malaria, especially in rural areas where injections cannot be given.

PROGNOSIS

Mortality rates of cerebral malaria in children, reported mainly from African countries, vary from 6 to over 50 percent, and up to 21 percent of patients have neurologic sequelae. In a study of 308 Gambian children, the mortality rate was 14 percent. Of those who survived, 32 (12 percent) had residual neurologic deficits, including hemiplegia, occipital blindness, aphasia, and cerebellar ataxia. Factors predisposing to sequelae included prolonged coma, protracted convulsions, and severe anemia.

OTHER NEUROLOGIC MANIFESTATIONS

Generalized tonic-clonic seizures and partial motor seizures are frequently observed in acute cerebral malaria. Epilepsy is a well-recognized late sequela of cerebral malaria. It has been suggested that the malarial granulomas of Dürck, formed by an astroglial reaction, may act as epileptogenic foci, giving rise to chronic epileptic seizures. Malaria is a common cause of febrile seizures in children in the tropics. A study in Congo showed that 9.6 percent of all children admitted to Brazzaville General Hospital between 1981 and 1983 presented with seizures. Status epilepticus occurred in 13.6 percent of the cases, and 67 percent of these were related to benign malaria. Febrile seizures occurred in 73.5 percent of all cases, and 81 percent of them were related to malaria. Approximately 60 percent of all seizure disorders between 1 month and 6 years of age in a large general hospital were related to benign or malignant forms of malaria, and seizures were the reason for admission in 10 percent of all children in that age group. In Nigeria 50 percent of cases of febrile convulsions are due to malaria.

Vascular lesions have been reported in association with malaria, including parenchymal and subarachnoid hemorrhages and cerebral arterial occlusions causing focal neurologic signs such as hemiplegia and aphasia. Extrapyramidal manifestations, including dyskinesias, myoclonus, chorea, athetoid movements, and even parkinsonism, may be seen in association with cerebral malaria or as late sequelae.

Benign intracranial hypertension was reported in an African woman with resistant malaria. Acute psychiatric disturbances, including schizophrenia-like and manic syndromes, depression, acute anxiety, amok and confusional states, hallucinatory delirium, amnesia, and twilight states, have been described in the course of malaria. Psychiatric features usually completely resolve after treatment with antimalarial drugs.

Some patients with falciparum malaria develop hypoglycemia, causing coma, decerebrate posturing, and seizures. Up to 52 percent of African children and about half the pregnant women with falciparum malaria treated with quinine have been found to have hypoglycemia. Pregnant women with mild malarial infections can become hypoglycemic without symptoms, but the fetus suffers severe distress or even death in utero. The hypoglycemia may develop hours or even days after admission. Quinine-induced hyperinsulinemia is probably the principal mechanism, but consumption of glucose by the parasite and increased peripheral utilization of glucose may be contributory. Clinical features characteristic of hypoglycemia, such as tremulousness, sweating, mydriasis, and tachycardia, may not be present. Hypoglycemia must be suspected and a blood glucose test performed in any patient who has convulsions, impaired consciousness, or unexplained neurologic symptoms or signs. Intravenous dextrose corrects hypoglycemia in children without difficulty. In quinine-treated adults, hyperinsulinemia may cause recurrent hypoglycemia despite continuous infusion of dextrose. A somatostatin analogue has proved effective in Thailand to treat this form of hypoglycemia.

A syndrome of isolated cerebellar ataxia following falciparum malaria has been recognized in Sri Lanka in patients without features of cerebral malaria. The ataxia occurs as the fever subsides, usually after an afebrile period of 2 to 4 days. The delay between onset of fever and ataxia is 3 to 4 weeks. Unsteadiness on walking is the first and the most noticeable symptom, reaching its maximum in 2 to 3 days, but in some cases the symptoms progress up to 2 weeks. Some patients may be bedridden because of the ataxia. On examination, abnormal heel-to-toe walking is a constant feature, and other cerebellar signs may be present. CSF examination, electroencephalogram, and computed tomographic (CT) brain scan are normal. Treatment consists of antimalarial drugs to clear any parasitemia, prednisolone, and supportive measures, including physiotherapy. Complete recovery usually occurs, taking a few weeks or up to 4 months.

Spinal cord syndromes resembling amyotrophic lateral sclerosis or combined system degeneration, as well as spastic and ataxic myelitides, have been reported in association with malaria. In cases of simultaneous cerebral and spinal disease, the clinical condition may resemble disseminated encephalomyelitis (e.g., spastic gait, tremor, and occasional nystagmus and speech disorders). On treatment with quinine these symptoms are reported to regress. Early literature refers to cases of neuritis, polyneuritis, Landry's paralysis, and cranial nerve palsies in association with malarial infections. More recently, cases of Guillain-Barré syndrome developing 2 to 3 weeks following vivax or falciparum malaria have been reported.

Transient muscular paralysis resembling periodic paralysis has been observed during febrile episodes of malaria. Following a shaking chill, the weakness first appeared in the lower limbs and soon spread, causing paralysis affecting the entire body except for the respiratory muscles. The patients remained conscious during the attack. Signs of improvement appeared in 4 to 6 hours, and the recovery was complete in 8 to 10 hours, the muscles that were affected first being the last to recover. Transient hypokalemia due to lysis of red cells and intense muscular contraction during rigors were suggested as the mechanism underlying the muscle paralysis.

ANNOTATED BIBLIOGRAPHY

Brewster DR, Kwiatkowski D, White NJ. Neurological sequelae of cerebral malaria in children. Lancet 1990;336:1039–43.

First clear documentation of neurologic sequelae in children.

Grau GE, Taylor TE, Molyneux ME, et al. Tumor necrosis factor and disease severity in children with falciparum malaria. N Engl J Med 1989;320:1586–91.

Tumor necrosis factor levels correlate well with disease severity.

Hien TT, White NJ: Qinghaosu. Lancet 1993;341:603–8.

A timely review of this promising therapy.

Molyneux ME, Taylor TE, Wirima JJ, Borgstein A. Clinical features and prognostic indlcators in paediatric cerebral malaria: a study of 131 comatose Malawian children. Q J Med 1989;71:441–59.

Excellent review of malaria in children.

Newton CR, Kirkham FJ, Winstanley PA, et al: Intracranial pressure in African children with cerebral malaria. Lancet 1991;337:573–6.

Demonstration of increased intracranial pressure.

Phillips RE. Hypoglycaemia is an important complication of falciparum malaria. Q J Med 1989;266:477–85.

Review of important factors in pathogenesis of neurologic complications.

Román GC. Cerebral malaria: the unsolved riddle. J Neurol Sci 1991;101:1–6.

Neuropathologic controversies.

Román GC, Senanayake N: Neurologic manifestations of malaria. Arq Neuropsychiat 1992;50:3–9.

Comprehensive review of the neurologic complications.

White NJ, Looareesuwan S, Phillips RE, et al. Single dose phenobarbitone prevents convulsions in cerebral malaria. Lancet 1988;2:64–6.

A simple treatment.

Wyler DJ. Malaria chemoprophylaxis for the traveler. N Engl J Med 1993;329:31–7.

Full review.

43
Cysticercosis

A. Spina-Franca

EPIDEMIOLOGY

The occurrence of epilepsy or the syndrome of raised intracranial pressure (intracranial hypertension) in a person living in or visiting a region where taeniasis (Greek: *tainai,* band, tape, tapeworm) is endemic or even in one living in close contact with people who have taeniasis should suggest a diagnosis of cysticercosis (Greek: *kystis,* bladder; *kerkos,* tail; a term used to describe the appearance of the larval form of the tapeworm) in the central nervous system (CNS).

The CNS form of the disease, known as *neurocysticercosis,* is the most common parasitic infection of the CNS. Susceptibility to the disease is universal, favoring neither sex and showing no racial predilection. The disease is most prevalent in the 20- to 40-year age range, although cases have been reported over the entire age range from 1 to 2 years on.

In endemic regions (i.e., all non-Islamic intertropical regions), the risk of infection is high from such common sources as ingesting the ova of *Taenia solium* by eating foods such as fresh vegetables and raw legumes contaminated by feces (night soil). Additionally, eating undercooked pork can result in absorption of larvae that develop into *Taenia solium.*

PATHOPHYSIOLOGY

Once ingested by the animal (including human) host, the ova liberate taenia embryos, which penetrate the host. Through the systemic circulation the embryos lodge in and infect a wide variety of organs, including brain and spinal cord, where they develop into their larval form, the *Cysticercus cellulosae* (cysticercus).

The cysticercus is a vesicular structure of approximately 1-cm diameter. Its interior is filled with a liquid in which the scolex (i.e., head) of the parasite is found invaginated. The survival of the cysticercus varies widely but on average is from 3 to 6 years. Clustered (macrocystic) cysticerci are sometimes found, as are the multivesicular form, known as *Cysticercus racemosus.*

Infestation of the CNS by multiple cysticerci is more common than single infestation. Usually they are lodged in the brain, in the ventricular system and/or the cranial subarachnoid space.

CLINICAL FEATURES

Neurocysticercosis may remain asymptomatic for months to years and is commonly a diagnosis made incidentally when neuroimaging is performed. However, the many symptomatic forms predominate.

Symptoms are related both to the parasite and to the inflammatory response that its presence generates. The sites occupied in the neuraxis play the same role expected in tumors of any kind: those remote from the main motor and sensory pathways evoke fewer symptoms for their size than those occurring in clinically more sensitive areas. The total number of parasites determines the amount of antigens they liberate, which governs the extent of the inflammatory response, a granulomatous reaction with secondary edema and vasculitis of adjacent vessels. In the brain parenchyma, the granulomatous response is more conspicuous around each of the cysticerci. The granulomatous reactions can be large enough to form space occupying lesions.

Once the cysticerci die, they tend to disintegrate or to be calcified. The calcified cysticerci and residua of the granulomas may persist for the rest of the patient's life.

Among the various clinical features, epilepsy and intracranial hypertension prevail. Secondary tonic-clonic generalized seizures are the most common type of epilepsy that occurs. Intracranial hypertension may occur in episodic fashion or be characterized by a persistent and progressively worsening picture. The association of epilepsy and intracranial hypertension is a common syndrome. Mental deterioration is another common feature and can be associated with the preceding manifestations.

Several distinctive but less common syndromes have become recognized from the tendency of cysticerci to occupy certain sites in the neuraxis. Hydrocephalus can result from mechanical blocking of cerebrospinal fluid (CSF) drainage when the parasite is located in the narrowed portions of the ventricular system or in the basal cisternae. The obstruction may also result from local inflammatory responses (ependymitis, arachnoiditis) or their sequelae. Focal arterial obstruction has been reported from cysticerci in the subarachnoid space at the base of the brain, mimicking the small, deep infarcts (lacunes) caused by microatheroma of small, penetrating arteries. Local compression syndromes from masses large enough to compress nerve roots, even the spinal cord, have been reported which are similar to those seen from other infections and from primary or metastatic tumors. Ocular, muscular, and subcutaneous cysticercosis can be associated and point to the diagnosis.

DIAGNOSIS

The diagnosis of neurocysticercosis is usually established by neuroimaging and by the CSF. Through neuroimaging, the cysticercus may be recognized in several forms: (1) as a vesicle, with the scolex in its interior; (2) as an inflammatory nodule; (3) as a poorly outlined vesicle, the scolex not always being visible; and (4) as a calcified structure, sometimes circumscribed by residual inflammation. These images are important for management, since the plan of treatment varies according to whether the cysticerci are living, active forms or inactive.

Detection of anti-*Cysticercus cellulosae* antibodies in the CSF is helpful in the diagnosis. Other CSF changes include increased cellularity, featuring lymphocytes and monocytes but marked by the presence of eosinophil cells, and an increase of γ-globulin, particularly immunoglobulin G, which can present ratios and indexes suggestive of local immune production. This set of changes plus the presence of anticysticercus antibodies is referred as the CSF syndrome of neurocysticercosis.

Relapses of the syndrome may occur, with an increase in the intensity of hypercytosis and eosinophil participation in the cytomorphologic profile. The exacerbation of the syndrome is related to degeneration of cysticerci and may contribute to evaluation of the effectiveness of adopted therapies.

TREATMENT

Parasiticidal drugs can be used in the treatment of neurocysticercosis, particularly in the active forms. Praziquantel (50 mg/kg/day) or albendazole (20 mg/kg/day) is given orally over the course of 2 or 3 consecutive weeks.

The treatment with parasiticides does not imply suspension of the treatment indicated for clinical manifestations, such as antiepileptic drugs for seizures and steroids for increased intracranial pressure. Corticosteroids or antihistaminics (dexchlorpheniramine) may be necessary to prevent side effects of the parasiticidal drug, particularly further increase in intracranial pressure by massive brain edema.

Some evidence suggests that the parasiticidal drugs now used are more effective on cysticerci lodged in the CNS parenchyma than in the subarachnoid space or in the ventricles. In the latter sites macrocystic and racemose cysticerci are usual. Neurosurgical removal is indicated for these forms of the parasite, particularly when single. Hydrocephalus from CSF obstruction should prompt early ventricular shunting to alleviate the resulting increase in intracranial pressure.

PROGNOSIS

In spite of the results obtained with medical or surgical treatment, the clinical sequelae of neurocysticercosis remain high. Prophylaxis is mandatory in endemic areas and within those regions to which susceptible persons might migrate. Basically, prophylaxis aims at interrupting the parasitic cycle by preventing humans from eating pork with viable cysticerci, thus giving rise to new taeniae. To prevent cysticercosis it is necessary to teach those at risk to avoid ingesting taenia ova with viable embryos. This is achieved by adequate burial of human feces and prevention of feces from entering the water supply and by avoiding the fertilization of vegetables with feces of persons with taeniasis or their irrigation with polluted water. Although prophylaxis is easy to carry out, poor socioeconomic and educational status are the main obstacles to adequate achievement in many of the endemic regions. Indeed, in some these regions, the incidence of neurocysticercosis is showing no signs of the desired decline.

ANNOTATED BIBLIOGRAPHY

Colli BO, Martelli N, Assirati JA Jr et al. Results of surgical treatment of neurocysticercosis in 69 cases. J Neurosurg 1986;65:309–15.

Details on surgical decision-making.

Cuetter AC, Guerra LC, Meza AD, Brower RD. Neurocysticercosis: a special problem of the southwestern United States. J Trop Geogr Neurol 1992;2:172–6.

Cases occurring in the United States.

Del Brutto OH. Diagnosis and management of cysticercosis. J Trop Geogr Neurol 1992;2:1–9.

Modern review.

Earnest MP, Reller LB, Filey CM, Grek AJ. Neurocysticercosis in the United States: 35 cases and a review. Rev Infect Dis 1987;9:961–79.

These cases occurred despite assumed adequate public health practices.

Machado LR, Nobrega JPS, Barros NG et al. Computed tomography in neurocysticercosis: a 10-year long evolution analysis of 100 patients with an appraisal of a new classification. Arq Neuropsiquiatr 1990;48:414–18.

Full details from a wide experience.

Monteiro L, Coelho T, Stocker A. Neurocysticercosis: a review of 231 cases. Infection 1992;20:61–5.

Of the 231 patients, 62 percent were symptomatic, while the remaining cases were diagnosed on imaging as incidental findings.

Schantz PM, Moore AC, Munoz JL et al. Neurocysticercosis in an Orthodox Jewish community in New York City. N Engl J Med 1992;327:692–5.

Health practices.

Scully RE, Mark EJ, McNeely WF, McNeely BU (eds). Case records of the Massachusetts General Hospital: a 63-year-old Cape Verdean woman with blurred vision, diplopia, a suprasellar mass and lymphocytic meningitis. N Engl J Med 1993;328:566–73.

Full details of a single case.

Sotelo J, Guerrero V, Rubio F. Neurocysticercosis: a new classification based on active and inactive forms. A study of 753 cases. Arch Intern Med 1985;145:442–5.

Extensive experience.

Spina-Franca A. Cysticercosis of the central nervous system. In Chopra JS, Jagannathan K, Sawhney IMS (eds). Advances in Neurology: Excerpta Med Int Congr Series 883. Elsevier, Amsterdam, 1990, pp. 283–91.

Textbook chapter.

Spina-Franca A, Livramento JA, Machado LR. Cysticercosis of the central nervous system and cerebrospinal fluid: immunodiagnosis of 1573 patients in 63 years (1929–1992). Arq Neuropsiquiatr 1993;51:16–20.

The development of these techniques.

Takayanagui OM, Jardim E. Therapy for neurocysticercosis: comparison between albendazole and praziquantel. Arch Neurol 1992;49:290–94.

Useful details.

Trelles JO, Trelles L. Cysticercosis of the central nervous system. In Vinken PJ, Bruyn GW (eds). Handbook of Clinical Neurology. Vol. 35. North Holland, Amsterdam, 1978, pp. 291–320.

A well-known clinical textbook chapter.

44

Schistosomiasis (Bilharziasis)

Michael Hoffmann

Schistosomiasis (Greek: *skhistos,* split; *soma,* body), or bilharziasis (Theodore Bilharz, German zoologist, who first described *Schistosoma hematobium* in 1851), causes neurologic involvement commonly enough to warrant inclusion in this book. Three schistosome species and several less prevalent species infect at least 200 million people worldwide. The estimated annual mortality from this trematode blood fluke is approximately 200,000. Tropism in geographical distribution as well as the organ involvement in humans differentiates these species.

Humans and intermediate amphibious snail hosts (*Biompheleria* and *Oncomelania* spp.) are required to complete the life cycle of this digenic trematode, whose habitat is restricted to the tropical and subtropical regions of the world. *Schistosoma mansoni* is found in South America (Brazil, Venezuela, Surinam), several Caribbean islands, parts of Africa, and the Middle East, with periportal fibrosis and portal hypertension the most important complications. *Schistosoma japonicum* is found in southeast Asia (mainly China and the Philippines) and causes disease similar to that produced by *S. mansoni* but a higher incidence of central nervous system (CNS) involvement. *S. hematobium* is extensive throughout Africa and the Middle East with a predilection for the veins of the urinary tract. Two schistosome species with restricted prevalence to date are *Schistosoma mekongi* (found in the Mekong river in Indochina), causing disease similar to *S. japonicum* disease, and *Schistosoma intercalatum* (only in west Africa). Schistosome dermatitis (swimmer's itch) follows body exposure to fresh water, as in swimming or bathing. It usually affects previously unexposed persons, causing a delayed hypersensitivity reaction. Nervous system involvement is most common with *S. hematobium* and *S. mansoni,* usually taking the form of various spinal cord presentations. Even among those populations where the various schistosome species are not native, such as those of North America and most of Europe, infections introduced by immigrants have contributed to making the problem worldwide.

BIOLOGY AND LIFE CYCLE

The schistosome life cycle is similar in all species, with minor differences accounting for the various pathophysiologies. Schistosomes even of the same species have recently been shown by restriction endonucleases to be genetically diverse and this is also thought to be an important factor in the development of granulomas and fibrosis.

By way of brief review, the eggs need to be deposited in fresh water. They hatch short-lived (8 to 12 hours) free-swimming miracidia, which infect the intermediate snail host. The miracidium multiplies via two stages of sporocysts, to produce numerous cerceriae, which when released into the water, target the human or other vertebrate host. The cerceriae are viable for only approximately 48 hours. Once a cerceria has penetrated the host, it is called a *schistosomula.* After journeying through the skin to the peripheral lymphatic and venous vessels, within a week the schistosomula reaches the right side of the heart and lung and thereafter follows an intravascular route to the liver portal vessels, feeding on the blood and eventually developing into an adult worm. Some female worms measure 20 to 26 mm long and 0.25 mm wide and produce up to 20 to 290 eggs per day. These sexually mature worms leave the liver once mated and migrate to the mesenteric vascular plexus in the case of *S. mansoni* or the vesicle vascular plexus in the case of *S. hematobium.* The female worms produce the eggs in passing through the bladder or bowel, so that the eggs are excreted via the urine or feces. Humans inhabiting and frequenting rivers and waterways are in this way able to complete the schistosome life cycle by their excreta finding their way back into the water.

657

PATHOPHYSIOLOGY

Three stages may be delineated. The initial invasion, termed *cercerial dermatitis* or *swimmer's itch,* is caused by penetration into the skin of cerceriae of human and nonhuman schistosomes. The second, or maturation, stage is termed *acute schistosomiasis* or *Katayama fever* (see below). This is an allergic response to a developing antigenic mass of ova and worms and presents as a serum sickness or an acute febrile illness, with pyrexia, urticaria, pulmonary and liver involvement, and lymphadenopathy. The third stage, *chronic schistosomiasis,* is a host immune reaction to the eggs in various organs, with the formation of edema, granulation tissue, fibrovascular obstruction, and calcification. It is this last stage that is of neurologic interest.

In individuals from endemic areas, initial infection is mostly unnoticed. Visitors to endemic areas may suffer an acute febrile illness as a manifestation of the immune response to the eggs and worms (Katayama fever), usually with an elevated eosinophil count and vigorous reaction of immune complexes to schistosome antigens. The development of disease in humans is a function of the worm load within the host and therefore of the number of eggs produced. It is the inflammatory and fibrotic response of host tissue that determines the severity of an individual's disease. Although protective immunity has been demonstrated in experimental animals, this has not been adequately documented in humans to date. The schistosomula is relatively susceptible to an immune attack in the first few days after infection and gradually becomes resistant with maturity.

The CNS disease is relatively rare and occurs via aberrant deposition of eggs in nervous tissue, either by migration of adult worms or by transport of eggs into nervous system circulation by collateral veins.

CLINICAL SYNDROMES

Systemic

Acute schistosomiasis presents as initial itching of the skin where the cerceriae penetrated and may be followed by several weeks of systemic illness, with pyrexia, weight loss, angioedema, cough, and headache, the syndrome complex called Katayama fever. The diagnosis is established by considering possible exposure and by a marked eosinophilia, increased immune complexes, antibodies to adult schistosome gut antigens, and eggs in the stool or eggs seen on microscopy from rectal biopsy. Other systemic illnesses include hepatic fibrosis (Symmers' fibrosis), as seen with infections of *S. mansoni, S. japonicum,* and *S. mekongi,* featuring hepatomegaly and obstruction of portal venous tracts with portal hypertension, hepatosplenomegaly,

esophageal and gastric varices, and hematemesis. Pulmonary hypertension is seen solely in patients also suffering from hepatic periportal fibrosis and portal hypertension, usually explained by obliteration of pulmonary arterioles by granulomatous inflammation secondary to embolization of schistosome eggs. Glomerulonephritis from immune complex disease is a complication that also occurs almost exclusively in people with periportal fibrosis. Anemia with protein-losing enteropathy is a consequence of inflammatory polyps, which develop in the large intestine owing to deposition of eggs, and cause the formation of an exudative granulomatous process associated with eggs, inflammatory cells, and fibrosis.

Central Nervous System Involvement

Involvement of the CNS was first reported in 1889 by Yamagiwa of Japan, who described intracerebral granulomas with *S. japonicum* ova. Overall, CNS complications from schistosomiasis have often been thought to be rare, but from postmortem as well as recent clinical studies it is apparent that nervous system involvement occurs in many more patients than is suggested by clinical symptomatology. Involvement occurs with *S. mansoni, S. hematobium,* and *S. japonicum,* with the former two species causing mainly spinal cord involvement and the latter mainly cerebral lesions (occurring in up to 3 percent of infections).

The Mechanism of Central Nervous System Invasion

The usual sites of infection and subsequent organ damage are the splenohepatic system and the urinary tract and bladder. Ectopic egg deposition is responsible for nervous system involvement, and the route by which eggs are deposited remains speculative and unproven. Batson's valveless plexus of veins connects the deep iliac veins and inferior vena cava with the veins of the spinal cord and brain. At times of increased intra-abdominal pressure (coughing, defecation, Valsalva maneuver, constipation, urinary retention), the abdominal venous flow can become reversed, and the eggs deposited normally in the portacaval system can then enter the spinal and subsequently cerebral veins. Other mechanisms include embolization to the brain via portal-pulmonary arteriovenous anastomoses and direct oviposition by adult worms residing adjacent to the cerebral or vertebral veins. It is also postulated that the smaller egg size of *S. japonicum* and its far greater daily egg production account for the more frequent cerebral involvement by this species.

Spinal Schistosomiasis

Spinal schistosomiasis is the most common form of CNS involvement. *S. mansoni* and *S. hematobium* have a predilection for the lower spinal cord. All the forms listed below arise from ectopic schistosome ova deposition, with host inflammatory responses and tissue damage following. Schistosomal spinal cord disease is almost solely due to *S. hematobium* and *S. mansoni*. In endemic areas schistosomiasis is a common cause of myelopathy of nontraumatic cause, as pointed out by Haribhai et al. (1991). The schistosomal myelopathies present with easily recognizable clinical syndromes based on the locus of the mass.

Intrathecal granuloma formation is nearly always low lumbar and sacral, with the most common level of involvement being the T12–L1, conus, and cauda equina regions. The clinical presentation evolves from acute to subacute over days to a few weeks as a radicular syndrome with flaccid, often asymmetric paraparesis. The syndrome is also characterized by hyporeflexia or areflexia associated with sphincter dysfunction, by low back pain, and by dermatomal sensory impairment attributed to lesions affecting the sacral, lumbar, and at times lower thoracic segments.

Transverse myelitis, with either an acute or a subacute presentation, constitutes the most common form of spinal cord involvement. As with the intrathecal granuloma form of affliction, the predilection is for the lower cord, unlike other forms of myelitis, which more commonly affect the midthoracic cord. The pathophysiology in this form is poorly understood; in some rare cases it has been postulated to be vasculitis of the spinal vessels with subsequent myelonecrosis. Clinical presentation is with symmetric or asymmetric flaccid paraparesis, sensory impairment, sphincter incontinence, and back and limb pain. It is a diagnosis of exclusion.

Radiculitis occurs when the granulomas impinge on a nerve root, with accompanying host reaction and inflammation and tissue fibrosis. Multiple nerve root involvement may occur and may eventually lead to spinal arachnoiditis, diagnosed from circumstantial evidence, myelography, computed tomography (CT) myelography, or magnetic resonance imaging (MRI).

Radiculomyelitis occurs in various forms corresponding to anatomic variations and varying extent of infection. Clinical signs of both upper and lower motor neuron involvement in the lower spinal cord, together with the necessary cerebrospinal fluid (CSF) pleocytosis, peripheral blood eosinophilia, and radiologic and serologic tests for schistosomiasis, are required for such a diagnosis.

Vascular involvement is the rarest form of spinal involvement, although it is possibly underreported. Rare instances of anterior spinal artery occlusion by schistosomiasis force recognition even of this entity in the wide differential diagnosis of acute anterior spinal artery occlusion.

Cerebral Schistosomiasis

Several subtypes of cerebral schistosomiasis occur, the two best know being mass lesions and focal epilepsy.

Focal deficits (i.e., mass lesions) occur with widely varying frequency. The frequency of infection with *S. japonicum* ranges from 2 to 5 percent, but no systematic studies are available. Almost any presentation consistent with mass lesions in the cortex, subcortical regions, basal nuclei, and white matter can occur, with the usual syndrome complex of long tract signs, namely weakness, primary sensory disturbances, visual abnormalities, ataxia, behavioral abnormalities, epilepsy, extrapyramidal presentations, and even isolated headache. A picture of behavioral change without long tract signs may occur. Anatomic brain imaging with CT scanning or MRI is usually diagnostic along with appropriate clinical and laboratory evidence. The electroencephalogram is particularly useful in the diagnosis of the encephalopathic forms.

Epilepsy may occur in generalized and focal Jacksonian seizure types, either as the sole symptom or associated with more widespread clinical deficits. Paroxysmal θ and δ slowing, asymmetric background rhythms, and spikes and sharp waves have been found on electroencephalography.

Encephalitis/encephalomyelitis and meningitis may present with a fulminating illness with spiking fever, behavioral changes, and long tract signs of motor, sensory and visual tract deficits, coma, meningeal irritation, and papilledema signifying raised intracranial pressure. Depending on the anatomic affliction of the gray and white matter and meninges, these are variously classified as encephalitis, encephalomyelitis, and meningitis, with most being a combination of two or three clinical descriptions (for the CSF, see below). The interval between exposure and first cerebral symptoms ranges from 6 weeks to 6 months, as compared with about 2 months to 1 year or longer in the schistomiasis subtype presenting as a slowly expanding mass lesion.

DIAGNOSIS

Diagnostic Tests

A peripheral eosinophilia ($> 700/mm^3$ absolute count) is invariable. Stool and urine specimens must be tested for the ova, while bearing in mind that with *S. hematobium*, midday urine specimens are most likely to yield eggs in patients harboring them. Rectal mucosal biopsy is useful if urine and stool specimens are negative and suspicion remains high. In endemic populations, urine, stool specimens, and rectal biopsies are frequently positive for ova in entirely asymptomatic persons.

Serodiagnostic tests were usefully employed in a comprehensive prospective myelopathy protocol by Haribhai et al. (1991), with the finding that enzyme-linked immunoabsorbent assay (ELISA) of the CSF helped to suggest the diagnosis. Comparison of the total immunoglobulin E, total eosinophil counts, ELISA, and the indirect immunofluorescence test indicates that ELISA has at best a specificity of 95 percent and a sensitivity of 96 percent. To date ELISA has been the most reliable test, with egg antigens giving better results than worm antigens. The indirect hemagglution test has relatively low sensitivity. The polymerase chain reaction is the most sensitive method to detect DNA. It has already been usefully applied to the diagnosis of toxoplasmosis, falciparum malaria, and Chagas' disease and may be a future tool for schistosomiasis testing.

CSF testing is important for the diagnosis as well as for excluding other spinal infections. The findings are relatively nonspecific and consist of a pleocytosis of about 100 cells/mm^3, with a lymphocyte or less commonly a neutrophil predominance and at times an eosinophilia. The eosinophilia is highly suggestive of parasitic diseases in general. Protein elevation is the rule, as are normal to slightly depressed glucose levels. CSF ELISA levels and intrathecal antibody production are useful diagnostic measurements, which decrease following appropriate praziquantel therapy.

Radiology

Most radiologic studies to date have used myelography and CT myelography with the characteristic features being an expanded lower spinal cord or conus medullaris, or the granulomatous mass lesions of the cord. Myelography typically shows a partial or at times a complete block having the vertical extent of about one vertebral body. Myelography is relatively insensitive to the smaller lesions and does not exclude the diagnosis when normal. Where MRI is available, the study is usually more sensitive, showing an irregularly enlarged conus or lower spinal cord with heterogeneous enhancement. With more advanced or long-standing disease, cord atrophy may be noted with CT or MRI scanning. In schistosomal transverse myelitis, early studies with CT myelography are usually normal with MRI scanning sometimes showing changes, none of which are specific.

THERAPY

Control of Schistosomiasis

Health education measures include the curbing of indiscriminate urination and defecation into streams and rivers. Intermediate host control involves use of molluscicides or destruction of the snail habitat. Such drastic measures, however, need to be assessed in terms of environmental impact and ecosystem homeostasis. At present management is, practically speaking, restricted to chemotherapeutic treatment of infected and or symptomatic individuals.

Chemotherapy

The mainstay of treatment for all forms of schistosomiasis, whether systemic or involving the nervous system is praziquantel, given in an oral dose of 40 mg/kg stat. Oxamniquine, 15 mg/kg in a single oral dose with food, is similarly effective. Metrifonate, not widely available, has the advantage of low cost but has an inconvenient dose regimen of 7.5 to 10 mg/kg administered biweekly for three doses.

Steroids

The use of steroids is controversial, but because of the inflammatory component of granulomatous and necrotic myelitis lesions, they are used in conjunction with praziquantel, especially in severe infections. Rapid resolution of clinical symptoms with steroids alone has been documented many times. A commonly used dose is 60 mg daily for 2 weeks.

Surgery

Laminectomy may be required in patients presenting with acute paraplegia, incontinence, and spinal granulomatous mass lesions on radiologic imaging.

PROGNOSIS

The majority of patients improve dramatically with chemotherapy, especially if treated early in the course of disease. Improvement has occurred within days to weeks after treatment with steroids as well as with praziquantel. With clinical improvement, concomitant normalization of the CSF glucose, protein, cell count, and ELISA titers, as well as spinal cord conus shrinkage (in those with documented swelling), can be expected, as shown by Haribhai et al. (1991) in their prospective myelopathy study. Scrimgeour et al. and Gajdusek (1985) reported a mortality decrease from 72 percent prior to 1965 to 11.5 percent or less in 1985 in patients with confirmed schistosomal myelopathy. With MRI and more accurate serodiagnostic techniques, this figure may well be lower at present. The current trend in treatment in patients with a schistosomal syndrome is early use of praziquantel and use of steroids in selected cases.

ANNOTATED BIBLIOGRAPHY

Blansjaar BA. Schistosomiasis. In Vinken PJ, Bruyn GW. (eds). Handbook of Clinical Neurology. North Holland, Amsterdam, 1988, pp. 535–43.

Comprehensive overview of central nervous system schistosomiasis with good treatise of pathogenesis and clinical syndromes.

Capron A, Dessaint JP. Immunologic aspects of schistosomiasis. Annu Rev Med 1992;43:209–18.

IgE levels and acquired resistance.

Cosnett JE, Van DJ. Schistosomiasis (bilharzia) of the spinal cord: case reports and clinical profile. Q J Med 1985;61:1131–9.

Myelopathy profiles described.

Haribhai HC, Bhigjee AI, Bill PL et al: Spinal cord schistosomiasis. A clinical, laboratory and radiological study, with a note on therapeutic aspects. Brain 1991;114:709–26.

Details on 14 patients with transverse myelitis, conus medullaris, or cauda equina lesions. A CSF bilharzia ELISA test, developed to indicate infection, proved sensitive for the diagnosis.

King CH, Mahmoud AA. Drugs five years later: praziquantel. Ann Intern Med 1989;110:290–6.

Literature review from 1983 to July 1988. Cost factors seem to limit the use of praziquantel for trematode and cestode infections.

Mahmoud AAF, Wahab MFA. Schistosomiasis. In Warren KS, Mahmoud AAF (eds). Tropical and Geographic Medicine. 2nd Ed. McGraw-Hill, New York, 1990, pp. 458–73.

Standard reference.

Massachusetts General Hospital Case Records. Weekly clinicopathologic exercises. Case 21-195. A 21-year old man with fever, diarrhoea and weakness of the legs during a sojourn in Kenya. N Engl J Med 1985;312:1376–83.

Warnings to Westerners. Details of the conus medullaris and cauda equina syndromes.

Scrimgeour EM, Gajdusek DC. Involvement of the central nervous system in *Schistoma mansoni* and *S. hematobium* infection. Brain 1985;108:1023–38.

S. hematobium is mainly responsible for myelopathy in Africa, *S. mansoni* in the rest of the world.

45
Trypanosomiasis

Ayrton S. Massaro

AMERICAN TRYPANOSOMIASIS (CHAGAS' DISEASE)

Transmitted by hematophagous triatomid insects or reduviid bugs, Chagas' disease is a zoonosis resulting from human infections by a flagellated protozoan *Trypanosoma cruzi* (named for O. Cruz, Brazilian physician, 1872–1917) and has been named after C. Chagas (Brazilian physician, 1879–1934), who was responsible for most of the descriptions of the major clinical forms.

Epidemiology

The disorder is found only in the Western Hemisphere, where the sylvatic cycle is widely distributed from the southern United States to Argentina. Chagas' disease is endemic throughout Central and South America where an estimated 16 to 18 million persons are infected. Only a few cases have been reported in the United States despite the presence of several species of reduvid bugs and mammals infected with *T. cruzi*. In Latin America, patients live mostly in rural area. The amplitude of human infection is associated with the poor socioeconomic conditions of the population and the domestic nature of the vector. The infection remains a leading cause of heart disease in the endemic regions, and neurologic sequelae are infrequent.

Pathophysiology

The organism is found in wild and domestic animals and humans. The disease is transmitted by blood-seeking flying insects (Hemiptera) of the Reduvidae family (*Rhodnius, Triatoma, Pastrongylus*), also known in Portuguese as "chupanca" or "barbeiro," in Spanish as "vinchuca," and in English as "kissing bugs" or "assassin bugs."

Natural transmission of *T. cruzi* occurs in human when the feces of the infected bug, containing metacyclic trypomastigotes, contaminate a bite wound. A common and distinctive reduvid subfamily is known as kissing bugs for their tendency to bite the patient at mucocutaneous junctions, particularly the border of the lip and the outer canthus of the eye. After invading host cells, parasites replicate as amastigotes (Fig. 45-1) and differentiate into trypomastigotes, which are released when infected host cells rupture. The life cycle can then be completed when these circulating trypomastigotes are drawn into the insect vector on a subsequent bite.

Although most cases of human *T. cruzi* infection are acquired through the vector bites, other means are becoming significant. Blood transfusion from infected donors has been reported to cause Chagas' disease, especially in immunocompromised patients, including those with the acquired immunodeficiency syndrome (AIDS). Emigration of infected hosts to other countries also raises the risk of spreading the disease. Congenital transmission and infection of laboratory workers have also been documented.

In the acute stage of the disease, skeletal and cardiac muscles are the most heavily parasitized. A severe myocarditis develops in a small proportion of patients. This phase usually resolves spontaneously in 4 to 6 weeks. The cardiac disease is a cause of cerebral embolism.

Direct central nervous system (CNS) involvement in acute Chagas' disease is being increasingly described in children and may exist with mild clinical manifestations. A meningoencephalitis and acute chagasic multifocal encephalitis can occur. Direct brain involvement by parasites has been seen in macrophages, glial cells, and neurons and is thought to be the cause of neuronal depopulation, which has been seen in autopsy specimens. Immunocompromised patients, in-

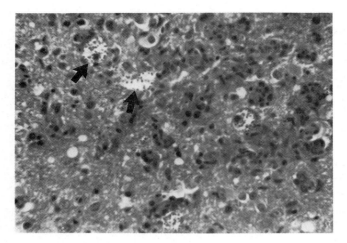

Figure 45-1. *T. cruzi* amastigotes forms *(arrows)* in the brain (parietal lobe).

cluding those suffering from AIDS, have shown diffuse meningoencephalitis affecting the hemispheric gray matter, basal ganglia, and cerebellum. Masses mimicking brain tumor have been reported biopsy-positive for *T. cruzi*. Even an obliterative arteritis is known to occur.

Clinical Features

The acute infection is usually not clinically evident or is present with only mild, nonspecific symptoms. In about one-third of newly inoculated patients, a distinctive inflammatory nodule, known as a chagoma, occurs and is usually associated with swollen satellite lymph nodes. There may be unilateral periorbital edema (Romana's sign). Fever, malaise, anorexia, mild limb edema, and hepatosplenomegaly may follow. After 2 weeks the parasites enter the circulation, favoring mesenchymal tissues, in which cysts form, degenerate, and burst open. Their bursting produces intense inflammatory reactions and releases organisms to invade even more widely, the nervous system being among the sites involved.

Neurologic involvement is uncommon, but the clinical syndromes are widely recognized. Episodes of mental confusion, somnolence, irritability, neck stiffness, and seizures may occur. Between 5 and 10 percent of patients die during the acute infection, often as the result of severe myocardial or cerebral involvement.

An indeterminate stage of Chagas' disease is characterized by the absence of symptoms, persistent antibody to *T. cruzi* and occult parasitemia. The majority of such patients never develop manifestations of chronic infection.

The chronic stage occurs in 10 to 30 percent of patients and may not develop for many years. Stroke is frequent in patients with severe cardiomyopathy from mural thrombi and ventricular dilation with apical aneurysms, usually demonstrable by echocardiography. The cardiac conduction system is also frequently affected, with bundle branch block a common finding. Muscle denervation and atrophy have been reported in chronic Chagas' disease and is probably explained by peripheral involvement by parasites. Neurologic symptoms have been described with cortical, pyramidal, and cerebellar signs.

Diagnosis

The diagnosis is made by demonstrating the organisms in a blood smear. If repeated attempts are unsuccessful, culture can be attempted. Polymerase chain reaction testing remains investigational.

Several tests are available for routine serologic diagnosis of chronic *T. cruzi* infection. The complement fixation, indirect hemagglutination, and indirect immunofluorescence tests are the most widely used in Latin America. Enzyme-linked immunosorbent assay (ELISA), when available, is now preferred.

The cerebrospinal fluid (CSF) in chronic infection shows increased numbers of lymphocytes and elevated protein and *T. cruzi* antibody levels. In immunosuppressed patients, bone marrow, pericardial fluid and CSF (Fig. 45-2) may contain parasites. Brain computed tomographic (CT) scan may show a contrast-enhancing, tumorlike mass with edema (Fig. 45-3).

Treatment and Prognosis

Benzimidazole and nifurtimox are the two best known drugs for acute Chagas' disease. There remain uncertainties about drug efficacy and the criteria for cure when these drugs are used in the acute stage of infection. Neurologic side effects of nifurtimox include restlessness, insomnia, and disorientation.

AFRICAN TRYPANOSOMIASIS (SLEEPING SICKNESS)

Trypanosoma brucei (named for D. Bruce, British surgeon, 1855–1931), a hemoflaggelate of the same genus as *T. cruzi*, is responsible for a fatal meningoencephalitis limited to Africa. Although known only in books to those in Western countries, sleeping sickness has been estimated to affect 20,000 annually of a population of over 50 million living in endemic areas.

Pathophysiology

Minor differences in clinical presentation and regional location have engendered belief that three subtypes exist: *T. brucei gambiense,* the best known of the dis-

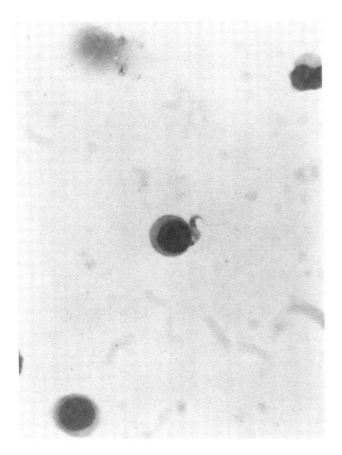

Figure 45-2. *T. cruzi* trypomastigote form in the CSF.

eases, endemic in Gambia and transmitted by the tsetse fly; *T. brucei rhodesiense,* also transmitted by the tsetse fly but differing from the subspecies responsible for Gambian trypanosomiasis; and *T. brucie brucie,* causing trypanosomiasis mainly in animals. The three subforms are currently recognized as variants of a single species, and it is likely the subspecies names will receive less use in future.

Humans, not domestic or wild animals, are thought to be the main reservoir except in Botswana, where the wild antelopes (known locally as bushbocks) are the main reservoir.

Parasites are directly injected into the patient during a blood meal. The bulk of the parasites remain initially at the inoculation site and form a chancre. Seeding through the bloodstream follows soon after, during which time the trypanosomes continue to multiply.

The neurologic manifestations arise from the clogging of small vessels in the brain, comparable with similar seeding in other organs. A meningoencephalitis occurs, together with perivascular cerebritis. This latter leads to widespread demyelination.

Clinical Features

The local chancre is tender and is accompanied by lymphadenopathy. The systemic signs include high fever, usually remitting, headache, subcutaneous nodules, lymphadenopathy, and splenomegaly. Distinctive syndromes have earned several eponyms not within the scope of this book. Hypogonadism has been described.

The neurologic symptoms in the early stages include severe headache, insomnia, and difficulty with concentration. The more serious stages occur later, months to many years after the initial inoculation. Thrombosis of many vessels can lead to sudden and severe neurologic deficits.

In the chronic stage of brain involvement, patients develop the syndrome that gave the disease the name sleeping sickness. Typically, they are inactive and appear mentally dulled. Electrophysiologic studies have documented a disorganization of the sleep-wake cycle, perhaps explaining the clinical appearance of sleep deprivation. More often, however, the clinical syndrome of widespread infection is that of an emerging dementia, accompanied by decline in activity and self-initiated behavior, accompanied by a vacant expression and drooping lids. Weight loss from lack of appetite, seizures, focal neurologic signs, and sustained high fever are among the signs appearing shortly before death.

Diagnosis

Wet mounts of the blood, CSF, or lymph node aspirate, allow direct demonstration of the parasites, which are best stained with Wright or Giemsa stain. Experience with an indirect fluorescent antibody test offers some hope for diagnosis when the wet mounts are negative.

Treatment and Prognosis

Untreated, the disease is fatal. Prior to the involvement of the nervous system, the current best treatment is with suramin. A test dose of 0.2 g IV is necessary to detect possible idiosyncratic reactions. If none is found, treatment can begin the next day with 1 g in 10 percent solution IV given on days 1, 3, 7, 14, and 21. This agent has poor penetration of the blood-brain barrier and for this reasons is not effective for patients with neurologic signs.

Melarsoprol, a form of British antilewisite, can be given in a dose of 1.8 to 3.6 mg/kg on 3 consecutive days, repeated again after days 10 and 21. A sudden aggravation of neurologic symptoms from death of parasites occurs in a minority of patients but can be severe enough to be fatal in some. Those with well advanced disease should be given lower doses. A Guil-

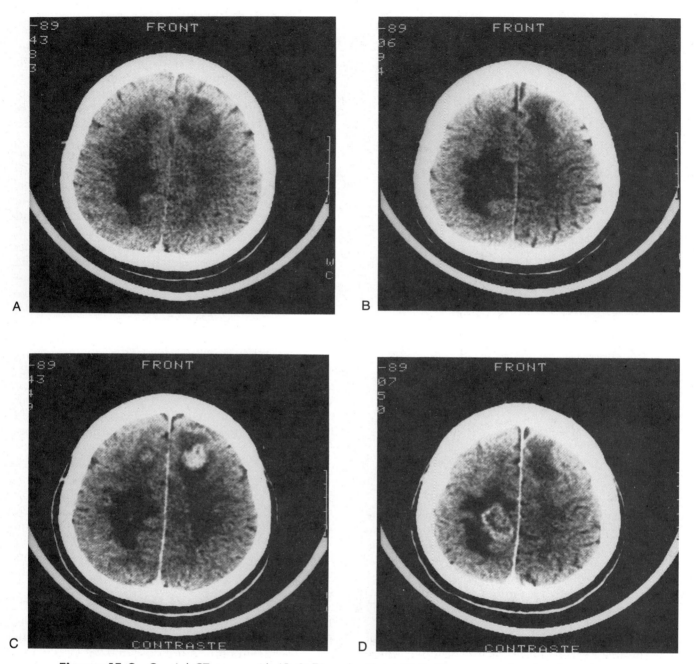

Figure 45-3. Cranial CT scans with (**A & B**) and without (**C & D**) contrast, showing the enhancing lesions with edema and mass effect in a patient with AIDS and reactivation of *T. cruzi* infection.

lain-Barré-like syndrome has been described with this therapy.

Recent reports have appeared of some success with the Gambian disease involving the nervous system by using nifurtimox, given at 30 mg/kg/day for 30 days in patients who are resistant to arsenicals. Those traveling to the endemic areas should have a single dose of pentamide 3 to 4 mg/kg IM, which will offer protec-

tion against Gambian sleeping sickness for more than 6 months.

ANNOTATED BIBLIOGRAPHY

Boa YF, Traore MA, Doua F et al: Les differents tableaux cliniques actuels de la trypanosomiase humaine africaine à T. b. gambiense. Analyse de 300 dossiers du foyer de

Daloa, Côte d'Ivoire. Bull Soc Pathol Exot Filiales 1988; 81:427–44.

Disorders of vigilance and sleeping disturbances in 69 percent, abnormal reflexes in 67 percent, tremor and movement disorders of choreoathetotic type in 35 percent, seizures in 35 percent, pareses or gait disorders in 15 percent, and psychiatric symptoms in 6 percent.

Chagas C. Nova tripanozomiaze humana. Estudos sobre a morfolojia e o cico evolutivo do *Schizotrypanum cruzi* n. gen., n. sp., ajente ediolojico de nova entidade morbida do homen. Mem Inst Oswaldo Cruz 1909;1:159–218.

The original article.

Kagan IG, Norman L, Allain D. Studies on *Trypanosoma cruzi* isolated in the United States. A review. Rev Biol Trop 1966;14:55–73.

Clinical classic.

Kirchoff IV. Current concepts: American trypanosomiasis (Chagas' disease)—a tropical disease now in the United States. N Engl J Med 1993;329:639–44.

Update.

Lyons M. African sleeping sickness: an historical review. Int J Study AIDS. 1991;2(suppl. 1):20–5.

Useful details.

Nothdurft HD, Taelman H, Boogaerts M et al. Schlafkrankheit bei deutschen Tropenreisenden. Dtsch Med Wochenschr 1989;114:1203–6.

Illness following a 2-day safari. Fever, lymphadenopathy and chancre led to blood smear, which made the diagnosis. Treatment with suramin sufficed. A risk of 0.3 per 100,000 was estimated for German travelers. (In German.)

Pepin J, Milord F, Meurice F et al: High-dose nifurtimox for arseno resistant Trypanosoma brucei gambiense sleeping sickness: an open trial in central Zaire. Trans R Soc Trop Med Hyg 1992;86:254–6.

Limited success with nifurtimox in arsenical-resistant disease.

Rosenberg S, Chaves CJ, Higuchi MI et al. Fatal meningoencephalitis caused by a reactivation of *Trypanosoma cruzi* infection in a patient with AIDS. Neurology 1992;42:640–2.

Single case report.

Spina-Franca A. Trypanosomiase americaine (maladie de Chagas) et le système nerveux. Bull Soc Pathol Exot Filiales 1988;81:645–9.

Review from an experienced Brazilian neurologist (in French).

Tapie P, Tabaraud F, Doua F et al. Sleep-wake cycle in human African trypanosomiasis. J Clin Neurophysiol 1993;10:190–6.

No hypersomnolence seen on 24-hour polysomnograms, only persistent disturbance of the sleep-wake cycles.

Villanueva MS. Trypanosomiasis of the central nervous system. Semin Neurol 1993;13:209–18.

Review of both American and African trypanosomiasis.

Zaniboni A. Suramin: the discovery of an old anticancer drug. Med Oncol Tumor Pharmacother 1990;7:287–90.

Experience with this agent.

46

Tuberculosis

M. Zuheir Al-Kawi

Although the first description of tuberculous meningitis in modern times is attributed to Sir Robert Whytt, it is clear that Avicenna (980–1037) was the first to give a detailed lucid description of meningitis. Tuberculosis was a major killer between the 17th and the early 20th centuries. The Industrial Revolution resulted in crowding in cities, which created favorable conditions for the spread of the disease. The mainstay of treatment was to boost the innate defenses of patients by improving their exposure to sun, open air, and good nutrition. Many sanatoria were built for that purpose in Europe and North America. Over 60 years passed between Koch's discovery of the pathogen and the advent of the antituberculous chemotherapy era, ushered by streptomycin in 1946. Since then, established cases have been easier to treat, and the incidence of new infections has declined.

Since the mid-1980s tuberculosis in general and central nervous system (CNS) tuberculosis in particular have regained some of their lost importance because of the influence of two major factors. Travel and migration have brought many people from endemic areas to low-incidence areas. The human immunodeficiency virus (HIV) epidemic has caused a surge in the active cases of tuberculous infection. As the pathology of the illness hangs in the balance between the load of organisms and the host's immune defense, a wide spectrum of interaction between the two brings in more cases, atypical presentations, or an immune reaction.

MICROBIOLOGY

The majority of human infections with mycobacteria is related to *Mycobacterium tuberculosis*. In the past, *Mycobacterium bovis* was responsible for some human cases, especially involving the gastrointestinal tract and joints (e.g., Pott's disease). Eradication of cattle disease and treatment of human cases have made this infection very rare. Patients with the acquired immunodeficiency syndrome (AIDS), however, are susceptible to infection with *Mycobacterium avium intracellulare*.

M. tuberculosis is a weakly gram-positive bacillus, which is aerobic and nonmotile and does not form spores. The bacilli are described as acid-fast or acid-alcohol-fast, and they require special staining such as the Ziehl-Neelsen stain, with which they appear as slightly curved red rods 2 to 4 μm long and 0.22 to 0.5 μm in width. Laboratories now use the auramine stain more frequently, with which the rod is easily distinguished by its yellow color against a blue background. Its growth is 20 times slower than that of *Escherichia coli*. This is probably related to the rate of synthesis of DNA, RNA, and proteins. The cell wall of the mycobacterium has a complex lipoid structure, which may play an important role in protecting it from natural bactericidal activity inside the macrophages.

EPIDEMIOLOGY

Tuberculous meningitis is always secondary to tuberculosis affecting other organs, the most common focus being in the lungs. It is generally stated that from 5 to 15 percent of people infected develop active tuberculosis. Only half of these cases become infectious (cavitary pulmonary), the other half being noncavitary or extrapulmonary. Only 5 to 10 percent of patients with active cases develop meningitis. Infection in childhood, miliary tuberculosis, malnutrition, alcoholism, and immuno deficiency or immunosuppression are predisposing factors. The morbidity of tuberculosis in patients with AIDS exceeds that in any other patient group.

PATHOLOGY

The CNS may be involved in one or more of three forms of tuberculosis: epidural (spinal or cranial) tuberculosis, intracranial tuberculomas, and tubercu-

669

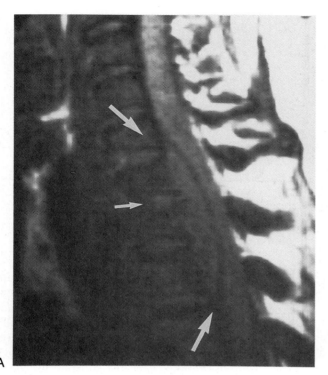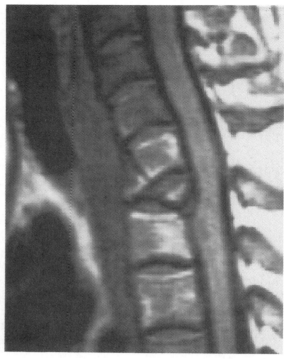

A

B

Figure 46-1. **(A)** Pott's disease at the cervicothoracic junction. Note the destruction of the disc space and the collapse of the anterior part of the vertebral body, as well as the epidural abscess causing posterior displacement and compression of the spinal cord *(arrows)* in a 25-year-old woman presenting with progressive paraplegia of a few months duration. **(B)** Following 12 months of antituberculous medications without surgery, the epidural abscess has resolved and pressure on the cord has been relieved, with marked clinical improvement. Note the residual vertebral body destruction and the high-intensity signal, which denotes healing changes.

lous meningitis. Epidural tuberculosis in the spinal column is usually secondary to infection of the cancellous bone in two adjacent vertebrae with destruction of the interposing disc. Granuloma or cold abscess may extend to the epidural space around the cord and cause cord compression and paraplegia (Fig. 46-1). On rare occasions, the epidural space may be the major site of involvement, with minimal bone destruction. Cord compression or thrombosis of a radicular artery may be responsible for paraplegia.

Intracranial tuberculomas are mass lesions, which can be found in different numbers and locations inside the parenchyma of the brain and occasionally under the surface of the meninges. A tuberculoma consists of granulation tissue and giant cells surrounding a center of caseation with a sparse population of mycobacteria. It is surrounded externally by a zone of gliosis with a variable amount of edema. Tuberculoma is to be distinguished from the rare tuberculous abscess; the latter contains pus with a large number of mycobacteria and indicates failure of the immune mechanism responsible for impeding the growth and proliferation of the organism.

In tuberculous meningitis there is predilection for the basal cisterns (prepontine, interpeduncular ambient, and chiasmatic) where inflammatory exudate accumulates. The normally transparent leptomeninges become opaque. A thick green exudate contains lymphocytes, plasma cells, and epithelioid cells. The penetrating arteries may undergo fibrinoid necrosis, which results in deep infarcts. Following treatment, the exudate thickens, becomes fibrous, and may compromise the function of cranial nerves by constriction, causing blindness or cranial palsies.

PATHOGENESIS

The organism never reaches the nervous system directly. Primary infection usually occurs in the lungs and spreads from the regional lymph nodes to the bloodstream via the thoracic duct. Primary hematogenous spread may result in disseminated miliary tuberculosis or produce a few metastatic foci. A caseous focus in the meninges, in the choroid, or near the surface of the brain may discharge its contents into the subarachnoid space, resulting in meningitis. On

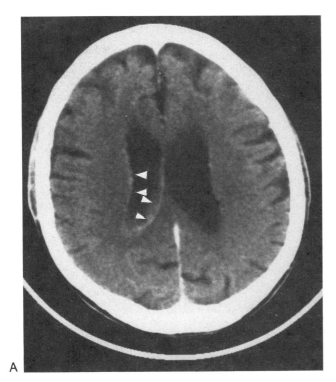 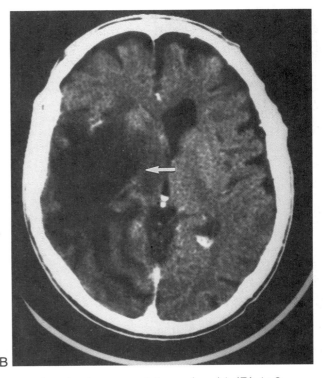

Figure 46-2. **(A)** Tuberculous ventriculitis. Note the ependymal enhancement *(arrowheads).* **(B)** At 2 months following initiation of treatment, the temporal horn of the right lateral ventricle was sequestered by ependymal adhesions (*arrow*), causing an acute unilateral hydrocephalus that required surgical shunting.

the other hand, late hematogenous tuberculosis may complicate chronic tuberculosis in any organ and be triggered by a compromise of cellular immunity. Progressive involvement of other organs, including the brain and the meninges, occurs. The complications of meningitis include hydrocephalus, which may be obstructive secondary to closure of the aqueduct by ependymitis or may be of the communicating variety secondary to basal meningitis. Isolated single ventricle entrapment and hydrocephalus may also occur (Fig. 46-2). Arteritis and phlebitis may lead to infarction or rarely to intracranial hemorrhage. Chronic inflammation may lead to arachnoiditis, with subsequent compromise of cranial nerves functions.

CLINICAL MANIFESTATIONS

Knowledge of patients' physical and social backgrounds may help in identifying them as belonging to the population at risk for tuberculosis. Prior residence in an endemic area or contact with an infected person should raise suspicion. Adverse living conditions, such as being homeless, incarcerated, malnourished, or alcoholic, increase the risk of active tuberculosis. Chronic illness such as AIDS, renal failure, or diabetes and treatment with corticosteroids and im-

munosuppression also favor dissemination and progression of infection. In persons infected with HIV, extrapulmonary tuberculosis, including that in the CNS, is common.

Symptoms and signs depend on the type and extent of infection; therefore, a wide spectrum is to be expected. Systemic symptoms such as fever and malaise are minimal or absent in tuberculoma but may be present in spinal tuberculosis and are most obvious in tuberculous meningitis. Fever, however, remains low-grade and rarely exceeds 39°C unless a complicating secondary infection, such as aspiration pneumonia, is present.

In *spinal tuberculosis,* back or neck pain is the initial symptom and may last for several months before progressive paraparesis sets in. Occasionally, sensory and motor signs in a radicular distribution suggest the level of epidural granuloma. *Intracranial tuberculoma,* on the other hand, presents with the general symptoms of a space-occupying lesion, such as headache and convulsions. Focal signs of motor or sensory disturbance may come late. Rarely, the tuberculoma may involve a critical area such as the hypothalamus, in which case endocrine abnormalities may be an early manifestation (Fig. 46-3). The salient clinical features of *tuberculous meningitis* include fever, headache, and vomiting, fol-

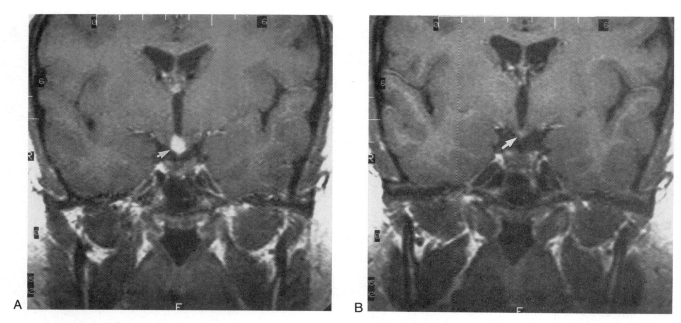

Figure 46-3. **(A)** An 18-year-old woman presenting with obesity, amenorrhea, and diabetes insipidus. Gadolinium-enhanced T₁-weighted images on magnetic resonance imaging (MRI) shows a hypothalamic tuberculoma. *(arrow)*. **(B)** After 15 month of antituberculous therapy, the tuberculoma resolved completely *(arrow)*.

lowed by lethargy and convulsions. Stiff neck and Kernig and Brudzinski signs can be minimal in children and are always much less marked than in pyogenic meningitides. Signs of raised intracranial pressure are common, and diplopia and decreased visual acuity may occur at any point during the course of the illness. Fundoscopy can show choroidal tubercles as ill-defined, yellowish, round or oval bodies. It may also show papilledema. Focal signs such as hemiplegia or aphasia occur later in unrecognized cases and suggest infarction secondary to arteritis. In miliary tuberculosis, involvement of the choroid with tubercles and phlyctenular keratitis (from the Greek for blisters on the cornea) are suggestive of the disease. An encephalopathic picture comes late and may be followed by rapid progression to coma and death.

DIAGNOSIS

Evidence for tuberculosis elsewhere in the body should be sought, and chest x-ray in particular is helpful. Skin tests for delayed hypersensitivity to tuberculin purified protein derivative (PPD) (Mantoux, Tine, Heaf) are of limited value, and their value decrease with increasing patient age, especially in endemic areas where positive skin test is commonplace. A positive skin test, however, is significant in populations with low exposure to tuberculosis or vaccination, while a negative test does not rule out the diagnosis. Imag-

ing studies are the essential modalities in investigating intracranial tuberculomas and spinal tuberculosis, while cerebrospinal fluid (CSF) examination is the major test in tuberculous meningitis.

Spinal tuberculosis presents with back pain, which may or may not be accompanied by radicular symptoms and signs. Radiographic evaluation of the clinically suspected region of the vertebral column is usually obtained first. Findings in the early stages may be subtle; narrowing of the disc space appears first, followed by involvement of the adjacent vertebral bodies manifested by irregular borders. Further destruction, especially anteriorly, causes wedging of the vertebral bodies and kyphosis. The characteristic gibbus is then formed. Paraspinal abscess appears as a soft tissue density shadow surrounding the involved area. Levels commonly involved are the thoracic followed by the lumbar and cervical region. Myelography shows an extradural defect in the contrast column or complete block at the involved level. Computed tomography (CT) gives further details about the destruction of vertebral bodies and abscess formation, especially if performed following myelography (CT-myelography). Magnetic resonance imaging (MRI) is even more effective in demonstrating anatomic details and may be more sensitive in early cases, showing signal changes in the vertebral bodies. A CT-guided biopsy of the involved area in experienced hands can retrieve material for pathologic and microbiologic confirmation. The differential diagnosis includes metastatic malignancies, lymphoma, and bacterial spondylitis with *E. coli, Brucella,* or *Staphylococcus.*

In the case of intracranial tuberculomas, a CT of the head with contrast enhancement shows a single or multiple mass lesions of varying size, typically with ring enhancement but no evidence of the enhancement typical of tumor found on CT or cerebral angiography. Helpful features in reaching the diagnosis in this case include the patient's residence in an endemic area or exposure to a known case, evidence of tuberculosis elsewhere in the body, multiplicity of lesions, and relatively less severe symptoms and signs than would be expected from a mass lesion of similar size and location if it were malignant. MRI with gadolinium enhancement is more sensitive and helps in detecting smaller tuberculomas, especially in the subpial location. Differential diagnosis includes intracranial neoplasms such as meningioma, glioma, lymphoma, metastatic malignancies, multiple abscesses, toxoplasmosis, and fungal infections. In the proper clinical setting, if the patient's condition permits and when follow-up imaging studies are obtainable, a therapeutic trial with antituberculosis drugs for 3 to 6 weeks may help clarify the diagnosis and spare the patient a craniotomy. Corticosteroids should be avoided during the therapeutic trial. In cases in which the diagnosis is uncertain, a stereotaxic or open biopsy is needed. Care is to be exercised to avoid disseminating the infection to the subarachnoid space (Fig. 46-4B) and to ensure adequate coverage with antituberculous drugs.

In *tuberculous meningitis,* imaging studies show the typical meningeal enhancement in the basal cisterns or the ependymal enhancement in the ventricles commonly associated with hydrocephalus. The combination of parenchymal lesions (tuberculoma), meningeal enhancement, and some degree of hydrocephalus is characteristic. The CSF characteristically shows lymphocytic pleocytosis and decreased glucose. Protein levels are rarely normal and may be very high. The diagnosis is usually based on identifying *M. tuberculosis* in the CSF by a direct smear or by culture in Löwenstein-Jensen medium. The organism may be difficult to see on acid-fast smear owing to the relatively low number of bacilli in the lumbar CSF. Ventricular fluid, if available, is more revealing. The detection rate is proportional to the time spent in

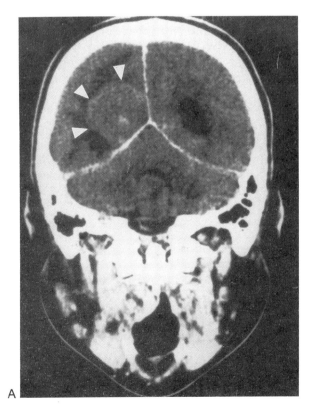
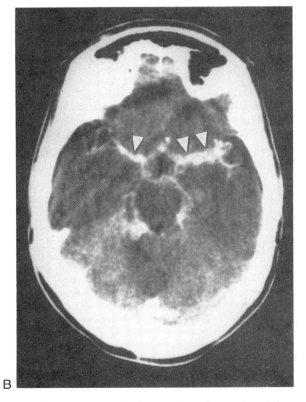

A

B

Figure 46-4. **(A)** A large tuberculoma in the medial part of the posterior right hemisphere *(arrowheads).* **(B)** Following biopsy, contamination of the subarachnoid space with tuberculosis resulted in meningitis and typical enhancement of the basal meninges *(arrowheads).*

examining the smear under the microscope. Growing *M. tuberculosis* takes a minimum of 3 weeks and usually 6 weeks. Positive results, however, may be obtained by smear or culture even days after therapy has been started. Indirect methods of testing the CSF have been reported to be helpful in rapid diagnosis. These include bromide partition and adenosine deaminase activity, although the latter may give similar titers in lymphoma or brucellosis. Newer methods allow the detection of antibodies against mycobacteria or Bacille Calmette-Guérin (BCG) antigens by enzyme-linked immunosorbent assay (ELISA) or detection of parts of the mycobacterial genome after amplification by the polymerase chain reaction. The diagnosis is not excluded by a normal peripheral white count, erythrocyte sedimentation rate chest x-ray, or CSF.

The differential diagnosis includes viral meningitis, fungal meningitis, postinfectious encephalomyelitis, and occasionally brucellosis or partly treated pyogenic meningitis. In the latter case C-reactive protein, lactate dehydrogenase, or N-acetylneuraminic acid in the CSF may show positive or increased titers.

MANAGEMENT

Antituberculous chemotherapy involves the use of drugs with good penetration into the CSF, and triple drug therapy is recommended, especially during the first 3 months of treatment. Table 46-1 lists the commonly used drugs in their order of importance. Since the majority of these drugs are available only in oral forms, severely sick patients have to be treated through a gastric tube. The duration of treatment should be individualized, depending on the extent of infection at the time of diagnosis and the rate of resolution of symptoms and signs. It generally ranges from 9 to 18 months. Shorter courses remain controversial in CNS tuberculosis and may not prevent recrudescence.

Adjunctive management includes supplemental pyridoxine (vitamin B_6), 10 to 25 mg/day, which should be added to isonicotinic hydrazide (INH) to prevent neuropathy. Supportive treatment should include attention to nutrition and fluid and electrolyte balance. Hyponatremia secondary to inappropriate secretion of antidiuretic hormone (SIADH) is very common and frequently requires fluid restriction, in addition to the use of hypertonic saline solutions with or without diuretics. The use of corticosteroids remains controversial, but it should be considered in severely ill patients and occasionally in children and in those with severe changes in the CSF that suggest an impending spinal block.

Common complications, such as convulsions, require careful management. Some antiepileptic drugs may increase the chance of hepatotoxicity when combined with antituberculous medications. Careful choice and proper attention to blood levels while monitoring the liver function tests is necessary. Many patients can be withdrawn from antiepileptic medications once the infection has resolved and convulsions have not recurred.

When meningitis is accompanied by significant hydrocephalus, a shunt procedure is indicated, especially when there are signs of increased intracranial pressure. Shunting is usually followed by improvement in the patient's level of alertness. Surgery has a limited role in the treatment of spinal tuberculosis, as chemotherapy is effective in the majority of patients, with surprising return of function after complete paraplegia in several cases.

PROGNOSIS

While return of function is expected with medical treatment in most cases of spinal tuberculosis and isolated intracranial tuberculoma, meningeal infection carries a worse prognosis. Severe disease at diagnosis is associated with high mortality and morbidity. Complications include cranial nerve palsies, hemiplegia,

Table 46-1. Drugs Commonly Used for Antituberculous Chemotherapy

Drug	Dosage, mg/kg	Average Adult Dose	Side Effects
Isoniazid	15	300–600 mg once daily	Polyneuritis Hepatotoxicity
Pyrazinamide	30	1.5–3 g daily	Hepatotoxicity, hyperuricemia, gastrointestinal intolerance
Rifampicin	10	600 mg once per day before breakfast	Liver dysfunction, contraceptive failure, body fluids discoloration
Ethambutol	15–25	1 g daily	Optic neuritis, teratogenic
Streptomycin	15–40	1 g daily IM	Eighth cranial nerve damage
Ethionamide	15	1 g daily	Hepatotoxic, gastrointestinal intolerance, hypoglycemia in diabetics

paraplegia, aphasia, seizures, loss of cognitive functions, hydrocephalus, and hydromyelia.

ANNOTATED BIBLIOGRAPHY

Al-Deeb SM, Yaqub BA, Sharif HS, Motaery KR. Neurotuberculosis: a review. Clin Neurol Neurosurg 1992;94 (suppl.):S30–3.

General review of tuberculosis around the world.

Goel A, Pandya SK, Satoskar AR. Whither short-course chemotherapy for tuberculous meningitis? Neurosurgery 1990;27:418–21.

Treatment for less than 2 years seemed insufficient, as recrudescence of meningitis and some more serious complications occurred. Longer therapy is recommended.

Harder EJ, Al Kawi MZ, Carney P. Intracranial tuberculoma: conservative management. Am J Med 1983;74: 570–76.

Saudi Arabian experience.

Leonard JM, Des-Prez RM. Tuberculous meningitis. Infect Dis Clin North Am 1990;4:769–87.

Thorough modern review.

Maniar P, Joshi L. ELISA—its evaluation in diagnosis of tuberculosis meningitis. Indian J Pediatr 1990;57: 667–72.

ELISA showed a sensitivity of 97.72 percent and a specificity of 95.35 percent for tuberculous meningitis.

Palur R, Rajshekhar V, Chandy MJ et al. Shunt surgery for hydrocephalus in tuberculous meningitis: a long-term follow-up study. J Neurosurg 1991;74:64–9.

In a study of 114 patients with tuberculous meningitis and hydrocephalus, the less affected patients seemed to respond better.

Parsons M. Tuberculous Meningitis, Tuberculomas and Spinal Tuberculosis. Oxford University Press, New York, 1988.

Standard book reference.

Pettersson T, Klockars M, Weber TH, Somer H. Diagnostic value of cerebnrospinal fluid adenosine deaminase determination. Scand J Infect Dis 1992;24:121–2.

Short report of comparison with viral and bacterial meningitis and other neurologic diseases, showing the highest adenosine deaminase activities in patients with tuberculous meningitis (median 21.3 units/L, range 20.0 to 23.0). Lymphoma was a close sceond.

Shankar P, Manjunath N, Mohan KK et al. Rapid diagnosis of tuberculous meningitis by polymerase chain reaction. Lancet. 1991;337:5–7.

PCR was more sensitive than conventional bacteriology and ELISA in confirming clinical diagnosis of tuberculous meningitis.

Snider DE Jr, Roper WL. The new tuberculosis (editorial). N Engl J Med 1992;326:668–72.

Modern editorial review.

Tandon PN, Bhatia R, Bhargava S. Handbook of Clinical Neurology. Vol. 52. 1988; p. 15.

Textbook chapter.

World Health Organization. Drugs used in mycobacterial disease. Model Prescribing Information 1991.

Details of options for therapy.

47
Brucellosis

M. Zuheir Al-Kawi

Humans become infected with brucellosis as secondary hosts since the disease is primarily a zoonosis. Malta fever, Mediterranean fever, and undulant fever are but a few of the names used to refer to this disease. Chronicity and intracellular infection give the disease a similarity to tuberculosis, while multiplicity and variety of symptoms make it a great mimicker similarly to syphilis.

MICROBIOLOGY

There are six species of the *Brucella* genus (D. Bruce, British surgeon, 1855–1911). Only the first three are known to cause significant human disease. In order of frequency, they are as follows: *Brucella melitensis* (primarily found in sheep and goats); *B. abortus* (infects cattle); *B. suis* (primarily infects swine and rodents); *B. canis* (infects dogs but rarely humans); and *B. neotomae* and *B. ovis*, which are not reported to infect humans.

The organisms are facultatively intracellular, small, nonencapsulated gram-negative short rods (bacilli or coccobacilli), 0.5 by 0.6 to 1.5 μm in size. They are aerobic and nonmotile and do not form spores. They withstand freezing for several weeks but require special media and long incubation for isolation in cultures. Human infection occurs by consumption of uncooked meat or unpasteurized dairy products, by contact with animal carcasses, or (in veterinarians) at the time of delivery of animals. Cheese or ice cream made of unpasteurized goat milk may maintain infective organisms for up to 8 weeks.

EPIDEMIOLOGY

The prevalence is variable and depends on the level of control of animal disease. No accurate figures for incidence of human cases exist from many countries where the disease is endemic. It is common in countries around the Mediterranean. The quoted incidence, per 100,000 is 12 per year, in Spain and 20 in Greece, compared with 0.1 in the United States. It is estimated that nearly 7 percent of the patients develop neurologic involvement.

PATHOGENESIS

Entry in humans usually occurs via the oral route. Rarely, the disease may be transmitted by blood transfusion or through the placenta to the fetus. Unusual routes include the skin in slaughterhouse workers, inhalation of aerosolized organisms by animal handlers, and contact with open wounds or injection of live vaccine by veterinarians. Stomach acidity may be the first natural barrier against infection. One of the author's patients developed the clinical infection while receiving an antacid H_2-blocker, but her family consuming the same food escaped.

After entry, polymorphonuclear leukocytes are attracted to phagocytize the organism. Depending on the virulence of the organism, it may either be killed or survive. Macrophages are also involved; interacting with T cells, they proliferate and take up the invading bacteria. Intracellular bactericidal activity requires fusion of phagosomes with the lysosomes, a process virulent strains can evade by virtue of containing some inhibitory compounds in the cell wall. *B. melitensis*, for example, is more resistant to intracellular bactericidal activity and consequently causes more infections in humans. The macrophages would then provide the organisms with a protected place to multiply and carry infection to other organs, including the liver, spleen, bone, and probably brain.

Humoral- as well as cell-mediated immunity is involved in the defense and pathogenesis. IgM antibodies arise earlier, and their susceptibility to precipitation by 2-mercaptoethanol (2-ME) is tested in separating titers related to IgG and to IgM antibodies on agglutination tests. IgG antibodies rise later. Both IgG and IgA antibodies may act as agglutinating or blocking antibodies. Blocking antibodies appear in long-standing chronic brucellosis, in which central nervous system (CNS) involvement commonly occurs, and cause problems in serologic diagnosis. Different types of T lymphocytes are stimulated by the brucella antigens, and they in turn activate macrophages through the balance of the different cytokines secreted by T cells. This intricate balance leads to variability and different intensity of clinical manifestations. Granuloma formation may occur in several tissues, including bones. Spondylitis, vertebral collapse, and abscess formation lead to cord compression. Chronic symptoms are probably related to a more complex mechanism, including vasculitis or an immune complex mechanism, it is poorly understood. Reported pathologic changes in the CNS include acute and chronic vasculitis, inflammatory cell infiltration in the meninges and perivascular spaces, encephalomalacia, and demyelination in the cord and roots.

CLINICAL MANIFESTATIONS

Headache and behavioral changes can be easily recognized as related to a meningoencephalitic process, especially when accompanied by nausea and vomiting. Other symptoms may show less obvious links. Psychiatric manifestations may range from simple lack of concentration to anxiety, agitation, depression, and frank psychosis with hallucinations. The patient may present with signs of raised intracranial pressure and papilledema. Deafness is frequent. Diplopia, facial paresis, and/or vertigo herald the involvement of other cranial nerves. Atypical brief transient episodes of unilateral numbness, akin to transient ischemic attacks (TIAs), may occur and may occasionally be associated with drop attacks. Myelopathy when associated with nystagmus or oculomotor abnormalities may mimic multiple sclerosis. In cases of myeloradiculopathy, root involvement may predominate early, raising suspicion of an acute inflammatory neuropathy and masking the signs of myelopathy. Radiculitis improves first after treatment and may give way to the appearance of myelopathic symptoms with spasticity and hyperreflexia. Epileptic seizures and psychiatric symptoms may be the presenting complaint; they frequently become exacerbated or appear de novo shortly after treatment is started. Abnormal movements such as myoclonus or tremor may appear, as well as focal neurologic deficits such as hemiplegia or aphasia. The paucity of systemic symptoms and signs

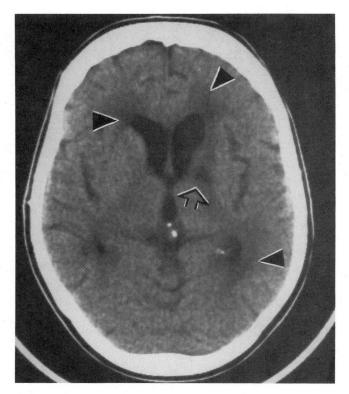

Figure 47-1. Spondylitis *(arrows)* in spinal brucellosis.

is not uncommon. Fever, lymphadenopathy, splenomegaly, and even nuchal rigidity may be absent.

IMAGING

Imaging studies in the case of spinal involvement show findings (Fig. 47-1) similar to those of tuberculous spondylitis (see Ch. 46). Brain imaging studies are frequently negative or nonspecific. Computed tomography (CT) may show focal hypodensities (Fig. 47-2) from infarction in the case of vasculitis or may show nonspecific calcifications. Cerebral angiography is usually negative in cases presenting with TIA-like symptoms but may show arterial occlusions. Magnetic resonance imaging (MRI) is more sensitive and may show multifocal or diffuse subcortical white matter changes (Fig. 47-3), which require differentiation from multiple sclerosis. Meningeal enhancement after gadolinium injection may be seen in meningoencephalitis.

DIAGNOSIS

A high index of suspicion is necessary, as the disease may present with protean symptoms. History of exposure should be actively sought when symptoms and signs are suggestive. Cerebrospinal fluid (CSF) analy-

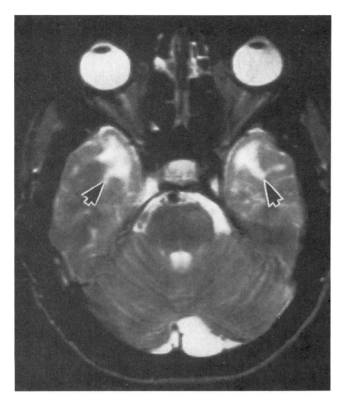

Figure 47-2. Ct scan showing multiple focal hypodensities *(arrows)* from infarction in a case of brucellosis.

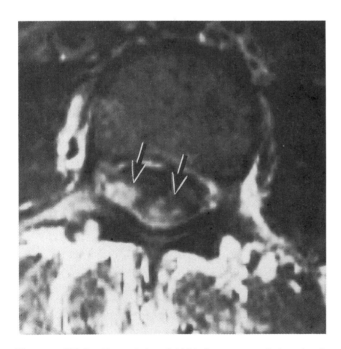

Figure 47-3. T₂-weighted MRI showing multifocal subcortical white matter changes *(arrows)* in a case of brucellosis.

sis shows moderate pleocytosis, commonly with lymphocytic predominance, hypoglycorrachia, and variable increase in protein content, usually less than that seen in tuberculous meningitis. Isolation of the organism by culture of blood, bone marrow, or CSF is definitive but not always successful. Chances of growth become less with the chronicity of the infection. Serologic studies are the mainstay of laboratory confirmation. The standard agglutination test remains useful and reproducible. A titer of 1:160 dilution or higher in the serum is supportive of the diagnosis. A titer of 1:80 is suspicious and requires repeating the test in 1 week. A low titer or false-negative is not uncommon and is attributed to blocking antibodies; in that case the anti-human globulin (Coombs) test or repetition of the agglutination test at higher dilutions to avoid the prozone phenomenon is helpful. Pretreatment of specimens with 2-mercaptoethanol allows differentiation between IgG and IgM antibodies. Recently, enzyme-linked immunosorbent assay (ELISA) has been adopted in a number of laboratories because of its sensitivity and specificity. The presence of agglutinating titers in the CSF is diagnostic, especially if a high ratio relative to the titers in the serum is present.

DIFFERENTIAL DIAGNOSIS

The list of diseases mimicked by neurobrucellosis is a long one. Back pain and radiculopathic symptoms should be differentiated from herniated intervertebral disc. Tuberculosis and viral and fungal infections are to be differentiated from brucella meningoencephalitis. Symptoms of polyradiculitis may be mistaken for Guillain-Barré syndrome. Neurobrucellosis should be considered in the etiology of psychosis, intracranial hypertension, and subarachnoid and intracerebral hemorrhage in endemic regions or when atypical features are present.

TREATMENT

At least two drugs with good intracellular activity and CNS penetration should be used (Table 47-1). The duration of therapy should be no less than 3 months. Some chronic infections require 6 to 9 months of therapy, guided by the persistence of CSF pleocytosis. A Jarisch-Herxheimer type of reaction has been reported in the early phase of treatment. It was usually mild or moderate and manifested by fever, arthralgia, tachycardia, and worsening headache. Interruption of treatment however was not necessary. Triple therapy with doxycycline, rifampicin, and cotrimoxazole is probably most effective. Doxycycline has the advantage of lipid solubility and infrequent doses, but it may produce gastrointestinal, photosensitivity, bone, and

Table 47-1. Drugs in the Treatment of Brucellosis

	Advantage	Disadvantage	Dose	Side Effect
Doxycyline	Lipid-soluble, infrequent doses		100 mg bid	Gastrointestinal Photosensitivity Bone and dental
Tetracycline		Frequent doses	500 mg qid	As above ?Nephrotoxic
Cotrimoxazole	Oral and intravenous forms	Relapse rate	160 mg tid	Nausea, vomiting
				Bone marrow suppression Skin rash
Rifampicin	Lipid-soluble		600–900 mg/daily	Nausea Vomiting Hepatotoxic Flushes
Ciprofloxacin		Not well tested		
Streptomycin		Intramuscular, painful	1 g daily	Ototoxicity

dental side effects. Tetracycline requires frequent doses, 500 mg qid, has side effects similar to those of doxycycline, and may be nephrotoxic. Cotrimoxazole, available in both intravenous and oral forms, given 160 mg tid, has the disadvantages of a high relapse rate, nausea, vomiting, occasional bone marrow suppression, and skin rash. Rifampicin, a lipid-soluble agent given 600 to 900 mg daily, may cause nausea, vomiting, hepatotoxic effects, and occasionally also flushing. Streptomycin must be given by a painful intramuscular injection, in a dose of 1 g daily and has a well-known ototoxicity. Ciprofloxacin has not been well tested.

ANNOTATED BIBLIOGRAPHY

Al-Deeb SM, Yaqub BA, Sharif HS et al. Neurobrucellosis. In Vinken PJ, Bruyn GW (eds). Handbook of Clinical Neurology. Vol. 8(52). Elsevier, Amsterdam, 1988.

Textbook chapter.

Bashir R, Al-Kawi MZ, Harder EJ, Jinkins J. Nervous system brucellosis: diagnosis and treatment. Neurology 1985; 35:1576–81.

Early experiences in Saudi Arabia.

Lulu AR, Araj GF, Khateeb MI et al. Human brucellosis in Kuwait: a prospective study of 400 cases. Q J Med 1988; 66:39–54.

Fully 77 percent of patients showed acute disease with fever, rigor, headache, sweating, arthralgia, myalgia, and low back pain. Neurobrucellosis occurred in 7 percent and hepatosplenomegaly in 41 percent. Raw milk was the usual source of infec-

tion. A relapse rate of 50 percent was seen with cotrimoxazole treatment. Streptomycin combined with either tetracycline, rifampicin, or doxycycline was more effective, but the best results were obtained with a combination of with streptomycin, tetracycline, and rifampicin.

Madkour MM (ed). Brucellosis. Butterworths, London, 1989.

Entire monograph on the subject.

McLean DR, Russell N, Khan MY. Neurobrucellosis: clinical and therapeutic features. Clin Infect Dis 1992;15: 582–90.

In 18 patients seen in Riyadh, 11 had meningitis alone or with papilledema, optic neuropathy, or radiculopathy. Meningovascular disease with stroke or hemorrhage occurred in four. Eleven recovered fully with treatment.

Mousa AM, Bahar RH, Araj GF et al. Neurological complications of brucella spondylitis. Acta Neurol Scand 1990; 81:16–23.

Spondylitis from brucellosis is common. In 15 of 22 patients, spondylitis was associated with neurologic complications.

Mousa AM, Muhtaseb SA, Reddy RR et al. The high rate of prevalence of CT detected basal ganglia calcification in neuropsychiatric (CNS) brucellosis. Acta Neurol Scand 1987;76:448–56.

CT-detected calcifications in the basal ganglia in 9 out of 65 patients with CNS brucellosis.

Sharif HS, Clark DC, Aabed MY et al. Granulomatous spinal infections: MR imaging. Radiology 1990;177:101–7.

MRI used in 81 patients with spinal granulomatous disease allowed prediction of the presence of neurologic complications in 93 percent. Healing was suggested by high signal intensity on T_1-weighted images.

48
Viral Infections

John J. Halperin

GENERAL FEATURES OF VIRAL INFECTIONS

Viral infections of the nervous system may involve the meninges (meningitis), the brain (encephalitis), the spinal cord (myelitis), or dorsal root ganglion neurons (neuronitis). Of these, dorsal root ganglion neuronitis is probably the most common, occurring frequently with the varicella-zoster virus. Meningitis is more common than encephalomyelitis. In each instance, the site of infection reflects a specific interaction between the virus and the host.

Some aspects of these infections are common to virtually all agents. The patient with viral (so-called aseptic) meningitis, a term implying meningeal inflammation and presumably infection, in the absence of a bacterial pathogen, typically presents with headache, mild to moderate meningismus, photophobia, and systemic symptoms indicative of infection, such as fever and malaise. Patients with encephalitis, who almost always have a concomitant meningitis, have varying levels of depressed consciousness, seizures, or focal abnormalities, depending on the location and severity of involvement.

Although some infectious agents have typical clinical presentations, the signs and symptoms are more commonly rather nonspecific, and laboratory and epidemiologic support for a specific diagnosis becomes necessary. Outbreaks of diseases that occur in late summer and fall are often enteroviral. Summertime clusters may be due to arboviral infection, something national public health surveillance networks generally can anticipate. In the prevaccination era, winter epidemics were typically related to mumps or measles. Exposure to pets should bring lymphocytic choriomeningitis virus infection to mind; exposure to rodents suggests leptospirosis. Animal bites raise the possibility of rabies; arthropod bites suggest arboviruses; monkey bites can cause myelitis as a result of monkey B (herpes simian) virus.

Approximately three-quarters of all cases of aseptic meningitis are attributable to enteroviral infection; the remainder are due to mumps, herpes, lymphocytic choriomeningitis virus, adenoviruses, California viruses, leptospirosis, and human immunodeficiency virus. In contrast, in approximately three-quarters of cases of encephalitis, the etiologic agent is never identified. One-quarter of encephalitis cases used to be due to mumps, but this entity has essentially disappeared with widespread vaccination, at least in Western countries.

General laboratory findings are typical of those seen in viral syndromes that affect almost any organ system, although some infections, such as herpes encephalitis, may more commonly be associated with a leukocytosis or hyponatremia. Cerebrospinal fluid (CSF) examination generally demonstrates a significant lymphocytic/ monocytic pleocytosis (100s to 1,000 or so cells), although in the first 24 to 48 hours of infection, a neutrophilic pleocytosis may predominate. The CSF protein concentration is usually modestly elevated; the glucose level is usually normal. In some infections, especially herpes, a moderate number of erythrocytes may be present.

The diagnosis of the specific etiologic agent generally involves a combination of epidemiologic considerations, clinical phenomena, and specific laboratory investigations, including viral culture of the CSF, measurement of specific immunoglobulin (Ig)M antibody or measurement of rising peripheral blood antibody titers over time, typically a fourfold rise in titer over 3 to 6 weeks. More recently, detection of viral genomic material with the polymerase chain reaction (PCR) has become useful in the diagnosis of some infections, particularly herpes.

In most instances, viral infection of the nervous system is an outgrowth of systemic infection. Although many organisms cause systemic infection, only a select few can breach the blood-brain barrier. The efficacy of this barrier is evidenced by the rarity of central nervous system (CNS) viral infection, averaging slightly more than 10,000 cases of aseptic meningitis and 1,000 cases of primary encephalitis per year in the United States. It is presumed that CNS invasion most commonly occurs by penetration of the blood-brain barrier at its weakest points, either the choroid plexus or by entry into peripheral nerves at their unprotected peripheral terminals, with subsequent axonal transport back into the CNS. Most diagnosable nervous system viral infections fall into one of the five following groups: (1) the human T-cell lymphotropic viruses (HTLV); (2) enteroviruses; (3) arboviruses; (4) herpesviruses; and (5) miscellaneous (rabies, rubeola, rubella, and mumps). (Table 48-1). The HTLV viruses are considered separately.

HERPES

Herpes (Greek: *herpein,* to creep—the same etymology as "serpent," as in the skin eruption from shingles) virus infections of the CNS, particularly herpes simplex (HSV) are important for several reasons. First, except for those occasions when arbovirus epidemics occur, they are the most common cause of encephalitis, causing 20 percent of all cases in the United States in which an etiologic agent can be determined. Second, their effects on the nervous system can be devastating; untreated, the mortality rate from HSV-1 encephalitis (which accounts for 95 percent of all adult herpes encephalitis cases) can exceed two-thirds of patients, with major sequelae in many of the survivors. Most important, if diagnosed and treated rapidly with acyclovir, the morbidity and mortality rates can be decreased substantially.

The herpesviruses are fairly large, enveloped viruses, with icosahedral symmetry, containing double-stranded DNA. This group includes herpes simplex types 1 and 2, human herpesvirus 6, cytomegalovirus, varicella-zoster, and Epstein-Barr virus.

Herpes Simplex

HSV-1, distributed worldwide, most commonly causes oral lesions but is the most common cause of HSV encephalitis. Patients with HSV encephalitis may or may not have an antecedent history of oral herpes. In one-third of patients with encephalitis, the infection is probably primary; in the remainder, it represents dissemination of previously acquired and dormant virus. There is no specific age predilection. HSV-1 encephalitis occurs sporadically throughout the year, sometimes beginning as a nonspecific febrile illness and other times as a febrile illness with abrupt development of focal neurologic signs. Experimental evidence indicates that this virus can enter the CNS through the olfactory nerve; other studies have suggested intracranial migration from the nucleus of the ophthalmic division of the trigeminal ganglion. Because either mechanism could account for its topography, the issue remains unresolved.

Although this agent has a predilection for the medial frontal and medial temporal lobes (limbic encephalitis), many patients do not have the classic presentation with headache, personality change, temporal lobe seizures, and memory loss. Patients may initially develop seizures, ataxia, cranial nerve palsies, hemiparesis, and the less well-recognized dysautonomia (reflected by gastrointestinal hypoactivity, urinary retention, and hypotension). The syndrome usually progresses over 1 to 2 weeks. The variation in the clinical picture makes precise diagnosis difficult. The results of computed tomographic scans, expected to show hemorrhagic medial temporal lobe lesions, may be negative early on, although ultimately, electroencephalography, magnetic resonance imaging, and even radionuclide brain scans usually implicate a temporal lobe focus. The CSF often demonstrates a neutrophilic pleocytosis early, rapidly evolving to a lymphocyte-predominant picture, frequently with a hemorrhagic component and occasionally with some depression of the CSF glucose level. In rare patients, the CSF may be completely normal.

Even in the best of centers, clinical assessment may lead to diagnosis of HSV encephalitis when other causes are responsible for the patient's difficulty. Therefore, brain biopsy has been widely recommended in the past for definitive diagnosis (Fig. 48.1). Pathologic study demonstrates a hemorrhagic necrotizing encephalitis with intranuclear Cowdry A inclusions. Immunostaining can identify specific viral antigens, and electron microscopy can demonstrate virions. Recent work suggests PCR analysis of the CSF may provide a rapid, reliable, and relatively noninvasive method of diagnosis if and when this technology becomes widely available.

Because treatment is most effective when started before the patient's level of consciousness is depressed, the mortality rate is 17 percent if acyclovir is begun while the patient is still conscious and reasonably neurologically intact compared with more than 60 percent if the drug is started when the patient is comatose. Acyclovir's toxicity is limited; therefore, it is now commonplace to initiate treatment rapidly and try to exclude other diagnoses by biopsy only if the patient does not respond appropriately to therapy. Treatment typically consists of 10 to 12.4 mg/kg IV, infused over 1 hour, and repeated every 8 hours for 10 days.

Table 48-1. Summary of Virus Classes and Major Clinical Characteristics

Group	Virus	Structure	Epidemiology	Syndrome	Severity	Notes
Herpesvirus		Icosahedral, large, enveloped, dsDNA	Sporadic	Encephalitis, meningitis, radiculitis		
	HSV-1			Encephalitis, temporal/ frontal	>50% mortality rate untreated	95% of HSV encephalitis
	HSV-2 Varicella-zoster			Neonatal encephalitis Radiculitis, myelitis, granulomatous angiitis		
	Human herpes 6, EBV, CMV			Immunocompromized		
Enterovirus		Icosahedral, small, nonenveloped, ssRNA	Late summer/ early fall	Meningitis, poliomyelitis	Benign meningitis to lethal polio	Three-quarters of aseptic meningitis
			Human is only host			
	Polio			Motor neuronitis	Variable	Almost eliminated by vaccination
	Coxsackie A, B and echoviruses			Meningitis, rare polio-like	Benign	
Arbovirus		Enveloped, ssRNA	Late summer/ early fall; epizootic + mosquito/ tick	Encephalitis; uncommon but severe		10% of human encephalitis
Togavirus α-Virus	Eastern equine	Icosahedral Northeast, Gulf of Mexico	Encephalitis	Most severe		
	Venezuelan equine		South and Central America, Florida, Texas	Encephalitis		
	Western equine		Rural western US	Encephalitis	Relatively mild	Most common α-virus
Flavivirus	St. Louis		US	Encephalitis		Most common in US
	Japanese Tick-borne encephalitis complex		Europe/Asia	Encephalitis Encephalitis		
Bunyavirus		Helical, enveloped, ssRNA	East/central US			
California group	LaCrosse			Encephalitis	Relatively mild	
	Snowshoe hare			Encephalitis	Relatively mild	
	California virus			Encephalitis	Relatively mild	Second most common in US
Rhabdovirus	Rabies	Helical/bullet, ssRNA	Europe, eastern US Animal bites	Encephalitis	Lethal	

Abbreviations: EBV, Epstein-Barr virus; CMV, cytomegalovirus; ds, double-stranded; ss, single-stranded; US, United States; HSV, herpes simplex virus.

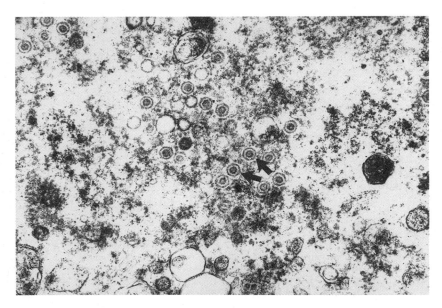

Figure 48-1. Electron micrograph of brain biopsy in a patient with herpes simplex encephalitis showing virions *(arrows)*.

Genital Herpes

HSV-2 most commonly causes genital herpes. HSV-2 meningitis is often preceded by pelvic or perineal radicular pain, with or without obvious herpetic lesions; so a careful history may be diagnostic. However, HSV-2 can also cause disseminated herpes, with an accompanying severe encephalitis in one-third, in newborns of mothers with genital herpes. This devastating encephalitis has a 20 percent mortality rate, with serious sequelae in many of the survivors. This infection also responds to acyclovir but is better avoided by avoiding vaginal deliveries in mothers known to be infected with HSV. Like cytomegalovirus and varicella-zoster, HSV-2 can also cause a significant encephalitis in immunocompromised patients. This too responds to high-dose acyclovir, although early aggressive treatment is essential.

Herpes Zoster

Although HSV can cause radicular symptoms and even zosterlike skin lesions, herpes zoster is the expected cause of shingles. In this disorder, the virus, which is normally dormant in the dorsal root ganglion, migrates peripherally, causing dermatomal radicular pain accompanied by a corresponding vesicular eruption. Often, the radicular pain or, on occasion, itching precedes the rash by several days. Normally, the entire syndrome subsides in 4 to 6 weeks. This disorder occurs commonly in elderly persons; 50 percent of individuals older than 80 will have had this disease at one time or another. It is also common in immunocompromised patients.

Although acyclovir shortens the duration of the rash, it is not clear that it has any impact on the most frequent long-term consequence of shingles, that is, postherpetic neuralgia, which occurs in up to one-third of patients over the age of 50, but rarely in younger individuals. Like other neuralgias, this may respond symptomatically to carbamazepine, phenytoin, or tricyclic antidepressants and related compounds. In elderly patients, the neuralgia is often poorly responsive to treatment and becomes a trial of the patient's fortitude. Recent use of capsaicin to deplete substance P from nociceptive neurons has elicited a more positive response from pain neurophysiologists than from patients with neuritic pain, but it may be worth trying. The role of steroids remains controversial, except in ophthalmic herpes, where their use may be essential to limit damage to the eye. In many cases, the central processes of sensory neurons may also be affected, with an accompanying CSF pleocytosis; in particularly severe instances, a segmental myelitis may also occur (see Ch. 31). Some patients with ophthalmic herpes have had a cerebral vasculitis develop, presumably as the virus migrated along the central portions of the trigeminal neurons, reaching the cerebral vessels. In some such patients, typical granulomatous angiitis has developed (see Ch. 38).

ENTEROVIRUSES

The enteroviruses (Greek: *enteron,* intestine) are the most commonly identified agents responsible for viral meningitis; they cause 70 to 80 percent of all cases of aseptic meningitis (90 percent of cases in which the etiologic agent is identified). They are also responsible for 10 to 20 percent of encephalitis cases.

These agents are picornaviruses—small, nonenveloped, single-stranded, RNA-containing viruses, with icosahedral symmetry. There are more than 68 different identified enteroviruses, subclassified as (1) polioviruses (3 types); (2) Coxsackie A (23 types) and B viruses (6 types), named for the town in upstate New York where they were first identified; (3) echoviruses (31 types)—an acronym for "enteric cytopathic human orphan" viruses; and (4) 5 recently identified types that do not fit any of these groups. All groups can cause encephalitis or meningitis. Although these agents constitute only a small subset of cases of encephalitis of identified cause, the most common subtypes to cause this disorder are ECHO 6 and 9 and Coxsackie A9, B2, and B5. A somewhat longer list can cause meningitis.

These viruses are generally transmitted by the fecal-oral route and occur most commonly in those areas where hygiene is suboptimal. Because humans are the only hosts for these organisms, it is reasonable to hope that widespread vaccination could eliminate these illnesses, just as smallpox appears to have been eradicated. Unfortunately, individuals may be asymptomatic gastrointestinal carriers, permitting perpetuation of these organisms when clinically obvious infection rates are low. Disease tends to occur in summertime epidemics, with incidence peaks from July to September. Children and young adults are those most commonly affected. All of these agents generally proliferate in the gastrointestinal tract and then disseminate hematogenously to the reticuloendothelial system and other specific target organs, be it the heart, skin, meninges, or nervous system.

Poliomyelitis

Thanks to widespread vaccination, poliovirus infection is now only rarely seen in developed countries; for example, fewer than 10 cases/year have occurred in the United States throughout the last decade (and then primarily in unvaccinated subpopulations), with no cases within the past 2 years. In many other parts of the world, this remains an important disease. For many patients, infection is asymptomatic, particularly in children younger than age 4. In underdeveloped regions with poor hygiene, in which most individuals are exposed as infants, true paralytic polio is rare, as most of the population is immunized by minor or asymptomatic natural infection in infancy. In regions with better hygiene but limited vaccination, infection occurs at a somewhat older age, but even so, most infections are asymptomatic.

As with other enterovirus infections, symptomatic patients (probably about 5 percent of infected individuals) may first have a minor febrile illness, often with headache, sore throat, myalgias, anorexia, nausea, and vomiting, presumably reflecting viral dissemination. In approximately 0.1 percent of infected individuals, major illness develops with nervous system involvement, typically with muscle pain, weakness, and meningismus. It is common teaching that the muscles destined to become involved are those that develop this pain. Although only a minority of patients with polio have the minor illness prodrome, virtually all have an acute febrile illness with meningitis either immediately before or at the time of development of paralysis. This major illness is self-limited, and the fever usually subsides within a few days.

It is presumed that the virus seeds the nervous system directly during dissemination by preferential binding to motor nerve terminals where the blood-nerve barrier is incomplete and where there probably are specific receptors to which the virus binds. The virus is probably then transported back to the CNS by retrograde axonal transport. This postulated process may be supported by old clinical observations that paralytic polio is more likely to affect limbs that have been exercised or injured (e.g., injections; bulbar polio occurs more frequently in patients who have undergone tonsillectomies), either of which might be expected to increase membrane turnover at the neuromuscular junction, with an increased likelihood of endocytosis of attached virions. Regardless of the mechanism, the virus preferentially invades motor neurons, causing a focal poliomyelitis in the motor nuclei of the spinal cord or brainstem (Greek: *polios,* gray, which differentiates this disorder from leukoencephalitis). This causes rapidly progressive weakness and muscle atrophy and fasciculations, affecting the limb or bulbar musculature, often asymmetrically and patchily. Although 5 to 10 percent of patients die acutely, for most patients, the course is a slow recovery over the subsequent months. The long-term sequelae are typically variable weakness and atrophy. Years later, patients may have progressive weakness in previously involved muscles (postpolio syndrome), often misdiagnosed as amyotrophic lateral sclerosis (see Ch. 32).

Other Enteroviruses

Although other enteroviruses may cause a poliolike syndrome, fortunately, this is rare. Coxsackie and ECHO viruses can cause a poliolike syndrome, rarely an encephalitis. Coxsackie B is typically more severe than A or echovirus. The diagnosis may be aided by accompanying symptoms. Coxsackie A infection is often accompanied by herpangina or painful lesions on the soft palate or in the tonsillar fossae; Coxsackie B more commonly causes pleurodynia or pericarditis. A rash may accompany many of these infections. Although all the enteroviruses are more likely to cause a relatively benign aseptic meningitislike picture, they are particularly troublesome in agammaglobulinemic individuals, in whom they can cause chronic meningitis and a dermatomyositislike illness.

Diagnosis and Treatment

The diagnosis of enteroviral infections can often be accomplished by CSF viral culture. In the absence of this method, demonstration of a fourfold rise in antibody titer or demonstration of IgM antibody by enzyme-linked immunosorbent assay (ELISA) can be diagnostic, although the large number of antigenically distinct viruses makes serologic testing cumbersome. Enteroviruses can frequently be isolated from stool samples; however, because asymptomatic carriage of these agents is so frequent, the diagnostic utility of this is limited. Treatment is generally supportive because recovery is the norm, with significant morbidity or mortality being uncommon. In light of the usually excellent prognosis, extensive diagnostic evaluations to identify the precise agent are usually unnecessary.

ARBOVIRUSES

The term "arbovirus" persists in common use because this classification remains useful to the clinician and infections with these organisms share many common clinical features not limited to the mode of transmission. (Most virologists prefer nomenclature based on intrinsic viral properties, rather than the rather arbitrary shared property of being arthropod-borne.) Typically, arbovirus encephalitis accounts for about 10 percent of human encephalitis cases in the United States and elsewhere each year.

Viral Groups

Arboviruses are generally divided into five families: Togaviridae, Reoviridae, Rhabdoviridae, Filoviridae, and Bunyaviridae. Most human arboviral encephalitis is caused by the Togaviridae and the Bunyaviridae. Togaviruses (which also include the more common rubella virus) are enveloped viruses that contain single-stranded RNA and have icosahedral symmetry. This large family is subdivided into two major genuses, originally referred to as groups A and B but now called α-viruses and Flaviviruses, respectively.

α-Viruses are mosquito borne; Flaviviruses are transmitted by mosquitoes, ticks, and possibly other vectors. α-viruses include Eastern, Western, and Venezuelan equine encephalitides; the Flaviviruses, which are slightly smaller than α-viruses (40 to 70 nm in diameter), include St. Louis and Japanese encephalitis and the tick-borne encephalitis complex, a cause of significant morbidity in Europe and Asia. Also included among the Flaviviruses are the agents responsible for yellow fever and dengue. Although the source of major epidemics, these two have few primarily neurologic manifestations and are not discussed in detail here.

Viruses of the other clinically important group, the Bunyaviridae, each contain three circular single-stranded RNA segments, are enveloped, and have helical symmetry. This group includes the California virus group, which in turn includes Lacrosse, snowshoe hare, and California encephalitis viruses. The remaining arboviruses are of considerable biologic interest, but either do not typically cause human neurologic disease or are of limited clinical importance in Europe or North America.

Pathophysiology

All arboviral infections are zoonoses, that is, infections occurring primarily in nonhuman species by which humans become infected as an incidental host. A primary host is required for all—an animal that becomes infected and survives for a period of time, despite significant viremia. An arthropod vector then feeds on an infected, viremic animal, ingesting virus particles that then proliferate in the arthropod's gut or salivary glands (this generally requires an incubation period of about 1 week in the arthropod), which can then be introduced into a new host with the next feeding. This cycle permits a continuous amplification and perpetuation of the virus. Any host, including a human, in which sustained viremia does not occur, is considered an incidental host and is of no value to the virus's reproductive cycle.

When arthropods feed on vertebrate hosts, they inject saliva containing a number of enzymes (such as anticoagulants) to facilitate feeding. Because arboviruses replicate and/or are stored in the arthropod's salivary glands, the injected saliva carries virus into the new, unwitting host where it rapidly gains access to capillaries. The organisms can then spread through the blood stream to the reticuloendothelial system (lymph nodes, spleen, and endothelium) where the virus can then replicate. After a variable incubation period (typically on the order of 1 to several weeks), the virus again disseminates hematogenously, this time potentially involving other organ systems, including the brain.

On occasion, conditions permit rapid proliferation of vectors (e.g., rainy weather facilitating mosquito proliferation). When this occurs, epidemics of arthropod-borne infections may ensue, and then large numbers of incidental hosts are at risk of infection. Because of this pattern, careful epidemiologic and ecologic studies, and monitoring of sentinel species that are at risk of becoming infected (horses, birds, and even sentinel chickens), can permit anticipation of epidemics and early institution of vector control measures before large numbers of humans become infected. Such measures have helped minimize epidemics. In 1992, only 45 cases of arboviral encephalitis were reported in the United States, with similar small numbers in countries practicing these preventive measures.

Although most arboviral infections follow this epidemic cycle, some, including St. Louis encephalitis and the California viruses, can behave somewhat differently. In these groups, the virus can be transmitted from a mosquito through its eggs to its offspring, permitting perpetuation of the virus without involving intermediate hosts. Therefore, unlike the other forms of epidemic arboviral disease, these can be endemic, maintaining a significant background infection rate without significant involvement of other species.

Diagnosis and Treatment

The diagnosis is often based on epidemiologic considerations and demonstration of rising antibody titers. Culture of these agents is rarely successful. Demonstration of IgM antibody by ELISA can be useful because these antibodies are normally only present during acute infection. No specific therapy is available for any of these infections, although careful supportive care, including careful fluid management, is often all that is necessary.

α-Viruses

Eastern Equine Encephalitis

This is the most severe form of arboviral encephalitis in the United States, but it is fortunately rare, with small outbreaks occurring every few years. It occurs most frequently in coastal regions of the northeast and along the Gulf of Mexico. Cases in horses tend to occur between May and September, preceding human cases by about 1 month. In Florida's more temperate climate, equine cases may occur year round. As with virtually all infections, subclinical cases outnumber clinical ones. However, this ratio is lower for this infection than for most other arboviruses, with about 29 subclinical cases for each clinical 1 in adults but 4 subclinical cases for each clinical 1 in children younger than 4 years of age. The principal mosquito vector, *Culiseta melanura,* lives in freshwater swamps and feeds exclusively on birds. Only when concurrent Aedes mosquitoes feed on infected birds do other species (horses and humans) become infected.

The clinical course is typically fulminant, with rapid progression to coma and seizures, frequent respiratory depression and autonomic dysfunction, proceeding in 1 to 2 weeks to death in about 50 percent of cases. The outlook is even worse in those younger than age 20 or older than 60, in whom the mortality rate approaches 75 percent. Of survivors, 30 percent have significant neurologic sequelae. Pathologically, the brain contains scattered areas of necrosis and hemorrhage, with no specific topographic distribution.

Venezuelan Equine Encephalitis

This is the most important arboviral infection in South and Central America, and it occurs sporadically in the Florida Everglades and in Texas. Outbreaks occur in rainy months, when the vectors proliferate in tropical coastal regions. Although many individuals in endemic areas have serologic evidence of exposure to this agent, in only a small proportion, does neurologic disease develop. Infection is rarely subclinical but often consists of little more than a febrile illness. Among those younger than 15 years of age who become infected, approximately 4 percent have encephalitis. This occurs in an even smaller proportion of infected adults. The basal ganglia and substantia nigra are involved particularly commonly. Among those in whom encephalitis develops, the mortality rate is typically about 20 percent, with neurologic sequelae occurring fairly commonly.

Western Equine Encephalitis

This is the most common α-virus encephalitis and the third most common cause of arboviral encephalitis (after St. Louis and California) in the United States, typically with 30 to 40 cases per year, occurring primarily in rural areas of the western states. As with other arboviral diseases, cases occur in the summer months, particularly if the preceding spring has been unusually damp. Although equine cases typically outnumber human ones, the horse is as much an incidental host as the human.

This illness is much less severe than Eastern equine encephalitis. Subclinical cases outnumber clinical ones by more than 1,000 to 1, although in children younger than 4 years of age, clinical cases may be relatively more frequent and more severe. Five to 10 days after infection, patients abruptly have headache, chills, nausea, vomiting, and malaise develop. Within a few days, mental confusion, somnolence, and meningismus develop and may evolve to coma and seizures. As with most other arboviral encephalitides, there is no particular topography to the CNS involvement, and in fact, the examination findings may well be nonfocal. Recovery typically occurs after several weeks, although 30 percent of children and 10 to 15 percent of adults may have neurologic sequelae. Case fatality rates have generally been 7 to 9 percent.

Pathologically, involvement is diffuse, although the basal ganglia may be preferentially involved. Some survivors have developed parkinsonism.

Flavivirus

St. Louis Encephalitis

This is the most common arboviral encephalitis in the United States, and it has been the cause of major epidemics. Annual incidence has ranged from 17 to 1,815 cases in recent decades. Disease severity varies widely, with mortality rates typically about 8 percent, although this is considerably higher (35 percent) in individuals older than age 60. The disease tends to be endemic in many areas, particularly in the western United States, although cases occur throughout the country. The vectors, Culex mosquitoes, breed in polluted or stagnant water, which occurs in both urban and rural areas. The principal vertebrate hosts for this infection are wild birds, the only hosts in which a sufficient viremia occurs to permit the virus amplifying cycle. Despite a viremia lasting weeks, the birds do not become particularly ill. In areas where St. Louis encephalitis is endemic, sentinel chickens are maintained to monitor for infection. Mosquitoes tend to feed on birds early in spring and summer and mammals later in the season. Hence, human disease incidence tends to increase late in the summer and in fall.

In most patients, infection causes nothing more than a flu-like illness. Even when the CNS is infected, one-quarter of patients may only have an aseptic meningitis develop. Because many infections are mild or subclinical, particularly in children, there tend to be high levels of immunity among individuals living in endemic areas, with immunity increasing with age. As a result, the ratio of subclinical to clinical cases has varied in different epidemics, depending on the local population at risk, between 19:1 and 470:1. In some parts of the country, there is little endemic activity. In such areas, there is little "herd immunity," and introduction of the infection can cause explosive epidemics.

The clinical phenomena are typical of all the arboviral encephalitides, with fever, headache, photophobia, nausea, and vomiting proceeding to altered mental status, focal signs, and occasionally, seizures. Intense muscle pain occurs frequently as does hyponatremia. Serum creatine kinase and aldolase concentrations may be elevated as a result of skeletal muscle involvement, and electromyographic results may be abnormal. CNS pathologic findings are comparable to those in the other arboviral encephalitides, varying in severity but with particularly prominent involvement of the brainstem, cortex, and substantia nigra.

The diagnosis is best made by specific IgM-capture ELISA. The symptoms typically resolve over several weeks, and long-term neurologic sequelae are relatively infrequent.

Japanese Encephalitis

This is rare in Western countries but is well known in the East from as far north as Eastern Siberia, Japan, and Korea through China, Guam, and Taiwan to the southern countries, such as Vietnam and Thailand and into Malaya, Singapore, and India. It occurs most often in late summer and fall where there is seasonal variation and all year in the tropics. The human is an incidental host for the mosquito-borne disease which mainly affects birds and domestic animals.

Severe rigors occur in almost all cases. In addition to the headache, fever, seizures, and hyperthermia, Japanese encephalitis has a higher frequency of focal neurological signs than the other arboviruses, hemiparesis especially featuring arm weakness being the most common. Fatal outcome is not rare, occurring in up to a third of cases. About 20% of those surviving who developed neurological signs retain them to some degree.

Bunyavirus

California Encephalitis

This group usually includes benign febrile illnesses, sometimes with a superimposed aseptic meningitis. However, the California encephalitis viruses can cause encephalitis and are in fact the second most common cause of arboviral encephalitis in the United States. The behavior of this infection is somewhat different from that of the other arboviral encephalitides because it is an endemic rather than an epidemic disease. In these viruses, there has been demonstration of transovarial and venereal transmission of infection (i.e., the infected Aedes mosquitoes are not only the vector for infection but also the reservoir, passing infection on to their offspring or their mates). In addition, small mammals such as squirrels and chipmunks can act as amplifying hosts. However, because a background level of infection is ensured among the principal vectors, there is a fairly constant number of human cases from year to year, without the epidemics that are dependent on sporadic surges in amplification.

Despite the name of this viral group, the disease occurs primarily in the east central states, with the Lacrosse virus (first isolated in Wisconsin) being responsible for most cases. The mosquito occurs primarily in small collections of water in hardwood forests. As with other arboviral infections, the peak incidence is in summer. Children are affected disproportionately frequently, with only 3 percent of reported cases occurring in individuals older than 20 years of age.

Cases may be mild or severe. Children with the mild form have a meningitis-like illness lasting about 1 week. In severely affected patients, a more protracted illness with altered sensorium develops. Focal signs develop in a significant number of patients, and seizures occur commonly. Case fatality rates are low, although neurologic sequelae, most commonly seizures, are seen in about one-third of children with the severe form.

RABIES

Widespread immunization in recent years has rendered rare the childhood exanthems that have been associated with a variety of forms of encephalitis. The one remaining encephalitis that is currently reappearing is rabies. This is a disease that has been well known—and greatly feared—at least since the days of Hippocrates. Although human rabies cases all but disappeared from the United States in recent decades because of near universal vaccination of household pets, this disease has undergone a resurgence, thought to be largely attributable to the inadvertent introduction of rabid raccoons from Europe in an effort to replenish depleted raccoon stocks in the southeast. This has given rise to an epidemic of rabies among wild raccoons along the eastern seaboard that has now reached the major population centers in the northeast, including the recent report of the first human case of rabies in New York state in years. In Western Europe, there has been an epidemic developing westward for some years. Northern France was involved with a regular outbreak each year. Recent data suggest that the epidemic is receding because wild animals have been provided feeds that contain vaccine.

Pathophysiology

The rabies virus is a rhabdovirus, a small bullet-shaped, enveloped virus with helical symmetry, containing single-stranded RNA. Infection occurs after bites by rabid animals. The virus ascends in peripheral nerves, apparently being taken up in sensory nerve endings and then transported back to the CNS by retrograde axonal transport. The incubation period varies widely but is in part a reflection of the site of inoculation; bites on the head lead to neurologic symptoms more rapidly than do those on the extremities. Typically, the incubation period is 20 to 60 days. On occasion, incubation periods of 1 year have been observed. The virus ultimately has a predilection for neurons in the limbic system, brainstem, and Purkinje cells.

Clinical Features

Typically, the illness begins with fever, headache, malaise, agitation, and anxiety, followed by dysphagia (with spasms of the throat muscles), dysarthria, and seizures. Often patients have severe dysesthetic pain. (In 10 to 15 percent of patients, the onset resembles the Guillain-Barré syndrome, with ascending but asymmetric paralysis.) It has been suggested that the agitation helps perpetuate the virus in that affected individuals are more likely to bite others around them. The painful difficulty swallowing has led to the notion of *hydrophobia*, a fear of swallowing anything, even saliva or water. Once begun, the illness progresses rapidly to coma, seizures, hypothalamic dysfunction, severe CNS damage, and death. The mortality rate is essentially 100 percent.

Diagnosis

The diagnosis is made by history and the clinical presentation. Laboratory support can include viral isolation from the CSF, saliva, or urine or immunofluorescence demonstration of virus in nerve endings in skin obtained from the neck. Pathologic study demonstrates typical intraneuronal intracytoplasmic inclusions, Negri bodies, consisting of clusters of virions, with particularly prominent involvement of the limbic system, hippocampus, pyramidal neurons, and Purkinje cells.

Treatment

Presymptomatic treatment consists of careful and immediate cleaning of the wound, local and systemic treatment with hyperimmune globulin, and immunization. Once symptomatic, even heroic measures rarely offer any hope. Interestingly, in Europe, rabies has been controlled by providing wild animals with feed that contains a vaccine. Whether such efforts will be needed in the United States is currently being debated.

ANNOTATED BIBLIOGRAPHY

Aslanzadeh J et al. Use of polymerase chain reaction for laboratory diagnosis of herpes simplex virus encephalitis. Ann Clin Lab Sci 1993;23:196–202.

Newer technology.

Fishbein DB, Robinson LE. Rabies. N Engl J Med 1993;329:1632–8.

Steps to take to control disease.

Gilden DH. Herpesvirus infections of the central nervous system, in Tyler KL, Martin JB (eds). Infectious Diseases of the Central Nervous System. FA Davis, Philadelphia, 1993, pp. 76–102.

Overview of herpes infections.

Irani DN, Hanley DF, Johnson RT. Acute viral encephalitis—diagnosis and clinical management. In Tyler KL, Martin JB (eds). Infectious Diseases of the Central Nervous System. FA Davis, Philadelphia, 1993, pp. 3–22.

Overview of viral encephalitis.

Lipton HL, Jubelt B. Enterovirus infections of the central nervous system, in Tyler KL, Martin JB (eds). Infectious Diseases of the Central Nervous System. FA Davis, Philadelphia, 1993, pp. 103–30.

Details of enteroviral CNS infections.

Mateos-Mora M, Ratzan KR. Acute viral encephalitis. In Schlossberg D (ed). Infections of the Nervous System. Springer Verlag, New York, 1990, pp. 105–34.

Full discussion of viral encephalitis.

Meyers BR, Gurtman AC. The aseptic meningitis syndrome. In Schlossberg D (ed). Infections of the Nervous System. Springer Verlag, New York, 1990, pp. 31–41.

Text for viral meningitis.

Whitley RJ et al. Vidarabine vs acyclovir therapy in herpes simplex encephalitis. N Engl J Med 1986;314:144–9.

Established efficacy of acyclovir and also demonstrated pitfalls of clinical diagnosis of HSV encephalitis.

49

AIDS and Opportunistic Infections

Allen J. Aksamit, Jr.

The acquired immunodeficiency syndrome (AIDS) epidemic has brought new challenges to the clinical neurologist. Now 14 years into the epidemic, specialists from neurology, internal medicine, and infectious diseases are learning new lessons about coping with human immunodeficiency virus (HIV)-related disease and the host of opportunistic infections that invade the brain as a consequence of the severe immunosuppression of AIDS.

The unique aspects of the immunosuppression of AIDS have brought formerly rare diseases, such as progressive multifocal leukoencephalopathy (PML), toxoplasmosis, and cryptococcal meningitis, to the forefront of neurologic practice.

Other diseases that were thought to be banished to antiquity have undergone a resurgence, including tuberculosis of the nervous system and neurosyphilis. Finally, a variety of new syndromes have emerged, such as primary HIV infection and cytomegalovirus (CMV) ascending polyradiculopathy/ependymitis. HIV infection of the nervous system required almost 4 years before it was recognized as a distinct clinical entity.

The neurologic syndromes produced by HIV and associated opportunistic infections are nonspecific, often not identifying the causative organism. Time-honored clinical neurologic skills can, for example, segregate a myelopathy from an ascending polyradiculopathy, but such separation does not fully distinguish the etiologic agent. Still, the use of a classical neurologic framework helps to narrow the differential diagnosis in the attempt to distinguish the myelopathy of lymphoma from an ascending polyradiculopathy caused by CMV.

Because clinical examination falls short in fully distinguishing the etiologic agent of various neurologic syndromes occurring in AIDS, neurologists are re-quired now to be familiar with and know the limitations of complex microbiologic testing. This includes the use of such techniques as in situ hybridization and the polymerase chain reaction (PCR) to fully evaluate the patient's clinical syndrome. Also, multiple simultaneous pathogens can occur, laying another level of complexity in interpreting patients' neurologic symptoms and abnormal laboratory findings. Finally, AIDS-related lymphoma in the nervous system can mimic several opportunistic infections and must be considered in many clinical circumstances because of the variety of neurologic symptoms it can cause.

When a patient presents with a history of HIV seropositivity and a neurologic syndrome, one approach would be simply to list all the possible central nervous system (CNS) pathogens, including HIV itself, and use laboratory testing to discriminate between them. However, a more reasonable approach is to categorize the AIDS-related CNS disease based on the clinical syndrome, keeping in mind the most common pathogen responsible for each syndrome, as outlined in Table 49-1. By segregation of the clinical syndrome into focal CNS disease, dementia, meningitis, myelopathy, or polyradiculopathy, the microbiologic investigations can be narrowed to specific microorganisms likely to be responsible, which can be followed with appropriate therapy. In each case, opportunistic lymphoma needs to be considered.

With this framework, patients with a variety of neurologic syndromes and HIV seropositivity can be evaluated in a systematic way. However, lessons were learned early in the AIDS epidemic about the variability of neurologic presentation of each of these opportunistic infections, and the possibility of new opportunistic infections or old ones presenting in new ways needs always to be kept in mind.

Table 49-1. AIDS-Related Clinical Central Nervous System Disease

	Focal CNS	Dementia	Meningitis	Myelopathy	Polyradiculopathy
Viral	PML VZV leukoencephalitis	HIV encephalitis/ leukoencephalopathy CMV PML	HIV HSV CMV VZV	Vacuolar myelopathy VZV HSV	CMV VZV HSV
Bacterial	*M. tuberculosis* *Nocardia* Syphilis	Syphilis *M. tuberculosis*	*M. tuberculosis*	Syphilis	Syphilis
Fungal	*Cryptococcus* *Aspergillosis*	*Cryptococcus*	*Cryptococcus* *Candida*		
Parasitic	Toxoplasmosis	Toxoplasmosis	Toxoplasmosis		
Neoplastic	Lymphoma Kaposi's sarcoma	Lymphoma	Lymphoma	Lymphoma	Lymphoma

Abbreviations: CMV, cytomegalovirus; CNS, central nervous system; HIV, human immunodeficiency virus; HSV, herpes simplex virus; PML, progressive multifocal leukoencephalopathy; VZV, varicella zoster virus.

NEUROLOGIC COMPLICATIONS OF HUMAN IMMUNODEFICIENCY VIRUS INFECTION OF THE BRAIN

Background

HIV-1 is an important cause of neurologic morbidity and death among patients infected with this virus. The prevalence of primary neurologic complications in the circumstance of AIDS varies with the report but ranges from 31 to 65 percent of all adult patients infected with HIV. Recent evidence has suggested HIV disseminates to the CNS early after primary systemic infection. In children with HIV infection, 50 to 90 percent may have CNS infection.

HIV-related disease can affect any part of the nervous system; so HIV-related disease of the nervous system can be included in virtually any neurologic differential diagnosis. The clinical syndromes of HIV infection are protean, but distinct syndromes have emerged in patients who are HIV seropositive. Many can be the presenting manifestation of AIDS. Therefore, part of the difficulty in determining whether HIV is contributing to neurologic illness is the identification of HIV infection. The patient may not be aware of past exposure, or patients are often reluctant to volunteer at risk behaviors. Therefore, HIV serologic testing should be considered in situations in which HIV syndromes fit the clinical circumstance.

There is debate about whether asymptomatic HIV-seropositive patients are neurologically normal by testing. Specifically, several studies have looked at subtle neurobehavioral changes by psychometric testing. Some studies suggest there are no significant neurologic abnormalities present in otherwise asymptomatic individuals, whereas others have correlated a change in neurobehavioral measures correlating with a reduction in CD4 counts. Further studies comparing homosexual HIV-seronegative controls with HIV-seropositive patients with a lymphadenopathy-associated syndrome found mild neurocognitive changes in 50 percent compared with 8 percent of the control group.

HIV has been found in the cerebrospinal fluid (CSF) of asymptomatic HIV-seropositive individuals with some associated CSF abnormalities. In one survey, a protein level greater than 40 mg/dl was found in 47 percent of asymptomatic patients and a mild pleocytosis was found in 7 percent. HIV was cultured from the CSF of asymptomatic individuals before zidovudine treatment in 42 percent of patients.

Other laboratory testing has revealed minor abnormalities in asymptomatic patients with HIV infection. A study found 30 percent of HIV-seropositive patients tested with electroencephalography (EEG) had mild abnormalities, despite no neurologic symptoms.

Early invasion of the nervous system after systemic exposure to HIV has been documented in a number of cases. In one circumstance, iatrogenic infection by HIV was followed 15 days later by appearance of HIV in the nervous system, as evidenced by mild inflammatory change and the presence of virus by culture and PCR findings. This particular case also suggested some HIV replication based on the presence of HIV proteins in brain by immunohistochemical analysis.

Meningitis

Acute "aseptic" meningitis has been associated with primary seroconversion and dissemination to the CNS. In addition, however, a more chronic syndrome has also been associated with "latent" infection, which is manifested only by headache, malaise, and chronic abnormalities on CSF examination. Other reports suggest an activation of inflammatory cells in the CSF as

HIV progresses to frank AIDS-related complex or as other opportunistic infections present themselves.

Cognitive Disorders

The clinical neurocognitive syndromes of HIV brain infection have been grouped under the rubric of HIV-associated cognitive-motor complex. Under this heading are included the more severe HIV-associated dementia complex and the less severe HIV-associated minor cognitive-motor disorder. The former designation has been associated with a disabling cognitive syndrome that causes impairment accompanied by motor dysfunction, disabling behavioral changes, or both.

These disorders are frequent in the circumstance of HIV infection and may be the primary presentation of AIDS. However, frank severe dementia in the absence of symptoms of systemic infection is rare. The neurocognitive complaints of HIV infection of the brain are typically of a "subcortical type" (see below) and, early on, can be confused with the effects of systemic illness or depression.

As in many clinical syndromes, exact quantitative pathologic correlates of neurocognitive HIV syndromes are lacking. However, qualitative pathologic correlates of neurocognitive disorders are well described and include HIV-1 encephalitis (with parenchymal inflammation) (Figs. 49-1 and 49-2), HIV-1 leukoencephalopathy (with white matter changes predominant) (Fig. 49-1), lymphocytic meningitis (when the inflammatory aspects are more meningeal), and poliodystrophy (when neuronal loss is the predominant finding).

Clinical Aspects of Human Immunodeficiency Virus-Associated Cognitive-Motor Complex

The first symptoms of cognitive involvement by HIV are difficulty with concentration, mental slowness, and a loss of mental precision. The most prominent symptoms are often behavioral, with apathy, abulia, loss of energy, reduced emotional responsiveness, social withdrawal, loss of interest in business, mental inflexibility in new environments, and irritability. This loss of integrative mental and behavioral abilities has been termed "subcortical" because of the relative preserva-

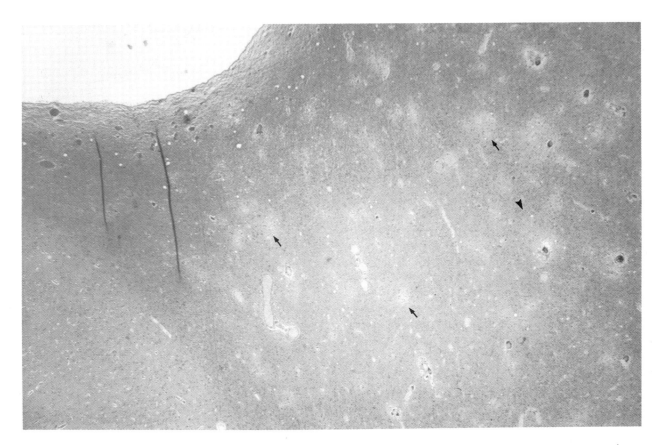

Figure 49-1. Low magnification of periventricular white matter of brain in a patient with HIV-associated cognitive-motor complex. There is patchy rarefaction (*arrows*) of the white matter, often in a perivascular distribution (*arrowhead*) (hematoxylin and eosin counterstain, original magnification ×25).

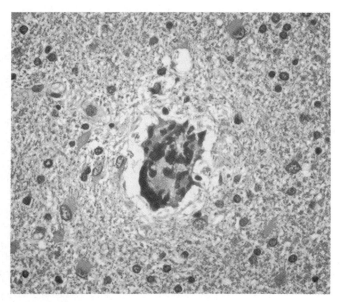

Figure 49-2. Multinucleate giant cell in a perivascular area from the same patient shown in Figure 49-1. This is the hallmark, although not universal, histologic change of HIV-1 encephalitis. These cells contain most of HIV-1 virus in the brain. (Hematoxylin and eosin counterstain, original magnification ×630).

tion of discrete higher cortical function modalities. Language changes are distinctly uncommon. Spatial and temporal disorientation can occur. Motor symptoms, although not necessarily motor signs, are common early. These are usually reported as imbalance, tremor, or a sense of lower extremity heaviness.

On mental status examination, early, there is typically an impairment in digit span testing forward and backward. There is slowed learning and often impaired recall, that is mild in degree. Frequently, a blunted affect may be apparent during the interview.

On neurologic examination, there is frequent hyper-reflexia, sometimes frontal release signs, slow alternating motor rate, a tendency for ataxic gait (affecting axial greater than appendicular musculature), and an increase in tone. These motor findings are often associated with signs of mild distal peripheral neuropathy on reflex and sensory testing. As the disease progresses, the patient has global dementia and anarthria and shows signs of spasticity, hyper-reflexia, wasting, immobility, and contractures.

Neuroimaging

Clinical dementia is most often accompanied by atrophy of the brain, as evidenced by widening of the cortical sulci and enlargement of the ventricles (Fig. 49-3). Apparent cerebral atrophy on imaging can occur in as short a time as 4 weeks. Magnetic resonance imag-

ing of the brain frequently shows T_2-weighted white matter changes affecting the centrum semiovale with a non-discrete increased T_2 signal. This abnormality is typically nonenhancing, bilateral, and predominant in the deep white matter or periventricular regions.

Cerebrospinal Fluid Findings

The abnormalities present on CSF examination do not predict the clinical state of the patient. The CSF may indeed be normal, even with significant injury to the brain because of HIV infection. However, more typically, the protein level is mildly increased, and a mild pleocytosis is seen. Markers in the CSF for inflammation are typically present with elevated levels of neopterin, β_2-microglobulin, and quinolinic acid.

Differential Diagnosis

Because of the nonspecific nature of the symptoms, other CNS infections need to be excluded. The main purpose of laboratory testing, such as CSF examination and imaging of the brain, is to exclude opportunistic infections or CNS lymphoma. Meningitis from indolent opportunistic infections such as cryptococcosis or tuberculosis can cause neurocognitive changes.

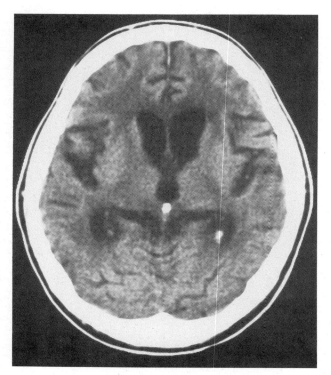

Figure 49-3. CT head scan of a patient with HIV-associated cognitive-motor complex. The sulci and the ventricles are enlarged from atrophy in this 42-year-old man. Periventricular white matter changes are obvious.

Bifrontal parenchymal disease from Toxoplasma, CNS lymphoma, PML, or CMV infection can cause subcortical neurocognitive symptoms. In addition, the clinician must exclude depression or withdrawal effects of substance abuse.

Clinical Course

Primary HIV CNS involvement that causes neurocognitive changes is generally regarded as inexorably progressive. However, in the early stages, the patient may have no definite symptoms or those that occur may be mild. Fluctuations in the degree of disturbance are frequent. In addition, the neurocognitive complaints can be associated with periods of long plateaus with no measurable changes in neurocognitive scores extending over months or years. Because toxic-metabolic factors and systemic illness affect neurobehavioral functioning, these may often contribute to symptoms or signs of neurocognitive change.

Human Immunodeficiency Virus-Associated Progressive Encephalopathy of Childhood

Clinically, diseases affecting the brain in HIV-seropositive children, who are usually congenitally infected, can begin as early as 2 months of age. The signs of disease typically are failure to acquire, or loss of, neurologic developmental milestones. The rate of separation of expected neurologic development from observed neurologic development curves defines the progression of neurologic disease. Progressive encephalopathy has been used to designate those children who have a progressively deteriorating course.

On examination, there is typically microcephaly in young children. Weakness, spasticity, hyper-reflexia, and ataxia are all common manifestations as the disease becomes more manifest. Worsening head circumference measured by loss of percentile rank and evidence of active HIV infection systemically make HIV progressive encephalopathy highly likely.

There is no single pathognomonic laboratory indicator of HIV associated progressive encephalopathy of childhood. Neuroimaging usually demonstrates cerebral atrophy. This finding is progressive on magnetic resonance imaging (MRI) or computed tomographic (CT) serial scans of the head. CT scan of the head commonly shows basal ganglia calcification, which correlates with the pathologic entity of calcific basal ganglia vasculopathy. CSF findings are typically normal, although protein level and cellular count elevations are well recognized as possible without another opportunistic infection present.

Pathologic examination of the brain most commonly shows calcific basal ganglia vasculopathy, characterized by both capillary and arteriolar calcifications. HIV encephalitis with multinucleated giant cells and inflammatory changes are relatively uncommon but possible in children, distinguishing this entity from adult forms of HIV primary infection of the brain. HIV leukoencephalopathy without inflammatory changes is relatively common in children. The cerebral atrophy inevitably present represents neuronal cell loss and loss of neuronal interconnections. In the spinal cord, degeneration of the corticospinal tracts is frequently observed.

Vacuolar Myelopathy

Vacuolar myelopathy associated with HIV infection may not be secondary to direct HIV infection of the spinal cord. The exact pathogenesis of that pathologic entity remains to be determined.

Clinically, symptoms of this disorder typically begin late in the course of HIV-related neurologic disease and are often associated with concomitant findings of the HIV cognitive-motor complex. The most common symptoms are those referable to the corticospinal tracts with increasing spasticity, weakness (especially in the lower extremities), and urinary incontinence. Sensory symptoms referable to the spinal cord are relatively uncommon.

The signs affect the lower extremities more than the upper. There is weakness in the upper motor neuron pattern that may rapidly or slowly progress. Spasticity is significant, and Babinski's sign is inevitably present as the disease progresses.

Laboratory investigations are designed to exclude other causes. Lymphoma, varicella-zoster virus, CMV, and syphilis can all cause myelopathy, although all of these tend to be of a more fulminant nature than that associated with vacuolar myelopathy.

Neuromuscular Disorders Associated With Human Immunodeficiency Virus Infection

A variety of peripheral neuropathic disorders can occur in the circumstance of HIV. The most common is the distal, painful, symmetric sensory neuropathy observed late in the course of HIV infection. The exact pathogenesis of this entity is unclear. This should be distinguished from other peripheral nerve disorders associated with opportunistic infections.

Acute inflammatory demyelinating polyneuropathy or the Guillain-Barré syndrome can occur coincidentally with HIV infection. Most commonly, this is an ascending polyradiculoneuropathy with a prominent demyelinating component on electrophysiologic examination that occurs early in the course of HIV infection. This is similar to the Guillain-Barré syndrome of patients without HIV, except there is inevitably a CSF pleocytosis. It must be distinguished from other opportunistic infections such as CMV polyradiculopathy. The usual range of CSF lymphocytosis in this HIV-related disease is 10 to 50 cells/mm^3.

A variety of other neuropathic disorders have been described in association with HIV. These include mononeuritis multiplex, cranial nerve mononeuropathies (Bell's palsy prominent among them), subacute sensory ganglioradiculoneuropathy (rare), and chronic inflammatory demyelinating polyneuropathy.

A symmetric proximal wasting syndrome ascribed to a myopathic disorder has been recognized in HIV-seropositive patients. Controversy remains in both the clinical realm and the area of muscle pathologic findings as to whether this represents a primary HIV-related myopathic disorder or whether some or all of these patients have a myopathy related to zidovudine therapy. It is clear that some patients have improvement in their proximal wasting and weakness after discontinuing zidovudine therapy.

PROGRESSIVE MULTIFOCAL LEUKOENCEPHALOPATHY

PML has become an important opportunistic infection because of the AIDS epidemic. It remains the prototypic human disease in which demyelination is the primary outcome of a direct viral lytic infection of oligodendrocytes in the brain. JC virus, the etiologic virus, causes a lytic infection of multiple oligodendrocytes, leading to microscopic demyelinated plaques. These multifocal lesions enlarge and coalesce to form macroscopic areas of demyelination, which accounts for the clinically apparent focal neurologic deficits and radiographic abnormalities.

Historically, PML was described as a unique neuropathologic entity in 1958. Early on, a viral cause was suspected because the disease was associated with clinical states of immunosuppression and "inclusions" were noted pathologically in oligodendrocytic nuclei, suggesting the accumulation of viral products. Early electron microscopic studies supported this hypothesis, but the viral etiologic agent was not proved until homogenates of PML brain were inoculated into human fetal glial cell cultures, yielding a unique papovavirus designated JC virus. Except for one early report associating PML with Simian virus 40, all subsequent cases of PML studied in detail have been related to JC virus infection of the CNS, including a few previously believed to be secondary to Simian virus 40.

The prevalence of this illness in the pre-AIDS era is difficult to determine; although it was a rare disorder, many cases were unreported. A review published in 1984 examined the features of 230 cases recorded since 1958. Most of those patients had an associated underlying defect in T-cell immunity. Soon after the onset of the AIDS epidemic in 1981, PML became recognized as an opportunistic infection associated with it.

The actual prevalence of PML among HIV-seropositive patients is controversial. Original estimates from pathologic series encompassing studies of patients seen in AIDS referral centers suggested an incidence of 4 to 8 percent of all patients who died of HIV-related disease. These estimates may be high, based on the referral nature of the reporting centers. Epidemiologic surveys estimating the prevalence of PML among the patient population with AIDS suggested that, in 0.8 percent of HIV-seropositive patients, PML develops. The latter study has been criticized because it may have had a low case ascertainment bias. In either case, whereas this disorder was a rare disease in the pre-AIDS era, it is much more commonly encountered in routine practice, especially in areas where AIDS-related disease is a significant problem. With more than 300,000 AIDS cases reported in the United States and a conservative prevalence rate of 2 percent, the estimated 6,000 cases of AIDS-associated PML since the onset of the AIDS epidemic is 26 times as many cases as in the pre-AIDS 25 years. As patients with AIDS live longer because of successful treatment of other opportunistic infections, it is likely more PML will occur because of persistent immune suppression.

Clinical Features

The clinical presentation of PML is of a subacute focal neurologic deficit occurring in the context of an immunosuppressive illness affecting cell-mediated immunity. The onset can be abrupt but more typically evolves over hours or days. Because of the abrupt onset of the clinical syndrome and the focal nature of the disorder, the disease has, at times, been clinically confused with stroke.

Although the name implies multifocal deficits, the typical clinical presentation at the time of onset is unifocal. However, multifocal deficits can evolve as the clinical syndrome progresses and may be a clue to the diagnosis. Eighty to 90 percent of patients present with cerebral syndromes, and 10 to 20 percent have signs and symptoms referable to the cerebellum or brainstem. Virtually any area of the brain white matter is vulnerable neurologically. Clinically important spinal cord involvement is virtually unheard of, and pathologic studies suggest that, rarely, the spinal cord can be involved. Changes in mentation and cognition are frequent and are the presenting manifestations of disease in 35 percent of patients. Clinically, the diagnosis may be obscured initially because of the seemingly nonlocalized nature of these neurologic deficits. These patients typically have frontal or multifocal lesions evident on neuroimaging.

Unlike infections of the nervous system in immunopreserved patients, there is no fever or headache associated with the onset or progression of PML. The usual cerebral signs of mass effect or meningeal irritation are conspicuously absent. Changes in the level of consciousness are dependent on the location and extent of the focal involvement. The progression of the clinical syndrome is insidious but may have plateaus along its course of days to weeks.

Some authors have found an occipital predominance of white matter lesions, with the clinical presentation of homonymous hemianopsia being the most common focal cerebral symptom at onset. A review of 67 patients with pathologically proved PML suggests that,. although a homonymous visual field defect is a common presenting manifestation, cerebral lesions are randomly distributed throughout the hemispheres. Hemiparesis, homonymous visual loss, and altered mentation are the three most common initial manifestations. The proportion of cerebral to cerebellar and brainstem involvement roughly parallels the proportion of brain blood flow and is likely related pathogenically to the dissemination of virus to the nervous system by a hematogenous route.

Before 1981, the most common reason for immunosuppression associated with PML was chronic lymphocytic leukemia or Hodgkin's disease. In general, any lymphoreticular malignancy can be associated with PML. However, a variety of other disorders, including granulomatous processes such as sarcoidosis, immunodeficiency states secondary to transplantation and immunosuppressive therapy, or collagen-vascular disorders such as systemic lupus erythematosus have been associated with a predilection to PML. The common factor shared among all of these disorders is a defect in cell-mediated immunity. However, the exact nature of the immune dysfunction responsible for JC virus infection of the brain remains unclear. Since 1981, the most common underlying immune defect associated with new cases of PML is AIDS.

Beyond the male predominance of patients with AIDS-associated PML, there is no gender predilection for PML. The age of onset of the illness reflects the age groups of patients affected by the underlying immunosuppressive illness. Children are only rarely affected, presumably because they are not exposed to JC virus until middle to late childhood. However, children as young as age 7 have been described who are HIV positive and have the clinical syndrome of PML. Whereas in the pre-AIDS era, the typical onset was in the sixth to seventh decade, the average age of patients has fallen proportionately to the number of patients with AIDS affected by this illness.

Diagnostic Evaluation

Laboratory testing is often nonspecifically abnormal. EEG may show focal slowing but is generally nonspe-

cific. CT scanning of the head shows focal demyelinated areas when they are severe but is insensitive. Early in the course of the disease, there may be a clinical-CT scan dissociation with clinically significant lesions not apparent on CT scan.

MRI scanning of the brain is the most sensitive method to detect focal demyelinated areas and may be diagnostic in the proper clinical context. Different from the periventricular predisposition of demyelinated areas associated with multiple sclerosis, the MRI lesions of PML are typically superficial, subcortical, and often apparently unifocal, beginning at the gray-white matter junction and spreading circumferentially or coalescing over time (see Pathology, below). Typically, the lesions show an increased T_2-weighted signal on MRI scanning with slight or no mass effect. Only rarely is significant edema or mass effect seen. Peripheral enhancement with gadolinium contrast material has been described. Contrast enhancement should raise the question of a different pathologic process. Focal deficits seen clinically are accompanied by abnormalities evident on head MRI scanning because the cause for neurologic dysfunction in PML is myelin destruction. The absence of abnormalities on a high-quality head MRI scan associated with focal neurologic deficits clinically virtually excludes the possibility of PML. The focal lesions of PML on MRI scan (Fig. 49-4) are usually easily distinguishable from CNS toxoplasmosis, brain abscesses from other opportunistic infections, and CNS lymphoma based on the lack of mass effect and absence of contrast enhancement on MRI scanning. HIV-related leukoencephalopathy can be confused with PML, but this entity is usually simultaneously bilateral, tends to occur deeper in the centrum semiovale, and has a less discrete appearance on T_2-weighted MRI scans (see above). Brain biopsy is the only definitive means to exclude confusion with these other neuropathologic entities in ambiguous cases.

CSF findings are usually normal. An elevation of the protein concentration to a level less than 100 mg/dl is seen in 30 percent of patients. The cell count is typically normal, but an elevation of the cell count to less than 30 cells/μl is present in 15 percent of patients. The mild elevations of protein level and cell count are more common among patients who are relatively immunopreserved or who have opportunistic. infections. An assay for antibodies against JC virus in the CSF is an insensitive means for confirmation of the diagnosis. Rarely, oligoclonal bands have been reported in the CSF of patients with PML.

New studies with PCR technology to amplify viral DNA from the CSF have been encouraging. Initially, PML in only 10 to 30 percent of patients could be

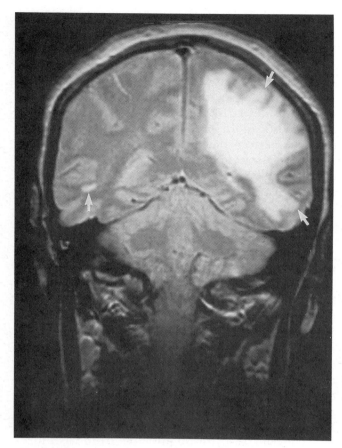

Figure 49-4. Coronal section MRI head scan of a patient with PML showing the increased T$_2$ signal without mass effect in the white matter of the cerebral hemisphere. The demyelination typically starts subcortical at the gray-white matter junction (*arrows*) and expands circumferentially.

isphere of the brain, accounting for the enlarging unifocal appearance on MRI scan (Fig. 49-4).

At the light microscopic level, oligodendrocytes infected by JC virus undergo nuclear morphologic changes with enlargement and effacement of the usual chromatin pattern. Nuclei take on a groundglass appearance. These changes in the oligodendrocytes are secondary to filling the nuclei with virions. The altered appearance of the affected oligodendrocytic nuclei have been referred to as inclusions. As the disease progresses, these inclusion-bearing oligodendrocytes typically ring a central area of severe demyelination devoid of oligodendrocytes (Fig. 49-5). Axons that traverse the white matter are largely spared. A prominent reactive astrocytosis is also characteristic. In some but not all cases, a striking bizarre astrocytic morphologic change is observed, particularly in the center of more chronic lesions with severe demyelination. These morphologically altered astrocytes have been shown to be infected by JC virus. There is macrophage infiltration as myelin degeneration progresses, with macrophages engulfing myelin debris.

In non-AIDS-related PML, the pathologic response is not inflammatory. However, in some circumstances, particularly in patients whose immune system is relatively preserved, there is a prominent perivascular lymphocytic infiltration, presumably representing an

detected by this method, but more recent studies suggest a 60 percent detection rate.

Pathology

The diagnosis of PML is based on the clinical circumstances and the characteristic changes present pathologically on brain biopsy or autopsy. Pathologically, the diagnosis is not difficult when adequate tissue is available for study. Grossly, demyelinating lesions are confined to the white matter of the brain, usually in the cerebral or cerebellar hemispheres or less often in other parts of the brainstem. No pathologically documented case of PML has been reported to involve the optic nerve. Spinal cord changes are exceedingly rare. The demyelinated lesions are frequently immediately subcortical or near the deep gray matter in the cerebral hemispheres. Early, the typical lesions are multiple and grossly millimeters in size and show coalescence. Although multifocal (and thus the name), the lesions are frequently confined to a single lobe or hem-

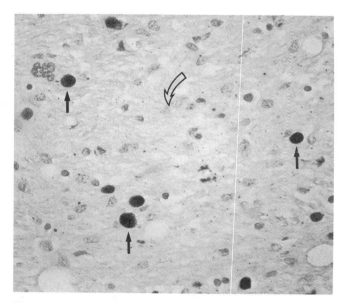

Figure 49-5. PML lesion in the subcortical white matter. The enlarged oligodendrocytic nuclei undergoing destruction by JC virus infection are accentuated in this figure by a dark stain for JC virus DNA. These nuclei (*solid arrows*) surround a more complete demyelinated core (*open arrow*) devoid of oligodendrocytes. Nonradioactive in situ hybridization for JC virus DNA (hematoxylin counterstain, original magnification ×630).

immune response to JC virus. On the other hand, scant perivascular inflammatory cells are commonly seen in the circumstance of AIDS-associated PML. It is also not uncommon to see coincident HIV infection of perivascular macrophages by HIV virus in a bed of surrounding demyelination related to PML.

Electron microscopy can be used to confirm the diagnosis on brain tissue. The presence of papovavirus-sized virions present in oligodendrocytic nuclei is diagnostic. Filamentous forms are sometimes seen in the nuclei of infected oligodendrocytes, although the relevance of these structures to progression of disease has not been firmly established.

Immunohistochemical staining for JC virus capsid proteins can be done by immunofluorescence or peroxidase methods, with specific antisera raised against JC virus. However, staining with a polyclonal antisera directed against antigens shared by the human polyomaviruses (JC and BK viruses) and Simian virus 40 is also diagnostic of PML.

In situ hybridization studies with biotin-labeled nonradioactive probes have been shown to be sensitive and specific for the detection of the JC virus genome in PML-involved brain tissue. The methodology has become standardized such that this means of detection of virus can be used to confirm the diagnosis. The JC virus genome is detected in the nuclei of infected oligodendrocytes and can also be seen in many of the bizarre astrocytes in the PML-involved brain.

Pathogenesis

JC virus is ubiquitous in the human population. Seventy percent of adults carry antibodies against the virus. The location of primary infection in the body and the timing of dissemination of virus to the nervous system relative to the development of PML remains controversial.

The frequent seroprevalence among the adult population suggests JC virus a weak pathogen under normal immune circumstances. Two lines of reasoning suggest the virus is hematogenously disseminated to the brain. First, the lesions of PML are typically found at the gray-white matter junctions similar to those of other hematogenously disseminated disorders such as brain abscess or metastatic neoplasm. Second, the proportion of cerebral to cerebellar involvement is roughly proportional to their respective blood flows. The initiation of PML, however, which requires a state of immunosuppression, may occur by one of two mechanisms. First, the virus may be disseminated to the brain during primary infection in childhood or adolescence. It may remain latent there until a state of immunosuppression leads to reactivation in infected oligodendrocytes. Second, the virus may be reactivated in a distant organ such as kidney or bone mar-

row and hematogenously disseminated to the brain just before active oligodendrocytic infection. These two mechanisms may not be mutually exclusive. If JC virus is latent in the brain, it may be reactivated during immunosuppression and lead to oligodendrocytic infection, or the virus may be reactivated in a peripheral site and also disseminate hematogenously.

Treatment

A variety of antiviral substances have been tried with little success. These include vidarabine, acyclovir, idoxuridine, zidovudine, tilorone, levamisole, and transfer factor without reported success.

Cytarabine has had limited success, with more reported among non-AIDS-related PML cases than in patients with AIDS. Doses have varied between reports, but most authors have used 2 mg/kg/day or 60 mg/m^2/day IV for 5 to 7 days. It is unclear whether coincident or exclusive intrathecal therapy offers any survival advantage. Systemic cytarabine is inevitably associated with bone marrow toxicity. Intrathecal therapy alone may provide less toxicity.

Both interferon-α and -β have been used either singly or in combination with other antivirals, with only a few scattered reports of success.

There are anecdotal reports that PML may rarely spontaneously remit, even in the context of AIDS. Improved systemic immune status is most correlated with prolonged survival.

TOXOPLASMOSIS

CNS toxoplasmosis is the second most frequent organism causing CNS opportunistic infection associated with AIDS. It has been estimated that 3 to 40 percent of all patients with AIDS will have CNS toxoplasmosis develop sometime during their illness. It is the most common cause of focal opportunistic infection of the brain in AIDS. Early on in the AIDS epidemic, cerebral biopsy was required for antemortem diagnosis. Currently, however, the diagnosis is based on the combination of clinical history, positive serologic findings, neuroimaging characteristics, and response to antimicrobial therapy.

Toxoplasma gondii is an obligate intracellular parasite. Although the organism is ubiquitous throughout the world and infects many species of animals, cats are thought to serve as the primary reservoir for transmission to humans. Ingestion of infected undercooked beef, lamb, or pork may transmit the disease, but the primary route of dissemination to humans presumably is oral-fecal caused by feline contamination of the environment.

Seroprevalence indicates exposure to the Toxoplasma organism and is highly dependent on geography. Estimates in different geographic locations have suggested that 5 to 70 percent of the general population are exposed. This range of differing seroprevalence may explain the varying incidence of toxoplasmosis of the CNS in AIDS among differing geographic locations in the world.

Clinical Features

The three main presentations of CNS toxoplasmosis brain abscess in the context of AIDS are as an acute mass lesion with focal symptoms, subacute encephalopathy with focal symptoms, or a subacute generalized encephalopathy without localizing findings. The most common presenting neurologic signs and symptoms of CNS toxoplasmosis in order of frequency are headache, global confusion, gait disorder, focal weakness, cerebellar symptoms and signs, language disturbance, seizures, and coma. Fever is also common. Toxoplasmosis has only rarely been associated with infection of the spinal cord.

There is a predilection of the Toxoplasma organism to cause focal brain abscess in brain parenchyma adjacent to ependymal surfaces. However, any area of the cerebrum, cerebellum, or brainstem is potentially vulnerable to infection, in that order of frequency. Some focal neurologic sign is present in 70 to 90 percent of patients. The quality of focal neurologic sign present is dependent on the location of brain involvement. A common syndrome complex is headache, hemiparesis, and lethargy, evolving acutely or subacutely. Because of the tendency for a periventricular location, focal brain lesions may alternatively present without dramatic focal changes on neurologic examination.

Diagnostic Evaluation

The diagnosis rests on the constellation of characteristic neuroimaging and serologic findings and the response to therapy. The CT scan is abnormal in 70 to 90 percent of patients, showing ring-enhancing lesions most often deep in the parenchyma along CSF pathways. Mass effect is usual. Less often, involvement of the cortex, particularly at the subcortical gray-white junction, can occur. The neurodiagnostic imaging of choice, however, is MRI scan of the head (Fig. 49-6). Because CNS toxoplasmosis is often not sampled for biopsy now, prospective sensitivity studies of MRI scans are not available. However, a comparative study of CT to MRI scanning of the head has suggested that MRI reveals lesions not apparent on the CT scan, both as additional lesions or as single lesions not seen on CT. On head MRI, focal lesions have a tendency to be periventricular in location, ring or irregularly enhance with gadolinium, and exhibit some associated edema or mass effect. MRI of the head shows multifocal lesions in 70 to 90 percent of patients.

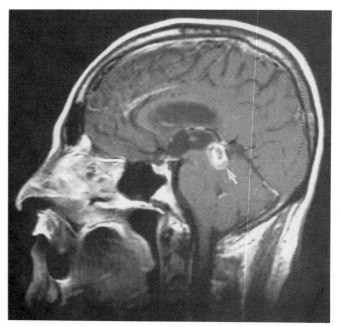

Figure 49-6. T_1-weighted sagittal view MRI head scan with gadolinium enhancement of a patient with CNS toxoplasmosis. A deep periaqueductal enhancing *Toxoplasma* abscess (*arrow*) is present, causing third nerve paresis and obstructive hydrocephalus. This lesion was one of two in the brain of this patient and responded to anti-Toxoplasma therapy in 1 week.

Toxoplasmosis of the brain is believed to be a reactivation infection. Therefore, serologic results should always be positive in the blood. Serologic titers greater than 1:1,024 or a fourfold increase in the titers is thought to be diagnostic. Lower titers of positive serologic analysis are more commonly seen in CNS toxoplasmosis and cannot distinguish active CNS infection from that of patients previously infected. Negative serologic findings in the past were used as a marker to exclude the diagnosis. However, a recent study suggests up to 16 percent of patients with bona fide CNS toxoplasmosis may be seronegative. Some debate has emerged on the insensitivity of the serotesting used for that study, but another explanation may be that serologic reactivity attenuates as AIDS and the immune system disease progresses, leading to lower levels of antibodies despite manifest infection.

CSF analysis may be helpful but may not be required for the confirmation of CNS toxoplasmosis. It is mainly useful to exclude other coincident pathogens. In CNS toxoplasmosis, leukocyte count of the CSF can be normal. In 27 to 42 percent, the leukocyte count is elevated to less than 70 nucleated cells/mm³. The CSF protein level is elevated (greater than 45 mg/dl) in 65 to 85 percent of patients. The glucose content is depressed in only 8 to 14 percent. Toxoplasma serologic results on undiluted CSF are reported to be positive in 62 to 88 percent of patients with active CNS toxoplasmosis. However, because mass effect may be prominent, CSF examination may be potentially dangerous. Neuroimaging should always precede CSF examination because the lack of focal signs on clinical examination may not exclude obstructive focal mass effect.

Brain biopsy in general is not required to make the diagnosis because most patients are treated empirically for CNS toxoplasmosis who have positive serologic findings and focal suggestive imaging results. However, biopsy may be required when there has been a lack of response to empiric therapy, suggesting the possibility of either CNS lymphoma or a brain abscess from a different organism. It must also be realized that, because lesions are at times ill defined, sampling error may make brain biopsy nondiagnostic.

Pathology

Pathologic findings from brain biopsy or autopsy specimens from patients with CNS toxoplasmosis show ill-defined necrosis and inflammation without the granulation tissue of other causes of brain abscesses. Severe infection is associated with central coagulative or hemorrhagic necrosis. Surrounding mononuclear inflammatory infiltrates and macrophages, often full of lipid debris, are present. Toxoplasma organisms encysted as bradyzoites or free organisms called tachyzoites are sometimes demonstrable on routine stains, typically at the advancing edges of brain lesions. As the disease progresses, a more organized "abscess," consisting of lipid-laden macrophages and residual reactive astrocytes, may be the only remnant of brain parenchymal inflammation, particularly after successful treatment. Less intense inflammatory reaction or even isolated encysted organisms without inflammatory response can also be encountered in the brain.

On routine stains of brain specimens, clusters of *Toxoplasma* tachyzoites are small and difficult to see. Immunohistochemical staining of brain samples with Toxoplasma antiserum enhances the detection of organisms in questionable cases.

Treatment

The accepted therapy for CNS toxoplasmosis is pyrimethamine and sulfadiazine, usually given concomitantly with folic acid. More recently, because of the high incidence of allergic reaction to sulfadiazine, pyrimethamine plus clindamycin has been suggested to be equally efficacious in treating this disorder. Short courses of corticosteroids are reserved for patients who have significant mass effect. Short-duration steroid therapy does not seem to have a negative influence on long-term survival.

Patients with a presumptive diagnosis by positive serologic and imaging findings receive therapy and are observed for clinical and radiographic response. Clinical response occurs in 75 percent within 10 days and radiographic response, in 2 weeks or less. Clinical or radiographic progression in the face of anti-toxoplasma therapy should raise the index of suspicion for other CNS pathologic conditions, often requiring brain biopsy for definitive diagnosis. Alternative differential diagnostic consideration include, most prominently, CNS lymphoma. However, brain abscesses from other opportunistic infections, such as aspergillosis, tuberculosis, or nocardiosis, should also be considered.

CRYPTOCOCCAL MENINGITIS

Among all opportunistic infections in AIDS, cryptococcal infection is the most frequent primary cause of meningitis (Figs. 49-7 to 49-9) (see also Ch. 42). It is the first manifestation of AIDS by opportunistic infection in 45 percent of patients. It has been estimated 7 percent of patients with AIDS will have cryptococcal meningitis during the course of their lifetime.

The most specific means for identification of infection is CSF culture. The specificity of a positive CSF culture is virtually 100 percent, and the sensitivity is high. However, the results from CSF culture for *Cryptococcus* typically takes 2 to 6 weeks. The most rapid sensitive diagnostic test is identification of cryptococ-

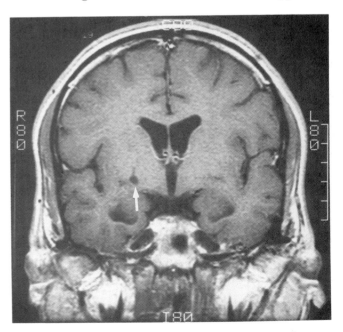

Figure 49-7. T$_1$-weighted gadolinium-enhanced coronal MRI head scan from a patient with AIDS and cryptococcal meningitis. The deep basal ganglia nonenhancing lesions (*arrow*) were proved to be cryptococcal microabscesses at autopsy.

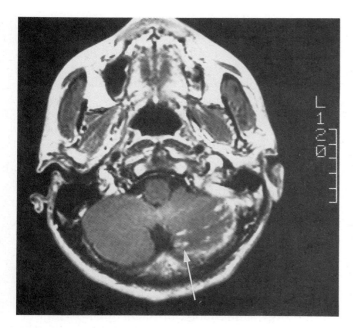

Figure 49-8. Gadolinium-enhanced MRI head scan of a patient with cryptococcal meningitis and a cerebellar syndrome. Parenchymal cerebellar folia enhancement (*arrow*) represents direct invasion by *Cryptococcus*.

cal antigen in the CSF. Although a variety of techniques are used to detect the polysaccharide capsule antigen, the most commonly used is the latex agglutination test. In one study of patients with AIDS, cryptococcal antigen was positive in 91 percent of patients who were later confirmed to have cryptococcal meningitis by culture. The 9 percent negative rate was equivalent to that in studies in other immunosuppressed individuals. In one study, patients with cryptococcal meningitis had blood findings that were positive for cryptococcal antigen in 98 percent. It is unclear why some patients have cryptococcal meningitis and had negative antigen in the CSF but positive antigen levels in the blood. However, this finding emphasizes the importance of checking for cryptococcal antigen in the blood and CSF of patients with AIDS.

Amphotericin B has been used as the mainstay for treatment of cryptococcal meningitis. Typically, 1.5 g IV given over 6 weeks has been used. In the AIDS population, this has been associated with a 79 percent 6-week survival rate. The use of coincident flucytosine 75 to 100 mg/kg/day has been associated with more bone marrow toxicity. There is controversy whether amphotericin B alone versus the addition of flucytosine is most appropriate in this AIDS infection. Chronic suppressive therapy, however, has been recommended. This includes either oral ketoconazole or weekly amphotericin B. Increasing experience with other imidazoles may lead to improved regimens for treatment of this disorder.

CYTOMEGALOVIRUS

Pathologically significant CMV is a common systemic infection in AIDS, estimated to occur in 62 to 76 percent of patients. It most severely affects the retina,

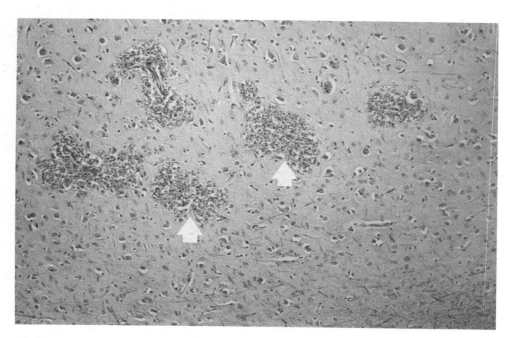

Figure 49-9. Perivascular parenchymal invasion by *Cryptococcus* (*arrows*) in a patient with AIDS and clinical meningitis (PAS-LFB stain, original magnification ×100).

liver, kidney, adrenal gland, pancreas, or lung. Dissemination to the nervous system is presumably through viremia. The incidence of CNS involvement by CMV in AIDS is unknown, but autopsy series estimate 16 to 26 percent. CMV probably represents the third most common opportunistic infection of the human nervous system in AIDS.

Neurologic manifestations of CMV infection in the AIDS population can be broken down into four categories. First, rare cases of transient acute "aseptic" meningitis can occur. This has been rarely documented by isolation of CMV. Second, a subacute encephalopathy characterized by microglial nodules affecting the cerebral cortex has been described. Third, CMV in AIDS causes an ascending prominent inflammatory polyradiculopathy. Finally, CMV can cause a disseminated diffuse ventriculitis and brainstem encephalitis associated with an encephalitic syndrome, which may coincide with polyradiculopathy or polycranial neuropathy.

The acute meningitis of CMV has no distinguishing characteristics. The usual syndrome of headache, fever, and stiff neck come on over hours to days. The index of suspicion is raised by the presence of an immunosuppressed state such as AIDS. Focal features are distinctly uncommon, although cranial nerve paresis has been reported.

The subacute encephalitis of CMV infection clinically presents as a diffuse encephalopathic illness. Concentrational, attentional, and cognitive complaints are prominent manifestations of the disease. These may be present in the context of systemic reactivation of CMV manifest as CMV viruria or more prominent infection of the retina or lungs. However, the extra-CNS manifestations of CMV may be completely inapparent. The illness progresses over weeks and causes a "subcortical" type of dementia, leading to impairment of motor skills, abulia, ataxia, and seizures. Focal neurologic deficits are infrequent, although frequent signs of cerebellar ataxia, apraxia of movement, diffuse hyper-reflexia, and profound global cognitive decline become prominent as the disease progresses. This syndrome is virtually indistinguishable from primary HIV encephalitis.

A common neurologic manifestation of CMV infection is an ascending polyradiculopathy, typically occurring in the context of clinical AIDS. Pre-existing CMV retinitis is a common but not necessary manifestation of CMV infection that precedes neurologic involvement. The syndrome of ascending polyradiculopathy mainly affecting the cauda equina is typically motor with prominent pain and sometimes prominent paresthesias. Bowel and bladder involvement with lower motor neuron type of urinary retention or fecal incontinence is frequent. Sensory manifestations can

be a prominent part of the presenting symptom complex, but findings are less common. The sacral dermatomes are most often affected when sensory signs are present. A clear-cut sensory level is often difficult to detect. The presentations of the motor symptoms are frequently asymmetric but rapidly evolve and are of a lower motor neuron variety. These typically present over hours to days, evolving into a flaccid paraparesis with areflexia. Upper extremity involvement can be seen but is relatively less frequent.

Progressive polyradiculopathy caused by ascending CMV infection is easily clinically distinguished from the more common distal symmetric polyneuropathy of HIV infection. The latter is more sensory and slowly progressive, infrequently produces weakness, and does not affect sphincter function. CSF parameters are frequently normal or show only mild elevation of protein levels or mononuclear cell count. CMV cauda equina polyradiculopathy can be mimicked more closely by ascending herpes simplex or zoster infection or CNS lymphoma.

The fourth profound manifestation of CMV is that of a diffuse ependymitis affecting the ventricular system and meningitis of the pial surface along the brainstem. Neuropathologic examination done on patients with the ependymitis-meningitis syndrome frequently

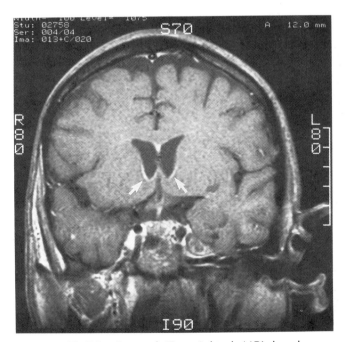

Figure 49-10. Coronal T$_1$-weighted MRI head scan shows subependymal gadolinium enhancement (*arrows*) along the surface of the lateral ventricle of this patient with AIDS and CMV polyradiculopathy. This finding may be present with or without cerebral symptoms suggestive of encephalitis.

also reveals coincident cauda equina involvement by the virus. The clinical manifestations of this disease are usually those of a meningitis, but the presentation is more subacute or chronic over days to weeks.

The most prominent changes on diagnostic evaluation affect the CSF in the circumstance of the ascending CMV polyradiculopathy or CMV-induced ependymitis and brainstem encephalitis. Typically, there is a prominent pleocytosis in the CSF. Unlike most other viral infections, this consists of a predominance of polymorphonuclear cells. The protein level elevation is often high, and the glucose content in the CSF is usually depressed. Because of these findings, confusion with bacterial or fungal infections is common. On the other hand, CSF study of CMV subacute microglial encephalitis associated with dementia and seizures is either associated with mild or no elevation in protein level and normal to slightly elevated lymphocyte count.

Neuroimaging of patients with the ependymitis and brainstem encephalitis by MRI scan with gadolinium enhancement shows an outlining of the ventricular system with gadolinium secondary to the prominent inflammatory response present along the ventricles and CSF pathways (Fig. 49-10). This pattern of subependymal enhancement on MRI can also be present when ascending CMV polyradiculopathy is the only clinical manifestation. Subependymal enhancement with gadolinium is characteristic of CMV infection. However, because of the multitude of infections that can occur in the context of AIDS, other pathogens should be sought by further diagnostic evaluation of the CSF. MRI of the spinal cord and cauda equina in CMV polyradiculopathy is usually normal. Likewise, myelographic results are usually normal but can show thickened or adherent roots. Neuroimaging of CMV encephalitis with microglial nodules is unrewarding. The findings on CT or MRI of the head are usually those of cerebral atrophy without focal abnormalities or gadolinium enhancement.

Electrophysiologic examination of CMV polyradiculopathy typically shows an axonal process affecting motor nerves predominantly. Paraspinal denervation early and prominent involvement of F-waves give a clue about the proximal nature of this disorder and distinguish it from the peripheral neuropathy associated with HIV infection or the toxicity of anti-HIV drugs.

The diagnosis of CMV infection in the nervous system is based on direct isolation of CMV, identification of viral products such as DNA, or pathologic examination showing characteristic cytomegalic inclusion cells (Fig. 49-11). CMV is difficult to culture from the CSF. The most sensitive means for detecting the virus in

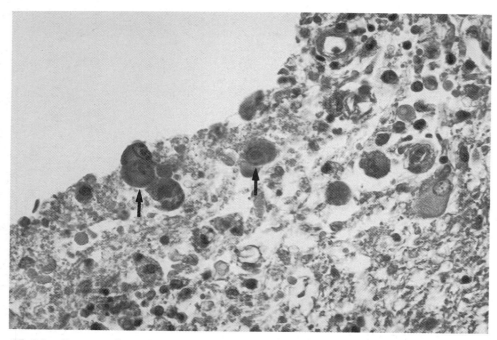

Figure 49-11. Cytomegalic inclusion cells (*arrows*) at the subependymal surface of the lateral ventricle from a patient with AIDS and CMV ependymitis and clinical encephalitis and meningitis (hematoxylin and eosin stain, original magnification ×630).

CSF specimens is the PCR. Recent studies have suggested that nearly all patients who have CMV ependymitis and brainstem encephalitis or CMV polyradiculopathy will have positive results by PCR. It is easy to understand why this might be so, given the ependymal, subependymal, and subpial location of viral infection in this syndrome. The sensitivity of PCR detection, however, in multifocal microglial nodule encephalitis or aseptic meningitis is unknown.

Ganciclovir is a specific antiviral agent that has been shown to be effective in controlling CMV infection systemically and the retinitis. There are scattered reports of success using ganciclovir, 2.5 mg/kg IV every 8 hours for 10 days to treat the CMV polyradiculopathy. Maintenance therapy has been suggested for patients with AIDS. Ganciclovir penetrates the blood-brain barrier and CSF levels are 40 to 50 percent of plasma levels. Chronic suppressive therapy is usually needed in view of the high incidence of relapse of patients with retinitis after therapy is discontinued.

TUBERCULOSIS IN THE CENTRAL NERVOUS SYSTEM

The frequency with which tuberculosis infects the CNS in the context of HIV-related disease is difficult to ascertain (see also Ch. 46). This presumably reflects the variability of tuberculosis occurring among different geographic and environmentally exposed groups who may also be at risk for HIV infection. It has been stated that HIV-positive patients are at an increased risk for CNS dissemination of pulmonary tuberculosis, particularly where it is endemic. One study suggested CNS infection by tuberculosis occurs in 2 percent. A better estimate of involvement of the nervous system comes from looking at a retrospective analysis of patients who have pulmonary tuberculosis and HIV seropositivity. In that group, it is estimated that 10 to 19 percent had CNS tuberculosis.

The clinical manifestations of tuberculous meningitis in HIV-related disease are similar to those in patients who do not have HIV-related disease. The typical syndrome evolves in a variety of temporal profiles and may be acute, subacute, or chronic, coming on over a period longer than 4 to 6 weeks. Cryptococcal infection and tuberculosis can be considered the most common causes for chronic meningitis in patients with HIV infection.

As in other patients with tuberculous meningitis, elevation of the CSF protein level is common, but among HIV-seropositive patients, the protein concentration may be normal in 17 to 43 percent. A low CSF glucose level in meningeal tuberculosis is common and is seen in 50 to 80 percent. CSF direct staining for acid-fast bacilli is negative in 77 to 80 percent of patients, despite their severe immunosuppression.

Skin testing for delayed hypersensitivity is usually negative for reaction to tuberculin proteins because of anergy. In HIV-seropositive patients with documented CNS tuberculosis, 71 to 100 percent of patients have no skin response. However, skin testing with a positive response and negative CSF cultures might still prompt empiric antituberculous therapy in the face of a chronic meningitis without other explanation. The PCR may be of some additional rapid diagnostic help for tuberculous meningitis. Some reports suggest positive results in patients when the CSF culture is negative. The sensitivity of this assay is yet to be fully determined in HIV-seropositive patients with tuberculosis involving the nervous system.

The pathologic findings of tuberculous meningitis or tuberculous parenchymal involvement in HIV are not distinctive compared with those in either nonimmunosuppressed patients who have tuberculous meningitis or immunosuppressed patients from other causes.

The treatment of tuberculous meningitis in association with HIV has been further complicated by the emergence of multiply drug-resistant tuberculosis organisms. Some strains in particular are resistant to isoniazid and rifampin, which are generally regarded as the two best drugs for tuberculosis. There are varying recommendations about the use of antituberculous drugs in association with meningitis or primary intraparenchymal brain involvement. At least three drugs should be used and possibly four. These should include a combination of isoniazid, rifampin, pyrazinamide, and/or ethambutol, and/or streptomycin. Pyridoxine should be given to all patients who are receiving isoniazid. Visual-evoked responses have been used to monitor for ethambutol toxicity in some patients. In monitoring for a response, it must be kept in mind that the CSF abnormalities take 1 to 2 months to improve significantly. The glucose level shows improvement first and should return to normal levels within 2 to 3 weeks.

The use of corticosteroids is somewhat controversial. Patients who present with a hydrocephalus, coma, or a marked mass effect clearly benefit by taking steroids in the short term. Focal cranial nerve involvement may also be improved by steroids. Patients who are ambulatory and fully conscious probably should not be treated with steroids. A decision to use steroids is more problematic in patients who have mild or moderate changes in level of consciousness, with or without nuchal signs, but no focal mass effect or signs of CSF obstruction. Close observation, repeated scanning, and frequent neurologic examination for signs of neurologic deterioration are required to determine whether antituberculous drugs alone are sufficient to reverse the potentially fatal effects of tuberculous meningitis.

MISCELLANEOUS ORGANISMS INVOLVING THE CENTRAL NERVOUS SYSTEM

Varicella-Zoster Virus

Varicella-zoster virus causes clinical herpes zoster (shingles) as a reactivation infection in AIDS and in other immunosuppressed states (see also Ch. 48). However, because of the greater compromise of the immune state in AIDS, varicella-zoster virus tends to disseminate or to involve parts of the nervous system other than the dorsal root ganglion and sensory nerves (Fig. 49-12).

Varicella-zoster virus can cause multifocal brain parenchymal disease in patients with AIDS. The disease clinically behaves as a subacute to chronic focal neurologic deficit and looks similar to progressive multifocal leukoencephalopathy on the CT scan, except for a greater tendency to involve the gray and the white matter. On MRI scan, however, there is intense gadolinium enhancement of these subcortical lesions as they advance, distinguishing them from PML. The leukoencephalitis caused by varicella-zoster virus can be subacute or chronic in its progression. Only biopsy or autopsy reveals the true cause with typical changes of intranuclear inclusions compatible with varicella-zoster virus infection.

Herpes Simplex Virus

Herpes simplex virus both types 1 and 2 has been reported to cause CNS infections in patients with AIDS (see also Ch. 48). Herpes simplex type 2 as a reactivation infection can start as only an anal-genital skin eruption, but it progresses to an ascending meningitis or cauda equina syndrome with an inflammatory reaction. The distinguishing feature is the accompanying skin eruption. Both types 1 and 2 have been associated with meningoencephalitis, and the usual temporal lobe predilection for herpes simplex virus can be present in AIDS.

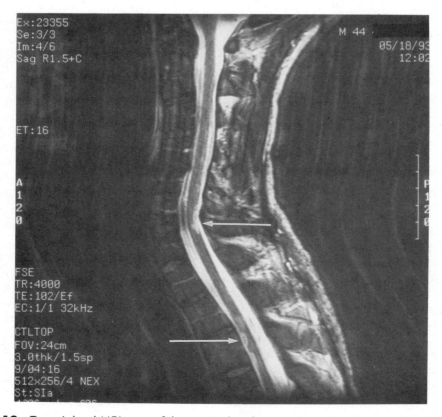

Figure 49-12. T$_2$-weighted MRI scan of the cervical and upper thoracic spinal cord. Multifocal lesions are seen in the lower cervical and thoracic spinal cord (*arrows*). Segmental paresis and myelopathy occurred in this patient with AIDS and clinical zoster. The myelopathy improved in response to steroids and acyclovir.

Nocardia

Nocardia, when it occurs in the nervous system in AIDS, usually presents as a brain abscess (see also Ch. 42). There are no clinically distinguishing features that segregate nocardial brain abscesses from other causes of brain abscesses. Gratefully, the occurrence seems to be infrequent.

Neurosyphilis

Neurosyphilis has enjoyed a resurgence in the AIDS era (see also Ch. 41). Its treatment has become more of a challenge because of the persistent immunosuppression and incomplete clearing of syphilis with standard antibiotic regimens of the past. Meningitis is the most common presentation of neurosyphilis clinically. Neurosyphilis can also present with strokelike episodes secondary to meningovascular involvement. Finally, neurosyphilis can cause an ascending polyradiculopathy. As with CMV polyradiculopathy, the CSF can show a marked pleocytosis with predominance of polymorphonuclear cells.

Aspergillosis

Aspergillosis, a common cause of brain abscess among transplant recipients, can also cause brain abscess in AIDS (see also Ch. 40). The vascular invasive nature of this fungus leads to a presentation often similar to a strokelike episode. Alternatively, subacute progression of focal neurologic deficit associated with a more generalized encephalopathy is a common presentation. Treatment is difficult, but a clue about the CNS disease may be gained by evaluating the primary pulmonary disease that may be coincident.

Candida

Candida can cause an acute or subacute evolving meningitis without distinguishing features (see also Ch. 40). However, it seems to be one of the rare causes of meningitis, despite its common occurrence in the oral cavity, pharynx, and esophagus. Usually, the CNS disease occurs as a consequence of much more widespread systemic dissemination, leaving the meningitis as only one facet of the overwhelming widespread infection.

ANNOTATED BIBLIOGRAPHY

Aksamit AJ. PCR detection of JC virus. In Persing DH (ed). Diagnostic Molecular Microbiology. American Society for Microbiology, Washington, D.C., 1993, p. 361.

Basic science techniques.

American Academy of Neurology AIDS Task Force. Nomenclature and research case definitions for neurologic manifestations of human immunodeficiency virus-type I (HIV-1) infection. Neurology 1991;41:778.

Description of cognitive disorders.

Anders KH, Guerra WF, Toniyasu U et al. The neuropathology of AIDS. Am J Pathol 1986;124:537–58.

The experience at th University of California at Los Angeles.

Astrom K-E, Mancall EL, Richardson EP. Progressive multifocal leukoencephalopathy. Brain 1958;81:93.

Initial report.

Behar R, Wiley C, McCutchan JA. Cytomegalovirus polyradiculoneuropathy in acquired immune deficiency syndrome. Neurology 1987;37:557–61.

Single case report.

Berenguer J, Moreno S, Laguna F et al. Tuberculous meningitis in patients infected with the human immunodeficiency virus. N Engl J Med 1992;326:668–72.

Twenty-one percent of 2,205 cases.

Berger J. Neurosyphilis in human immunodeficiency virus type 1-seropositive individuals. Arch Neurol 1991;48:700–2.

Prospective studies.

Berger JR, Kaszovitz B, Donovan Post J, Dickinson G. Progressive multifocal leukoencephalopathy associated with human immunodeficiency virus infection. Ann Intern Med 1987;107:78–87.

Review of cases to that time.

Davis LE, Hjelle BL, Miller VE et al. Early viral brain invasion in iatrogenic human immunodeficiency virus infection. Neurology 1992;42:1736–9.

Evidence of HIV replication.

Hollander HH, Levy JA. Neurologic abnormalities and recovery of human immunodeficiency virus from cerebrospinal fluid. Ann Intern Med 1987;106:692–5.

Latent infection.

Janssen RS, Cornblath DR, Epstein LG et al. Human immunodeficiency virus (HIV) infection and the nervous system. Neurology 1989;39:119–22.

Reports on frequency of neurologic involvement in AIDS.

Koralnik IJ, Beaumanoir A, Hausler R et al. A controlled study of early neurologic abnormalities in men with asymptomatic human immunodeficiency virus infection. N Engl J Med 1990;323:864–70.

Thirty percent had EEG abnormalities.

Lanska MJ, Lanska DJ, Schmidley JW. Syphilitic polyradiculopathy in an HIV-positive man. Neurology 1988;38:1297–301.

A 22-year-old man.

Morgello S, Cho E-S, Nielsen S et al. Cytomegalovirus encephalitis in patients with acquired immunodeficiency syndrome. Hum Pathol 1987;18:289–97.

Report of 30 cases.

Petito CK, Cho E-S, Lemann W et al. Neuropathology of acquired immunodeficiency syndrome (AIDS): an autopsy review. J Neuropathol Exp Neurol 1986;45:635–46.

Review of 153 cases.

Porter SB, Sande MA. Toxoplasmosis of the central nervous system in the acquired immunodeficiency syndrome. N Engl J Med 1992;327:1643–8.

Case reports.

Sharer LR. Pathology of HIV-1 infection of the central nervous system: a review. J Neuropathol Exp Neurol 1992;51:3–11.

Review article.

Tartaglione JA, Collier AC, Coombs RW et al. Acquired immunodeficiency syndrome: cerebrospinal fluid findings before and during long-term oral zidovudine therapy. Arch Neurol 1991;48:695–9.

No correlations between findings and clinical improvement.

50

Creutzfeldt-Jakob Disease and Related Disorders: Transmissible Spongiform Encephalopathies

Edward P. Richardson, Jr.

Creutzfeldt-Jakob disease (CJD) is the generally accepted name of the most frequent human variety of a group of relentlessly progressive, devastating cerebral disorders of humans and animals that are now known to be due to the presence of prions. This term (pronounced pree-on) was introduced in 1982 by Stanley Prusiner to designate the infectious agent that induces scrapie, a cerebral disease that mainly affects sheep and goats. Prusiner suggested in addition that CJD, which had already been shown to be transmissible to nonhuman primates, might likewise be a prion disease. The pathogenic agent was thought originally to be a form of virus. Prusiner and his coworkers (Prusiner, 1993) showed, however, that unlike viruses, the scrapie-inducing agent contains no demonstrable nucleic acids. To bring out its special properties and to emphasize that it is not a virus, Prusiner suggested that it be called prion, defined as "small proteinaceous infectious particles which are resistant to inactivation by most procedures that modify nucleic acids."

As far as is known, prions have no pathogenic effects on organ systems other than the central nervous system (CNS), but they result in devastating changes in the CNS, particularly in gray matter structures of the brain. These characteristically consist of neuronal loss, gliosis, and a diffuse fine-meshed vacuolation of the neuropil that is commonly referred to as a spongiform state. Because of this, and the fact that prion diseases can be transmitted in the manner of infections, these disorders are frequently referred to collectively as transmissible spongiform encephalopathies. Several of the prion diseases affect human beings, and these are the main topic of the present discussion. Several others occur in various animal species (e.g., scrapie, referred to above, and bovine spongiform encephalopathy, (which affects cattle).

Much progress has been made in understanding the nature and molecular biology of prions. (For comprehensive reviews, see Prusiner, 1993; DeArmond and Prusiner, 1993.) The pathogenic protein (prion), which is protease resistant, is derived from a precursor protein, (PrP), a normal protease-sensitive structural protein in brain tissue and other organs, for which the human encoding gene, PRNP, on the short arm of chromosome 20, has now been cloned. Formation of prions is a post-translational event that produces what apparently is solely a conformational change in the PrP molecule, a change that often includes production of an amyloid-forming molecular configuration. Just how the change is brought about in the precursor protein still is not understood. Once it has occurred, the resulting prions in the brain induce production of yet more prions from PrP, so that increasing amounts of the pathogenic agent are thus formed. Just how prion replication occurs is not known. The effect of this replicative process is to bring about lethal damage to CNS neurons. This is what occurs when prions are inoculated into the brain or tissues of a susceptible animal host, as in experimental scrapie, or as has happened accidentally to humans in iatrogenic CJD (see below). In sporadic CJD, which is by far the most frequent form of human prion disease, it is not known what brings about conversion of PrP to prion protein; the possibility of a genetic predisposition is discussed below.

There is strong evidence now, largely based on experiments with transgenic mice, that there are differing strains, or isolates, of prions for which there are distinct species barriers. These observations indicate that, for successful transmission of prion disease to occur, there must be a match between the particular isolate of inoculated prions and the animal's PrP. As has been stated, PrP is a normal structural protein; its function, however, is not yet known. Recent experiments have shown that it is possible, by genetic manipulation, to produce strains of mice that have no PrP whatsoever, and yet, as far as can be judged by their general health, behavior, and life span, they are none the worse for its absence. In one important respect, however, they differ from ordinary mice; they are invulnerable to prion inoculations. These experimental results provide strong support for the hypothesis that prion-induced disease requires the presence of the appropriate PrP.

There is yet another way in which prion diseases can occur: by mutations in the encoding gene for PrP. The mutant PrP apparently has an abnormally enhanced susceptibility to transformation into prions. Several mutant forms of human PrP have now been identified, most of them characterized by single amino acid substitutions. These PrP mutations run in families as a dominantly inherited trait. As is brought out below, most of them result in what can be classified as hereditary CJD, but others, as will be seen, induce clinicopathologic syndromes that differ from classic CJD.

The known human prion diseases (transmissible spongiform encephalopathies) are the following:

CJD
    Sporadic form
    Inherited form
    Iatrogenic form
    Gerstmann-Sträussler-Scheinker syndrome (GSS)
Familial fatal insomnia (FFI)
Kuru

CREUTZFELDT-JAKOB DISEASE

General Considerations

CJD is the most frequent prion disease that affects human beings. It is nevertheless a relatively rare disease, with a yearly incidence of about 1 per 1,000,000. (For comparison, the yearly incidence of Alzheimer's disease after the age of 60 has been reported to be 127 per 100,000.) The name of the disease derives from case reports by H. G. Creutzfeldt and A. M. Jakob, who, in the early 1920s, gave detailed clinico-pathologic descriptions of several patients with a rapidly evolving progressive disorder characterized by dementia and varying degrees of spasticity, ataxia, and involuntary movements. Postmortem examination showed diffuse degenerative changes in the cerebral cortex and other gray matter structures. The first report, by Creutzfeldt, presented the case of a young woman who died at the age of 22 after a 1-year remitting and relapsing illness characterized by dementia and a spastic gait disorder. In retrospect, judging from the clinical details of the case and the character of the neuropathologic lesions, it is doubtful that Creutzfeldt's case would now be classified as CJD, but Jakob, who later described a somewhat similar illness in five middle-aged adults, thought that all of these patients had the same disease. Review and re-evaluation of the neuropathologic specimens from Jakob's cases, however, indicate that not all of them represent CJD as the term is now understood, although some clearly do. In any event, whatever may be its historical accuracy, the term CJD is now so universally accepted that it is pointless to try to replace it.

Varieties

As indicated in the listing above, CJD occurs in various forms, depending on the circumstances under which it makes its appearance. Nevertheless, the disease itself, in its clinical and pathologic expression, is the same in all of these varieties.

Sporadic Form

As already stated, this is by far the most frequent variety of CJD. Here, the disease comes on spontaneously, without any contributory preceding factors. It is not transmitted from person to person, nor is it related to any particular environmental exposure, noxious or not. The resemblance of CJD to scrapie has raised the question as to whether the human disease might ensue on ingestion of, or continued contact with, sheep or products made from them, but the evidence at present indicates that the disease does not arise in this way. There is now, however, a suggestion that there may be a genetic predisposition to sporadic CJD: homozygosity for either amino acid at codon 129 (which codes for methionine or valine) was found to be considerably more frequent in patients with sporadic CJD than in the general population, in which homozygosity and heterozygosity are about evenly balanced.

Familial Form

Epidemiologic studies have shown that CJD occurs as a familial disorder in more than 15 percent of patients, in whom it is transmitted as an autosomal dominant genetic trait. Family groups in many parts of the world have now been identified in which a point mutation in the gene encoding PrP results in the development of CJD. Examples are a mutation at codon 178, with production of asparagine instead of aspartic acid, found in families in the United States and several European countries, and a relatively widespread mutation at codon 200, giving a substitution of lysine for glutamic acid, which affects families in the Near East, Europe, South America, the United States, and as has recently been disclosed, in Japan. The literature on the molecular genetics of CJD and other prion diseases has become so extensive that adequate presentation of it is beyond the scope of this chapter; Prusiner's review (1993) provides good access to these new developments.

Iatrogenic Form

In a number of tragic instances, material infected with CJD prions has been unknowingly introduced into the tissues of patients, resulting in their acquiring CJD. This has happened with corneal transplants and with dural grafts. In addition, CJD occurred in two young people who had undergone investigation for intractable seizures; in these instances, the electrodes that were used for intracerebral electroencephalographic (EEG) recordings had been inadequately sterilized. The largest number of iatrogenic cases of CJD (in more than 40 patients, ranging in age from 10 to 41 years) occurred among the recipients of human growth hormone, given because of growth failure. The hormone was derived from pituitary glands obtained at postmortem examinations; some of these glands apparently were contaminated with CJD prions. Study of these cases indicated that the incubation period ranges from 4 to 30 years. Fortunately, synthetic growth hormone is now available, so that there is no need ever again to administer cadaver-derived hormone. With iatrogenic CJD, as with the sporadic form, there is now evidence for a genetic predisposition, in that homozygosity at codon 129 is overrepresented in these patients.

Clinical Aspects

Clinically, CJD in its typical form is characterized by rapidly advancing progressive dementia, accompanied by varying degrees of other neurologic abnormalities such as ataxia, derangements of posture and movement, myoclonic muscular contractions, disturbances of vision, and seizures. Meanwhile, there is no evidence of any associated response of the immune system. More specifically, an analysis of a consecutive series of 230 neuropathologically verified cases (Brown et al., 1986) brings out the following points (borne out on the whole by our own experience): CJD is a disease of adults, mostly of middle age or older. The age at onset in this large series ranged between 19 and 83 years, with a mean of 61.5. Men and women are equally affected. About one-third of the patients have prodromal symptoms (asthenia and disturbances of sleeping and eating patterns), usually beginning a few weeks before the appearance of overt neurologic illness. This prodromal state in most patients gradually merges with the manifestations of the CNS disorder. In about one-fifth of cases, the onset of the neurologic illness is rapid or even sudden. The most frequent abnormality referable to the nervous system at the beginning (in two-thirds of the patients surveyed) is in the sphere of mental functioning, sometimes occurring as cognitive or other higher-function disturbances, sometimes as disorders of behavior. These mental changes are followed (or occasionally preceded) by derangements of motility, muscle tone or posture, special senses, or (rarely) peripheral sensation (mainly in the form of paresthesias).

As the illness evolves into its fully developed state, the already established abnormalities become worse, and others make their appearance. A broad range of manifestations of neurologic disease is the result. The mental abnormalities develop into dementia in most cases. Ataxia of cerebellar type, involving gait and limb movements, is frequent (appearing early in one-third of the patients and, ultimately, in nearly two-thirds); it is so regular a manifestation of CJD that it seems unnecessary to suggest a special ataxic variety, as has been done in the past. Some patients (about 10 percent) have vertigo.

Somewhat less frequent than ataxia, yet prominent in many cases of CJD, is disturbance of vision, referable to lesions in vision-related regions of the cerebral cortex. The disturbance sometimes takes the form of hemianopic or generalized loss of vision; sometimes it consists of visual hallucinations, or bizarre alterations of perception—as in one of our patients, who insisted that the rugs in his living room were askew when actually they were not. In the past, patients with prominent visual symptoms and extensive occipital lesions have been classified as having the Heidenhain variant of CJD (following a clinicopathologic report in 1929), but these patients have so much in common with other patients with CJD that it no longer is necessary to assign them to a special group. Other neuro-ophthalmologic manifestations, occurring in some patients, are derangements of ocular motility: nystagmus, periodic alternating nystagmus, and slowness of saccadic movements.

With progression of CJD, movement disorders of many kinds can appear, including tremors and choreoathetoid movements, and development of a lead-pipe kind of rigidity in about one-half of the patients. Perhaps the most frequent and striking movement abnormality, regularly observed in patients with CJD, is the presence of myoclonic jerk-like contractions of the musculature, often spontaneous, but often also brought on by sudden sensory stimuli, such as a loud noise or even a touch (startle myoclonus). Typical as it is for CJD, myoclonus is a manifestation of the late phases of the disease, rather than its onset or early stages.

Another clinical feature of CJD deserving emphasis is the occurrence of seizures. These developed in 8 percent of the above-cited series of patients. The seizure patterns are extremely variable, generalized or focal, major or minor. They are characteristic of the late phases of the illness.

After Jakob's description of a patient with signs of lower motor neuron disease and lesions in the spinal cord suggestive of amyotrophic lateral sclerosis, the thought prevailed for many years that the spinal cord might be significantly involved in CJD. Subsequent experience has indicated, however, that any evidence of disease in the spinal cord is at most slight and occurs only in the terminal phases. The concept, therefore, of an "amyotrophic form" of CJD can be discarded.

In general, the course of the illness is relatively short in comparison with the long duration of Alzheimer's disease. This rather rapid evolution is reflected in one of the terms that has been used to designate CJD: subacute spongiform encephalopathy. In the series cited above, progressive mental and physical decline led to death within 1 year of onset in 90 percent of the patients. Another 5 percent died within the next year; the remaining 5 percent survived longer (up to 10 years). Some of the patients with an unusually prolonged course underwent more or less extended periods in which the disease remained on a plateau of severity, although progression eventually occurred in the long run.

Pathologic Aspects

As has already been mentioned, a characteristic feature of the prion diseases in general, including CJD, is a fine-meshed spongy vacuolation of the neuron-containing structures. This is due to multiple minute intracytoplasmic fluid accumulations in neurons, an appearance that has become known as spongiform change and has led, as previously stated, to designation of CJD and related disorders as spongiform encephalopathies. Study of a broad range of cases, with attention to the relationship of the pathologic changes to the clinical stage of the disease, suggests that, in the earliest lesions, the first visible neuropathologic change is cytoplasmic vacuolation without evidence of neuronal loss. As the disease progresses, the death of neurons becomes increasingly evident, accompanied by astrocytic enlargement and proliferation and consequent fibrillary gliosis.

Meanwhile, at no time is there any evidence of inflammation or alterations in the blood vessels or meninges.

These destructive changes tend to be most pronounced in the cerebral cortex, especially in the deeper layers, but they are present also, and often to a severe degree, in the caudate nucleus, putamen, thalamus, and cerebellar cortex. Rarely, there has been concomitant severe destructive disease of the white matter of the cerebral hemispheres. The upper brainstem may show evidence of damage (which, together with the abnormalities in the cerebellum, may account for the derangements of ocular motility seen in some cases). The lower brainstem and spinal cord are only slightly, and very infrequently, affected.

Another lesion that is characteristic of the spongiform encephalopathies (prion diseases) is the presence of amyloid plaques, found mainly in the cerebral or cerebellar cortex. They were first recognized in kuru (see below) and so are often called kuru plaques, but they are also frequent in CJD, as indicated by their presence in nearly one-half of the patients in a well-studied CJD series. They are universally found in GSS. In their morphologic and staining properties, these prion-associated plaques closely resemble the amyloid plaques occurring in Alzheimer's disease, but unlike those, they generally are not surrounded by rings of abnormal neurites. Moreover, with immunostaining, kuru plaques are positive for prion protein and negative for β-amyloid; the Alzheimer's disease plaques are prion negative but β-amyloid positive.

Laboratory Studies in Diagnosis

The laboratory investigations generally used in neurologic diagnosis are mostly helpful in a negative sense. All blood studies so far undertaken have been unhelpful, and the cerebrospinal fluid, in keeping with the lack of inflammation in the brain or meninges, is normal.

The EEG may, however, show abnormalities that can lead to a correct diagnosis. Approximately 80 percent of a well-studied series of patients with clinical and pathologic evidence of CJD showed an EEG pattern characterized by runs of periodic sharp wave complexes that became evident within 3 months of the onset of the illness and persisted thereafter. The remaining patients, in some of whom the course was unusually prolonged, had other EEG abnormalities that were not distinctive. Evoked-potential studies have been found to be normal until after the disease is far advanced, with much destruction of brain tissue, so that they do not help in early diagnosis.

Computed tomographic scanning, and particularly magnetic resonance imaging (MRI), occasionally are helpful in arriving at a diagnosis of CJD. MRI can show high signal intensity in the basal ganglia and thalamus late in the illness; it nevertheless can be normal, even in the presence of severe clinical manifestations. These imaging methods do serve to exclude neoplasms and other space-occupying lesions, and focally destructive processes (e.g., infarcts and demyelinative plaques). Moreover, they can help in eliminating Alzheimer's (or Pick's) disease, because, in these disorders, the brain is visibly atrophic by the time dementia is evident; in CJD, the brain may appear perfectly normal in the presence of overt clinical disease.

Although one can reasonably suspect CJD in the presence of typical symptoms and signs, and consistent findings with ancillary studies, the only certain way to establish the diagnosis is by neuropathologic examination of brain tissue, either obtained during life by surgical biopsy, or after death by postmortem examination. If it is thought by the physician and family that the necessity of making a diagnosis is such as to warrant a biopsy, an attempt should be made to obtain definitely diseased tissue, as indicated by asymmetric or focal findings on clinical examination, or possibly by MRI abnormalities. A finding of normal tissue morphology does not exclude the disease; the pathologic features of CJD are, however, when present, sufficiently distinctive to eliminate other disorders from consideration. Formerly, proof of a transmissible spongiform encephalopathy required transmission of the disease by inoculation of brain tissue into the brains of susceptible animals (mostly primates). Current work with specific antiprion antibodies suggests that the outlook for their use in accurately and rapidly making a diagnosis of CJD and other prion diseases is most promising.

Treatment

Unfortunately, at present there is no effective treatment for CJD or any of its variants. It pursues its relentless course uninfluenced by anything anyone can do. The most that can be done is to make the patient as comfortable as possible. Death is the inevitable outcome.

Other Human Prion Diseases

Compared with CJD, the remaining prion diseases are very rare. Furthermore, it may be somewhat artificial at present to retain these separate designations because increasing experience with the prion diseases suggests that they may represent points along a spectrum of clinicopathologic manifestations, rather than separable nosologic entities. This continuum is especially evident in the group of hereditary prion diseases in which the same precursor protein mutation can give rise to greatly varying disease pictures, although the same clinical manifestations can occur with differing mutations. Nevertheless, the disorders to be mentioned have a place in the historic development of ideas regarding this set of diseases, and they are often referred to in the contemporary literature. As in the case of CJD, there is no effective treatment for any of them.

Gerstmann-Sträussler-Scheinker Syndrome

It still is customary to set aside under this heading some rare cases of prion disease that clinically and pathologically differ considerably from the classic pattern of CJD as described above. The original case reports, from Vienna in 1936, emphasized dominant inheritance, a very chronic course, prominent ataxia of cerebellar type, dementia in the late stages, and neuropathologically, plaque-like deposits in the cerebral and cerebellar cortex. Subsequent experience has shown that there are two clinical variants, one in which ataxia is predominant (the ataxic form) and one in which mental changes appear early and become severe, although ataxia is less pronounced (the telencephalic form). The average course is 5 years. Myoclonus generally does not occur, and there is no distinctive EEG pattern. On neuropathologic examination, the plaques, which are composed of prion-amyloid, are more numerous and clustered than in CJD or kuru. Widespread neuronal loss and gliosis are evident, but the spongiform change, although characteristically present to some degree, may be absent.

Much knowledge has lately been gained as to the molecular genetics of GSS. The original Austrian patients, and others in Europe and the United States (mostly with ataxic GSS), have a mutation at codon 102, resulting in a substitution of leucine for proline. In some other families, in the United States and France, with dementing GSS (the telencephalic form), a mutation at codon 117 leads to the production of valine instead of alanine, and still other mutations, producing GSS-like syndromes, have been identified.

Familial Fatal Insomnia

In this dominantly inherited prion-induced syndrome, the distinctive features are intractable insomnia, with peculiar dreamlike states, and autonomic nervous system dysfunction, with absence of dementia until the terminal phases. During the latter course of the illness, which has shown a duration of 7 to 25 months, ataxia and myoclonus develop. Neuropathologic examination has shown selective neuronal loss and gliosis in the anterior and medial-dorsal nuclei of the thalamus and in the inferior olivary nuclei in the brainstem, relative preservation of the cerebral cortex throughout, and spongiform change in only two of eight cases examined. FFI has now been shown to be associated with a mutation of the precursor protein gene at codon 178, with substitution of asparagine for aspartic acid, a mutation that has already been mentioned above as the genetic basis for families with inherited CJD. Reference has also been made to the predisposing effect of homozygosity at codon 129 in cases of sporadic and iatrogenic CJD. Recent studies show that homozygosity for the allele coding for methionine is associated with FFI; homozygosity for valine at codon 129 predisposes to familial CJD.

Kuru

This disorder, which now is largely of historic interest, was found to be a major cause of death among the Fore people of Papua New Guinea. Clinically, it resembles GSS in the prominence of ataxia, the prolonged course, and the absence of dementia until the late phases but differs from it in the lack of evidence for genetic transmission. Pathologically, it is characterized by severe cerebellar involvement, spongiform change, and prion-amyloid plaques (first seen in kuru and thus, as already indicated, often called kuru plaques; these incidentally show some morphologic differences from GSS plaques).

Kuru was the first of the prion diseases that was found to be transmissible to animals. The disease is now thought to have been spread by the practice of ritual cannibalism (although the oral route has been found experimentally to be a very inefficient way of transmitting prion diseases). It affected chiefly women and children, who had the greatest exposure to the prion-infected brain tissue. The incubation period was found to be as long as 30 years. With the discontinuation of cannibalism in the affected tribal group, the disease is disappearing.

ANNOTATED BIBLIOGRAPHY

Barboriak DP, Provenzale JM, Boyko OB. MR diagnosis of Creutzfeldt Jakob disease. AJR Am J Roentgenol 1994; 162:137.

Details of brain imaging.

Büeler H, Aguzzi A, Sailer A et al. Mice devoid of PrP are resistant to scrapie. Cell 1993;73:1339–47.

Precursor protein may be required for susceptibility to scrapie.

Brown P, Cathala F, Castaigne P, Gajdusek DC. Creutzfeldt-Jakob disease: clinical analysis of a consecutive series of 230 neuropathologically verified cases. Ann Neurol 1986;20:597–602.

Clinical review demonstrating rigidity, myoclonus, and characteristic EEG changes may occur rather late, although cerebellar and visual signs occur early.

Brown P, Cervenakova L, Goldfarb LG et al. Iatrogenic Creutzfeldt Jakob disease: an example of the interplay between ancient genes and modern medicine. Neurology 1994;44:291–3.

Case histories of 56 iatrogenic cases show 52 homozygous at codon 129, suggesting susceptibility is important for successful transmission.

Brown P, Rogers-Johnson P, Cathala F et al. Creutzfeldt-Jakob disease of long duration: clinicopathological characteristics, transmissibility, and differential diagnosis. Ann Neurol 1984;16:295–304.

Early clinical reports.

De Armond SJ, Prusiner SB. The neurochemistry of prion diseases. J Neurochem 1993;61:1589–601.

Current details of basic biology.

Esmonde TFG, Will RG. Magnetic-resonance imaging in Creutzfeldt Jakob disease. Ann Neurol 1992;31:230–1.

Case reports.

Gajdusek DC. Unconventional viruses and the origin and disappearance of kuru. Science 1977;197:943–60.

Review of biologic features of unconventional agents.

Gertz H-J, Henkes H, Cervos-Navarro J. Creutzfeldt-Jakob disease: correlation of MRI and neuropathologic findings. Neurology 1988;38:1481–2.

With autopsy data.

Gibbs CJ Jr, Gajdusek DC, Asher DM et al. Creutzfeldt-Jakob disease (spongiform encephalopathy): transmission to the chimpanzee. Science 1968;161:388–9.

Original transmission of CJD to a nonhuman primate.

Goldfarb LG, Petersen RB, Tabaton et al. Fatal familial insomnia and familial Creutzfeldt-Jakob disease: disease phenotype determined by a DNA polymorphism. Science 1992;258:806–8.

Examples of two distinct disease phenotypes linked to a single pathogenic mutation.

Grant MP, Cohen M, Petersen RB et al. Abnormal eye movements in Creutzfeldt-Jakob disease. Ann Neurol 1993; 34:192–7.

Three patients who showed periodic alternating nystagmus and slow vertical saccades early in the course of the disease.

Inoue I, Kitamoto T, Doh-ura K et al. Japanese family with Creutzfeldt-Jakob disease with codon 200 point mutation of the prion protein gene. Neurology 1994;44:299–301.

Latest report; heterozygous point mutation at codon 200, suggesting the mutation is not race specific.

Levy SR, Chiappa KH, Burke CJ, Young RR. Early evolution and incidence of electroencephalic abnormalties in Creutzfeldt-Jakob disease. J Clin Neurophysiol 1986;3: 1–21.

Classic work on EEG findings.

Masters CL, Gajdusek DC. The spectrum of Creutzfeldt-Jakob disease and the virus-induced subacute spongiform encephalopathies. In Smith WT, Cavanagh JB (eds). Recent Advances in Neuropathology. Churchill Livingstone, Edinburgh, 1982, p. 139.

Textbook chapter, with review of brain sections from Jakob's laboratory.

Masters CL, Gajdusek DC, Gibbs CJ Jr. The familial occurrence of Creutzfeldt-Jakob disease and Alzheimer's disease. Brain 1981;104:535–58.

Masters CL, Richardson EP Jr. Subacute spongiform encephalopathy (Creutzfeldt-Jakob disease). The nature and progression of spongiform change. Brain 1978;101: 333–44.

Pathologic features of 21 cases.

Medori R, Montagna P, Tritschler HJ et al. Fatal familial insomnia: a second kindred with mutation of prion protein gene at codon 178. Neurology 1992;42:669–70.

Report of a second kindred.

Palmer MS, Dryden AJ, Hughes JT, Collinge J. Homozygous prion protein genotype predisposes to sporadic Creutzfeldt-Jakob disease. Nature 1991;352:340–2.

In 21 of 22 sporadic CJD cases, homozygosity was found at the polymorphic amino acid residue 129.

Prusiner SB. Novel proteinaceous particles cause scrapie. Science 1982;216:136–44.

Older review but still informative about unconventional agents.

Prusiner SB. Neurological review. Genetic and infectious prion diseases. Arch Neurol 1993;50:1129–53.

Update of earlier work.

Richardson EP Jr. Myoclonic dementia. In Rottenberg DA, Hochberg FH (eds). Neurological Classics in Modern Translation. Hafner Press, New York, 1977, p. 95.

English translations of papers by Creutzfeldt and Jakob.

Rocca WA, Amaducci LA, Schoenberg BS. Epidemiology of clinically diagnosed Alzheimer's disease. Ann Neurol 1986;19:415–24.

Salazar A, Masters CL, Gajdusek CJ, Gibbs CJ. Syndromes of amyotrophic lateral sclerosis and dementia: relation to transmissible Creutzfeldt-Jakob disease. Ann Neurol 1983;14:17–26.

Clinical and pathologic details.

Serban D, Taraboulos A, DeArmond SJ, Prusiner SB. Rapid detection of Creutzfeldt-Jakob disease and scrapie prion proteins. Neurology 190;40:110–7.

Enzyme-linked immunosorbent assay studies.

Watanabe R, Duchen LW. Cerebral amyloid in human prion disease. Neuropathol Appl Neurobiol 1993;19:253–60.

Association found between prion disease and amyloid deposition in the brain.

51
Introduction to Neoplasms

Lisa M. DeAngelis

Primary intracranial neoplasms (Greek: *neos*, new; *plasmein*, formation or new growth) can arise from any of the structures and cell types present in the cranial vault. These structures include not only the brain with all of its cell types but also the meninges, blood vessels, pituitary gland, and skull. Tumors can also arise from residual embryonic tissue. Metastatic (from the Greek for displacement) tumors can involve the brain, lepto-meninges, dura, or skull.

The clinical features of each tumor are discussed in the following chapters.

As an overall principle, treatment should be based on a pathologically confirmed diagnosis. Although characteristic clinical and radiographic features may strongly suggest a specific tumor diagnosis, there is no substitute for histologic review. Except for patients whose discovered primary tumor makes the secondary brain lesion almost certainly a metastasis, every patient harboring an intracranial neoplasm should be considered for a diagnostic procedure. Few exceptions will be found to this general approach.

EPIDEMIOLOGY

Around the world, the incidence of intracranial neoplasms varies from 6 to 14.4 per 100,000/year. Based on a national survey done in 1973–1974, the incidence of primary intracranial tumors and of metastatic tumors is roughly identical at 8.2 to 8.33 per 100,000 in the United States. Metastatic tumors are thus as common as all primary intracranial neoplasms combined, making them twice as common as gliomas. Although brain tumors are relatively uncommon compared with other neoplasms such as lung, breast, and colon cancer, the incidence of brain tumors has been steadily rising; this has been associated with an increasing mortality rate attributed to brain tumors, particularly among elderly patients.

Overall, there is a slight male preponderance for both primary and secondary tumors, except for me-ningiomas and pituitary tumors, which are more common in women.

The incidence rate of primary intracranial neoplasms increases steadily with advancing age until the eighth decade when it begins to fall (Table 51-1). The types of neoplasms differ by age groups. Cerebellar astrocytomas, medulloblastomas, and ependymomas are tumors of childhood or young adulthood; malignant gliomas, meningiomas, and acoustic neuromas occur in middle to late life.

In most studies, gliomas (i.e., tumors that arise from the glial tissues), are the most common primary intracranial neoplasm (Table 51-2) save for the consistent reports from the epidemiologic studies from Mayo Clinic, which have shown a higher incidence of meningiomas than gliomas. This difference may be due to the high rate of autopsies performed in that popula-

Table 51-1. Annual Incidence Rate of Primary Intracranial Neoplasms in the United States

	Incidence Rate per 100,000		
	Total	Male	Female
All ages	8.2	8.2	8.1
Under 5	2.5	2.9	2.1
5–4	2.1	2.3	2.0
15–24	3.1	2.9	3.3
25–34	4.5	1.9	6.9
35–44	5.7	4.5	6.8
45–54	17.3	17.9	16.7
55–64	20.4	23.6	17.4
65–74	20.4	26.0	16.2
75+	15.4	17.3	14.2

(Adapted from Walker et al., 1985, with permission.)

Table 51-2. Incidence of Primary Intracranial Neoplasms

	Percentage	
	n = 13,720[a]	n = 223[b]
Glioma	57.8	35
Glioblastoma	20.0	—
Medulloblastoma	2.2	0.9
Other astrocytomas	35.7	—
Meningioma	19.5	39
Neurinoma	6.9	4.0
Pituitary adenoma	14.4	13
Other	1.4	7.6

[a] Data from Walker et al., 1985.

[b] Data from Annegers et al., 1981.

tion, with the frequent identification of an unsuspected meningioma at death. Far less frequent are pituitary tumors (about 15 percent) and acoustic neuromas (about 5 percent).

GENETIC AND ENVIRONMENTAL FACTORS

Cancer is a genetic disease whereby the accumulation of cellular mutations permits uncontrolled cell growth. For brain tumors, putative genetic factors have yet to be defined, and tumor development almost certainly represents acquired somatic mutations. Clearly defined heritable factors play only a minor role in the genesis of brain tumors. Only 5 percent of patients with a glioma have a family history of brain tumor, and most do not fall into an obvious autosomal dominant or recessive pattern. Certain inherited diseases, such as tuberous sclerosis or neurofibromatosis type I, predispose the patient to the development of brain tumors, but these tumors tend to occur in children or young adults and do not account for most primary brain tumors, which develop in later years. In Turcot's syndrome, a rare autosomal recessive disease that causes multiple polyposis of the colon and brain tumors, the brain tumor is usually a glioma.

Several environmental factors have been tentatively linked to the development of brain tumors, but they apply to few patients. Cranial irradiation may predispose the patient to a variety of intracranial neoplasms, specifically meningiomas and gliomas. The doses required to achieve tumor development tend to be high, making incidental skull radiographs or even repeated imaging during frequent angiograms an unlikely source of tumor development. Women with breast cancer have an increased incidence of meningiomas.

Workers in petrochemical factories and their families and those in the aerospace industry are said to have an increased incidence of brain tumors, but this is not definite. Brain tumors are not associated with lifestyle characteristics, such as smoking or alcohol use. All told, it is unusual for a patient with a brain tumor to have a specific predisposing factor identified.

ANNOTATED BIBLIOGRAPHY

Annegers JF, Schoenberg BS, Okazaki H, Kurland LT. Epidemiologic study of primary intracranial neoplasms. Arch Neurol 1981;38:217–19.

Meningiomas are slightly more frequent than gliomas but many are incidental.

Davis DL, Schwartz J. Trends in cancer mortality: US white males and females, 1968–83. Lancet 1988;1:633–636.

Rising incidence of brain tumors, particularly with advancing age.

Hochberg F, Toniolo P, Cole P. Non-occupational risk indicators of glioblastoma in adults. J Neurooncol 1990;8: 55–60.

There is no association with lifestyle characteristics.

Ikizler Y, van Meyel DJ, Ramsay DA et al., Gliomas in families. Can J Neurol Sci 1992;19:492–97.

Only 6.7 percent of patients with gliomas had a family history of brain tumor. No consistent inheritance pattern.

Newton HB, Rosenblum MK, Malkin MG. Turcot's syndrome. Cancer 1991;68:1633–9.

Rare genetic syndrome associated with brain tumors.

Olshan AF, Breslow NE, Daling JR et al. Childhood brain tumors and paternal occupation in the aerospace industry. J Natl Cancer Inst 1986;77:17–19.

A small epidemiologic study suggesting a slightly increased risk.

Schlehofer B, Blettner M, Becker N et al., Medical risk factors and the development of brain tumors. Cancer 1992; 69:2541–7.

No association with head injury, family history, or cranial or dental radiographs.

Walker AE, Robins M, Weinfeld FD. Epidemiology of brain tumors: the national survey of intracranial neoplasms. Neurology 1985;35:219–26.

Rates for metastases approach those for all primary tumors.

Waxweiler RJ, Alexander V, Leffingwell SS et al., Mortality from brain tumor and other causes in a cohort of petrochemical workers. J Natl Cancer Inst 1983;70:75–81.

A mortality study suggesting petrochemical workers have a higher incidence of death as a result of brain tumors than expected.

52
Primary Brain Tumors

Lisa M. DeAngelis

Intracranial tumors can arise from any of the cells that constitute the central nervous system. Regardless of the specific type of tumor, most primary brain tumors have common clinical features. The presence of a neoplasm is usually established by computed tomography (CT) or magnetic resonance imaging, (MRI) but treatment is based on a pathologically verified diagnosis. A discussion of the clinical features is followed by a discussion of each tumor type.

Brain tumors produce both specific and nonspecific symptoms and signs. The nonspecific symptoms include headache, seen in about one-half of patients, and symptoms of increased intracranial pressure with nausea and vomiting, which are observed in 25 percent. Because of the widespread availability of CT and MRI scans, papilledema is now seen in less than 10 percent of patients, even when symptoms of raised intracranial pressure are present. Most patients with these symptoms as a result of a brain tumor also have specific or lateralizing neurologic symptoms, suggesting a structural process. Lateralizing signs are determined by the location of the tumor and commonly include hemiparesis, sensory loss, visual field defects, and aphasia. The presence of any one of these necessitates evaluation with a cranial CT or MRI scan. Seizures are a common presenting symptom in patients with brain tumors, particularly low-grade gliomas. Seizures from brain tumors may be either generalized or partial; generalized seizures may have a focal onset, reflecting the underlying mass. Hemorrhage into the tumor may present like a stroke; intratumor hemorrhage occurs primarily in glioblastoma multiforme and oligodendroglioma.

MRI scan is the most sensitive method to establish the diagnosis of a brain tumor. If possible, it should be the first test obtained in a patient with symptoms or signs that suggest an intracranial mass. The more commonly available CT scan is usually accurate for the diagnosis of a brain tumor but may give negative results in patients with a low-grade glioma presenting as an isolated seizure. Contrast enhancement using intravenous iodinated compounds for CT scan or gadolinium contrast for MRI scan greatly improves the tumor detection rate. Malignant primary brain tumors usually appear as contrast-enhancing mass lesions with edema extending throughout the peritumor white matter. Low-grade malignancies, such as astrocytomas, typically do not enhance by either method and are best appreciated on T_2-weighted MRI.

GLIOMAS

Glial tumors are the most common primary brain tumor. They arise from the glial (from the Greek for glue) cells (astrocytes or oligodendrocytes), which support the neurons, and the tumors are of varying malignancy.

The pathologic grade of glial neoplasms is one of the most important prognostic factors for patients and also determines their treatment.

Gliomas are graded pathologically according to the World Health Organization criteria, using a three-tier system histologically based on increasing deviation from normal microscopic cellular appearance, implying increased malignancy. For the most common gliomas, the astrocytomas are divided into astrocytoma (from the Greek for star-shaped cell + tumor), anaplastic (Greek; *ana*, lacking; *plasma,* shape or form) astrocytoma, and glioblastoma multiforme (from the Greek for glial germ cell tumor with many shapes). The grading system is based on pathologic features, such as cellular pleomorphism, mitoses, and endothelial proliferation; when present, necrosis establishes the diagnosis of glioblastoma multiforme.

The less common tumors arising from the oligodendroglia (Greek: *oligo,* few; *dendros,* tree [limbs]) are divided into low-grade oligodendrogliomas and the uncommon anaplastic oligodendroglioma.

Low-Grade Gliomas

Most low-grade gliomas, either *astrocytomas* or *oligodendrogliomas,* present in the third to fifth decades of life with a peak incidence at 40 years of age. There is a 3:2 male preponderance. Low-grade gliomas are not discrete lesions. They are highly infiltrative and do not destroy the underlying brain tissue until late in their course. They may arise in any region of the brain, although they usually occur in the cerebral hemispheres. They are slow-growing tumors, a characteristic that correlates with the absence of mitoses, cellular pleomorphism, and necrosis seen histopathologically.

Astrocytomas and oligodendrogliomas frequently present with seizures in an otherwise neurologically normal patient. Often, the lesion has been present for years before the diagnosis, and many persist for years before producing neurologic disability. However, all low-grade gliomas eventually grow, and transformation into a high-grade glioma is a common and unpredictable outcome.

Low-grade gliomas are identified on CT or MRI scans as nonenhancing masses, which are hypodense on CT and hyperintense on T_2-weighted MRI (Figs.

52-1 and 52-2.) The development of enhancement on follow-up studies in a previously diagnosed low-grade tumor suggests malignant transformation. This change is usually, but not always, associated with worsening clinical symptoms.

The treatment of choice is surgical extirpation. Complete removal may be curative but is rarely possible; subtotal resection is the alternative. If the lesion cannot be resected even in part because of its location in vital brain structures, stereotactic biopsy is performed for diagnosis. After surgery, additional treatment may include cranial radiotherapy or chemotherapy. The best timing for adjuvant radiotherapy has not been established, but it benefits those patients with progressive neurologic signs or increased seizure frequency. Chemotherapy has little effect and is not used routinely in the initial treatment of astrocytomas but may be beneficial for oligodendrogliomas. Chemotherapy may enable the physician to defer radiotherapy, a particularly important issue in the young patient, or to reduce the size of the brain treated through the radiotherapeutic port, thus minimizing exposure of normal brain to irradiation.

In many patients who undergo cranial radiotherapy, deleterious effects may occur on memory and cognitive status, which may not be evident for months to years after completion of therapy. Such effects are

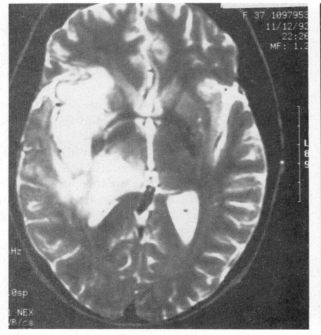
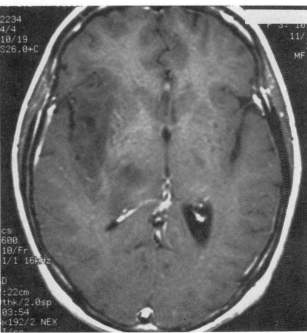

Figure 52-1. MRI scan of a low-grade oligodendroglioma. **(A)** T_2-weighted image demonstrates diffuse hyperintensity throughout the insula and extending into the right thalamus. **(B)** Postgadolinium image does not show enhancement. Diffuse hypodensity and mass effect are evident in the regions corresponding to increased signal on the T_2-weighted image.

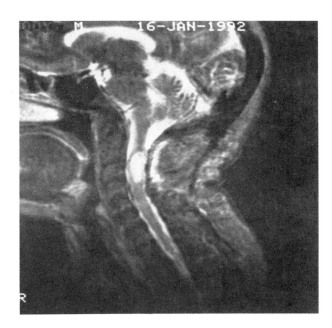

Figure 52-2. Spinal cord glioma shown on T_2-weighted MRI scan in the cervical region.

irreversible and may be progressive. Rarely, radiation necrosis can develop within the irradiated port, which can act as a mass lesion and be indistinguishable from tumor recurrence on CT or MRI scans. These complications of radiotherapy are directly related to the total dose delivered as well as the daily dose. Because of the late delayed effects of radiotherapy and the frequently benign clinical course of many low-grade astrocytomas, such patients may be followed while receiving anticonvulsants alone, often for several years, before a change in their clinical condition mandates definitive treatment. There are no data to guide the decision regarding the timing of radiotherapy, but a prospective study currently being performed will shed some light on this issue in the future.

The overall prognosis for patients with low-grade gliomas is approximately 50 percent surviving for 5 years. Because of the high incidence of long-term survival and the fact that many patients are neurologically normal at the time of diagnosis and most are young, the issue of long-term treatment-related complications becomes important (see section on treatment).

In addition to the typical low-grade gliomas already discussed, there are a few other low-grade lesions that have an even better prognosis but are extremely rare. The *pilocytic astrocytoma* typically develops in the cerebellum of children, the so-called cerebellar astrocytoma, but it may arise in any region of the brain throughout young to midadulthood. Unlike most low-grade gliomas, the pilocytic astrocytoma may enhance

prominently on CT or MRI scan and is often associated with cystic changes, which may be both macroscopic and microscopic. Often, an enhancing mural nodule is seen in association with a cyst. The prominent enhancement may suggest a malignant lesion. Pathologically, the pilocytic astrocytoma may be highly cellular, but necrosis and endothelial proliferation are absent. This lesion is cured with surgery in most patients, and postoperative radiotherapy is not indicated. Occasionally, the tumor may recur, but prolonged survival can still be seen after reresection if there has been no biologic transformation to a higher grade of malignancy, an unusual occurrence.

The second benign glioma is the *pleomorphic xanthoastrocytoma* (Greek: *xantho,* yellow). Like the pilocytic astrocytoma, it may enhance vigorously. It is often seen in the temporal lobes of young adults. Cellular pleomorphism and high cellularity are seen pathologically, but these features, which suggest malignancy, do not carry the ominous prognosis usually associated with them. The pathologic hallmark of this neoplasm is the presence of fat-laden cells, which should suggest this diagnosis. This tumor can also be cured with surgery alone, and adjuvant radiotherapy is not necessary despite the frightening histologic appearance. Because these tumors are rare, they are infrequently encountered and difficult to recognize. Nevertheless, their excellent prognosis makes their consideration imperative.

High-Grade Gliomas

Anaplastic astrocytomas, anaplastic oligodendrogliomas, and glioblastomas multiforme are highly malignant and aggressive neoplasms that require prompt diagnosis and treatment. High-grade gliomas may arise from a prior low-grade lesion, but they may also arise de novo. This change can be seen pathologically in lesions that have varying grades of glioma present within them. Low-grade astrocytoma may be evident in one region of the tumor, but glioblastoma multiforme is present in a separate area. A lesion is graded and behaves biologically according to the highest grade evident in the tumor, but the classification is obviously derived from the material available from biopsy. Hence some high-grade gliomas may be misclassified early.

Malignant gliomas occur in any age group, but their peak incidence is in the fifth and sixth decades of life. There is a 2:1 male predominance.

For all malignant gliomas, the patient's outcome is strongly related to several prognostic factors, which are independent of treatment. Performance status or the patient's overall functional capacity directly influences survival. The better the patient's condition is the longer the survival, and usually, these patients remain functional for a longer period. Age and pathologic grade are indirectly related to outcome. Epidemiologic studies have established that age older than 60 years strongly predicts a poor outcome as does high pathologic grade. With treatment, patients with an anaplastic astrocytoma have a median survival of 3 years, but those with a glioblastoma multiforme have a median survival of only 1 year.

Clinically, patients often present with a single seizure similar to those with low-grade gliomas. More obvious are those with progressive hemiparesis or symptoms of increased intracranial pressure. Radiographically, these tumors almost always appear as single ring-enhancing lesions on CT or MRI, a finding that may also occur with metastatic tumors, abscesses, or resolving hemorrhage. Multiple lesions often satisfy clinicians as to metastases, but a word of caution is warranted because 5 percent of malignant gliomas are multifocal at diagnosis.

When a lesion of this type is identified and a routine physical examination, chest radiograph, stool guaiac analysis, and blood work do not reveal a potential primary malignancy, the patient should undergo biopsy at least. If the location of the tumor is favorable, craniotomy should be performed with the purpose of removing as much tumor as possible. Patients who present with a single lesion with these clinical and radiologic characteristics rarely have metastatic disease, and they should not undergo an extensive search for a primary that does not exist.

Treatment of malignant gliomas includes surgery, radiotherapy, and chemotherapy in all patients. Even with the best current treatment, the outcome for a malignant glioma is suboptimal. Although many patients may have undergone what appears initially to be complete resection or a complete response after cranial irradiation, the tumor will recur and claim the life of the patient in virtually all cases. Despite the poor outlook, therapeutic advances through clinical research point toward future advances that are being tested actively in the stages of clinical trials. Because primary brain tumors are a relatively rare neoplasm, it is important that any patient with this diagnosis be considered for entry into a clinical study. The following paragraphs discuss each therapeutic modality and the author's best recommendation for treatment.

Surgery is important diagnostically and therapeutically. Although partial or complete removal is the recommended approach for all patients with primary brain tumors, emergency surgery has become a rarity. It is necessary only when patients are in imminent danger from herniation. Making a judgment about impending herniation is clinical, by seeking signs of obtundation or pupillary asymmetry; the decision should not be based solely on the radiographic images because some degree of midline displacement is common.

Most patients benefit from a few days of corticosteroid therapy before the surgical procedure, and this also permits the physician to take time to consider the best surgical approach. Complete resection of MRI-visible tumors can often be achieved and is the surgical goal. Removal of large portions of the tumor facilitate an appropriate tissue diagnosis. Furthermore, the extent of resection is an independent prognostic factor, and patients have longer survival if a grossly complete resection has been achieved. Depending on the location and extent of the tumor, resection is not always possible. Stereotactic biopsy is the preferred approach for tissue diagnosis when the lesion is deep, involving the basal ganglia or thalamus, or large, especially when it is bilateral or crosses the corpus callosum.

After surgery, radiotherapy is given to all patients with malignant gliomas. Radiotherapy is administered to the involved areas of the tumor, usually to a total dose of about 6,000 cGy. Radiotherapy produces tumor regression and clinical improvement in most patients and delays recurrence in all.

Chemotherapy is usually used as adjuvant treatment to radiation. Carmustine (BCNU) is the standard drug used for anaplastic astrocytoma and glioblastoma multiforme. Although it does not produce a response in most patients, there appears to be a subset of patients who have prolonged survival (more than 18 months) when BCNU is added to surgery and irradiation. Many clinical trials have been conducted to examine the efficacy of other agents, drug combinations, or means of drug delivery (such as intra-arterial chemotherapy), but none have proved superior to BCNU. Furthermore, BCNU is well tolerated by most patients, and therefore, the author includes it as treatment in all newly diagnosed patients. At the time of recurrence, patients may be considered for reresection if the lesion is surgically accessible, and reoperation prolongs the patient's life a median of 6 additional months. Chemotherapeutic options include other agents, such as procarbazine or intra-arterial cisplatin. Additional radiotherapy can be administered with brachytherapy or stereotactic radiosurgery. Both methods deliver high-intensity focused irradiation, which can be safely delivered, even after standard external beam radiotherapy.

Brachytherapy is the temporary implantation of iodine-125 seeds into the tumor, which delivers approximately 6,000 cGy over 6 days. The seeds are then removed. Brachytherapy is followed by focal radionecrosis, usually several months after implantation, in approximately 50 percent of patients. Surgical resection of the necrosis is often required.

Stereotactic radiosurgery delivers about 1,600 cGy

by external beam irradiation using photons or heavy particles to a well-focused area in a single dose. No surgical procedure is required, and the incidence of radionecrosis requiring surgical debulking is probably lower. With current technology, stereotactic radiosurgery is limited to relatively small lesions (less than 3 cm), whereas brachytherapy can be used in larger tumors. Both offer improved local control after recurrence. However, only a minority of patients are eligible for these techniques, and these candidates tend to be better-risk patients.

Although often treated the same as glioblastoma multiforme, the anaplastic oligodendroglioma may be considered a separate entity. Here, surgical resection should also be done for diagnosis and treatment, and radiotherapy and chemotherapy are used. However, recent reports have changed therapy by demonstrating the particular sensitivity of this tumor to the chemotherapeutic combination of procarbazine, lomustine, and vincristine. As part of the initial treatment, chemotherapy given before radiotherapy can substantially shrink the lesion, facilitating a more limited port for radiotherapy. If given at recurrence, most patients respond with partial or complete resolution of visible tumor. Although this tumor is rare compared with the much more common anaplastic astrocytoma or glioblastoma multiforme, its unique sensitivity to chemotherapy requires a different and potentially more optimistic approach. Recurrent anaplastic oligodendrogliomas after procarbozine, lomustine, and vincristine chemotherapy and radiotherapy often respond to other agents, such as melphalan, although bone marrow toxicity is frequently limiting (Fig. 52-3).

Brainstem Glioma

Benign and malignant gliomas can arise anywhere there is glia. When the brainstem is the site, the unique clinical presentation and uniformly poor response to treatment warrants considering this glioma as a separate entity.

Most brainstem gliomas develop in the second decade of life, but they can present up through the fourth decade and rarely in the older population. Although both histologically benign and malignant tumors are seen, there is no definite relationship between histologic type and prognosis; specifically, benign tumors do not do better than malignant lesions.

The overwhelming majority of brainstem gliomas develop in the pons, and patients present with oculomotor paresis, facial weakness, ataxia, and bulbar difficulties, often without "long tract" signs of hemiparesis or sensory change. Despite the diffuse enlargement of the pons caused by this expansile and infiltrative tumor ("pseudohypertrophy of the pons"), obstruction of the fourth ventricle or aqueduct causing hydrocephalus is rare, and patients infrequently have symptoms of increased intracranial pressure. Symptoms usually develop subacutely over weeks, but occasionally, an adult patient may have subtle symptoms that resolve and then reappear over a several-year period. MRI scan is necessary to diagnose this tumor and to distinguish it from other brainstem processes, such as a cavernous angioma or arteriovenous malformation. CT scanning is often nondiagnostic until the mass is large. On the MRI scan, a diffusely enlarged brainstem is evident. Small foci of enhancement may be apparent, but prominent enhancement is uncommon. Diffuse hypointensity on T_1-weighted images is often a striking feature and is thought to confer a poor prognosis.

Because of its location, resection is not feasible. For similar reasons, only the minority of patients can safely undergo biopsy, making the diagnosis dependent on the characteristic radiographic image. Radiotherapy is the primary treatment and can prolong survival for a median of 1 year. Chemotherapy has not been useful.

There are occasional patients who have a more indolent and prolonged course; these are often adults with a long history of mild symptoms who can be successfully weaned off corticosteroids after completion of radiotherapy.

EPENDYMOMA

Ependymomas (from the Greek for second layer) arise from the ependymal cells that line the ventricular cavities and central canal. Pathologically, they consist of fusiform cells that form true rosettes. Occasionally, they have more malignant characteristics, but these features do not clearly confer a worse prognosis. In the intracranial cavity, they occur most commonly in the fourth ventricle but are rarely seen in the supratentorial compartment, usually in the pediatric population. They may also occur at any level of the spinal canal, often originating from the filum terminale.

The clinical presentation varies according to the location. Tumors in the fourth ventricle cause obstructive hydrocephalus with symptoms of increased intracranial pressure and local symptoms with vertigo and ataxia. Spinal tumors cause back pain, which may be the only symptom for many months before the diagnosis is made. Leg weakness and sensory and sphincter symptoms may follow.

Treatment consists primarily of attempted gross surgical removal followed by focal radiotherapy. Although there has been concern about spread of the tumor through the cerebrospinal fluid (CSF) pathways, this spread is rarely clinically important, and radiotherapy to the length of the neuraxis is not necessary.

With treatment, the 5-year survival rate is 30 to 40 percent. The myxopapillary variant of the ependymoma has a more benign course. It usually occurs in the filum terminale and may be cured by compete resection, particularly if this is accomplished en bloc. Postoperative radiotherapy is not necessary.

Medulloblastoma

The term *medulloblastoma* (Greek: *medullo,* marrow) was coined by Bailey and Cushing in 1925 to describe a particular tumor that occurred in the fourth ventricle and cerebellum of children. This tumor is clearly a discrete entity, but it is unfortunately named because there is no embryonal cell identified as a medulloblast. The cell of origin is in dispute, but the tumors appear to arise from primitive embryonic rests.

The tumor usually occurs in childhood with a peak onset in the second decade; however, medulloblastomas also arise in young adults. They typically present as a mass filling the fourth ventricle and causing obstructive hydrocephalus. The patient presents with symptoms of increased intracranial pressure, and because of the frequent nausea and vomiting, gastroin-

testinal disease is often the first diagnosis. Adults tend to have tumors that originate in the cerebellar hemisphere and present with unilateral cerebellar signs.

Like other primary brain tumors, medulloblastomas should be resected with every effort made for a total removal. Postoperatively, the patient needs a staging evaluation because there is a high incidence of leptomeningeal seeding and even, occasionally, bone marrow involvement. Spinal MRI scan with gadolinium, CSF analysis, and bone marrow biopsy should be performed in every patient. If an initial CSF cytologic examination reveals malignant cells and the spinal MRI scan is negative, the CSF analysis should be repeated several weeks after surgery because a few cells can be seen after resection. However, this does not put the patient into a poor-risk subgroup.

After surgery, all patients are treated with neuraxis radiotherapy to a total of 3,600 cGy plus an additional boost to the posterior fossa for a total dose of approximately 5,500 cGy. Recent work has shown that poor-risk patients, those with disseminated disease at diagnosis or large tumors with local invasion, have improved survival with the addition of chemotherapy to radiotherapy. In addition, standard-risk patients may also benefit from chemotherapy, but this is more con-

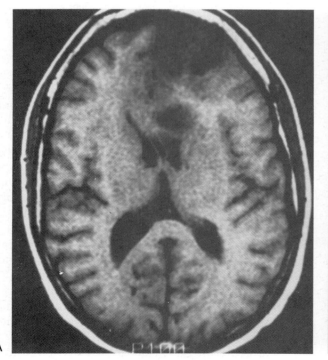
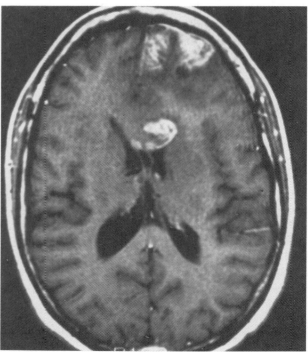

A   B

Figure 52-3. **(A)** Pre- and **(B)** Postgadolinium MRI scans of an anaplastic astrocytoma. Enhancement is evident in the left frontal lobe, and the tumor extends into and crosses the corpus callosum. Mass effect on the frontal horn of the lateral ventricle is apparent. Although the enhancing regions appear separate, they are connected by infiltrative tumor seen pathologically.

troversial. With the current therapeutic approach, the 5-year survival rate is 50 to 60 percent. This success is partially tempered by the high incidence of delayed sequelae of treatment, including growth retardation, cognitive impairment, and endocrinologic disturbances.

PRIMARY CENTRAL NERVOUS SYSTEM LYMPHOMA

Formerly a rare brain tumor, primary lymphoma of the nervous system has attracted attention because it is associated with a variety of immunodeficiency states, particularly acquired immunodeficiency syndrome, (AIDS), but is also increasing in frequency in apparently immunocompetent patients. It usually involves the deep periventricular structures and is multifocal in about one-half of patients. It can also involve the eye and leptomeninges in 20 and 35 percent of patients, respectively.

Patients usually present with a rapid change in their level of alertness or cognitive state along with lateralizing signs, similar to those associated with other intracranial masses. Only about 10 percent of patients present with seizures. Ocular lymphoma presents with floaters or visual blurring and is frequently diagnosed as uveitis when cells are seen on slit-lamp examination.

A characteristic CT or MRI appearance with prominent and diffuse enhancement is seen in more than 90 percent of patients (Fig. 52-4).

A unique feature of cerebral lymphoma is its sensitivity to corticosteroids. These drugs can cause tumor regression and disappearance of the lesions as a result of direct cytotoxicity. This may obscure the opportunity to establish a tissue diagnosis, and if the patient is clinically stable, steroids should be withheld until a biopsy has been obtained. Unlike other primary brain tumors, primary central nervous system lymphoma is not treated with surgical resection. Stereotactic biopsy is the procedure of choice to establish the diagnosis, but resection does not improve survival rates. The standard treatment had been cranial irradiation, which produced a median survival of 15 to 18 months. Recent work has focused on the addition of chemotherapy, particularly high-dose methotrexate, before radiotherapy. This combined modality treatment has become the most promising approach, yielding a median survival of 44 months. Unfortunately, those with AIDS and primary central nervous system lymphoma do not fare as well.

The median survival with cranial irradiation alone is 2 to 5 months, primarily because patients die of systemic opportunistic infections. Most patients with AIDS and this disease are not candidates for chemotherapy; however, there may be a subgroup who will benefit from a more vigorous approach.

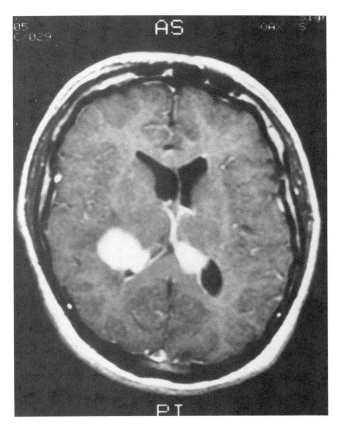

Figure 52-4. Gadolinium-enhanced MRI scan of a primary central nervous system lymphoma. The tumor is bilateral. Periventricular tumor extends into the ventricular system, and subependymal spread of tumor is apparent bilaterally. Note the diffuse and brisk enhancement of the lesions with minimal surrounding edema.

COLLOID CYST OF THE THIRD VENTRICLE

Colloid cyst of the third ventricle is a benign neoplasm derived from vestigial ependymal cells. It arises from the anterior roof of the third ventricle and can reach several centimeters in size (Fig. 52-5). It is composed of epithelial cells surround by a capsule and is filled with a gelatinous substance. This is a congenital structure, but symptoms develop in adulthood.

Patients present with intermittent symptoms of elevated intracranial pressure. Headache, obtundation, ataxia, paresthesias, leg weakness, and poor vision are the common symptoms. It is commonly taught that the tumor can hang from a stalk, and changes in head position can result in sudden obstruction of the foramen of Monro with obstruction of the lateral ventricles and severe headache when the cyst abruptly blocks the flow of CSF. Although a change in body position may precipitate the crisis, proof of such an obstruction is rare, and few patients have these presenting features. Occasionally, a patient may not develop acute

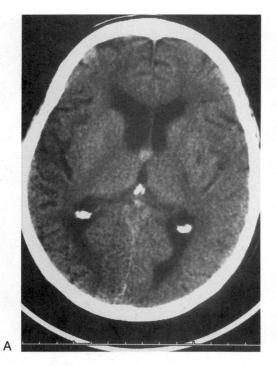 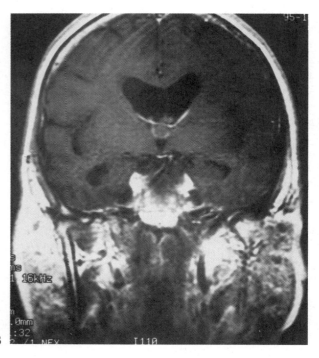

Figure 52-5. **(A)** Noncontrast CT scan and **(B)** postgadolinium MRI scan of a patient with an incidental colloid cyst. The lesion is dense preconstrast on CT scan, but a rim of enhancement is evident on the MRI scan (linear-enhancing structures on MRI scan are veins). The colloid cyst caused moderate obstructive hydrocephalus, although the patient was asymptomatic.

attacks but usually presents with chronic hydrocephalus. Some colloid cysts are found incidentally and do not appear to be symptomatic.

Treatment has been surgical excision, but surgery may be difficult in this area. Stereotactic aspiration and drainage of the cyst is feasible and safe in selected patients. Many advocate shunting alone with no attempt to remove the benign growth; this relieves the symptoms in virtually all patients.

BIBLIOGRAPHY

Gliomas

Bernstein M, Laperriere N, Leung P, McKenzie S. Interstitial brachytherapy for malignant brain tumors: preliminary results. Neurosurgery 1990;26:371–80.

Burger PC, Green SB. Patient age, histologic features, and length of survival in patients with glioblastoma multiforme. Cancer 1987;59:1617–25.

Cairncross JG, Macdonald DR. Successful chemotherapy for recurrent malignant oligodendroglioma. Ann Neurol 1988;23:360–4.

Cairncross JG, Macdonald DR. Chemotherapy for oligodendroglioma. Arch Neurol 1991;48:225–7.

Clark GB, Henry JM, McKeever PE. Cerebral pilocytic astrocytoma. Cancer 1985;56:1128–33.

Florell RC, MacDonald DR, Irish WD et al. Selection bias, survival, and brachytherapy for glioma. J Neurosurg 1992;76:179–83.

Garcia DM, Fulling KH, Marks JE. The value of radiation therapy in addition to surgery for astrocytomas of the adult cerebrum. Cancer 1985;55:919–27.

Glass J, Hochberg FH, Gruber ML et al. The treatment of oligodendrogliomas and mixed oligodendroglioma-astrocytomas with PCV chemotherapy. J Neurosurg 1992; 76:741–5.

Gutin PH, Leibel SA, Wara WM et al. Recurrent malignant gliomas: survival following interstitial brachytherapy with high-activity iodine-125 sources. J Neurosurg 1987; 67:864–73.

Laws ER Jr, Taylor WF, Clifton MB et al. Neurosurgical management of low grade astrocytoma of the cerebral hemispheres. J Neurosurg 1984;61:665–73.

Leibel SA, Sheline GE, Wara WM et al. The role of radiation therapy in the treatment of astrocytomas. Cancer 1975; 35:1551–57.

Loeffler JS, Alexander E, Shea WM et al. Radiosurgery as part of the initial management of patients with malignant gliomas. J Clin Oncol 1992;10:1379–85.

Palma L, Guidetti B. Cystic pilocytic astrocytomas of the cerebral hemispheres. J Neurosurg 1985;62:811–5.

Walker MD, Green SB, Byar DP et al. Randomized comparisons of radiotherapy and nitrosoureas for the treatment of malignant glioma after surgery. N Engl J Med 1980; 303:1323–9.

Wallner KE, Gonzales MF, Edwads MSB et al. Treatment results of juvenile pilocytic astrocytoma. J Neurosurg 1988;69:171–6.

Wood JR, Green SB, Shapiro WR. The prognostic importance of tumor size in malignant gliomas: a computed tomographic scan study by the Brain Tumor Cooperative Group. J Clin Oncol 1988;6:338–43.

Brainstem Gliomas

Freeman CR, Krischer J, Sanford RA et al. Hyperfractionated radiation therapy in brain stem tumors. Cancer 1991;68:474–81.

Grigsby PW, Garcia DM, Simpson JR et al. Prognostic factors and results of therapy for adult thalamic and brainstem tumors. Cancer 1989;63:2124–9.

Jenkin RDT, Boesel C, Ertel I et al. Brain-stem tumors in childhood: a prospective randomized trial of irradiation with and without adjuvant CCNU, VCR, and prednisone. J Neurosurg 1987;66:227–33.

Mantravadi RVP, Phatak R, Bellur S et al. Brain stem gliomas: an autopsy study of 25 cases. Cancer 1982;49: 1294–96.

Pompili A, Riccio A, Jandolo B et al. CCNU chemotherapy in adult patients with tumors of the basal ganglia and brain stem. J Neurosurg 1980;53:361–3.

Recht LD, Lew R, Smith TW. Suspected low-grade glioma: is deferring treatment safe? Ann Neurol 1992;31:431–6.

Zorzi F, Facchetti F, Baronchelli C et al. Pleomorphic xanthoastrocytoma: an immunohistochemical study of three cases. Histopathology 1992;20:267–9.

Ependymoma

McCormick PC, Torres R, Post KD et al. Intramedullary ependymoma of the spinal cord. J Neurosurg 1990;72: 523–32.

Ross GW, Rubinstein L. Lack of histopathological correlation of malignant ependymomas with postoperative survival. J Neurosurg 1989;70:31–6.

Schweitzer JS, Batzdorf U. Ependymoma of the cauda equina region: diagnosis, treatment, and outcome in 15 patients. Neurosurgery 1992;30:202–7.

Sonneland PRL, Scheithauer BW, Onofrio BM. Myxopapillary ependymoma: a clinicopathologic and immunocytochemical study of 77 cases. Cancer 1985;56:883–93.

Whitaker SJ, Bessell EM, Ashley SE et al. Postoperative radiotherapy in the management of spinal cord ependymoma. J Neurosurg 1991;74:720–8.

Medulloblastoma

Evans AE, Jenkin RDT, Sposto R et al. The treatment of medulloblastoma. J Neurosurg 1990;72:572–82.

Hazuka MB, DeBiose DA, Henderson RH et al. Survival results in adult patients treated for medulloblastoma. Cancer 1992;2143–8.

Krischer JP, Ragab AH, Kun L et al. Nitrogen mustard, vincristine, procarbazine, and prednisone as adjuvant chemotherapy in the treatment of medulloblastoma. J Neurosurg 1991;74:905–9.

Olshan JS, Gubernick J, Packer RJ et al. The effects of adjuvant chemotherapy on growth in children with medulloblastoma. Cancer 1992;70:2013–7.

Packer RJ, Finlay JL. Medulloblastoma: presentation, diagnosis and management. Oncology 1988;2:35–49.

Packer RJ, Sutton LN, Goldwein JW et al. Improved survival with the use of adjuvant chemotherapy in the treatment of medulloblastoma. J Neurosurg 1991;74:433–40.

Silverman GL, Palkes H, Talen B et al. Late effects of radiotherapy on patients with cerebellar medulloblastoma. Cancer 1984;54:825–9.

Primary CNS Lymphoma

Baumgartner JE, Rachlin JR, Beckstead JH et al. Primary central nervous system lymphomas: natural history and response to radiation therapy in 55 patients with acquired immunodeficiency syndrome. J Neurosurg 1990;73: 206–11.

DeAngelis LM, Yahalom J, Rosenblum M et al. Primary CNS lymphoma: managing patients with spontaneous and AIDS-related disease. Oncology 1987;1:52–9.

DeAngelis LM, Yahalom J, Thaler HT et al. Combined modality therapy for primary CNS lymphoma. J Clin Oncol 1992;10:635–43.

Hochberg FH, Miller DC. Primary central nervous system lymphoma. J Neurosurg 1988;68:835–53.

Schaumburg HH, Plank CR, Adams RD. The reticulum cell sarcoma-microglioma group of brain tumours. Brain 1972;95:199–212.

Colloid Cyst

Kondziolka D, Lunsford LD. Stereotactic management of colloid cysts: factors predicting success. J Neurosurg 1991;75:45–51.

53

Central Nervous System Metastases

Lisa M. DeAngelis

Metastatic disease can involve the nervous system at any level. The most common locations for metastases are the brain, the epidural spinal space, the leptomeninges, and the brachial and lumbar plexi. Less common sites include the dura, spinal cord parenchyma, and peripheral nerve. Metastases to the nervous system are common and affect at least 25 percent of all patients with disseminated cancer. They profoundly affect a patient's quality of life and often shorten survival. Early diagnosis and appropriate therapy often ameliorate the neurologic symptoms and restore or maintain a patient's independent function.

BRAIN METASTASES

Brain metastases are the most common metastatic complication in the nervous system, occurring in about 15 percent of patients with systemic cancer. Lung and breast cancers and melanoma are the most common solid tumors that metastasize to the brain, although any tumor can form a metastatic cerebral deposit. Some tumors, such as melanoma and testicular and choriocarcinoma, have a disproportionately high incidence of brain metastases, probably as a result of specific features of the tumor cell and the cerebral microenvironment, which may foster implantation and growth of tumor emboli in the brain. Brain metastases can be the first presentation of systemic cancer. Most of these patients have lung cancer as the underlying primary tumor. If a primary source cannot be detected by physical examination, routine blood work, urinalysis, and chest radiography, it is unlikely that an extensive systemic evaluation will reveal the primary. Frequently, a primary cannot be identified even at autopsy. In these patients, the histologic diagnosis must be obtained from biopsy or resection of the cerebral mass.

Brain metastases form as a consequence of hematogenous dissemination from the primary tumor. Generally, they are distributed throughout the brain in proportion to its volume and blood flow, resulting in approximately 90 percent of metastases forming in the supratentorial compartment. This distribution applies to brain metastases from most primaries. However, some tumors that arise in the pelvic region preferentially metastasize to the cerebellum in about 50 percent of patients.

Because brain metastases arise from tumor emboli in the circulation, it has been presumed that they are always multiple, whether numerous lesions can be identified at diagnosis or not. However, both radiographic and autopsy studies show that one-half of patients have only a single brain metastasis, and additional microscopic foci of tumor are not seen on autopsy specimens.

Leptomeningeal metastases (see below) can develop in association with brain metastases. Fifteen percent of patients with brain metastases in the posterior fossa develop leptomeningeal tumors, but only 3 percent of those with supratentorial lesions develop this complication.

The presenting symptoms and signs of brain metastases are determined by their location within the brain and are identical to those of any other space-occupying cerebral lesion. Focal or generalized seizures are the presenting symptom in 15 to 20 percent, and more than one-half of patients have lateralizing signs with hemiparesis, visual field deficits, or language problems. About 75 percent also have some impairment in their level of alertness or cognitive processes. The symptoms usually develop subacutely, but occasionally they begin with a strokelike presentation, sometimes as a result of an intratumor hemorrhage. Brain metastases from renal or thyroid cancers, melanomas, and choriocarcinomas have a propensity to bleed.

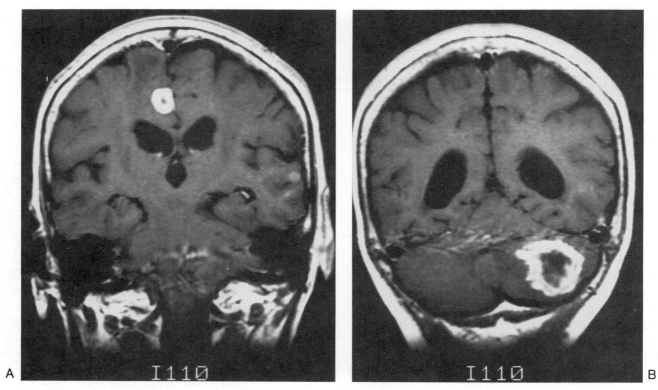

Figure 53-1. (A & B) Gadolinium-enhanced MRI scans of a patient with multiple brain metastases from breast carcinoma. Note the ring-enhancing pattern, particularly in the cerebellar lesion.

The diagnosis is established by computed tomographic (CT) or magnetic resonance imaging (MRI) scan. Where available, MRI is more sensitive, even though the radiographic image of brain metastases is usually similar on the CT and MRI scans. By either technique, most metastases appear as ring-enhancing lesions surrounded by edema, which extends into the white matter (Fig. 53-1). Metastases rarely involve the corpus callosum or extend into a contralateral hemisphere as primary brain tumors do. Rarely, the lesions are calcified. Calcification usually occurs after cranial irradiation.

Treatment includes supportive and definitive measures. Definitive treatment is directed against the tumor and includes surgery, radiotherapy, and chemotherapy. Supportive treatment includes corticosteroids (to control cerebral edema and reduce mass effect) and anticonvulsants. Each is discussed separately.

Corticosteroids are usually the first therapeutic intervention and are often administered immediately after the initial CT or MRI scan that demonstrates metastatic lesions. Steroids usually have a dramatic and rapid effect, producing clinical improvement within hours in most patients. They diminish edema by restoring the integrity of the leaky blood vessels

associated with metastatic disease. Dexamethasone is the corticosteroid of choice because of its limited mineralocorticoid activity. Although the starting dose is usually 16 mg/day, the dose should be adjusted according to the patient's symptoms. Every effort should be made to taper dexamethasone as quickly as possible to minimize the significant side effects that develop with chronic use, including steroid-induced myopathy, diabetes, insomnia, and psychologic changes. After completing definitive treatment, corticosteroids can be tapered off in most patients with brain metastases.

Anticonvulsants are used in every patient who has had a seizure. In some countries, especially in the United States, they are frequently administered prophylactically. Although no prospective study has been done, retrospective data raise serious questions concerning the benefit of prophylactic anticonvulsants. Efficacy has not been established, and all anticonvulsants carry the risk of side effects. Specific toxicities seen in patients with brain tumors include Stevens-Johnson syndrome, with phenytoin or carbamazepine, and phenobarbital-induced rheumatism. Except in patients with brain metastases from melanoma (who have a 50 percent incidence of seizures) or those who have had craniotomy and receive a brief postoperative course of anticonvulsants, the author and the editors do not routinely prescribe prophylactic anticonvulsants.

Surgical treatment is primarily reserved for patients with single lesions whose systemic disease is under control. Patients eligible for surgery should have a cranial MRI scan with gadolinium to ensure there is only one lesion. In two recently completed randomized prospective studies, patients who had a complete resection followed by whole-brain radiotherapy (WBRT) had a significantly prolonged survival (median of 40 versus 15 weeks) compared with patients treated with WBRT alone. Equally important, the surgically treated patients had improved neurologic function and remained independent for a longer duration. Although surgical therapy is superior to standard treatment with cranial radiotherapy alone, only about 30 percent of all patients with brain metastases are eligible for this approach.

Cranial radiaotherapy is the mainstay of treatment for most patients with brain metastases. WBRT is usually administered in a rapid fractionation scheme (300 cGy × 10 fractions) to achieve quick palliation. This program is effective, but the median survival from the time of diagnosis is only 4 to 6 months, primarily because patients die of their systemic cancer. For patients with limited disease, a radiosensitive primary (such as breast cancer), and those whose disease may allow prolonged survival, consideration should be given to a more protracted course of WBRT (e.g., 200 cGy × 20 fractions) to reduce the potential for delayed radiation toxicity, resulting in dementia; the late delayed toxicities of WBRT are related to high daily fractions and to the total dose. Recurrence of brain metastases after WBRT may be treated with a second course of WBRT, or if the number of recurrent lesions is small (one to two), brachytherapy (see below) or stereotactic radiosurgery may be additional options. The role of these newer techniques in the primary treatment of brain metastases is being defined.

Patients with brain metastases from chemosensitive primaries, particularly breast cancer, choriocarcinoma, and small cell lung cancer, often respond to systemic chemotherapeutic regimens. Chemotherapy is used for the treatment of recurrent brain metastases when surgery or further radiotherapy are no longer options.

EPIDURAL SPINE METASTASES

Epidural spine metastases are fairly common, occurring in approximately 5 percent of patients with cancer. They are important because they cause severe disability, much of which can be prevented with early diagnosis. Most epidural spine metastases develop as a consequence of a vertebral body metastasis growing into the epidural space, resulting in spinal cord compression. Some tumors, such as lymphoma, may grow along the paravertebral gutter, invade the neural foramina, and grow in the epidural space without destroying bone. The most common tumors that cause epidural spinal cord compression are lung, breast, and prostate cancers, although any tumor resulting in vertebral metastases can produce this complication. Approximately 70 percent of epidural metastases occur in the thoracic spine, 20 percent in the lumbar spine, and 10 percent in the cervical spine (Fig. 53-2). Regardless of the spinal location, the clinical presentation is similar. The initial symptom is back or neck pain in at least 95 percent of patients. Pain is usually the first and may be the only symptom for weeks or months. At diagnosis, 75 percent of patients are also

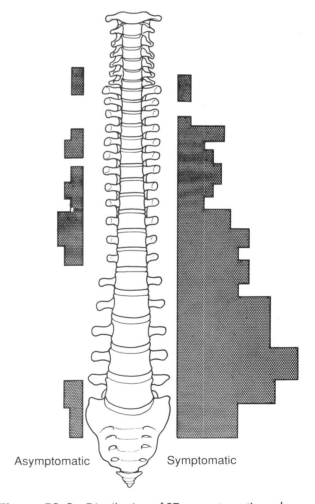

Asymptomatic   Symptomatic

Figure 53-2. Distribution of 87 asymptomatic and symptomatic spinal epidural metastases. Level L4 is involved most frequently. (From Boogerd et al., 1992, with permission.)

weak, but weakness is rarely the first symptom. Sensory loss and sphincter dysfunction are seen in about one-half of patients at diagnosis. Although back pain may be a chronic symptom, weakness and autonomic and sensory impairment can develop subacutely, and paraparesis or paraplegia may develop abruptly even without antecedent neurologic signs. It is this potential for acute myelopathy that makes early diagnosis and prompt treatment of epidural disease critical. Furthermore, the patient's clinical state at diagnosis is important prognostically with respect to the preservation or restoration of neurologic function after treatment of the epidural tumor. If patients are ambulatory at diagnosis, they will probably remain so after treatment, but if they are not, the chance of regaining independent ambulation is small even with the best therapy.

The diagnosis is suggested by radiographs of the spine, particularly when vertebral collapse is seen in association with vertebral metastases, or by bone scans, which visualize vertebral metastases. However, neither of these tests can distinguish between epidural metastases and the more common simple vertebral bone metastasis. Demonstration of an epidural tumor must be done by myelography or MRI scan of the spine. Where available, spine MRI has largely replaced myelography and is the superior test (Fig. 53-3). The complete spine can be imaged noninvasively, delineating the rostrocaudal extent of the epidural lesion and identifying those patients (5 to 10 percent) with multiple sites of epidural tumor. However, if MRI is not available, myelography is an excellent alternative diagnostic test. The entire spinal column must be visualized, even if a cervical puncture is required, when a complete block is seen from below. Once diagnosed, epidural metastases must be treated promptly.

The first intervention is usually administration of corticosteroids. Dexamethasone promptly relieves

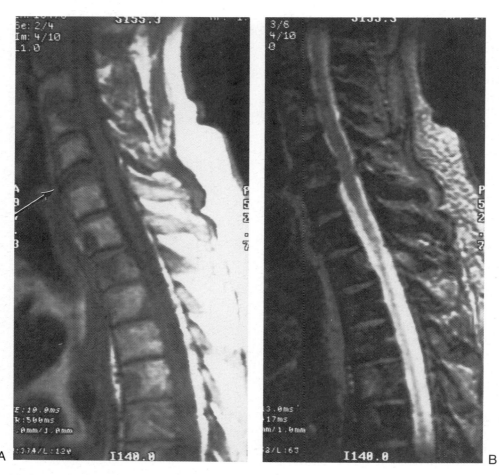

Figure 53-3. (A & B) MRI scans of the spine revealing compression of the C6 vertebral body (*arrow*) by prostate cancer with epidural extension of tumor and distortion of the cervical cord. There are multiple other vertebrae involved by bony metastases but not causing epidural compression.

back pain, and there are data to suggest that high-dose corticosteroids (100 mg/day of dexamethasone) relieve pain more effectively and rapidly than standard regimens. However, high-dose steroid dosing does not enhance neurologic recovery. Particularly with these regimens, dexamethasone must be tapered quickly to minimize corticosteroid toxicity. Definitive treatment consists of radiotherapy or surgery. Radiotherapy is at least as effective as laminectomy for most patients with epidural metastases. It usually produces tumor regression with the relief of spinal cord compression. Sustained pain relief is often achieved, but only a minority of patients have marked neurologic improvement with treatment. Certain situations demand a surgical approach. Tissue diagnosis is essential in the patient who presents with epidural compression as the first manifestation of cancer. Patients with highly radioresistant tumors, such as renal carcinomas, or those with intractable back pain after radiotherapy may benefit from surgery. The standard operative approach has been laminectomy, but these tumors typically arise anteriorly from the vertebral body. Anterior vertebral body resection is the preferred approach for definitive resection of tumor and has been associated with an increased incidence of neurologic recovery; however, it is a more complicated surgical undertaking, particularly when the tumor is in the thoracic spine. Laminectomy may still be appropriate for a tumor that lies posteriorly. There are no data to suggest that laminectomy reverses the neurologic deterioration that may develop during radiotherapy.

LEPTOMENINGEAL METASTASES (CARCINOMATOUS MENINGITIS)

Metastases to the leptomeninges may occur in isolation or accompany brain metastases. They develop as a consequence of hematogenous dissemination of tumor, but once established, tumor can circulate freely

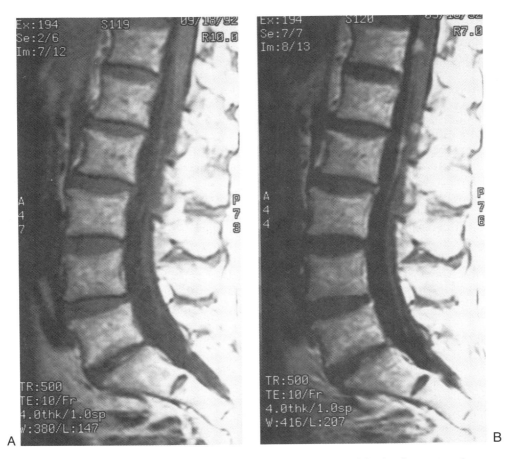

Figure 53-4. **(A)** Pre- and **(B)** postgadolinium-enhanced MRI scans of the lumbar spine demonstrating leptomeningeal metastases to the cauda equina. Multiple nodules and coating of the nerve roots by tumor can be seen after gadolinium administration.

within the subarachnoid space, leading to multiple deposits along the neuraxis. They occur in about 5 percent of patients with cancer, and breast and lung cancers and lymphomas are the most common primaries.

Leptomeningeal metastases can produce a wide range of neurologic symptoms and signs. Multiple lumbar and cervical radiculopathies, usually painful, cranial neuropathies, and communicating hydrocephalus with symptoms of increased intracranial pressure are the most common clinical manifestations. Patients may have one or any constellation of these symptoms at presentation. The diagnosis is established by the demonstration of malignant cells in the cerebrospinal fluid (CSF) or by visualization of subarachnoid nodules on gadolinium-enhanced MRI scans or myelography (Fig. 54-4). Frequently, multiple lumbar punctures are required to identify malignant cells, and MRI scans of the brain or spine are often negative. CT scanning plays only a minor role, and the results are usually negative, even when contrast enhancement is used.

Routine CSF analysis may support the diagnosis when an elevated protein concentration, reduced glucose concentration, and pleocytosis are seen. Tumor markers are occasionally helpful but are not a substitute for an unequivocal cytologic specimen that reveals the tumor.

Treatment is directed toward the entire CSF and the clinically affected region. Radiotherapy is administered to the symptomatic area, such as WBRT for cranial neuropathies or lumbar spine radiotherapy for radiculopathy. Intrathecal chemotherapy, usually with methotrexate or cytarabine, is given to treat the disease circulating within the CSF. Intrathecal chemotherapy can be administered by repeated lumbar punctures, but placement of an Ommaya reservoir is safer, more efficient, and ensures better drug distribution. Corticosteroids are not helpful in the symptomatic management of leptomeningeal metastases, except temporarily for patients with increased intracranial pressure, which often requires a shunt for correction.

BRACHIAL AND LUMBOSACRAL PLEXOPATHY

Tumor can infiltrate either the brachial or lumbosacral plexus. It may involve a plexus by contiguous growth, such as a Pancoast tumor (H. Pancoast, 1875–1939, American radiologist) invading the brachial plexus, or by hematogenous dissemination. Breast and lung cancers and lymphomas are the most common causes of brachial plexopathy, whereas colon and breast cancers, sarcomas, and lymphomas typically involve the lumbosacral plexus.

Metastatic plexopathy, either brachial or lumbosacral, is almost always painful. In brachial plexopathy, patients present with pain and primarily lower trunk involvement with dysesthesias and weakness in the distribution of C7, C8, and T1. Lumbosacral plexus involvement is painful in 95 percent of patients, and weakness or sensory symptoms occur with equal frequency in both upper and lower plexus distributions. In contrast to tumor plexopathy, radiation-induced plexopathy is less likely to be painful and is associated with lymphedema of the affected limb. When radiotherapy damages the brachial plexus, it tends to affect the upper plexus preferentially because of the ports used in this area, but radiotherapy can affect any region of the brachial or lumbosacral plexus. Radiation-induced plexopathy is the major differential diagnostic consideration in any patient with cancer whose prior radiotherapeutic port overlapped either plexus. Either brachial or lumbosacral plexopathy may coexist with an epidural tumor because of direct growth of the tumor into the adjacent spinal canal. These patients may have bilateral signs, evidence of a myelopathy, or a Bernard-Horner syndrome (in brachial plexopathy), all of which suggest epidural involvement. These patients must be evaluated with a spine MRI scan or myelogram to ascertain the extent of local disease. Plexopathy is a clinical diagnosis that can usually be confirmed by CT or MRI scan of the brachial or lumbosacral plexus.

Typically, the tumor appears as a mass or infiltrative lesion of the plexus on the CT or MRI scan. The main entity in the differential diagnosis, radiation-induced fibrosis, obliterates the normal tissue planes but rarely appears as a mass lesion. Occasionally, microscopic infiltration by the tumor is not evident on the CT or MRI scan. In this circumstance, alternative diagnoses must be excluded, such as leptomeningeal tumor mimicking a plexopathy, but occasionally, surgical exploration and biopsy of the plexus and surrounding tissues is necessary. The treatment of tumor plexopathy is primarily radiotherapy. Systemic chemotherapy is useful, particularly in patients with lymphomas or breast cancers, which are chemosensitive neoplasms. Corticosteroids do not improve neurologic function in patients with metastatic plexopathy.

ANNOTATED BIBLIOGRAPHY

Brain Metastases

Boogerd W, Dalesio O, Bais EM et al. Response of brain metastases from breast cancer to systemic chemotherapy. Cancer 1992;69:972–80.

Brain metastases from breast cancer respond to combination therapy.

Cairncross JG, Kim J-H, Posner JB. Radiation therapy for brain metastases. Ann Neurol 1980;7:529–41.

A classic article on radiotherapy for brain metastases.

Cohen N, Strauss G, Lew R et al. Should prophylactic anticonvulsants be administered to patients with newly-diagnosed cerebral metastases? A retrospective analysis. J Clin Oncol 1988;6:1621–4.

Prophylactic anticonvulsants do not clearly reduce the incidence of seizures.

Delattre JY, Krol G, Thaler HT et al. Distribution of brain metastases. Arch Neurol 1988;45:741–4.

Brain matastases tend to form in the "watershed" regions.

Galicich JH, Sundaresan N, Arbit E et al. Surgical treatment of single brain metastasis: factors associated with survival. Cancer 1980;45:381–6.

Resection improves survival rates.

Gelber RD, Larson M, Borgelt BB et al. Equivalence of radiation schedules for the palliative treatment of brain metastases in patients with favorable prognosis. Cancer 1981;48:1749–53.

Multiple radiotherapeutic schedules offer equal efficacy.

Loeffler JS, Kooy HM, Wen PY et al. The treatment of recurrent brain metastases with stereotactic radiosurgery. J Clin Oncol 1990;8:576–82.

Radiosurgery is beneficial in some patients.

Patchell RA, Tibbs PA, Walsh JW et al. A randomized trial of surgery in the treatment of single metastases to the brain. N Engl J Med 1990;322:494–500.

A prospective study that addresses the issue of surgery.

Posner JB, Chernik NL. Intracranial metastases from systemic cancer. Adv Neurol 1978;19:579–92.

Excellent overview.

Zimm S, Wampler GL, Stablein D et al. Intracerebral metastases in solid-tumor patients: natural history and results of treatment. Cancer 1981;48:384–94.

Comprehensive survey.

Epidural Spine Metastases

Delattre J-Y, Arbit E, Rosenblum MK et al. High dose versus low dose dexamethasone in experimental epidural spinal cord compression. Neurosurgery 1988;22:1005–7.

Animals that received high-dose steroids did better.

Gilbert RW, Kim J-H, Posner JB. Epidural spinal cord compression from metastatic tumor: diagnosis and treatment. Ann Neurol 1978;3:40–51.

Detailed study.

Greenberg HS, Kim J-H, Posner JB. Epidural spinal cord compression from metastatic tumor: results with a new treatment protocol. Ann Neurol 1980;8:361–6.

High-dose steroids improve pain but not neurologic function.

Rodichok LD, Harper GR, Ruckdeschel JC et al. Early diagnosis of spinal epidural metastases. Am J Med 1981;70:1181–8.

A study of back pain in patients with cancer.

Sarpel S, Sarpel G, Yu E et al. Early diagnosis of spinal-epidural metastasis by magnetic resonance imaging. Cancer 1987;59:1112–6.

MRI scanning is the most sensitive.

Siegal T, Siegal T. Surgical decompression of anterior and posterior malignant epidural tumors compressing the spinal cord: a prospective study. Neurosurgery 1985;17:424–32.

Anterior decompression is the treatment of choice.

van der Sande JJ, Kroger R, Boogerd W. Multiple spinal epidural metastases; an unexpectedly frequent finding. J Neurol Neurosurg Psychiatry 1990;53:1001–3.

High incidence of multiple level cord compression.

Leptomeningeal Metastases

Blaney SM, Balis FM, Poplack DG. Pharmacologic approaches to the treatment of meningeal malignancy. Oncology 1991;5:107–16.

Review of chemotherapy.

Little JR, Dale AJD, Okazaki H et al. Meningeal carcinomatosis. Arch Neurol 1974;30:138–43.

One of the first.

Olson ME, Chernik NL, Posner JB. Infiltration of the leptomeninges by systemic cancer. Arch Neurol 1974;30:122–37.

Clinical classic.

Rodesch G, Van Bogaert P, Mavroudakis N et al. Neuroradiologic findings in leptomeningeal carcinomatosis: the value interest of gadolinium-enhanced MRI. Neuroradiology 1990;32:26–32.

Enhanced MRI may demonstrate the tumor.

Schold SC, Wasserstrom WR, Fleisher M et al. Cerebrospinal fluid biochemical markers of central nervous system metastases. Ann Neurol 1980;8:597–604.

Defines the utility of tumor markers.

Shapiro WR, Young DF, Mehta BM. Methotrexate: distribution in cerebrospinal fluid after intravenous, ventricular and lumbar injections. N Engl J Med 1975;293:161–6.

Disturbution of methotrexate by Ommaya reservoir or lumbar puncture injection.

Plexopathy

Bagley FH, Walsh JW, Cady B et al. Carcinomatous versus radiation-induced brachial plexus neuropathy in breast cancer. Cancer 1978;41:2154–7.

Clinical clues in differential diagnosis.

Jaeckle KA, Young DF, Foley KM. The natural history of lumbosacral plexopathy in cancer. Neurology 1985;35: 8–15.

Pelvic tumors and colon cancers are the principal causes.

Kori SH, Foley KM, Posner JB. Brachial plexus lesions in patients with cancer: 100 cases. Neurology 1981;31: 45–50.

The definitive study.

Lederman RJ, Wilbourn AJ. Brachial plexopathy: recurrent cancer or radiation? Neurology 1984;34:1331–1335.

Differentiating points.

Thomas JE, Cascino TL, Earle JD. Differential diagnosis between radiation and tumor plexopathy of the pelvis. Neurology 1985;35:1–7.

Clinical and radiologic features.

54

Neurologic Paraneoplastic Syndromes

Lisa M. DeAngelis

Neurologic paraneoplastic syndromes or "remote effects" of cancer on the nervous system refer to a group of disorders associated with an identifiable or occult cancer but not resulting from metastasis to the nervous system, metabolic or nutritional disorders, or treatment effects. Despite the intense interest in them, paraneoplastic syndromes are rare, occurring in less than 1 percent of patients with cancer. In one-half to two-thirds of patients, the neurologic syndrome precedes and prompts the diagnosis of systemic cancer. Because specific paraneoplastic syndromes are associated with particular cancers, the diagnosis of a paraneoplastic syndrome can direct the search for the underlying malignancy to one or a few organs. In many cases, the paraneoplastic neurologic syndrome has its onset at a time when there is limited oncologic disease and the cancer may be relatively easy to control or even cure. However, most patients with paraneoplastic syndromes are left with significant neurologic disability.

DIAGNOSIS

Although there is variability in clinical presentation, certain clinical features may suggest a paraneoplastic syndrome, and several of these syndromes have a stereotypic presentation. Most paraneoplastic syndromes are severe, progress steadily over weeks to months, and then stabilize. Syndromes that come on acutely, are mild, or are characterized by exacerbations and remissions are less likely to be paraneoplastic. Often paraneoplastic syndromes are associated with an inflammatory cerebrospinal fluid (CSF) profile, including pleocytosis, elevated protein or myelin basic protein level, or oligoclonal bands. Leptomeningeal metastasis needs to be excluded with a CSF cytologic examination. Finally, most patients with paraneoplastic syndromes present with a clinical syndrome that predominantly affects one region of the nervous system, although patients diagnosed with paraneoplastic encephalomyelitis show clinical evidence of widespread nervous system dysfunction. In some patients with other paraneoplastic syndromes, there is pathologic evidence of diffuse involvement throughout the neuraxis. In recent years, the diagnosis of at least some of the paraneoplastic syndromes has been aided by the detection of characteristic autoantibodies. With the exception of the antibody found in Lambert-Eaton myasthenic syndrome, the etiologic significance of most of these autoantibodies is unknown. However, their presence helps confirm the clinical diagnosis of a paraneoplastic syndrome and further focuses the search for an underlying malignancy.

SPECIFIC SYNDROMES

Paraneoplastic Cerebellar Degeneration

Paraneoplastic cerebellar degeneration (PCD) presents clinically as a pancerebellar disorder (i.e., affecting all cerebellar function), usually with a subacute onset over weeks to months and subsequent stabilization. The predominant clinical findings are appendicular and truncal ataxia, dysarthria, diplopia, and nystagmus (which is often downbeating). The cerebellar syndrome is typically severe and functionally devastating, leaving the patient wheelchair dependent and frequently unable to write or speak intelligibly.

Associated findings at other levels of the neuraxis, when present, are generally mild. Although dementia has been reported fairly frequently, accurate evaluation of cognitive function is often limited by dysarthria and ataxia and probably does not contribute significantly to the clinical syndrome in most patients. Diplopia is a common complaint, although detection of oculomotor abnormalities is less common. Dysphagia, sensorineural hearing loss, neuropathy, and extrapyramidal and spinal cord signs have also been reported.

Pathologically, there is extensive and often complete loss of Purkinje cells in the cerebellum. Inflammatory infiltrates, if present, are usually mild and limited to the leptomeninges, although in a minority of patients, there is an associated prominent diffuse infiltrating encephalomyelitis.

PCD has been most often associated with lymphomas and lung, ovarian, and breast cancers, although isolated cases have been reported with a great variety of tumor types. In more than one-half of patients, the onset of neurologic symptoms precedes the diagnosis of cancer. Overall, the sex incidence is roughly equal between men and women, and the age distribution reflects that of the underlying malignancies.

Computed tomographic (CT) or magnetic resonance imaging (MRI) scans may be normal or may demonstrate cerebellar atrophy, particularly later in the disease process. Autoantibodies, specifically YO, which cross reacts with Purkinje cells, and HU, which cross reacts with all neurons, have been associated with PCD. Identification of these autoantibodies may be helpful diagnostically, but not all patients with PCD have autoantibodies.

Treatment has been unsuccessful. There are isolated reports of responses to immunosuppression, plasmapheresis, or treatment of the underlying cancer, but most patients with PCD remain neurologically disabled.

Opsoclonus-Myoclonus

The syndrome of opsoclonus-myoclonus may occur as a complication of encephalitis, trauma, increased intracranial pressure, thalamic hemorrhage, toxic encephalopathies, or hyperosmolar coma. It is rarely seen as a paraneoplastic syndrome.

Paraneoplastic opsoclonus-myoclonus occurs most often as a complication of neuroblastoma in children. Two percent of children with neuroblastoma have it, although 50 percent of children with opsoclonus-myoclonus are found to have neuroblastoma. The prognosis of neuroblastoma is better in children who have opsoclonus-myoclonus and there is a higher than expected incidence of tumors with benign histologic types.

The disorder usually improves or resolves with treatment of the underlying tumor, although it may be unresponsive to treatment of the tumor or to immunosuppressive therapy. The opsoclonus-myoclonus syndrome has been rarely reported as a complication of adult tumors, most commonly lung cancers. It has also been associated with breast cancer and a specific autoantibody, anti-RI, which is distinct from other autoantibodies seen in paraneoplastic diseases.

Limbic Encephalitis

Paraneoplastic limbic encephalitis presents typically with the subacute onset of personality and mood changes, with severe impairment of recent memory. Occasionally, there are associated findings of encephalopathy, including agitation, confusion, hallucinations, or seizures. The dementia is usually progressive. Limbic encephalitis may be seen in isolation or may be associated with diffuse nervous system involvement in the syndrome of encephalomyelitis or with the syndrome of subacute sensory neuronopathy (see below).

It occurs rarely as a complication of lung (particularly small cell) or other cancers, although a similar syndrome can occur without a neoplasm. Its incidence is equal in men and women. The CSF is typically inflammatory, and CT and MRI scans are typically normal, although they may show mild atrophy and hyperintensity in the medial temporal lobes on MRI. The autoantibody HU may be associated with limbic encephalitis. Pathologically, there is extensive loss of neurons with reactive gliosis, perivascular lymphocytic cuffing, and microglial proliferation, usually restricted to limbic and insular cortex.

No treatment has been successful, but there are occasional reports of spontaneous remissions or improvement with treatment of the underlying tumor.

Retinal Degeneration

Paraneoplastic retinal degeneration, also called cancer-associated retinopathy, is a rare syndrome that usually presents with episodic visual obscurations, characterized by blurring, glare, and photosensitivity, that progress to painless visual loss. The symptoms begin unilaterally but become bilateral. Visual testing shows scotomas and loss of visual acuity. Funduscopic examination may reveal arteriolar narrowing and abnormal mottling of the retinal pigment epithelium.

Cancer-associated retinopathy occurs in association with small cell lung cancer. Typically, visual symptoms precede the diagnosis of cancer. The electroretinogram is abnormal. Pathologically, there is loss of photoreceptors and ganglion cells; on electron microscopy, melanin granules are evident. Serum antibodies that react immunohistochemically with antigens in retinal photoreceptor and ganglion cells have been found in some patients with this disorder, suggesting an immune-mediated mechanism. No treatment exists.

Necrotizing Myelopathy

This rare syndrome has caused a few well-documented frenzied attempts at diagnosis for patients presenting with rapidly ascending flaccid paraplegia.

Back or radicular pain are not prominent features, distinguishing this entity from metastatic spinal cord compression. Often, there is progressive compromise, leading to respiratory failure and even death. Compressive spinal cord lesions, a more likely cause of progressive paraparesis, need to be excluded in the initial evaluation. The CSF usually shows an inflammatory formula, and myelography or MRI may show spinal cord swelling, often leading to a diagnosis of acute infarction or myelitis but rarely the correct entity.

At autopsy, there is widespread spinal cord necrosis, involving all components of the cord but with some white matter predominance. Inflammatory lesions are not typical.

The mechanism of this syndrome is unknown. Necrotizing myelopathy may be seen in association with lymphoma, leukemia, or lung cancer, although it may also occur in previously healthy patients or in those without an identifiable neoplasm. The onset of the disorder may precede or follow the diagnosis of cancer. No treatment has been successful.

Subacute Motor Neuronopathy

Paraneoplastic subacute motor neuronopathy occurs as a rare complication of Hodgkin's and other lymphomas and, occasionally, other cancers. The disorder is characterized by gradually progressive weakness and bulbar dysfunction. All patients have lower motor neuron signs, but approximately one-third also have definite upper motor neuron signs. The rate of progression may be slow enough to mislead the clinician to diagnose amyotrophic lateral sclerosis. The clinical course is typically benign or remitting.

The CSF is generally acellular with a mildly elevated protein. Oligoclonal bands may be present. Electrical studies show denervation with normal nerve conduction velocities. Multifocal conduction block is occasionally seen. This syndrome may occur at any time in the course of the oncologic illness, but most often, it occurs when the patient is in remission. In a few cases, a paraproteinemia has been found, which may lead to the diagnosis of lymphoma in the patient who presents with neurologic symptoms and has no history of cancer. In these patients, neurologic improvement may occur with treatment of the lymphoma. At autopsy, the usual pathologic changes are noninflammatory loss of anterior horn cells and demyelination of ventral roots, although there may be more extensive myelopathic changes. Corticospinal tract involvement may be seen in patients with upper motor neuron involvement.

By electron microscopy, Walton et al. (1968) found viral particles in the anterior horn of spinal cord in a patient with this syndrome. It has been suggested that a viral mechanism may be an important factor, although the exact mechanism is not known.

No treatment exists, and the clinical course is variable. Some patients experience a complete recovery, but others remain neurologically disabled.

Subacute Sensory Neuronopathy

Sensory neuronopathy, known to the French as the Gougerot-Sjögren syndrome, is a rare syndrome that can occur in previously healthy individuals and with a variety of underlying conditions, including Sjögren's syndrome. Probably, in fewer than one-half of patients, it is a paraneoplastic syndrome.

The symptoms typically begin in middle age, and men and women are about equally affected. The initial symptoms are dysesthetic pain and numbness in the distal extremities, which progresses over days to several weeks to involve the limbs, trunk, and rarely, the face and causes a severe sensory ataxia. Deep tendon reflexes are lost, but motor function is preserved. The syndrome may occur in pure form or be a part of a more diffuse encephalomyelitis.

The CSF typically has an inflammatory appearance. Sensory nerve action potentials have a low amplitude or are absent. Motor nerve action potentials are normal, and there is no electromyographic evidence of denervation. Autopsies have shown the early pathologic changes are mostly limited to the dorsal root ganglia, where there is loss of neurons and lymphocytic inflammatory infiltrates. As the disease progresses, the inflammatory process may involve the dorsal root, posterior columns, and peripheral nerve.

Paraneoplastic sensory neuronopathy may occur as a pure syndrome or as part of a more diffuse encephalomyelitis. The HU antibody is frequently associated with it. At least two-thirds of patients with paraneoplastic sensory neuronopathy have lung cancer, usually small cell. In most, the neurologic syndrome precedes the diagnosis of cancer, which is of limited extent at the time of diagnosis.

Treatment of the underlying tumor, plasmapheresis, or immunosuppressive therapy does not improve the course of the neurologic disease.

Subacute Sensorimotor Neuropathy

Because subacute sensorimotor neuropathy can be induced by many known etiologic mechanisms, including diabetes mellitus, nutritional deficiency of alcoholism or chronic illness, vitamin B_{12} deficiency, exposure to toxins, and chemotherapeutic agents (vincristine and cisplatin, in particular), the rare diagnosis of paraneoplastic sensorimotor neuropathy should be made with caution and only after other causes are excluded. As a true paraneoplastic syndrome, it is most frequently associated with lung cancer and may precede the diagnosis of cancer by up to 5 years. The course is variable, with a few patients having stable disease or a remission with treatment of the underlying tumor. Patients typically present with a slowly progressive distal symmetric polyneuropathy.

The CSF is usually normal or has a mildly elevated protein, and electrical testing reveals small amplitude potentials, with denervation on electromyography. Axonal degeneration is generally the major pathologic finding, although occasionally, segmental demyelination is seen. The cause of this disorder is unknown. There have been reports of response to corticosteroid therapy, particularly in patients with prominent demyelination and elevated CSF protein levels.

Acute Polyradiculoneuropathy

Paraneoplastic acute polyradiculoneuropathy is a remote effect, usually associated with Hodgkin's disease, in which the clinical and pathologic features are similar to typical Guillain-Barré syndrome. The neurologic symptoms can begin either during active disease or when the disease is in remission. The clinical course is independent of that of the lymphoma and may respond to plasmapheresis.

Lambert-Eaton Myasthenic Syndrome

The Lambert-Eaton myasthenic syndrome occurs in patients without cancer, although in more than one-half, cancer develops during the course of the illness and is usually a small cell lung cancer. Patients present with proximal weakness and fatigability, which is progressive but, unlike myasthenia gravis, rarely involves the bulbar musculature. Respiratory weakness can occur. Power increases with continued use of the muscles; so the patient's report of weakness may be greater than the examiner's findings. Cholinergic dysautonomia occurs in more than one-half of patients, causing dry mouth and impotence.

Characteristic abnormalities are found on electrophysiologic testing, including very low compound muscle action potentials, which may increase to normal after brief exercise. Repetitive stimulation causes a decrement of the compound muscle action potentials at low rates of stimulation and an increment at high rates of stimulation. Lambert-Eaton myasthenic syndrome is thought to be a disorder of reduced release of acetylcholine from presynaptic nerve terminals, and in almost one-half of patients, there are detectable antibodies that react with the voltage-dependent calcium channel at the nerve terminal. Evidence that Lambert-Eaton myasthenic syndrome is actually an autoimmune disease includes its association with other autoimmune diseases, the clinical response to immunosuppression, and most compellingly, the results of passive transfer experiments in which the

disorder has been induced in experimental animals after injection of immunoglobulin G from patients with Lambert-Eaton myasthenic syndrome. Rare patients develop Lambert-Eaton myasthenic syndrome in conjunction with paraneoplastic cerebellar degeneration, without cerebellar-directed antibodies. Distinct from most of the other paraneoplastic syndromes, Lambert-Eaton myasthenic syndrome is often responsive to plasmapheresis or immunosuppressive therapy. Other treatments include guanidine hydrochloride, which mobilizes calcium, and 4-aminopyridine, which acts on potassium channels, but both have significant side effects. The drug 3,4-diaminopyridine also facilitates release of transmitter but with fewer side effects. Cholinesterase inhibitors show minimal benefit in most patients.

Treatment of the underlying malignancy in some instances improves the neurologic syndrome.

Polymyositis-Dermatomyositis

Despite clinical claims for decades, the association of cancer with polymyositis and dermatomyositis is not entirely established, but particularly in older patients, there is evidence to suggest that the disorders are related.

Patients present with painful proximal muscle weakness, an elevated serum creatine kinase level, and characteristic skin changes. Progression of the disease occasionally leads to respiratory failure. Myopathic electromyographic abnormalities support the diagnosis. Inflammation is seen on muscle biopsy.

The onset of myositis precedes the diagnosis of cancer in most patients in whom they occur together, and although there have been a variety of tumor types reported, breast, ovary, lung, and gastric tumors are most common.

In some patients, the skin and muscle abnormalities improve with treatment of the underlying tumor. However, spontaneous improvements occur, and some patients respond to corticosteroid therapy, chemotherapeutic agents, or immune globulin. The disorder is a result of complement-mediated vasculopathy, although the exact pathogenic mechanism is unknown.

ANNOTATED BIBLIOGRAPHY

Anderson NE, Cunningham JE, Posner JB. Autoimmune pathogenesis of paraneoplastic neurological syndromes. Crit Rev Neurobiol 1987;3:245–99.

A comprehensive review of all neurologic paraneoplastic diseases.

Corsellis JAN, Goldberg GJ, Norton AR. "Limbic encephalitis" and its association with carcinoma. Brain 1968;96:481–96.

A classic article.

Dalmau J, Graus F, Rosenblum MK, Posner JB. Anti-HU associated paraneoplastic encephalomyelitis/sensory neuronopathy. A clinical study of 71 patients. Medicine 1992;71:5972.

The definitive study of encephalomyelitis and the HU antibody.

Graus F, Vega F, Delattre J-Y et al. Plasmapheresis and antineoplastic treatment in CNS paraneoplastic syndromes with antineuronal autoantibodies. Neurology 1992;42:536–40.

Plasmapheresis is not useful in most patients.

Hildebrand J. Signs, symptoms, and significance of paraneoplastic neurological syndromes. Oncology 1989;3:57–68.

A good overall review of the topic.

Kissel JT, Halterman RK, Rammohan KW et al. The relationship of complement-mediated microvasculopathy to the histologic features and clinical duration of disease in dermatomyositis. Arch Neurol 1991;48:26–30.

Autoimmune vasculitis may be the mechanism of dermatomyositis.

Leys K, Lang B, Johnston I, Newsom-Davis J. Calcium channel autoantibodies in the Lambert-Eaton myasthenic syndrome. Ann Neurol 1991;29:307–314.

Autoantibodies are likely to be responsible for the disease.

Luque FA, Furneaux HM, Ferziger R et al. Anti-RI: an antibody associated with paraneoplastic opsoclonus and breast cancer. Ann Neurol 1991;29:241–51.

Describes the association between RI antibodies and opsoclonus.

O'Neill JH, Murray NMF, Newsom-Davis J. Lambert-Eaton myasthenic syndrome: a review of 50 cases. Brain 1988;111:577–96.

The best clinical overview of Lambert-Eaton myasthenic syndrome.

Schold SC, Cho E-S, Somasundaram M, Posner JB. Subacute motor neuronopathy: a remote effect of lymphoma. Ann Neurol 1979;5:271–87.

Describes the clinical features of motor neuropathies.

Thirkill CE, Fitzgerald P, Sergott RC et al. Cancer-associated retinopathy (CAR syndrome) with antibodies reacting with retinal, optic-nerve, and cancer cells. N Eng J Med 1989;321:1589–94.

A convincing article on the significance of autoantibodies in cancer-associated retinopathy.

Walton JN, Tomlinson BE, Pearce GW. Subacute "poliomyelitis" and Hodgkin's disease. J Neurol Sci 1968;6:435–45.

Viral particles were seen in the anterior horn cells.

Younger DS, Rowland LP, Latov N et al. Lymphoma, motor neuron diseases and amyotrophic lateral sclerosis. Ann Neurol 1991;78:86.

Nine new patients and literature review of relationship between lymphoma and motor neuron disease.

55
Meningiomas

Lisa M. DeAngelis

Meningiomas are usually benign neoplasms arising from mesenchymal cells of the leptomeninges. Some 60 percent occur in women, predominately in middle to late life. They are multiple in at least 1 to 2 percent of patients, with an incidence as high as 8 to 16 percent reported in autopsy and computed tomographic (CT) scan studies. They appear to be more frequent in women with breast cancer, although this epidemiologic association is controversial.

PATHOLOGY

Most meningiomas are histologically benign lesions, with rare instances of atypical and malignant variants. Several histologic subtypes of meningioma exist: meningothelial, transitional, fibroblastic, and psammomatous (Greek: *psammos,* sand), but they all have the same clinical behavior, and the pathologic distinction has no impact on treatment or prognosis.

The exception is the angioblastic (Greek: *angio,* vessel; *blastos,* germ) meningioma, which is now usually recognized as being a distinct tumor by the term *hemangiopericytoma.* The hemangiopericytoma typically occurs in younger patients, has an aggressive clinical course, and frequently leads to disseminated metastases.

Despite the benign pathologic appearance of most meningiomas, a few have an aggressive clinical course because of frequent recurrences. Rarely, a meningioma breeches the pia-arachnoid and invades the underlying brain tissue; cortical invasion indicates malignant behavior, whether or not pathologic features of malignancy are evident. Because of their aggressive behavior, these tumors should be treated as malignant lesions (see below). Most meningiomas grow as a discrete mass, but occasionally, they can grow as a sheet (meningioma en plaque) along a dural surface.

Meningiomas are slow-growing neoplasms and may be present for many years before producing neurologic dysfunction. They may be found at autopsy in patients who never had neurologic symptoms, and they are occasionally discovered accidentally when a CT or magnetic resonance imaging (MRI) scan is done for another purpose. Asymptomatic meningiomas do not always require treatment, particularly in elderly patients.

Approximately 90 to 95 percent of meningiomas contain progesterone receptors and about 35 percent, estrogen receptors. The presence of these hormonal receptors may partially explain the relatively higher incidence of this tumor in women. They may also account for the occasional patient who develops explosive growth, usually of a previously asymptomatic meningioma, during pregnancy.

CLINICAL FEATURES

Meningiomas are extra-axial and produce symptoms and signs by compressing the underlying brain or cranial nerves. They can develop in any location, but because they grow from arachnoid cells of the arachnoid villi, through which cerebrospinal fluid is resorbed into the sinuses, the most common sites include the convexity of the brain, particularly adjacent to the falx, the sphenoid wing, and the cavernous sinus. They can also develop in the spinal canal, particularly in the thoracic region. The clinical symptoms and signs are dependent on the location of the tumor.

Convexity lesions may present with seizures and a slowly progressive hemiparesis. Contralateral leg weakness may be the predominant or only manifestation of a lesion of the falx. Cavernous sinus and sphenoid wing tumors may present with ocular motility dysfunction, visual impairment, ptosis, proptosis, and headache. Tumors that arise from the olfactory groove may cause personality changes and headache and result in unilateral impairment of smell. Intraspinal meningiomas may produce painless, progressive leg weakness or sensory dysfunction. Sphincter problems are a late sign.

DIAGNOSIS

When central nervous system symptoms develop in a patient, cranial CT or MRI scan is usually the first test performed. On CT scan and T_1-weighted pregadolinium MRI scans, most meningiomas are isodense or isointense to normal brain tissue. After contrast administration, they enhance prominently and diffusely (Fig. 55-1). Edema of the underlying brain tissue is usually, but not always, absent and tends to be seen with histologically malignant or biologically aggressive tumors but not specifically related to tumor size. Calcification is frequent and is best appreciated on the CT scan (Fig. 55-2). The proximity of the lesion to a dural surface and evidence that the lesion is extra-axial as opposed to intra-axial (compression of underlying brain and absence of brain parenchyma surrounding the lesion) strongly suggest a meningioma. Meningiomas adjacent to bone frequently cause hyperostosis. This is a specific sign and can be seen on the CT scan, particularly the bone windows. It is less clear on the MRI scan and occasionally is evident on plain skull

films. It should be detectable by palpation of the skull, a too-often missed part of the clinical examination.

Spinal meningiomas are best identified on MRI scans where they appear as enhancing intradural extramedullary lesions. In the absence of a MRI scan, a myelogram will also visualize the tumor.

Unlike other primary central nervous system tumors, angiography, where available, is often important in the diagnosis and surgical treatment of meningiomas. Because meningiomas arise from a dural surface, they are fed by the external carotid artery. Angiographic demonstration of a tumor blush originating from the external carotid circulation establishes the diagnosis of meningioma and excludes further consideration of other primary brain tumors, such as gliomas. It does not exclude a dural-based metastasis if this is a clinical consideration, particularly in patients with breast carcinoma. Tumors that arise near the cavernous sinus or optic nerve may be difficult to differentiate from an aneurysm on a CT or MRI scan. Angiography excludes an aneurysm and reveals the tumor blush characteristic of a meningioma. With tumors of the sphenoid wing, it is important to determine the relationship of the tumor with the middle cerebral artery. Tumors adherent to the falx may invade the superior sagittal sinus. Often, angiography is necessary to delineate the extent of the tumor before

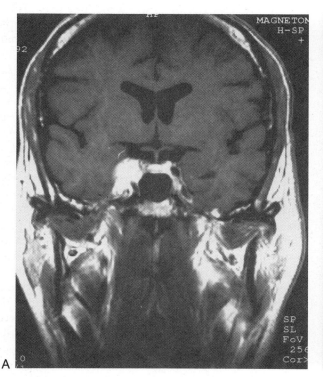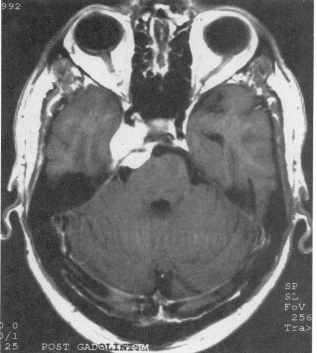

Figure 55-1. **(A)** Coronal and **(B)** axial images of cavernous sinus meningioma. There is prominent and diffuse enhancement of the tumor after gadolinium on these T_1-weighted images.

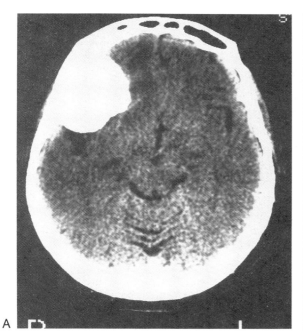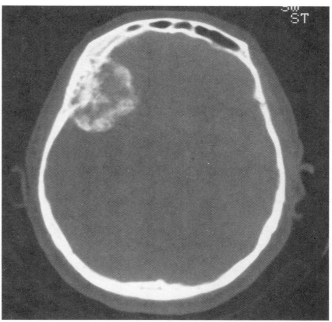

Figure 55-2. Noncontrast CT scan of a large meningioma. **(A)** Calcification is evident throughout the tumor, which has a density similar to that of the neighboring bone. A broad dural-based attachment is apparent, and there is no edema of the surrounding brain. **(B)** Bone windows reveal hyperostosis in the skull underneath the meningioma.

surgical excision. In many of these circumstances, magnetic resonance angiography provides the necessary preoperative information, sparing the patient the potential risk of arterial puncture and iodinated contrast. Spinal meningiomas do not require angiography preoperatively.

TREATMENT

Surgical extirpation remains the definitive therapy for meningiomas. Complete resection results in a high cure rate, with 93 percent of patients being recurrence free at 5 years, 80 percent at 10 years, and 68 percent at 15 years.

The feasibility of surgical removal is dependent on the location of the lesion. Tumors over the convexity can be completely removed in 96 percent of patients. Parasellar tumors are completely removed in 57 percent and sphenoid ridge lesions in only 28 percent. The remaining patients undergo varying degrees of subtotal excision. Recurrent meningiomas can be treated effectively with reresection. However, those patients in whom multiple recurrences develop often exhaust the surgical route after four to five craniotomies.

Radiotherapy is not administered routinely to patients after surgery, including those known to have a subtotal resection. The rate of tumor growth and the expected time to recurrence is very variable, and patients with a subtotal excision may not have recurrent tumor develop for several years. Radiation therapy is frequently given after a second resection when residual disease was left behind, particularly if the lesion is in a critical area, such as the cavernous sinus or optic nerve. Radiotherapy can produce some shrinkage of the lesion, although significant resolution of the mass is uncommon. Although tumor regression is modest at best, radiotherapy does appear to slow the rate of recurrence and delay the time to next relapse.

The pathologic diagnosis of malignancy can be difficult because some meningiomas show bizarre, hyperchromatic nuclei. Patients with malignant meningiomas should receive postoperative radiotherapy even if a complete resection has been achieved. Malignant meningiomas always recur, usually within 1 to 2 years of the initial craniotomy. Atypical meningiomas have a course between the typical benign and malignant tumors. Radiation therapy is occasionally advised after initial surgery, but many physicians wait for recurrence and irradiate after a reoperation. Stereotactic radiosurgery has been effective for some meningiomas. This technique has the advantage of delivering highly focused radiotherapy in a single dose, usually about 1,600 cGy. It may be used as the initial radiotherapy but it can also be used for recurrence after conventional irradiation because normal brain tissue is spared. The tumor must be small (less than 3 cm) to be treated with stereotactic radiosurgery, and critical structures such as the optic nerve should not be included in the radiosurgery port. Unfortunately, this limits the applicability of the technique, but it nonetheless affords an additional therapeutic option for eligible patients.

Conventional chemotherapy is ineffective against meningiomas of any grade. Because of the high incidence of sex steroid receptors on meningiomas, hormonal manipulation has been tried. There has been recent enthusiasm for the antiprogestational agent, mifepristone. However, it had only a modest effect on recurrent meningiomas that were progesterone-receptor positive and was ineffective against the few malignant meningiomas tested.

ANNOTATED BIBLIOGRAPHY

Adegbite AB, Khan MI, Paine KWE et al. The recurrence of intracranial meningiomas after surgical treatment. J Neurosurg 1983;58:51–6.

Relationship between extent of resection and recurrence.

Boylan SE, McCunniff AT. Recurrent meningioma. Cancer 1988;61:1447–52.

Recurrences are common.

Carella RJ, Ransohoff J, Newall J. Role of radiation therapy in the management of meningioma. Neurosurgery 1982; 10:332–9.

Radiotherapy can help control growth.

Firsching RP, Doz P, Fischer A et al. Growth rate of incidental meningiomas. J Neurosurg 1990;73:545–7.

Many incidental meningiomas remain unchanged for years.

Grunberg SM, Weiss MH, Spitz IM et al. Treatment of unresectable meningiomas with the antiprogesterone agent mifepristone. J Neurosurg 1991;74:861–6.

Some meningiomas appear to stabilize with this new agent.

Haak HR, deKeizer RJW, Hagenouw-Taal JCW et al. Successful mifepristone treatment of recurrent, inoperable meningioma. Lancet 1990;336:124–5.

This antiprogestational agent has modest activity against meningiomas.

Jacobs DH, Holmes FF, McFarlane MJ. Meningiomas are not significantly associated with breast cancer. Arch Neurol 1992;49:753–6.

Continues the controversy, which remains unresolved.

Kondziolka D, Lunsford LD, Coffey RJ et al. Stereotactic radiosurgery of meningiomas. J Neurosurg 1991;74: 552–9.

A new therapeutic approach.

Kondziolka D, Lunsford LD, Coffey RJ et al. Gamma knife radiosurgery of meningiomas. Stereotact Funct Neurosurg 1991;57:21.

The technique is useful for some patients.

Miralbell R, Linggood RM, de la Monte S et al. The role of radiotherapy in the treatment of subtotally resected benign meningiomas. J Neurooncol 1992;13:157–64.

Radiation therapy can delay recurrence.

Mirimanoff RO, Dosoretz DE, Linggood RM et al. Meningioma: analysis of recurrence and progression following neurosurgical resection. J Neurosurg 1985;62:1824.

An excellent analysis of recurrence rates after resection, depending on location.

Moguilewsky M, Pertuiset BF, Verzat C et al. Cytosolic and nuclear sex steroid receptors in meningioma. Clin Neuropharmacol 1984;7:375–81.

Most meningiomas have sex steroid receptors.

Schoenberg BS, Christine BW, Whisnant JP. Nervous system neoplasms and primary malignancies of other sites. Neurology 1975;25:705–12.

The breast cancer-meningioma controversy: a pro association.

Sheehy JP, Crockard HA. Multiple meningiomas: a long-term review. J Neurosurg 1983;59:1–5.

About 5 percent of patients have multiple meningiomas.

Solero CL, Fornari M, Giombini S et al. Spinal meningiomas: review of 174 operated cases. Neurosurgery 1989; 25:153–60.

A comprehensive review.

56
Pituitary Tumors

Lisa M. DeAngelis

Pituitary tumors are benign endocrinologic neoplasms that arise from cells of the anterior pituitary gland. Metastasis outside the sella is almost unknown. It is the location of the gland intracranially at the base of the brain that allows otherwise small pituitary adenomas to compress or invade intracranial structures, resulting in neurologic symptoms. Thus, they are classified as intracranial neoplasms. Pituitary tumors are common and represent at least 10 percent of all symptomatic intracranial neoplasms. In addition, they are identified in 8 to 13 percent of all autopsies, with some reports giving an incidence as high as 27 percent. Most tumors discovered at autopsy are asymptomatic microadenomas.

Pituitary adenomas are classified according to size (macroadenoma or microadenoma; the latter is less than 1 cm) and the hormone secreted. The tumor may be secretory or nonsecretory (null cell). Secretory tumors may secrete prolactin (PRL), growth hormone (GH), corticotropin (ACTH), thyrotropin, or gonadotropin. In the days when histopathologic examination was the main source for tumor classification, tumors were labeled according to their staining characteristics; the most common was the chromophobe adenoma, which was acidophilic and associated with GH, and basophilic (which was associated with ACTH). Chromophobe tumors include lesions that secrete PRL, GH, and even ACTH, so that this histologic classification was proved to be inadequate to cope with the tumor type and is no longer used, although it is found throughout the older literature.

TUMOR TYPES

Prolactinoma

This is the most common pituitary tumor. It is more common in women, at a 4:1 ratio, with a peak incidence in the fourth decade. Prolactinomas often produce serum PRL levels above 200 ng/ml (normal, less than 20ng/ml) and even into the 1,000-ng/ml range. Nonprolactinomas can also cause an elevation of the serum PRL level by disrupting the dopamine inhibitory pathway from the hypothalamus, which controls PRL secretion. However, serum PRL levels are usually below 200 ng/ml when caused by disinhibition. Therefore, the serum PRL level may differentiate between these two possibilities.

The clinical presentation of prolactinomas differs by sex. Women have amenorrhea and galactorrhea, which may be the only symptoms. In men, the initial symptom is usually impotence, although this may be ignored for many years, particularly in elderly patients. Occasionally, galactorrhea is also seen. Men infrequently seek consulation for the impotence but more often consult the physician for visual symptoms (see below) from a tumor that has extended into the suprasellar compartment.

Growth Hormone Adenomas

These are the second most common pituitary adenoma. There is a male predominance of 2:1.

Somatostatin, the hypothalamic peptide that inhibits pituitary GH release, is released in a pulsatile fashion, causing GH release to be pulsatile, even in the presence of an adenoma. Thus, a random GH level may be normal, even in an acromegalic patient. Overproduction of GH results in increased serum levels of somatomedin-C and insulin-like growth factor-1, which plays a role (poorly understood) in adding to the GH effect on its target tissues.

GH adenomas are associated with acromegaly (Greek, *acro*, extremity of the body; *megaly*, large) in adults and gigantism in children. These signs are often present for many years before the patient comes to medical attention because the physical changes can be insidious. Patients also have insulin resistance with diabetes mellitus, hypertension, arthritis, and cardiac disease, which accounts for the increased mortality rate associated with GH excess. The tumors are usually macroadenomas when detected, and visual symptoms often bring the patient to medical attention, at which time the features of acromegaly are apparent.

Corticotropin-Secreting Tumors

These account for about 5 percent of pituitary adenomas. They cause Cushing's disease (Harvey Cushing, 1869–1939, American surgeon), and patients present with symptoms of hypercortisolism, including mental changes, obesity, striae, hypertension, and diabetes mellitus. Because the symptoms of excess glucocorticoid are so severe and characteristic, most of these tumors are identified when they are microadenomas. There is a significant female predominance with a 4:1 ratio.

Thyrotrophic Adenomas

Such tumors are very rare, making up about 1 percent of pituitary adenomas, and they cause hyperthyroidism. These tumors are often macroadenomas at diagnosis.

NEUROLOGIC FEATURES

Regardless of the hormone secreted by a pituitary tumor, when the mass extends into the suprasellar compartment, neurologic symptoms develop. Compression of the optic chiasm, leading to a bitemporal hemianopia, is often the first manifestation. However, if this develops slowly, patients may be unaware of loss of their peripheral vision; occasionally, an incident such as an automobile accident may bring the deficit to attention. If there is progressive growth, the optic nerves are compressed, causing visual loss, and there may be extension into the cavernous sinus with ophthalmoplegia. In patients who have not been seen regularly by a physician, the degree of shrinkage of the visual fields before the patient becomes aware of the disturbance is often surprising.

Headache is a common symptom and may be directly related to the pituitary tumor, particularly in those with significant suprasellar extension or invasion of the cavernous sinus, but it may also be independent of the tumor, as in those with microadenomas.

Pituitary apoplexy is an unusual presenting symptom but eventually occurs in about 5 percent of patients with pituitary adenomas. Apoplexy is due to acute hemorrhage or infarction of the adenoma, resulting in acute headache, visual loss, ophthalmoplegia, and frequently, coma. Acute hypopituitarism also occurs. Apoplexy may occur in any patient with an adenoma, but the pregnant patient is more vulnerable to this acute event because pituitary neoplasms often enlarge rapidly during pregnancy.

DIAGNOSIS

The diagnosis of pituitary tumors has been greatly facilitated by magnetic resonance imaging (MRI) scans. Microadenomas, the optic nerve, and chiasm are easily identified on coronal MRI scans of the sella turcica (Fig. 56-1). Although often used when MRI is not available, a computed tomograph scan is often inadequate for the visualization of small pituitary lesions. Intrapituitary hemorrhage can be seen in some patients with apoplexy but may also be evident in some patients without the clinical apoplectic syndrome. In severe apoplexy with coma, blood extravasates into the subarachnoid space, leading to meningeal irritation and often a misdiagnosis of aneurysmal subarachnoid hemorrhage. Rarely, a large hemorrhage can extend into the brain parenchyma or the ventricular system.

In patients suspected of having a pituitary tumor, serum should be assayed for pituitary hormones. Somatomedin-C and insulin-like growth factor-1 are measured in GH-secreting tumors, and an oral glucose tolerance test is occasionally necessary. ACTH-secreting tumors may be difficult to diagnose because they may be very small and not visible on MRI scan. Provocative hormonal testing (such as the dexamethasone suppression test, the metyrapone test, or the corticotropin-releasing factor stimulation test) is often useful. In some patients, bilateral sampling of the inferior petrosal sinus for ACTH is helpful.

TREATMENT

The first therapeutic consideration for any patient with a pituitary neoplasm is surgery. Transsphenoidal resection of pituitary tumors is effective and associated with minimal morbidity. Microadenomas and small macroadenomas restricted to the sellar contents can be completely removed. Larger tumors that extend into the suprasellar space can also be removed through the transsphenoidal approach, although partial resection is more frequent in this situation. Complete resection can cure this tumor and usually leaves the patient intact endocrinologically. In patients who have visual loss at the time of surgery, about 75 percent will improve or have full recovery of vision after transsphenoidal removal. The complications from transsphenoidal resection include cerebrospinal fluid rhinorrhea (about 4 percent), diabetes insipidus (which is usually transient), and infection.

Medical therapy with bromocriptine is an alternative for some patients with prolactinomas. Bromocriptine is a dopamine agonist that inhibits PRL secretion.

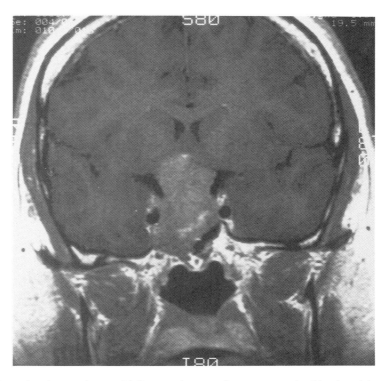

Figure 56-1. A prolactinoma in a middle-aged man who presented with visual loss. Postgadolinium T₁-weighted coronal MRI scan of a macroadenoma filling the sella turcica, invading the cavernous sinus, and extending into the hypothalamus and floor of the third ventricle. Most of the tumor enhances homogeneously, except for a small area inferiorly.

It shrinks an adenoma and normalizes the serum PRL level by reducing cell size and decreasing hormone synthesis. For patients with only amenorrhea and galactorrhea, this may completely reverse their symptoms. However, withdrawal of the medication results in rising PRL levels and the reappearance of the adenoma on imaging studies. Therefore, as an exclusive treatment, bromocriptine is a long-term commitment, and many patients cannot tolerate the drug because of frequent side effects, including nausea, headache, and dizziness. Bromocriptine is useful for patients with large prolactinomas, which can be reduced with medication to facilitate complete surgical removal, or for temporary shrinkage of an adenoma that enlarged during pregnancy and will likely regress spontaneously after gestation. Bromocriptine has occasionally been reported to be useful in patients with nonfunctioning and GH-secreting tumors, although the mechanism of action in these cases is uncertain.

Radiotherapy is used for patients who have had recurrent tumors or who have residual disease after surgery, particularly those with invasive tumors. It produces regression, often with prolonged control of tumor growth. Delayed effects of radiotherapy are common after several years. In most patients, panhypopituitarism develops, which must be sought in their long-term follow-up.

An advance in the treatment of GH-secreting adenomas is the use of octreotide, an analogue of somatostatin. Octreotide is used in patients who have not responded to surgery and radiotherapy, but it has been effective with reduction of GH levels in more than 90 percent, with shrinkage of the tumor mass in about 44 percent of patients. It must be administered subcutaneously and can produce intolerable gastrointestinal side effects.

ANNOTATED BIBLIOGRAPHY

Cardoso ER, Peterson EW. Pituitary apoplexy: a review. Neurosurgery 1984;14:363–73.

A comprehensive review.

Cohen AR, Cooper PR, Kupersmith MJ et al. Visual recovery after transsphenoidal removal of pituitary adenomas. Neurosurgery 1985;17:446–52.

Many patients experience visual improvement.

Grigsby PW, Simpson JR, Emami BN et al. Prognostic factors and results of surgery and postoperative irradiation in the management of pituitary adenomas. Int J Radiat Oncol Biol Phys 1989;16:1411–7.

Many patients have a successful complete removal.

Klibanski A, Zervas NT. Diagnosis and management of hormone-secreting pituitary adenomas. N Engl J Med 1991; 324:822–31.

A comprehensive review.

Leavens ME, McCutcheon IF, Samaan NA. Management of pituitary adenomas. Oncology 1992;6:69–79.

An up-to-date review.

McCollough WM, Marcus RB, Rhoton AL Jr et al. Long-term follow-up of radiotherapy for pituitary adenoma: the absence of late recurrence after > 4500 cGy. Int J Radiat Oncol Biol Phys 1991;21:607–14.

Radiotherapy is a useful adjunct to surgery.

Oldfield EH, Doppman JL Nieman LK et al. Petrosal sinus sampling with and without corticotrophin-releasing hormone for the differential diagnosis of Cushing syndrome. N Engl J Med 1991;325:897–905.

A useful diagnostic method for tumors poorly visualized on MRI scan.

Randall RV, Scheithauer BW, Laws ER Jr et al. Pituitary adenomas associated with hyperprolactinemia: a clinical and immunohistochemical study of 97 patients operated on transsphenoidally. Mayo Clin Proc 1985;60:753–62.

A comprehensive analysis of the most common pituitary tumor.

Reincke M, Allolio B, Saeger W et al. The "incidentaloma" of the pituitary gland. JAMA 1990;263:2772–6.

Pituitary adenomas are frequently found on computed tomographic or MRI scans done for another purpose.

Russell DS, Rubinstein LJ. Secondary tumours of the nervous system. In Pathology of Tumours of the Nervous System. 5th Ed. Williams & Wilkins, Baltimore, 1989, pp. 809–54.

Details of pathologic findings.

Snyder PJ, Fowble BF, Schatz NJ et al. Hypopituitarism following radiation therapy of pituitary adenomas. Am J Med 1986;81:457–62.

Most patients experience delayed hypopituitarism.

Tindall GT, Oyesiku, NM, Watts NB et al. Transsphenoidal adenomectomy for growth hormone secreting pituitary adenomas in acromegaly: outcome analysis and determinants of failure. J Neurosurg 1993;78:205–15.

The transsphenoidal approach is effective for GH-secreting adenomas.

Vance ML, Harris AG. Long-term treatment of 189 acromegalic patients with the somatostatin analog octreotide. Arch Intern Med 1991;151:1573–8.

The latest advance for the treatment of acromegaly.

Zervas NT, Martin JB. Management of hormone-secreting pituitary adenomas. N Engl J Med 1980;302:210–4.

A basic review.

57
Acoustic Neuromas

Lisa M. DeAngelis

Acoustic neuromas are benign neoplasms that arise from the Schwann cells (Theodore Schwann, 1810–1882, German anatomist) that surround the vestibular portion of the eighth cranial nerve. They are more accurately called vestibular schwannomas, but the technically incorrect term of acoustic neuroma is firmly fixed in medical nomenclature. Although schwannomas can develop in many sites, acoustic neuromas are the most common, accounting for 5 to 10 percent of all intracranial neoplasms and most of the tumors in the cerebellopontine angle. They develop with equal frequency in men and women and are usually identified in the fourth and fifth decade of life, although they can develop at any time throughout adulthood. Acoustic neuromas are more common in patients with von Recklinghausen's disease (neurofibromatosis type I). The unusual occurrence of bilateral acoustic neuromas is the hallmark of central neurofibromatosis or neurofibromatosis type II.

PATHOLOGY

Acoustic neuromas are firm and encapsulated. Small lesions are usually spherical, whereas large lesions are lobulated. The site of tumor development is difficult to predict and may occur within the internal auditory canal where it can adhere to the facial nerve, making resection difficult.

CLINICAL FEATURES

They are slow-growing neoplasms and may be present for many years before they produce symptoms. Because they are extrinsic to brain tissue and grow slowly, they may reach considerable size before becoming clinically apparent.

The earliest symptom is usually hearing loss, with or without tinnitus. Dizziness, vertigo, gait imbalance, and headache are less common and usually late symptoms; diplopia, hoarseness, dysphagia, facial pain or numbness, and progressive ataxia may also develop in patients with large tumors that compress or distort the brainstem. The classic syndrome, described in the days when the lesions were not discovered until they were large, featured ipsilateral hearing loss, ipsilateral abolition of the corneal reflex, peripheral facial weakness, and cerebellar incoordination with contralateral paresis and brisk reflexes.

On examination, for patients encountered in modern times, hearing impairment is evident in more than 95 percent of patients. Audiometry usually reveals a high-frequency hearing loss, but more severe loss and other patterns may also be found.

DIAGNOSIS

Magnetic resonance imaging (MRI) has greatly simplified the diagnosis of acoustic neuroma. The cerebellopontine angle is well visualized by MRI, and acoustic neuromas enhance briskly after gadolinium administration. Where available, MRI scans should be the first test when the diagnosis of acoustic neuroma is considered. It is usually the only test necessary; a normal MRI scan excludes the diagnosis.

With the use of high-quality MRI scans, there is no need for cerebrospinal fluid (CSF) analysis to look for an elevated protein concentration (which may be normal with small tumors), as described in the older literature. Likewise, brainstem auditory-evoked responses used in diagnosis demonstrate prolongation of wave I-III and wave I-V interwave latencies in 98 percent of patients; however, this is nonspecific and no substitute for MRI. Computed tomographic scan with contrast is less desirable because of the frequent artifacts that may obscure small lesions in the posterior fossa.

If MRI is not available, these other steps in diagnosis must be used, recognizing their shortcomings.

TREATMENT

The treatment for acoustic neuromas is surgical. Complete removal is a curative procedure, and no additional therapy is necessary. The choice of surgical approach and the feasibility of a complete resection depends on the size of the lesion. A primary therapeutic consideration is preservation or restoration of facial and cochlear nerve function with surgery. Hearing is more likely to be preserved when the tumor is small, the patient has a normal or near-normal brainstem auditory-evoked response, and the tumor does not extend to the fundus of the internal auditory canal. Only about 20 percent of patients have significantly useful hearing at diagnosis and a tumor small enough so that preservation of hearing is a possibility.

Even with microsurgical techniques, only 33 percent of these patients have intact hearing postoperatively. Most patients with significantly impaired or absent hearing before surgery do not improve after resection. If the lesion is unilateral, this rarely limits the patient's functional capacity; however, bilateral lesions can produce deafness.

Preserving facial nerve function is more important to patients than preserving hearing. In a survey of 541 patients who had resections of acoustic neuromas, facial weakness was considered the most serious long-term complication from surgery, and it affected, in varying degrees, 80 percent of patients. Small tumors more often lend themselves to definitive resection without a disruption in facial nerve function. Ninety-five percent of patients with small tumors have good facial nerve function postoperatively. Even 50 to 60 percent of patients with the largest tumors can have relatively intact facial nerve function postoperatively, but the remainder frequently have permanent paralysis.

Facial impairment can be a consequence of severing the facial nerve during surgery, but many patients with anatomically preserved facial nerves have significant facial weakness postoperatively. Less than 10 percent of those with facial weakness immediately after surgery have significant postoperative improvement. Many patients are unable to return to full activity because of severe facial weakness. Difficulty with mouth closure can impair chewing, and most commonly, difficulty with eye closure can lead to corneal abrasions and infection. If the patient is unable to close the eyelids in the immediate postoperative period, the cornea must be protected with local measures, such as artificial tears and an appropriate eye patch (one that does not rest on the open eye). If facial paresis is severe and

permanent, a tarsorrhaphy may be necessary. Even patients with incomplete facial weakness who can close their eyes with effort may have dryness, pain, abrasions, and infections. They often require constant local care of the eye.

Because the consequences of cochlear and facial damage can be devastating, surgeons may elect to perform a subtotal resection to minimize nerve damage. This is particularly important in elderly patients or those with bilateral acoustic tumors. The evidence suggests these patients do well and rarely experience tumor regrowth. They do not require adjuvant therapy but should be followed closely to assess possible recurrences.

Apart from cochlear and facial nerve damage, additional postoperative complications include CSF leaks, meningitis, and wound infections. CSF leaks develop in approximately 14 percent of all patients with acoustic neuromas. Meningitis occurs in 5 percent. Rarely, intracranial hemorrhage, stroke, or hydrocephalus develops after acoustic neuroma surgery. Subjectively, patients frequently experience other postoperative difficulties, such as headache, which is seen in approximately 35 percent of all patients.

An alternative treatment to surgical resection is radiosurgery. Radiosurgery uses highly focused irradiation from gamma particles, photons, or other sources to deliver high-intensity radiotherapy, usually in a single dose. The treatment is noninvasive, can be done on an outpatient basis, and is fairly easy to administer in experienced hands. Therapy is designed to deliver about 2,000 cGy to the margins of the tumor. This technique eliminates the risks of surgical complications, such as CSF leaks, but patients are still at risk for hearing and facial nerve dysfunction.

Despite the obvious attractions of radiosurgery, the incidence and long-term prognosis of cranial nerve dysfunction after this treatment has not been established. Hearing loss and facial paresis may appear acutely after radiosurgery or may be delayed by several months. Other potential limitations of radiosurgery include the size of the lesion; tumors greater than 3 cm cannot be effectively treated with this technique. Radiosurgery appears to halt progression of the tumor but not to produce significant shrinkage of the lesion. Although the exact role of radiosurgery for the treatment of acoustic neuromas must be defined with additional clinical studies and long-term follow-up, it offers an alternative therapeutic approach, which is useful, particularly in patients unable to undergo surgery.

Tumor recurrence is uncommon after either surgery or radiosurgery. Relapses may develop months or usually years after initial therapy. The treatment of recurrence must be individualized but may include reoperation or radiosurgery. Conventional radiotherapy may also be used, although it has limited efficacy. Chemotherapy is not useful.

ANNOTATED BIBLIOGRAPHY

Bryce GE, Nedzelski JM, Rowed DW, Rappaport JM. Cerebrospinal fluid leaks and meningitis in acoustic neuroma surgery. Otolaryngol Head Neck Surg 1991;104:81–7.

CSF leaks occurred in 13.4 percent of patients.

Flickinger JC, Lunsford LD, Coffey RJ et al. Radiosurgery of acoustic neurinomas. Cancer 1991;67:345–53.

A promising technique.

Glasscock ME, Kveton JF, Jackson CG et al. A systematic approach to the surgical management of acoustic neuroma. Laryngoscope 1986;96:1088–94.

Most tumors can be definitively treated.

Kartush JM, Lundy LB. Facial nerve outcome in acoustic neuroma surgery. Otolaryngol Clin North Am 1992;25:623–47.

Good preoperative facial nerve function can often be preserved.

Kemink JL, Langman AW, Niparko JK, Graham MD. Operative management of acoustic neuromas: the priority of neurologic function over complete resection. Otolaryngol Head Neck Surg 1991;104:96–9.

Subtotal resection is sometimes preferable.

Linskey ME, Lunsford LD, Flickinger JC. Radiosurgery for acoustic neurinomas: early experience. Neurosurgery 1990;26:736–45.

One of the first reports on this technique for this tumor.

Selesnick SH, Jackler RK. Clinical manifestations and audiologic diagnosis of acoustic neuromas. Otolaryngol Clin North Am 1992;25:521–51.

Reviews audiograms and evoked response data.

Shelton C. Hearing preservation in acoustic tumor surgery. Otolaryngol Clin North Am 1992;25:609–21.

New techniques can facilitate resection with preserved hearing.

Wallner KE, Sheline GE, Pitts LH et al. Efficacy of irradiation for incompletely excised acoustic neurilemomas. Neurosurgery 1987;67:858–63.

Radiotherapy offers modest improvement.

Wiegand DA, Fickel V. Acoustic neuroma—the patient's perspective: subjective assessment of symptoms, diagnosis, therapy, and outcome in 541 patients. Laryngoscope 1989;99:179–87.

The true incidence of symptoms and therapeutic complications.

58
Radiotherapy and Chemotherapy

Lisa M. DeAngelis

RADIOTHERAPY

The principal use for radiotherapy is in the treatment of tumors, with far more limited use for arteriovenous malformations.

Methods of Treatment

Standard external beam radiotherapy is administered through ports to the areas involved by the tumor, usually to a total dose of about 5,000 to 6,000 cGy. It is delivered in approximately 200-cGy/day fractions. Whole-brain radiotherapy is given for tumors that are often multifocal, such as brain metastases or primary central nervous system lymphomas, whereas radiotherapy directed at the focus of tumor is used most often to treat primary brain tumors because they are localized to a particular region of brain. The dose of radiotherapy is limited by the tolerance of the normal brain tissue included in the radiated field. Tolerance is usually reached with the initial course of treatment and reirradiation with conventional radiotherapy is rarely possible.

Radiotherapy can also be administered with brachytherapy or stereotactic radiosurgery. Both methods deliver high-intensity focused irradiation, which can be safely delivered even after standard external beam radiotherapy. *Brachytherapy* is the temporary implantation of iodine-125 seeds into the tumor, which delivers approximately 6,000 cGy over 6 days. The seeds are then removed. Brachytherapy is followed by focal radionecrosis, usually several months after implantation. Surgical resection of the necrosis is required in approximately 50 percent of patients.

Stereotactic radiosurgery delivers about 1,600 cGy by external beam irradiation with photons or heavy particles to a well-focused area in a single dose. No surgical procedure is required, and the incidence of radio-necrosis that requires surgical debulking is probably lower. With current technology, stereotactic radiosurgery is limited to relatively small lesions (less than 3 cm), whereas brachytherapy can be used in larger tumors. Both offer improved local control after recurrence. However, only a minority of patients are eligible for these techniques, and these candidates tend to be better-risk patients. Stereotactic radiosurgery is also a frequent choice for the treatment of small, surgically inaccessible arteriovenous malformations. The full value of this therapy for such malformations remains unsettled.

Side Effects

The acute effects of cranial irradiation primarily affect extracerebral tissues and include hair loss, conjunctivitis, otitis media, acute parotitis, xerostomia, bitter taste in the mouth, and accelerated tooth decay and loss.

Acute neurologic deterioration can occur with headache, nausea, vomiting, and worsening of the neurologic deficit. Although headache is common with conventional fractions of approximately 200 cGy/day, severe neurologic compromise is uncommon and tends to occur when high daily fractions are administered to patients with pre-existing increased intracranial pressure. Steroids can reduce acute neurologic toxicity and ameliorate symptoms if they develop.

Chronic effects are usually delayed at least 1 year before they become clinically obvious. A poorly understood *leukoencephalopathy* has been described in survivors of prophylatic brain irradiation given up to a 3,500-cGy total dose of radiation in fractionated doses, especially those given large daily fractions of 400 cGy or more and those also given chemotherapy. The steadily progressing syndrome features apathy, abulia, memory loss, gait ataxia, and later, urinary incontinence. Radiographically, a striking widespread high signal change in the centrum semiovale is seen by magnetic resonance imaging (MRI), and less striking low-attenuation foci in the same locations are seen on computed tomographic (CT) scans. Leukoencephalopathy is more likely to develop when cranial radiotherapy is combined with some chemotherapeutic agents, particularly methotrexate.

In many patients who undergo cranial radiotherapy, a milder memory impairment and cognitive disturbance occurs, which may not be evident for months to years after completion of the treatment. Such effects are irreversible and may be progressive. Rarely, patients can develop *radiation-induced necrosis* within the irradiated port, which can act as a mass lesion and be indistinguishable from tumor recurrence on CT or MRI scan. Occasionally, a positron emission tomographic scan can help differentiate recurrent tumor (usually showing hypermetabolism) from radionecrosis (hypometabolism), but biopsy or resection may be necessary for diagnosis and therapy. Corticosteroids can alleviate symptoms caused by radiation-induced necrosis.

Delayed complications of radiotherapy are directly related to the total dose delivered and the daily dose. Because of the late delayed effects of radiotherapy and the frequently benign clinical course of many low-grade astrocytomas, such patients may receive anticonvulsants alone and be followed, often for several years, before a change in their clinical condition mandates definitive treatment (see Ch. 52). There are no data to guide the decision regarding the timing of radiotherapy, but a prospective study currently being performed will shed some light on this issue.

CHEMOTHERAPY

Settings for Use

Chemotherapy is used primarily in the treatment of systemic cancer, but it is also used for brain tumors and occasionally for nonmalignant processes, such as multiple sclerosis and the vasculitides of the nervous system.

For brain tumors, chemotherapy is usually used as adjuvant treatment to radiotherapy. The nitrosoureas, particularly carmustine, are the standard drugs used for anaplastic astrocytomas and glioblastomas multiforme. Carmustine is well tolerated by most patients and has no neurotoxicity. Additional chemotherapeutic options include such agents as procarbazine, intra-arterial cisplatin, or investigational drugs. For primary brain tumors, at the time of recurrence, patients may be considered for surgical reresection if the lesion is surgically accessible. Reoperation prolongs life a median of 6 additional months.

The combination of procarbazine, lomustine, and vincristine is being popularized for the initial treatment of anaplastic oliogodendrogliomas. This regimen, given before radiotherapy, can substantially shrink the lesion, facilitating a more limited port for therapy. If given at recurrence, most patients respond with partial or complete resolution of visible tumor. Recurrent anaplastic oligodendroglioma after such chemo- and radiotherapy often responds to other agents, such as melphalan, although bone marrow toxicity is frequently limiting.

Side Effects

The most common complication of all forms of chemotherapy is a *peripheral neuropathy*. The vinca alkaloids, particularly vincristine, cause a dose-related sensimotor neuropathy that is characterized by paresthesias, extensor weakness of the fingers and toes, and areflexia. It is predominantly an axonal neuropathy, and motor nerve conduction velocities may be normal. The neuropathy is dose related and largely reversible.

Cisplatin causes a predominantly large fiber *sensory neuropathy*. It is related to the cumulative dose of cisplatin and is characterized by prominent loss of vibration sense, loss of position sense, and a sensory ataxia. Cutaneous sensation is relatively preserved. The deep tendon reflexes are lost early. Nerve biopsies show loss of large-diameter fibers. The neuropathy may progress for several months after the drug is discontinued and is not readily reversible.

Antimetabolites form the treatment plan in many cancers. 5-Fluorouracil, especially when combined with thymidine, may cause a *subacute cerebellar degeneration* that has its onset within days after treatment has begun, is dose related, and is usually reversible. High-dose cytarabine can also cause a dose-related pancerebellar syndrome, usually after a cumulative dose of about 24 g/m^2, but this can occur after a single dose of 3 g/m^2. It usually reverses with discontinuation of the drug. The folic acid antagonist methotrexate may cause a subacute or acute multifocal *encephalopathy* within 1 week or more after high-dose therapy, which may present with focal signs, such as hemiparesis, and even progress to coma. Patchy low densities may be scattered throughout the white matter on CT scans. Although there is no adequate therapy, withholding methotrexate is the usual recommendation.

Drugs administered intrathecally or in an Ommaya reservoir can also produce neurotoxicity. Methotrexate and cytarabine can both produce an acute aseptic meningitis with headache, fever, meningismus, and an abnormal cerebrospinal fluid, including elevated protein concentration and cell count and even depressed glucose concentration. These changes usually occur within 24 hours of injection and are self-limited. More seriously, intrathecal chemotherapy can cause a leukoencephalopathy, even in the absence of cranial radiotherapy. Rarely, a permanent severe myelopathy occurs.

Little neurotoxicity has been encountered with the nitrosoureas (carmustine and lomustine), antipurines (6-mercaptopurine), alkylating agents, and antibiotics used in chemotherapy.

ANNOTATED BIBLIOGRAPHY

Allen JC, Rosen G, Mehta BM, Horten B. Leukoencephalopathy following high-dose IV methotrexate chemotherapy with leucovorin rescue. Cancer Treat Rep 1980;64:1261.

A discouraging leukoencephalopathy may develop after methotrexate.

Casey EG, Jellife AM, Le Quesne M, Millett YC. Vincristine neuropathy: clinical and electrophysiological observation. Brain 1973;96:69.

Sensorimotor neuropathy is expected after plant alkaloid therapy.

Hadley WG, Lassman LP, Pearce GW. Neuropathy of vincristine in man. J Neurol Sci 1970;10:107.

Mainly sensory and not readily reversible.

Marks JE, Baglan RJ, Prassad SC, Blank WF. Cerebral radionecrosis: incidence and risk in relation to dose time fractionation and volume. Int J Radiat Oncol Biol Phys 1981;7:243.

Attempt to delineate the factors responsible for delayed radiation-induced necrosis.

Roelofs RI, Hrushesky W, Rogin J, Rosenberg L. Peripheral sensory neuropathy and cisplatin chemotherapy. Neurology 1984;34:934.

Early and severe sensory neuropathy in 92 percent of patients.

59

Hydrocephalus

J. P. Mohr and J. C. Gautier

Hydrocephalus (from the Greek for water in the head) can be defined as an abnormal increase in the amount of cerebrospinal fluid (CSF) within the skull. It is the accumulation of CSF beyond the limits of its absorption or brain compliance to the extra pressure created by its increased presence that leads to the clinical syndromes.

CEREBROSPINAL FLUID PATHWAYS

CSF is produced by the choroid plexi (known to Galen and so named because their appearance seemed similar to the richly vascular membranes covering the fetus at birth), which cling like a grape vine to the walls of the lateral ventricles of the cerebral hemispheres and to the roof of the fourth ventricle just in front of the cerebellum. (The ventricles were so named because they resembled the stomach or belly; Latin: *venter.*)

Daily CSF production, some 150 ml, is pumped out of the cerebral ventricles and washes through the interhemispheric foramina adjacent to the septum. The foramina are named after Alexander Monro (Scottish anatomist, 1733–1817), who described them in 1797. From there, the CSF gains the third ventricle and thence passes through the aqueduct of Sylvius (Dutch or French anatomist, F. Sylvius, 1614–1672) down through the fourth ventricle, where it is joined by that produced by the choroid plexus in the fourth ventricle. The combined output reaches the subarachnoid space by way of the lateral exits adjacent to the pons, the foramen of Luscka (H. von Luscka, German anatomist, 1820–1875), and in the midline, through the caudally placed foramen of Magendie (F. Magendie, French physiologist, 1783–1855) at the base of the cerebellum. From these outflow sites, the CSF bathes the lower brainstem, pooling in the large space at the base of the brain near the foramen magnum known as the cisterna magna (from the Latin for reservoir of large size).

Some of the CSF migrates downward to the spinal canal, but most of it is carried upward over the brainstem and cerebellum. The ventral flow passes through the prepontine cistern and the posterior through the cerebellar cisterns, upward through the narrow spaces constrained by the tentorium cerebelli, which force the CSF around the midbrain in patterns of flow that seem almost unpredictable through the space known as the cistern ambiens (from the Latin for reservoir going around [the midbrain]). Much of it passes through the cleft in front of the midbrain known as the incisura (from the Latin for a cut into), finally gaining the supratentorial compartment.

From this level, the CSF passes laterally through the sylvian fissure, medially and anteriorly through the interhemispheric fissure, posteriorly behind the callosum and over the convexities, following the major sulci (see Fig. 9-1). For generations, it was accepted that CSF passed over the cerebral hemispheres and was reabsorbed entirely through the superior and lateral sinuses by specialized filters rather like the renal glomeruli, the pacchionian granules (A. Pacchioni, Italian anatomist, 1665–1726). More recent evidence indicates that much of the CSF is absorbed through the Virchow-Robin spaces as it passes up over the hemispheres.

PATHOPHYSIOLOGY

As the CSF volume increases in those brain cavities affected by the site of the block, pressure slowly increases in the system as the brain's compliance is gradually consumed and finally exceeded. In conditions of sudden and severe obstruction, CSF is forced through the single cell layer of the ventricular wall and causes an increase in extracellular space in the brain regions close to the ventricles.

Some degree of accumulation of CSF occurs over

the years as the ventricular size slowly increases with age. The compliance of the brain to the effects of compression by increased ventricular volume also declines over the years, and elderly brain cavities do not revert as rapidly or completely after removal of a given volume of CSF as they do in younger individuals.

Diseases That Cause Obstruction

This complex path of CSF is subject to a variety of disorders, both congenital and acquired, which result in some degree of obstruction of this flow. If the obstruction is severe enough, the continued production of fluid eventually inflates the brain walls, which attempt to contain the growing fluid volume and uses up the available compliance of the adjacent brain tissue, and symptoms result from a combination of compression and ischemia of the affected tissues. Relief of the obstruction before permanent injury may occur results in reversal of the symptoms.

Tumors

The most easily understood causes of obstruction along the CSF pathways are tumors that arise near one of the many smaller channels. The lateral ventricles of the cerebrum are so large that no tumors arising from the brain can block them completely, but tumors arising from the choroid plexus may rarely do so. However, tumors near the foramen of Monro may obstruct one or both foramina, causing accumulation of CSF and secondary enlargement of one or both cerebral ventricles. Most are malignant growths arising from the adjacent septum pellucidum (Latin for transparent partition), but rarely, a colloid cyst arising from adjacent structures may grow large enough to block the foramina. It has long been said that the colloid cyst, when on a stalk or pedicle, can swing about in the third ventricle, transiently blocking one or both foramina of Monro, causing sudden and severe hydrocephalus with headache and even loss of consciousness. However colorful and memorable the description, neither of the authors has actually seen or heard of such a case, and real examples have been hard to find in the literature.

Tumors growing in the walls of the third ventricle usually cause far more symptoms from involvement of the brain than they do from distortion of the ventricle, but those arising from the pineal body and posterior midbrain can block the aqueduct of Sylvius early enough to balloon the third and lateral ventricles and make hydrocephalus a major part of the clinical picture. Tumors arising from the floor of the fourth ventricle or from the meninges near the foramina of Luschka or Magendie and even large tumors arising from cranial nerves near these outlets may obstruct the fourth ventricle, causing hydrocephalus that also affects the aqueduct and third and lateral ventricles. All such diseases that block CSF outflow are known as obstructive hydrocephalus. Found more often in children but also in a few young adults, the Arnold-Chiari malformation may play a role in obstructing the outflow at the base of the cerebellum because of downward traction on the brainstem and cerebellum through the foramen magnum, reducing the volume of the cistern.

Meningeal Diseases

Diseases of the subarachnoid space, especially meningitis, subarachnoid hemorrhage, and even extensive subarachnoid involvement by parasitic cysts, may so thoroughly clog the CSF pathways at the base of the brain as to trap CSF in the fourth ventricle, causing the same retrograde obstruction. However, because the CSF pathways are intact up to the subarachnoid space, such forms of hydrocephalus are known as *communicating hydrocephalus*. When severe, subarachnoid hemorrhage in the supratentorial cisterns can clot CSF pathways below. Occlusion of the large venous sinuses would be expected to impair CSF reabsorption through the pacchionian granules, but this usually causes so much brain injury from infarction that the role of hydrocephalus is not a prominent part of the clinical picture.

Other Causes

Less easily understood is the process of aging or loss of competence of the pacchionian granules, resulting in gradual accumulation of CSF in the subarachnoid space. Their causes are difficult to prove; they have not been as readily accepted as have those from the more obvious causes.

Clinical Features

At first, brain compliance allows the enlargement of the ventricles and the compression of the brain parenchyma without causing symptoms. With time and when the rate of ventricular enlargement is rapid, symptoms develop, the most well-recognized and distinctive of the symptoms being imbalance, incontinence, and mental changes. For those already bedridden from an acute illness, signs of imbalance are not sought, and catheterization often prevents the detection of incontinence. Therefore, mental changes are the most obvious. For those initially ambulatory, imbalance and incontinence have a chance to be noticed more readily.

Imbalance

The imbalance begins as an unsteady gait with faulty foot placement and frequent falls. The broad-based gait typical of peripheral neuropathy or cerebellar disease is not prominent. Instead, the leg position usually remains in the narrow width typical of normal people, but the stride shortens, the steps become halting, and often the placement of the foot is inaccurate enough that the weight is not easily borne. Unexplained falls occur, sometime backward. Because such gaits are commonly seen among elderly people, it has long been assumed that such deficiencies are part of growing old, but no obvious features separate the gait of the old from those with active hydrocephalus. In addition, the ventricular system is usually enlarged in elderly people with gait problems. In the extremes of hydrocephalus, the length of the step can be so short that the patient seems to make almost no forward progress while the number of steps involved in turning around increases well beyond the usual three to four quick foot position movements. The authors have experience with one patient who required 27 separate progressive changes in positions of the feet before successfully turning fully around. The uncertainty of foot placement and the imprecise sequencing of steps creates the impression of a loss of planning, an apraxia, rather than mere incoordination or ataxia (see also Ch. 22).

Incontinence

A common associated complaint is incontinence, usually only urinary but, occasionally, fecal. The events occur as a surprise, are embarrassing and distressing, and more often prompt a visit to the physician than does the imbalance. Analysis of urodynamic functions shows hyperactivity of bladder contraction, which may revert to normal after reduction of the elevated CSF pressure. Levels of vasoactive intestinal peptide, polypeptide YY, somatostatin, and δ-sleep-inducing peptide are all low in hydrocephalus and improve after successful therapy.

Mental Changes

When the hydrocephalus is severe or prolonged, mental changes occur, which feature a slowing in the rate of responsiveness. Patients often show a decline in sustained motor and verbal activity. Conversation is often not initiated, and when forced by an observer, the response tends to be brief, a condition known as dynamic aphasia, referred to by some as transcortical motor aphasia. Compared with normal people, the patient's head and eyes are abnormally directed toward movements from irrelevant environmental stimuli, a condition termed easy distractibility. Interruptions in speech and other motor behaviors occur often, and the patient may remain passively immobile and expressionless for seconds to minutes. Despite the delays in responsiveness, the utterances show no signs of impaired memory or disordered selection of words

or use of grammar, but the slow rate of responding and interruptions may cause low scores on timed tests of higher cerebral function, making it difficult to separate the low scores from those caused by an actual dementia. When the disorders are far advanced, the level of activity may be so low that the patient is akinetic and mute.

Clinicoanatomic Correlations

Considering the issue of the mechanism by which hydrocephalus produces its distinctive symptoms, it is a disappointment more is not known of the precise correlation between the regions affected by hydrocephalus and the symptoms produced. When confined to one lateral ventricle (unilateral hydrocephalus) from obstruction of one of the foramina of Monro, the usual complaint is headache without imbalance, incontinence, or mental changes. One example of diverticulum of the aqueduct, producing impaired upward gaze during periods of hydrocephalus, suggests the symptoms may be explained by stretching effects on the relevant pathways. The impression has been used to explain the gait disturbance from stretching of motor fibers, mainly affecting movements of the leg, passing adjacent to the ventricular walls, yet the most striking examples of imbalance have been reported in hydrocephalus especially involving the fourth ventricle, suggesting pressure against the cerebellum is important. Incontinence has been postulated from stretch effect on the walls of the hypothalamus, but there is little certainty on this point. For the mental changes, stretching of the walls of the frontal ventricles might suffice, but similar stretch in the posterior horns does not seem to produce visual symptoms. Therefore, the explanation might be found in the reduced cerebral blood flow described from high intracranial pressure (see below).

Laboratory Studies

In the days before adequate brain imaging, high intracranial pressure was inferred from findings of elevated lumbar CSF pressure, with values over 180 to 200 mmH$_2$O, and was attributed to brain mass or hydrocephalus. The diagnosis of brain mass or clogging of the CSF pathways as a cause of hydrocephalus has never been the major issue in explaining hydrocephalus. The real problem has always been separating the clinically important hydrocephalus from that secondary to brain atrophy, so-called hydrocephalus ex vacuo (from the Latin for hydrocephalus due to emptiness, i.e., absence of brain tissue) and predicting the beneficial effects of CSF drainage as treatment for hydrocephalus with no obvious cause.

In some instances, clinically important hydrocephalus was discovered to exist in patients whose CSF pressures on lumbar puncture were slightly above the upper range of normal values. Reference was made to the pascalian principle of the hydraulic press in explaining increased force applied to brain walls by the large ventricular volume in patients whose pressure was only slightly elevated above normal. Functionally important hydrocephalus in patients with slightly elevated pressure came to be known as "normal-pressure hydrocephalus," a term quickly popularized by its acronym, NPH.

When radioisotopes were invented, they were quickly put to use to estimate the extent of stagnant flow in a test known as radionuclide cisternography. In normal people, after instillation of a small volume of radioisotope in the lumbar space, the tracer quickly accumulates over the superior sagittal sinus, proof the CSF was being reabsorbed. In clinically important hydrocephalus, the flow was stalled, little of it accumulated along the sinus, and some of it could even be seen diffusing retrograde up the fourth ventricle and aqueduct by 48 hours, even gaining the lateral ventricles in the cerebral hemispheres. Most of patients with such a stagnant CSF system improved after shunting, but some did not, causing restless interest in more definitive testing.

After the development of computed tomography made brain imaging popular, measurements of the CSF pressure became less popular and were replaced by estimates of ventricular volume, as measured at several points along the CSF pathways. After it was discovered that the mere presence of hydrocephalus did not predict the response to CSF drainage, further

studies indicated the best predictors were enlargement of the third ventricle and the temporal horns. The advent of magnetic resonance imaging (MRI) added another dimension (Fig. 59-1). Not only an accurate picture of the hydrocephalus was obtained, but also the involvement of the adjacent brain structures and the movement of CSF through the ventricular pathways was observed. The movement of CSF through the aqueduct is usually rapid enough to create a flow void on MRI scanning, and in hydrocephalus, this flow rate is reduced. Hydrocephalus, when prolonged or severe enough, also causes the transudation of CSF through the monocellular cuboidal endothelium of the ependyma lining the ventricular walls, causing signals that reflect the accumulated CSF in the adjacent brain. These findings have had little predictive value for the effects of shunting.

It has long been assumed that structural brain injury from severe or sustained hydrocephalus explains the failure of shunt therapy in some cases. This assumption has led to the development of tests to show impaired brain metabolism or reduced bloods flow in the parenchyma affected by hydrocephalus. Low flows have been seen in the basal parts of the brain, although clinical improvement has not reliably been correlated with improved flows after shunting. Given the rapid development of such testing, it should not be long before a reliable predictor to the effects of shunting will be found. Such studies may eventually shed light on the mechanism of the distinctive symptoms.

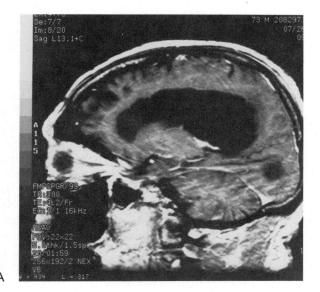 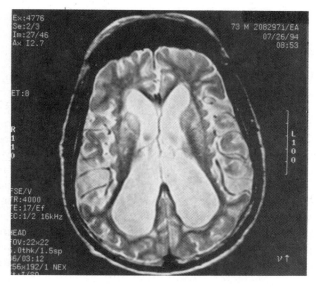

A   B

Figure 59-1. (A) T_1-weighted sagittal MRI scan showing great dilation of the lateral ventricles. (B) T_2-weighted axial scan showing widely dilated lateral ventricles.

Therapy

As suggested above, the issue is not so much arriving at a diagnosis as predicting the response to shunt therapy. In many cases in which hydrocephalus is due to temporarily clogged CSF pathways, the hydrocephalus fades on its own. When it does not, simple CSF drainage by repeated lumbar puncture can often relieve symptoms, at least temporarily. If the relief of symptoms occurs from lumbar puncture, followed by relapse, shunting can be done in hopes of permanent relief. Although a simple procedure, it is not entirely harmless. Done in elderly patients with reduced brain compliance, complications occur in up to 20 percent of cases. The big danger, usually not experienced, is lobar hemorrhage in the brain route chosen for shunt placement. If the pressure-sensitive valve in the shunt tubing has too low a pressure, the CSF can drain off too efficiently with collapse of the brain, which is also uncommon. More often, annoying and sometimes serious complications arise from sepsis in the shunt tubing, blockage in the tubing, obstruction of the superior vena cava, pulmonary emboli, bowel perforation, and even renal failure. Given that the shunt may not reverse a syndrome easily diagnosed as Alzheimer's disease in an elderly person, it is no wonder few physicians rush to put in a shunt until the diagnosis of functional hydrocephalus is clearer.

Medical therapy has received little attention, but it has long been known that the use of acetazolamide reduces CSF production by the choroid plexi. It has been assumed that such effects would prove transient, as are the effects of acetazolamide on renal acid-base balance, but recent work, using doses of 250 to 500 mg daily, has produced sustained improvements in gait and bladder disturbances for as long as 1 year.

ANNOTATED BIBLIOGRAPHY

Adams RD, Fisher CM, Hakim S et al. Symptomatic occult hydrocephalus with "normal" cerebrospinal fluid pressure (a treatable syndrome). N Engl J Med 1965;273: 117.

The article that prompted modern interest in the syndrome.

Ahlberg J, Norlen L, Blomstrand C, Wikkelso C. Outcome of shunt operation on urinary incontinence in normal pressure hydrocephalus predicted by lumbar puncture. J Neurol Neurosurg Psychiatry 1988;51:105–8.

Bladder hyperactivity may be reduced by shunting.

Aimard G, Vighetto A, Gabet JY et al. Acetazolamide: une alternative à la dérivation dans l'hydrocéphalie à pression normale? Resultats préliminaires. Rev Neurol (Paris) 1990;146:437–9.

Reversed many symptoms in 10 of 15 patients for as long as 1 year.

Bradley WG Jr, Whittemore AR, Kortman KE et al. Marked CSF void: indicator of successful shunt in patients with suspected normal-pressure hydrocephalus. Radiology 1991;178:459–66.

Pulsation void at the aqueduct correlates with shunt outcome.

Fisher CM. The clinical picture in occult hydrocephalus. Clin Neurosurg 1977;24:170.

The fine details of the clinical states, sequence of onset, and severity of deficit in personally studied cases.

Hasan D, van Peski J, Loeve I et al. Single photon emission computed tomography in patients with acute hydrocephalus or with cerebral ischaemia after subarachnoid haemorrhage. J Neurol Neurosurg Psychiatry 1991;54:490–3.

Correlations between low regional cerebral blood flow in basal brain regions and hydrocephalus.

Kaye JA, Grady CL, Haxby JV. Reversibility of metabolic and cognitive deficits in normal pressure hydrocephalus following shunt surgery. Ann Neurol 1987;22:124.

Detailed computed tomographic and positron emission tomographic study.

Larsson A, Wikkelso C, Bilting M, Stephensen H. Clinical parameters in 74 consecutive patients shunt operated for normal pressure hydrocephalus. Acta Neurol Scand 1991;84:475–82.

Large series (74 patients) detailing lack of good predictors from clinical and radiologic factors and the frequency and type of complications.

Mampalam TJ, Harsh GR 4th, Tien RD et al. Unilateral hydrocephalus in adults. Surg Neurol 1991;35:14–9.

Headache the most common symptom in 14 patients, 7 caused by tumor; others included venous angioma, ependymal cyst, and postinflammatory gliosis but was idiopathic in four patients.

Vannests JAL. Three decades of normal pressure hydrocephalus: are we wiser now? J Neurol Neurosurg Psychiatry 1994;57:1021–5.

Diagnosis no longer an issue; management still is.

60
Alzheimer's Disease

J. P. Mohr and J. C. Gautier

Dementia should be added to heart disease, cancer, and stroke as one of the great dreads of those facing advancing age. A variety of toxins, viruses, traumatic injuries, strokes, endocrine and metabolic disorders, systemic and intracranial infections or tumors, subdural hematomas, and depression can cause impairment of higher cerebral function, but it is the more common condition, known as Alzheimer's disease, that has so much of the population worried. This condition, long thought to be attributable to widespread atrophy of the brain, is yielding somewhat to intense study. Although atrophy is common, no substantative correlation has been found between Alzheimer's disease and the extent of atrophy. Furthermore, although it has been popular to claim that no causes have been found, epidemiologic studies have shown at least more than a chance association with head injuries, an avoidable environmental risk factor, and some forms of the disease have a genetic substrate. Despite these advances, no definitive therapy has yet been developed. The condition affects higher cerebral function far more than the main sensorimotor systems and does its damage over a period of years. Those around victims must adjust to their ever-declining skills and bear heavy custodial demands into the predictable future.

Alzheimer's disease is the common baseline condition against which the many less common forms of atrophies and dementia are compared. They are dealt with in the following chapters.

EPIDEMIOLOGY

There is no doubt as to the worldwide importance of dementia in elderly people, females more so than males, whether labeled Alzheimer's disease or senile dementia of the Alzheimer type. In former times, an arbitrary separation was made between those patients whose dementia began after age 65 (senile) versus those younger than that age (presenile), a separation point no longer recognized. In America, Alzheimer's disease is estimated to affect 1.2 to 5.0 percent of the population older than 65, rising steeply with each decade. Similar rates from 2.5 percent in Canada to 4.61 percent in Shanghai indicate a worldwide distribution of this disease. Some 750,000 to 1 million in America are estimated to be in the advanced stage of the disease. In the European Community, these figures mean some 1.5 to 2.5 million people are afflicted, and they account for some 200,000 to 250,000 new hospitalizations annually. With advancing age, the incidence rises dramatically, approaching 20 to 30 percent in those older than age 80. Those diagnosed with the condition have a life expectancy reduced by about one-half of that of the nonaffected people of similar age.

Its high prevalence in elderly people has attracted theses that it represents the accumulation of years of some sort of exposure. Yet case-control studies, comparing affected individuals with normal people who share the same known risk factors save the one under investigation, have been unable to find a clear connection for many of the proposed toxins. Highest on the list has been aluminum, a common contaminant in drinking water. Although the aluminum content in the brain of cases with Alzheimer's disease is not known to be elevated compared with that of controls, the amount of aluminum is elevated in the neurofibrillary tangles, a histologic correlate of Alzheimer's disease. However, no correlations have been found between memory deficiency in elderly people and aluminum levels in drinking water. This polyvalent ion attracted attention because acute aluminum intoxication produced a syndrome of dementia in the early days of hemodialysis for renal disease and because zinc, another polyvalent ion, is heavily concentrated in the limbic system, which is a preferential site for this disease.

Another popular idea was that mild dementia after major head injury could mean that Alzheimer's disease follows minor head injury. The evidence here is conflicting. In an extensive review of Olmstead County, Minnesota by Mayo Clinic researchers, no evidence was found for a role of trauma in Alzheimer's disease. The standardized morbidity ratio was a mere 1.06 compared with controls. However, in studies from the United Kingdom, there has been a correlation between head injuries and earlier onset of Alzheimer's disease and a correlation between the histologic appearance of the brains from patients with Alzheimer's disease and from those with dementia pugilistica (see Ch. 61).

Although there is a gross similarity in the appearance and microscopic changes in brains with Alzheimer's disease and those of normal elderly individuals, which has suggested that the process may be the normal aging process somehow deranged or exaggerated, the detailed findings in Alzheimer's disease are rather distinctive to the disease. The heavy involvement of the parietal, temporal, and frontal lobe association systems, compared with the sparing of the major motor and sensory pathways, raised speculations that the disease falls on the phylogenetically newer portions of the brain, regions perhaps more susceptible than the older regions to toxic effects. A popular speculation is that the increased concentration of oxidative proteins in the brains of older animals suggests there is some accumulated effect of damage by free radicals, which could be prevented by treatment with free-radical scavengers. A more persistent idea has been the overproduction or some defect in the proper disposal of the end products of cellular metabolism, itself perhaps deranged because of a basic disease in one or more regions of the brain. Epidemiologic models of the distribution of incubation periods for this disease support some prenatal factor. Although familial cases are rare, enough evidence has accumulated to prognosticate a risk for the disorder that is 7 to 8 percent for those whose parent or sibling is affected compared with 2 to 3 percent for the population older than 65.

The occurrence of similar lesions in those with Down syndrome has added impetus to the genetic explanation. The problem is not the age of the parents. Although Down syndrome is more common among births from older mothers, no such relationship has been found for Alzheimer's disease among the offspring. Instead, attention has focused on attempts to relate disorders at specific gene locations to the neuropathologic findings, here with some success, but the significance of the discoveries is still unknown. Recent evidence also suggests the association between chro-mosome 19 and late-onset Alzheimer's disease may be related to the apolipoprotein E type 4 allele(s), with those homozygotic for this allele having a high enough frequency by age 80 for the association to be considered causal.

Progress on the discovery of a cause remains slow, in part for lack of an animal model. As recently as 1992, announcement of the long-awaited model had to be retracted for insufficient evidence.

PATHOLOGY

Gross and Microscopic Anatomy

In 1907, Alzheimer described the index case of the condition that was to bear his name, that is, a 51-year-old woman whose clinical course ran 5 years, beginning with impaired memory, delusions, and hallucinations and, finally, ending in a severe dementia. Severe atrophy and the histologic features that came to be associated with his name were the main findings. Alzheimer's report was prompted by his impression that the patient was rather young for this clinical picture of dementia with atrophy, which theretofore had been thought of as senility.

The brain in patients with Alzheimer's disease shows atrophy, usually symmetric, which is most prominent in the parietal and temporal lobes, especially affecting the hippocampus. This distribution of atrophy accounts for the disturbances in higher cerebral function and loss of memory that are the main clinical features of the condition. The density of large neurons was long thought to decline throughout the cortex with age, but recent evidence argues such losses are hard to quantify. If so, Alzheimer's disease stands as a disease, not simply an intensification of the aging process.

In some neurons in elderly people, a distinctive silver-staining histologic formation, known as the neurofibrillary tangle, is found. In the neuropil, silver-staining, so-called senile, plaques are encountered. In the center of the plaques, there is β/A4 protein, which is a 4-kD peptide derived from an amyloid precursor protein. The plaques are often encountered in the brains of elderly people, more often in females, yet the frequency of such findings is low (roughly 30 percent). In those with Alzheimer's disease, the frequency is more than 60 percent.

Another common finding is amyloid deposits around and in the walls of arteries (congophilic angiopathy), which has also been taken as an almost-constant feature of the disease (see below under Basic Biology).

Basic Biology

Detailed chemical analysis of neurofibrillary tangles has shown them to be paired helical filaments that contain mainly τ protein, ubiquitin, and other neuro-

Large amounts found in primates, related to age, and seemingly produced by neurons.

McKhann G, Drachman D, Folstein M et al. Clinical diagnosis of Alzheimer's disease. Neurology 1984;34:939.

Broad overview of criteria for diagnosis.

Murphy M. The molecular pathogenesis of Alzheimer's disease: clinical prospects. Lancet 1992;340:1512–4.

Brief but updated overview.

Parent M, Delacourte A, Defossez A et al. Maladie d'Alzheimer: étude de la distribution des proteines tau constitutives des paires de filaments en hélice dans le tissu nerveux central humain. C R Acad Sci III 1988;306: 391–7.

Tau proteins are present in cortical gray matter but not easy to find in the white matter.

Peterson C, Ratan RR, Shelanski ML, Goldman JE. Cytosolic free calcium and cell spreading decrease in fibroblasts from aged and Alzheimer donors. Proc Natl Acad Sci U S A 1986;83:7999–8001.

Evidence that Alzheimer's disease is systemic.

Rapaport SI. Brain evolution and Alzheimer's disease. Rev Neurol (Paris) 1988;144:79.

Detailed thesis arguing that rapid evolution of the human brain, especially in the association areas, basal nucleus of Meynert, amygdala, and hippocampus, have made these regions susceptible to Alzheimer's disease effects through disease-specific genomic character function.

Rocca WA, Amaducci LA, Schoenberg BS. Epidemiology of clinically diagnosed Alzheimer's disease. Ann Neurol 1986;19:415.

Prevalence of 1.9 to 5.6 cases per 100,000 age 65 and older and incidence of 2.4 per 100,000.

Schaumburg HH, Suzuki K. Non-specific familial presenile dementia. J Neurol Neurosurg Psychiatry 1968;31: 479–86.

Familial dementia with cortical cell loss but no histologically specific findings.

Sevush S, Guterman A, Villalon AV. Improved verbal learning after outpatient oral physostigmine therapy in patients with dementia of the Alzheimer type. J Clin Psychiatry 1991;52:300–3.

Some signs that physostigmine can improve scores.

St. George-Hyslop PH, Tanzi RE, Polinsky RJ et al. Absence of duplication of chromosome 31 genes in familial and sporadic Alzheimer's disease. Science 1987;238:664.

No evidence to support the hypothesis that Alzheimer's disease has overexpression or duplication of one or more genes. This thesis was initially put forward based on Alzheimer-like neuropathologic changes in the brains of some cases of Down syndrome and gene mapping of familial Alzheimer's disease and amyloid B protein to this autosome. No evidence yet that specific gene defects are the cause of Alzheimer's disease.

Steiner B, Mandelkow EM, Biernat J et al. Phosphorylation of microtubule associated protein tau: identification of the site for $Ca^{2(+)}$ calmodulin dependent kinase and relationship with tau phosphorylation in Alzheimer tangles. EMBO J 1990;9:3539–44.

Phosphorylation of τ at serine 405 in the C-terminal tail of the protein changes its properties.

Tamminga CA, Foster NL, Fedio P et al. Alzheimer's disease: low cerebral somatostatin levels correlate with impaired cognitive function and cortical metabolism. Neurology 1987;37:161–5.

Somatostatin-like immunoreactivity found low in cases of Alzheimer's disease compared with age-matched controls.

Teri L, Borson S, Kiyak HA, Yamagishi M. Behavioral disturbance, cognitive dysfunction, and functional skill. Prevalence and relationship in Alzheimer's disease. J Am Geriatr Soc 1989;37:109–16.

The caregivers report frequent problems.

Waltregny A, Maula AA, Brucher JM. Contribution of stereotactic brain biopsies to the diagnosis of presenile dementia. Stereotact Funct Neurosurg 1990;54:409–12.

Many clinical examples of Alzheimer's disease have another condition on biopsy.

Wetterling T. Alzheimersche Krankheit. Uberblick uber den aktuellen Stand der Forschung. Fortschr Neurol Psychiatr 1989;57:1–13.

Thorough review.

Williams DB, Annegers JF, Kokmen E et al. Brain injury and neurologic sequelae: a cohort study of dementia, parkinsonism, and amyotrophic lateral sclerosis. Neurology 1991;41:1554–7.

No evidence for head trauma as a cause of Alzheimer's disease.

Wurtman RJ, Corkin S, Growdon JH, Ritter-Walker E (eds). Alzheimer's Disease. Advances in Neurology. Vol. 51. Raven Press, New York; 1990.

Useful general reviews.

61

Other Degenerative Diseases Featuring Dementia

J. P. Mohr and J. C. Gautier

In the heyday of light microscopy, several diseases were described with dementia as a prominent feature, each separated from the other or from Alzheimer's disease by a seemingly unique or at least distinctive location of the disease process or histologic features. In the years since their initial description, detailed studies of the genetics and cellular biology of many of these conditions have blurred these once-clear distinctions by adding other layers of information, with some confirming the differences but others showing similarities. Adherence to tradition prompts a continued attempt to distinguish some of these disorders from one another, but further research advances may threaten their existence as entities in the years ahead. The conditions are listed in rough order of their frequency. All are rare.

PICK'S LOBAR SCLEROSIS

In 1892, Arnold Pick (Czech neurologist, 1851–1924), described a 71-year-old man with a progressive decline in mental function that featured antisocial behavior, memory loss, and aphasia. Severe atrophy of the temporal lobes was found. Pick was impressed by the focal atrophy, a finding that was contrary to the view then popular that atrophies were diffuse and symmetric.

The number of reported cases remains small. Some estimates have been made that Alzheimer's disease occurs more than 10 times more frequently than does Pick's disease, even though the two share the same age range of occurrence. Women are more often affected, and up to 20 percent of cases have been familial, with autosomal dominant inheritance.

By macroscopic and light microscopic criteria, this condition is different from Alzheimer's disease. Alzheimer's disease is usually bilateral and roughly symmetric, most often affecting the parietal region and remaining confined to the cortical gray matter. Pick's disease may also be bilateral, but in roughly one-half of the cases, the atrophy is predominantly asymmetric (usually affecting the left side). It affects the temporal and frontal lobes more than the parietal and seems to affect the white matter almost as much as the gray matter. Characteristically, the posterior two-thirds of the first temporal gyrus are spared. When severe, the atrophy is more striking than that of Alzheimer's disease, with the affected parts shrunken to a small portion of their normal size, producing a knife-edged appearance of the gyri, which is easily visible on computed tomography or magnetic resonance imaging.

The microscopic findings show few of the neurofibrillary tangles and plaques that are typical of Alzheimer's disease. Pick's disease falls heavily on the upper layers of cortical neurons. Many neurons have a swollen (ballooned) appearance with silver-staining inclusions in the cytoplasm (Pick bodies), a combined change known as the Pick globose cell. In some cases of lobar atrophy, these histologic changes are not present, a point that has left the diagnosis of such cases unclear.

Pick's and Alzheimer's diseases have been shown to have a number of additional differences. Studies of the content of the intracellular inclusions in the former have found them to be composed of straight fibrils, not the coiled pairs found in Alzheimer's disease. The distribution of monoamine oxidase activity also differs between the two diseases. In other findings, some similarities have been uncovered. The regulatory protein ubiquitin has been found in both the neurofibrillary tangles of Alzheimer's disease and in the Pick bodies; high ratios of chromogranin A to synaptin/synaptophysin have been found in both diseases. The importance of these similarities is unknown. To add to the difficulties, one case report of a 75-year-old demented woman demonstrated Pick bodies in a setting of pathologic findings otherwise consistent with striatonigral degeneration and olivopontocerebellar atrophy, all in the same patient.

The clinical diagnosis of Pick's disease is difficult. Patients with lobar atrophy usually show apathy, abulia, reduction of speech, bulimia, and bouts of irrational behavior. In contrast with the behavior in Alzheimer's disease, those with Pick's disease usually do not show an early disorder of memory or disorientation in time and space. Aphasia may be a prominent feature, typically with relative sparing of repeating aloud, a syndrome complex also seen in Alzheimer's disease. Those with anterior temporal lobe atrophy may show severe behavior derangements, such as the Klüver-Bucy syndrome (featuring hypersexuality, loss of normal fear, and tendency to swallow all objects at hand) early in the course, whereas such changes are rather rare in Alzheimer's disease. Psychiatric disorders can include paranoia, delusions, and obsessive-compulsive behavior, which are seen less often in Alzheimer's disease. When testable in the early stages, memory function has often been far superior to language function, a point in favor of the diagnosis on clinical grounds. The course of the disease may be a few years, but it may last well beyond a dozen. As in Alzheimer's disease, weakness, sensory loss, and blindness are not an expected feature of the disease.

No treatment has been discovered.

CREUTZFELDT-JAKOB DISEASE

See Chapter 50.

NEURONAL ACHROMASIA (CORTICOBASAL DEGENERATION)

This rare entity, first described by Rebeiz, Kolodny, and Richardson in 1968 as corticodentatonigral degeneration with neuronal achromasia, has been described in few patients but is distinctive enough that it has earned its own place in clinical neuropathology. Insufficient numbers of cases have been reported to guess at their epidemiology and frequency of occurrence.

The gross pathologic findings in the small number of cases have expanded the findings of the original material. Focal, sometimes unilateral, rarely general, cortical atrophy has been described. The appearance to the naked eye does not distinguish it from Alzheimer's disease. Microscopy shows many neurons that do not take conventional stains (achromasia) and are usually swollen. Neurofibrillary tangles, senile plaques, Pick bodies, and other histologic signs of other dementing disease are often absent. In some of the cases, the degeneration has been cortical only and, in some, corticonigral. When combined degeneration has been encountered, neurofibrillary tangles and even lobar white matter gliosis have been described in some cases with neuronal achromasia, arguing by microscopic criteria that Alzheimer's and Pick's diseases may coexist with achromasia, making it difficult to claim neuronal achromasia as a unique entity. However, the immunochemical characteristics of the phosphorylated epitopes of the neurofilaments have not been those forms unique to Alzheimer's or Pick's disease. Instead, the ballooned neurons resemble those caused by neurotoxins, which interfere with axonal transport. As yet, no specific toxin has been identified.

The variety of areas affected has made it difficult to create a reliable clinical picture. For the few instances of predominantly right hemispheral atrophy, a prominent left-sided dyspraxia with alien hand sign (see Ch. 25, Frontal Lobe) has been the striking feature and has been used by some clinicians to suggest the diagnosis in life. In others, features of aphasia have suggested the lobar atrophy of Pick's disease, while in others, the dementia has had all of the features of Alzheimer's disease. The evolution of this disease over several years puts it in the same time frame with Alzheimer's and Pick's diseases.

No treatment is known.

DEMENTIA PUGILISTICA

This Latinized title for disturbance in higher cerebral function after repeated boxing matches (see also Ch. 6) has been the strongest link between brain injuries and Alzheimer's disease. Large numbers of neurofibrillary tangles are common in the brains of boxers but are usually not accompanied by the neuritic plaques also typically found in Alzheimer's disease. The once-distinctive absence of plaques, however, has been found to be something of an artifact because immunocytochemical methods have found evidence of the same β-amyloid protein regions comparable to that found in Alzheimer's disease, even though typical silver-staining plaques are infrequently seen. The neurofibrillary tangles react to the same antigens as do those found in Alzheimer's disease. It has bee argued that the Alzheimer's disease-type changes are set in motion by the neuronal injuries in boxing and that such injuries could be one of the precipitating factors in Alzheimer's disease. Striking amounts of β-A4 amyloid have been found in the cortex of patients dying within days of severe head injury, indicating the head injury itself may quickly generate such changes.

The disorder is most often found in boxers who have borne up under many heavy punches, some of them famous fighters said to be able to take "heavy punishment" and many second-rate boxers who have been knocked out often in their careers.

Psychiatric symptoms are common in the early stages; a flattened affect occurs more often than emotional lability. Within 2 or 3 years, extrapyramidal symptoms mimicking parkinsonism appear, related to neuronal loss in the substantia nigra. A more global dementia soon follows. Fighters who continue in the ring when the syndrome appears are more susceptible to serious injuries, which include shearing of the midbrain and injuries to the cervical spine.

ATROPHIES WITH DEMONSTRATED CAUSE

These conditions were classified among the atrophies for generations until modern investigations uncovered their cause. They are described in other chapters in detail and are here named only for attempts at completeness to link this book with those that have gone before. These entities include Creutzfeldt-Jakob disease, Gerstmann-Sträussler disease, and Hallervorden-Spatz disease.

OTHER AND SUBCORTICAL ATROPHIES

These conditions have an uncertain nosology. They received attention as part of a classification scheme that tried to sort atrophies into functional systems or anatomic areas in the days before much work had been done on the molecular biology. In many instances, the clinical syndromes were proved at autopsy to be explained by clinically unsuspected focal infarction, hemorrhage, and even indolent neoplasms, findings that blurred the attempts to develop distinctive syndromes for atrophy alone. In some instances, atrophy alone was the main finding. In the classification that follows, Huntington's disease, which features atrophy of the striatum, mainly the caudate, and Parkinson's disease, which features atrophies of the substantia nigra and related projection systems, are only briefly described. Their main presentations are found in chapters devoted to the main clinical manifestations as movement disorders (see Chs. 22 and 75 to 77).

Non-Pick Lobar Atrophy

Known as progressive aphasia without dementia, these unusual cases have been followed in life as the aphasia slowly intensified, and at autopsy none of the features distinctive for Alzheimer's, Pick's, or other diseases were found. In one case, spongiform changes were seen but without other features sufficient to diagnose Creutzfeldt-Jakob disease. Some of the clinical features have made it impossible to separate them from Pick's disease. Isolated progressive apraxias are commonly seen (see Subcortical Gliosis below).

Subcortical Gliosis

Formerly known as type II Pick's disease, this condition is now thought to be a separate disorder. Only a few instances have been described in which considerable subcortical gliosis is seen, usually confined to a single lobe, parietal more than others. It is separated from Pick's disease by the absence of Pick bodies and from Creutzfeldt-Jakob disease by the absence of spongiform change. The course may be rather prolonged. Its occurrence suggests a link to other focal atrophies, although no genetic or underlying cause has been found.

Huntington's Disease

This degenerative disease (see Ch. 77) has been the subject of intense research because it is surprisingly common, affecting some 5 to 10 per 100,000 people in the general population. It is genetically determined and is transmitted in an autosomal dominant pattern the penetrance of which is almost complete, thus affecting almost everyone at risk.

The striatum is heavily affected, with prominent shrinkage of the head of the caudate nucleus. Histologically, the main cell loss is among the small neurons, less so among the larger neurons in the striatum, and there is an associated gliosis. The neurons of the frontal and temporal lobe are also affected but to a lesser degree.

The condition develops slowly, usually making its appearance in patients in their 40s or 50s, after procreation has created another generation at risk. The involvement of the striatum is responsible for the chorea that attracted Huntington's attention and led to his discovery of the familial inheritance patterns. It is believed that the cortical atrophy accounts for the accompanying dementia, which shares many features with Alzheimer's disease. Disorders of behavior, which are unusual for Alzheimer's disease, often accompany the condition, including changes of personality to paranoid, hypersexuality, impulsivity, antisocial acts, drug and alcohol dependence, and gross psychosis. The suicide rate is higher in this group.

Parkinson's Disease

This worldwide disease (see Ch. 75) affects some 100 per 100,000 persons, making it the most common form of movement disorder encountered in clinical neurology. It develops from loss of neurons in the pigmentary nuclei in the upper brainstem, with the zona compacta of the substantia nigra and the locus ceruleus of the pons being especially heavily affected. Lewy bodies, a form of intracytoplasmic hyaline inclusions, are a distinctive but not unique finding in many neurons. Although the major cell loss is in these sites, making Parkinson's disease mainly a local atrophy of specific cellular groups in the basal ganglia and brainstem, in some cases, atrophy may also affect the cortical surface.

Tremor, rigidity, and hypokinesia are the main manifestations; dementia also occurs in those with associated cortical atrophy. Dementia affects roughly 20 percent of those with Parkinson's disease.

Thalamic Atrophies

In 1939, Stern described the case of a 40-year-old man with a rapid decline in memory, comprehension, and hypersomnia; apathy; primitive reflexes; and loss of pupillary responses. At autopsy, mild atrophy was found over the convexities, but the thalamus was strikingly atrophic, save for the ventral posterior and reticular nuclei and medial and lateral geniculate bodies.

The few cases reported since have also shown disproportionate atrophy of the thalamus in all but a few cases. The thalamus has been found to be grossly shrunken, with widespread neuronal loss and gliosis. The dorsomedial and centromedial nuclei have been found to be the most often affected. The histologic changes typical of Alzheimer's or Pick's disease have been inconspicuous. The involvement of the neothalamus instead of the paleothalamus and archithalamus have given rise to speculation that the condition affects regions in the thalamus comparable to the involvement of association systems of the cortex typically affected in Alzheimer's disease. Such speculations also indicate the degree of ignorance of the causes of thalamic atrophy. Some reports have shown the atrophy involving these structures.

The clinical course is brief, months to a few years, and features a steadily evolving dementia, in some instances with myoclonus. All of these features together have more often suggested a diagnosis of Creutzfeldt-Jakob disease, and the lack of such findings at autopsy seem to be one reason for the case reports. In one case, the thalamic atrophy was associated with motor neuron disease.

ANNOTATED BIBLIOGRAPHY

Cummings JL, Duchen LW. Klüver-Bucy syndrome in Pick disease: clinical and pathologic correlations. Neurology 1981;31:1415.

Anterior temporal lobe lesions may produce this effect.

Deymeer F, Smith TW, DeGirolami U, Drachman DA. Thalamic dementia and motor neuron disease. Neurology 1989;39:58–61.

A 46-year-old patient whose course was 30 months. Attempts to transmit the disease to animals were unsuccessful.

Dickson DW, Yen SH, Suzuki KI et al. Ballooned neurons in select neurodegenerative diseases contain phosphory-lated neurofilament epitopes. Acta Neuropathol (Berl) 1986;71:216–23.

Ballooned neurons contained phosphorylated epitopes but not of the types seen in Alzheimer's or Pick's disease. The swollen neurons resembled changes caused by neurotoxins.

Gibb WRG, Luthert PJ, Marsden CD. Corticobasal degeneration. Brain 1989;112:1171–92.

Three more cases resembling neuronal achromasia.

Goecke Hoyer G, Reuther R, Schmitt HP. Primare Degeneration des Thalamus mit Demenz Zwei Beobachtungen mit familiarem Hintergrund. Fortschr Neurol Psychiatr 1990;58:262–9.

Thalamic atrophy in two patients clinically suspected to have Creutzfeldt-Jakob disease.

Kirschner HS, Tanridag O, Thurman L, Whetsell WO. Progressive aphasia without dementia: two cases with focal spongiform degeneration. Ann Neurol 1987;22:527–32.

Not Creutzfeldt-Jakob disease.

Leger JM, Levasseur M, Benoit N et al. Apraxie d'aggravation lentement progressive: étude par IRM et tomographie à positons dans 4 cas. Rev Neurol (Paris) 1991;147:183–91.

Four well-documented cases of parietal lobe atrophy.

Lippa CF, Cohen R, Smith TW, Drachman DA. Primary progressive aphasia with focal neuronal achromasia. Neurology 1991;41:882–6.

A 69-year-old man with progressive aphasia, autopsy signs of focal cortical degeneration of the left superior frontal gyrus, and microscopy showing neurons with achromasia but no signs of Alzheimer's, Pick's, or other dementing disorders.

Mansvelt J. Pick's disease: A Syndrome of Lobar Cerebral Atrophy. Enschede, Netherlands, 1954.

The study documenting asymmetric atrophy in one-half of the cases, usually involving the left side.

Mesalum MM. Slowly progressive dysphasia without generalized dementia. Ann Neurol 1982;11:592–8.

A case of lobar atrophy featuring aphasia but without distinctive features suggesting Alzheimer's, Pick's, or other diseases.

Morris JC, Cole M, Banker BQ, Wright D. Hereditary dysphasic dementia and the Pick-Alzheimer type. Ann Neurol 1984;16:455–66.

Dysphasia may be the initial sign.

Neumann MA, Cohn R. Progressive subcortical gliosis: a rare form of presenile dementia. Brain 1967;90:405–18.

The type II Pick's disease, affecting the parietal lobe, with predominantly subcortical gliosis.

Pick A. Über die Bezeihungen der senilen hirnatrophie zur Aphasie. Prager Med Wochenschr 1892;17:165.

The index case.

Rebeiz JJ, Kolodny EH, Richardson EP Jr. Corticodentatonigral degeneration with neuronal achromasia. Arch Neurol 1968;18:20.

The first case. The nondominant hemisphere was the more affected.

Roberts GW, Allsop D, Bruton C. The occult aftermath of boxing. J Neurol Neurosurg Psychiatry 1990;53:373–8.

β-protein was found in plaques immunologically comparable to that found in Alzheimer's disease.

Roberts GW, Gentleman SM, Lynch A, Graham DI. BA4 amyloid protein deposition in brain after head trauma. Lancet 1991;1:1422–3.

Within days.

Signoret JL, Hauww JJ. Maladie d'Alzheimer et Autres Démences. Vol. 1. Médecine—Sciences. Flamm, Paris, 1991, p. 511.

A good clinicopathologic update of rare dementias.

Sjögren T, Sjögren H, Lindgren AGH. Morbus Alzheimer and morbus Pick. A genetic, clinical and patho-anantomic study. Acta Psychiat Neurol Scand Suppl 1952;82:1.

Apparently transmitted by an autosomal dominant gene.

Sparks DL, Woeltz VM, Markesbery WR. Alterations in brain monoamine oxidase activity in aging, Alzheimer's disease and Pick's disease. Arch Neurol 1991;48:718–21.

Monoamine oxidase activity differs in different brain regions between those with Alzheimer's disease compared with those with Pick's disease.

Stern K. Severe dementia associated with bilateral symmetrical degeneration of the thalamus. Brain 1939;62:157–71.

The first fully described case.

62
Clinical Disorders of the Autonomic Nervous System

E. Oribe and O. Appenzeller

CLASSIC DISORDERS

Autonomic Failure With Multiple System Atrophy and Pure Autonomic Failure

As experiments in nature, the classic forms of primary autonomic failure offer a unique opportunity to understand autonomic nervous system function. The classic primary illnesses of the autonomic nervous system that cause autonomic failure can be divided into central and peripheral forms (Table 62-1). In the central forms, such as autonomic failure with multiple system atrophy (MSA), autonomic failure is due to lesions affecting preganglionic neurons located in the central autonomic network, brainstem, and spinal cord. In the peripheral forms, such as pure autonomic failure (PAF), autonomic failure is a disorder of peripheral ganglia and postganglionic neurons (see Ch. 34).

MSA encompasses a group of neurodegenerative diseases, including the Shy-Drager syndrome, olivopontocerebellar atrophy (OPCA), and striatonigral degeneration (SND). In MSA, failure of the autonomic nervous system is accompanied by somatic neurologic abnormalities. Cell loss and gliosis is present in different combinations mainly in the putamen, substantia nigra, locus ceruleus, pontine nuclei, inferior olive, cerebellar cortex, dorsal vagal nuclei, spinal cord intermediolateral cell column (IML), and Onuf's nucleus. Oligodendroglial and neuronal cytoplasmic and intranuclear argyrophilic inclusions, which are thought to be specific to MSA, may be present not only in those areas that are most affected by cell loss and gliosis but in areas that are relatively spared. The sympathetic ganglia are usually normal. The dysfunction of central biochemical mechanisms present in MSA is reflected by decreased norepinephrine and do-pamine and other neurotransmitters and peptides in postmortem brains.

Different clinical forms of MSA have been described, depending on the degree of involvement of extrapyramidal, cerebellar, or pyramidal systems accompanying autonomic failure. In MSA with SND, there is predominance of extrapyramidal features with rigidity, postural abnormalities, and akinesia. In OPCA with autonomic failure, cerebellar features predominate with ataxia; in the pyramidal form, pyramidal dysfunction is prominent. Often, as the disease progresses, the clinical distinction between forms becomes less evident, reflecting an overlap in pathologic lesions.

The cause of MSA is not known. Among several possibilities, a viral cause has been suggested by reports of patients with OPCA-MSA clinically in association with human T-cell lymphotropic virus type II retroviral infection (see Ch. 49). In other instances, the link with specific causes is more tenuous. It is possible that MSA is an entity of varied pathogenesis.

MSA is more frequent than previously thought. Its incidence is in the range of 5 to 15 per 100,000, and it may account for 10 percent of patients with clinically idiopathic parkinsonism. The age of onset is 5 to 10 years younger than that of idiopathic Parkinson's disease. Survival in MSA is rarely more than 5 to 6 years after diagnosis.

The diagnosis of MSA depends on the presence of suggestive clinical features and laboratory findings. As in the peripheral forms of autonomic failure, orthostatic and postprandial hypotension occur frequently as the initial presentation of the illness. Urinary frequency, urgency, and a reduced stream that resembles bladder outflow obstruction are prominent early on (up to 40 percent of men with MSA undergo surgery

Table 62-1. Autonomic Dysfunction

Classic disorders
  Pure autonomic failure
  Multiple system atrophy
    Striatonigral degeneration
    Olivopontocerebellar atrophy
  Parkinson's disease with autonomic failure
Common dysfunction
  Orthostatic hypotension of the elderly (see Ch. 34)
  Reflex syncope
  Deconditioning and postural tachycardia syndrome
  Dysautonomia associated with mitral valve prolapse
  Migraine and cluster headache
  Drug induced
    Nitrovasodilators
    Sympatholytics
    Phenothiazines
    Tricyclic antidepressants
    Insulin
  Diabetic autonomic neuropathy
  Landry-Guillain-Barré syndrome
  Infectious causes
    Human immunodeficiency virus disease
    Leprosy
    Chagas' disease
    Botulism
  Toxic autonomic neuropathies
    Alcohol
    Vincristine
    Cisplatin
    Heavy metals
    Solvents
  Metabolic
    Uremia
    Liver disease
  Nutritional deficiencies
    Subacute combined degeneration

Connective tissue diseases
  Rheumatoid arthritis
  Systemic lupus erythematosus and mixed connective tissue diseases
Raynaud's syndrome
Erythromelalgia
Hirschprung's disease
Uncommon dysfunction
  Acute and chronic panautonomic neuropathy (pandysautonomia)
  Chronic autonomic neuropathies
    Peripheral neuropathies
    Distal small-fiber neuropathy
    Distal sympathetic neuropathies
  Amyloid neuropathy
    Sporadic systemic amyloid neuropathy
    Multiple myeloma-associated amyloid neuropathy
  Paraneoplastic
    Acute paraneoplastic autonomic neuropathy
    Sensory neuronopathy with autonomic failure (may be paraneoplastic)
    Lambert-Eaton myasthenic syndrome
  Hereditary neuropathies
    Familial amyloidotic polyneuropathy
    Hereditary sensory and autonomic neuropathy (types I, II and IV)
    Hereditary motor and sensory neuropathy (types I and II)
    Friedreich's ataxia
    Porphyria
    Fabry's disease
    Navajo neuroarthropathy
  Adie's syndrome
  Paroxysmal or intermittent acral dysautonomia
  Chronic idiopathic anhidrosis
  Paroxysmal hyperhidrosis

for suspected prostatism). Later on, urge incontinence is followed by detrusor dysfunction and large residual urine volumes. In women, denervation of the urethral sphincter causes stress incontinence. Nocturia is present in most patients. In men, impotence also occurs early, with erectile and later ejaculatory failure. Inability to sweat may cause heat intolerance. Vocal cord paralysis may be the only somatic feature present early in the illness. Later on in the course of the illness, swallowing difficulties and abnormalities in respiratory control (an important cause of death in MSA) become prominent. Patients have daytime gasping, nocturnal laryngeal stridor as a result of vocal cord abductor muscle paralysis, and snoring because of pharyngeal muscle dysfunction. (Snoring is a common symptom of limited clinical consequence when it occurs alone.) In advanced stages of the illness, there is severe motor disability, loss of bladder control, and speech and swallowing difficulties. Mental functions, however, are preserved, and decisions regarding tracheotomy and life support pose ethical considerations.

Autonomic testing (see Ch. 16) at the time of diag-nosis frequently reflects widespread autonomic involvement. Cardiovascular autonomic testing reveals orthostatic hypotension, loss of the normal heart rate variability, and subnormal increases in plasma norepinephrine levels in response to standing or tilting. In advanced illness, supine hypertension and exaggerated pressor responses to vasoconstrictor drugs occur as a result of denervation supersensitivity. Urodynamic studies show uninhibited detrusor contractions in response to bladder filling, loss of ability to initiate voluntary micturition, loss of proximal urethral sphincter tone with bladder incontinence, and inability to contract the distal urinary sphincter to prevent urine leakage. Urethral sphincter electromyography may show polyphasic long-duration motor units, which are manifestations of peripheral sprouting caused by a loss of Onuf's nucleus neurons. Polysomnography, important to evaluate in sleep-related respiratory dysrhythmias, may disclose recurrent episodes of obstructive central or mixed apnea, which are prominent during non-rapid eye movement stages I and II and rapid eye movement sleep (see Chs. 11 and

79). Responses to hypoxia and hypercapnia can be impaired. The plasma concentration of vasopressin does not increase in response to hypotension but does increase normally in response to changes in osmolarity, reflecting dysfunction of central autonomic connections. Also, the increases in plasma concentrations of corticotropin and β-endorphin in response to hypoglycemia are subnormal. Anemia may be present in advanced illness.

Brain imaging in MSA shows varying patterns and degrees of atrophy of the brainstem, middle pontine, and cerebellar peduncles and the cerebellum. In OPCA, atrophy of the vermis and cerebellar cortex may be prominent. Posterolateral putaminal hypointensity present on T_2-weighted magnetic resonance imaging (MRI) sequences (matching pathologic cell loss) is considered unique to MSA. Positron emission tomography (PET) scanning using fluorine-18-labeled 6-fluorodopa and carbon-11-labeled nomifensine reveals severe loss of caudate putaminal radionuclide storage and reuptake capacity in MSA, indicating dopaminergic dysfunction. The relative preservation of caudate dopaminergic function in Parkinson's disease may help to distinguish it from MSA.

The clinical distinction between MSA and Parkinson's disease with autonomic failure may be subtle (Table 62-2). The true incidence of autonomic failure in Parkinson's disease is not clear due to the contribu-

tion of treatment with dopaminergic and anticholinergic drugs, which can cause hypotension and bladder dysfunction. In Parkinson's disease, Lewy bodies are frequently detected in the autonomic hypothalamic nuclei, dorsovagal nucleus, and sympathetic ganglia, whereas these are infrequently present in MSA (the incidence is similar to that in controls). The most consistent pathologic finding in patients with Parkinson's disease and autonomic failure is significant cell loss in intermediolateral cell columns (which is of lesser degree than in MSA). Patients with Parkinson's disease may have symptoms of autonomic dysfunction similar to those present with MSA, including orthostatic and postprandial hypotension (Fig. 62-1), sexual dysfunction, constipation, sialorrhea, and sweating abnormalities.

Features that suggest MSA as opposed to Parkinson's disease include earlier age of onset, antecollis, history of impotence or incontinence, cerebellar or pyramidal involvement, and perhaps most importantly, lack of consistent response or loss of response to levodopa. Early and severe autonomic failure is much more common in MSA than in Parkinson's disease. An important feature differentiating the incontinence of MSA from that of Parkinson's disease is the presence of a normal sphincter electromyogram in Parkinson's disease. Brain PET and MRI studies help differ-

Table 62-2. Autonomic Dysfunction or Failure (Shy-Drager-Like) Syndromes

Autonomic Failure With	Clinical Features	Laboratory Features	Pathology
MSA	Prominent autonomic failure: orthostatic hypotension, genitourinary, respiratory symptoms, poor response to levodopa, decreased survival, preservation of intellect	Subnormal increase in arginine vasopressin in response to hypotension; abnormal urethral sphincter electromyogram; caudate, putaminal, and cerebellar atrophy on MRI; caudate and putaminal abnormalities on PET	Intracytoplasmic and neuronal inclusion bodies
SND	Rigidity and akinesia more prominent than tremors; antecollis, pyramidal tract signs		
OPCA	Cerebellar ataxia, intention tremors	Prominent cerebellar and pontine atrophy on CT/MRI	
Parkinson's disease	Rigidity, akinesia, resting tremors, response to levodopa, frequent dementia	Relatively spared caudate function on PET	Lewy bodies predominantly in substantia nigra
Diffuse Lewy body disease	Rigidity and akinesia prominent, poor response to levodopa, dementia	Not well documented	Lewy bodies diffusely including cortical neurons

Abbreviations: MSA, multiple system atrophy; SND, striatonigral degeneration; OPCA, olivopontocerebellar atrophy; MRI, magnetic resonance imaging, PET, positron emission tomography; CT, computed tomography.

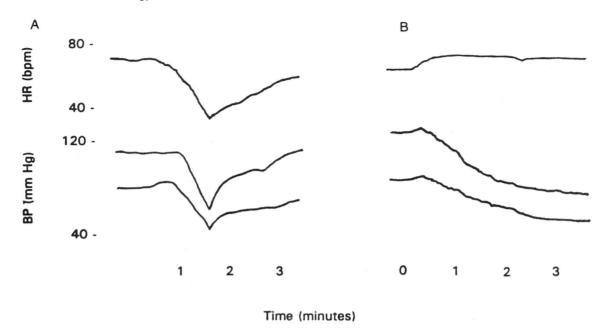

Figure 62-1. **(A)** Blood pressure (BP) (upper trace, systolic pressure; lower trace, diastolic pressure) and heart rate (HR) changes in a patient with neurocardiogenic syncope induced by a passive 60-degree head-up tilt. Hypotension due to reflex-mediated vasodilation is accompanied by paradoxic slowing of the HR (see Ch. 34). **(B)** Changes in BP and HR in a patient with autonomic failure with multiple system atrophy. There is a rapid fall in BP in response to the upright posture, indicating sympathetic vasomotor failure. The minimal increase in HR despite the marked fall in BP indicates parasympathetic and sympathetic cardiomotor failure.

entiate MSA from Parkinson's disease with autonomic failure in some instances.

The classic peripheral form of primary autonomic failure, pure autonomic failure (PAF) (also known as Bradbury-Eggelston syndrome, idiopathic orthostatic hypotension) is characterized by widespread autonomic failure occurring in isolation without somatic neurologic findings. Pathologic, biochemical, and pharmacologic findings indicate that PAF is a disorder mainly of postganglionic autonomic neurons. There is marked loss of ganglionic neurons, and some of the remaining neurons contain Lewy bodies. Cell loss in the spinal cord intermediolateral column may result from retrograde neuronal death. Preservation of central autonomic circuits in patients with PAF is reflected by the normal concentration of norepinephrine transmitter metabolites in the cerebrospinal fluid, normal increase of the plasma concentrations of vasopressin in response to hypotension, and of corticotropin and β-endorphin in response to hypoglycemia. Brain imaging study results are normal.

The differential diagnosis between MSA and PAF is important because of the different prognosis of these disorders. Whereas the prognosis in MSA is poor (most patients are completely dependent in advanced illness and do not survive beyond 6 years), survival of up to 15 to 20 years with a relatively functional life is not uncommon in PAF. The clinical distinction be-

tween PAF and MSA with somatic neurologic abnormalities is straightforward. The distinction between "early" MSA (when somatic neurologic findings are absent) and PAF is particularly difficult. It is said that a 5-year waiting period is prudent before making a clinical diagnosis of PAF and excluding MSA. Different neuroendocrine responses to hypotension and administration of clonidine have been reported to help distinguish MSA, in which central autonomic pathways are involved, from PAF in which these are spared. In MSA, hypotension does not induce a normal rise in plasma vasopressin concentration, whereas in PAF, the rise is normal (Fig. 62-2). Similarly, a normal increase in plasma growth hormone concentration in response to administration of clonidine is present in PAF but is subnormal in MSA. Administration of L-threo-DOPS (a synthetic aminoacid that is decarboxylated within neurons to form norepinephrine) may also help differentiate MSA from PAF because it increases blood pressure when given to patients with MSA but not when given to patients with PAF (where postganglionic adrenergic neurons are dysfunctional).

COMMON DISORDERS OF AUTONOMIC FUNCTION
Autonomic Neuropathies

Peripheral nerve disorders can involve afferent or efferent autonomic nervous system pathways. Autonomic dysfunction is usually present when small nerve

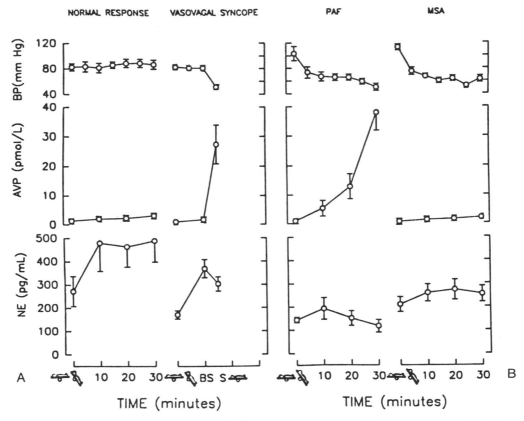

Figure 62-2. Mean arterial pressure (BP) and plasma concentration of vasopressin (AVP) and norepinephrine (NE) before and during upright tilt in **(A)** normal subjects (normal response, n = 5; vasovagal syncope, VVS, n = 9) and **(B)** patients with autonomic failure (pure autonomic failure, PAF, n = 4; multiple system atrophy, MSA, n = 9). Tilt started at time zero. In the subjects with VVS, the baseline values, the values before syncope (BS), and the values at the time of syncope (S) are shown. In response to similar degrees of hypotension, vasopressin increased in patients with intact afferent and central baroreflex pathways (VVS and PAF) but did not increase in patients with degeneration of central pathways (MSA). In patients with MSA, vasopressin increases normally in response to increases in plasma osmolarity (not shown in this figure). Data are mean ± standard error. (From Kaufmann et al, 1992, with permission.)

fibers that are part of baroreflex and efferent sympathetic pathways or parasympathetic or sympathetic nerve fibers are affected by a neuropathic process. With small-fiber neuropathies, there is pain and temperature sense loss accompanied by sympathetic failure. Many autonomic neuropathies are suspected to be immune mediated.

With rare exceptions (e.g., diabetic peripheral neuropathy), most peripheral neuropathies do not have overwhelming autonomic failure. As a rule, autonomic dysfunction in peripheral neuropathies is symptomatic in the acute stages or in the chronic stages when autonomic nervous system mechanisms are stressed. For example, asymptomatic orthostatic hypotension may become symptomatic after prolonged standing; exercise; exposure to heat, cold, or altitude; or as a result of medications.

Diabetic autonomic neuropathy is the most frequent cause of autonomic neuropathy. Ten to 20 percent of all diabetic patients have abnormalities in autonomic testing. The incidence is slightly higher for insulin-dependent diabetes mellitus compared with noninsulin-dependent diabetes mellitus. Most patients with diabetic autonomic neuropathy, however, are asymptomatic. The presence of antibodies against the vagus and other nerves suggests that autoimmune mechanisms may cause this disorder. Recent reports suggest that diabetic neuropathy may result in part from defective autonomic innervation of blood supply to peripheral nerves. Those patients who are symptomatic may have orthostatic hypotension, sweating abnormalities, gastrointestinal motility symptoms, diarrhea, and impotence. In some patients, orthostatic hypotension may be exacerbated by administration of insulin, which has been reported to reduce right atrial pressure and cardiac output. Sweating may be absent (diabetic anhydrosis) in the lower limbs and may be accompanied by a compensatory excess of sweating in the upper body. Gustatory sweating (profuse facial and neck sweating during meals) is typical of diabetic autonomic neuropathy. Constipation is frequent, and as many as 20 percent of diabetic patients with gastrointestinal symptoms have radiologic evidence of gastric retention. Symptoms of delayed gastric emptying (gastroparesis) include early satiety and postprandial nausea and vomiting. Diabetic diarrhea (which can be explosive, watery, and steatorrheic) may result indirectly from bacterial overgrowth. Lack of awareness of hypoglycemia in some diabetic patients may be due in part to a reduction in the autonomic response to hypoglycemia (hypoglycemia-associated autonomic failure). The presence of diabetic autonomic neuropathy has been associated with increased mortality rates (mainly as a result of renal failure).

Loss of normal heart rate variability and resting tachycardia (vagal denervation) are the most frequent initial laboratory abnormalities. Later on, sympathetic denervation follows, and eventually, in advanced diabetic autonomic neuropathy, the heart is "denervated," and the heart rate may respond only to circulating catecholamines and hormones.

Neuropathic foot problems in diabetes closely mimic those found in leprosy with ulceration, subsequent osteomyelitis, neuropathic edema, fractures and destruction of bone, and ultimately Charcot (neuroarthropathic) foot. Underlying these disastrous complications of diabetes is the neuropathy that causes impairment of pain and temperature sensation (early) and autonomic failure, without which foot lesions do not occur. Clinically apart from the obvious foot lesions, there are hemodynamic abnormalities (raised arterial systolic pressures and reduced transit times) and extensive medial vascular calcifications (Mönckeberg's sclerosis), even in young patients. Similar calcifications may occur after lumbar sympathectomy, suggesting a link between the autonomic degeneration and medial damage. Because of this degeneration, there is also an increase in bone blood flow (bone blood vessels have a rich autonomic innervation), which can be demonstrated even in radiologically normal bone. This increase in blood flow leads to bone reabsorption with osteopenia, which is also found in the bones of the hands of diabetic patients. The development of neuroarthropathy requires both somatic and autonomic neuropathic dysfunction; either alone is not sufficient for this syndrome.

In painful diabetic neuropathy, the sympathetic denervation is incomplete. The increased blood flow also present in this variety can temporarily be normalized by sympathetic activation, such as coughing.

In the diabetic neuropathic foot, there is also loss of sweating in a stocking distribution, but this usually follows demonstrable abnormalities in autonomic cardiovascular control. The mechanisms involved in antidromic vasodilation (flare component of the triple response of Lewis) (T. Lewis, English physician, 1881–1945) and in cutaneous vascular reflexes and neurogenic inflammation are interesting in the development of diabetic foot complications. Quantitative measures of the flare and other vascular reactions on the soles of the feet show a clear reduction in these responses in diabetic patients with foot lesions. The loss of nociception predisposes patients to injury (impairment of afferent protective pain sensation), and impairment of effector function (the neurogenic vascular response to injury) together with autonomic dysfunction usually are deciding factors in the development of the diabetic foot.

The autonomic manifestations of the *Landry-Guillain-Barré syndrome* (GBS) reflect the relative involvement of various afferent and efferent autonomic feedback loops by demyelinating lesions. Segmental demyelination of cranial nerves IX and X, the sympathetic chains, and white rami communicantes explain cardiac arrhythmias (usually tachycardia) and hypertensive or hypotensive episodes that are present in 50 percent of patients with Landry-Guillain-Barré syndrome. Hypertension, which can be severe enough to cause retinal or cerebral hemorrhage, is attributed to dysfunction of the afferent limb of the baroreflex and loss of the ability of the reflex to buffer blood pressure and heart rate changes. Hypotension, which may be sudden and follow episodes of hypertension, is due to acute vasodilation. Orthostatic hypotension, anhydrosis, constipation, gastroparesis, bladder incontinence (in up to one-third of patients), and rectal incontinence can be present. Autonomic disturbance tends to correlate with the severity of somatic involvement. Autonomic nervous system dysfunction is uncommon in chronic inflammatory demyelinating polyradiculoneuropathy.

Acute pandysautonomia, an autonomic neuropathy that produces autonomic failure of acute or subacute onset has been described after viral-like illnesses. In some cases, there is isolated cholinergic and adrenergic failure. Recovery is slow and may be incomplete.

Less common causes of autonomic neuropathy include numerous inherited and acquired disorders. In *porphyria,* tachycardia, abdominal pain, nausea and vomiting, diarrhea, constipation, and urinary retention reflect brainstem, spinal cord, vagal, and sympathetic nerve involvement. *Hereditary sensory and autonomic neuropathies* (HSAN) are accompanied by autonomic symptoms. Blood pressure lability, hyperhidrosis, decreased tearing, and gastrointestinal and taste disturbances are present together with sensory symptoms (lack of pain and temperature sensation) in familial dysautonomia (Riley-Day syndrome, HSAN type III). This autosomal recessive disorder affects Ashkenazi Jews and has been suggested to result from defective nerve growth factor function. *HSAN type IV* (Swanson), with loss of small myelinated and unmyelinated autonomic and somatic nerve fibers, is accompanied by loss of pain sensation and anhidrosis, causing hyperthermia. The disorder has autosomal recessive inheritance. There is mild autonomic impairment in HSAN type I. With hereditary motor and sensory neuropathy *types I, II,* and *III,* autonomic involvement is usually not clinically significant. In Navajo neuroarthropathy, Charcot joints are accompanied by thermoregulatory dysfunction.

In *Hirschprung's disease,* or congenital aganglionosis, absence of enteric ganglia presents in newborns as intestinal obstruction. This disorder is present in one of every 5,000 to 8,000 births and may be related to a neural crest disorder.

In sporadic *systemic amyloid neuropathy,* there is severe autonomic failure and pain accompanied by small-fiber sensory loss. Orthostatic hypotension, abnormal sweating, and impotence are frequent and are accompanied by selective loss of pain and temperature senses. There is amyloid deposition in nerves and autonomic ganglia with loss of unmyelinated and small myelinated somatic and autonomic nerves and IML cells. In *familial amyloid polyneuropathy,* autonomic failure is also severe and accompanied by sensory abnormalities similar to those of the sporadic form. This disease usually begins in young adulthood and follows a dominant inheritance. There is accumulation of amyloid, usually as a result of a point mutation of the transthyretin prealbumin gene on chromosome 18. There is no treatment, and death, which is due to cardiac or renal failure, occurs after 10 to 15 years of illness. Autonomic involvement may be present in some cases of multiple myeloma-associated amyloid neuropathy.

Various infectious disorders cause autonomic dysfunction. With *acquired immunodeficiency syndrome,* autonomic dysfunction usually accompanies peripheral nerve involvement. Autonomic symptoms include orthostatic hypotension, loss of sweating, urinary dysfunction, and impotence. Some gastrointestinal manifestations of this disease, such as diarrhea, may be due in part to autonomic neuropathy. Usually, autonomic nervous system dysfunction follows that of other human immunodeficiency virus-related neurologic findings. Autonomic nervous system involvement, however, can also be asymptomatic and be detected only by autonomic testing. *Leprosy* can result in hypohidrosis in the territory of affected nerves and orthostatic hypotension together with a variety of auto-

nomic abnormalities that may be subclinical. In *Chagas' disease* (see Ch. 45), infection with *Trypanosoma cruzi* causes sympathetic and peripheral nerve destruction through an autoimmune process. Destruction of myenteric plexi and autonomic nervous system ganglia produces gastrointestinal motility dysfunction (megaesophagus and megacolon), and destruction of myocardium and conduction systems causes arrhythmias. *Botulinum toxin,* produced by *Clostridium botulinum,* results in acute autonomic dysfunction by interfering with the neuronal release of acetylcholine. Symptoms of sudo- and secretomotor failure accompany gastrointestinal and urinary dysfunction. Autonomic nervous system dysfunction appears to be more severe with type B botulism in which neuromuscular weakness is less prominent than with type A. Generalized *tetanus* produces severe autonomic overactivity (tachycardia, hypertension, diaphoresis, and fever accompanied by elevated catecholamine levels). Autonomic overactivity is probably due to a direct effect of the tetanus toxin as it persists after curarization.

Vitamin B$_{12}$ deficiency may cause autonomic nervous system dysfunction with severe postural hypotension, gustatory sweating, impotence, ptosis, and pupillary abnormalities accompanied by tremors (all patients with suspected MSA should be screened for vitamin B$_{12}$ deficiency). Orthostatic hypotension, sometimes an initial presentation of vitamin B$_{12}$ deficiency, usually responds well to vitamin supplementation. Alcoholic patients may have a predominantly vagal autonomic neuropathy with abnormal heart rate variability tests. Because sympathetic vasomotor and sudomotor loss occurs late in *alcoholic polyneuropathy,* orthostatic hypotension is present only in severely affected patients. *Uremia* and *liver failure* may be accompanied by autonomic dysfunction.

Toxic neuropathies that feature autonomic failure include those caused by cisplatin, vincristine, amiodarone, perhexiline maleate, heavy metals, N-3-pyridylmethyl-N'-p-nitrophenylurea acrylamide, and organic solvents.

Symptoms of autonomic neuropathy may be present with rheumatoid arthritis, systemic lupus erythematosus, mixed connective tissue diseases, and Gougerot-Sjögren's syndrome. Paraneoplastic neuropathies may manifest with sweating, orthostatic hypotension, genitourinary dysfunction, and intestinal pseudo-obstruction. Antineuronal nuclear antibodies (anti-Hu) have been detected in several patients with paraneoplastic autonomic dysfunction and should be sought when patients are evaluated who have unexplained autonomic failure. Symptomatic cholinergic and sympathetic autonomic failure may be present in the Lambert-Eaton myasthenic syndrome.

Reflex Syncope

Reflex syncope results from a reflex mechanism that triggers withdrawal of sympathetic outflow and increases parasympathetic activity, causing hypotension (and sometimes slowing of the heart) with symptomatic cerebral hypoperfusion. The reflex is activated by excessive afferent discharges that originate from various sensory receptors (e.g., the carotid sinus and cardiac and visceral mechanoreceptors) or directly from the cortex and limbic system (in syncope induced by emotion and pain).

On clinical grounds, syncopal events are reflex in origin when a particular precipitating maneuver can be identified. In those who are susceptible, coughing, laughing, swallowing, defecating, bladder emptying, and other maneuvers that activate mechanoreceptors (i.e., cardiac, arterial, bronchial, esophageal, gastric, rectal, and bladder) can induce reflex syncope. Frequently, a combination of factors act together to precipitate syncope. For example, micturition syncope in elderly men with prostatic hypertrophy occurs while they stand and force urine flow against an obstructed bladder outlet. In this situation, bladder mechanoreceptor activation occurs in the setting of an already decreased cardiac output (caused by increased intrathoracic pressure and dependent blood pooling) and increased intracranial pressure (as a result of the strain during efforts to void). Reflex syncope is usually brief, and recovery is prompt. Frequently, formes frustes occur when blood pressure falls cause symptoms, but hypotension is not sufficient to cause loss of consciousness (presyncope).

Neurocardiogenic syncope (Fig. 62-1), mainly thought to be triggered by excessive afferent cardiac and vascular mechanoreceptor discharges, is a frequent cause of syncope in all age groups. It is usually accompanied by prodromal symptoms that reflect autonomic activation, such as pallor, sweating, pupillary dilation, nausea, vomiting, and abdominal discomfort, together with symptoms of cerebral hypoperfusion, such as lightheadedness and visual and auditory disturbances followed by alteration of consciousness. Neurocardiogenic syncope usually occurs while the patient is upright and in conditions that are associated with vasodilation in various vascular beds, such as after exercise, a meal, or ingestion of alcohol.

The differential diagnosis of reflex syncope relies on a careful history and reports from those present during an attack. The initial objective is to exclude seizures, cardiac disease, and arrhythmias as a cause of transient loss of consciousness. The absence of a residual confusional state is the norm and helps distinguish reflex syncope from an epileptic seizure. Clonic movements that resemble epileptic seizures (convul-

Table 62-3. Mechanisms That Cause Decreased Cerebral Perfusion and Syncope

Decreased cardiac venous return
    Hypovolemia
    Diversion of blood to splanchnic circulation
    Maneuvers that obstruct venous return
Decreased vascular tone
    Acute vasodilation (reflex syncope)
    Lack of vasoconstriction (autonomic failure)
Cardiac pump failure
    Obstruction to flow
    Arrhythmia
    Ischemia
Increased intracranial pressure
    Maneuvers (Valsalva)
    Space-occupying lesions

sive syncope), however, can occur with reflex syncope as a result of cerebral ischemia and may mislead the clinician in the diagnosis.

Because the common denominator of syncope is a symptomatic fall in cerebral perfusion, the differential diagnosis is broad. Disorders that produce a fall in cardiac venous return, vascular tone, or cardiac pump failure can result in syncope by promoting falls in cardiac output and blood pressure (Table 62-3). A fall in venous cardiac return may result from hypovolemia, excessive venous pooling, or diversion of blood to different vascular beds (e.g., the gut, varicose veins, and so-called third spaces) and maneuvers that increase intra-abdominal or intrathoracic pressure, such as straining and the Valsalva maneuver (which also produce a concomitant increase in intracranial pressure and impede cerebral blood flow). Dysfunction of the baroreflex as a result of autonomic failure can cause orthostatic hypotension, leading to syncope. Syncope can occur because of falls in cardiac output produced by severe aortic or pulmonary flow obstruction, arrhythmias, and episodic reflex mechanisms. Numerous medications produce vasodilation and diversion of blood to splanchnic capacitance circulations. On occasion, poorly understood mechanisms can precipitate syncope in the setting of a psychiatric disorder (*psychiatric syncope*).

A cause of syncope cannot be found in up to one-half of syncopal patients (i.e., *unexplained syncope*), despite a detailed history and physical examination, including supine and upright blood pressure measurements and electrocardiography. In many cases, further investigations are unrevealing. The frequent absence of abnormalities during evaluation may be explained by the sporadic nature of syncope. Valuable diagnostic clues can be obtained from reproducing maneuvers (e.g., carotid sinus massage, Valsalva maneuver, hyperventilation, and vigorous exercise) that precipitated spontaneous syncope. In some instances, the cause of syncope can be determined when syncope is reproduced or when a potential cause can be demonstrated in a laboratory setting. The prolonged head-up tilt test is used as a provocative "diagnostic test" (there is no "gold standard" for the diagnosis of unmonitored syncope) for the diagnosis of neurocardiogenic syncope in patients with unexplained syncope. Prolonged upright tilt with the lower limbs immobilized stresses autonomic cardiovascular reflexes by producing enhanced blood pooling and filtration of fluid into the dependent tissues and triggers this type of syncope in the susceptible individual. To be diagnostic, this test must not only trigger neurocardiogenic syncope but also reproduce the patient's typical symptoms. If patients recognize the symptoms induced during tilt as being similar to those present during spontaneous syncope, it is assumed that a neurocardiogenic reflex mechanism caused the patient's spontaneous syncope. The usefulness of the unmedicated head-up tilt test is based on its noninvasive nature, relative safety, and high specificity (around 90 percent). The head-up tilt test has been reported to induce neurocardiogenic syncope in 25 to 75 percent of patients with a history of unexplained syncope. The relatively low sensitivity reported in some studies can be increased at the expense of a lower specificity when the test is combined with the administration of β-adrenergic or vasodilating drugs. In one-half of the patients with unexplained syncope in whom neurocardiogenic syncope is not diagnosed, the test elicits blood pressure and heart rate responses that indicate a possible cause of syncope (e.g., orthostatic hypotension or exaggerated heart rate response as a result of hypovolemia).

The usefulness of other tests such as prolonged electrocardiographic (Holter) monitoring has been limited by their low sensitivity and specificity. On the other hand, in patients with recurrent unexplained syncope, prolonged event-triggered electrocardiographic monitoring (cardiac "loop" or event recorders) has been reported to determine whether an arrhythmia has caused syncopal symptoms. In selected patients (e.g., those with left ventricular dysfunction, spontaneous ventricular ectopy, or abnormal signal-averaged electrocardiograms) and elite athletes, invasive cardiac electrophysiologic studies can be done to determine whether a susceptibility to develop certain cardiac arrhythmias causing syncope is present.

Deconditioning and Postural Tachycardia Syndrome

The frequent presence of orthostatic symptoms as a result of postural intolerance in chronically bedridden patients can be explained by cardiovascular deconditioning produced by bed rest. Exercise capacity is diminished, and resting heart rate is increased. Baroreflex responses and parasympathetic tone are decreased, and sympathetic tone is enhanced. Deconditioning caused by bed rest appears to be related to the combined effects of reduced hydrostatic pressure on the cardiovascular system and reduced physical activity, which result in reduced plasma volume and heart size, impaired vasomotor tone, decreased red blood cell mass, and decreased carbohydrate metabolism.

Exaggerated heart rate increases (usually more than 30 beats/min) in response to standing (i.e., postural tachycardia), akin to those produced by deconditioning, are present in some active individuals despite their lack of recent bed rest or immobility. Presenting symptoms include orthostatic lightheadedness, palpitations, headaches, and recurrent syncope. Routine autonomic test results are usually normal other than for exaggerated heart rate (and sometimes an increase in diastolic pressure) on assuming the upright posture. The increases in norepinephrine levels to standing are sometimes exaggerated. Some patients have "hyperadrenergic" responses to infusion of catecholamines, suggesting adrenoceptor denervation supersensitivity. Decreased blood volume and red blood cell mass and excessive venous blood pooling in the lower limbs have been reported in some subsets of patients. Small-fiber autonomic neuropathy (suggested by the presence of decreased pain thresholds and sudomotor and gastrointestinal dysfunction) has been implicated as a causative mechanism in some patients. Mitral valve prolapse is frequently associated with postural tachycardia, increased β-adrenoceptor sensitivity, and the presence of "idiopathic" hypovolemia.

Changes in autonomic patterns similar to those produced by deconditioning on earth can be reproduced by exposure to microgravity during space flight. The effects of exposure to microgravity on autonomic cardiovascular and other functions have been studied during actual space flights and simulation of microgravity conditions on earth by maneuvers such as prolonged six-degree head-down tilt, prolonged bed rest, and whole-body water immersion. Microgravity is believed to produce changes in body fluid distribution that result in a decreased plasma volume, baroreceptor sensitivity, and adrenergic responses. Early neuroendocrine responses to microgravity include increased atrial natriuretic factor and decreased arginine vasopressin, renin, angiotensin, and aldosterone, which promote a decrease in plasma volume. Decreased plasma volume and increased leg compliance (and blood pooling) that occur during exposure to microgravity account for some of the orthostatic hypotension and increased resting heart rate that astronauts suffer from on re-entry into earth's gravity. Countermeasures developed to prevent hypotension in astronauts returning to earth rely on increasing intravascular volume and tone. These include a combination of periods of in-flight lower body negative pressure (reproducing some of the cardiovascular effects of gravity) and exercise (to reinforce the pumping action of muscles) together with fluid loading just before return to gravity. Lessons learned from space flight may have value in treating earthbound disorders of the autonomic nervous system, such as MSA and PAF.

MISCELLANEOUS DISORDERS

Disorders of Central Autonomic and Spinal Cord Pathways

Autonomic syndromes can reflect the location of central nervous system lesions involving autonomic pathways and, thus, may have localizing value to the clinician. For example, infarctions of the medial frontal lobe may produce urinary incontinence and thermoregulatory and cardiac abnormalities, and infarctions of the operculum may produce contralateral hyperhidrosis. Seizures originating in several frontal regions can trigger cardiac arrhythmias, syncope, pain, and vomiting. Disorders that affect the hypothalamus lead to various autonomic disturbances, depending on the site and extent of the lesions. Thermoregulatory dysfunction with hyperthermia (anterior hypothalamus), hypothermia (posterior hypothalamus), or circadian temperature variation abnormalities (suprachiasmatic nucleus) may be present either alone or combined with disorders of endocrine and sexual function. Lesions of the suprachiasmatic area of the hypothalamus may affect sleep-wake and temperature cycles and behavior. Lesions of the dorsomedial and anteroventral thalamic nuclei, thought to interrupt pathways connecting the amygdala and prefrontal cortex with the hypothalamus, are found in fatal familial insomnia. This rare prion-related autosomal dominant degenerative disorder presents in the third or fourth decade of life with progressive insomnia, sympathetic overactivity, and endocrine and motor disturbances such as ataxic gait and myoclonus. In this disorder, increased sympathetic activity is thought to result from degeneration of the thalamic nuclei, which may remove the hypothalamus from inhibitory cortical control. Lesions of the parabrachial region can manifest as intractable vomiting. Medullary lesions, by affecting the nucleus tractus solitarii, rostral ventrolateral medulla, the nucleus ambiguus, the lateral medullary reticular formation, or cranial nerves IX and X, may manifest as disorders of cardiac, vascular, and respiratory regulation. Cerebellar lesions can produce hypotension or hypertension.

Some lesions cause a syndrome of autonomic over-activity (*autonomic storm*) by releasing the hypothalamus from inhibitory cortical control. Examples of central nervous system lesions that may be associated with autonomic storm include subarachnoid and intracerebral hemorrhage, head trauma, cerebral infarction, tumors, meningitis, increased intracranial pressure, and extensive white matter diseases.

Various thermoregulatory, vasomotor, sudomotor, genitourinary, and gastrointestinal abnormalities reflect the anatomic distribution of spinal cord lesions. Spinal cord lesions above the T5 segment produce orthostatic hypotension because spinal sympathetic efferent fibers to the large splanchnic vascular bed are not activated when blood pressure falls. In some cases, however, specially with lesions above the C6 segments that free local vascular reflexes from central autonomic nervous system control, massive release of norepinephrine occurs in response to viscus distention and noxious stimuli. In this situation, there is severe hypertension, diaphoresis, and piloerection (autonomic storm), probably as a result of denervation supersensitivity and lack of baroreflex compensation. Patients with lesions below the midthoracic spinal segments are usually spared from autonomic storm because they have relatively intact splanchnic sympathetic function. High spinal cord lesions that interrupt cardiac sympathetic innervation can result in severe bradycardia and cardiac standstill during maneuvers that produce vagal activation, such as tracheal stimulation (e.g., intubation and suctioning). High cord lesions produce upper motor neuron bladder dysfunction in which bladder volumes are small and the detrusor muscle is overactive. Complete destruction of the cord below the T12 segment results in lower motor neuron bladder dysfunction with distention and overflow incontinence. A similar presentation occurs with destruction of the sacral cord, anterior roots, or peripheral nerves, but in this situation, bladder and sacral sensation are spared. Acute cord lesions that produce spinal shock and lesions that affect the sacral parasympathetic innervation of the gut result in fecal retention. Autonomous lower bowel function may be restored in the chronic phases. High cervical cord lesions may result in poilkilothermia-like states (some patients require stable-temperature air-conditioned environments). Autonomic dysfunction in multiple sclerosis (hypohidrosis of the body with compensatory hyperhidrosis of the face and neck) may be associated with lesions at the level of the spinal cord.

Hypertension

Chronic hypertension may result and be maintained in part from the effects of sympathetic overactivity. Sympathetic overactivity may cause increased vasoconstriction, trophic effects on blood vessels, and retention of sodium ion (Na+) by the kidney. Increased sympathetic tone also stimulates the release of epinephrine from the adrenal glands, which in turn, further increase the release of norepinephrine through prejunctional stimulation in a positive feedback loop (this mechanism may also be a cause of sustained hypertension in pheochromocytoma).

In *essential hypertension*, the role of enhanced sympathetic activity, with its trophic effects on blood vessel smooth muscle, appears to be more significant in early rather than later stages when cardiac and vascular smooth muscle hypertrophy are already present. Sympathetic nerve activity and plasma norepinephrine concentrations are also increased in insulin resistance with hyperinsulinemia.

The release of endothelium-derived vasoactive factors, regulated in part by the autonomic nervous system, appears to play an important role in chronic hypertension. Indeed, endothelium-derived nitric oxide, which is the major determinant of vascular tone (and blood pressure) under physiologic conditions, has been reported to be decreased in some forms of hypertension. The role of endothelin-1, a powerful vasoconstrictor with mitogenic effects on blood vessels, remains to be established. Evidence suggests that autonomically mediated hypertension results from a complex interplay between neural, endothelial, and hormonal factors.

Dysfunction of the baroreflex may result in hypertension or hypotension. Baroreflex failure, a condition of unknown cause in which there is marked blood pressure lability accompanied by inappropriate heart rate responses that may last up to several days, may be easily confused with pheochromocytoma because catecholamine levels may be elevated.

Cerebral and spinal cord lesions can present with acute hypertension (e.g., in the setting of autonomic storm) by interrupting certain autonomic nervous system pathways.

Hyperthermia

Hyperthermia occurs when normal or defective heat loss mechanisms are overwhelmed by heat production or exposure to excessive ambient temperatures. Exertional hyperthermia (during vigorous exercise when heat production is maximal) manifests as muscle cramps and heat exhaustion, which may progress to heat stroke when central temperatures rise above 41°C and is accompanied by an acute onset of an encephalopathy. Hypotension; tachycardia; and fluid, electrolyte, and metabolic derangements are usually present. Muscle enzymes are elevated if rhabdomyolysis occurs. Exertional heat stroke usually occurs in young and healthy individuals who exert themselves excessively (sometimes wearing heavy clothing) or have poor physical conditioning, are not acclimated to high ambient temperatures and humidity, and are dehydrated. Classic heat stroke, on the other hand, usually occurs in the very young or elderly and results from exposure to high ambient temperatures. Risk factors include underlying illness, immobility, use of medication (with anticholinergic and vasoconstrictor effects and diuretics), dehydration, and habitation in poorly ventilated dwellings. The mortality rate from heat stroke is as high as 10 percent despite optimal treatment.

Hyperthermia may occur as a result of cerebral lesions that affect thermoregulatory pathways (e.g., lesions in the region of the tuber cinereum). *Central fever* without recognizable causative hypothalamic lesions may be due to the effects of various local and circulating thermogenic factors. Before reaching a diagnosis of central fever, more common causes of fever and the presence of defective peripheral heat loss mechanisms should be excluded.

Hyperthermia and autonomic dysfunction together with movement disorders (usually rigidity) and encephalopathy are present in the *neuroleptic malignant syndrome*. Severe forms are accompanied by metabolic derangements and failure of multiple organs. The use of neuroleptics, tricyclic antidepressants, lithium, cocaine, and amphetamines with other agents and the withdrawal of antiparkinson medication have been linked to this disorder. The treatment of this syndrome includes withdrawal of offending drugs and the administration of dopaminergic agents (e.g., bromocriptine) and muscle relaxants (e.g., dantrolene).

Dopamine β-Hydroxylase Deficiency

In dopamine β-hydroxylase deficiency, there is diffuse sympathetic autonomic dysfunction because of the patient's inability to convert dopamine to norepinephrine. The diagnosis of this rare congenital disorder is made by finding low norepinephrine levels together with abnormally elevated dopamine plasma concentrations. At birth, patients may be hypothermic and have delayed eye opening, hypoglycemia, and hypotension. In adulthood, there may be severe orthostatic hypotension, ptosis, defects in sweating, and retrograde ejaculation. Treatment of this deficiency involves administering L-threo-DOPS, a nonphysiologic precursor of norepinephrine, which is decarboxylated to norepinephrine by neuronal dopa decarboxylase to bypass the enzymatic defect.

TREATMENT OF AUTONOMIC NERVOUS SYSTEM DYSFUNCTION

Orthostatic Hypotension

Because treatment of the underlying cause of autonomic dysfunction is not usually possible, the clinician's efforts should be directed at treating the patient's symptoms. This is particularly important when orthostatic hypotension is treated, in which the symptoms rather than the blood pressure values should be followed to assess the patient's response. Indeed, in many patients with chronic autonomic failure, effective cerebral perfusion occurs with remarkably low arterial pressures as a result of an adaptation of cerebral autoregulation. In these patients, even modest increases in systemic blood pressure are sufficient to reduce orthostatic symptoms.

The objectives of treatment are to increase upright brain perfusion by (1) reducing venous pooling in the lower body and splanchnic circulations and through (2) volume expansion. Altered circadian blood pressure rhythms and the effects of meals on blood pressure should be taken into account when treatment of orthostatic hypotension is planned in patients with autonomic failure. For example, in such patients with autonomic failure, blood pressure is lowest in the early morning and increases as the day goes on to reach a maximum at night, and the blood pressure may decrease after meals, exercise, and alcohol intake. This also should be kept in mind when the effects of treatment are assessed.

As a general guideline, nonpharmacologic treatment should be instituted first; if this is not effective in relieving symptoms, pharmacologic therapy should be added. Patients should avoid maneuvers and environments that lower blood pressure and make orthostatic symptoms worse, such as exercise, straining, and standing up suddenly; warm weather; and hot baths. Antihypertensive agents such as diuretics and α-adrenoceptor blocking and psychotherapeutic drugs should be avoided. When postprandial hypotension is present, smaller and more frequent meals with a lower carbohydrate content and institution of postprandial recumbent rest periods are effective measures that reduce postprandial blood pressure falls. Caffeine (two cups of coffee or 250 mg) in the morning and after lunch helps to prevent postprandial blood pooling in the gut circulation.

Initial treatment strategies aimed at decreasing venous pooling and increasing extracellular fluid volume should also combat the effects of physical deconditioning caused by recumbency and inactivity. Patients should be instructed to perform maneuvers such as squatting, bending over, crossing the legs, and assuming a knee-chest position, which by increasing venous return and by lowering the head, have an immediate effect in reducing symptoms because they produce small but useful increases in systemic blood pressure. Elevating the upper body by head-up body tilting during the night (12-inch blocks placed under the feet at the head of the bed) has been shown to increase blood pressure and orthostatic tolerance during the day in those patients with autonomic failure that retain the ability to secrete renin (i.e., have intact pressure-volume diuresis mechanisms). The decrease in renal artery pressure produced by the upright posture stimulates the release of renin from the juxtaglomerular apparatus of the kidney and promotes increased intravascular volume through angiotensin and aldosterone effects. A head-up tilt at night also decreases the excessive nocturnal diuresis and sodium loss in these patients.

Moderate exercise training (if tolerated) is beneficial because it may result in an increase in extracellular fluid volume and an increase muscle tone, which improves the pumping action of limb and abdominal muscles (vis a tergo). This is particularly useful when carried out in a swimming pool with special support to allow upright underwater leg movement. External compression garments, such as elastic stockings and abdominal binders, although an effective short-term remedy, have the potential to depress compensatory neurohumoral responses and lower abdominal muscle tone and may, in the long term, be counterproductive.

When nonpharmacologic measures and coffee fail, fludrocortisone acetate is used in conjunction with nocturnal head-up tilt as an initial pharmacologic treatment of orthostatic hypotension. Fludrocortisone acetate has two effects, depending on the doses used. At low doses (less than 0.1 mg/day), it produces a rise in blood pressure by an increase in peripheral resistance. This effect is thought to be due to increased sensitivity of vascular adrenoceptors to circulating norepinephrine and to increased rigidity of arteriolar walls. At higher doses (more than 0.1 mg/day), it also promotes extracellular fluid volume expansion. If a combination of physical maneuvers and fludrocortisone acetate are not sufficient to control disabling orthostatic symptoms, a variety of drugs may be added in an attempt to increase blood pressure by increasing extracellular fluid volume and vascular resistance (Table 62-4). The α-adrenoceptor agonists increase blood pressure by increasing peripheral resistance. Not infrequently, sympathomimetics are poorly tolerated because of their side effects (e.g., anxiety, tremor, and insomnia). The vasoconstrictor effect of prostaglandin synthetase inhibitors is attributed to decreased formation of vasodilatory prostaglandins. The β-blockers are reported to decrease postural hypotension by blocking vascular α-2-adrenoceptors, which produce vasodilatation. Yohimbine, by antagonizing central (and perhaps peripheral) α-2-adrenoceptors, enhances sympathetic efferent activity, increasing blood pressure in patients with autonomic failure. In those patients with autonomic failure and orthostatic hypotension who have symptomatic postprandial hypotension, the synthetic vasopressin and somatostatin

Table 62-4. Treatment of Neurogenic Orthostatic Hypotension

Objective	Mechanism	Drug/Intervention
Expand blood volume	Stimulate renin release	Head-up tilt
	Mineralocorticoid effects	Fludrocortisone (>0.1 mg/day) + dietary salt
	Antidiuretic effects (V_2 agonist)	Desmopressin
	↑ Red cell mass	Erythropoietin
		Interval hypoxic training
Enhance vasoconstriction	↑ α-Adrenoceptor sensitivity	Fludrocortisone (<0.1 mg/day)
	α-Agonists	Phenylpropranolamine, ephedrine, methylphenidate, tyramine, ergotamine, midodrine
	α_2-Antagonists	Yohimbine
	Norepinephrine precursors	L-threo-DOPS
	β-Antagonists	Propranolol, pindolol, xamoterol
	Dopamine antagonists	Metoclopramide
	Gut vasodilatory peptide antagonists[a]	Octreotide
	Adenosine antagonists[a]	Caffeine
	Vasodilatory prostaglandin antagonists[a]	Indomethacin, ibuprofen

Abbreviations: DA, dopamine; NA, norepinephrine; DDAVP, desmopressin; L-threo-DOPS, l-3, 4-dihydroxyphenylserine; V_2, vasopressin receptor; ↑, increased.

[a] Suited for treatment of postprandial hypotension.

analogues desmopressin and octreotide may be used to prevent regional extracellular fluid volume shifts seen during the night and after meals. Caffeine, perhaps by inhibiting the vasodilation produced by adenosine, helps in ameliorating postprandial hypotension. Metoclopramide is thought to improve orthostatic hypotension through inhibition of the vasodilatory and natriuretic effects of dopamine. Recently, erythropoietin, a growth factor, has been reported to be effective in increasing blood pressure in patients with hypotension caused by autonomic dysfunction. A similar effect can be obtained by hypoxic interval training, a method used to increase erythropoietin by intermittent short-term hypoxia. Administration of L-threo-DOPS, a synthetic amino acid precursor of norepinephrine, is the treatment of choice in dopamine β-hydroxylase deficiency because it bypasses the enzymatic defect. In patients with MSA, this agent may increase blood pressure through a central effect by increasing vasoconstrictor sympathetic outflow to muscle.

Supine hypertension, which results from the added effects of baroreceptor reflex dysfunction, denervation supersensitivity, and hypertensive drug therapy, is present in many patients. Blood pressure should be monitored closely because severe supine hypertension, particularly in the evening, may result in intracerebral and retinal hemorrhage. Even mildly elevated supine blood pressure may contribute to excessive nocturnal polyuria and sodium loss and aggravate orthostatic blood pressure falls present in the morning. Usually, preventing recumbency and elevating the

head are sufficient to prevent complications from supine hypertension. Some patients control the tendency to have supine hypertension by having an alcoholic drink at bedtime, but others require antihypertensive agents before going to sleep. Over-the-counter medications such as sympathomimetic-containing eye drops, diet pills, and cold remedies should be avoided because they may precipitate hypertension as a result of denervation supersensitivity in some patients. For this reason also, when treating bladder dysfunction, α-agonists should be used with extreme caution. Patients with autonomic failure are at high risk during anesthesia because of exaggerated vasodilation in response to anesthetic drugs, supersensitivity to pressor agents, and the inability of baroreflex mechanisms to counteract decreases in venous return (and blood pressure) produced by positive pressure ventilation. For these reasons, invasive hemodynamic monitoring with pulmonary capillary wedge pressure determinations is indicated during general anesthesia.

Neurocardiogenic Syncope

The treatment of hypotension caused by recurrent neurocardiogenic (or vasovagal) syncope poses a problem because of the sporadic nature of this syndrome and the lack of experimental data regarding the effectiveness of different treatments. Low doses of β-adrenoceptor blocking agents are thought to prevent recurrences of neurocardiogenic syncope by "blunting" the sympathetically mediated increase in myocardial contractility and resulting mechanoreceptor discharges that trigger syncope. In addition, inhibition of β-adrenoceptor-induced vasodilation counteracts dependent venous pooling. Fludrocortisone acetate, by increasing extracellular fluid volume and sensitizing adrenoceptors to the vasoconstrictor effect of catecholamines, is effective in some cases. In small studies, α-adrenoceptor agonists have been reported to prevent recurrence of neurocardiogenic syncope. Theophylline, which is thought to act by blocking adenosine receptors, has been reported to decrease the rate of recurrence of neurocardiogenic syncope when given in low doses. Cardiac pacing is not effective in preventing neurocardiogenic syncope, confirming the minor role of bradycardia as a cause of hypotension in this syndrome. Furthermore, an increase in heart rate in the setting of low right atrial pressure can further decrease filling pressures and will not be effective in increasing cardiac output.

Genitourinary Dysfunction

Treatment of urinary dysfunction includes catheterization and anticholinergic and sympathomimetic medication, depending on the pathophysiology and severity of the symptoms. Measurement of bladder volumes is valuable to guide treatment of urinary retention. Intermittent catheterization is helpful when residual volumes of more than 100 ml are present. In general, volumes should be kept below 500 ml. If residual urinary volume is approximately 300 ml, catheterization is done three times a day; if more than 400 to 500 ml, catheterization is done more frequently. In those with advanced illness, permanent catheterization or the use of a urosheath is necessary. Drugs with anticholinergic effects are helpful in treating detrusor hyperreflexia (e.g., propantheline) but can result in urinary retention. Cholinergic agents are not helpful in improving bladder contractility in autonomic failure. Urinary leakage (a characteristic finding in multiple system atrophy with autonomic failure caused by inability to contract the distal urethra) frequently requires catheterization. Although α-adrenoceptor agonists increase urethral resistance, they should be avoided in patients with syndromes of generalized autonomic failure in which there is a risk of hypertensive crises as a result of denervation supersensitivity. Nocturnal head-up tilt and, when ineffective, addition of nasal desmopressin spray reduce the nocturnal polyuria present in many patients with autonomic failure.

Erectile impotence can be treated with intracorporeal injections of vasodilator drugs such as papaverine (alone or together with α-adrenoceptor blockers such as phentolamine) or prostaglandin E₁. Additional treatment modalities include a variety of penile prostheses. There are no satisfactory practical treatments for neurogenic ejaculatory failure.

Gastrointestinal Dysfunction

Hydrophyilic colloids and bulk-forming agents are used as a first line of treatment in diabetic gastroparesis. If these are ineffective, prokinetic agents such as domperidone and metoclopramide (given before meals and at bedtime) accelerate gastric emptying after meals (through a local effect), relieving gastroparesis and constipation. Metoclopramide also inhibits vomiting (through a central effect). Cisapride, which enhances local release of acetylcholine from myenteric plexus neurons, appears to increase gut contractility and decrease transit time in gastroparesis and intestinal pseudo-obstruction. Erythromycin accelerates gastric emptying by stimulating gut motilin receptors. Broad-spectrum antibiotics (tetracycline, doxycycline, metronidazole, or ampicillin) may be used to treat diarrhea when bacterial overgrowth is suspected as a cause. Octreotide, a somatostatin analogue that inhibits the release of gut neuropeptides, has been reported to increase gut transit and improve abdominal distention in patients with diabetic diarrhea, intestinal pseudo-obstruction, and bacterial overgrowth.

Autonomic Storm

Various disorders, including neuropathies (e.g., Landry-Guillain-Barré syndrome, porphyria, and diphtheria), tetanus, delirium tremens, and central nervous system lesions can, by disturbing autonomic pathways, result in a syndrome of acute autonomic overactivity (autonomic storm). In this syndrome, hypertension, tachycardia, sweating, and pallor and massive release of catecholamines into the circulation may be accompanied by subendocardial damage and cardiac arrhythmia, neurogenic pulmonary edema, and cerebral and retinal hemorrhages. In some instances, severe bradycardia is present due to uncontrolled parasympathetic outflow.

Intensive monitoring and aggressive management of hypertension using nitrovasodilators and α-adrenoceptor-blocking agents may be required. Treatment of severe neurogenic pulmonary edema includes ventilatory support, oxygen supplementation, and measures aimed at treating the underlying cause (e.g., reducing intracranial pressure with cerebral mass lesions). Patients with high thoracic spinal cord lesions in whom sympathetic storm develops may require a combination of local anesthetics (to block excessive afferent stimulation), ganglion or α-adrenoceptor blockers, and anticholinergic drugs to control symptoms. In many cases, however, identifying and eliminating precipitating factors (e.g., visceral and cutaneous stimulation) results in prompt resolution and prevention of autonomic storm.

Hyperthermia

The treatment of hyperthermia involves cooling of the body and, in many instances, intensive supportive care. Cooling is best achieved by evaporation of water sprayed on the body by fanning with warm air (warm air spray). Cold water immersion appears to be less effective than warm air spray, perhaps because of increased cutaneous vasoconstriction. Massaging the limbs helps by increasing skin circulation. Phenothiazines can be used to reduce shivering that may occur during cooling. The β-adrenoceptor agonists (isoproterenol) should be used to treat hypotension rather than α-adrenoceptor agonists because these cause cutaneous vasoconstriction and thus limit heat loss. Seizures should be treated with diazepam.

Essential Hyperhidrosis

Treatment of essential hyperhidrosis involves local measures to avoid maceration and infection and decrease sweating. If axillary sweating is severe and disabling enough despite topical aluminum chloride hexahydrate (20 percent) treatment, sweat gland excision and T2–T3 sympathectomy (the definitive treatment) may be considered. Palmar and plantar hyperhidrosis usually responds to tap water iontophoresis. Biofeedback has been reported to be useful in some instances of essential hyperhidrosis.

ANNOTATED BIBLIOGRAPHY

Appenzeller O. The Autonomic Nervous System. An Introduction to Basic and Clinical Concepts. 4th Ed. Elsevier, Amsterdam, 1990.

Standard text.

Appenzeller O. Peripheral autonomic neuropathies. In Robertson D, Biaggioni I (eds). Disorders of the Autonomic Nervous System. Vol. 13. Churchill Livingstone, London, 1995

Review chapter.

Bannister R, Mathias CJ (eds). Autonomic Failure. A Textbook of Clinical Disorders of the Autonomic Nervous System. 3rd Ed. Oxford University Press, Oxford, 1992.

Textbook.

Cortelli P, Parchi P, Contin M et al. Cardiovascular dysautonomia in fatal familial insomnia. Clin Auton Res 1991; 1:15–21.

Details in two cases.

Costa C, Duyckaerts C, Cervera P, Hauw JJ. Les inclusions oligodendrogliales: un marquer de atrophies multisystématisées. Rev Neurol (Paris) 1992;148:284–280.

Argyrophilic oligodendroglial inclusions in sporadic OPCAs.

Cowley AW Jr. Long-term control of arterial blood pressure. Physiol Rev 1992;72:231–300.

Lengthy review.

Cryer PE. Iatrogenic hypoglycemia as a cause of hypoglycemia-associated autonomic failure in IDDM. A vicious cycle. Diabetes 1992;41:255–60.

Three syndromes described.

Eckberg DL, Sleight P. Human Baroreflexes in Health and Disease. Oxford University Press, Oxford, 1992.

Textbook.

Freeman R, Miyawaki E. The treatment of autonomic dysfunction. J Clin Neurophysiol 1993;10:61–82.

Review article.

Freeman R, Saul JP, Roberts MS et al. Spectral analysis of heart rate in diabetic autonomic neuropathy. Arch Neurol 1991;48:185–90.

Studies on 15 patients showed a usefulness of power-spectral analysis.

Hoeldtke RD, Streeten DHP. Treatment of orthostatic hypotension with erythropoietin. N Engl J Med 1993;329: 611–5.

Benefits using 50 units/kg three times a week for 6 to 10 weeks.

Kaufmann H, Oribe E, Miller M et al. Hypotension-induced vasopressin release distinguishes between pure autonomic failure and multiple system atrophy with autonomic failure. Neurology 1992;42:590.

Lipsitz LA. Orthostatic hypotension in the elderly. N Engl J Med 1989;321:952–7.

Review article.

Low PA (ed). Clinical Autonomic Disorders. Evaluation and Management. Little, Brown, Boston, 1993.

Textbook.

Robertson D. Orthostatic hypotension. In Melmon KL, Morelli H (eds). Clinical Pharmacology. McGraw-Hill, New York, 1992, p. 84.

Standard text.

63

Amyotrophic Lateral Sclerosis and Related Diseases

Lewis P. Rowland

AMYOTROPHIC LATERAL SCLEROSIS

Definition and Terminology

Motor neuron diseases (plural) consist of several different disorders that are characterized by degeneration and loss of motor neurons. *Motor neuron disease* (singular) is the adult-onset form and, in turn, includes several different syndromes. *Amyotrophic lateral sclerosis* (ALS) includes both upper and lower motor signs. *Progressive spinal muscular atrophy* (PMSA) is manifested by lower motor neuron signs alone. *Primary lateral sclerosis* includes upper motor neuron signs alone. *Motor neuropathy* is defined by finding slow motor nerve conduction velocity or block of conduction in physiologic tests. In most countries, motor neuron disease and ALS are equivalent terms, encompassing spinal muscular atrophy but not the neuropathies or lateral sclerosis. The cause and pathogenesis are unknown, except for heritable forms and rare conditions from intoxication with lead (see Ch. 72), accidental lightning strikes (see Ch. 31), radiotherapy (see Ch. 58), and paraneoplastic syndromes (see Ch. 54). This section is concerned only with the adult-onset forms. Childhood spinal muscular atrophy is usually inherited.

Epidemiology

ALS occurs worldwide at roughly the same prevalence of about 50 per 100,000. On the Pacific island of Guam, the incidence was originally much higher than any other place in the world, but with modernization and changing environment, the disease has become less common, reaching the levels seen elsewhere. Risk factors were not identified reproducibly in Guam or elsewhere. A local plant, the cycad, was suspected of

containing an excitatory neurotoxin but that was not substantiated.

Men are affected more often than women in ratios of 1.5 to 3.0 to 1. There is an increasing frequency with rising age until age 80, when there is a fall-off. Only 5 percent of cases appear before age 30. An adolescent form is rare in most countries but is seen more often in Tunisia, where it is an autosomal recessive trait. A familial form maps to chromosome 21 at the site of the gene for superoxide dismutase.

Pathology

The hallmark of the disease is degeneration and loss of motor neurons in the cerebral cortex, motor nuclei of the brainstem, and anterior horn cells of the spinal cord. Inclusion bodies may be seen, but not consistently. If the upper motor neurons are affected, there is degeneration of the corticospinal tracts in the spinal cord. Sensory tracts are usually spared.

Clinical Manifestations

By definition, patients with motor neuron disease must show lower motor neuron signs (weakness, wasting, and fasciculation). If there are also upper motor neuron signs, the syndrome is properly called ALS. If there are Babinski signs or clonus, there is no doubt that upper motor neuron signs are present. If these signs are lacking, most experienced clinicians regard the presence of active tendon jerks in a limb with wasted, twitching muscles as an upper motor neuron sign. However, this has become a point of uncertainty because some patients with motor neuropathy show this combination.

In general, patients with ALS account for 90 percent of all patients with motor neuron disease. Those with purely lower motor neuron or purely upper motor neuron disorders are equally infrequent, and some experts consider them different diseases. However, more than one-half of adult patients with spinal muscular atrophy show degeneration of the corticospinal tracts at autopsy (which is the reason PSMA is considered a form of ALS and not a separate disease). Primary lateral sclerosis is considered below.

Progressive bulbar palsy is another traditional classification, which is the name for a syndrome of dysarthria and dysphagia resulting from a lower motor neuron disorder that is manifest by wasting of the tongue and loss of the pharyngeal reflex. This term, however, is losing favor because almost all patients with dysarthria and dysphagia also show fasciculations in limb muscles or overactive reflexes and Babinski's signs. That is, they already have signs of ALS.

There are two main categories of symptoms: weakness or spastic gait. Weakness may commence in the arms or hands first and then involve the legs, the legs may come first, or there may be dysarthria, usually accompanied later by dysphagia. Ultimately, all limbs are affected. Spastic gait disorder may be the first symptom.

The signs conform to the symptoms. That is, limb weakness is accompanied by wasting and fasciculations (see Ch. 22). Dysarthria is accompanied by scalloping of the margins of the tongue and fasciculations are seen at the margins or dorsum. Whether tendon jerks are present or absent depends on the balance of the lower and upper motor neuron pathologic findings. Babinski's sign may be present even when knee and ankle jerks cannot be elicited, and it may be absent if the great toe is paralyzed. Other common early manifestations are muscle cramps and weight loss.

As the disease progresses, there is increasing disability from loss of hand functions, inability to walk, loss of independence in activities of daily living, malnutrition from dysphagia, and finally, inability to breathe without support. Eye movements and autonomic functions are spared unless life is prolonged for years by mechanical ventilation. Then there may be ophthalmoplegia and urinary sphincter problems.

If there is bilateral involvement of the corticospinal tracts, there may be the syndrome of *pseudobulbar palsy* in addition to the lower motor neuron signs of true palsy. This combination is seen in only a few patients. The upper motor neuron lesions are identified by emotional lability (inappropriate laughing and crying) in combination with a more vigorous response of the uvula in the pharyngeal reflex (gag reflex) than on volitional innervation. There may also be snout and jaw reflexes and upper motor neuron signs in the limbs. There is no sensory loss, a clinical hallmark for ALS.

Dementia and parkinsonism appear in some pa-

tients. Familial ALS is similar, except for a slightly younger age at onset and sometimes longer duration.

Prognosis

The mean duration of symptoms is about 4 years, with extremes from 6 months to 25 years. About 20 percent of patients live longer than 5 years. A poor prognosis is associated with advancing age at onset, bulbar symptoms, and respiratory failure. It is difficult to predict survival in an individual patient, and for ethical reasons, no patient should be told that he or she "has 6 months to live."

Diagnosis

The clinical diagnosis of ALS is usually accurate because there is no other condition that causes the unique combination of upper and lower motor neuron signs. There are few other conditions in which widespread fasciculation is evident. The main problems now are cervical spondylotic myelopathy and multifocal motor neuropathy with conduction block.

Cervical spondylotic myelopathy can cause spastic paraplegia with no sensory loss. Whether it can also cause widespread fasciculation in the arms with wasted hands is widely believed but may not be correct; 5 to 10 percent of all patients with ALS have had cervical laminectomies that did not arrest progression of the disease. The syndrome of "numb clumsy hands" helps to identify spondylosis. As a general rule, there should be some sensory loss to make the diagnosis of spondylotic myelopathy.

Motor neuropathy with conduction block is difficult to identify clinically but progresses more slowly, is more likely to affect the hands first, and is more often grossly asymmetric. The patients are apt to be younger and the disease more slowly progressive. The defining and required feature is evidence of multiple conduction blocks in physiologic studies. About 75 percent of these patients have antibodies to the ganglioside GM1. The condition is important to recognize because it responds to treatment with immunosuppressive drugs or intravenous immunoglobulin therapy.

Myasthenia gravis is another major cause of dysarthria and dysphagia, but fasciculations identify ALS. Ophthalmoplegia is common in myasthenia but exceptional in ALS.

Benign fasciculation is important to recognize; motor neuron disease is almost never manifested as fasciculation without accompanying weakness. Cramps are frequent in patients with benign fasciculation, a combination called the Denny-Brown, Foley syndrome.

Pseudobulbar palsy can be caused by multiple sclerosis, or bilateral strokes, as well as ALS. Patients with pseudobulbar palsy in motor neuron disease, by definition, also show fasciculation in the tongue or limbs; these lower motor neuron signs are not seen in other conditions. History, examination, and where necessary, magnetic resonance imaging (MRI) help to differentiate these syndromes, which are only rarely the source of diagnostic confusion.

Laboratory Studies

There is no pathognomonic laboratory test for ALS. Electromyography is needed to bolster the clinical diagnosis by showing signs of denervation in at least three limbs. Nerve conduction velocity is usually normal; slowing or block of conduction identifies motor neuropathy. The cerebrospinal fluid is usually normal in ALS except for a protein content of 50 to 75 mg/dl; values higher than 75 mg/dl may increase the likelihood of monoclonal paraproteinemia, which is found in about 10 percent of all cases. Antibodies to ganglioside GM1 are found in about 10 percent of patients with motor neuron disease, not only those with motor neuropathy; very high titers seem less frequent in patients with definite upper motor neuron signs.

Treatment

There is no known treatment that arrests the progression of ALS but immunosuppressive therapy or intravenous immunoglobulin therapy may reverse motor neuropathy with conduction block. Failed agents include immunosuppressive drugs, gangliosides, plasmapheresis, antiglutamate regimens, selegiline, and nerve growth factors. That is why it is so important to identify motor neuropathy with conduction block, which may simulate motor neuron disease clinically but can be reversed by immunosuppressive drug therapy or intravenous immunoglobulin therapy.

Symptomatic treatment is often effective, directed first to maintaining function in occupation and activities of daily living. Posterior leaf orthoses assist walking when there is foot-drop. Special tools can aid in eating and dressing. Communication aids vary from pointing boards to voice-activated computers. Anticonvulsant drugs can relieve cramps but are rarely accepted by patients. Gastrostomy may be needed to maintain nutrition. The decision to use a tracheostomy is a major concern; once there is a tracheostomy, long-term use of a respirator is likely to follow. Patients should discuss a living will and views about resuscitation.

PRIMARY LATERAL SCLEROSIS

It is uncertain whether this disorder is a form of motor neuron disease or an independent disease, which cannot be proved even at autopsy. It is a diagnosis of exclusion, and in former days, it was a diagnosis to be eschewed because compressive lesions could not be excluded until an autopsy was performed. Now, however, there are better tests for multiple sclerosis, and MRI can evaluate the possibility of compressive lesions, syringomyelia, or Chiari malformation.

The condition begins after age 40 with a spastic gait. There is no weakness of leg muscles, but alternating movements and skilled movements are impaired in the feet. The arms and hands may be similarly but less severely affected, and there may be pseudobulbar palsy. By definition, there are upper motor neuron signs in all cases: overactive reflexes, Hoffmann's and Babinski's signs, clonus. There is no sensory loss, and the sphincters are usually spared.

Laboratory Tests

The most common cause of isolated spastic paraparesis in middle life is multiple sclerosis. Therefore, tests must include MRI with gadolinium of brain and cervical spinal cord. Cerebrospinal fluid analysis, including oligoclonal bands and gamma globulin synthesis, and evoked responses for vision, hearing, and somatic sensation. As indicated earlier, MRI also evaluates cervical spondylosis, extramedullary tumors, or malformations. Rare causes are excluded by measurement of very long chain fatty acids (for adrenoleukodystrophy) and titers of human T-cell lymphotropic virus type I antibodies (for tropical spastic paraplegia) (see Ch. 31).

Prognosis

Although ALS ought theoretically to start as primary lateral sclerosis, this is rarely seen, even when electromyelography shows evidence of lower motor neuron disease that is not seen clinically. It is exceptional for primary lateral sclerosis to be the first stage of ALS. Most patients with primary lateral sclerosis live more than 10 years. Treatment is symptomatic.

SPINAL MUSCULAR ATROPHY OF CHILDHOOD

Autosomal recessive motor neuron diseases of childhood have been the subject of heated debates about classification. It is convenient to consider three types. The infantile or Werdnig-Hoffman type is manifest before age 6 months and is fatal in about 85 percent of patients before age 2 years. The survivors do not walk. A childhood form begins later, and the children usually walk. This form is compatible with a long life, but there may be progression and loss of ability to walk. A juvenile type is also called the Kugelberg-Welander syndrome. Here, proximal limb weakness begins late in childhood or in adolescence.

The clinical features are similar in all three groups

but vary in severity and the age at onset. In Werdnig-Hoffmann disease, the limbs are flail and areflexic. Fasciculation is seen only in the tongue, not in the limbs. Respiration is affected within a few months in fatal cases. In later-onset syndromes, limb weakness is mostly proximal, resulting in waddling gait as the main disorder. Upper limb weakness may be mild or severe, and there are usually no bulbar signs. There is, however, a disorder in which dysphagia and dysarthria are the major manifestations (Fazio-Londe syndrome).

All three of the main forms map to chromosome 5 and seem to be allelic variants of the same disorder. The gene product has not yet been identified. Treatment is symptomatic.

ANNOTATED BIBLIOGRAPHY

Ben Hamida M, Hentati F, Hamida CB. Hereditary motor system disease (chronic juvenile amyotrophic lateral sclerosis). Brain 1990;113:347–63.

An exotic form of a juvenile form of ALS, studied well in Tunisia.

Brzustowicz LM, Lehner T, Castilla LH et al. Genetic mapping of chronic childhood-onset spinal muscular atrophy to chromosome 5q11.2-13.3. Nature 1990;344:520.

Historic paper mapping all three forms of childhood spinal muscular atrophy to the same gene on chromosome 5, indicating that they are allelic disorders.

Lange DJ, Trojaborg W, Latov N et al. Multifocal motor neuropathy with conduction block: is it a distinct clinical entity? Neurology 1992;42:497–505.

A study of the physiologic definition of conduction block, applied to a population of clinically different forms of motor neuron disease. Conduction block seems to be uncommon in patients with definite upper motor neuron signs.

Norris FH Jr. Adult progressive muscular atrophy and hereditary spinal muscular atrophies. Handbook Clin Neurol 1991;59:13–34.

A comprehensive review of pure lower motor neuron syndromes.

Pestronk A, Cornblath DR, Ilyas AA et al. A treatable multifocal motor neuropathy with antibodies to GM1 ganglioside. Ann Neurol 1988;24:73–8.

Not the first article to describe motor neuropathy with conduction block but the one that had prominent impact because the patients improved with cyclophosphamide therapy.

Pringle CE, Hudson AJ, Munoz DG et al. Primary lateral sclerosis. Clinical features, neuropathology, and diagnostic criteria. Brain 1992;115:495–520.

Review and analysis of a series of patients with purely upper motor neuron signs.

Rowland LP (ed). Amyotrophic Lateral Sclerosis and Other Motor Neuron Diseases. Raven Press, New York, 1991.

A comprehensive multiauthored review of cause, pathogenesis, epidemiology, manifestations, differential diagnosis, pathologic findings, and treatment of ALS and related syndromes.

Rowland LP. Surgical treatment of cervical spondylotic myelopathy: time for a controlled trial Neurology 1992;42:5–13.

A critical review of the literature indicates the problems of defining cervical spondylotic myelopathy, especially the differentiation from multiple sclerosis and ALS.

Smith RA (ed). Handbook of Amyotrophic Lateral Sclerosis. Marcel Dekker, New York, 1992.

A practical manual to guide clinicians in the management of patients with ALS.

Williams DB, Windebank AJ. Motor neuron disease (amyotrophic lateral sclerosis). Mayo Clin Proc 1991;66:54–82.

A comprehensive review of the modern literature.

Younger DS, Chou S, Hays AP et al. Primary lateral sclerosis. A clinical diagnosis reemerges. Neurology 1988;45:1304–7.

A statement of the modern recognition of primary lateral sclerosis, which has re-emerged as a legitimate clinical diagnosis because imaging of brain and spinal cord eliminates many structural lesions that might cause the syndrome and because cerebrospinal fluid analysis, MRI, and evoked responses can evaluate multiple sclerosis. Laboratory diagnosis is emphasized.

Younger DS, Rowland LP, Latov N et al. Lymphoma, motor neuron diseases, and amyotrophic lateral sclerosis. Ann Neurol 1991;29:78–86.

The association of ALS with lymphoma is rare, but the combination is no longer regarded as an accident.

64

Hereditary and Nonhereditary Ataxias and Hereditary Paraplegias

J. C. Gautier and J. P. Mohr

HEREDITARY AND NONHEREDITARY ATAXIAS

In clinical neurology, the term ataxia (Greek: *a-taxis,* without order) is restricted to disordered movements in the absence of weakness. Ataxia thus can result either from proprioceptive loss, cerebellar disease, or both (see Chs. 22 and 23). Peripheral disease, for example, tabes dorsalis, which was originally described as "ataxie locomotrice" by Duchenne de Boulogne (French neurologist, 1806–1875), or some polyneuropathies (Ch. 32) can cause ataxia.

By tradition, however, any chapter on hereditary and nonhereditary ataxias covers diseases in which the lesions are most obvious in the cerebellum, either on the cerebellar cells or on their axons in the cerebellipetal tracts in the spinal cord or brainstem. Within that cohort, lesions occur in quite a few other systems (e.g., the posterior columns of the spinal cord, the pigmented cells in the brainstem, and most often the corticospinal tracts). The whole group is a highly heterogeneous kaleidoscope of many diseases.

Although rare in adults, hereditary and nonhereditary ataxias are important in neurologic practice because they raise difficult problems of early diagnosis, prognosis, and in many cases, genetic counseling. Some of these disorders are hereditary, others are sporadic, and still others are due to toxins, deficiencies, or the remote effects of cancers. The box below outlines this broad classification, which in addition, points to the main differential diagnoses when such ataxias first occur in adulthood.

Congenital and Early-Onset Ataxias

Congenital ataxias and ataxias that occur in infancy are not within the scope of this book, but to give the reader a basis for further information, they are listed in the four boxes below. Detailed accounts of these rare diseases can be found in the book by A. E. Harding (1984). Those that allow survival into adolescence and adult age are briefly described here.

Several congenital ataxias are probably dysgenetic in origin. In very rare cases (e.g., in granule cell hypoplasia), survival into adulthood has been reported. In the diseases listed in in the second box, the ataxia is intermittent, presumably because it results from the accumulation of a noxious substance, such as ammonia. In some (e.g., in Hartnup disease), neurologic disorders can appear during adolescence. In others (e.g., Leigh's disease), rare adult cases have been reported. In still another group of hereditary ataxias, which is seen mainly in infants and children, the course of the disease is usually progressive (see box).

Abetalipoproteinemia (Bassen-Kornzweig Syndrome)

This autosomal recessive disorder has as its basic defect a lack of apolipoprotein of β-lipoproteins that carry chylomicrons and very low-density lipoproteins.

HEREDITARY AND NONHEREDITARY ATAXIAS

Hereditary
Sporadic
Toxic
    Alcohol
    Anticonvulsivant therapy
    Methyl bromide
Deficiencies
    Hypoparathyroidism
    Vitamin E deficiency
Paraneoplastic

CONGENITAL ATAXIAS

Joubert's syndrome
Granule cell hypoplasia
Pontoneocerebellar hypoplasia
Gillespie's syndrome
Dysequilibrium syndrome
Paine's syndrome
Unclassified cases ("ataxic cerebral palsy")

INTERMITTENT ATAXIAS WITH A
KNOWN METABOLIC DEFECT

With hyperammonemia and ornithine trans-
    carbamylase deficiency
        Citrullinemia
        Arginosuccinicaduria
        Arginase deficiency
        Hyperornithinemia
With aminoaciduria but no hyperammo-
    nemia
        Intermittent branched chain ketoaci-
            duria
        Isovaleric acidemia
        Hartnup disease
Pyruvate and lactate metabolic defects
        Pyruvate dehydrogenase deficiency
        Pyruvate carboxylase deficiency
        Subacute necrotizing encephalomyelo-
            pathy (Leigh's disease)
        Biotin-dependent carboxylase defects
        Mitochondriopathies

PROGRESSIVE ATAXIAS

Abetalipoproteinemia
Hypobetalipoproteinemia
Hexosaminidase deficiency
Cholestanolosis
Mitochondriopathies
Gamma glutamyl cysteine synthetase defi-
    ciency
Glutamate dehydrogenase deficiency
Partial hypoxanthine guanine phosphoribo-
    syl transferase deficiency
Ataxia telangiectasia
Xeroderma pigmentosum
Cockayne's syndrome

There is an associated severe deficit in fat-soluble vitamins. Some workers think it is probably the secondary
vitamin E deficiency that is mainly responsible for the
neurologic disorders (see Ch. 71).

The earliest symptom, steatorrhea, appears during
infancy, years before the neurologic dysfunction.
Neurologic symptoms and signs develop during childhood and are usually completed by the age of 20. The
earliest neurologic sign is areflexia. The full clinical
picture includes in addition ataxia, dysarthria, sensory
loss, pes cavus, and scoliosis, all features that resemble
Friedreich's ataxia (see below). Extensor plantar responses and external ophthalmoplegia may occur.
The patient's stature is short, probably a reflection of
the malabsorption syndrome. Night blindness caused
by pigmentary retinal degeneration, possibly related
to vitamin A deficiency, can antedate ataxia or be clinically absent.

The presence of acanthocytes (Greek: *acantha*,
thorn), that is, red blood cells with thornlike projections, is a major feature because of an abnormal lipid
content in the cell membrane. It should be noted that
acanthocytes are also present in adult-onset ataxic
neuropathy and in a few hereditary syndromes with
ataxia and involuntary movements in which serum
lipid levels are normal.

As the term abetalipoproteinemia implies, serum
levels of cholesterol, triglycerides, and free fatty acids
are very low. Chylomicrons can be absent. Additional
investigations include electroretinography, which can
detect preclinical retinopathy, and electromyography,
which shows low sensory action potentials and denervation as a result of peripheral neuropathy. A possible
cardiac involvement may be uncovered by cardiac
evaluation.

Large doses of vitamin E have been reported to slow
or arrest the progressive nervous disorders. Other fat-
soluble vitamins can be useful.

Hexosaminidase Deficiency

This defect causes accumulation of GM_2 gangliosides
in body tissues, including the brain. A few cases have
been reported in which ataxia, spasticity, dysarthria,
dysphagia, chorea, and distal wasting developed as
late as in the third decade.

Cholestanolosis or Cerebrotendinous Xanthomatosis

This is a rare disorder inherited in autosomal recessive
fashion, featuring the accumulation of cholestanol, a
metabolite of cholesterol, in the central nervous system and tendons. The basic metabolic defect is unknown.

Tendinous xanthomas, particularly in the Achilles
tendon, occur with zonular cataracts in childhood.
Ataxia, spasticity, and pseudobulbar palsy usually de-

velop as late as the second or third decade. Palatal myoclonus has been reported. There is often some degree of mental defect. A peripheral neuropathy can be associated. In the serum, the cholestanol level is high, but the cholesterol concentration is normal.

Ataxia Telangiectasia (Louis-Bar Syndrome)

This is a relatively frequent autosomal recessive disorder. This disease is explained by a gene defect that has been localized to chromosome 11q22-33 and is closely related to members of the immunoglobulin-gene superfamily. There is a brittleness and a defective repair of DNA.

Ataxia is obvious as soon as the infant walks. Later, choreoathetosis and dysarthria appear. The face becomes impassive. There is a peculiar disorder of gaze called oculomotor apraxia (see Ch. 28). Intellectual deterioration of variable degree is usually present.

The telangiectasias are made of a web of venules. They generally appear later than the ataxia, about age 5, first in the outer parts of the conjunctiva and then on the pinna, bridge of the nose, and cheeks (butterfly pattern) and creases of the skin at the elbow. There is growth retardation.

A major feature of ataxia telangiectasia is the profound immunologic disorder, affecting lymphocytes and immunoglobulins. The number of circulating lymphocytes is frequently reduced, the thymus is atrophic and lacks cortex and Hassall's corpuscles, and the lymph nodes lack follicles. Delayed hypersensitivity is absent or reduced. There is a deficiency in most types of immunoglobulins, which is particularly severe for immunoglobulin A. Patients are highly sensitive to infections and prone to develop malignancies.

Pathologically, there is a diffuse loss of Purkinje and granule cells and a loss of cells in the dorsal part of the inferior olive, substantia nigra, anterior horn, and sympathetic ganglia. In addition, there is degeneration of the posterior columns and spinocerebellar tracts.

Death usually occurs during the second or third decade of life as a result of bronchopulmonary infections or cancer, often lymphoma.

Xeroderma Pigmentosum

This is another rare autosomal recessive disorder in which cells are unduly sensitive to ultraviolet light and chemical carcinogens as a result of their inability to achieve excision repair of DNA. Cell death and mutations are consequently frequent.

This is primarily a skin disease with keratosis, telangiectasia, and a variety of skin cancers. The neurologic syndromes include microcephaly, mental retardation, and areflexia. Ataxia, choreoathetosis, spasticity, and peripheral neuropathy can appear later. A few cases

with mild neurologic deficits have been reported, and some patients can have a normal life expectancy.

Cockayne's Syndrome

This is usually so severe a disease that death occurs before age 20 years, but a few instances of late onset with a benign course have been reported.

Hereditary Ataxias in Adults

Those starting out in neurology are somewhat frustrated by the complexity of the hereditary ataxias in adults. It is probably in this part of neurology that a classification system seems to be most needed. Unfortunately, none that would be wholly satisfactory can yet be proposed because of a lack of insight into the causal processes.

Clinical classifications cannot account for the countless clinical variations of the many types of diseases. Pathologic classifications, once the "gold standard" in neurology, do not suffice either because the number of detailed studies is still small and most have reported a single case in a family. Furthermore, the lesions vary from case to case, even with a similar clinical picture and even in the same family. These nonuniform presentations reflect the well-known variable phenotypic expression of autosomal dominant genes.

It can be surmised that the hereditary ataxias in adults result from an inborn error of metabolism, but as yet, none has been firmly established. Progress in molecular genetics has already shed some light on a few clinical subtypes and more advances can reasonably be expected in the forthcoming years. It is hoped that such progress will have therapeutic consequences, which is particularly awaited in a field in which, for the time being, no effective therapy is available.

Granted that there is no current satisfactory classification, at least some effort at clarification can be gained by a chronologic review of the pioneer studies that are, as it were, successive pieces of the puzzle. This short historic review shows that the hereditary ataxias (1) cover a vast span from peripheral nerves to cerebral cortex with central core lesions in the spinal cord and cerebellum and (2) are intricate diseases (i.e., individual cases often show lesions that trespass the bounds of traditional "diseases" in that one patient can have lesions that pertain both to Friedreich's ataxia and Charcot-Marie-Tooth disease).

In this review, sporadic cases (Greek: *speirein,* to disperse) are also considered, namely, those cases that have no family history. This can result either from an inadequate family investigation or from a fresh mutation. Like those attributable to heredity, sporadic cases are due to an inborn error of metabolism, and they are truly inherited. Moreover, for each type of sporadic disease, there is a hereditary, obviously familial, counterpart.

Historic Review

In 1863, Nikolaus Friedreich (German neurologist, 1825–1882) first reported on a hereditary ataxia with onset around puberty. The bulk of the lesions affected the spinal cord, particularly Clarke's columns, the direct spinocerebellar tract, and the posterior columns. This is known as Friedreich's disease or Friedreich's ataxia (see below). It became obvious later that lesions of the peripheral nerves and corticospinal tract are often associated. The description of this disorder became a classic in clinical neurology, the recall of the elements of which has taxed the memories of generations of neurologists.

In 1886, J. M. Charcot (1825–1893) and Pierre Marie (1853–1940) in France and H. H. Tooth (1856–1925) in England described peroneal muscular atrophy, a heterogeneous group of hereditary diseases in which lesions mainly involve the peripheral nerves and roots (see Chs. 12 and 80). Members of the same family can have either Charcot-Marie-Tooth or Friedreich's disease.

In 1893, Pierre Marie grouped under the term of "hérédo-ataxie cérébelleuse," that is, hereditary cerebellar ataxia, cases that differed from Friedreich's disease chiefly by a later onset and retained or even brisk reflexes. The new and significant idea in Marie's concept was that the main lesions were presumed to be cerebellar. Marie stressed the probable heterogeneity of this group, and this was amply confirmed later. However, the term hereditary cerebellar ataxia is still used by many clinicians as a first working diagnosis.

In 1900, the French neurologists, J. Dejerine (1849–1917) and André-Thomas (1867–1962) reported two cases of sporadic olivopontocerebellar atrophy (OPCA) in which the main lesions involved the middle cerebellar peduncles and the inferior olives, that is, they affected the afferent (cerebellipetal) fibers to the cerebellum. OPCA is usually sporadic, but there is also a familial form first described by the German neurologist Menzel in 1891 in which, it must be noted, lesions of Friedreich's disease were also present. In the two cases described by Dejerine and Andre-Thomas, only one had a postmortem examination, and the spinal cord was not properly examined. This probably is the origin of the concept of the so-called "pure" OPCA, which is at least very rare.

Either sporadic or familial, OPCA is usually associated with various other lesions (e.g., of pigmented cells of the brainstem and of the spinal cord, such as the posterior columns, spinocerebellar tracts, corticospinal tracts, anterior horn cells, lateral horn cells, and sympathetic ganglia). These many and various associations are at the origin of the concept of multiple system atrophy.

Since OPCA is usually only a part of an intricate array of lesions, it has been cogently argued that it is no longer a useful clinical diagnosis. Most neurologists, however, have kept OPCA as a first working diagnosis inasmuch as magnetic resonance imaging (MRI) provides clear evidence of middle cerebellar atrophy of the pons and peduncles.

In 1921, J. Ramsay Hunt (American neurologist, 1872–1937) reported on six cases of a disease termed asynergia cerebellaris myoclonica: four single ones and two twin brothers, in which features of Friedreich's ataxia were later associated with myoclonus and epilepsy. The distinctive feature was atrophy of the dentate nucleus and superior cerebellar peduncle (dentatorubral atrophy). In members of a family with this syndrome, OPCA has been reported.

In 1922, Pierre Marie, Charles Foix (1882–1927), and T. Alajouanine (1890–1980) in France described four patients with a particular pattern of cerebellar atrophy. There was a loss of Purkinje cells restricted to or heavily predominant on the superior vermis and adjacent hemispheres. The cases were sporadic and of late onset. In 1907, G. M. Holmes (British neurologist, 1876–1965) described familial cases with the same pattern of atrophy and an early onset. In 1959, it was shown that lesions of the Marie-Foix-Alajouanine type are similar to those caused by alcoholic cerebellar degeneration.

In 1926, the French pathologist G. Roussy (1874–1948) and neurologist G. Lévy (1886–1935) reported on seven patients from a family with Friedreich's ataxia in whom tremor and distal wasting had developed with an early onset (hereditary areflexic dystasia). It is now known that instances of the Roussy-Lévy syndrome, Friedreich's, and Charcot-Marie-Tooth diseases can appear in members of the same family. It is generally considered that the Roussy-Lévy syndrome is a variant of a subtype of Charcot-Marie-Tooth disease (HHMSM type 1, see Ch. 80).

In 1938, a diffuse loss of Purkinje cells was identified by the Dutch neurologists Brouwer and Biemond and was related to the remote effects of cancers.

Friedreich's Ataxia

With a prevalence of 1 in 50,000, Friedreich's ataxia is the most common hereditary ataxias. It is usually autosomal, but many patients lack a family history. The responsible gene has been assigned to chromosome 9 without evidence of genetic heterogeneity.

Pathologically, there is loss of cells in Clarke's column with degeneration (i.e., demyelination fiber atrophy and replacement gliosis) in the spinocerebellar tracts, chiefly the direct (dorsal) one. There is also loss of cells in the dorsal root ganglia with degeneration of the posterior columns and distal degeneration of the corticospinal tract. Besides these essential or core lesions, there can be degeneration of the dentate nucleus and superior cerebellar peduncle and optic atrophy. In a few cases, there is loss of anterior horn cells, which makes a transition with Charcot-Marie-Tooth disease. There is often a cardiomyopathy.

Clinically, the disorders usually appear during the teen-age years first, with an ataxia of stance and gait, loss of ankle and knee jerks, loss of sense of position and vibration, Romberg's sign, and bilateral Babinski's sign. Dysarthria is constant later. After a few years, in the full-fledged picture, there is kyphoscoliosis and pes cavus (clubfoot). In about one-half of the cases, there is, in addition, optic atrophy, deafness, distal wasting, and diabetes. Cardiomyopathy can be detected by early electrocardiography or echocardiogram.

The course is progressive, and patients are wheelchair bound by their 20s and die in their 30s, often of cardiomyopathy.

Mild forms restricted to one or two features (e.g., pes cavus and absent ankle and knee jerks) are not rare. They should be sought in the families of patients with the classic form. In such cases, a near-normal life span can be expected. The heart, however, should be regularly evaluated. Hereditary motor and sensory neuropathy if often associated (see Ch. 80).

Hereditary Cerebellar Ataxia

This is an autosomal dominant disorder with a late onset during the 40s to 60s. Sporadic cases occur.

Clinically, the patients are distinct from those with Friedreich's ataxia by the absence or mildness of joint position sense and vibration sense disorders. Consequently, the reflexes are brisk with extensor plantars. Optic atrophy and ocular palsies are frequent.

Pathologic reports are few. Some cases are variants of Friedreich's ataxia. Others have shown degeneration, mainly of the ventral spinocerebellar tracts; still others showed pontocerebellar-associated lesions that could have the significance of transitional forms with OPCA.

Olivopontocerebellar Atrophy

Most cases of OPCA are sporadic, but many of them could be autosomal recessive The onset is in the 40s to 60s. There is a dominantly inherited form with an onset around age 30 and a less severe course than the recessive or sporadic cases. In the dominant form, the gene has been assigned to chromosome 6p near the human lymphocyte antigen complex. Oligodendroglial argyrophilic inclusions were absent in one domi-

nant case compared with nine cases of multiple system atrophy. A deficiency in glutamate dehydrogenase has been reported in some recessive inherited cases.

Clinically, there is a progressive incoordination of trunk and limbs, with uncertain gait and dysarthria. Commonly, sometimes prominent at the onset, extrapyramidal signs are present: rigidity, akinesia, and mask-like facies. Ankle and knee jerks are normal, although occasionally, they can be either absent or brisk with extensor plantars. Some intellectual impairment is frequent. Autonomic dysfunction, including sphincter incontinence and postural hypotension, is not rare.

MRI shows nicely the atrophy of the pons, middle cerebellar peduncles, and cerebellum.

Pathologically, the core lesion is the degeneration of pontocerebellar fibers with atrophy of the basis pontis, brachium pontis, and white matter of the cerebellum. The degeneration of olivocerebellar fibers is less severe. In most cases, there are associated lesions in the substantia nigra, striatum, and anterior and lateral horns of the spinal cord. In the familial form, the spinal lesions of Freidreich's disease are associated.

Joseph, Machado-Joseph, or Azorean Disease

Several families of Portuguese descent, several of which lived in the Azores, were affected by related autosomal dominant degenerative diseases. Joseph and Machado were the family names of two of them. The disease has now been reported from Portugal and Japan.

The clinical onset is about age 25, with early disorders of gait and rigidity soon superseded by spasticity with brisk reflexes and Babinski's signs. Dysarthria and difficulties in swallowing are common. Vertical gaze and convergence are impaired. Nystagmus is prominent. Facial and lingual fasciculations are usual. Cerebellar incoordination can be present and peripheral neuropathy with wasting. Death usually occurs within 15 years.

Pathologically, there are OPCA lesions with various associations of degeneration of the substantia nigra, striatum, dentate nuclei and superior cerebellar peduncles, corticospinal tract, nuclei of cranial nerves, anterior spinocerebellar tracts, and lateral horns of the spinal cord.

Restricted Cortical Cerebellar Atrophies

Sporadic cases of late onset were described by Marie-Foix-Alajouanine (see above), but similar lesions result from chronic alcoholic intoxication. It is generally believed that most cases of Marie-Foix-Alajouanine type were due to alcohol, although there is some evidence of an associated genetic predisposition. A rare autosomal dominant form has also been described with onset around the fifth decade.

Clinically, there is a progressive ataxia of gait and instability of the trunk, most obvious when the patient walks. Movements of the upper limbs are remarkably spared. In familial cases, the course is progressive. In alcoholic cases, the evolution usually stabilizes (see Ch. 67). More than a direct toxic action of alcohol, malnourishment is probably responsible for the cerebellar lesions.

Pathologically, there is a loss of Purkinje cells, strikingly restricted or predominant on the upper vermis and nearby hemispheres.

Ramsay Hunt's Syndrome

Sporadic cases are associated with myoclonus and epilepsy and later cerebellar ataxia. Familial cases resemble Friedreich's ataxia, with myoclonus and epilepsy appearing about the third decade. This syndrome is heterogeneous. It has been shown recently that many cases are due to mitochondrial encephalomyelopathy (see Ch. 82), although a number of Scandinavian origin are similar to Unverricht-Lundborg progressive myoclonic epilepsy (Baltic myoclonus). Still other cases await a more precise diagnosis.

Paraneoplastic Cerebellar Degeneration

Clinically, ataxia of gait, trunk, and limbs with dysarthria and nystagmus develop subacutely in weeks or months. The onset can be so rapid as to suggest vascular disease. The presence of cancer might be revealed by the neurologic disorders. Most of the cancers are either ovarian or oat cell lung carcinomas or Hodgkin's disease.

Treatment of the cancer can bring improvement of the cerebellar disorders, lending support to the autoimmune pathogenic hypothesis. Anti-Purkinje cell antibodies have been reported in some cases.

Pathologically, there is a diffuse loss of Purkinje cells, with various degrees of perivascular lymphocytic cuffing (i.e., inflammatory signs). The latter can be most severe and be part of a paraneoplastic subacute polioencephalomyelitis, chiefly with oat cell lung carcinoma.

Miscellaneous

A small number of identified causes may explain ataxia, most of them in the form of a toxin.

Anticonvulsants. Acute intoxication with most anticonvulsants causes ataxia and nystagmus. Chronic intoxication, particularly with phenytoin, can cause incoordination of movements, dysarthria, and nystagmus. As a result of an often associated neuropathy, ankle and knee jerks are depressed. Pathologically, there is a diffuse loss of Purkinje cells. Anoxia accompanying epileptic fits can also cause loss of Purkinje cells.

Mercury. Organic mercury in the form of methyl mercury can be ingested with fish (Minamata disease, named for the site in Japan where major industrial waste dumping poisoned large numbers of people), treated seeds, or meat from animals fed with treated grain. Inorganic mercury can be an industrial hazard. Clinically, methyl mercury poisoning causes a severe ataxia, affecting gait and movements of the trunk and limbs. The association with a concentric constriction of the visual fields, caused by a selective involvement of the calcarine cortex, is diagnostic. Pathologically, there is loss of granule cells in the cerebellar cortex. Peculiar lesions of the dendrites of Purkinje cells have also been reported.

Methyl Bromide. Accidents have been reported as industrial hazards or from leaking fire extinguishers. Clinically, there were epileptic fits, myoclonus, and cerebellar disorders, although the latter were often qualified of "atypical" because of association with "oppositionist spasms." The authors do not know of detailed pathologic accounts.

Vitamin E Deficiency. As a result of chronic fat malabsorption, vitamin E deficiency can cause a spinocerebellar degeneration in adults (see Abetalipoproteinemia, above), as it does in children.

Hypothyroidism. Whether primary or secondary, hypothyroidism can cause and can be revealed by incoordination of movements. There can be dysarthria and nystagmus. Other evidence of myxedema is present. Replacement therapy should bring improvement. In evaluating ataxia ascribed to hypothyroidism, one should be wary to evaluate also the consequences on movement of a possible associated myopathy.

THE HEREDITARY PARAPLEGIAS

The "pure form" (see below) of this usually autosomal dominant disorder was described by Strümpell in Germany and Lorrain in France in the 1880s. The age of onset is variable from childhood to old age. The predominant disorder is spasticity not weakness. There is a progressively disabling spastic paraparesis with brisk reflexes and extensor plantars. There are no sensory signs and generally no sphincteric disturbances. In the upper limbs, the tendon reflexes are brisk, and some patients have difficulties in fine manipulative tasks. The course is progressive.

Pathologically, there is degeneration of the crossed and uncrossed corticospinal tracts in the spinal cord. There can be some demyelination of the fasciculi graciles.

The differential diagnosis should exclude compression of the spinal cord, multiple sclerosis, and myelitis, particularly caused by human T-cell lymphotropic virus type 1. The familial history of course is of major significance, but there are sporadic cases.

Hereditary or familial spastic paraplegia is in fact a vast and heterogeneous group that can be associated with progressive bulbar palsy of childhood (Fazio-Londe syndrome), here mentioned because it can appear in young adults; amyotrophy, spinocerebellar and ocular palsies (Ferguson-Critchley syndrome); optic atrophy (Behr's syndrome); retinal degeneration (Kjellin syndrome); retinal degeneration and ophthalmoplegia (Barnard-Scholz syndrome); extrapyramidal disorders; and polyneuropathy. This grouping is based on the clinical common denominator of the presence of a bilateral pyramidal syndrome, but most probably, molecular genetics will help to discern many specific entities.

ANNOTATED BIBLIOGRAPHY

Costa C, Duyckaerts C, Cervera P, Hauw JJ. Les inclusions oligodendriogliales, un marqueur des atrophies multisystematisées. Rev Neurol (Paris) 1992;148:274–80.

Evidence that autosomal dominant OAPC does not belong to multiple system atrophies.

Escourolle R, Gray F, Hauw JJ. Les atrophies cérébelleuses. Rev Neurol (Paris) 1982;138:953–65.

A clear and concise history of cerebellar atrophy.

Hanauer A, Chery M, Fujita R et al. The Friedreich ataxia gene is assigned to chromosome 9q13-q21 by mapping of tightly linked markers and shows linkage disequilibrium with DqS15. Am J Hum Genet 1990;46:133–7.

Neurogenetics in detail.

Harding AE. The Hereditary Ataxias and Related Disorders. Churchill Livingstone, Edinburgh, 1984.

A thorouqh review of hereditary ataxias and paraplegias and an attempt at classification.

Jacobs JM, Le Quesne PM. Toxic disorders. In Hume Adams J, Duchen LW (eds). Greenfields Neuropathology. 5th Ed. E. Arnold, London, 1992.

An account of the cerebellar disorders caused by mercury poisoning.

Landrieu P. Le conseil génétique en neurologie. Rev Neurol (Paris) 1992;148:97–106.

A review of advances and technical and ethical problems in genetic counseling.

Marie P. Sur l'hérédo-ataxie cérébelleuse. Sem Med 1893; 13:444–7.

The seminal article on the concept of cerebellar atrophies.

Marsden CD, Harding AE, Obeso JA. Progressive myoclonic ataxia (the Ramsay Hunt syndrome). Arch Neurol 1990; 47:1121–5.

The syndrome can be due to mitochondrial encephalomyelopathy or Unverritcht-Lundborg disease or be still idiopathic.

Oppenheimer DR. Diseases of the basal ganglia cerebellum and motor neurons. In Hume Adams J, Duchen LW (eds). Greenfield's Neuropathology. 5th Ed. E. Arnold, London, 1992.

Classic neuropathology.

Peterson RDA, Funkhouser JD. Ataxia-telangiectasia: an important clue. N Engl J Med 1990;332:122–3.

A review of the advances in genetics.

Poirier J, Gray F, Escourolle R. Manuel de Neuropathologie. 3rd Ed. Masson, Paris, 1989.

A lucid pathologic account of cerebellar and spinal degenerations.

Reynaud P, Loiseau H, Coquet M et al. Un cas adulte d'encéphalomyélite nécrosante subaigue de Leigh. Rev Neurol (Paris) 1988;144:259–65.

A case in a 35-year-old patient and a review of juvenile and adult cases.

Rogelet P, Gerard JM, Michotte A. Xanthomatose cérébrotendineuse. Rev Neurol (Paris) 1992;148:541–45.

Two cases with MRI results and a review of the clinical and biologic features.

Savoiardo M, Strada L, Girotti F et al. Olivopontocerebellar atrophy: MR diagnosis and relationship to multisystem atrophy. Radiology 1990;174:693–6.

Full details, including pontine changes.

Sorbi S, Piacentini S, Fani C et al. Abnormalities of mitochondrial enzymes in hereditary ataxias. Acta Neurol Scand 1989;80:103–10.

Enzymes in circulating platelets, which are measurable during the patient's life.

Staal A, Meerwaldt JD, van Dongen KJ et al. Non-familial degenerative disease and atrophy of brainstem and cerebellum. Clinical and CT data in 47 patients. J Neurol Sci 1990;95:259–69.

No relationship between clinical syndrome, its duration and severity, and the degree of atrophy on computed tomography.

Victor M, Adams RD, Mancall EL. A restricted form of cerebellar cortical degeneration occurring in alcoholic patients. Arch Neurol 1959;1:579–88.

Lesions caused by alcohol are similar to those of Marie-Foix-Alajouanine cortical degeneration of late onset. The same year, Alajouanine et al. reported on six cases caused by alcohol without postmortem examination in Sur six cas d'atrophie cérébelleure du type cortical tardif (Pierre Marie, Foix, Alajouanine) observés chez des alcooliques chroniques. Rev Neurol (Paris) 1959;100:411–39.

Yokota T, Wada Y, Furukawa T et al: Adult-onset spinocerebellar syndrome with idiopathic vitamin E deficiency. Ann Neurol 1987;22:84.

Slowly evolving syndrome in a man and his uncle.

65

Syringomyelia and Syringobulbia

J. P. Mohr and J. C. Gautier

The term *syringomyelia,* that is, a cavity in the spinal cord (Greek: *syrinx,* a tube or a flute), was coined in 1824 by the French physician Ollivier d'Angers. It is a rare disease. Its mechanism has been incompletely elucidated despite recent advances from magnetic resonance imaging (MRI), but it is an archetypal neurologic disorder because it epitomizes the symptoms and signs of a lesion in the center of the cord. In syringomyelia, the cavity is entirely or for the most part distinct from the central canal. Distentions of the latter are termed *hydromyelia.*

PATHOLOGY

Because of the (relative) simplicity of the anatomy of the cord and of the lesions, there is a close correspondence between pathologic and clinical features, which explains why syringomyelia is so often a topic for demonstrations to students.

The cavity extends through several segments of the cord, usually in the lower cervical and upper thoracic segments. It can extend rostrally into the medulla (*syringobulbia*) and, in rare cases, into the pons or even as high as the internal capsule. However, the first cervical segment is usually spared, a fact not taken into account in some hypotheses of the pathogenesis of syringomyelia (see below). Caudally, the syrinx can develop into the lower thoracic and lumbar cord. Rare cases span the entire length of the cord.

The cavity may be divided into two parts, one on each side of the cord, throughout or only for part of the length of the lesion. The lesion(s) may be unilateral but commonly are bilateral and may be cruciform (i.e., have the shape of a cross on transverse cuts).

In the *cord* (Fig. 65-1), the cavity is primarily located in the gray commissure behind the central canal (interruption of spinothalamic fibers as they decussate in the posterior commissure causes anesthesia for tem-perature and pain) (see Fig. 31-5) and extends mainly in the dorsal horns (which explains the clinical observation of areflexia). The syrinx is lined by glial tissue and, where there is a large cavity that has engulfed the central canal, by ependymal cells. The cavity is filled with a clear or yellowish fluid. It is close to cerebrospinal fluid (CSF) in composition when it communicates with the central canal and is more proteinaceous when it is separate. This fluid-filled cavity causes damage to the neighboring structures, namely the anterior horns (which causes wasting of muscles supplied by these segments), the intermediolateralis (autonomic) horn (which explains autonomic disorders such as neuropathic arthropathies, painless ulcers, and sometimes an oculosympathetic syndrome), the lateral corticospinal tract (weakness, exaggerated tendon reflexes, and Babinski's sign), and more rarely, the dorsal columns (loss of position and vibration sense).

In some cases, the cavity empties when the patient is head down and refills when the head is elevated, a point of diagnosis differential with central cord tumors (see below).

In the *medulla,* the shape of the lesions is more that of a cleft than of a cavity. The most frequent cleft starts from below the floor of the fourth ventricle, lateral to the nucleus of cranial nerve XII, and runs ventrolaterally to the nucleus ambiguus (which explains paralysis of palate, larynx, and pharynx) and the sensory nucleus of the cranial nerve V (anesthesia and facial pain). This type of cleft can be bilateral and is usually asymmetric. Another type of cleft is more median in location, interrupting the connections of the vestibular nuclei with the medial longitudinal fasciculus (nystagmus). In rare cases, a cleft located between the pyramid and inferior olive cuts the fascicular fibers of cranial nerve XII (atrophy of the ipsilateral half of the tongue).

807

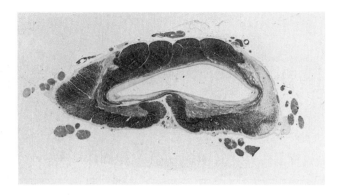

Figure 65-1. Syringomyelia. Tranverse section of the cervical spinal cord. Large syrinx. Note the degeneration of the left lateral tract (see text). (Loyez stain for myelin; × 7.) (Courtesy of Professor J. J. Hauw, Laboratoire de Neuropathologie, la Salpêtrière, Paris, France.)

Neurologic and craniospinal malformations are frequently present: Chiari malformation, platybasia, and fusion of vertebrae (Klippel-Feil syndrome) (see Ch. 31).

PATHOGENESIS

Dysraphism

This term means disturbed fusion. In the case of syringomyelia, it has been proposed that there might have been an incomplete closure of the embryonic central canal. Together with delay in opening the outlets for CSF in the fourth ventricle (foramina of Magendie and Luschka) or herniation of the cerebellar tonsils in a Chiari malformation, this closure would obstruct CSF flow and cause syrinx formation as a consequence of elevated CSF pressure. This possibility was strongly advocated by the American neurosurgeon W. Gardner who reported, among 74 operated syringomyelias, 68 Chiari malformations, 3 Dandy-Walker malformations, and 3 congenital cysts that blocked CSF flow. This type of syringomyelia with obstruction in the vicinity of the foramen magnum is labeled type I in Barnett's classification. Decompressive surgery was the logical consequence of such a view and is still practiced, but the suggestion that the canal be plugged to block a linkage between the syrinx and the CSF at the foramen magnum is no longer heeded.

Obviously, there are cases of syringomyelia without obstructive lesions on the CSF flow pathways (Barnett type II, see box), which provides a major alternative explanation to the preceding hypothesis. Moreover, recent studies have demonstrated that CSF pressure within the central canal, even in a setting of obstruction, is too low to generate enough force to disrupt

---

BARNETT'S CLASSIFICATION OF SYRINGOMYELIA

Type I   Syrinx with obstruction of the foramen magnum and dilation of the central canal.
          A With type I Chiari malformation.
          B With other obstructive lesions of the foramen magnum.
Type II   Syrinx without obstruction of the foramen magnum (idiopathic type).
Type III Syrinx with other diseases of the spinal cords.
          A Spinal cord tumors.
          B Traumatyic myelopathy.
          C Spinal arachnoiditis.
Type IV   Pure hydromyelia with or without hydrocephalus.

---

the central canal. Instead, it has been theorized that pressure may be transmitted from the CSF outside the cord to the cord parenchyma via the Virchow-Robin spaces, which is possibly sufficient to cause cavity formation.

MRI studies have recently suggested two mechanisms of cavity formation. First, lesions obstructing the CSF outlets of the fourth ventricles would cause the cavities of hydromyelia. Second, lesions obstructing the upper end of the central canal or its continuity with the subarachnoid space would appear to produce a syrinx that does not communicate with the central canal. These findings suggest that syrinxes associated with obstructive lesions in the region of the fourth ventricle are not explained by a caudalward flow of CSF into the central canal, as originally postulated by Gardner.

In the present state of knowledge, it would seem safe to conclude that the pathogenesis of syringomyelia is still far from clear. The Gardner hypothesis currently appears consistent with hydromyelia; the pressure-from-outside hypothesis would be consistent with syringomyelia.

Idiopathic Syringomyelia

These cases correspond to Barnett's type 2. Little is understood of their formation, except they are consistent with dysraphism without CSF pressure disorders. They are often associated with other tokens of dysraphism such as spina bifida, meningoceles, myelomeningoceles, and other abnormalities such as syndactyly, pes cavus, thoracic malformations, and cervical ribs so often that some authors gather them together in the concept of "status dysraphicus."

Acquired Diseases

Lesions located in the center of the cord can cause symptoms and signs similar to those of syringomyelia or, in some cases, perhaps cavity formation. Alternatively, they can be considered as special types of syringomyelia or as syringomyelic syndromes (Barnett's type III, see box) to distinguish them from idiopathic syringomyelia.

Intramedullary Tumors

Intramedullary tumors, especially astrocytomas and ependymomas (see Ch. 52) may pursue a long and indolent course, mimicking every detail of syringomyelia. Furthermore, such lesions may have associated cavities or cysts that may create a syringomyelic syndrome superimposed on the syndrome caused by the tumor or distinguishing them from the tumor itself.

Trauma

Trauma, usually years before, is followed by syringomyelia more often than was believed in the pre-MRI era and is seen most often in paraplegic or tetraplegic patients. Post-traumatic syringomyelia of course raises medicolegal issues. The cavity seems to develop from cores of infarcted tissue (see pencil infarcts, Ch. 31) rather than from lysis of hematomas. The mechanism of extension of the cavities is unexplained. Spinal arachnoiditis, an ill-defined condition, is thought to cause syrinx formation by hampering CSF drainage in the region of the upper cord.

CLINICAL FEATURES

The course of the disease is generally chronic with possible, unpredictable exacerbations. The onset is most often insidious, although acute onsets (paraplegia and acute respiratory distress caused by bilateral vocal cord paralysis) have been reported. Syringomyelia is more frequent in men. The clinical onset is generally between age 25 and 40 years, but a fair number of cases are known in children and also reported in the sixth and seventh decades.

Syringomyelia

Patients usually seek advice because they have burnt a finger without noticing it, they have noticed areas that do not feel normally hot and cold in the tub or shower, there is wasting of the hand, or trophic disorders occur such as painless ulcers of the hand, an arthropathy (that can have an acute onset), or (and which is diagnostic of syringomyelia) hypertrophy of the whole hand termed cheiromegaly (from the Greek for big hand).

Neurologic examination shows a characteristic level or suspended syndrome associated with a below-the-level syndrome (see Ch. 31).

The *suspended syndrome* involves one or both upper limbs, usually with extension on the chest in the shape of a cuirass or small sweater. There is loss of pain and hot and cold sensation, with sometimes a difference in severity between the three modalities. Touch, position of limbs, and vibration are spared. This is often so characteristic for syringomyelia that this sensory loss pattern has been termed the syringomyelic dissociation. At the onset, the sensory disorders are not as extensive. They are unilateral and involve the ulnar side of the hand, forearm, arm, and chest in "half-cuirass." This pattern is also very suggestive of the diagnosis. It should also be remembered that the sensory root of the trigeminal nerve runs down low in the cervical cord (see Ch. 29, cranial nerve V), so that there can be facial loss of sensation in cervical syringomyelia and, as a corollary, that facial sensory loss does not necessarily mean syringobulbia.

Pain is rare but may exist in syringomyelia. Lightning or burning pains can mimic brachial neuralgia or shoulder rheumatism.

Loss of tendon reflexes usually involves all reflexes of the upper limbs. Loss of the brachioradialis with a spared or exaggerated flexion of the fingers is said to be highly suggestive of syringomyelia.

Wasting involves mainly the muscles of the hand, and as a result of unequal involvement of muscular groups, the hand often assumes particular positions; such as claw hand or preacher's hand. In long-standing cases, wasting may involve the forearm, arm, and shoulder. Weakness is usually less than that suggested by wasting. There are few or no fasciculations.

The paravertebral muscles are severely involved early; hence kyphoscoliosis is observed. In children and adolescents, the latter should raise the possibility of the diagnosis.

Trophic disorders are frequent, including dry coarse skin; painless indolent ulcers; and painless neuropathic joints, mainly osteolytic in the shoulder and mainly hypertrophic in the elbow; cheiromegaly is diagnostic (see above).

Below the lesion, there is a spastic paraparesis, rarely a paraplegia. There are few or no sphincteric disorders. In some cases, there are sensory disorders below the lesion (believed to be due to compression or destruction of tracts by the syrinx), but usually they are separated from the suspended deficit by normal regions.

MRI has shown that syrinxes often do not cause the

full-blown syndrome described above and that cases with few clinical signs are probably frequent.

Syringobulbia

Facial pains can resemble essential trigeminal neuralgia (see cranial nerve V, Ch. 29), but some features are distinctive. Pain can involve all three trigeminal branches, and sooner or later anesthesia appears, which first involves the skin around the mouth and nostrils. The lips and tongue are the last to be involved.

Nystagmus is usually horizontal-rotatory. Unilateral paralysis of the soft palate, pharynx, and larynx is characteristic of the retro-olivary clefts. As mentioned, an acute paralysis of the glottis dilators (Gebhardt's syndrome, see cranial nerves IX and X, Ch. 29), is possible. Atrophy of one-half of the tongue is often isolated as is the cleft between the pyramid and inferior olive that causes it. A Bernard-Horner syndrome is sometimes observed (see Ch. 27).

INVESTIGATIONS

MRI is the best tool currently available (Fig. 65-2), demonstrating the lesion in most instances. With MRI, as mentioned, it has been something of a surprise to find that the severity of the clinical syndrome is not correlated with the dimensions of the syrinx, a point against basing therapy on the size of the cyst. MRI has also revealed instances of asymptomatic cavities. Spinal cord *arteriovenous malformations* have even been found in which the clinical diagnosis seemed to be syrinx.

When MRI is not available for visualization of the cavity, other means of visualization have been used with varying degrees of success. *Computed tomographic myelography,* with metrizamide, oil contrast, or air can be performed in the hope there is a communication between the cavity and the central canal and that the contrast medium will find its way into the cavity. Demonstration that the cerebellar tonsils lie below the foramen magnum points to a Chiari malformation but, of course, is not diagnostic evidence of a syrinx.

The major differential diagnosis is a *tumor,* which MRI usually resolves. Without MRI and where contrast has not entered the cavity, advantage can be taken of the collapse of the syrinx when the patient is head down on a tilt table under fluoroscopic observation. When successful, this maneuver helps to rule out a tumor.

Plain spine films are of no use to demonstrate a syrinx, but they can assist in showing platybasia or osseous abnormalities of the craniospinal junction or the cervical spine (see above and Ch. 31).

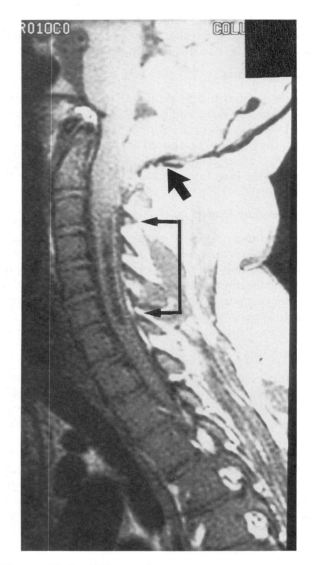

Figure 65-2. MRI scan demonstrating syrinx (*small arrows*) and foramen magnum *(large arrow).*

TREATMENT

The natural course of the disease, with long plateaus and unpredictable aggravations, and its possible spontaneous arrest make it difficult to evaluate any form of therapy. For patients whose illness seems relentlessly progressing, good results of syringoperitoneal shunting have been reported. Where there is hydrocephalus, ventricular shunting may precede syrinx shunting.

Prevention of dysraphic states might reduce the already-small incidence of syringomyelia. Recent studies indicate an inverse relationship between folate and cyanocobalamin levels during pregnancy, and neural tube defects at birth suggest that pre-emptive treatment with these vitamins might reduce the frequency of such defects. The evidence is strong enough that plans are underway in some countries to ensure adequate levels of folate in baked bread.

ANNOTATED BIBLIOGRAPHY

Ball MJ, Dayan AD. Pathogenesis of syringomyelia. Lancet 1972;2:799–801.

CSF pressure is too low to cause syrinx; view opposing Gardner (see below).

Barnett H, Jousse A. Post-traumatic syringomyelia. In Vinken PJ, Bruyn GW (eds). Handbook of Clinical Neurology. Vol 26. North-Holland, Amsterdam; 1976, pp. 113–57.

Review of traumatic syrinx and its relation to syringomyelia.

Barnett HJM, Foster J, Hudgson P. Syringomyelia. WB Saunders, Philadelphia; 1973.

Extensive review of syringomyelia with detailed references.

Cambier J, Lhuillier M, Levesque M. Syringomyelie. Medicine Interne 1973;8:739–54.

Clear review with clinical wisdom.

Donauer E, Rascher K. Syringomyelia: a brief review of ontogenetic, experimental and clinical aspects. Neurosurg Rev 1993;16:7–13.

Utility of MRI without and with gadolinium.

Gardner W. Hydrodynamic mechanism of syringomyelia: its relationship to myelocele. J Neurol Neurosurg Psychiatry 1965;28:247.

This hypothesis is now largely ignored.

Grant R, Hadley DM, MacPherson P et al. Syringomyelia: cyst measurement by magnetic resonance imaging and comparison with symptoms, signs and disability. J Neurol Neurosurg Psychiatry 1987;50:1008–14.

No clear correlation between cystic diameter and length and syndrome.

Hackney DB. Magnetic resonance imaging of the spine. Normal anatomy. Top Magn Reson Imaging 1992;4:1–6.

Normal anatomy.

Heller JG. The syndromes of degenerative cervical disease. Orthop Clin North Am 1992;23:381–94.

Useful account of differential diagnoses.

Hughes JT. Syringomyelia and syringobulbia. In Blackwood W, Corsellis JAN (eds). Greenfield's Neuropathology. 3rd Ed. E. Arnold, London, 1976.

Sound, basic pathology.

Iqbal JB, Bradey N, Macfaul R, Cameron MM. Syringomyelia in children: six case reports and review of the literature. Br J Neurosurg 1992;6:13–20.

Update of the syndrome in children.

Jonesco-Sisesti N. La Syringobulbie. Masson, Paris, 1932.

Great classic.

Maroon JC, Abla AA, Wilberger JI et al. Central cord syndrome. Clin Neurosurg 1991;37:612–21.

Detailed clinical syndrome review.

Milhorat TH, Miller JI, Johnson WD et al. Anatomical basis of syringomyelia occurring with hindbrain lesions. Neurosurgery 1993;32:748–54.

Autopsy-MRI correlations.

Mills JL, Simpson JL. Prospects for prevention of neural tube defects by vitamin supplementation. Curr Opin Neurol Neurosurg 1993;6:554–8.

As little as 4 mg of folate daily appears to prevent 72 percent of expected neural tube defects. The Public Health Service currently recommends that women at risk for becoming pregnant take 0.4 mg of folate daily.

Poser C. The Relationship of Syringomyelia and Neoplasm. Charles C. Thomas, Springfield, IL, 1956.

Early account emphasizing tumors as a cause of syringomyelia syndrome.

Squire MV, Lehr RP. Post-traumatic syringomyelia. J Neurol Neurosurg Psychiatry 1994;57:1095–8.

An autopsy study of 20 cases, showing an incidence 20 percent, approximating that found by MRI. The syrinx seemed to develop from cores of old infarcts. Syrinxes would develop from pencil infarcts rather than from hematomas.

Stevens JM, Serva WAD, Kendall BE et al. Chiari malformation in adults: relation of morphological aspects to clinical features and operative course. J Neurol Neurosurg Psychiatry 1993;56:1072–7.

The most severe ataxia was correlated with the greatest descent of the cerebellar tonsils; motor weakness and atrophy correlated best with brainstem compression.

Tashiro K, Fukazawa T, Morikawa F et al. Syringomyelic syndrome: clinical features in 31 cases confirmed by CT myelography or magnetic resonance imaging. J Neurol 1987;235:26–30.

Few signs in many cases.

Wilson SAK. Syringomyelia, syringobulbia. In Bruce AN (ed). Neurology. 2nd Ed. Butterworth (Publishers), London, 1954, pp. 1184–202.

Classic clinical description.

Zager EL, Ojemann RG, Poletti CE. Acute presentations of syringomyelia. Report of three cases. J Neurosurg 1990;72:133–8.

Useful reminder.

66

Neuro-Behçet's Disease

M. Zuheir Al-Kawi

This unusual disorder was first described in the Middle East. Over many years, cases were reported from countries of the Mediterranean basin, Japan, and neighboring countries. In 1937, the Istanbuli dermatologist Hulusi Behçet published his observations on a syndrome characterized by a clinical triad of oral aphthous ulcers, genital ulcers, and uveitis. The syndrome is now known to have a variety of manifestations, affecting multiple organs and including the eyes, skin, vascular system, nervous system, joints, and intestines. Few advances in laboratory diagnosis have been made, and the diagnosis remains clinical. Neuro-Behçet's can take many forms and has many differential diagnoses, including idiopathic intracranial hypertension and multiple sclerosis.

EPIDEMIOLOGY

The cause remains obscure, but it is considered to result from some factor(s) in the environment that work on a background of genetic predisposition. This view is based on the variability of prevalence with geographic location. Most patients are of the histocompatibility antigen HLA-B5(51) group. The areas in which the disease occurs frequently trace the ancient silk routes along which the genetic susceptibility was transmitted. Lack of familiarity probably contributes to underdiagnosis in other countries. For reasons still unclear, neurologic involvement occurs in 14 to 49 percent of patients, depending on the clinical series.

CLINICAL PRESENTATIONS

Neurologic manifestations can be grouped into three categories. The first is an *aseptic meningitis* or meningoencephalitis presenting with headache, fever, mild nuchal rigidity with or without confusion, lethargy, or disturbances in concentration or conversational interaction. The cerebrospinal fluid shows mild to moderate pleocytosis with normal sugar levels and only minor changes in the protein content. Cultures are negative. Another form is *parenchymatous foci secondary to small vessel vasculitis*, which tends to involve the basal parts of the brainstem, diencephalon, and spinal cord. The symptoms develop subacutely and may mimic multiple sclerosis (see Chs. 38 and 73). The third form, *vascular involvement*, commonly presents as thrombosis of the dural sinuses with the syndrome of intracranial hypertension (Ch. 35). Less commonly, arterial involvement leads to ischemic cerebral infarcts or aneurysmal bleeding.

Systemic manifestations feature the three elements of the originally described triad. The *oral aphthous ulcers* have no special distinguishing features from common canker sores. They are usually painful, superficial, whitish, well-demarcated spots surrounded by an erythematous mucosa (Plate 66-1). The painful *genital ulcers* are often concealed by the patient for fear of the stigma of venereal disease. In the active phase, they are usually punched-out erosions on the scrotum or the labia. After healing, they may leave a scar, which helps to confirm the history of ulceration. However, scarring is not a constant feature. The *ocular signs* may present as uveitis with hypopyon or as retinal vasculitis with or without anterior uveitis. Optic neuritis, optic atrophy, episcleritis, and conjunctival ulcers may occur. Retinal involvement may be detected in presymptomatic patients by demonstrating leakage from retinal vessels on fluorescein angiography.

Other manifestations include erythema nodosum, acneiform lesions, skin vasculitis with small infarcts, arthritis, superficial and deep thrombophlebitis, pulmonary embolism, intracardiac thrombi, and colitis.

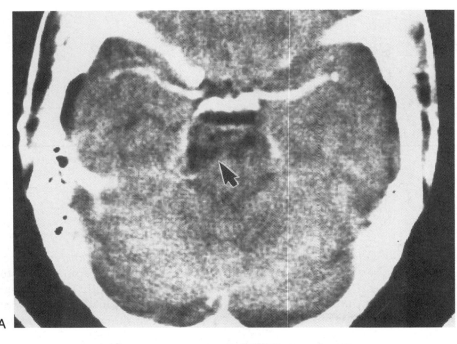

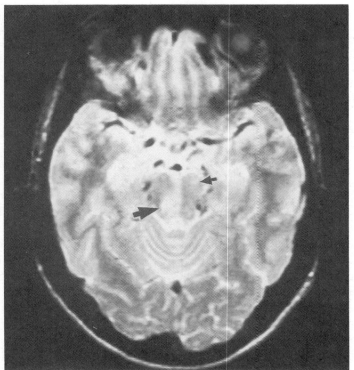

Figure 66-1. **(A)** Computed tomographic scan showing areas of hypodensity *(arrow)* in the pons in a 28-year-old man with neuro-Behçet's disease. **(B)** Magnetic resonance image showing high signal areas in the midbrain *(arrows).*

DIAGNOSIS

The diagnosis of neuro-Behçet's disease is clinical and based on recognition of the syndromic cluster. Signs of involvement of the nervous system may occasionally precede the systemic manifestations and cause a diagnostic problem. The International Study Group for Behçet's disease recently proposed a set of criteria for the clinical diagnosis, but unfortunately, neither neurologic symptoms nor vascular thrombosis were included (Table 66-1). The skin reaction to needle prick, that is, the formation of a sterile vesicular lesion at the site of the needle prick (pathergy test), may be helpful, but a positive result may simply reflect the extent of traumatization to the skin with the needle; more positive results are supposedly obtained if a blunt needle is used with multiple punctures through the skin.

The erythrocyte sedimentation rate is usually but not invariably elevated; it may correlate with disease activity. Unlike in multiple sclerosis, it is unusual to find oligoclonal bands on cerebrospinal fluid protein electrophoresis.

Magnetic resonance imaging is the most sensitive brain imaging method for the detection of lesions, which characteristically cluster around the basal part of the brainstem and thalamic regions. Typically, they show as foci of high signal intensity on T_2-weighted images in the acute phase (Fig. 66-1). They may be associated with focal swelling and regress after the attack is over or after treatment.

TREATMENT

During the acute phase of the disease, high-dose pulsed methylprednisolone is helpful to suppress meningeal or parenchymal exacerbations. Frequently, oral prednisone at a dose of 1 to 2 mg/kg/day is used as a primary treatment or to follow pulsed steroids. Azathioprine reduces the need for long-term corticosteroids and has been proved to be effective in placebo-controlled double-blind trials at a dose of 2.5 mg/kg/day. Colchicine was also shown to be effective, especially with joint and skin manifestations. Other drugs that have been used include cyclosporine, cyclophosphamide, chlorambucil, and methotrexate. Vascular involvement may require antiplatelet or anticoagulant therapy.

ANNOTATED BIBLIOGRAPHY

Al-Kawi MZ, Bohlega S, Banna M. MRI findings in neuro-Behçet's disease. Neurology 1991;41:405–8.

Six cases with central nervous system involvement.

International Study Group for Behçet's Disease. Criteria for diagnosis of Behçet's disease. Lancet 1990;335:1078–80.

Serdaroglu P, Yazici H, Ozdemir C et al. Neurologic involvement in Behçet's syndrome. A prospective study. Arch Neurol 1989;46:265–9.

Study of 323 consecutive patient seen in a 1-year period, only 17 percent of whom had neurologic findings.

Wechsler B, Godeau P (eds). Behçet's disease. Excerpta Medica, Amsterdam, 1993.

Standard text.

Yazici H, Pazarli H, Barnes CG et al. A controlled trial of azathioprine in Behçet's syndrome. N Engl J Med 1990; 322:326–8.

Results of a trial in Turkish men.

Yazici H, Barnes CG. Practical treatment recommendations for pharmacotherapy of Behçet's syndrome. Drugs 1991; 42:796–804.

Treatment suggestions for each element of the syndromes, including arteritis and the use of azathioprine, cyclosporine, colchicine, and corticosteroids.

Table 66-1. Criteria for Diagnosis of Behçet's Disease

Oral ulceration	Minor aphthous, major aphthous, or herpetiform ulceration that recurred at least three times in one 12-month period.
Plus 2 of the following:	
Eye lesions	Recurrent genital ulceration or scarring. Anterior uveitis, posterior uveitis, or cells in the vitreous on slit-lamp examination, or retinal vasculitis.
Skin lesions	Erythema nodosum, pseudofolliculitis, or papulopustular lesions, or acneiform nodules in postadolescent patients not receiving corticosteroid treatment.
Positive pathergy test	Findings applicable only in the absence of other clinical explanations.

(From International Study Group for Behçet's Disease, 1990, with permission.)

67

Ethanol Abuse

John C. M. Brust

"Problem drinkers" include both alcoholic people (i.e., those who are psychically or physically dependent on ethanol) and those who drink more sporadically and get into trouble when they do. So defined, in the United States, problem drinkers constitute 7 percent of adults and account for more than 100,000 deaths annually, roughly 5 percent of the American mortality rate. Ethanol contributes to disease and death by diverse means.

ETHANOL OVERDOSE

The pervasiveness of drunkenness in society makes it easy to forget that it can be a direct cause of death. Because of tolerance, blood ethanol concentrations are an unreliable indicator of intoxication in chronic drinkers. In novices, blood levels of 50 to 150 mg/dl produce euphoria or dysphoria, impaired judgment, and incoordination. At 150 to 250 mg/dl, there is slurred speech and gait ataxia, drowsiness, and labile mood or behavior. A level of 300 mg/dl produces incoherent speech or stupor with heavy breathing. At 400 mg/dl, there may be coma, and at 500 mg/dl, death may occur from respiratory arrest. Ethanol metabolism (to acetaldehyde and, ultimately, carbon dioxide and water) proceeds independently of blood levels, which fall 10 to 25 mg/dl/hr. A level of 200 mg/dl thus requires roughly 10 hours to reach zero, and no practical pharmacologic agent hastens the process. Apart from metabolism, ethanol is slightly eliminated by the lungs, the basis for the breath tests popular with the police in many countries.

Variants of ethanol overdose include *pathologic intoxication,* in which drinking, sometimes in small amounts, precipitates extreme excitement and irrational or even violent behavior, and "blackouts," in which the drinker appears awake and behaviorally normal yet the following day has no recall of the episode. The mechanisms of these conditions are disputed.

Management of ethanol overdose includes consideration of other possible causes of stupor or coma in an alcoholic person, including hypoglycemia, meningitis, subdural hematoma, and liver failure. Respiratory support in an intensive care unit is the principal treatment. Sedatives should be avoided in obstreperous or violent patients, and stimulants are contraindicated in those with a depressed sensorium. Gastric lavage is of no use unless additional drugs have been taken. Hemodialysis or peritoneal dialysis can be used for patients with extremely high blood ethanol levels, metabolic acidosis, or additional drug ingestion (e.g., methanol or ethylene glycol) and for severely intoxicated children.

Ethanol is often taken with other drugs, especially opioids and other sedatives, sometimes in suicide attempts. Effects on alertness and respiration can be additive or even synergistic.

ETHANOL DEPENDENCE AND WITHDRAWAL

Physical dependence on ethanol leads to a variety of withdrawal symptoms and signs. Within hours or a few days of abstinence, there are tremors, hallucinations, and seizures, alone or in combination. After 48 hours or more of abstinence, there may be delirium tremens, which may or may not be preceded by tremor, hallucinations, or seizures.

Tremor can appear on awakening after only a few days of drinking and is promptly relieved by more ethanol. It is rapid and distal, but if drinking cannot continue, it becomes coarse and accompanied by insomnia, easy startling, agitation, flushing, sweating, nausea, vomiting, tachypnea, and tachycardia. Mentation is usually intact, however. The tremor may last for up to 2 or 3 weeks.

Perceptual disturbances include illusions and hallucinations, which are visual, auditory, tactile, olfactory, or combinations. Insight as to their unreality is often preserved, and the subject is not delirious. Hallucinations are usually fleeting and fragmentary, clearing within a few days, but patients with repeated bouts have evolved into a more chronic schizophrenic-like state.

Ethanol withdrawal can precipitate seizures in epileptic patients. Ethanol-related seizures in nonepileptic patients without other predisposing factors often occur within a few days of abstinence but sometimes happen during active drinking or more than 1 week after the last drink. They usually consist of a single major motor seizure or a cluster of seizures within a period of a few hours. Status epilepticus occurs in a small minority of cases, and focal features are sometimes present even in patients without known earlier head injury or other cerebral pathologic conditions.

Delirium tremens is overdiagnosed. In addition to tremor and hallucinations, patients have delirium with extreme inattentiveness and usually agitation, plus sympathetic overactivity, with fever, tachycardia, blood pressure swings, and profuse sweating. The mortality rate is as high as 15 percent, mostly the result of pneumonia, sepsis, or other associated disease, but sometimes apparently the result of the delirium tremens itself.

The management of ethanol withdrawal depends on the aim: to prevent or treat either early abstinence symptoms or delirium tremens. Tremor can be treated and other symptoms perhaps averted by giving sedatives that are cross tolerant with ethanol, usually benzodiazepines in titrated dosage. Neuroleptics are best avoided, even in hallucinating patients, because they lower seizure threshold. Ethanol itself has a low margin of safety when used parenterally and is potentially toxic to many organs. β-Adrenergic blockers can reduce withdrawal tremor.

Unless status epilepticus is present, seizures usually do not require treatment. If their cause is uncertain, an anticonvulsant can be given until the diagnosis is established. Phenytoin is probably ineffectual in ethanol-related seizures; phenobarbital has the theoretic advantage of cross tolerance with ethanol. Status epilepticus is treated no differently than in other settings. When the diagnosis of ethanol-related seizures is made, based on the history and a negative workup, including electroencephalography, the use of long-term anticonvulsants is not indicated.

Hypomagnesemia is common during early withdrawal and merits replacement therapy. Hypokalemia and hypocalcemia may also be present, and most patients are nutritionally deficient. The nutritional deficiencies also include vitamin B_1. Thiamine 100 mg intramuscularly is a safeguard against the precipitation of Wernicke-Korsakoff syndrome (see Ch. 71), which is one of the conditions that require emergency treatment in the care of alcoholic patients (see below).

The treatment of delirium tremens is a medical emergency; once present, the symptoms cannot be abruptly reversed by any agent. The mainstay of treatment is sedation with a parenteral benzodiazepine, usually diazepine, sometimes requiring very large doses (e.g., up to several hundred milligrams daily). In patients with hepatic failure, such treatment may unavoidably precipitate hepatic coma. General medical management includes fluid and electrolyte replacement, blood pressure and cardiac monitoring, and consideration of other alcohol-related systemic or neurologic diseases.

Abstinence is common in controlled environments such as hospitals or jails, sometimes revealing an alcohol problem not volunteered by the patient on admission. In some settings, physicians allow small and declining doses of alcohol in hopes of preventing full-blown delirium tremens, a practice frowned on by more austere physicians.

WERNICKE-KORSAKOFF SYNDROME

Alcoholic patients are often deficient in protein and vitamins, and the limited storage capacity of thiamine means that symptoms can appear after only a few weeks of inadequate intake. Although Wernicke's and Korsakoff's syndromes are pathologically similar, they are clinically distinct. *Wernicke's syndrome* consists of altered mentation, abnormal eye movements, and ataxic gait, evolving subacutely over a few days. The mental symptoms include inattentiveness, lethargy, indifference, psychomotor slowing (abulia), and impaired memory and cognition. Abnormal eye movements usually begin with nystagmus, abduction or horizontal gaze paresis then appears and progresses to complete external ophthalmoplegia. Ptosis is rare, and pupillary reactivity is nearly always preserved. Truncal ataxia may prevent walking or standing, but ataxia of the limbs and dysarthria is unusual.

Patients often have additional signs of nutritional deficiency, including skin changes and peripheral neuropathy. Beriberi heart disease is rare, but autonomic abnormalities are common, including cardiac arrhythmia, postural hypotension, and hypothermia. (Fever suggests infection.) Sudden circulatory collapse can follow even mild exertion. Untreated patients progress to stupor, coma, and death.

Frequently present are elevated serum pyruvate levels that fall with treatment. More specific is a decreased erythrocyte content of transketolase. Cerebrospinal fluid is normal, except for occasional mild protein elevation.

Korsakoff's syndrome is a more purely amnestic disorder, both retrograde and anterograde. It often emerges as other mental abnormalities of Wernicke's syndrome are responding to treatment; early in the course, there may be striking confabulation, which, however, is nonspecific. Alertness, attentiveness, and behavior are relatively preserved, but there may be a striking lack of insight (anosognosia) to the disturbance.

The pathologic lesions of Wernicke-Korsakoff syndrome consist of neuropil degeneration, often with relative preservation of neurons, plus prominent blood vessels, macrophages, and sometimes petechiae, affecting the medial thalamus, hypothalamus (including the mammillary bodies), periaqueductal gray matter, and periventricular pons and medulla. With chronicity, gliosis becomes increasingly prominent. Cerebellar lesions affect largely the anterosuperior vermis and consist of multilayer neuronal loss, especially involving Purkinje cells.

The clinicopathologic correlation of the eye movement abnormalities is thus straightforward; both cerebellar and vestibular compromise probably contribute to gait ataxia. The basis of the amnesia is more controversial. Current evidence favors damage to the dorsomedial nucleus of the thalamus.

Treatment of Wernicke's syndrome is with parenteral thiamine 50 to 100 mg daily plus multivitamins. Cardiovascular instability requires strict bed rest. Hypomagnesemia and other electrolyte disturbances are corrected. Protein replenishment requires caution in the presence of abnormal liver function. With treatment, eye movements begin improving within a few hours and, usually, are full within a week; horizontal nystagmus often persists. Mentation also improves, but more than 80 percent of patients then demonstrate Korsakoff's amnesia. In most of these, memory impairment is permanent. Ataxia also tends to improve incompletely.

ALCOHOLIC CEREBELLAR DEGENERATION

Cerebellar ataxia frequently affects alcoholic patients without other evidence of Wernicke's syndrome, and this dissociation, plus the different nature of the cerebellar pathologic findings compared with the periventricular diencephalic and brainstem changes, suggests deficiencies other than thiamine might contribute. The symptoms evolve over days, weeks, or months, sometimes stabilizing even with continued drinking. As in Wernicke's syndrome, limb ataxia is less prominent than gait disturbance, and dysarthria is rare. The treatment is thiamine and multivitamins. Improve-

ment is less predictable when Wernicke's syndrome is not present. Cerebellar degeneration is often found at autopsy or on computed tomography in alcoholic people without clinical ataxia.

ALCOHOLIC POLYNEUROPATHY

Like cerebellar ataxia, peripheral sensorimotor neuropathy is present in most patients with Wernicke-Korsakoff syndrome but most often occurs alone. Paresthesias initially affect the feet and then the hands; there may follow burning or lancinating pain and severe tenderness of the soles or calves. Impaired vibratory sensation and decreased or absent ankle tendon reflexes are early signs; proprioception is usually preserved until other sensory modalities are markedly affected. Weakness, beginning distally, can appear at any time, and eventually even proximal limb muscles become weak. Autonomic symptoms are less common than with diabetic neuropathy, but there may be postural hypotension, cardiac arrhythmia, urinary or fecal incontinence, hypothermia, dysphagia, dysphonia, or abnormal sweating. The cerebrospinal fluid may contain a mildly elevated protein level but is otherwise normal.

Electromyographically, there is denervation and moderately severe reduction of nerve conduction velocities. Pathologically, there is degeneration of myelin and axons. Although a toxic role of ethanol has been proposed, nutritional deprivation is the likelier cause of alcoholic polyneuropathy; the responsible nutrient (e.g., thiamine with or without other vitamin deficiencies) has not been identified, however. Symptomatic improvement follows abstinence, multivitamins, and resumption of an adequate diet.

Alcoholic people are subject to pressure palsies. The radial and peroneal nerves are most often affected, and weakness often exceeds sensory loss. Recovery takes days or weeks, during which time splints can prevent contractures.

PELLAGRA

In alcoholic patients who are deficient in niacin, pellagra develops, with characteristic skin and gastrointestinal symptoms and altered mentation, ranging from dementia to psychosis (see Ch. 71). The symptoms improve with vitamin replacement.

ALCOHOLIC AMBLYOPIA

Visual impairment progressing over days or weeks was formerly called "tobacco-alcohol amblyopia," but the cause appears to be nutritional deficiency, not toxicity. The responsible nutrient is uncertain. On examination, there are central or centrocecal scotomas and pallor of temporal disc margins. Pathologically, demyelination affects the maculopapular bundle especially. Abnormalities are always bilateral, vision is rarely if ever totally lost, and improvement, albeit often incomplete, occurs with vitamin replacement even when drinking continues.

ALCOHOLIC MYOPATHY

Muscle injury in alcoholic people can produce asymptomatic elevation of serum creatine kinase levels; progressive proximal weakness, resembling polymyositis; or acute rhabdomyolysis with marked weakness, swelling, tenderness, and myoglobinuria with renal shutdown. Cardiomyopathy sometimes coexists, and the likely cause is ethanol toxicity rather than nutritional deficiency. Symptoms sometimes emerge during a binge. Treatment consists of abstinence and, if myoglobinuria is present, forced fluids. Strength usually improves within days.

MARCHIAFAVA-BIGNAMI DISEASE

The pathologic changes of Marchiafava-Bignami disease (i.e., demyelination of the midcorpus callosum) do not readily explain the devastating symptoms (i.e., dementia, often progressing over a few weeks or months to coma and death). The diagnosis can sometimes be made premortem by magnetic resonance imaging, and some cases have undergone spontaneous reversal. The disease nearly always affects alcoholic patients. Its cause is unknown.

ALCOHOLIC DEMENTIA

A controversial issue is whether ethanol causes lasting cognitive impairment in the absence of nutritional deficiency, head trauma, hepatic failure, or other indirect means. Radiographically, enlarged cerebral ventricles and widened sulci reportedly paralleled "dementia" in alcoholic patients without other signs of Wernicke-Korsakoff disease, and both symptoms and radiographic abnormalities allegedly improved with abstinence. Opposing the concept of alcoholic dementia are those who maintain that additional brain pathologic findings have not been ruled out in reported cases; moreover, true brain "atrophy" would not be reversible. The question is of obvious importance, for if ethanol is directly toxic to neurons, a safe threshold dose has not been defined.

ALCOHOLIC KETOACIDOSIS

By unclear mechanisms, heavy drinking sometimes leads to accumulation of β-hydroxybutyrate and ketoacidosis. Typically, a binge is interrupted by anorexia, vomiting, dehydration, obtundation, and Kussmaul

respirations (A. Kussmaul, German physician, 1822–1902). The blood glucose level may be normal, high, or low. A large anion gap is present, but the nitroprusside test, which does not detect β-hydroxybutyrate, may be negative. Treatment consists of glucose and multivitamins and correction of dehydration, hypotension, electrolyte imbalance, and bicarbonate level as needed. Other possible causes of acidosis (e.g., methanol or ethylene glycol poisoning and sepsis) must be excluded.

ETHANOL AND STROKE

Similar to coronary artery disease, epidemiologic studies suggest that modest doses of ethanol decrease the risk for stroke, whereas higher doses increase it. The relationship is complex. Confounding factors include tobacco, and there may be differences between hemorrhagic and occlusive stroke, between ethnic groups, and between acute and chronic drinking. Acutely and chronically, ethanol causes hypertension, and it variably affects lipoproteins, platelets, clotting factors, and cerebrovascular reactivity. Alcoholic cardiomyopathy predisposes to embolic stroke.

OTHER INDIRECT EFFECTS OF ETHANOL

Acute alcoholic hepatitis and cirrhosis are common in alcoholic patients, and liver failure accounts for considerable alcohol-related mortality. Hepatic encephalopathy must be considered in any alcoholic patient with altered mentation. Alcoholic people are also subject to dementia, myoclonus, and myelopathy after portocaval shunting and, in those who have had repeated bouts of hepatic encephalopathy, to a chronic state of dementia, dysarthria, ataxia, tremor, asterixis, and choreoathetosis.

Ethanol requires nicotinamide adenine dinucleotide for metabolism, and the resulting cofactor deficiency, plus nutritional deprivation and inadequate hepatic glycogen stores, sets the stage for hypoglycemia, especially during binges. The symptoms include abnormal behavior, coma, and seizures. Treatment consists of intravenous 50 percent dextrose followed by admission to the hospital and close observation; relapses are common.

Alcoholic people are frequently immunosuppressed and thus prone to infection. Bacterial, tuberculous, and other infectious meningitides must be ruled out in any alcoholic patient with fever or altered mentation.

Trauma, including automobile accidents, homicide, and suicide, is common among alcoholic people. Chronic subdural hematoma must be considered in any drinker with an abnormal mental status.

Although not specific to alcoholism, drinkers are

especially prone to central pontine myelinolysis. The cause is overvigorous correction of hyponatremia.

FETAL ALCOHOL SYNDROME

More than one-third of infants born to alcoholic mothers have fetal alcohol syndrome, consisting of microcephaly; mental retardation; poor coordination; decreased weight and length; distinctive facial anomalies; and less consistently, abnormalities of skeleton, heart, skin, muscle, kidney, and genitals. First-trimester exposure is the most critical factor, and partial expression of the syndrome (e.g., mental deficiency without other characteristic anomalies) may be even more common. A safe dose has not been identified. Ethanol thus may be the leading teratogenic cause of mental retardation in the Western world.

ANNOTATED BIBLIOGRAPHY

Alldredge BK, Lowenstein DH, Simon RP. A placebo-controlled trial of intravenous diphenylhydantoin for short-term treatment of alcohol withdrawal seizures. Am J Med 1989;87:645–8.

An emergency room study showing that phenytoin does not prevent ethanol-related seizures.

Brust JCM. Stroke and substance abuse. In Barnett HJM, Mohr JP, Stein BM, Yatsu FM (eds). Stroke. Pathophysiology, Diagnosis, and Management. 2nd Ed. Churchill Livingstone, New York, 1992, p. 875.

A review of stroke associated with ethanol, tobacco, and illicit drugs.

Brust JCM. Ethanol. In Neurological Aspects of Substance Abuse. Butterworths, Stoneham, MA, 1993.

Comprehensive text addressing both licit and illicit drugs.

Centers for Disease Control. Alcohol-related mortality and years of potential life lost—United States. MMWR 1990; 39:173.

Centers for Disease Control estimates in the United States show annual ethanol-related deaths exceed 100,000.

Charness ME, Simon RP, Greenberg DA. Ethanol and the nervous system. N Engl J Med 1989;321:442–54.

A short review that encompasses both clinical phenomena and pathophysiology.

Day NL, Jasperse D, Richardson D et al. Prenatal exposure to alcohol: effect on infant growth and morphologic characteristics. Pediatrics 1989;84:536–41.

A balanced review of a controversial subject.

Gorelick PB. The status of alcohol as a risk factor for stroke. Stroke 1989;20:1607–10.

A brief survey of an often inconsistent literature.

Jensen GB, Pakkenberg B. Do alcoholics drink their neurons away? Lancet 1993;342:1201–10.

An autopsy-based study suggests apparently not; most of the volume loss is in the white matter and may be reversible.

Ng SKC, Hauser WA, Brust JCM, Susser M. Alcohol consumption and withdrawal in new-onset seizures. N Engl J Med 1988;319:666.

A case-control study that quantifies the amount of ethanol associated with seizures and suggests that mechanisms other than withdrawal might be operative in some patients.

Sellers EM, Kalant H. Alcohol intoxication and withdrawal. N Engl J Med 1976;294:757.

Although nearly two decades old, useful descriptions of two common problems.

Urbano-Marquez AM, Estruch R, Navarro-Lopez F et al. The effects of alcoholism on skeletal and cardiac muscle. N Engl J Med 1989;320:409.

Persuasive evidence that ethanol is directly toxic to skeletal and cardiac muscle.

Victor M. Persistent altered mentation due to ethanol. In Brust JCM (ed). Neurological Complications of Drug and Alcohol Abuse. Neurol Clin 1993;11:639.

A skeptical review of the concept of "alcoholic dementia."

Victor M, Adams RD, Collins GH. The Wernicke-Korsakoff Syndrome. 2nd FA Davis, Philadelphia, 1989.

A classic monograph based on the authors' own clinical experience.

68
Drug Dependence

John C. M. Brust

Drug dependence is of two types. *Psychic dependence* refers to craving and drug-seeking behavior. *Physical dependence* is an adaptive state in which discontinuation of a drug or administration of an antagonist produces somatic withdrawal symptoms and signs. Depending on the drug and the circumstances of administration, psychic and physical dependence can exist alone, or together. *Addiction* refers to psychic dependence.

The term *drug abuse* is a social judgment that might reflect either a drug's perceived harm or simply its illegality. In some countries, the legal status of a drug has little to do with its potential harmfulness.

Below is a list of the major classes of drugs that can cause psychic dependence, physical dependence, or both.

OPIOIDS

Opioid agonists include morphine, heroin, methadone, fentanyl, meperidine, hydromorphone, propoxyphene, and codeine. Their antagonists include naloxone and naltrexone. Mixed agonist/antagonists include pentazocine and buprenorphine.

Taken as intended, agonists produce drowsy euphoria, analgesia, cough suppression, and miosis. There is also often nausea, vomiting, sweating, pruritus, hypothermia, postural hypotension, constipation, and decreased libido. Parenterally, opioid agonists produce an ecstatic "rush" followed by euphoria and either relaxed "nodding" or garrulous hyperactivity. With overdose, there is coma, pinpoint (but reactive) pupils, and respiratory depression. Treatment of overdose includes ventilatory support and naloxone, given in small bolus doses (0.4 to 2.0 mg, up to 20 mg) to avoid precipitation of florid withdrawal symptoms. Because the antagonist may wear off sooner than the agonist, hospitalization and careful observation are advisable.

Opioid withdrawal produces craving, irritability, lacrimation, rhinorrhea, sweating, yawning, mydriasis, myalgia, muscle spasms, piloerection, nausea, vomiting, abdominal cramps, fever, hot flashes, tachycardia, hypertension, and orgasm. Seizures and delirium are not features of opioid withdrawal, at least in adults, and their presence mandates a search for other causes. In contrast to withdrawal from sedatives or ethanol, the syndrome is rarely dangerous. It can be prevented or treated with methadone 20 mg once or twice daily. (In newborns, opioid withdrawal can be life threatening; treatment is with either methadone, paregoric, or if additional drug withdrawal is suspected, barbiturates.)

PSYCHOSTIMULANTS

Psychostimulants include amphetamine, methamphetamine, methylphenidate, ephedrine, phenylpropanolamine (which is sold over the counter as a de-

---

DRUGS ASSOCIATED WITH PSYCHIC
OR PHYSICAL DEPENDENCE

Opioids
Psychostimulants
Sedatives/hypnotics
Marijuana
Hallucinogens
Inhalants
Phencyclidine
Anticholinergics
Ethanol
Tobacco
Caffeine

congestant or a diet pill), and cocaine. Cocaine hydrochloride is usually taken intranasally or parenterally. Alkaloidal cocaine (sold as "crack" in some countries) is smokable, as is a methamphetamine preparation known as "ice."

Psychostimulants produce euphoria and psychomotor hyperactivity. With parenteral use or smoking, there is a euphoric rush that is different from that of opioids. Repeated use leads to the emergence of abnormal movements (at first, stereotypy and then bruxism, frank chorea, or dystonia) and psychic changes (paranoia progressing to frank psychosis with auditory, visual, or tactile hallucinations). Overdose causes headache, chest pain, hypertension, fever, sweating, and tachycardia or cardiac arrhythmias. Agitation progresses to delirium or even coma, and there may be seizures, myoglobinuria, metabolic acidosis, shock, and death. Treatment includes, as needed, benzodiazepines for sedation, bicarbonate, cooling, antihypertensives, anticonvulsants, respiratory and blood pressure support, and antiarrhythmic agents. Withdrawal from psychostimulants produces fatigue, hunger, and depression. There are no life-threatening signs, but suicidal ideation can necessitate hospitalization and treatment.

SEDATIVES/HYPNOTICS

Sedative agents include barbiturates (e.g., phenobarbital, pentobarbital, and secobarbital), benzodiazepines (e.g., diazepam, chlordiazepoxide, and alprazolam), and miscellaneous agents (e.g., glutethimide, methaqualone, and ethchlorvynol).

Acute effects resemble those produced by ethanol: euphoria or dysphoria, impaired judgment, and incoordination. Overdose causes coma and respiratory depression, although the latter is far less pronounced with benzodiazepines than with other sedatives.

Treatment of an overdose is supportive. Urinary alkalinization and forced fluids are given for long-acting barbiturates. A specific benzodiazepine antagonist, flumazenil, is available but has a much shorter duration of action than benzodiazepines themselves.

Sedative withdrawal also resembles that of ethanol, with tremor, seizures, or frank delirium tremens. Mild withdrawal symptoms can be prevented or treated with titrated doses of barbiturates or benzodiazepines. Delirium requires intensive care.

MARIJUANA

The hemp plant, *Cannabis sativa,* contains more than two dozen cannabinoid compounds, of which Δ-9-tetrahydrocannabinol is the principal psychoactive ingredient. Marijuana refers to preparations made from cut leaves and tops. Hashish (from the Arabic for grass) is made from the plant resin, which contains high concentrations of psychoactive cannabinoids. Smoked or eaten in desired amounts, marijuana produces a relaxed euphoria, often with disinhibition, silliness, depersonalization, subjective time slowing, conjunctival injection, tachycardia, and postural hypotension. Paradoxic reactions consist of anxiety or panic, and overdose causes confusion or psychosis with auditory and visual hallucinations. Accidents can occur during intoxication, but true fatal overdose has not been documented. Withdrawal can produce craving, headache, jitteriness, and anorexia; physical signs are difficult to discern.

HALLUCINOGENS

Hallucinogenic plants have been used for religious or recreational purposes throughout the world for millennia. In Western countries, the most popular agents are the phenylalkylamine mescaline (from peyote cactus), the indolalkylamines psilocybin and psilocin (from the mushroom *Psilocybe*), and the synthetic ergot drug *d*-lysergic acid diethylamide (LSD). Other phenylalkylamine agents produce amphetaminelike and hallucinatory effects; one of these, methylenedioxymethamphetamine ("ecstasy"), became popular among American students during the 1980s. (Some drugs that can cause hallucinations, e.g., cannabinoid psychostimulants or anticholinergics, are not classified as hallucinogens because they are not usually taken for that purpose and hallucinogenic doses also tend to produce delirium.)

The acute effects of hallucinogens cause altered perception (i.e., illusions, or hallucinations, usually visual, formed, and elaborate). Associated symptoms include altered mood or depersonalization, dizziness, tremor, paresthesias, and rare instances of death. Some users experience anxiety, paranoia, or panic ("bad trips"), which can lead to self-mutilation or suicide. Others have "flashbacks," the spontaneous recurrence of symptoms days to months after use. High doses can cause hypertension, obtundation, and seizures, but fatal overdose per se has not been reported.

Treatment of overdose consists of calm reassurance in a quiet environment. Benzodiazepines can be given in severe cases. There are no withdrawal symptoms.

INHALANTS

Recreationally used inhalants include aerosols (e.g., refrigerants, bronchodilators, hair sprays, and deodorants), bottled fuel gas, fire-extinguishing agents, glues, lighter fluid, spot removers, paints, marker pens, and gasoline. These products contain variable mixtures of aliphatic hydrocarbons (e.g., *n*-hexane), aromatic hydrocarbons (e.g., toluene), and halogenated hydrocarbons (e.g., trichlorethylene). In addition, nitrous oxide is sniffed from whipped cream canisters and butyl or amyl nitrite from "room fresheners." In the United States, most inhalant abusers are children and adolescents.

Despite their chemical diversity, the acute desired effects produced by these agents are remarkably similar, resembling ethanol intoxication. There is euphoria, impaired judgment, and incoordination. High doses, however, cause hallucinations and seizures. Death can result from coma and apnea (an unusual occurrence because loss of consciousness usually interrupts further sniffing). More often, fatalities are the result of accidents, cardiac arrhythmias, aspiration of vomitus, or in those sniffing from plastic bags, suffocation.

Treatment consists of respiratory and cardiovascular monitoring. Symptoms tend to clear within a few hours. Aside from craving, there are no predictable withdrawal symptoms.

PHENCYCLIDINE

Nicknamed "angel dust," phencyclidine, a N-methyl-d-asparte antagonist with potent neuronal suppressor effects, is known as a *dissociative anesthetic* because subjects appear awake with staring eyes. It is not used commercially because it causes psychosis. In recreational use, it is usually smoked, often with marijuana. Low doses produce euphoria or dysphoria with a feeling of numbness. With increasing intoxication there is burst nystagmus, ataxia, tachycardia, hypertension, fever, and sweating. Paranoia progresses to agitation or psychosis, and there may be hallucinations, catatonia, myoclonus, rhabdomyolysis, seizures, coma, respiratory failure, and death.

Treatment consists of benzodiazepine sedation and restraints as needed. Attempts to reassure the patient usually aggravate symptoms. Patients may require forced diuresis, cooling, antihypertensives, anticonvulsants, and cardiovascular and respiratory monitoring. Neuroleptics carry the risk of aggravating fever and myoglobinuria but may be necessary for dangerous psychosis. The symptoms persist for hours or days. There are no withdrawal symptoms other than craving.

ANTICHOLINERGICS

The most popular form of anticholinergic abuse is ingestion of the plant *Datura stramonium* ("jimsonweed"), which grows ubiquitously in many parts of the world and contains atropine and scopolamine. Users are often children and adolescents. Also ingested for their anticholinergic effects are antiparkinsonian drugs and the antidepressant amitriptyline. Intoxica-

tion produces euphoria, often with a dry month, decreased sweating, and tachycardia. With overdose, there are delirium, hallucinations, dilated unreactive pupils, and in severe cases, myoclonus, seizures, coma, and death.

Treatment includes intravenous physostigmine 0.5 to 3 mg, repeated as needed every 30 minutes to 2 hours, plus gastric lavage, cooling, bladder catheterization, respiratory and cardiovascular monitoring, and as needed, anticonvulsants. Neuroleptics, which have anticholinergic actions, are contraindicated. Withdrawal symptoms do not occur.

MEDICAL AND NEUROLOGIC COMPLICATIONS OF ILLICIT DRUGS

Infection

Acquired immunodeficiency syndrome (AIDS) is now the most common cause of death in American parenteral drug abusers. By 1994, heterosexual parenteral drug abusers constituted 25 percent of cases of AIDS reported to the United States Centers for Disease Control; homosexual drug abusers constituted 6 percent more. In New York City, a surrogate for large cities elsewhere, nearly two-thirds of patients receiving methadone maintenance therapy are human immunodeficiency virus (HIV) antibody positive, and the fear of AIDS has altered patterns of use, e.g., encouraging heroin sniffing and crack cocaine smoking. (Crack use, however, is also an AIDS risk factor through associated promiscuous behavior and coexisting sexually transmitted disease.) Parenteral drug abusers are subject to the same neurologic complications of HIV infection that affect members of other risk groups, and asymptomatic HIV-seropositive drug abusers are no likelier than others to develop mental abnormalities or to become symptomatic with AIDS.

Even before the AIDS epidemic, parenteral drug abusers were prone to an array of local and systemic infections, many of which produced neurologic symptoms. These included infectious hepatitis (leading to encephalopathy or hemorrhagic stroke), cellulitis, pyogenic myositis, osteomyelitis (including vertebral, with root or spinal cord involvement), endocarditis (with meningitis, cerebral infarction, cerebral abscess, or septic ["mycotic"] aneurysm), tetanus (usually severe), wound botulism, and malaria. Fungal infections affect the heart or brain. Sinus botulism occurs in cocaine snorters.

Trauma

Acute drug intoxication can lead to trauma (e.g., automobile accidents in marijuana users, violence in cocaine or phencyclidine users, falls in elderly people receiving sedatives, and self-mutilation in users of hallucinogens). However, most of the injuries that affect illicit drug users are the consequence of illegal trafficking and procurement. Before the AIDS epidemic, such trauma was the major cause of morbidity and mortality in heroin users.

Seizures

Depending on the drug, seizures can be secondary to acute intoxication, withdrawal, or an indirect consequence of trauma or infection. With sedatives (including benzodiazepines), seizures are a feature of withdrawal. Anecdotal reports suggest that they occur during intoxication with methaqualone or glutethimide.

Although opioids used experimentally lower the seizure threshold, seizures infrequently complicate acute intoxication, and in adults, they are not a feature of withdrawal. A metabolite of meperidine (normeperidine) is more epileptogenic, and seizures and myoclonus sometimes occur in patients receiving even recommended doses. Seizures also are common in parenteral users of pentazocine combined with the antihistamine tripelennamine ("Ts and blues").

Seizures can occur in cocaine users without other signs of overdose. In chronic users, seizures sometimes emerge in a pattern that resembles electrical kindling. Cocaine seems to be more epileptogenic than amphetamine or other similar psychostimulants, perhaps because of its local anesthetic actions. Seizures have also occurred in users of the over-the-counter psychostimulant phenylpropanolamine.

A case-control study found that marijuana is protective for new-onset seizures, perhaps related to the nonpsychoactive cannabinoid, cannabidiol, which is an anticonvulsant in animals. Such observations, coupled with identification of endogenous brain marijuana receptors and ligands, raises the possibility of a new class of anticonvulsant pharmaceuticals.

Stroke

Some drugs (e.g., ethanol and tobacco) have been identified as risk factors for occlusive and hemorrhagic stroke through epidemiologic studies, both case-control and prospective cohort. With other drugs (e.g., heroin, amphetamine, or cocaine), an association with stroke is based on cumulative case reports. There are many potential mechanisms for any agent. For example, in parenteral drug users, strokes develop through such systemic complications as hepatitis, endocarditis, and AIDS. In heroin users, nephropathy develops with hypertension, uremia, and bleeding. Heroin also causes stroke through less identifiable mechanisms, perhaps toxic or immune vasculitis. "Ts and blues" users develop pulmonary embolization of

foreign material, in turn creating arteriovenous shunts that set the stage for embolization to the brain.

Amphetamine and methamphetamine are especially likely to cause intracerebral hemorrhage. Acute severe hypertension is probably operative in many cases, and hyperthermia may contribute. In users of amphetamine and methamphetamine, vasculitis develops, in some cases affecting medium-sized arteries and resembling polyarteritis nodosa and, in others, affecting smaller arteries and veins and resembling allergic vasculitis.

Including neonates, more than 300 strokes have been reported in cocaine users. Among adults, infarcts and hemorrhages occur with roughly equal frequency, and among those with hemorrhages, more than one-half have had angiographic or autopsy evidence of vascular malformations or saccular aneurysms. Occlusive and hemorrhagic strokes have occurred with roughly equal frequency among alkaloidal cocaine users. Strokes affecting users of cocaine hydrochloride have been predominantly hemorrhagic. A possible mechanism of some cocaine strokes is vasospasm. Cocaine and some of its metabolites are cerebral vasoconstrictors, and hemorrhage might occur when vasospasm subsides in the presence of marked hypertension.

Stroke has been reported in users of either LSD and phencyclidine, each of which is vasoconstrictive.

Chronically Altered Mentation

That users of illicit drugs have lasting cognitive or behavioral disturbance is undisputed. What is controversial is whether such changes occur independently of ethanol abuse, head injury, malnutrition, or infection (including HIV). Moreover, the predrug mental status is often difficult to determine, and although no cognitive or behavioral pattern defines or predicts drug use (i.e., there is no such thing as an "addictive personality"), a variety of mental disturbances are overrepresented among illicit drug users. At the present time, the weight of evidence is against heroin or other opioids having lasting direct adverse mental effects. Despite anecdotal claims to the contrary, the same can be said for marijuana and hallucinogens. With psychostimulants, especially cocaine, two types of ill effect have been claimed, namely lasting psychic depression (perhaps from permanent depletion of dopamine in the brain "reward circuit") and impaired intellectual function, allegedly correlating with cerebral atrophy and irregularly reduced cerebral blood flow. The acute effects of phencyclidine resemble schizophrenia, and lasting schizophrenic illness has been observed in some chronic users. Toluene sniffers have had dementia with cerebral white matter lesions. Gasoline sniffers have developed lead encephalopathy. Sedatives, including benzodiazepines, are a common cause of cognitive impairment in elderly people, but permanent compromise is difficult to document. Barbiturates, given as anticonvulsants, cause developmental delay in small children.

Miscellaneous Effects

Rhabdomyolysis, myoglobinuria, and renal failure without other signs of overdose have affected users of heroin and cocaine. In phencyclidine users, rhabdomyolysis tends to occur in obviously toxic patients.

Heroin users are subject to traumatic peripheral nerve injuries (including pressure palsies during coma). They also develop, probably on an immune basis, polyneuropathy of the Guillain-Barré type and brachial or lumbosacral plexopathy resembling neuralgic amyotrophy. Brachial plexopathy has also resulted from septic aneurysm of the subclavian artery.

Sensorimotor polyneuropathy occurs in sniffers of glue that contains n-hexane; severely affected patients have become quadriplegic. With improvement, pyramidal signs sometimes become unmasked, implying central nervous system damage too.

In nitrous oxide sniffers, myeloneuropathy develops, which is clinically indistinguishable from that caused by cobalamin deficiency. Anemia is absent (although, interestingly, short-term high-dose nitrous oxide exposure can produce megaloblastic anemia without myeloneuropathy). The cobalamin-dependent enzymes, methylmalonyl coenzyme A mutase and methionine synthetase, are inactivated by nitrous oxide. Clinical improvement follows cessation of use.

In a number of Californians who took a synthetic meperidine-like opioid, severe parkinsonism developed. The responsible toxin was a byproduct of manufacture, 1-methyl-4-phenyl-1,2,3,6-tetrahydropyridine, a metabolite of which damages cells of the substantia nigra. The symptoms responded to levodopa therapy but recurred if the drug was discontinued. Positron emission tomographic studies of asymptomatic subjects exposed to the drug revealed decreased striatal dopamine receptors, raising the possibility that, with aging, these patients will become parkinsonian.

European smokers of "heroin pyrolysate" have developed a syndrome of dementia, ataxia, quadriparesis, blindness, and death, and autopsies have shown white matter spongiform changes. The responsible toxin has not been identified.

A heroin user whose mixture contained quinine became blind; vision improved when be resumed heroin minus the quinine.

Cocaine has precipitated symptoms in patients with Gilles de la Tourette's syndrome.

Chronic ataxia is a complication of toluene sniffing; white matter changes are seen in the cerebellum.

Marijuana inhibits luteinizing and follicle-stimulating hormones. In men, impotence and sterility develop, and women have menstrual irregularities. The symptoms clear with abstinence.

Fetal Effects

Similarly difficult to define are the effects of illicit drugs on intrauterine development because drug-using pregnant women often abuse ethanol, smoke tobacco, are malnourished, and receive no prenatal care until delivery. Infants exposed to heroin in utero have reportedly been small for gestational age, at risk for respiratory distress, and prone to developmental delay later in life. Cocaine exposure has reportedly caused abruptio placentae, decreased birth weight, microcephaly, congenital anomalies, tremor, perinatal stroke, and delayed milestones. Marijuana exposure has been associated with decreased birth weight and length. Carefully controlled studies will be required to define the specificity of these purported associations.

ANNOTATED BIBLIOGRAPHY

Brust JCM. Neurological Aspects of Substance Abuse. Butterworth-Heinemann, Stoneham, MA, 1993.

A comprehensive text that includes both licit and illicit agents, addressing pharmacology and animal studies, historic background, overdose and withdrawal, medical and neurologic complications, fetal effects, and pharmacology.

Chiriboga CA. Fetal effects. In Brust JCM (ed). Neurological Complications of Drug, and Alcohol Abuse. Neurol Clin 1993;11:707.

A critical review of adverse effects attributed to various abused substances.

Gautier JC. L'angiopathie cérébrale moniliforme des toxicomanes. Signification physiopathologique. Role possible du spasme. Bull Acad Natl Med 1988;172:87.

A brief review that questions the role of vasculitis in psychostimulant-related stroke.

Khantzian EJ, McKenna GJ. Acute toxic, and withdrawal reactions associated with drug use, and abuse. Ann Intern Med 1979;90:361.

Although a decade and a half old, a useful summary.

Levine SR, Brust JCM, Futrell N et al. Cerebrovascular complications of the use of the "crack" form of alkaloidal cocaine. N Engl J Med 1990;323:699.

Twenty-eight cases, including infarction, intracerebral hemorrhage, and subarachnoid hemorrhage.

Levine SR, Brust JCM, Futrell N et al. A comparative study of the cerebrovascular complications of cocaine: alkaloidal versus hydrochloride—a review. Neurology 1991;41:1173.

A literature review that suggests different pathophysiologic effects of alkaloidal cocaine and cocaine hydrochloride.

Lowenstein DH, Massa SM, Rowbotham MC et al. Acute neurologic, and psychiatric complications associated with cocaine abuse. Am J Med 1987;83:841.

The view from a municipal hospital emergency room.

Ng SKC, Brust JCM, Hauser WA, Susser M. Illicit drug use, and the risk of new onset seizures: contrasting effects of heroin, marijuana, and cocaine. Am J Epidemiol 1990;132:47.

A case-control study that unexpectedly identified heroin use as an independent risk factor and cannabis as protective.

Pascual-Leone A, Dhuna A, Anderson DC. Cerebral atrophy in habitual cocaine abusers: a planimetric CT study. Neurology 1991;41:34.

Radiographic evidence for possible long-term brain damage.

Sloan MA, Kittner SJ, Rigamonti D, Price TR. Occurrence of stroke associated with use/abuse of drugs. Neurology 1991;41:1358.

Eleven cases involving cocaine, phencyclidine, heroin, phenylpropanolamine, and pseudoephedrine.

Stolerman I. Drugs of abuse: behavioral principles, methods, and terms. Trends Pharmacol Sci 1992;13:170.

A short basic review.

Weinrieb RM, O'Brien CP. Persistent cognitive deficits attributed to substance abuse. In Brust JCM (ed): Neurologic Complications of Drug, and Alcohol Abuse. Neurol Clin 1993;11:663.

A thorough and critical review of a difficult subject.

69
Fluid and Electrolyte Disturbances

J. P. Mohr and J. C. Gautier

Disturbances in sodium, potassium, and calcium metabolism are the most important abnormalities of fluid and electrolyte balance in clinical neurology. The neurologic consequences of disordered water balance are often equated with those of sodium metabolism because changes in serum sodium values are the most obvious among the routinely measured electrolytes.

HYPONATREMIA AND WATER INTOXICATION

Excess sweating, with attendant salt loss and replacement by heavy drinking of tap water or other low-sodium liquids, accounts for most instances of water intoxication or functional hyponatremia. In hospital practice, hyponatremia in a setting of cerebral aneurysmal subarachnoid hemorrhage may occur despite normal fluid treatment for reasons of elevated plasma atrial naturetic factor and vasopressin levels. Cerebral infarction is more common in this group of patients. In severe meningitis and after major head injury, hypothalamic injury may also cause hyponatremia, but this portion of the clinical picture is often of secondary importance. Chronic intoxication is also possible from inappropriate antidiuretic hormone secretion in a setting of adrenal insufficiency or myxedema, and it may be the first sign of an antidiuretic hormone-secreting bronchogenic carcinoma.

In the days before the risks were well known, iatrogenic causes included rapid administration of 5 percent dextrose and water solutions; excessive irrigation of the bladder with water; injudicious use of hypotonic fluids in patients with impaired renal function; and therapy with tricyclic antidepressants, neuroleptic agents, carbamazepine, diuretics, oral hypoglycemic agents, analgesics, and antineoplastic agents in high doses. Occasional psychotic patients may drink themselves into an acute state of severe water intoxication.

The *acute clinical picture* features lightheadedness, imbalance, and mild weakness, which disappears within hours of correction of the deficiency. Although the effects of water overload might be expected to differ from those attributable to hyponatremia alone, few studies document the differences in clinical syndromes in the two conditions. In all cases, the severity of the syndrome depends on how rapidly the excess occurs. When the sodium level falls rapidly and, in most instances, when it is below 120 mEq/L, the clinical picture, although highly variable, may include headache, generalized weakness, vomiting, delirium, stupor, and even myoclonus or seemingly focal signs, such as dysphasia, hemianopia, and hemiparesis. If the disorder progresses to coma and seizures, there is a poor prognosis for functional recovery.

The recommended *treatment* for acute states is intravenous furosemide at a dose of 1 mg/kg and 3 percent saline and potassium. Once the sodium level reaches 130 mEq/L, efforts may cease. Correction back toward normal should not proceed too quickly. When this is achieved within 24 hours, a certain number of patients suffer central pontine myelinolysis, the lesions appearing acutely on a magnetic resonance imaging scan. Slower correction is recommended, spanning 48 hours or so. If the condition is mild or chronic, water restriction suffices.

HYPERNATREMIA

A gradual evolution of stupor, even to the point of coma, occurs when water deprivation or other conditions lead to hyperosmolality. The two most common causes are heat stroke and nonketotic hyperglycemic hyperosmolality, but untreated diabetes insipidus and other, iatrogenic, causes, including excessive solute loads from hypertonic fluids, tube feedings, and peritoneal or hemodialysis dialysis, are on the list. Rarely, the sodium bicarbonate used during cardiac arrest has precipitated such states.

When the serum sodium level exceeds 160 mEq/L, consciousness is depressed. There are few distinctive syndromes other than stupor and coma.

Treatment by hasty correction of hypernatremia (within hours) using dilute fluids can produce a syndrome of water intoxication despite elevated serum sodium levels. As in hyponatremia, it is recommended that the abnormality be corrected over a period of 48 hours.

HYPOKALEMIA

Potassium loss from renal or gastrointestinal disorders is the most common cause of hypokalemia. Many diuretics promote renal loss of potassium, as does the uncommon syndrome of renal tubular acidosis. Gastrointestinal conditions that cause potassium loss are headed by diarrheal diseases, less often by protracted vomiting, and only occasionally, by the chronic use of laxatives. Serum potassium may be decreased by some antacids, penicillins, and steroids.

Although disorders of sodium feature changes in levels of alertness, weakness, most often in the limbs, is the first and most prominent sign of changes in serum potassium concentrations, whether increased or decreased. The prominent weakness may lead to a misdiagnosis of acute polyneuritis, polymyositis, and rarely, amyotrophic lateral sclerosis.

In addition to weakness, hypokalemia may exaggerate clinical problems in several other disease states. In anesthesia, skeletal muscle-blocking agents such as curare often have an exaggerated effect with hypokalemia. Total body potassium stores are frequently depleted in chronic alcoholic people, making them at risk for intravenous fluid therapy. Hypokalemia has helped precipitate hepatic encephalopathy in a setting of chronic hepatic insufficiency because the alkalosis accompanying hypokalemia increases ammonia diffusion into the portal circulation and hypokalemia, leading to more renal ammonia production.

Rapid replacement of potassium can be risky and has precipitated hyperkalemia in some patients, especially those undergoing therapy with agents interfering with the renin-aldosterone axis.

HYPERKALEMIA

Hyperkalemia is uncommon. The few clinically important instances are found in a setting of the liberal use of potassium-sparing diuretics; ingestion of salt substitutes; altered renin-aldosterone interactions from drugs such as β-blocking agents, indomethacin, and ibuprofen; and in hospital settings with the use of succinylcholine, hypertonic agents, heparin, and rarely, hyporeninemic hypoaldosteronism.

Cardiac arrhythmias are the major serious risk. The initial clinical picture, as in hypokalemia, begins as diffuse skeletal muscle weakness.

Calcium gluconate is used acutely to reverse life-threatening hyperkalemia, given intravenously in a 10 percent solution in doses of 10 to 30 ml over 3 to 4 minutes. Reversal of the potassium levels to normal requires exchange resins, diuretics, and in some instances, dialysis.

HYPOCALCEMIA

The common causes of hypocalcemia are hypoparathyroidism (occasionally after accidental removal of all the parathyroid glands during thyroid or parathyroid surgery), disorders of vitamin D metabolism, and chronic therapy with phenytoin (which converts vitamin D to an inactive metabolite).

Although often cited in the popular press as a cause for easy fatigability, emotional lability, impaired memory, and other behavioral disorders, hypocalcemia usually causes annoying muscle twitches, paresthesiae, spasms of the wrists and ankles, and rarely, seizures. Isolated papilledema has been reported.

The spontaneous discharge of motor (and sensory) peripheral nerves, known as *tetany*, may present clinically as unprovoked cramps or painful spasms, most often of the wrists or ankles (carpopedal spasm). The evidence of instability of the neuronal axonal membrane thought responsible for the spasm can be evoked by special tests. Trousseau's sign (A. Trousseau, French physician, 1801–1867) is a cramp-like carpal spasm produced by inflating a blood pressure cuff on the arm to levels above systolic pressure, inducing ischemia. Chvostek's sign (F. Chvostek, Austrian surgeon, 1834–1884) can usually be elicited, that is, a light reflex hammer tap just anterior to the external auditory meatus excites the facial nerve and triggers orbicularis oris or oculi muscles.

The acute symptoms can usually be abolished within minutes by intravenous infusion of 10-ml ampules of calcium gluconate over a 10-minute period diluted in 50 ml of 5 percent dextrose and water. The use of vitamin D in the form of dihydrotachysterol 0.75 mg is commonly required. It enhances intestinal absorption of calcium but is not an acute treatment because it takes several weeks for an effect to appear.

HYPERCALCEMIA

Primary hyperparathyroidism, neoplasms metastatic to bone or those that produce parathyroid hormone, and immobilization are the usual causes of this uncommon condition.

In the usual cases, impaired nerve conduction occurs with hypercalcemia, leading to generalized weakness and chronic constipation. In some, behavioral disorders resembling bifrontal tumor or hydrocephalus are the predominant signs, with headache, delirium, reduction in spontaneity, and in extreme cases, coma. The diagnosis is often made by inspection of the serum electrolyte pattern.

In acute states, lowering of calcium levels by the use of furosemide in doses up to 100 mg every 1 to 2 hours accompanied by generous or rapid infusion of saline usually leads to excretion of calcium. Plicamycin, used as an intravenous bolus dose of 25 μg/kg body weight or by infusion over 3 hours, usually lowers calcium within 6 to 12 hours. For long-term therapy, aspirin and indomethacin may help lower calcium through prostaglandin inhibition, but in·the more refractory cases, dialysis is necessary.

HYPERMAGNESEMIA

Rarely, this state has been reported to precipitate a degree of neuromuscular, autonomic, and pupillary paralysis that suggests severe brainstem dysfunction. The full explanations for the syndrome are unknown, but the treatable clinical state prompts inclusion of magnesium among those electrolytes studied in acute, unexplained coma.

ANNOTATED BIBLIOGRAPHY

Arieff AI, Llach F, Massry SG. Neurological manifestations and morbidity of hyponatremia: correlation with brain water and electrolytes. Medicine (Baltimore) 1976;55: 121.

Still a classic.

Brunner JE, Redmond JM, Haggar AM et al. Central pontine myelinolysis and pontine lesions after rapid correction of hyponatremia: a prospective magnetic resonance imaging study. Ann Neurol 1990;27:61–6.

The occurrence of central pontine myelinolysis was more frequent among those with the lowest serum sodiums (below 100 mmol/l) and those whose correction to normal was achieved within 24 hours (1.25 mmol/l · hr) compared with one-half that rate).

Castelbaum AR, Donofrio PD, Walker FO, Troost BT. Laxative abuse causing hypermagnesemia, quadriparesis and neuromuscular junction defect. Neurology 1989;39: 746–7.

Prolonged use.

Ghaznawi HI, Ibrahim MA. Heat stroke and heat exhaustion in pilgrims performing the Haj (annual pilgrimage) in Saudia Arabia. Ann Saudi Med 1987;7:323.

Details of extremes of dehydration.

Hahn TJ. Drug-induced disorders of vitamin D and mineral metabolism. Clin Endocrinol Metab 1980;9:107.

Useful advice.

Juan D. Hypocalcemia: differential diagnosis and mechanisms. Arch Intern Med 1979;139:1166.

A full account.

Nathan DM. Long-term complications of diabetes mellitus. N Engl J Med 1993;328:1676–85.

Modern review.

Pasman JW, Gabreels FJ, Semmekrot B et al. Hyperkalemic periodic paralysis in Gordon's syndrome: a possible defect in atrial natriuretic peptide function. Ann Neurol 1989;26:392–5.

Hypertension, tubular acidosis and hyperkalemia with a normal glomerular filtration rate accounted for hyperkalemia in a 14-year-old boy.

Rizzo MA, Fisher M, Lock JP. Hypermagnesemic pseudocoma. Arch Intern Med 1993;153:1130–2.

Extreme hypermagnesemia (9.85 mmol/l) caused neuromuscular and parasympathetic blockade with fixed and dilated pupils.

Seliger G, Cosman F, Abrams GM, Lindsay R. Hypercalcaemia causing declining cognitive function in a head-injured patient. Brain Inj 1989;3:315–8.

Caused by immobilization.

Wijdicks EF, Ropper AH, Hunnicutt EJ et al. Atrial natriuretic factor and salt wasting after aneurysmal subarachnoid hemorrhage. Stroke 1991;22:1519–24.

Plasma atrial naturetic factor and vasopressin levels are initially as high as two to three times normal in patients with subarachnoid hemorrhage and correlate with a negative sodium balance. Ischemic strokes occur more often in this group.

70
Organ Failure

J. P. Mohr and J. C. Gautier

HEPATIC ENCEPHALOPATHY

Hepatic encephalopathy usually occurs at the end stage of hepatocellular failure; it may be precipitated by a sudden rise in gut protein levels (from heavy feeding or from the protein contained in the blood after gastrointestinal bleeding) and frequently follows portacaval shunting for esophageal bleeding. The relationship to protein loads seems suitably explained by the findings that the dysfunctional liver could not metabolize the chemical it faces and excess amounts of chemical released in the blood somehow have a toxic reaction in the brain.

Pathophysiology

Brain disease after severe hepatic disease is seen in many species and has led to many animal model attempts to clarify the underlying cause for so-called hepatic encephalopathy. No single mechanism has been found to be responsible, but among the candidates are the long-suspected direct neurotoxic effect of the elevated serum ammonia levels; the elevated levels of phenols, mercaptans, and fatty acids (especially the short- and medium-chain varieties, which suppress midbrain reticular formation activity in animals); and the wide variations from normal in the concentration of circulating amino acids (especially phenylalanine). More recently discovered are altered concentrations of neurotransmitters, including dopamine, norepinephrine, and γ-aminobutyric acid; increased cerebral concentrations of serotonin and its amino acid precursor tryptophan, especially in the basal ganglia and thalamus; the presence of false neurotransmitters, including phenylethanolamine and octopamine; increased levels of benzodiazepine receptor ligands; and disturbances in glutamate-mediated excitatory amino acid neurotransmission. The therapeutic attempts to alter ammonia and amino acid levels have

a long history. Attempts to correct benzodiazepine receptor and glutamate-mediated neurotransmitters are only now underway. Finally, with improved brain imaging, a potentially important role for brain edema in the encephalopathy is becoming better understood.

Clinical Features

The early signs of developing encephalopathy appear as changes in the level of interaction with the environment. At first, the patient shows delays of seconds before replies, giving the appearance of being confused. Mild disorientation is evident on questioning. Within hours to days, delirium develops, usually without hallucinations or excessive motor activity, known as a quiet or somnolent delirium. The most prominent motor sign, which may occur in isolation but usually accompany the delirium, is asterixis (from the Greek for lacking a fixed position). It is best demonstrated by having patients stretch their arms and hands and watching them for sudden lapses in posture. As evidence, it is not a disorder of the arms, per se, but of posture, it has also been described in the feet and even in the oropharynx.

When cerebral edema becomes prominent, many signs suggesting impending herniation have been described, including asymmetric pupils and Cheyne-Stokes respirations, and more focal signs suggesting to some observers the patient has had a stroke. Included in the latter are clonus, hemiparesis, dysconjugate eye movements, and ocular bobbing (see Ch. 28). For patients who are successfully treated, all of these signs can disappear. Patients in whom neurologic symptoms develop within 7 days of the onset of jaundice have the highest incidence of cerebral edema and are thought to have the best response to treatment.

For comments concerning portocaval myelopathy (encephalomyelopathy, see Ch. 31).

Laboratory Diagnosis

Tests of concern to the neurologist include the brain images, electroencephalogram (EEG), and evoked cerebral potentials. Increased signals in T_1-weighted magnetic resonance imaging have been seen in the basal ganglia and have returned toward normal after successful treatment; the explanation is still unknown.

Classically, the conventional EEG shows a triphasic waveform (see Ch. 11) in well-established hepatic encephalopathy, but its appearance only late in the course makes it of limited prognostic value. Spectral analysis has permitted the identification of these waveforms against the background EEG before they are visible to naked-eye inspection. Visual- and somatosensory-evoked potential show increased latencies and gradual diminution of the individual waves as the hepatic encephalopathy syndrome progresses. The brainstem portions of the auditory-evoked potentials show no changes.

Transcranial Doppler (see Ch. 13) and intracranial pressure monitoring are useful in following the course of the cerebral edema.

Therapy

The first step is to reduce available ammonia by limiting dietary protein. The use of nonabsorbable antibiotics (neomycin 2 to 4 g/day orally) has long been popular, but benefits have not always been seen in double-blind studies. Special diets of branched-chain amino acids have met with modest success. Liver transplants still have a high incidence of neurologic complications; seizures occur in some 25 percent. Phenytoin is usually effective in controlling the seizures, but monitoring of blood levels is advised.

RENAL FAILURE AND HEMODIALYSIS

Neurologic disturbances in the wake of acute or chronic renal failure and dialysis remain important clinical problems still awaiting adequate therapy.

Pathophysiology

The chemical basis for the neurologic complications of chronic renal failure and dialysis are still unsettled, but especially for those undergoing dialysis, aluminum remains a prime candidate. The main source appears to be aluminum hydroxide gels, not aluminum in the diet. Most of the latter accumulates in bones. There is a correlation between the rapidity of rise in the serum aluminum concentration and the occurrence and severity of disturbances in consciousness. When the elevations in aluminum levels occur slowly, over years, the main deposition occurs in bones, not the brain. The bone aluminum concentration does not predict neurologic syndromes. How the aluminum reaches the brain is unclear, but some evidence suggests it is transported by a glutamate-sensitive mechanism. How aluminum causes brain disturbances is also unclear, but recent work suggests it does not accomplish its effects by promoting the occurrence of Alzheimer's disease-like neurofibrillary plaques or tangles, which contain aluminum (see Ch. 60).

Clinical Features

Neurologic disorders occur in three settings of renal disease: acute renal failure, chronic renal failure, and dialysis.

In *acute renal failure,* neurologic disturbances typically begin as a severe agitated delirium, usually accompanied by cortical (occipital) blindness. The neurologic symptoms are often established for hours before evidence of the renal abnormalities appear in blood or urine tests. Once treatment has begun for the acute renal failure, the neurologic disorder returns toward normal, usually requiring several days for total clinical recovery. The patients seen by the authors have been amnestic for the entire episode.

Acute brain imaging with computed tomography or magnetic resonance imaging has not shown lesions, although signs of edema have been seen in those with acute hypertensive encephalopathy. The explanation for the syndrome in acute renal failure is still unknown.

Chronic renal insufficiency (failure) has long been associated with a generalized sensorimotor polyneuropathy (see Ch. 32) with loss of reflexes in the lower extremities and impairment of balance and gait. Late in the course of renal failure, before the days of dialysis, it was common to discover that the patient slowly develops less interest, with declining spontaneous activity, reduced conversation, poor memory, and decline in appetite. These behavioral changes are usually accompanied by generalized weakness, which is followed later by tremulousness, asterixis, myoclonic jerks, and in some instances, tetany. Seizures also occur. These late complications of renal failure are mainly seen nowadays in patients with obstructive uropathy from cancer or those who for other reasons are not undergoing dialysis.

Dialysis Complications

The widespread use of dialysis has allowed many patients to live well beyond their expected life span without this treatment. Two types of neurologic complications have become well recognized. The first is the *disequilibrium syndrome,* which features a subacute development of severe headache, seizures, impaired memory, and delirium without agitation. The usual cause is an excessively rapid institution of hemodialysis, and it has also been documented from rapid correction of dehydration with fluid intravenous therapy. Although the exact cause is unclear, the syndrome generally subsides within days by slowing the program of dialysis to three times a week. More serious is *progressive dialysis encephalopathy,* which has been tied to the use of aluminum hydroxide gel as an antacid (see above). After institution of dialysis, symptoms have occurred in as quickly as 4 days, but most cases occur 3 months to 7 years after therapy has begun. The clinical syndrome has a gradual onset with some fluctuations in severity but usually becomes steadily progressive to the fatal outcome. Disturbed speech is prominent with stuttering, dysnomia, and even global dysphasia and mutism. Dementia may be a separate syndrome, presenting with disorientation and impaired memory, mimicking many clinical features of Alzheimer's disease. In a few patients, the disorder takes the form of agitation, hallucinations, and paranoid delusions. Once started, dialysis encephalopathy usually progresses inexorably to a fatal outcome within 3 to 15 months. No program of hemodialysis has yet been found to avoid this risk.

Therapy

Abandonment of dialysis in favor of renal transplants has been tried with some success. Thus far, none of the many treatments that hoped to reverse or correct the putative imagined abnormalities have shown success. No value has been seen from vitamins, steroids, penicillamine, dimercaprol, antibiotics, anticonvulsants, or levodopa therapy.

ANNOTATED BIBLIOGRAPHY

al-Mardini H, Harrison EJ, Ince PG et al. Brain indoles in human hepatic encephalopathy. Hepatology 1993;17:1033–40.

Brain serotonin levels are higher in patients dying with hepatic encephalopathy compared with matched controls.

Bommer J, Ritz E. Water quality—a neglected problem in hemodialysis. Nephron 1987;46:1–6.

The water supply is a source of aluminum.

Candy JM, McArthur FK, Oakley AE et al. Aluminium accumulation in relation to senile plaque and neurofibrillary tangle formation in the brains of patients with renal failure. J Neurol Sci 1992;107:210–8.

No clear correlation between the presence and intensity of β/A4 amyloid precursor immunostaining or senile plaques with aluminum concentrations in the cerebral cortex.

Davies MG, Rowan MJ, Feely J. EEG and event related potentials in hepatic encephalopathy. Metab Brain Dis 1991;6:175–86.

Review of clinical neurophysiology in hepatic encephalopathy.

Dawson AM, Mclaren J, Sherlock S. Neomycin in the treatment of hepatic coma. Lancet 1957;2:1263.

The classic article but less clear evidence for effects today.

De-Deyn PP, Saxena VK, Abts H et al. Clinical and pathophysiological aspects of neurological complications in renal failure. Acta Neurol Belg 1992;92:191–206.

Modern review including dialysis dementia and dysequilibrium syndromes.

English A, Savage RD, Britton PT. Intellectual impairment in chronic renal failure. B M J 1978;1:888–90.

The EEG is normal in chronic dialysis.

Knudsen GM, Schmidt J, Almdal T et al. Passage of amino acids and glucose across the blood brain barrier in patients with hepatic encephalopathy. Hepatology 1993;17:987–92.

Phenylalanine passage correlates with the severity of the clinical syndromes.

Merrill JP, Legrain M, Hoigne, R. Observations on the role of urea in uremia. Am J Med 1953;14:519.

Elevated urea alone is not the explanation for the mental changes.

O'Grady JG, Schalm SW, Williams R. Acute liver failure: redefining the syndromes. Lancet 1993;342:273–5.

New clinical names for syndrome subtypes based on the time of onset.

Plauth M, Egberts EH, Hamster W et al. Long term treatment of latent portosystemic encephalopathy with branched chain amino acids. A double blind placebo controlled crossover study. J Hepatol 1993;17:308–14.

Long-term branched chain amino acid supplementation was superior to placebo in patients with mild encephalopathy.

Rakela J, Mosley JW, Edwards VM et al. A double blinded, randomized trial of hydrocortisone in acute hepatic failure. The Acute Hepatic Failure Study Group. Dig Dis Sci 1991;36:1223–8.

No value of 400 or 800 mg of hydrocortisone per day compared with placebo.

Rozga J, Podesta L, LePage E et al. Control of cerebral oedema by total hepatectomy and extracorporeal liver support in fulminant hepatic failure. Lancet 1993;342:898–9.

A method for reducing cerebral edema while awaiting a liver transplant.

Sprague SM, Corwin HL, Tanner CM et al. Relationship of aluminum to neurocognitive dysfunction in chronic dialysis patients. Arch Intern Med 1988;148:2169–72.

Higher aluminum levels were associated with greater number of neurologic observed abnormalities.

Yurdaydin C, Gu ZQ, Nowak G et al. Benzodiazepine receptor ligands are elevated in an animal model of hepatic encephalopathy: relationship between brain concentration and severity of encephalopathy. J Pharmacol Exp Ther 1993;265:565–71.

Elevated levels of benzodiazepine receptor agonists are present in animal models and in humans with hepatic encephalopathy.

71
Vitamin Deficiencies

J. P. Mohr and J. C. Gautier

Vitamins (Latin: *vita*, life; + amines), those compounds that are indispensable to normal human metabolism but not manufactured by it, are present in large amounts in the usual Western diet. In such conditions, the faddist public consumption of vitamins is a waste. However, there are still many regions all over the world where episodic or chronic famine or substarvation as a result of socioeconomic conditions or wars causes many cases of vitamin deficiencies. It is also important to realize that, even in Western countries, there are still cases of vitamin deficiencies in some communities.

Apart from the basic lack of vitamins in the diet, vitamins can be lacking because their absorption is hindered (i.e., by digestive diseases or surgery), their requirements are increased by some abnormality in the diet (i.e., alcoholism), or their metabolism is deranged by some additional factor, such as some forms of drug therapy. In some settings, for instance, chronic malabsorption syndromes or starvation, there may be a multivitamin deficiency.

Overall, deficiencies in vitamins in the B group are the most important in pathologic conditions of the nervous system.

VITAMIN B₁

Thiamine, a water-soluble, widely available vitamin, is found in all foods, except fats, oils, and sugar. The shells of cereal grains and rice are rich in the vitamin but have far lower levels after they are milled. Cooking temperatures above 100°C destroy much of the vitamin in natural foods. Alcoholism, malabsorption states, folate deficiency, and chronic malnutrition reduce its intestinal absorption. Some fish preparations popular in Asia contain thiaminases that deplete the available thiamine. Thiamine depletion can occur within a few weeks in thiamine-poor diets.

Pathophysiology

Thiamine diphosphate is a coenzyme involved in oxidative carboxylation. Axonal membranes contain the vitamins, and thiamine and its esters are involved in neurotransmission, a function separate from its role as a coenzyme.

Thiamine deficiency is thought to impair the chains of relevant metabolic reactions, but how the nervous system is injured is not clear. In the peripheral nervous system, a deficiency mainly affects the axons of the longer nerve fibers. In the central nervous system, incomplete foci of necrosis are seen in the perimesencephalic gray matter of the midbrain, the thalamus adjacent to the third ventricle, and also in the mammillary bodies in patients who die with Wernicke-Korsakoff syndrome (see below). In some, because there is hyperplasia of the capillaries, the lesions have been hemorrhagic.

The occurrence of a sensorimotor peripheral neuropathy in thiamine-deficient subjects has prompted speculation that disordered thiamine metabolism might be involved in the occurrence of Friedreich's ataxia and the olivopontocerebellar ataxia syndromes. Although slightly lower levels of spinal fluid thiamine are found in these conditions, blood levels are the same as those in controls.

Clinical Disorders

The various forms of thiamine deficiency are all known as beriberi (a Singhalese term meaning extreme weakness). In so-called wet beriberi, cardiac disease with congestive failure is a prominent feature as is a subacute sensorimotor peripheral neuropathy. The edematous limbs may be tender to palpation.

In dry beriberi (no cardiac disease), there is no peripheral edema, and the neuropathy is chronic, symmetric, and predominantly distal, clinically similar to many other deficiency states. The maximal nerve conduction velocities are somewhat unusual in that they may be normal for both motor and sensory fibers.

The more distinctive neurologic disorder is the *Wernicke-Korsakoff syndrome* (see Ch. 67), also known as cerebral beriberi. This syndrome, sometimes precipitated by intravenous glucose therapy in a severely thiamine-depleted patient, usually a chronic alcoholic patient but sometimes a patient with hyperemesis gravidarum or pyloric stenosis, evolves within hours to days and features changes in alertness, often accompanied by a severe amnesia (Korsakoff's psychosis, see Chs. 21 and 67); extraocular disturbances with prominent nystagmus, disturbances in horizontal gaze, and occasionally as severe as complete ophthalmoplegia; and ataxia, especially affecting the trunk, including difficulties in standing. Polyneuropathy also occurs in most cases.

Treatment

Treatment is nothing short of a medical emergency. Intramuscular injection of 50 mg of thiamine daily is a good plan for all patients admitted with any suspicion of dietary deficiency, especially those with cardiac symptoms. After a few days, oral therapy with as little as 2.5 to 5 mg/day suffices. For Wernicke-Korsakoff syndrome, this program is also sufficient treatment to stabilize and reverse those elements that are treatable. Larger doses are not absorbed. The extraocular movement disorders improve within hours. The ataxia improves over days and weeks. The severe amnestic state may be permanent.

VITAMIN B₂

Riboflavin deficiency is likely to play a role in some nutritional polyneuropathies.

VITAMIN B₃

Nicotinic acid (also known as niacin) deficiency causes pellagra (Italian: *pelle* skin; *agro* rough), also known as St. Ignatius' itch. It is a disease of people consuming diets limited to corn (maize) and of alcoholic persons.

The fully developed disease includes skin, gastrointestinal, and blood disorders. The nervous system involvement features an encephalopathy with depression, irritability, memory impairment, apathy, and insomnia.

Pathologically, the axonal reaction (i.e., a rounded aspect with loss of Nissl bodies and eccentric nuclei, classically explained as a reaction to axonal interruption), is seen in a wide array of large cells (from the Betz cells to the anterior horn cells) with a predominance of such changes in the pontine reticular formation. In pellagra, it would seem that this histopatho-

logic change is due to a direct effect of niacin deficiency on the cell body.

VITAMIN B₅

A deficiency in pantothenic acid is likely to play a role in some nutritional neuropathies.

VITAMIN B₆

The metabolism of pyridoxine can be disrupted by drugs such as isoniazid and hydralazine, given, respectively, for tuberculosis and hypertension. The former causes an excess excretion of pyridoxine, and the latter leads to hydrazones that make pyridoxine unavailable.

Both cause a neuropathy beginning with tingling and burning pains in the feet, followed by weakness and loss of ankle jerks. Treatment consists in preventative intake of pyridoxine and discontinuation of the drug.

Pyridoxine *overload,* not deficiency, can cause a sensory polyneuropathy with distal paresthesias, numbness, and even Lhermitte's sign (see Ch. 31). Dysautonomia has been reported. Ankle jerks are absent and position sense is disturbed. Biopsy shows axonal loss, chiefly in the large myelinated fibers. The toxicity to the dorsal spinal ganglia of pyridoxine in large amounts has been demonstrated. The prognosis for the corrected overload is usually good.

VITAMIN B₁₂

To neurologists, this vitamin deficiency has long been the best-known example of a combined system disease, affecting both the blood and the nervous system. The history of its discovery and studies into the mechanisms of disease rank among the classics of clinical neurology.

Pathophysiology

The basis for the well-known white matter lesions in the nervous system is thought to be a defect in myelin formation. At least three mechanisms are involved. First, methionine is essential for methylation of myelin basic protein. Vitamin B₁₂ deficiency means a lack of the methylcobalamin vitamin cofactor needed to produce methionine from dietary homocysteine. Second, the lack of cyancobalamin also prevents adenylcyancobalamin formation, a step in the production of succinyl coenzyme A from methylmalonyl coenzyme A, the defective step resulting in the formation and accumulation of nonphysiologic fatty acids in nervous system lipids. Third, choline and its phospholipid derivatives are also not formed.

Although the histopathologic changes showed distention and degeneration of myelin sheaths in a diffuse fashion throughout the white matter of the spinal cord, the most affected parts are the heavily myelinated fibers of the posterior and lateral columns of the cord, the cervical and thoracic spinal cord more so than other regions.

Pernicious anemia, the name originally given to the deficiency state, is most often the result of an autoimmune gastritis coupled with antibodies directed against intrinsic factor, which is responsible for vitamin B_{12} absorption. Other autoimmune endocrine deficiencies, among them thyroiditis and idiopathic adrenal insufficiency may occur with the malabsorption syndrome. Other causes of poor absorption include loss of intestinal surface area from gastrectomy or ileal resection; inflammatory diseases, such as regional enteritis or tuberculous enteritis; malabsorption secondary to scleroderma; and even the poor intake of the vitamin, which occurs in some strict vegetarian diets. The presence of an abnormal vitamin B_{12}-binding protein has been described. Vitamin B_{12} deficiency seems to occur more often than expected in patients with acquired immunodeficiency syndrome. The Imerslund-Grasbeck syndrome, featuring megaloblastic anemia, proteinuria, and multiple focal neurologic findings, has been considered part of this disease complex.

Clinical Picture

The classic clinical picture (see also Ch. 31) was established in the days before widespread availability of vitamin B_{12} therapy, when symptoms were understood to reflect the damage to the spinal cord and peripheral nerves. The sensory paresthetic complaints affected the legs before the arms (because the fibers were longer in the legs) and were symmetric in the "stocking-glove" distribution with "pins and needles sensation" with diminished vibration and proprioceptive sensation from disease of the posterior columns. Involvement of the lateral spinal tracts produced weakness and stiffness, especially in the legs. The syndrome of spasticity, weakness, and sensory ataxia was considered diagnostic of combined system disease in former times. If the vitamin deficiency-induced polyneuropathy was marked, reflexes could be absent or greatly diminished. In advanced cases, the demyelination also affected the optic nerves and cerebrum. Optic atrophy occurred late and was associated with a loss of visual acuity and the development of centrocecal scotomata. In the most advanced cases, cerebral demyelination occurred with a clinical picture of lethargy, psychosis, and paranoia (*megaloblastic madness*), leading in long-standing cases to an irreversible dementia. Even coma occurred.

The largest modern series reviewed the illness in 143 patients over a 17-year period. Neurologic complaints were more frequent than medical, consisting mainly of paresthesias or ataxia. Multiple complaints were common, included among them were loss of cutaneous sensation, muscle weakness, diminished or hyperactive reflexes, spasticity, urinary or fecal incontinence, orthostatic hypotension, loss of vision, dementia, disturbances of mood, and psychoses. The most common finding on examination was diminished vibratory sensation and proprioception in the lower extremities. About 4 months passed between the first symptoms and institution of treatment. In this series, the severity of neurologic dysfunction before treatment was clearly related to the duration of symptoms before diagnosis.

Sensory-evoked potentials are usually slowed in the clinically affected limbs. Visual-evoked potentials can be abnormal in patients without clinical visual disorders.

Diagnosis

The diagnosis of vitamin B_{12} deficiency can be confirmed by determining serum vitamin B_{12} levels. Levels less than 100 pg/ml are diagnostic. A Schilling's test with the administration of radioactive vitamin B_{12} can determine whether the vitamin B_{12} deficiency reflects malabsorption or inadequate intake. A normal hematocrit has been noted in many cases with neurologic symptoms and signs, and the serum cobalamin concentration may be only moderately decreased. Overall, the hematocrit inversely correlates significantly with the severity of the neurologic findings.

Defects in folic acid metabolism have not yet become fully accepted to produce a neurologic syndrome comparable to that of pernicious anemia.

Treatment

Parenteral vitamin B_{12} injections are mandatory immediately after the diagnosis is established. Administration of exogenous intrinsic factor corrects the malabsorption abnormality on the Schilling's test. If the malabsorption is due to disease or surgery of the ileum, the findings in the Schilling's test remain abnormal even after administration of intrinsic factor. After replenishing hepatic stores, monthly injections of 1 mg are adequate therapy because daily requirements are about 2.5 μg. In modern series, all patients responded to therapy, and in almost one-half of them, clinical recovery was complete.

VITAMIN A

Overload, not deficiency, of this lipid-soluble vitamin can cause elevated intracranial pressure in infants and headaches from elevated pressure in adults. Vomiting blurred vision, and diplopia may be part of the clinical picture. Bone pain and new periosteal bone formation on radiographs are suggestive of the diagnosis.

VITAMIN E

Awareness that vitamin E, in its active form of D-α-tocophorol, may stabilize membranes through an antioxidant effect has fueled interest in its possible role as a neuroprotectant therapy against unspecified and unknown neurotoxins. Theses have been put forward that vitamin E could retard the aging process through its role as an antioxidant.

Clinical examples of deficiency seem extremely rare for this fat-soluble vitamin, which is present in many foods and requires bile for its absorption. Vitamin E deficiency is thought to be one of the causes of a progressive peripheral neuropathy with ataxia in patients with severe malabsorption states. A relationship between the neuropathies of diseases with acanthocytes has been suggested.

Thus far, all attempts to show vitamin E as a therapy for neurologic disease has been disappointing failures. Little effect was found when it was used as an anticonvulsant. It has had some success in limiting the process of infarction in animal models. Changes in glutathione levels in patients with multiple sclerosis have prompted untested speculations of a therapeutic value. It showed little benefit compared with selegiline for Parkinson's disease.

ANNOTATED BIBLIOGRAPHY

Albin RL, Albers JW, Greenberg HS et al. Acute sensory neuropathy—neuronopathy from pyridoxine overdose. Neurology 1987;37:1729–32.

High doses of pyridoxine for toadstool ingestions.

Fahn S. The endogenous toxin hypothesis of the etiology of Parkinson's disease and a pilot trial of high dosage antioxidants in an attempt to slow the progression of the illness. Ann N Y Acad Sci 1989;570:186–96.

No benefit.

Hardie RJ. Acanthocytosis and neurological impairment: a review. Q J Med 1989;71:291–306.

Acanthocytes occur in abetalipoproteinemia, progressive spinocerebellar ataxia, and malabsorption of vitamin E, raising questions whether the latter could be involved in the first two.

Hauw JJ, DeBaecgue C, Hausser-Hauw C, Serdaru M. Chromatolysis in alcoholic encephalopathies. Pellagra-like changes in 22 cases. Brain 1988;111:843–56.

Lesions of pellagra are common in alcoholic encephalopathy.

Healton EB, Savage DG, Brust JC et al. Neurologic aspects of cobalamine deficiency. Medicine (Baltimore) 1991;70:229–45.

Detailed review of 143 patients seen over 17 years.

Jenner P, Dexter DT, Sian J et al. Oxidative stress as a cause of nigral cell death in Parkinson's disease and incidental Lewy body disease. Ann Neurol 1992;32(suppl):82–7.

Despite evidence of enhanced substantia nigra lipid peroxidation in patients with Parkinson's disease, catalase and glutathione peroxidase activity and vitamin C and E concentrations are normal. Reduced glutathione levels are decreased, paralleling the severity of the Parkinson's disease, suggesting glutathione changes may be involved in the pathology of Parkinson's disease.

Kayden HJ. The neurologic syndrome of vitamin E deficiency: a significant cause of ataxia. Neurology 1993;43:2167–9.

Syndrome mimicking Friedreich's ataxia.

Kieburtz KD, Giang DW, Schiffer RB, Vakil N. Abnormal vitamin B_{12} metabolism in human immunodeficiency virus infection. Association with neurological dysfunction. Arch Neurol 1991;48:312–4.

Higher frequency in patients with acquired immunodeficiency syndrome.

Minot GR, Murphy WP. Treatment of pernicious anemia by a special diet. JAMA 1926;87:470.

The classic article. In those days advised ingesting raw liver.

Pant SS, Asbury AK, Richardson EP Jr. The myelopathy of pernicious anemia. Acta Neurol Scand 1968;44(suppl 5:1–36.

Details of the neuropathology.

Pedraza OL, Botez MI. Thiamine status in inherited degenerative ataxias. J Neurol Neurosurg Psychiatry 1992;55:136–7.

Blood thiamine levels are the same in patients with ataxia compared with controls, but spinal fluid levels are a bit lower.

Russell JSR, Batten FE, Collier JE. Subacute combined degeneration of the spinal cord. Brain 1900;23:39.

Classic article.

Soria ED, Fine EJ. Somatosensory evoked potentials in the neurological sequelae of treated vitamin B_{12} deficiency. Electromyogr Clin Neurophysiol 1992;32:63–71.

Slowed sensory-evoked potentials.

72
Poisons and Toxins

Steven Gulevich and Neil L. Rosenberg

Neurotoxic injuries caused by abused substances and iatrogenic sources are common worldwide, not only from occupational exposures but also incidental to the likes of water contamination from industrial pollutants and chemicals used in farming. However, unless large numbers of affected individuals are seen, as in epidemics (e.g., eosinophilia myalgia syndrome caused by contaminated L-tryptophan), recognition of a toxic disorder may be difficult. Correct diagnosis is necessary to differentiate a naturally occurring disorder from a disorder caused by a neurotoxin. This may be particularly true for occupational neurotoxic disorders in which the diagnosis is essential to be able to prevent recurrence of the disease and to determine whether other workers are at similar risk.

Few neurotoxic disorders present with pathognomonic clinical, laboratory, or radiologic findings, and most tend to mimic metabolic, degenerative, nutritional, or demyelinating disorders.

This chapter deals with recognition of neurotoxic disorders caused by industrial and agricultural chemicals, most of which are work-related and biologic toxins. Basic principles of neurotoxicology are essential to develop an approach to the evaluation of the patient with a possible neurotoxic disease, and these are also presented.

BASIC PRINCIPLES OF NEUROTOXICOLOGY

Acute and Chronic Neurotoxicity

Understanding the difference between these two forms of poisoning with the resultant neurotoxicity is of even more importance in neurotoxicology than in other areas of toxicology because of the issue of reversibility. Some neurotoxic effects are reversible, and others are not. Such effects for some compounds occur at all sites they reach in the neuraxis; others are site dependent. For agents the main effects of which are

on the central nervous system (CNS), the lack of ability of the CNS to regenerate indicates that most injuries will be permanent. However, for those agents the effects of which are chiefly on the peripheral nervous system (PNS), the capacity of the latter for regeneration permits some significant pathologic injuries to be followed by recovery of most or all of the function.

Proximity to Exposure and Improvement With Removal of Toxin

Maximum symptoms generally occur with maximum exposure with little delay in the onset. The reasons are that the acute neurotoxic effects, commonly caused by physiologic effects, do not involve pathologic changes or degeneration of neuronal elements and are rapidly reversible. Examples would be those effects resulting from pharmacologic modification of excitable neuronal membranes or from a neurotransmitter system.

Strong Dose-Response Relationship

The dose-response relationship is a fundamental concept in toxicology and simply states that, within certain limits, under controlled conditions, there is a positive relationship between the amount (e.g., *dose*) of a chemical that an individual or group of individuals is exposed to and the toxic effect (e.g., *response*). The greater the duration of exposure is, the more likely it is that irreversible symptoms will occur. With neurotoxins, there is very little variability in the effects on different individuals, with the exceptions of extremes of age or health (especially severe liver disease). In regard to the dose-response relationship for neurotoxic effects, for most neurotoxins, the variability of response is less than that for other toxic effects. The reasons are not entirely clear, but this variability has been a consistent observation in clinical practice.

Neurotoxins are typically not associated with allergic (including hypersensitivity reactions) or idiosyn-

841

cratic reactions. Allergic effects are not dose related, and even subthreshold levels may produce a clinical response. Chemical idiosyncrasy is a genetically determined abnormal reaction to a chemical. A well-known example occurs in individuals with a genetically determined atypical pseudocholinesterase. Inheriting this abnormal enzyme will cause an individual to have a very prolonged, potentially fatal, effect after exposure to succinylcholine, which is used to induce skeletal muscle relaxation during surgery. Chemical idiosyncrasy, like chemical allergy, does not follow normal dose-response effects and is uncommon with neurotoxic exposures.

Multiple Syndromes From a Single Toxin

A feature of neurotoxins is the development of widely different neurologic syndromes, depending on the level and duration of exposure (i.e., the dose-response relationship). Examples include the transient nonspecific encephalopathy from acute high level exposure to n-hexane, which features euphoria, disorientation, and a cerebellar ataxia. By contrast, chronic, lower level exposure is associated with a peripheral neuropathy and a conspicuous lack of CNS dysfunction. This principle emphasizes the need to know not only what an individual is exposed to but also the general level of exposure.

Chemical Formula May Not Predict Toxicity

Chemicals with similar structure may not have similar toxicities. Toluene (methylbenzene) produces a dramatic clinical syndrome with chronic exposure characterized by dementia, anosmia, and cerebellar ataxia. Removing the methyl group from toluene produces benzene, a chemical with no clear chronic neurotoxicity but which may be carcinogenic at some levels of exposure.

Enhancement of Neurotoxicity by "Innocent Bystanders"

Individuals may be exposed to multiple chemicals and/or chemical mixtures, particularly in an occupational setting. Although neurotoxicity may be known for an individual chemical, its interaction with others in a mixture and how the interaction may contribute to or enhance neurotoxicity is rarely known. Mixtures are generally thought to be more neurotoxic than individual chemicals, but evidence is lacking. Few examples of enhancement of neurotoxicity caused by chemical innocent bystanders have been described, but the best known is enhancement of n-hexane neurotoxicity by

methyl ethyl ketone (see n-hexane below), which may be a model for others as yet incompletely understood.

Limits of Clinical Laboratory Testing

The clinical laboratory is only occasionally useful in diagnosis. The best results are in acute exposures to assess the degree of exposure, but usually, the history will identify the substance to which the individual was exposed because acute exposures are usually associated with completely reversible neurotoxic injuries and the neurologist is usually not involved in the diagnosis.

Chronic lower levels of exposure, often associated with neurotoxicity, may occur at such low levels that clinical laboratory tests do not establish a body burden for that particular chemical. Establishing a link between exposure and chronic clinical dysfunction also relies on a focused history of exposure and a neurologic examination more than on the clinical laboratory.

Nonfocal Syndromes

Neurotoxins most often affect the CNS and PNS in a diffuse or bilaterally symmetric fashion. Examples of diffuse injury include the distal axonopathy produced from acrylamide or n-hexane or the diffuse CNS white matter changes caused by chronic toluene abuse. Bilaterally symmetric focal injuries are primarily related to those toxins that have specific cell targets, such as the effect of 1-methyl-4-phenyl-1,2,3,6-tetrahydropyridine on the dopaminergic neurons of the substantia nigra.

Selective Neurotoxicity

Selectivity refers to the notion that a chemical produces injury to one type of tissue or organism without harming some other tissue or organism, even though the two may exist in intimate contact. It can also refer to a toxin that produces injury to a specific cell type or even a particular part of a cell without damaging another part of the cell. The cell type or part of the cell affected will determine the type of clinical effect that a neurotoxin may produce and whether there will be recovery of function or irreversible damage.

SPECIFIC NEUROTOXINS

Metals

Nearly all metals are neurotoxic, mostly in their ionic forms. Systemic symptoms of acute intoxication nearly always accompany neurologic manifestations, which tend to be nonfocal (e.g., encephalopathy). Chronic metal neurotoxicity, by contrast, usually has a distinct

Table 72-1. Toxic Metals

| Metal | Toxic Forms | Target Tissue | Acute Toxicity | Chronic Effects | | Treatment |
				Systemic	Neurologic	
Lead	Lead acetate, lead carbonate	Myelin, brain (especially hippocampus)	Gastroenteritis	Facial pallor, anemia gingival lines	Encephalopathy (children), neuropathy motor (adults)	Oral sulfates, penicillamine, zinc, atropine
Mercury	Elemental vapor, salts ($HgCl_2$), organic	Uncertain	Gastroenteritis, acute tubular necrosis	Acrodynia, chronic renal failure	Ataxia, encephalopathy to dementia (severe)	Penicillamine
Arsenic	Arsine gas (AsH_3), organic arsenate, inorganic arsenite	Liver, lungs, spleen, brain, $-SH$ groups	Gastroenteritis, cerebral edema	Abdominal pain, hyper-pigmentation	Encephalopathy (Wernicke-like), sensory neuropathy	Dimercaprol, penicillamine
Cadmium	Elemental metal	Kidney	Fever, headache, dyspnea, sore throat, pulmonary edema (severe)	Nephropathy	None	Calcium edetate
Aluminum	Aluminum hydroxide, aluminum phosphate	Bone, brain	Hypercalcemia, anemia	Bone pain, osteodystrophy	Dementia (?), myopathy (?)	Deferoxamine
Tin	Triethyltin, trimethyltin	Hippocampus, liver	Weakness, tremors, convulsions	Abdominal pain, headache	Visual disturbances, memory loss	Supportive
Thallium	Thallium, thallium salts	Axon, brain	Nausea cerebral edema convulsions,	—	Ataxia, peripheral neuropathy	Supportive
Manganese	$KMnO_4$, oxide, Manganese fumes	Globus pallidus	Methemoglobinemia, parethesias, incoordination, "Mn madness"	—	Parkinsonian syndrome	Edetate calcium disodium
Barium	Barium acetate, carbonate, chloride, etc. (acid-soluble)	Neuromuscular junction	Weakness, cardiac arrhythmia, hypokalemia	—	—	Sodium thiosulfate, cathartic

clinical picture specific to the particular metal (e.g., lead-induced motor neuropathy).

Metals can be thought of as *toxic* (Table 72-1), that is, possessing no essential biologic function, or *essential* (Table 72-2), that is acting as essential elements in trace concentrations but as toxins at higher concentrations. Mercury and plutonium are examples of the former and copper and chromium, of the latter. The essential metals may act as ligands (e.g., iron), enzyme cofactors (e.g., magnesium), or ionic solutes (e.g., potassium). A few, such as sodium, are so abundant that they lack the potential for permanent toxicity.

When there is a history of ingestion, the diagnosis is fairly straightforward. The diagnosis of chronic toxicity, however, often is more challenging. Fortunately, blood levels can be obtained on nearly all metals, and this is one of the few areas in clinical toxicology where the clinical laboratory is useful to confirm the diagno-

sis. With early diagnosis, treatment of metal intoxication is generally satisfactory. Supportive care and discontinuation of exposure alone are often adequate. For those susceptible, removal of the offending metal by chelation is indicated. Penicillamine, initially developed to remove the excess copper accumulation in Wilson's disease, is also an effective chelator of lead, mercury, and arsenic. Deferoxamine chelates aluminum and iron.

Lead

The classic metal intoxicant, lead, has been used in plumbing since ancient Roman times. Its more recent uses include paints and automobile batteries. The most toxic forms are lead acetate and lead carbonate. Lead exerts its toxic effects by damage to the cell membrane, probably mediated by inhibition of oxidative

Table 72-2. Toxicity of Essential Metals

Metal	Site of Toxic Action	Symptoms/Signs	Treatment
Chromium	Gastric/renal toxicity, skin and lung sensitizer	"Blackjack disease" (dermatitis, conjunctivitis), acute gastroenteritis, acute tubular neurosis	Symptomatic
Copper	Lysosomal membrane, erythrocyte membrane	Hepatic/renal failure Lethargy to Coma	Edetate calcium disodium, dimercaprol, penicillamine
Iron	Vascular membranes	Gastrointestinal hemorrhage, hepatic failure, lethargy	Deferoxamine
Magnesium	Neuromuscular junction	Paralysis, cardiac arrhythmia	Lavage, calcium gluconate
Potassium	Heart	Weakness, cardiac arrhythmia	Calcium gluconate
Selenium	Uncertain	Nausea, fatigue, irritability	Supportive
Zinc	Uncertain	Fatigue, fever, chills, dyspnea (fumes), abdominal pain, incoordination (ingestion)	Edetate calcium disodium, gastric lavage, N-acetylcysteine

enzymes (e.g., superoxide dismutase and glutathione peroxidase).

Acute ingestion produces a severe gastroenteritis and may proceed to circulatory collapse and death in extremely high level exposures. Chronic lead ingestion leads to characteristic systemic symptoms (facial pallor, gingival lines, and anemia, with "target" red cells), which may aid diagnosis in cases of occult exposure. Lead poisoning manifests itself more frequently among children because of their more efficient absorption from the gastrointestinal tract (50 percent in children versus 10 percent in adults) and the greater lead permeability of the immature blood-brain barrier.

In children, especially young toddlers, lead salts cross the blood-brain barrier to damage the CNS, primarily the hippocampus, probably by interrupting active transport in cerebral capillaries. The resulting encephalopathy may be complicated by cerebral edema and is 50 percent fatal. In adults, on the other hand, little lead crosses the blood-brain barrier and the peripheral nerves are the principal targets. Clinically, lead neuropathy affects mainly motor function. By electrophysiologic criteria, the neuropathy is primarily of the demyelinating type (see Chs. 32 and 80).

Prompt chelation with penicillamine may reverse lead toxicity. However, repair of CNS damage is incomplete, and lead-induced encephalopathy in children often results in permanent neurologic damage.

Mercury

The most toxic forms of this metal are its organic compounds and salts (e.g., $HgCl_2$). Although elemental mercury vapors are toxic when inhaled, liquid mercury has surprisingly low toxicity when ingested, and quicksilver was once touted for its imagined medicinal value (hence the term "quacksalver"). Organic mercury compounds become concentrated in tissue as they ascend the food chain, and thus fish pose the greatest potential exposure. Indeed, it was mercury-tainted fish from Minamata Bay in Japan that led to the most publicized outbreak of mercury poisoning (Minamata disease).

Mercury produces cerebellar ataxia and encephalopathy, which ranges from cognitive impairment to profound dementia. If prompt chelation with penicillamine is not undertaken, the neurologic deficit becomes permanent.

Arsenic

Arsenic is toxic as arsine gas (AsH_3) and as organic arsenate or inorganic arsenite. Sulfhydryl groups represent the probable target. Severe toxicity results from ingestion of 1 mg/kg. Doses exceeding 2 mg/kg are usually fatal. Acutely, poisoning causes cerebral edema and severe gastroenteritis, which may lead to shock and death. In addition, acute high-level exposure damages the proximal axons and myelin in the PNS, producing a picture that resembles the Guillain-Barré syndrome. Chronic arsenic exposure to sublethal doses results in a Wernicke-like encephalopathy and a mostly sensory neuropathy. Arsenic was a time-honored method of criminal poisoning. In chronic intoxication, arsenic can be found in hairs (see Ch. 80).

Other Metals

Several other toxic metal syndromes that occur infrequently deserve mention for their distinctive neurologic presentations. *Manganese* exposure may present with parkinsonism. *Thallium* toxicity manifests itself as cerebellar ataxia with peripheral neuropathy (see Ch.

88). The toxicity of *aluminum* for the nervous system remains uncertain. Aluminum's role in Alzheimer's disease has been largely discounted, although it may be partly responsible for dialysis-related dementia. Most of the essential metals possess minimal neurotoxicity. A notable exception is copper in Wilson's disease (see Ch. 80), although ordinary copper toxicity produces only nonspecific CNS depression. The remaining essential metals (Table 72-2) cause principally systemic symptoms.

Industrial Gases

These substances have a wide range of potency and sites of action. They share a high volatility and common route of entry—through inhalation—although a few (e.g., cyanide) have ingestible forms. Because of their volatility, sublethal exposures usually resolve promptly with supportive care alone, although certain specific measures are often indicated (Table 72-3).

Carbon Monoxide

Produced during inadequately oxygenated combustion, its irreversible binding to hemoglobin causes generalized cerebral hypoxia, which primarily damages the basal ganglia. In the case of carbon monoxide, the initial damage occurs in the globus pallidus. Further exposure may lead to generalized cerebral injury. Oxygen therapy promptly converts carbon to carbon dioxide. Where available, treatment in a hyperbaric chamber may be useful and in severe cases.

Nitrous Oxide

This compound retains its use as an anesthetic gas, principally for dental procedures. Because of the concentrations required, medically serious toxicity is uncommon, except in cases of chronic abuse of "laughing gas." In large doses, acutely, nitrous oxide produces a nonspecific encephalopathy. Chronic nitrous exposure leads to demyelination in the spinal cord and brain, myelopathy, and dementia, with a clinical picture similar to vitamin B_{12} deficiency. Nitrous oxide interferes with vitamin B_{12} metabolism and acts by creating a de facto vitamin B_{12} deficiency. Cessation of exposure and administration of vitamin B_{12} alleviates the symptoms over several months. Prolonged demyelination, however, can cause neuronal loss, with permanent neurologic residua in some cases of nitrous oxide poisoning.

Other oxides of nitrogen (predominantly nitric oxide and nitrogen dioxide) are common industrial pollutants, formed during combustion of fossil fuels. They possess minimal neurotoxicity at the usually encountered concentrations.

Carbon Disulfide

Carbon disulfide is used primarily as a solvent in the manufacture of rayon. Its other uses include as an insecticide and as a corrosion inhibitor. This substance is a potent neurotoxin, both centrally and peripherally. Ingestion of as little as 15 ml of the liquid may be fatal, and it has numerous sites of action within the cell. An acute sublethal exposure produces an enceph-

Table 72-3. Industrial Gases

Toxin	Action	Acute Effects	Chronic Effects	Treatment
Carbon monoxide	Binds to hemoglobin, prevents oxygen release	Unconsciousness, convulsions, death	Headache, fatigue, dizziness	100% oxygen, hyperbaric oxygen
Cyanide	Binds to cytochrome, inhibits aerobic metabolism	Cerebral anoxia, unconsciousness	None	100% oxygen, thiosulfate and nitrites
Hydrogen sulfide	Inhibits cytochrome oxidase	Anoxia with seizures	Headache, nausea, weight loss	Oxygen, nitrites
Carbon disulfide	Reacts with several nucleophilic agents	Hepatitis, headache, tremors, fatigue	Parkinsonism, distal axonopathy	None
Nitrous oxide	Interferes with vitamin B_{12} metabolism	Confusion, memory loss	Dementia, myelopathy	Vitamin B_{12}
Aliphatic hydrocarbons	Simple asphyxiants	Lightheadedness, dizziness, headache	None	Removal of exposure

alopathy characterized by mania, hallucinations, and memory loss. Parkinsonism may result in those who survive acute intoxication. In the peripheral system, carbon disulfide poisoning bears a striking resemblance to hexacarbon toxicity, by producing a distal demyelinating neuropathy (see Ch. 80). Other than supportive measures, no treatment for carbon disulfide is available.

Other Industrial Gases

Cyanide exists as a gas (HCN) or a solid (KCN). Occult sources of cyanide include sodium nitroprusside and the cassava nut. Cyanide binds to cytochrome aa3, inhibiting aerobic metabolism and causing systemic hypoxia. Treatment is the immediate administration of 100 percent pure oxygen, followed by sodium thiosulfate and hydroxycobalamin. Hydrogen sulfide, similar to cyanide, inhibits cytochrome oxidase and causes hypoxia. Treatment is likewise with oxygen and nitrates. Gaseous aliphatic hydrocarbons (e.g., methane and propane) act as asphyxiants.

Neurotoxic Hydrocarbons

Although most hydrocarbons possess systemic toxicity, only relative few (Table 72-4) are associated with specific neurologic syndromes. These are considered here. Other classes of hydrocarbons produce nonspecific mental status depression, for example, halogenated hydrocarbons (carbon tetrachloride, trichloroethylene, and others). The CNS depression is transient; prolonged exposure seldom results in anything more serious than subjective cognitive complaints. Dihydroxy compounds (ethylene glycol and propylene glycol) also produce transient CNS depression.

Alcohols

Methanol, like most compounds in this class, causes CNS depression, which may be severe (coma or convulsions). Its metabolites, formaldehyde and formic acid, induce severe acidosis, blindness, and in some survivors, permanent parkinsonism. However, methanol itself has minimal toxicity. Therein lies the rationale behind the antidote, ethanol, which has a greater affinity for alcohol dehydrogenase and prevents the conversion of methanol to its toxic metabolites (see Ch. 67). Methanol can be removed by dialysis.

Isopropanol, in addition to producing CNS and cardiovascular depression, is a powerful gastric irritant. Complications associated with higher doses include acute renal tubular necrosis, hemolytic anemia, and myoglobinuria. No antidote is available.

n-Hexane

Aliphatic hydrocarbons that contain 5 to 15 carbons are liquids at room temperature. Many are used as industrial solvents or fuels. All can produce CNS depression at high concentrations and severe chemical pneumonitis when aspirated. Hexane (C_6H_{14}) represents the prototype neurotoxicant hydrocarbon. A weak neurotoxin itself, when ingested it undergoes biotransformation to methyl-n-butyl ketone; 2,5-hexanediol; and 2,5-hexanediane. All possess far more neurotoxic potential than n-hexane. Only aliphatic hydrocarbons with 1,4 spacing of the carbonyl groups (γ-diketones) possess neurotoxicity. Hexane neuropathy is manifested as axonal neuropathy and, microscopically, as neurofilament accumulation near the nodes of Ranvier with resultant axonal swelling.

Non-neurotoxic hydrocarbons potentiate the neurotoxicity of n-hexane. Both 2-butanone (methyl ethyl ketone) and 4-methyl-4-pentanone (methyl isobutyl ketone), induce cytochrome P-450 mixed function oxidases and thus speed the biotransformation of n-hexane to the more potent neurotoxin, 2,5-hexanediol.

Removal of exposure remains the only available treatment. Slow, sometimes incomplete, relief of symptoms over 6 to 18 months is the rule.

Toluene

Toluene is a solvent used in many glues and paints. Although absorbed through the skin and gastrointestinal tract, most exposure is by inhalation. Acutely, toluene exposure causes CNS depression with lightheadedness, nausea, and headache. With chronic exposure, cognitive impairment, personality changes, and incoordination may develop. No remedy is available. Toluene does not cause neuropathy. The peripheral neuropathy once attributed to toluene was probably due to contaminants such as n-hexane. No therapy exists.

Pesticides

Substances used to kill insects and plants have deleterious effects when humans share the metabolic pathway on which the pesticide acts. Most commercially

Table 72-4. Neurotoxic Hydrocarbons

Type	Mode of Toxicity	Neurologic Effects
n-Hexane	Metabolized to γ-diketone, several modes of action (see text)	Distal axonopathy
Toluene	Central nervous system depressant	Dementia, cerebellar ataxia
Methanol	Metabolized to formaldehyde	Blindness, parkinsonism

Table 72-5. Pesticides by Class

Class	Examples	Mode of Action	Symptoms (Ingestion)	Treatment
Chlorinated hydrocarbons	DDT, lindane, Hexachlorocyclohexanes, chlorocyclodines	Block axonal transmission	Nausea, salivation, abdominal pain, seizures, CNS excitation	Supportive
Organophosphates	Malathion, parathion	Inhibit acetylcholinesterase (irreversible)	Salivation, CNS stimulation, seizures, sweating, delayed neurotoxicity	1. Atropine 2. Pralidoxime
Carbamates	Aldicarb	Inhibite acetylcholinesterase (reversible)	Salivation, CNS stimulation, seizures, sweating, delayed neurotoxicity	1. Atropine 2. Pralidoxime
Dipyridy herbicides	Paraquat, diquat	Produce superoxide from O_2	Dermatitis, conjunctivitis, pulmonary fibrosis	Supportive
Rodenticide alkaloids	Strychnine	Antagonizes CNS Glycine	Muscle twitching and spasm, seizures, coma	Supportive anticonvulsants
Polychlorinated biphenyls	Aroclor	Uncertain, induces cytochromes P-450?	Rash, nausea, distal paresthesias	Supportive

Abbreviation: CNS, central nervous system.

used pesticides cause illness when ingested (see Table 72-5), although they seldom produce symptoms in the small doses inhaled after appropriate use. Except for organophosphates and carbamates, no specific treatment is available for pesticide neurotoxicity.

Chlorinated Hydrocarbons

This class includes DDT, the chlorocyclodines, and hexachlorocyclohexanes. Lindane, which is used in scabies infection, also falls into this class. Chlorinated hydrocarbons, among other actions, slow closure of the sodium channels. This action manifests itself clinically as CNS hyperexcitability with excess salivation, tremor, and seizures. Although no antidote is available, supportive therapy, with vigorous treatment of seizures, provides satisfactory results.

Organophosphates

Organophosphates remain widely used as insecticides, herbicides, and rodenticides. They operate by irreversibly inhibiting acetyl cholinesterase by phosphorylation. Many central and most peripheral nervous functions rely on at least one cholinergic synapse; so organophosphates expectedly have a wide range of toxic effects. In the CNS, hyperexcitability progresses to seizures and coma with increasing dose. Peripherally, diaphoresis, muscle twitching, and salivation are seen. Deaths that occur usually result from respiratory failure as a result of bronchoconstriction, excessive secretions, and diaphragmatic paralysis. Assay of serum

butyrylcholinesterase activity measures the degree of organophosphate poisoning. When serum butyrylcholinesterase is inhibited to less than 10 percent of normal, severe toxicity results, and the likelihood of delayed neurotoxicity increases.

In addition to respiratory support, the symptomatic patient should receive intravenous atropine at a dose of 1 mg every 15 minutes as needed to reverse the anticholinergic effects of organophosphates over a period of 48 hours. Immediately after atropine, pralidoxime should be administered at a dose of 1 g intravenously, which is repeated every 12 hours as needed to reactivate acetylcholinesterase (by dephosphorylation). Pralidoxime produces immediate recovery; without it, cholinesterase activity may take 2 weeks to recover fully. Moreover, prolonged acetylcholinesterase inhibition in the CNS may produce delayed neurotoxicity. Organophosphate-induced delayed neurotoxicity manifests itself as ataxia and weakness 1 to 2 weeks after organophosphate exposure. Neuropathologically, wallerian degeneration is seen in the medulla, spinal cord, and peripheral nerve. The presumed mechanism is organophosphate inhibition of specific esterases (neurotoxic esterases or neuropathy target esterases) within the nervous system. Because of the CNS involvement, patients may have complete recovery from the neuropathy but have residual ataxia and spasticity.

Carbamates, such as aldicarb, are similar to organophosphates but their acetylcholinesterase inhibition is reversible. Treatment is the same as for organophosphate ingestion.

Naturally Occurring Toxins

The most potent poisons are not synthetic; they occur in nature. Through natural selection, most naturally occurring toxins have become receptor specific. These substances were useful in the early study of neurophysiology and even lent their names to certain receptor types (e.g., nicotinic). Several have valuable medicinal properties, such as, atropine, curare, and botulinum toxin. Favored sites of action of naturally occurring toxins include the neuromuscular junction and the cholinergic system. In addition to aiding diagnosis, this receptor specificity facilitates treatment in many cases.

A few natural toxins are produced by microbes (e.g., the organisms that cause diphtheria and tetanus), but the principal ones are derived from plants and animals. Table 72-6 contains a partial list. Plants that contain systemic and neurologic toxins tend to be shrubs, mushrooms, or other plants that grow low to the ground, with the toxins functioning to keep the plant from being eaten. Examples of neurotoxic plants include tobacco (nicotine), jimsonweed (atropine), and the Amanita species of mushrooms (muscarine).

Unlike plant toxins, animal toxins tend to be injected into their victims, not ingested. For the most part, neurotoxins derived from animals are proteins; because they cannot cross the blood-brain barrier, they must exert their toxicity peripherally (or by anaphylaxis). For neurotoxins, this leaves three principal sites: acetylcholine receptors, the neuromuscular junction, and the voltage-dependent sodium channels within the neuron. Table 72-6 shows examples of all three.

Marine Toxins

Neurotoxins are common among marine animals: pufferfish, jellyfish, sea anemones, and so forth. No specific antidotes are available for any of these toxins. The three major forms of toxins associated with seafood are cigua toxin, tetrodotoxin, and saxitoxin. *Cigua toxin* is produced by a free-swimming protozoan *Gambiendiscus toxicus,* attached to flora or algae in tropical reefs and ingested by a wide variety of fish. Storms, reef dredging, and shipwrecks on reefs seem to encourage "blooms," which increase the availability of the toxin. The toxin survives any method of food storage or preparation. No chemical analysis detects the toxin. The symptoms appear within a few hours or later as dysesthesias, paresthesias, cramps, dizziness, and ataxia, passing off over 1 day in mild cases. Paralysis, hallucinations, and autonomic failure have been reported in severe intoxications. Subsequent eating of fish (even uncontaminated fish) or nuts or engaging in vigorous exercise may precipitate the recurrence of symptoms months afterward. *Tetrodotoxin* is a potent nonpeptide neurotoxin produced in the tissues of wide variety of fish, especially puffers and ocean sunfish, and certain newts and frogs. Like ciguatoxin, it is not destroyed by cooking. Vomiting and diarrhea occur within a few minutes of ingestion from its stimulation of the chemoreceptor trigger zone on the floor of the fourth ventricle and the sodium channel-blocking effects include paresthesias and even paralysis in

Table 72-6. Common Naturally Occurring Neurotoxins

Toxin	Found in	Action	Clinical Effects	Antidote
Muscarine	*Amanita Muscaria, A. Phalloides*	Mimics ACh	Increased sweating, salivation, and bronchial secretions, bradycardia and bronchoconstriction	Atropine
Atropine	Jimsonweed	Antagonizes ACh	Dryness, delirium, convulsions	Physostigmine
Nicotine	Tobacco	Mimics ACh (nicotinic sites)	Salivation, abdominal cramps, mydriasis, tachycardia	Atropine
Tubocurarine	Many	Competes with ACh	Paralysis	None
Tetrodotoxin	Pufferfish	Binds axonal sodium channel	Paralysis	None
Muscimol	Various mushrooms	GABA-agonist	Drowsiness, tremors, delusions	None
α-Burgarotoxin	Snake venoms	Binds to nicotinic muscorinic receptors	Paralysis	None

Abbreviations: ACh, acetylcholine; GABA, γ-aminobutyric acid.

the severe cases. *Saxitoxin* comes from the "red tide" protozoa associated with shellfish and produces a syndrome like tetrodotoxin. It can be neutralized by boiling shellfish in water that contains 1 teaspoon of sodium bicarbonate per quart. Unhappily, this act also destroys most of the taste of the shellfish.

Land Toxins

The chief land animals that use neurotoxic venom are snakes and arachnids. Snake venoms contain peptide toxins that block presynaptic release of acetylcholine, bind postsynaptically with acetylcholine receptors, or bind to membrane sodium channels. Fanged snakes produce *presynatic venoms* the main effects of which are on clotting. The rapidly ascending paralysis of *postsynaptic venoms* from coral snakes and cobras is rarely fatal; impaired respiration, oculomotor dysfunction, and dysphagia may be prominent. Antivenom is the only treatment. Antivenom is available for pit viper and coral snake bites. Morphine is not recommended. Doses of five vials (50 ml) of antivenom should suffice for minor bites, but up to 40 vials may be needed for serious envenomations. Because horse serum is the basis for these antivenoms, hypersensitivity reactions are common, even anaphylaxis. The reaction can be controlled with intravenous antihistamines given concurrently. In the United States, a call to the National Poison Control Center (405-271-5454) often helps settle the management of bites from the rarer snakes.

ANNOTATED BIBLIOGRAPHY

Abou-Donia MB. Biochemical toxicology of organophosphorous compounds. In Blum K, Manzo L (eds). Neurotoxicology. Marcel Dekker, New York, 1985, pp. 423–444.

Mechanisms of toxicity and treatment.

Abou-Donia MB, Makkawy HM, Graham DG. The relative neurotoxicities of n-hexane, methyl n-butyl ketone, 2,5 hexanedione following oral or intraperitoneal administration in hens. Toxicol Appl Pharmacol 1982;62: 369–89.

Study of common hydrocarbon neurotoxins, including innocent bystanders.

Allsop JL, Martini L, Lebris H. Les manifestations neurologiques de la ciguatera. Rev Neurol (Paris) 1986;142:590.

Tropical fish poisoning.

Ballantyne B, Sullivan JB. Basic principles of toxicology. In Sullivan JB Jr, Krieger GR (eds). Hazardous Materials Toxicology. Williams and Wilkins, Baltimore, 1992, pp. 9–23.

Bower DJ, Hart RJ, Matthews PA. Non-protein neurotoxins. Clin Toxicol 1981;18:813.

Red tide.

Coburn RF. Mechanisms of carbon monoxide toxicity. Prev Med 1979;8:310–22.

Finkel AJ (ed). Hamilton and Hardy's Industrial Toxicology. 4th Ed. John Wright PSG, Boston, 1983, pp. 53–142.

Standard text.

Hilmey MI, Rahim SA, Abbas AH. Normal and lethal lead levels in humans. Toxicology 1976;5:155–9.

Hine CH, Pinto SS, Nelson KW. Medical problems associated with arsenic exposure. J Occup Med 1977;19:391–6.

Klaassen CD. Principles of toxicology. In Klaassen CD, Amdur MO, Doull J (eds). Cassarett and Doull's Toxicology. The Basic Science of Poisons. 3rd Ed. Macmillan, New York, 1986, pp. 11–32.

LaCoutre PG, Lovejoy FH. Methanol. Clin Toxicol Rev 1981;3:1–3.

Lampe KF. Toxic effects of plant toxins. In Classen CD, Amdur MO, Doull J (eds). Cassarett and Doull's Toxicology: the Basic Science of Poisons. 3rd Ed. Macmillan, New York, 1986, pp. 519–581.

Lange WR. Travel and ciguatera poisoning. Arch Intern Med 1992;152:2049–53.

Good advice.

Marcus SM. Hydrogen sulfide. Clin Toxicol Rev 1981;3: 1–3.

Review of diagnosis and treatment.

Murphy SD. Toxic effects of pesticides. In Classen CD, Amdur MO, Doull J (eds). Cassarett and Doull's Toxicology: The Basic Science of Poisons. 3rd Ed. Macmillan, New York, 1986, pp. 519–81.

Covers organophosphates, carbamates, hydrocarbons, and others.

Pettigrew LC, Glass JP. Neurologic complications of a coral snake bite. Neurology 1985;35:589.

Ptosis, dysphonia, dysphagia, and limb weakness.

Rosenberg NL. Neurotoxicology. In Sullivan JB, Krieger GR (eds). Hazardous Materials Toxicology. Williams and Wilkins, Baltimore, 1992, pp. 145–53.

Rosenberg NL, Kleinschmidt-DeMasters BK, Davis KA et al. Toluene abuse causes diffuse central nervous system white matter changes. Ann Neurol 1988;23:611–4.

Evidence of permanent neurotoxicity by bedside examination and magnetic resonance imaging.

Russell FE. Snake Venom Poisoning. Philadelphia, JB Lippincott, 1980.

Harrowing experiences.

Russell FE. Toxic effects of animal toxins. In Classen CD, Amdur MO, Doull J (eds). Cassarett and Doull's Toxicology: The Basic Science of Poisons. 3rd Ed. Macmillan, New York, 1986, pp. 706–56.

Covers envenomations by snakes, insects, and marine animals.

Schaumburg HH, Spencer PS. Recognizing neurotoxic disease. Neurology 1987;37:276–8.

Silbergeld EK. Developing formal risk assessment methods for neurotoxins. In Gilioli R, Cassitto MG, Foa V (eds). Neurobehavioral Methods in Occupational and Environmental Health. Pan American Health Organization, Washington, DC, 1988.

Torda TA, Sinclair E, Ulyatt DB. Puffer fish (tetrodotoxin) poisoning. Clinical record and suggested management. Med J Aust 1973;1:599.

Near fatality for a boy.

Vogel SN, Sultan TR. Cyanide poisoning. Clin Toxocol 1981;18:367–83.

Symptoms and treatments.

73
Multiple Sclerosis

Antonio Uccelli and Stephen L. Hauser

Multiple sclerosis is the prototypic demyelinating disease of the central nervous system (CNS). In the United States and Europe, multiple sclerosis is second only to trauma as a cause of acquired neurologic disability arising in young adulthood. Although the exact cause of multiple sclerosis is unknown, existing data support an autoimmune pathogenesis, triggered by some environmental exposure in a genetically susceptible host. Pathologically, this disease is characterized by perivenular and parenchymal inflammation, loss of the myelin sheath, relative sparing of axons and neurons, and severe gliosis. From a clinical perspective, multiple sclerosis is one of the most complex neurologic disorders because of the diversity of symptoms and signs that may occur. Its chronic nature and its often unpredictable clinical course may result in complications to many organ systems and extract an emotional toll on patients and their families. Hence optimal treatment often requires a multidisciplinary approach.

EPIDEMIOLOGY AND GENETICS

Multiple sclerosis is approximately twofold more common in females than in males. Onset is unusual before adolescence, but its incidence then increases steadily reaching a peak at approximately age 35 and declines thereafter. Rare cases of onset as early as age 2 or as late as the eighth decade of life are well documented. The mean age of onset is slightly older in men than in women.

Multiple sclerosis is in general a disorder of temperate climates. In North America and Europe, geographic gradients have been described, with prevalence rates decreasing with decreasing latitude. Prevalence is particularly high in Scandinavia and the northern British isles. The highest known prevalence of multiple sclerosis (250 per 100,000) is in the Orkney Islands located north of the Scottish mainland. North-south gradient effects support the hypothesis that an environmental exposure might influence multiple sclerosis.

Migration studies and identification of apparent point epidemics provide the strongest evidence in support of an effect of environment on multiple sclerosis. Migration from a high- to a low-risk area results in a lowering of the risk in the subsequent generation. For example, Japanese Americans living in Hawaii have a higher prevalence for multiple sclerosis than do Japanese who live in Japan. Other migration data support the concept that the environmental effect operates before the age of adolescence. The second line of evidence for an environmental effect on multiple sclerosis is derived from descriptions of apparent point epidemics. Perhaps the most convincing occurred in the Faroe Islands, located off of the coast of Denmark, after the British military occupation during World War II.

In addition to an effect of environment, evidence also supports a genetic influence on susceptibility to multiple sclerosis. Familial aggregation is known to occur, and the risk of disease is increased in relatives of an affected individual. Twin studies provide the most compelling support for a genetic effect. In various studies, the incidence of multiple sclerosis was found to be five- to sixfold higher in monozygotic twins of individuals with multiple sclerosis (25 to 30 percent concordance) than in dizygotic twins of affected patients (5 percent concordance).

Pedigree studies of multiply affected members of families suggest that multiple unlinked genes contribute to the risk for multiple sclerosis. The major histocompatibility complex (MHC) locus on chromosome 6 has been identified as one probable susceptibility region for multiple sclerosis. Linkage dysequilibrium studies suggest that the MHC class II HLA-DR locus is most closely associated with risk of disease. In most studies of northern Europeans, the HLA-DR2 allele was found to be most strongly associated with multiple sclerosis. Some reports suggested that HLA-DR3 is also associated with disease in some individuals. The HLA complex contributes only a minor genetic effect to multiple sclerosis, less than the effect of this locus on other chronic inflammatory diseases, for example, insulin-dependent diabetes mellitus or myasthenia gravis. The class II MHC region encodes proteins that function in the presentation of antigens to T cells, hence genetic associations of the MHC with multiple sclerosis suggest that a T-cell response contributes to the disease (see below). Other, non-MHC-linked loci reported to play some genetic role in multiple sclerosis include the T-cell receptor β chain, the immunoglobulin heavy chain, and the myelin basic protein gene. The most important genetic influences on multiple sclerosis remain to be defined. It is likely that it is not only a polygenic disorder but also that genetic heterogeneity is present, further complicating the search for susceptibility genes to multiple sclerosis.

PATHOLOGY

The pathologic hallmark of multiple sclerosis is the plaque, a well-demarcated gray or pink lesion, generally in white matter, that is characterized histologically by complete myelin loss, an absence of oligodendrocytes, and relative sparing of axons. Plaques are multiple, generally asymmetric, and tend to concentrate in deep white matter near the lateral ventricles, corpus callosum, floor of the fourth ventricle, deep periaqueductal region, optic nerves and tracts, corticomedullary junction, and the cervical spinal cord. The acute lesion in multiple sclerosis is characterized by perivascular and parenchymal infiltration by mononuclear cells, both T cells and macrophages, and by myelin breakdown that appears to be mediated by the infiltrating cells. Only rare B cells and plasma cells are present. As the lesions evolve, axons traversing the lesion show marked irregular beading. Proliferation of astrocytes occurs, and lipid-laden macrophages containing myelin debris are prominent. Progressive fibrillary gliosis ensues, and mononuclear cells gradually disappear. Proliferation of oligodendrocytes is also present initially, but these cells appear to be destroyed as the gliosis progresses. Gliosis is more severe in multiple sclerosis than in most other neuropathologic conditions. In chronic lesions, complete or nearly complete demyelination, dense gliosis, and loss of oligodendroglia are found. In some chronic active lesions, gradations in the histologic findings from the center to the edge of the lesion suggest that lesions expand by concentric outward growth. Axonal preservation is relative rather than absolute in multiple sclerosis. In approximately 10 percent of lesions, there is significant axonal destruction. In rare cases, complete destruction of the neuropil and cavitation occur.

Plaques are typically more numerous than anticipated on the basis of clinical findings. Approximately 35 percent of plaques are clinically silent with evidence of multiple sclerosis detected only on magnetic resonance imaging (MRI) or at autopsy.

PATHOPHYSIOLOGY

Loss of the myelin sheath may disrupt axonal saltatory conduction and result in either negative or positive functional consequences. Negative conduction abnormalities consist of slowed axonal conduction, frequency-related conduction block that limits the transmission of high-frequency impulse trains, and total conduction block. Changes in metabolic status and raised body temperature may profoundly influence the conduction properties of demyelinated axons. Positive conduction abnormalities include ectopic impulse generation, abnormal "cross-talk" between adjacent denuded axons, and increased sensitivity to mechanical stress. Conduction block may result in the characteristic fluctuations in function experienced by many patients and in the worsening that follows exercise or an elevation in core body temperature. Ectopic impulse generation or cross-talk may give rise to Lhermitte's sign, paroxysmal symptoms, or paresthesias (see below). Experimental therapies based on postulated conduction abnormalities in multiple sclerosis have included the use of calcium blockers to reduce the threshold for impulse generation and pharmacologic blockade of potassium channels (4-aminopyridine) that are exposed in the internodal axon membrane after myelin loss.

IMMUNOLOGY

A T-cell-mediated autoimmune mechanism appears to be important in the pathogenesis of multiple sclerosis. Support for immune mediation is derived from the histologic findings of the lesion, the similarity of multiple sclerosis to the animal model experimental allergic encephalomyelitis (EAE), and the detection of specific immune response in patients.

EAE is an autoimmune disease induced by immunization of genetically susceptible animals with whole myelin or purified myelin proteins, including myelin basic protein, proteolipid protein, or myelin oligodendrocyte protein. Pathologically, EAE is characterized by CNS inflammation, and in some chronic forms of EAE, striking demyelination also occurs. EAE is mediated by class II restricted T lymphocytes that recognize proteins of myelin. Sensitized T cells from an animal with EAE can be shown to be encephalitogenic by their ability to produce disease when transferred into a healthy, genetically identical, recipient. In some chronic forms of EAE, demyelination may require, in addition to effector T cells, the additional presence of autoantibodies.

Molecular dissection of the T-cell response to myelin basic protein in EAE has clarified the identity of the cells that mediate brain inflammation. T lymphocytes recognize antigen fragments bound to MHC molecules on the surface of specialized cells, which are termed antigen-presenting cells. The antigen recognition molecule, termed the T-cell receptor, is present on the surface of mature T cells. The T-cell receptor has evolved a genetic mechanism for the generation of diversity; thus the T-cell receptor molecules are different on different populations of lymphocytes. In rodents, EAE-inducing T cells express only limited numbers of different T-cell receptor genes and recognize only limited regions of the myelin basic protein molecule. This limited heterogeneity of T-cell receptor genes expressed by disease-inducing T cells in EAE has been exploited for therapeutic purposes, for example, by administration of peptides that resemble disease-inducing fragments of myelin basic protein but do not activate T cells or by immunization (vaccination) with synthetic peptides corresponding to T-cell receptor sequences present on encephalitogenic T cells. It appears that the T-cell populations that induce acute EAE are different in different rodent strains, and chronic forms of EAE are associated with an increase in the diversity of disease-inducing T cells.

In humans with multiple sclerosis, the frequency of myelin basic protein- or myelin oligodendrocyte protein-reactive T cells in peripheral blood is increased under some assay conditions, suggesting that T cells specific to myelin proteins may result in this disease. Furthermore, higher frequencies of myelin basic protein-, myelin oligodendrocyte protein-, and proteolipid protein-reactive T cells were found in cerebrospinal fluid, compared with peripheral blood, in multiple sclerosis, suggesting that these cells may home selectively to the CNS. One recent study suggested that T-cell receptor molecules similar to those expressed by EAE-inducing T cells were present in some brain lesions in this disease. These data provide additional support for an EAE-like response in multiple sclerosis.

MULTIPLE SCLEROSIS AND INFECTIONS

As noted above, epidemiologic evidence supports a role for an environmental exposure in multiple sclerosis. The risk also correlates with high socioeconomic status, which may reflect improved sanitation and delayed exposure to infectious agents. Some viruses, poliomyelitis and measles, for example, result in neuro-logic sequelae that are more common when the age of initial infection is delayed. In mice, a chronic demyelinating disease can result from infection with Theiler's virus, a murine coronavirus similar to measles. In multiple sclerosis, more than 20 different infectious agents have been reported at some time to be involved in the pathogenesis, but none, thus far, has withstood follow-up scrutiny. Serum antibody levels to measles virus have been consistently found to be elevated in patients, but multiple sclerosis may also occur in the apparent absence of prior measles infection. Recently, attention has focused on reports that a human lymphotropic virus type 1-(HTLV-1)-like retrovirus may cause multiple sclerosis; these claims, based on detection of virus-specific antibodies or nucleic acids, have not been confirmed.

CLINICAL MANIFESTATIONS

The onset of multiple sclerosis varies from an acute onset of symptoms, resembling the tempo of a stroke, to a slow, insidious progression over months or years. Often a careful review of the history reveals earlier episodes that had been forgotten or considered unimportant. The most common presenting symptoms reflect involvement of white matter tracts, resulting in weakness in one or more limbs (40 percent), optic neuritis (22 percent), sensory disturbances (21 percent), diplopia (12 percent), vertigo (8 percent), and bladder dysfunction (5 percent).

Motor weakness may present as insidiously as fatigue with exertion, imbalance, or loss of dexterity. Early in the disease, weakness may not be detected. Hyper-reflexia, absent superficial abdominal reflexes, or an extensor plantar response may be present. Occasionally, a tendon reflex may be lost because of a focal lesion in the dorsal root entry zone, simulating a peripheral nerve lesion.

Sensory symptoms may include paresthesia (tingling, pins and needles, or pain) or hypesthesia (numbness or a dead or anesthetic feeling). In acute myelopathy, tingling or numbness may begin in one foot, in the course of hours or days ascend, may cross to involve the other side, and subsequently, may spread to the perineum and lower trunk. In such cases, involvement of the trunk with a cord level is helpful because it distinguishes the sensory attack from acute peripheral neuropathy as a result of Guillain-Barré syndrome or other causes. In patients with established sensory deficits, unpleasant complaints of "swollen," "wet," or "tightly wrapped" body parts are common. Pain in multiple sclerosis may be burning or lancinating (pseudotabetic) in quality. Lhermitte's sign may occur with lesions of the cervical cord, which consists of electric shock-like sensations radiating down the spine (or less commonly up the occiput or down the arms) evoked by neck flexion. While common in multiple sclerosis, Lhermitte's sign may occur with a variety of spinal cord diseases, including cervical disc disease (see Ch. 31).

Cerebellar manifestations, nystagmus, caused by involvement of the vestibular pathways in the brainstem or cerebellum, are common. Also prominent are ataxia of gait and limbs and scanning speech. In individual patients, it may be difficult to distinguish the contribution of cerebellar involvement to specific symptoms when coexistent weakness, spasticity, vertigo, or sensory loss is present.

Optic neuritis, a common presenting manifestation of multiple sclerosis, results in visual loss of variable severity. Single attacks are typically unilateral but may be bilateral. They generally begin with visual blurring that may remain mild or progress to severe visual loss or, rarely, to complete loss of light perception. The patient may first detect visual loss on awakening or report its progression over hours or days. Pain, either of the globe or lateral supraorbital region, is commonly present. Pain may worsen with eye movement, and photophobia may be present. Examination may reveal an afferent pupillary defect, diminished visual acuity, impaired color vision, or a paracentral scotoma. Funduscopic examination may be entirely normal (retrobulbar neuritis), or the disc may be swollen (papillitis). Venous sheathing of the retinal vessels, when present, is an important sign of optic nerve disease associated with multiple sclerosis. Residual temporal pallor of the optic disc (optic atrophy) commonly follows bouts of optic neuritis (see Ch. 26).

Diplopia is another important cause of visual blurring in multiple sclerosis. Diplopia most often results from either a cranial nerve VI palsy or an internuclear ophthalmoplegia (INO). Ocular muscle palsies from involvement of the third or forth cranial nerves are rare. An INO consists of a delay or a failure of adduction on attempted horizontal gaze to one side that is accompanied by nystagmus in the abducting eye. INO results from a lesion of the median longitudinal fasciculus that connects the contralateral third and sixth cranial nerve nuclei; the lesion is usually contralateral to the direction of gaze that results in the INO. Bilateral INO in an awake patient is usually due to multiple sclerosis. Other gaze abnormalities include horizontal gaze palsies from ipsilateral lesions of the lateral pontine tegmentum and the "one-and-a-half" syndrome, consisting of a gaze palsy to one side and an INO to the other (see Ch. 28).

Other brainstem syndromes occur commonly in multiple sclerosis. Trigeminal neuralgia, a lancinating, shock-like facial pain, is one. Clinical features that should raise a question of multiple sclerosis in this setting include the onset of trigeminal neuralgia symptoms at a young age, bilateral involvement, associated objective signs of facial sensory loss, or underlying prolonged pain in addition to the brief paroxysms of shooting pain. Isolated facial palsy resembling idiopathic Bell's palsy may also occur. In multiple sclerosis, facial palsy is uncommonly accompanied by an ipsilateral decrease of sense of taste and may be associated with objective facial sensory loss, vertigo, or other signs of brainstem disease. Facial myokymia, characterized by repetitive twitching contractions of the facial musculature, is also possible.

Vertigo may present as gait unsteadiness and vomiting. A diagnosis of labyrinthitis is frequently considered in such cases, but the presence of other neighborhood signs that point to a brainstem, rather than an end-organ, cause are diagnostically helpful. Hearing loss is unusual in multiple sclerosis but may occur. Hemiplegia, aphasia, and hemianopia are distinctly rare.

A variety of paroxysmal symptoms have been described. These are most often stereotyped events, often triggered by movements or sensory stimuli. Trigeminal neuralgia is a lancinating shocklike facial pain (see Ch. 25).

Urinary bladder, and less frequently bowel, urgency or incontinence occurs in most patients with multiple sclerosis at some time and may be present at disease onset. Impotence from a failure to achieve erection is common in men.

Cognitive dysfunction may present as memory loss, emotional instability, and impaired reasoning. Measurable cognitive abnormalities are present in approximately one-third of patients with multiple sclerosis early in the disease course. Cognitive dysfunction correlates imperfectly with the disease burden measured by MRI.

Heat sensitivity may result in a marked worsening of symptoms during the course of a febrile illness or after a hot bath. Uthoff's phenomenon consists of transient visual blurring after exercise or heat exposure.

Severe or abnormal fatigue is reported by up to 88 percent of patients. The fatigue correlates poorly with disability and must be distinguished from depression.

A variety of paroxysmal symptoms have been described in multiple sclerosis. These are most often brief stereotyped events that may occur spontaneously or be triggered by specific movements or sensory stimuli. Paroxysmal dysarthria, diplopia, and ataxia have been reported, as have "tonic seizures," consisting of sustained tonic contractions of a limb.

COURSE AND PROGNOSIS

Multiple sclerosis is typically described as disseminated in time and space, meaning that the disease pursues a chronic course and affects multiple sites of the neuraxis. Although the course is variable and to some degree unpredictable, it is useful to distinguish several clinical forms. Relapsing-remitting multiple sclerosis is characterized by discrete attacks or flares of disease. Deficits may persist or be followed by partial or complete recovery within weeks to several months. The mean attack rate for patients with the relapsing-remitting form is approximately 1 to 1.5 per year. Chronic progressive multiple sclerosis results in gradual worsening of disability without recovery or pause. In most patients, progressive paraparesis or quadriparesis is the major functional consequence. Multiple sclerosis may begin with a primary progressive course, or secondary progression may evolve in patients with existing relapsing-remitting multiple sclerosis. Acute exacerbations can also occur in patients with progressive symptoms (progressive relapsing form). In most patients, significant disability develops during a 25-year follow-up period, but in 10 to 15 percent, a benign or mild course is present. Favorable prognostic factors include a benign course during the initial 5 years of disease and few attacks (e.g., less than two over 3 years) in the early years after onset. Unfavorable prognostic factors include a chronic progressive course, a high frequency of early attacks, or an early development of disability. The course of multiple sclerosis appears to be slightly more severe in males than in females. Several presenting symptoms have also been reported to correlate with the course. A favorable prognosis is associated with a monosymptomatic onset, isolated optic neuritis, or pure sensory presentation. By contrast, the presence of motor or cerebellar signs at onset is associated with a poor prognosis.

Life expectancy in multiple sclerosis is only modestly decreased compared with that in age-matched controls. By contrast, work capacity is greatly affected by the disease; 15 years after onset, only 25 percent of patients with multiple sclerosis remain capable of meaningful work.

Pregnancy may influence the course of multiple sclerosis. During pregnancy, patients experience fewer relapses compared with the nonpregnant population but have more attacks in the first 3 months postpartum. These opposing effects on the disease course tend to neutralize each other. It has been hypothesized that high serum levels of prolactin, a hormone with multiple systemic effects including immunostimulation, might underlie the increase in the risk of postpartum attacks. Elevated prolactin levels are sustained postpartum only with breast feeding, yet one retrospective study did not identify an effect of breast feeding on the incidence of postpartum flares.

DIAGNOSIS

In young adults, a history of relapsing and remitting symptoms, suggesting multifocal and asymmetric involvement of white matter tracts, leads easily to a correct diagnosis. In cases of explosive onset, primary progressive disability, or other unusual presentations, arrival at a correct diagnosis may be exceedingly difficult. In such situations, a history of prior attacks initially not recalled is most helpful. In many cases, examination reveals unexpected abnormalities suggestive of disseminated disease.

Various diagnostic criteria for multiple sclerosis have been proposed; some incorporate both clinical and paraclinical (e.g., laboratory) data to arrive at a "definite," "probable," or "possible" level of diagnostic confidence. Sound clinical judgment remains the cornerstone of correct diagnosis. A critical approach limits the chance of misdiagnosis, in particular when the onset is progressive or when symptoms unusual for multiple sclerosis, for example, aphasia, extrapyramidal syndromes, amyotrophy with fasciculations, peripheral neuropathy, seizures, or coma, occur.

Differential Diagnosis

The differential diagnosis of multiple sclerosis most often includes other diseases that result in multifocal CNS inflammation. Systemic lupus erythematosus, Behcet's disease, and sarcoidosis may be considered, but the characteristic systemic features of these disorders generally point to the correct diagnosis. Among infectious disorders, Lyme disease may involve the optic nerve, brainstem, and spinal cord and, thus, mimic multiple sclerosis, in particular, when the usual features of rash, meningoradiculitis, or fever are absent.

In young adults, the acute onset of focal neurologic signs may raise the question of cerebrovascular disease. Progressive focal deficits should always prompt consideration of a compressive lesion. Primary CNS lymphomas may produce solitary or multiple lesions that enhance by MRI and may resemble acute lesions of multiple sclerosis. The development of a progressive or relapsing brainstem disturbance may be due to a vascular malformation in the posterior fossa. Pontine glioma is distinguished from multiple sclerosis by its tendency to produce progressive deficits that involve contiguous structures. Adult Chiari malformation may also be considered in the setting of ataxia, nystagmus, and corticospinal tract disease.

Primary progressive myelopathy mimicking multiple sclerosis may be due to cervical spondylosis, extramedullary or intramedullary tumors, vascular malformations, or vitamin B_{12} deficiency. HTLV-1-associated myelopathy (or tropical spastic paraparesis) is a chronic disease characterized by progressive spasticity affecting the lower limbs in particular, with bladder dysfunction and back pain. It is caused by a human retrovirus that is endemic to tropical regions and Japan, areas where multiple sclerosis is uncommon. HTLV-1 is also an agent of acute T-cell leukemia, but the coexistence of myelopathy and leukemia is rare. Detection of specific antibodies to HTLV-1 should be followed by detection of viral nucleic acid or direct virus isolation, which are diagnostic for HTLV-1-associated myelopathy. Recently, cases of progressive myelopathy associated with infection with the HTLV-2 virus have been described.

On occasion, inherited degenerative diseases have been reported to resemble multiple sclerosis. These include mitochondrial disorders (including Leigh's disease, MELAS syndrome, and Leber's hereditary optic neuropathy), spinocerebellar ataxias, and leukodystrophies, including X-linked adrenoleukodystrophy.

Acute disseminated encephalomyelitis typically occurs in association with viral infections or vaccination. In acute disseminated encephalomyelitis associated with acute viral exanthems of childhood, the neurologic disorder may begin as the rash fades and the fever remits. It is characterized by the rapid development of multiple symptoms and signs, indicating extensive disruption of white matter pathways. Pathologically, the CNS is peppered with disseminated perivenous demyelinating lesions. In its most severe form, lesions are hemorrhagic because of a hyperacute immune response that results in destruction of vascular endothelium (acute hemorrhagic encephalitis of Weston-Hurst).

Neuromyelitis optica (Devic's syndrome) is characterized by the development of acute bilateral optic neuritis, followed within days to weeks by transverse myelitis, in a previously healthy individual. On occasion, myelitis may precede the development of optic neuritis. CNS lesions may be necrotizing and severe. Cerebrospinal fluid (CSF) findings are variable but, in some cases, consist of polymorphonuclear pleocytosis and raised protein content. Neuromyelitis optica is a common form of multiple sclerosis in Japan but is rare among white populations. An identical syndrome may occur in systemic lupus erythematosus or Behçet's disease.

Laboratory Diagnosis

Laboratory testing may support a diagnosis of multiple sclerosis and exclude other diseases that mimic the multiple sclerosis phenotype. In most situations, the most useful tests are CSF analysis, MRI studies, and evoked-response testing. CSF abnormalities consist of pleocytosis and an increase in the immunoglobulin (IgG) content. Modest CSF mononuclear pleocytosis (more than 5 cells/μl) is present in approximately 25 percent of patients. Counts above 50 cells/ml are unusual but may occur early in the disease course. Pleocytosis of more than 75 cells/ml or the presence of polymorphonuclear leukocytes in the CSF makes the diagnosis of multiple sclerosis unlikely. In approximately 80 percent of patients, the CSF content of IgG is increased in the setting of a normal total protein because of selective production of IgG in the CNS. Elevated CSF IgG is often expressed as a ratio of CSF IgG/albumin levels. Two or more bands of oligoclonal IgG (see above) are detected by agarose gel electrophoresis in CSF of most patients with multiple sclerosis, and the presence of oligoclonal bands correlates with raised CSF IgG levels. Oligoclonal bands may not be present at the time of initial presentation of MS.

MRI scanning has assumed an increasingly important role in the diagnosis and longitudinal clinical assessment of patients with multiple sclerosis. MRI abnormalities are present in more than 90 percent of patients with clinically definite multiple sclerosis. On inversion-recovery (T_1) imaging, the CNS appears normal or may reveal punctate areas of dark signal in white matter regions. The most characteristic MRI changes consist of multiple areas of bright signal on spin-echo (T_2) sequences (Fig. 73-1). Abnormal T_2 bright regions tend to be multiple, asymmetric, and periventricular in location. Some lesions may appear to extend in a linear fashion outward from the ventricular surface, corresponding to the pattern of perivenous demyelination observed pathologically (Dawson's fingers). T_2-bright-signal areas may also be detected in the spinal cord by MRI. Administration of the contrast agent gadolinium is used to detect "active" lesions in which the blood-brain barrier is disrupted and extravasation of the injected contrast agent into brain parenchyma occurs. Serial MRI studies in relapsing-remitting multiple sclerosis indicate that new abnormal foci appear 7 to 10 times more frequently than predicted on the basis of clinical criteria alone. A similar frequency of new lesions appear in chronic progressive multiple sclerosis, although abnormal foci in these patients tend to be more confluent than in patients with relapsing-remitting disease.

Evoked-response testing may detect slowing or interruption of conduction in visual, auditory, somatosensory, or motor pathways. Although it is assumed that the slowing in multiple sclerosis results from loss of saltatory conduction secondary to demyelination, in fact, slowed evoked responses are noted in many other diseases of the nervous system. It is thus a non-

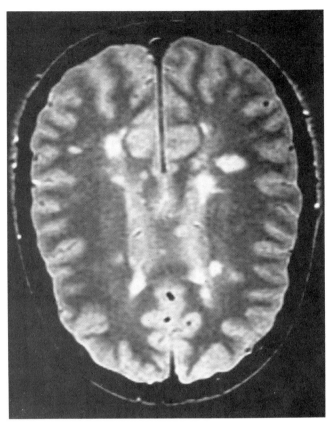

Figure 73-1. Spin-echo MRI sequence in multiple sclerosis demonstrates extensive bright signal abnormalities in periventricular white matter.

specific finding. Evoked responses are most useful when they differ between sides, suggesting an asymmetric disease process; when they document a second abnormality in the setting of a single clinically apparent lesion; or when they indicate an objective finding in a patient with subjective complaints only.

TREATMENT

Therapy for multiple sclerosis can be divided into interventions useful for (1) acute relapses, (2) prophylaxis of relapses, (3) chronic progressive type, and (4) symptomatic treatment (Fig. 73-2).

Acute relapses may be treated with intravenous methylprednisolone or adrenocorticotropic hormone. Pulse therapy with these agents speeds the tempo of recovery from acute attacks and may modestly improve the degree of recovery noted to occur over a short follow-up period. The use of these drugs is generally reserved for patients with moderate or severe attacks. In a recent trial of methylprednisolone for acute optic neuritis, therapy was associated with a reduction in the subsequent development of multiple sclerosis compared with placebo or oral prednisone

therapy. This result has raised the possibility that short-term treatment with methylprednisolone may retard the evolution of an initial attack to multiple sclerosis. MRI findings in patients with optic neuritis or other monosymptomatic presentations (e.g., transverse myelitis or brainstem encephalomyelitis) have prognostic implications relevant to the likelihood of evolution to multiple sclerosis over a 2- to 3-year period. MRI evidence of disseminated lesions at presentation are associated with a 35 to 45 percent evolution to multiple sclerosis compared with 5 to 10 percent in patients with normal or single-lesion MRI scans. Thus, methylprednisolone might be generally indicated for initial attacks when the MRI scan indicates multifocal disease.

Interferon-β (IFN-β) has been recently found to be effective in the prophylaxis of relapses in multiple sclerosis. Subcutaneous injections reduced the relapse rate by one-third and reduced severe relapses by one-half. Treatment was also associated with a marked reduction in the evolution of abnormalities detected by MRI scan, confirming the clinical effect on relapse rate. IFN-β treatment was also associated with a tendency for reduced accumulated disability, but this finding did not reach statistical significance. The drug was well tolerated in most patients; a transient flu-like syndrome may occur with initiation of therapy. Based on these results, IFN-β should be considered for patients with multiple sclerosis who ambulate independently and have relapsing-remitting disease with two or more relapses in the preceding 2 years. The mechanism responsible for the effect of IFN-β on this disease is unknown. It might work by reducing the expression of MHC molecules on the surface of antigen-presenting cells in the brain or elsewhere, by other immunosuppressive effects, or by an antiviral effect. MHC expression induced by IFN-γ can be blocked by IFN-β, and it is noteworthy that IFN-γ administration appeared to trigger attacks of multiple sclerosis in an earlier study.

Chronic immunosuppression has been advocated as therapy for some patients with chronic progressive disease. The antimetabolite azathioprine given orally is a relatively safe and well-tolerated form of chronic immunosuppression. Its beneficial effect is modest in controlled trials and must be weighed against potential risks that include hepatitis, susceptibility to infection, and a theoretical cancer risk. Methotrexate is another antimetabolite that has been used in progressive multiple sclerosis, and additional clinical trials of this drug are in progress. Pulse therapy with the alkylating agent cyclophosphamide is beneficial to young (younger than 40 years of age) ambulatory patients with rapidly progressive multiple sclerosis. The side effects associated with treatment are considerable and

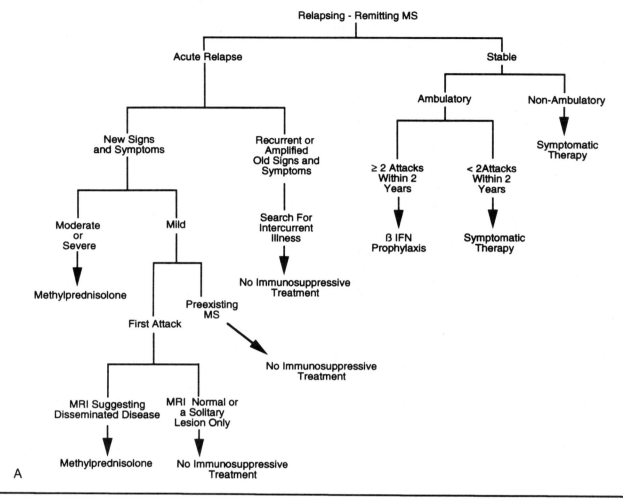

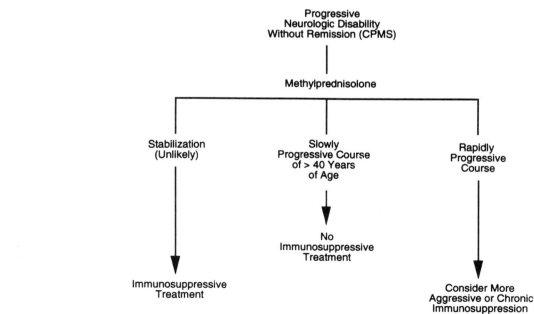

Figure 73-2. (A & B) Therapeutic strategies in multiple sclerosis. Methylprednisolone regimen consists of intravenous methylprednisolone, 1,000 mg IV daily for 3 days, followed by oral prednisone, 1 mg/kg/day PO for 14 days.

include nausea, hair loss, a risk of hemorrhagic cystitis, and temporary profound immunosuppression. Cyclosporine has also been shown to have a modest effect on the course of chronic progressive multiple sclerosis, but side effects, notably hypertension and reversible renal dysfunction, have limited its widespread use.

Symptomatic therapy is an often neglected but critical component of a comprehensive care plan for patients with multiple sclerosis. Paroxysmal symptoms are effectively treated with acetazolamide (125 to 250 mg three times a day) or carbamazepine (200 to 1,200 mg/day in divided doses). Lancinating pain may respond to carbamazepine, amitriptyline (50 to 200 mg/day), or phenytoin (300 mg/day). Spasticity may be treated with baclofen (15 to 80 mg/day, with dosages as high as 240 mg/day or by intrathecal administration in refractory cases). A single bedtime dose of diazepam (2 mg) may be useful for the treatment of nocturnal spasms. The distinction between dysesthesias caused by multiple sclerosis and radiculopathy from lumbar disc disease may be difficult in patients with unilateral leg pain, and nonsurgical therapy is often justified in the absence of convincing evidence of nerve root compression. Bladder hyper-reflexia is treated with anticholinergics (oxybutynin 5 mg two to three times a day or propantheline 7.5 to 15 mg four times a day). Urinary retention from bladder hyporeflexia may respond to the cholinergic drug bethanecol (10 to 50 mg three to four times a day). Dyssynergia between detrusor and external sphincter muscles is common in multiple sclerosis, is difficult to treat, and may require a combination of anticholinergic medications to inhibit bladder contractions, with intermittent catheterization. Ascorbic acid may reduce the risk of urinary tract infections. In patients with severe fatigue, an afternoon nap may be beneficial, and amantadine (100 mg twice a day) may benefit a small proportion of patients. Emotional lability responds to amitriptyline (25 to 75 mg/day) or to other tricyclic medications. Signs of depression need to be recognized and treated appropriately.

Care is maximized in settings that bring together teams of health care professionals experienced with the biology of multiple sclerosis and with the medical and social consequences of the disease. Chronic pain; spasticity; bowel, bladder, or sexual dysfunction; rehabilitation; challenges to job and family; and psychiatric issues are best managed in comprehensive care settings geared to the special problems of the population with multiple sclerosis.

ANNOTATED BIBLIOGRAPHY

Adams CWM, Poston RN, Buk SJ. Pathology, histochemistry and immunocytochemistry of lesions in acute multiple sclerosis. J Neurol Sci 1989;92:291–306.
Studies of 20 cases.

Beck RW, Cleary PA, Anderson MM Jr et al. A randomized, controlled clinical trial of corticosteroids in the treatment of acute optic neuritis. N Engl J Med 1992;326:581–8.
Intravenous followed by oral therapy is effective.

Goodkin DE, Doolittle TH, Hauser SS et al. Diagnostic criteria for multiple sclerosis research involving multiply affected families. Arch Neurol 1991;48:805–7.
Details of criteria provided.

The IFNB Multiple Sclerosis Study Group. Interferon beta-1b is effective in relapsing remitting multiple sclerosis. I: Clinical results of a multicenter, randomized, double-blind, placebo-controlled trial. Neurology 1993;43:655–61.
Effect of interferon-β on relapse rate and MRI.

The IFNB Multiple Sclerosis Study Group. Interferon beta-1b is effective in relapsing remitting multiple sclerosis. II: MRI analysis results of a multicenter, randomized, double-blind, placebo-controlled trial. Neurology 1993;43:662–7.
MRI findings in a large trial.

Martin R, McFarland HF, McFarland DE. Immunological aspects of demyelinating diseases. Annu Rev Immunol 1992;10:153–87.
Detailed review.

Miller A, Hafler DA, Weiner HL. Immunotherapy in autoimmune diseases. Curr Opin Immunol 1992;3:936–40.
Review article.

Oksenberg JR, Panzara MA, Begovich AB et al. Selection for T-cell receptor Vb-Db-Jb gene rearrangements with specificity for a myelin basic protein peptide in brain lesions of multiple sclerosis. Nature 1993;362:68–70.
T-cell receptors and gene rearrangements.

Olsson T, Zhi WW, Hojeberg B et al. Autoreactive T lymphocytes in multiple sclerosis determined by antigen-induced secretion of interferon. J Clin Invest 1990;86:981–5.
T cells and myelin autoantigens.

Paty DW, Oger JJ, Kastrukoff LF et al. MRI in the diagnosis of MS: a prospective study with comparison of clinical evaluation, evoked potentials, oligoclonal banding and CT. Neurology 1988;38:180–5.
The sensitivity of MRI in the diagnosis of multiple sclerosis.

Poser CM, Paty DW, Scheinberg L et al. New diagnostic criteria for multiple sclerosis: guidelines for research protocols. Ann Neurol 1983;13:227–31.
Still in force.

Prineas JW. The neuropathology of multiple sclerosis. In Koetsier JC (ed). Handbook of Clinical Neurology. Elsevier Science Publishers, Amsterdam, 1985.
Textbook chapter.

Raine CS, Scheiberg L, Waltz JM. Multiple sclerosis. Oligo-dendrocyte survival and proliferation in an active established lesion. Lab Invest 1981;45:534–46.

Oligodendroglia not primarily depeleted; the main attack is on myelin.

Sadovnick AD, Ebers GC. Epidemiology of multiple sclerosis: a critical overview. Can J Neurol Sci 1993;20:17–29.

Update.

Sadovnick AD, Macleod PMJ. The familial nature of multiple sclerosis: empiric recurrence risks for first, second, third degree relatives of patients. Neurology 1981;31:1039–41.

Review article.

Sears TA, Bostock H, Sheratt M. The pathophysiology of demyelination and its implications for the symptomatic treatment of multiple sclerosis. Neurology 1978;28:21–6.

Classic hypothesis.

Yudkin PL, Ellison GW, Ghezzi A et al. Overview of azathio-prine treatment in multiple sclerosis. Lancet 1991;338:1051–5.

A modest effect of azathioprine therapy.

74

Optic Neuritis

Antonio Uccelli and Stephen L. Hauser

Optic neuritis is an inflammatory demyelinating disease of the optic nerve. It is in general a disease of early to middle adulthood and occurs either as an isolated neurologic finding or in the setting of established multiple sclerosis. Most patients with isolated optic neuritis subsequently have multiple sclerosis. Other features of optic neuritis also support its classification as a monosymptomatic presentation of multiple sclerosis. In both, there is a twofold increased risk in females compared with males, a peak onset at 30 years of age, and an association with the histocompatibility antigen HLA-DR2. Finally, epidemiologic data indicate concordant geographic variation in the prevalence of both optic neuritis and multiple sclerosis.

CLINICAL FEATURES

The typical clinical presentation of optic neuritis consists of unilateral visual impairment, progressing over hours to several days. In occasional cases, visual loss may progress over 2 weeks or longer. Visual loss may be accompanied or preceded by retro-orbital or lateral supraorbital pain that may worsen with eye movement. Visual impairment ranges from mild to severe. The loss of visual acuity accompanying acute optic neuritis is associated with impaired color vision (dyschromatopsia) and in many cases with a visual scotoma, decreased contrast sensitivity, or movement phosphenes (brief flashes of light in one eye induced by eye movement). Some patients complain of photophobia or of improvement of vision in dim, as opposed to bright, light.

On examination, the most sensitive sign of optic nerve disease is the presence of an afferent pupillary defect, which is elicited by a swinging flashlight test. The affected pupil may be enlarged or irregular. Funduscopic examination may reveal swelling of the optic disc and rarely peripapillary hemorrhages (papillitis).

More often, the disc appears normal because of the distance of the lesion from the optic nerve head (retrobulbar neuritis, i.e., involvement of cranial nerve II behind the lamina cribrosa, where the optic fibers become myelinated). Some authors report retinal venous sheathing in up to 25 percent of patients, but others found the incidence to be lower. This finding consists of a white exudate, thought to include lymphocytes, surrounding retinal veins. Venous sheathing may be associated with inflammation in the vitreous or anterior chamber, and by abnormal vascular permeability demonstrated by fluorescein angiography. In two separate studies, retinal sheathing accompanying isolated optic neuritis was positively associated with subsequent progression to multiple sclerosis.

DIAGNOSIS

The diagnosis of optic neuritis is often not difficult in a young woman who complains of monocular visual impairment, which was progressive over 1 week and is accompanied by pain and funduscopic findings of papillitis. By contrast, diagnostic challenges may be present in older patients with suspected optic neuritis or in cases of bilateral visual loss.

Laboratory testing is valuable in patients with suspected optic neuritis, both to exclude other diseases and to provide prognostic information relative to the risk of subsequent development of multiple sclerosis. Documentation of formal visual acuity and fields, color vision, and contrast sensitivity is essential. Lumbar puncture is not routinely performed in cases of isolated optic neuritis, but the presence of oligoclonal banding increases the chances of subsequent development of multiple sclerosis. Visual-evoked potentials are abnormal in as many as 95 percent of patients with acute optic neuritis. Abnormalities consist of delayed conduction and a decrease in the amplitude of the

P100 waveform. Magnetic resonance imaging (MRI) may visualize abnormalities of the optic nerve in a proportion of patients and exclude compressive lesions that mimic the optic neuritis syndrome. In addition, MRI may detect disseminated, clinically silent, white matter abnormalities in more that one-half of patients with acute optic neuritis. Not surprisingly, the presence of multifocal MRI abnormalities in isolated optic neuritis is strongly associated with subsequent evolution to clinically definite multiple sclerosis (see below).

The differential diagnosis of optic neuritis may include a variety of vascular, hereditary, toxic, compressive, inflammatory, and infiltrative disorders (see also Ch. 21). Anterior ischemic optic neuropathy is a common cause of monocular visual loss. Compared with optic neuritis, anterior ischemic optic neuropathy generally presents at a later age; the onset of visual loss is more acute; and an altitudinal field defect, a pale disc, and flame-shaped peripapillary hemorrhages may be present. Compressive optic neuropathies caused by a tumor or associated with chronic sinus disease, on occasion, may mimic optic neuritis. The most common infectious causes of acute optic neuropathy are Lyme disease, neurovascular syphilis, and human immunodeficiency virus. In suspected bilateral optic neuritis, the possibility of neuromyelitis optica (Devic's disease) associated with multiple sclerosis, systemic lupus erythematosus, Behçet's disease, or other conditions may be raised. On rare occasions, pseudotumor cerebri or other causes of raised intracranial pressure may present as rapidly progressive bilateral visual loss and as papilledema mimicking papillitis. In some clinical settings, other diagnostic considerations include optic neuropathy associated with vitamin B_{12} or other nutritional deficiencies, tobacco-alcohol use, the little understood Jamaican optic neuropathy (see Chs. 69 and 73), and the mitochondrial disorder Leber's disease (see Ch. 26).

COURSE

In most cases of optic neuritis, good to excellent visual recovery can be expected. Two-thirds or more of patients regain visual acuity of at least 20/30. After recovery, residual deficits in visual fields, color vision, or sensitivity to contrast may persist even when visual acuity returns to normal. Uhthoff's sign, consisting of transient visual obscuration induced by exercise or an elevation in body temperature, may follow symptomatic or subclinical bouts of optic neuritis. In approximately 20 percent of patients with acute optic neuritis, one or more recurrences develop over a 3-year period. Similarly, an estimated 20 percent of patients have clinically definite multiple sclerosis within 3 years of acute optic neuritis. The incidence of multiple sclerosis continues to increase as the time of follow-up lengthens, and it is likely that 75 percent or more of patients with optic neuritis will ultimately have multiple sclerosis.

TREATMENT

In 1992 and 1993, Beck et al. reported the results of a multicenter trial to evaluate intravenous methylprednisolone (1 g/day for 3 days) followed by oral prednisone (1 mg/kg/day for 11 days) versus oral prednisone alone (1 mg/kg/day for 14 days) in the treatment of acute optic neuritis. Four hundred fifty-seven patients entered this placebo-controlled trial. The trial was single blinded only because patients randomized to receive intravenous methylprednisolone were hospitalized and aware of the treatment they received. In the intravenous methylprednisolone group, faster recovery of visual acuity, field defects, and contrast sensitivity occurred. A modest benefit of intravenous therapy persisted at the 6-month follow-up point but was no longer present at the 1-year point. The most surprising finding of this study related to a treatment effect on the long-term disease course. During a 2-year follow-up period, oral prednisone alone was associated with an increase in the risk of new episodes of optic neuritis compared with either the intravenous methylprednisolone or placebo groups. Furthermore, during a follow-up period of up to 3.5 years, there was a significant decrease in the development of multiple sclerosis in patients who had received intravenous methylprednisolone compared with those who had received oral prednisone alone or placebo. The protective effect of intravenous methylprednisolone appeared to be present for a 2-year period. As noted earlier, MRI was a predictor of the evolution to multiple sclerosis in this study. A normal MRI scan at entry was associated with a 2-year risk of clinical multiple sclerosis of approximately 5 percent compared with 35 percent in patients with MRI evidence of disseminated disease at entry.

Based on these results, oral steroids alone should probably not be used for the treatment of uncomplicated optic neuritis. Intravenous methylprednisolone followed by oral prednisone represents the best current therapy for acute optic neuritis and should be considered in patients with moderate or severe episodes or when MRI indicates the presence of disseminated disease.

ANNOTATED BIBLIOGRAPHY

Beck RW, Cleary PA, Anderson MM Jr et al. A randomized, controlled trial of corticosteroids in the treatment of acute optic neuritis. N Engl J Med 1992;326:581–8.

Intravenous followed by oral therapy has effects not seen with oral treatment alone.

Beck RW, Cleary PA, Trobe JD et al. The effect of corticosteroids for acute optic neuritis on the subsequent development of multiple sclerosis. N Engl J Med 1993;329: 1764–9.

Benefits from a 3-day course of intravenous methylprednisolone.

Compston D, Batchelor J, Earl C, McDonald WI. Factors influencing the risk of multiple sclerosis developing in patients with optic neuritis. Brain 1978;101:495–511.

Two seasonally based environmental factors, with the winter more likely and the summer less likely to precipitate multiple sclerosis.

Ebers GC. Optic neuritis and multiple sclerosis. Arch Neurol 1985;42:702–4.

Review article.

Francis DA, Compston D, Batchelor JR, McDonald WI. A reassessment of the risk of multiple sclerosis developing in patients with optic neuritis after extended follow-up. J Neurol Neurosurg Psychiatry 1987;50:758–65.

HLA-DR3 combined with HLA-DR2 increased the risk of multiple sclerosis 26-fold.

Frederiksen JL, Larsson HB, Henriksen O, Olesen J. Magnetic resonance imaging of the brain in patients with acute monosymptomatic optic neuritis. Acta Neurol Scand 1989;80:512–7.

Those with central nervous system findings on imaging had a higher risk of clinical multiple sclerosis later.

Optic Neuritis Study Group. The clinical profile of optic neuritis: experience of the Optic Neuritis Treatment Trial. Arch Ophthalmol 1991;109:1673–8.

Study of 448 patients.

Perkin CD, Rose FC. Optic Neuritis and Its Differential Diagnosis. Oxford University Press, Oxford, 1979.

Standard textbook.

Rizzo JF III, Lessel S. Risk of developing multiple sclerosis after uncomplicated optic neuritis: a long prospective study. Neurology 1988;38:185–90.

Study of 60 white patients showing 3.4 times the risk for women compared with men.

75

Parkinson's Disease

A. Lieberman

"Shaking palsy" was described in 1817 by James Parkinson (British neurologist, 1755–1824) and is now called Parkinson's disease. It is an idiopathic disorder and is one of the most common clinical problems in neurologic practice. Its diagnosis is essentially clinical and usually easy, except in the incipient stages. The current treatment is effective for a few years, and then gradually, control of the disorder is lost in most patients.

The incidence of Parkinson's disease is about 20 per 100,000 with a prevalence of 200 per 100,000 in Western countries. A substantial number of cases may be misdiagnosed as old age and thus escape inclusion in the census. There is evidence that the disease is less frequent in Asia and Africa for unclear reasons.

PATHOPHYSIOLOGY

The anatomic and physiologic aspects of the basal ganglia that provide a background to understanding Parkinson's disease have been considered in Chapter 26. The essential lesion in Parkinson's disease is the disappearance of melanin-containing cells in the substantia nigra pars compacta, particularly in its ventrolateral region, which projects particularly to the putamen. The normal concentration of dopamine in the putamen and caudate, the so-called dopaminergic nigrostriatal pathway, is reduced by at least 80 percent in Parkinson's disease. This reduction provides the basis for dopamine therapy.

However, Parkinson's disease is not merely a disease of the dopaminergic pathway. Many other cell populations are also decreased. The locus ceruleus, the main source of noradrenergic innervation in the central nervous system, and the dorsal motor nucleus of the vagus nerve are usually partially depopulated. In addition, lesions are usually found in nonpigmented cell groups, such as the basal nucleus of Meynert, the chief source of cholinergic innervation of the neocortex; the

substantia innominata; the hypothalamus; the mammillary bodies; the mesencephalic reticular formation; and the dorsal nucleus of the raphe. This last is a source of serotoninergic innervation. Lesions are also found, to a variable extent, in the tractus intermediolateralis of the spinal cord (the origin of sympathetic fibers) and in the sympathetic ganglia. Such a dissemination of the lesions shows that Parkinson's disease is a multisystem and multitransmitter disorder, and the general view that the pathophysiologic findings are based on dopamine deficit alone is too simplistic, although it explains the limited efficiency of levodopa therapy. Despite the multisystem nature of the disorder, it is curious there are no significant striatal lesions.

The histopathologic hallmark of Parkinson's disease is the presence of intraneuronal inclusions; the Lewy bodies, the origin of which is unknown, are almost diagnostic. They have, however, rarely been reported in other conditions, such as postencephalitic parkinsonism, clinically normal aged subjects when they preclinical parkinsonism is suspected (see below), in some parkinsonism plus syndromes (see Ch. 76), and in rare diseases, such as Hallervorden-Spatz disease, infantile neuroaxonal degeneration, or progressive dementia with quadriplegia in flexion.

Lewy bodies contain ubiquitin, phosphorylated neurofilaments, phospholipids, and cytoskeletal elements. They are distinct from Pick's bodies and the neurofibrillary tangles of Alzheimer disease (see Ch. 60).

A number of demented patients with Parkinson's disease have many Lewy bodies in the cortex (Lewy body dementia).

ETIOLOGY

The cause of Parkinson's disease is unknown. Inheritance, in the simple mendelian genetic sense, is not a major factor, as demonstrated by studies of monozygotic twins.

Environmental factors may play a role. A dramatic demonstration was brought about by drug abusers in whom a contaminant of meperidine, 1-methyl-4-phenyl-1,2,3,6-tetrahydropyridine (MPTP), caused parkinsonism with lesions and clinical disorders similar to those of Parkinson's disease. The MPTP model suggested several hypotheses. Could Parkinson's disease result from exposure to an unknown MPTP-like agent? If so, no such poison is currently known. Could long exposure to small quantities of this hypothetical poison or early exposure in life explain the delayed clinical onset of Parkinson's disease. Although attractive, this thesis is not supported by the absence of concomitant disease in monozygotic twins and spouses and the absence of clusters of Parkinson's disease. MPTP exerts its noxious activity because its catabolite MPP+ binds to neuromelanin, a derivative of catecholamine metabolism. Could a (hypothetical) noxious agent cause excessive formation of free radicals in the substantia nigra in Parkinson's disease? Such an effect would be consistent with the excess iron and decreased ferritin that is detected in the substantia nigra of patients with Parkinson's disease. Free radicals are generated by oxidative stress that harms by causing peroxidation of lipids. In Parkinson's disease, this could be supported by the low quantities of reduced glutathione or by mitochondrial complex I activity reduction. Selegiline hydrochloride inhibits the chief catabolic enzyme of dopamine, monamine oxidase B, and thus aims at preventing free radical production from dopamine catabolism. It is actually used with some success in Parkinson's disease, but whether its effect is in blunting an unknown source of oxidative stress remains elusive.

CLINICAL FEATURES

Parkinson's disease rarely begins before the age of 40; the peak incidence is the sixth decade. The primary clinical features include tremor, rigidity, bradykinesia or akinesia, and postural instability.

Primary Clinical Features

Tremor (see Ch. 22) is present in about 70 percent of patients. It is typically seen at rest and is decreased by movement. Although bilateral onset is possible, as a rule, it begins on one side, first affecting the fingers and hand. It can remain localized for months or years, but in most cases, it gradually involves the ipsilateral lower limb or then the opposite side. In some patients, it involves the tongue, lips, and jaw. A postural tremor may antedate the resting tremor (see Ch. 22). Tremor is the clinical feature of Parkinson's disease that is the least sensitive to treatment, but patients in whom it is prominent usually have a longer and less severe course than those without tremor.

Rigidity is an increased resistance to passive stretch. It is of the "lead pipe" type (as in the steady resistance to bending typical of a lead pipe) without the "clasp-knife" phenomenon typical of spasticity (see Ch. 22). In most cases, it is regularly interrupted by the 4- to 6-Hz tremor, thus giving the "cogwheel" phenomenon. It predominates on the flexors, causing the stooped ("simian") posture. When rigidity is the presenting disorder, it is unilateral, and may be difficult to distinguish from spasticity from upper motor neuron lesions. It must be remembered that, in Parkinson's disease, tendon reflexes and the plantar response are normal.

Bradykinesia or akinesia includes both slowness and poverty of movement and involves delay in initiating movements, arrests of ongoing movement, and inability to execute sequential movements (e.g., filliping or tapping with the foot). It is typically accompanied by an expressionless face ("masklike facies," often diagnosed clinically as depression) and a notable reduction in the frequency of blinking. The "parkinsonian stare" is often an immediate clue to the diagnosis. Bradykinesia encompasses slowness of speech, chewing, and swallowing. Unlike paralysis, bradykinesia can be suspended by intense excitement (e.g., a fire; kinesia paradoxica).

Postural instability results from impairment of postural or righting reflexes (see Ch. 22). Patients fall easily without adaptive reactions. In some, it is a distressing characteristic of the disease and does not respond to levodopa. Patients have difficulties turning about when walking.

Gait disturbances (see Ch. 22) are characterized by short, shuffling steps. Freezing is used to describe the sudden cessation of movement or the failure to initiate expected movements in a timely fashion. It typically occurs through doorways. Conversely, visible marks on the ground or the examiner's foot placed in front of the patient's foot can suppress the inhibition to a certain extent. Festinations (Latin: *festinare,* to hasten) are short episodes during which the patient hurries forward or backward as if chasing the body's center of gravity to avoid falling. Festination can be an early and an isolated sign for a time.

Secondary Clinical Features

These are either consequences of a combination of primary disorders and occur in less than 50 percent of the patients.

A certain number of disorders result from autonomic dysfunction or of dystonias. *Orthostatic hypotension* is infrequent but can cause syncope. It may be aggravated by therapy with levodopa and dopamine agonists. *Speech difficulties* include a diminution in volume and a tendency for words to run together. Chewing and dysphagia can be severe enough to require a feeding tube. *Urinary problems* usually take the form of urgency or hyperactive detrusor function with decreased capacity. In aging men, it is first necessary to rule out prostatism. *Constipation* is frequent and could be aggravated by anticholinergics and amantadine. *Impotence* is frequent. Most of these disorders can be ascribed to autonomic dysfunction (see Pathophysiology above). *Respiratory difficulties* can be due to a combination of chest wall rigidity, bradykinesia, and drug-induced dyskinesia. They manifest as shortness of breath, which is unrelated to effort. In Parkinson's disease (as contrasted to multiple system atrophy, see Ch. 76), vocal cord paralysis with stridor and inability to breath, a medical emergency, is rare. Respiratory difficulties cause added hazards in Parkinson's disease when surgery is contemplated.

Cognitive impairment can lead to *dementia* (a word that is avoided with patients). It occurs in up to 30 percent of the cases; its prevalence increases with age. It may be heralded by sleep disturbances, such as daytime drowsiness and nocturnal wakefulness. Of practical importance is that cognitive deterioration may be exacerbated by treatment with levodopa and especially anticholinergics and amantadine. These drugs usually induce a confusional state with delusions or hallucinations.

Depression occurs in 50 to 70 percent of patients and can be the presenting symptom. It can be a harbinger of cognitive decline. Many patients have an apathetic state that differs from depression in that it is not accompanied by sadness and guilt and does not clearly respond to antidepressant drugs.

Miscellaneous complaints are also common. *Sialorrhea* is generally thought to result from bradykinetic swallowing. *Seborrhea* gives the immobile face a characteristic shiny, glossy look. *Sensory symptoms,* such as burning paresthesias, cold sensations, and deep aches in the limbs, are often present.

The combination of primary and secondary clinical features in advanced cases produces a characteristic clinical picture, with the stooped patient walking hesitantly with frequent freezing spells. The face is immobile, drooling needs the help of a handkerchief, and speech is reduced to an unintelligible mumbling. In patients with early disease the condition may be difficult to diagnose. In such patients, the following signs help: the absence of swinging an arm on walking, difficulties in turning about in bed, micrographia (i.e., small writing that moreover can accentuate from the beginning to the end of a sentence), and inexhaustible blinking in response to a tap on the glabella (in normal subjects, the reflex is suppressed after a few taps). Clues to the reinforcement of tremor and cogwheel movement were mentioned in Chapter 22.

Early-Onset Parkinson's Disease

Rarely, Parkinson's disease begins in patients younger than age of 40 years, but such cases usually come to the neurologist's attention. In the series of Quinn et al. (1987), the cases with onset after the age of 21 had no significant history and responded well to levodopa therapy, although dyskinesias and response fluctuations occurred early. The incidence of dementia was nil or very low. In contrast, four cases beginning in patients younger than age 21 were all familial. All secondary cases were first-degree relatives, and all had had a young disease onset. The data suggested an autosomal recessive inheritance. No patient was demented. Familial Parkinson's disease with an autosomal dominant transmission has been reported in two large families. In both, there was an early onset and rapid worsening. Cases have also been reported from Japan, but it is not certain that they represent classic idiopathic Parkinson's disease.

Preclinical Parkinson's Disease

The observations of a substantial loss of nigral neurons (50 percent or more) and the severe putaminal dopamine depletion (80 percent or more) in overt Parkinson's disease suggest a long preclinical period of the disease, perhaps exceeding 10 years. Besides, in otherwise asymptomatic individuals whose brain specimens show incidental Lewy bodies, there is usually evidence of some substantia nigra pars compacta degeneration. The frequency of incidental Lewy bodies increases with age, and for every patient with patent Parkinson's disease, there are about 10 with incidental Lewy bodies. The possible existence of a large cohort of people who may develop Parkinson's disease if they live long enough has prompted efforts to develop methods to identify them so that treatment can be started before dopamine depletion has reached the clinical threshold.

LABORATORY STUDIES

Although the diagnosis of Parkinson's disease is essentially a clinical one, computed tomography or magnetic resonance imaging (MRI) may be useful to exclude the uncommon causes of parkinsonian syndromes, such as mass lesions, hydrocephalus, and multiple infarcts. MRI is especially useful in excluding brainstem and cerebellar atrophy that should point to parkinsonism plus conditions (see Ch. 76). Normally, iron deposits appear after age 20 as diminished intensity signals in the pallidum on T_2-weighted high field (1.5 T) MRI scans. Iron deposits in the putamen would suggest parkinsonism plus.

DIFFERENTIAL DIAGNOSIS

Parkinson's disease must be differentiated from parkinsonian syndromes, drug-induced parkinsonism, and parkinsonism plus syndromes (Fig. 75-1 and Ch. 76).

TREATMENT

Newly Diagnosed Parkinson's Disease

The monamine oxidase B inhibitor selegiline (see above) may slow the progression of Parkinson's disease somewhat. It is thus widespread clinical practice for newly diagnosed patients to start therapy with 5 mg twice a day and receive the drug throughout the entire course of treatment, even for some in the disabling phase (see below).

Disabling Parkinson's Disease

Therapeutic options include levodopa, dopamine agonists, anticholinergics, and miscellaneous other agents.

Levodopa is the first-choice drug. The dose should be kept as low as possible. The effective dose of levo-

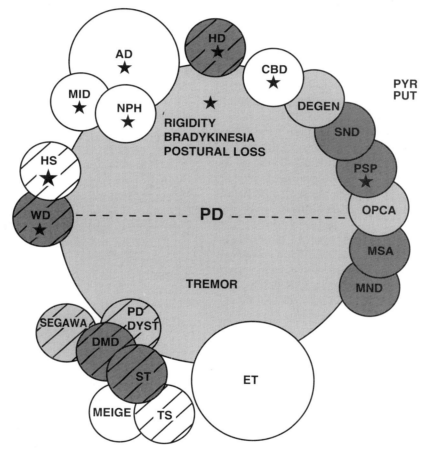

Figure 75-1. The spectrum of movement disorders and their main clinical manifestations. HD, Huntington's disease; CBD, corticobasilar degeneration; SND, striatonigral degeneration; PSP, progressive supranuclear palsy; OPCA, olivopontocerebellar atrophy; MSA, multisystem atrophy; MND, moton neuron disease; ET, essential tremor; TS, Gilles de la Tourette's syndrome; Meige, Meige syndrome; ST, spasmodic torticollis; DMD, dystonia musculorum deformans; PD dyst, Parkinson's disease dystonia; WD, Wilson's disease; NPH, normal progressive hydrocephalus; MID, multi-infarct dementia; AD, Alzheimer's disease; PD, Parkinson's disease.

dopa in early Parkinson's disease is between 300 and 500 mg given in three divided doses. To block extracerebral dopamine decarboxylase and allow the drug to enter the brain, it is combined with 50 to 75 mg decarboxylase inhibitors, either carbidopa or benserazide. Levodopa is available in controlled-release tablets that aim at a smooth sustained release of the drug into the blood. Some neurologists use these controlled-release tablets as their initial drug preparation. For maximum effect, the levo/carbidopa is given on an empty stomach 1 hour before meals, but nausea can prevent this approach. Where it is available, domperidone, a drug that blocks peripheral dopamine receptors, can alleviate this unwanted effect.

Some protein-containing foods may block levodopa absorption through the gut or its passage from the blood to the brain. These foods contain large amounts of the amino acids phenylalanine, leucine, and isoleucine. A low-protein diet can improve the efficiency of levodopa in some patients.

There is a controversy whether levodopa might be withheld in early Parkinson's disease for fear of a causal role in dyskinesias and response fluctuations (see below). Currently, it is agreed that the long-term prognosis is unaffected by early levodopa treatment.

Levodopa treatment is at first very effective in most patients, chiefly in regard to rigidity and akinesia, so that this response is taken by some as a diagnostic criterion. Such a "honeymoon" lasts only a few years. Whatever the benefits of selegiline, degeneration of cells continues, and after a few years, fluctuations in response and dyskinesias appear in about 80 percent of patients. Nigral degeneration presumably continues.

Response fluctuations and dyskinesias are at least partly related to peaks and troughs of plasma levodopa levels. They can occur as a wearing off between doses of levodopa (on-off episodes), representing an abrupt loss of efficacy and temporary excessive medication effect, usually causing dyskinesias. The dyskinesias are involuntary movements of the choreic, ballic, dystonic, and stereotypic type and are often very disabling. Fractionating the doses of levodopa according to the timing of the disorders with controlled-release preparations and adding a dopamine agonist (see below) while observing the patient in on–off phases is recommended.

In patients with severe response fluctuations and dyskinesias, drug holidays of 3 to 14 days have been proposed but are not widely popular. The improvement is at best temporary, and during the so-called holiday, Parkinson's disease disastrously worsens. Complications, such as aspiration pneumonia, phlebitis, and high fever resembling the malignant neuroleptic syndrome, can occur. Such therapeutic trials must be done only in a hospital. Of practical importance is that patients with Parkinson's disease who are admitted to a hospital for surgery should not have their medication discontinued and that, in such patients, general anesthesia remains a significant risk.

Dopamine agonists are drugs that stimulate dopamine receptors. Bromocriptine is begun at a dose of 1.25 to 2.5 mg/day, which can be built up gradually, according to the clinical improvement, in increments of 1.25 to 2.5 mg/day each week, to a maximum of 15 to 40 mg/day. Pergolide is begun at a dose of 0.05 to 0.10 mg a day and can be increased gradually in increments of 0.25 mg/day each week to a maximum of 1.5 to 3.0 mg per day. Many neurologists maintain the dose of levodopa at 500 to 750 mg/day and add a dopamine agonist before the response to levodopa declines. Dopamine agonists are more likely to cause nausea, orthostatic hypotension, and confusion than is levodopa.

Amantadine is an antiviral agent that also has antiparkinsonian activity. It is sometimes prescribed in newly diagnosed Parkinson's disease, usually at doses of 100 to 200 mg twice a day. Possible side effects include edema of the legs, confusion, hallucinations, nightmares and, falls.

Anticholinergics are structural analogues of atropine. They aim at counterbalancing the predominance of cholinergic systems caused by the deficit of dopamine. For many years, they were the only form of medical therapy. Several drugs are available, among which are trihexyphenidyl and benztropine mesylate. Anticholinergics may have a frank activity against tremor in some patients. They should be given very gradually and avoided in glaucoma and prostatism (urinary retention). They cause dry mouth and constipation and have frequent unwanted effects: confusion, hallucinations, and dysmnesia, particularly in patients with a cognitive deficit, should be avoided.

Propranolol, a β-blocker, can alleviate Parkinson's disease-related tremor. Depression can be treated with tricyclic antidepressants, trazodone, or fluoxetine. The doses are generally one-half those recommended for depressed patients without Parkinson's disease. Selegiline, at its usual dose, 10 mg/day, is a selective monoamine oxidase B inhibitor; although not contraindicated theoretically in association with tricyclic antidepressants, selegiline use should be avoided with antidepressants. Bupropion is an antidepressant that, by blocking the reuptake of dopamine, may also have a mild antiparkinson effect.

Surgery in Parkinson's Disease

There are two kinds of surgery in Parkinson's disease. One aims at compensating the deficit in dopamine (i.e., brain transplant); the other aims at suppressing or alleviating the clinical disorders, mainly tremor.

Brain transplants with fetal mesencephalon has superseded adrenal medulla as the graft. Currently, the graft is stereotactically implanted into the putamen-caudate in the hope that it will produce dopamine and trophic factors that could promote the build-up of adequate connections. Initial reports raised reservations, but recently, the results seem more encouraging. The procedure is indicated only in the most severe cases. The following issues are under investigation: the age of the human fetal tissue; the best position of the implant, either in the caudate or the putamen, currently the preferred site; single versus multiple, unilateral versus bilateral implants; and the coadministration of trophic factors and immunosuppressors. There is of course a debate about the ethics of using aborted human fetal tissue for grafting.

In regard to *palliative surgery*, there is a rationale for suppressing some neural relays in the basal ganglia circuitry (see Ch. 22) that exhibit hyperactivity in response to the striatal dopamine deficiency. Hyperactivity of these regions, including the globus pallidus, subthalamic nucleus, and some of the thalamic nuclei, are thought to result in inhibition of the supplementary motor cortex that induces rigidity and tremor. Rigidity and tremor are easily viewed as "positive" disorders (see Ch. 22). Bradykinesia could also be a positive trouble. Except in rare cases, the operations are unilateral because bilateral lesions carry a high risk of speech, balance, and cognitive disorders.

Pallidotomy was superseded by ventrolateral thalamotomy, but more precise pallidotomies, targeting the ventroposterior portion of the pallidum, have alleviated bradykinesia. Ventrolateral thalamotomy abolishes contralateral tremor in up to 90 percent of patients. Rigidity is decreased, but bradykinesia is unaffected. Such interventions are obviously indicated in highly selected patients with severe tremor that is refractory to medication. Thalamotomy and pallidotomy have risks of cerebral hemorrhage, infarction, or infection, in about 1 in 200 patients.

An alternative to destructive surgery is the use of high-frequency (100-Hz) stimulation by an implanted electrode in the thalamus. The stimulation can be interrupted during sleep. Results are reported to be excellent in 85 percent of patients. Destructive lesions have not been done on the nucleus subthalamicus for fear of causing hemiballismus (see Ch. 22). Recently, high-frequency (130-Hz) stimulation of the nucleus subthalamicus has alleviated contralateral bradykinesia and involuntary movements in selected patients.

ANNOTATED BIBLIOGRAPHY

Benabid AL, Pollak P, Gervason C et al. Long-term suppression of tremor by stimulation of the ventral intermediate thalamic nucleus. Lancet 1991;1:403–6.
Success in contralateral tremor suppression in 85 percent of patients.

Brooks DJ. Functional imaging in relation to parkinsonian syndromes. J Neurol Sci 1993;115:1–17.
Functional imaging (positron emission and single-photon emission computed tomography) has shown specific patterns related to subtypes of the Parkinson's disorders.

Goetz CG, Diederich NJ. Dopaminergic agonists in the treatment of Parkinson's disease. Neurol Clin 1992;10:527–40.
One of several excellent reviews in this volume.

Gray F. Neuropathologie des syndromes parkinsonieus. Rev Neurol (Paris) 1988;144:229–68.
Clear and detailed review of Parkinson's disease, parkinsonian syndrome, and parkinsonism plus pathologic conditions.

Lieberman A. Dopamine agonists used as monotherapy in de novo PD patients: comparisons with selegiline. Neurology 1992;42:37–40.
Selegiline, a monoamine oxidase type B inhibitor, slows progression of Parkinson's disease and delays the need for levodopa.

Marsden CD. Parkinson's disease. Lancet 1990;1:948–52.
Excellent modern review article.

Quinn N, Critchley P, Marsden CD. Young onset Parkinson's disease. Mov Disord 1987;2:73–91.
A series of 60 cases with review of the literature.

Pollack P, Benabid AL, Gross C et al. Effets de la stimulation du noyeau sous-thalamique dans la maladie de Parkinson. Rev Neurol (Paris) 1993;149:175–6.
Severe contralateral akinesia ameliorated.

Raypert AH. Environmental causation of Parkinson's disease. In Riggs JL (ed). The Neuroenvironmental Basis for Rising Mortality from Parkinson's Disease. Controversies in Neurology. Arch Neurol 1993;50:651–6.
Marshalling the evidence for both hypotheses.

Tsui JK, Ross S, Poulin K et al. The effect of dietary protein on the efficacy of L-dopa: a doubleblind study. Neurology 1989;39:549–52.
The findings suggest high dietary protein may affect the efficacy of levodopa at a central level.

Weiner WJ, Factor SA, Sanchez Ramos JR et al. Early combination therapy (bromocriptine and levodopa) does not prevent motor fluctuations in Parkinson's disease. Neurology 1993;43:21–7.
Disagreements with some earlier studies.

Yahr MD. Parkinson's disease. The L-dopa era. Adv Neurol 1993;60:11–7.
The impact of levodopa.

76
Parkinsonism Plus Conditions

A. Lieberman

STRIATONIGRAL DEGENERATION

Striatonigral degeneration (SND) is the degenerative disorder most commonly mistaken, for Parkinson's disease.

Pathologically, the brain shows a distinctive shrinkage and brown discoloration of the putamen and, to a lesser extent, of the caudate nucleus and globus pallidus. Microscopically, there is nerve cell loss and gliosis in the putamen, caudate nucleus, globus pallidus, subthalamic nucleus, substantia nigra, locus ceruleus, pontine nuclei, and the inferior olives.

Clinically, SND has almost the same picture as Parkinson's disease, with rigidity, bradykinesia, and postural instability. Rarely, there may be a rest tremor. These patients are usually not demented. Autonomic insufficiency may be a feature, but it is not as prominent a one as in multisystem atrophy (MSA see below).

It is the transient or poor response to levodopa that helps suggest the patient's condition in life and separates this disorder from Parkinson's disease.

PROGRESSIVE SUPRANUCLEAR PALSY

Progressive supranuclear palsy (PSP), the syndrome described by Steele, Richardson, and Olszewski and known also by their names, begins at approximately the same age as Parkinson's disease. It is one of the more common parkinsonism plus syndromes, with a prevalence approximately 1 percent that of Parkinson's disease.

The pathologic findings consist of neuronal loss associated with neurofibrillary changes and gliosis in the substantia nigra, subthalamic nucleus, globus pallidus, dentate nucleus, locus ceruleus, periaqueductal gray matter, and variably and less prominently, other brainstem nuclei. The degenerating neurons in the nigra are pale and swollen and contain featureless inclusion bodies.

PSP progresses clinically more rapidly than Parkinson's disease with significant disability occurring after 3 to 10 years. Typically, the condition begins with falls, impairment in full eye movements, and slurred speech. Initially, if the eye movement abnormalities are absent, PSP may be hard to distinguish from Parkinson's disease. The presence of ocular paresis, postural instability, axial rigidity, and pseudobulbar palsy are the features that make the diagnosis less difficult when all are present together.

The ocular movement abnormalities consist of an inability voluntarily to look up or down with preservation of eye movements on passive head movement or forced eyelid closure (Bell's phenomenon). The fast component of opticokinetic nystagmus is absent. Eventually, voluntary eye movements in all directions become paralyzed, the basis for the syndrome's name of supranuclear gaze palsy. Tremor is usually absent, and axial rigidity is more marked than appendicular rigidity, the opposite of the typical findings in Parkinson's disease. Gait disturbances are common. Patients with PSP walk precariously because of postural instability, and they fall readily when stopping or turning. Stepping movements, unlike those in Parkinson's disease, are done well. They compensate well for the postural instability when asked to walk on their knees or crawl. There may also be striking retrocollis, in contrast to the anterocollis of MSA (see below). In approximately 50 percent of patients, personality changes or dementia develop.

No treatment has yet been devised, but it is common for such patients to be put through the full gamut of medications for parkinsonism without benefit.

MULTISYSTEM ATROPHY

Shy and Drager (see also Ch. 62) described a distinct syndrome manifested by autonomic insufficiency in combination with neurologic abnormalities caused by degenerative changes in the basal ganglia, cerebellum, spinal cord, and peripheral sympathetic ganglia.

MSA appears at approximately the same age as Parkinson's disease and PSP, making early differential diagnosis difficult. Patients may have parkinsonism, intention tremor, ataxia, dysarthria, and anterocollis. Depression and emotional lability are common, but dementia is rare. Central nervous system (CNS) dysfunction may, occasionally, precede the autonomic dysfunction. There are two CNS syndromes: a parkinsonian syndrome, resembling SND and consisting of bradykinesia, postural instability, and rigidity out of proportion to tremor, and a cerebellar syndrome, resembling olivopontocerebellar atrophy (OPCA) and consisting of truncal ataxia, dysmetria, intention tremor, and slurred speech.

Many patients have features of both syndromes, hence the name MSA. There is confusion about nomenclature, with some neurologists using Shy-Drager syndrome and MSA interchangeably, as in this chapter, and others using MSA only for patients who exhibit a combination of autonomic nervous system insufficiency, parkinsonism, and cerebellar features. If MSA is used interchangeably with Shy-Drager syndrome then its prevalence is less than that of PSP. If MSA is used to encompass Shy-Drager syndrome, SND, and OPCA, then the prevalence is more than PSP.

The clinical features that help mark MSA are those of autonomic nervous system insufficiency, such as impaired sweating, impotence, vocal cord paralysis, and urinary and rectal incontinence. Vocal cord paralysis is a common occurrence, leading to hoarseness. In some patients, it requires a tracheotomy to relieve stridor. Sleep apnea, aspiration pneumonias, and cardiac arrhythmias are the usual causes of death, 5 to 10 years after diagnosis.

Levodopa may, in part, improve some of the parkinsonian features, but it exacerbates the orthostatic hypotension. Management of the orthostatic hypotension is a major undertaking and consists of using combinations of support hose, fluodrocortisone, salt tablets, and occasionally midodrine, a presynaptic α_2-adrenoreceptor antagonist (for further details of treatment, see Ch. 62).

CORTICOBASILAR DEGENERATION

Also known as *neuronal achromasia,* (see Ch. 61) the main movement disorders that occur are progressive rigidity, apraxia, and corticospinal tract dysfunction. Corticobasilar degeneration may be viewed a parkinsonism plus syndrome on which has been grafted cortical dysfunction.

The gross pathologic results of the small number of cases have expanded the findings of the original material. Focal, sometimes unilateral, rarely general, cortical atrophy has been described. The appearance to the naked eye does not distinguish it from Alzheimer's disease. Microscopy shows many neurons that do not take conventional stains (achromasia) and are usually swollen. Neurofibrillary tangles, senile plaques, Pick's bodies, and other histologic signs of other dementing disease are often absent. In some of the cases, the degeneration has been cortical only and, in some, corticonigral. When combined degeneration has been encountered, neurofibrillary tangles and even lobar white matter gliosis have been described in some cases with neuronal achromasia, arguing by microscopic criteria that Alzheimer's and Pick's diseases may coexist with achromasia, making it difficult to claim neuronal achromasia is a unique entity. However, the immunochemical characteristics of the phosphorylated epitopes of the neurofilaments have not been those forms unique to Alzheimer's or Pick's disease. Instead, the ballooned neurons resemble those caused by neurotoxins that interfere with axonal transport. As yet, no specific toxin has been identified.

To the extent that a typical clinical picture can be said to exist, patients show normal power who cannot voluntarily use the affected limbs. Attempts at using a limb may result in an appropriate movement or postures, sometimes with the development of marked rigidity. The inappropriate movements represent combinations of apraxia, rigidity, and sensory ataxia. Mental deterioration (see Ch. 61) is a late feature when it occurs.

No treatment exists.

OLIVOPONTOCEREBELLAR ATROPHY

OPCA (see also Ch. 64) is the name given to a heterogeneous group of syndromes the only common factor of which is a loss of neurons in the pons and cerebellum. There are both inherited and sporadic forms of OPCAs.

Pathologically, changes occur in the inferior olives, the ventral pontine and arcuate nuclei, and the deep and superficial cerebellar nuclei, including the Purkinje cells. Neuronal loss in these areas leads to demyelination and fibrillary gliosis of brainstem and cerebellar white matter. Occasionally, the spinal cord is also involved.

The disease onset ranges from less than 1 year in familial OPCA to 70 years in sporadic OPCA. The mean age of onset is 30 years for familial OPCA and 50 years for sporadic OPCA. The course is indolent for familial OPCA, with significant disability resulting in patient's becoming wheel-chair bound after 10 to

20 years. The course is more rapid for sporadic OPCA with significant disability after 5 to 10 years.

Cerebellar ataxia, postural instability, tremor, and dysarthria are prominent and defining characteristics. The dysarthria is characterized by combinations of scanning, bulbar, or pseudobulbar features. Myoclonus, torticollis, chorea, and athetosis may occur, more commonly in familial OPCA. Magnetic resonance imaging has greatly improved the possibilities of making the diagnosis in life.

The parkinsonian features may respond to levodopa. Some patients may even exhibit dyskinesias while taking levodopa.

HYPERKINETIC MOVEMENT DISORDERS

In addition to the parkinsonism plus syndromes, which are interesting because of their resemblance to and confusion with Parkinson's disease, there are several other movement disorders that can usually be distinguished from Parkinson's disease. Because of the association of these disorders with excessive movement: tremor, chorea, athetosis, dystonia, tic, and myoclonus, they are referred to as hyperkinetic movement disorders.

Essential tremor (see Ch. 22) is 4 to 10 times more common than Parkinson's disease. Because essential tremor usually is not disabling, it has received less attention than Parkinson's disease.

ANNOTATED BIBLIOGRAPHY

Bannister R. Treatment of autonomic failure. Curr Opin Neurol Neurosurg 1992;5:487–91.

Updated advice on management.

Eidelberg D, Takikawa S, Moeller JR et al. Striatal hypometabolism distinguishes striatonigral degeneration from Parkinson's disease. Ann Neurol 1993;33:518–27.

Caudate and putamen showed significant reductions in glucose metabolism compared with normal subjects and patients with Parkinson's disease.

Fearnley JM, Lees AJ. Striatonigral degeneration. A clinicopathological study. Brain 1990;113:1823–42.

Ten cases, one-half misdiagnosied as Parkinson's disease. Caudate and putamen involvement confirmed.

Friedman DI, Jankovic J, McCrary JA 3d. Neuro-ophthalmic findings in progressive supranuclear palsy. J Clin Neuro Ophthalmol 1992;12:104–9.

Vertical supranuclear ophthalmoparesis and instability of visual fixation more common among the 104 patients with PSP compared with those with Parkinson's disease, despite paresis of downgaze being thought a classic sign.

Karbe H, Holthoff V, Huber M et al. Positron emission tomography in degenerative disorders of the dopaminergic system. J Neural Transm Park Dis Dement Sect 1992;4: 121–30.

Alzheimer's and Parkinson's diseases share different topographies from PSP.

Rebeiz JJ, Kolodny EH, Richardson EP. Corticodentatonigral degeneration with neuronal achromasia. Arch Neurol 1968;18:20.

The first case. The nondominant hemisphere was the more affected.

Testa D, Savoiardo M, Fetoni V et al. Multiple system atrophy. Clinical and MR observations on 42 cases. Ital J Neurol Sci 1993;14:211–6.

Difficulties in the diagnosis of 42 cases because of admixtures with Parkinson's disease, SND, and OPCA.

77
Other Forms of Movement Disorders

A. Lieberman

CHOREA

Sydenham's Chorea

As far back as the Middle Ages, a suddenly appearing dancelike movement disorder affecting mainly children and adolescents was recognized. Then, it was thought to be a form of conversion hysteria. According to Gowers (1888), this distinctive disorder acquired the name "St. Vitus's dance" in the fourteenth century in Strasbourg, where youths afflicted by the movement disorder were sent by the magistrate to the chapel of St. Vitus in hopes of a cure. The reasons for a relationship to this boyhood saint, martyred in 303 A.D., has escaped many authors, including the recent reviewer, P. A. Nausieda (1985). Two centuries later, Thomas Sydenham (English physician, 1624–1689), who described many illnesses and originated the term scarlet fever, separated a disorder he termed minor chorea from St. Vitus's dance (major chorea). Soon, however, the term Sydenham's chorea was popularized and is frequently considered synonymous with St. Vitus's dance. Although as early as 1840, J. B. Bouillaud (French physician, 1796–1881) suggested a relationship between chorea and rheumatic fever (known in France as Bouillaud's disease), the relationship was firmly established only late in the nineteenth century through the writings of William Osler (Canadian-American physician, 1849–1919). Gowers himself, writing in 1888, while admitting many cases were related to heart disease, considered many others to be caused by "fright."

The disorder is most prevalent in children 5 to 15 years of age, is rare in younger children, and has slightly different features in older patients. In the high-prevalence group, it affects both sexes with equal frequency. It occurs most often in the spring in the Northern Hemisphere. In most cases, there are no other signs of rheumatic fever, but the relationship is clear enough that it is now accepted as a single sign of rheumatic fever. With improvement in the control of streptococcal infections and the decline in rheumatic fever in Western countries, there has also been a decline in the incidence of Sydenham's chorea.

Pathophysiology

The pathophysiology is now better known than in former times. For years it was taught that there were no lesions of the central nervous system, but repeated studies have shown widespread overt arteritis, petechial hemorrhages, and perivascular infiltrates, especially in the caudate and putamen. Abnormalities of these regions have recently been documented in life with magnetic resonance imaging and single-photon emission computed tomographic studies.

Clinical Features

The clinical features are distinctive. The movements typically develop acutely, at first affecting the face and hands and, less often, the legs. The trunk, even the diaphragm, may be affected. The syndrome progresses within a few weeks to its peak, but in mild cases, the diagnosis may be overlooked for months. The movements are quick, and their rhythm is irregular and of small amplitude, deflecting the lip, a finger, or the wrist, sometimes interfering with voluntary movements so as to cause objects to be dropped or handwriting to be scrawled. The sudden alterations in respirations may interfere with normal speech rhythms. Slight hypotonia is common. When extended, the fingers classically curve upward (spooning), and pronator drift is seen. Although the disorder may spread within days to affect a wide number of muscle groups, asymmetry is the rule, and as many as 60 percent of cases are limited to one side (hemichorea). No other findings are evident; language, memory, vision, and sensation are all normal.

The disorder lasts from a few weeks to several months, with rare instances of persistence. Recurrence is not rare, and sometimes happens with an interval of years.

Treatment

Treatment with penicillin prophylaxis is recommended for at least 5 years but plays no role in therapy of the chorea. Major tranquilizers have had some effect in reducing the severity of the chorea.

Chorea Gravidarum

This unusual disorder appears during the course of an otherwise normal pregnancy. A prior history of Sydenham's chorea in present in one-third of cases, and rarely, systemic lupus erythematosus is found. In some cases, there is no pregnancy, but the use of oral contraceptives is found.

Huntington's Disease

The essential features of this disorder were first described in 1841 by C. O. Waters, an American physician, in Franklin (eastern Long Island), New York as a hereditary disorder. As ably laid out by G. W. Bruyn (1968), the disorder seems to have been well known to those living in the area, including to the physician father and grandfather of George Huntington (Long Island internist, 1850–1916), whose name has been associated with the disease. Drawing on notes from his father and grandfather and his own observations, he detailed the elements in a lecture in 1872 but only as a particular form of Sydenham's chorea. The disease became important because of its high frequency, inherited character, and recently demonstrated genetic basis.

Huntington's disease is an autosomal dominant disorder with complete penetrance that occurs in 5 to 10 per 100,000. Among the disorders broadly classified as movement disorders, Huntington's disease is about 1 percent as frequent as Parkinson's disease. Although its greatest description was from the Long Island cases, writers in Scandinavia in the mid-1800s described a similar syndrome, and it is now known to be worldwide.

The gene has been found to be located on the short arm of chromosome 4, location D4S10, near the tip of the arm. Since this initial discovery, the literature on Huntington's disease has been dominated by the intense search for an even more precise gene location. Despite the incomplete knowledge concerning exact location, using DNA samples from family members through linkage studies, it is possible to estimate the probability that a given individual has the Huntington's disease trait. The current availability of such testing has brought about an equally worldwide controversy concerning the advisability of screening for presymptomatic individuals and prenatal testing with plans for abortion to eradicate the disease.

Pathophysiology

The pathophysiology of Huntington's disease stems from the basal ganglia lesions that characterize the disease. The most severely affected portions are the caudate nucleus and putamen. The atrophy that gradually occurs begins along that portion of the head of the caudate that abuts the ventricular wall, resulting in the flattening of the head of the caudate, which gives a distinctive appearance on computed tomographic and MRI scans. Changes also occur in the globus pallidus and the frontal cortex. There are significant neurochemical changes in most of the neurotransmitters used by intrinsic striatal neurons, including the central neurotransmitter for the striatum, γ-aminobutyric acid, and also for enkephalin, dynorphin, and substance P. There are also losses of these neurotransmitters in the globus pallidus and substantia nigra.

Clinical Features

The clinical features are easily recognized in well-established cases. Before DNA testing, descendants of those affected watched carefully for the first signs. The infrequent juvenile form is usually inherited through the fathers, suggesting that several factors influence the expression of the Huntington's disease gene. Although the onset can range from 2 to 80 years, in most patients, the disease develops in their 30s and 40s, allowing many with the disease to become parents before knowing that they are destined to become symptomatic. None of the many purely clinical attempts to detect the disease in its presymptomatic state have succeeded, but impaired oral agility many be an early sign.

For most patients, the initial symptoms are either personality changes, chorea, or a combination of both. The chorea is often very subtle at first, taking the form of frequent, minor adjustments in posture, often incorporated into a voluntary movement, giving the impression the patient is slightly uncomfortable and disinclined to sit still or afflicted by tendencies to facial grimacing. At this stage, even the patient may be unaware these are signs of illness and accepts them as personality traits. As Huntington's disease progresses, the chorea becomes more pronounced and less easily suppressed. Unhappily, the patient is often also in the early stages of cognitive impairment and memory loss, which frequently deny the victim insight into the evolving condition. Even at this time, a diagnosis of Huntington's disease may be difficult to make unless there is a family history.

A variety of psychiatric disturbances may accompany this disease. In some patients, the presenting diagnosis may be psychiatric. Antisocial behavior, paranoid ideation, or affective disorders may overshadow the slowly developing chorea for months or even years. Depression and suicide are frequent.

Once fully developed, the chorea is commonly accompanied by movement abnormalities, dysarthria, and dysphagia. Patients lose weight because of severe chorea and dysphagia; aspiration is a common cause of death. In the advanced stages of the disease, the chorea may fade slowly to a rigid and dystonic state. In juvenile Huntington's disease, with an onset of symptoms before age 20, rigidity, bradykinesia, and postural instability simulate Parkinson's disease, the Westphal variant (see below). Cerebellar signs and seizures occur in the juvenile form.

Huntington's disease is progressive; death occurs 10 to 30 years after the diagnosis.

A predominantly rigid form of the disease is known as the *Westphal variant* (K.F.O. Westphal, German neurologist, 1833–1890). Often seen in younger patients and often occurring in all patients near the end of their course, the clinical picture is of rigidity and hypokinesia. Roughly 6 percent have this variant as the only clinical syndrome.

Treatment

Treatment is symptomatic and not very satisfactory for any of the main features, including the chorea, depression, or psychotic changes.

Chorea and Stroke

Occlusion of small, deep arteries penetrating into the brain to supply the subthalamus or striatum has been the cause of a few instances of sudden-onset chorea. It is the locus and selective site of the lesion, not the process of infarction, which produces these syndromes; so it is not surprising that a handful of reports have appeared in which the cause of chorea was a small hematoma.

Of the several types of movement disorders described with small, deep lesions from stroke, the most frequently documented has been hemichorea, at times so violent as to be labeled *hemiballismus*. This violence is due to the predominance of involuntary movements affecting the proximal muscles; it has been proposed they are involuntary postural movements. The lesions that cause them have occurred sometimes in the subthalamic nucleus and the subthalamus and other times in the head of the caudate nucleus and adjacent corona radiata. Typically, the diagnosis of stroke is suggested by the abrupt onset, and the syndrome is usually unaccompanied by other complaints. The diagnosis rests on the chorea being limited to one side. It usually involves the shoulder, arm, forearm, hand,

and fingers. The course is usually brief, fading within days, but some have lasted for months. Hemiparesis has also occurred and brought about a termination of the ballic movements.

Treatment

Treatment is recommended with a butyrophenone (haloperidol). Beginning doses of 1 to 2 mg three times a day are a common approach, but the dose may have to be increased over several days to as high as 5 mg three times a day, and even then, a few patients have not responded.

Drug-Induced Chorea

Almost any movement disorder can be induced by a drug, but some drugs are more likely to induce movement disorders than others.

Many neuroleptic agents can cause chorea or dyskinesias, complex stereotyped behavior, or multifocal tics resembling Gilles de la Tourette's syndrome. Stimulant-induced dyskinesia usually consists of facial, buccal, and lingual movements. Rarely, generalized chorea associated with other manifestations of central nervous system stimulation may occur in drug abusers. Levodopa may induce chorea, athetosis, or dystonia when used in high doses to treat Parkinson's disease. These manifestations are a frequent complication after some years of treatment for Parkinson's disease.

Cessation of the offending drug, when possible, is usually followed by subsidence of symptoms gradually over days, but a few patients may have persisting chorea.

DYSTONIA

Dystonia (see Ch. 22) is a term that refers to involuntary, sustained, contractions, resulting in a sustained repetitive movement, that may be slow or rapid or in a sustained abnormal posture. It may occur as a separate disease entity, in which case it can be generalized, segmental, or focal. Alternatively, dystonia may occur as a symptom of another disease; prominent among these are Parkinson's disease and Wilson's disease (see Chs. 72 and 75).

Although it is easy to visualize uncontrollable tightening of muscles (mislabeled as cramping) confined to a few isolated muscles as originating locally rather than in the CNS, the evidence, despite the absence of pathologic findings in most patients, is that dystonia is of central origin. Dystonia may follow birth injury ("cerebral palsy"), anoxia, and severe head trauma; hemidystonia may follow hemorrhages in the contralateral putamen; and craniocervical dystonias may follow brainstem lesions produced by infarcts, multiple sclerosis, or encephalitis. Dystonia may also occur with other CNS diseases, such as spasmodic torticollis (see below) and juvenile-onset Parkinson's disease. Finally, CNS active drugs, such as levodopa, phenothiazines, and butyrophenones, may induce dystonia, especially in young people. The predilection of dystonia for the cranial, cervical, and truncal muscles suggests that dystonia originates in "centers" that link agonist-antagonist muscles on one side with agonist-antagonist muscles on the other. These centers, presumed to be located in the basal ganglia, brainstem, or upper cervical spinal cord, allow simultaneous complex movements involving muscles on both sides of the body, such as blinking, chewing, swallowing, speaking, and head turning. Abnormalities presumed to occur in these centers result in prolonged or inappropriate contraction of the relevant muscles.

Spasmodic Torticollis

This is the most common focal dystonia. In addition to turning (torticollis) and flexion (anterocollis) or extension (retrocollis) of the neck, the head may tilt toward one shoulder. Frequently, a shoulder is elevated and displaced forward toward the side on which the chin is pointing. The head deviation may be constant, or there may be spasmodic contractions of the neck muscles, resulting in coarse rhythmic jerking or tremor of the head in the direction of action of the most active muscle. The active muscles hypertrophy and can be readily identified by palpation. In about 50 percent of patients, spasmodic torticollis is associated with muscular pain, which is sometimes severe. The abnormal neck position may be associated with cervical spondylosis and radiculopathy. Spasmodic torticollis varies in intensity and is exacerbated by stress or fatigue. It may be relieved by relaxation; various "tricks," such as lightly holding the chin in the direction of the greatest pull; or by lying down.

The mechanisms responsible for spasmodic torticollis are unknown, but some studies suggest a disturbance in the vestibular system.

Segmental Dystonia

In this unusual set of disorders, contiguous body parts are affected, including craniocervical dystonia and Meige syndrome (characterized by blepharospasm and facial, mandibular, lingual, pharyngeal, and laryngeal dystonia often with torticollis). Focal dystonia affects a single body part and includes blepharospasm, spasmodic dysphonia, torticollis, writer's cramp, and foot dystonia. Multifocal dystonia affects two or more noncontiguous body parts, such as a combination of torticollis and foot dystonia. The intensity of dystonia can be influenced by activities, such as walking, running, writing, and talking, or changing position, such as lying down. Dystonia often increases with stress and fatigue. It may be relieved by rest, self-hypnosis, and various "tricks." A set of muscles or motor acts may be involved in dystonia, usually in a task-specific, focal dystonia such as writer's cramp. These focal dystonias are often associated with other segmental dystonias or spasmodic torticollis. For example, a dystonic foot may initially twist into an equinovarus position during running or walking, eventually developing a fixed posture. Truncal dystonia may initially manifest itself as tonic movement during walking, resulting in a bizarre or animal-like gait, becoming fixed in time, and resulting in scoliosis, lordosis, kyphosis, tortipelvis, and opisthotonic posturing. Dystonia may occur at rest, the so-called nonkinesigenic paroxysmal dystonia, or be precipitated by movement, the so-called kinesigenic paroxysmal dystonia.

In some patients, dystonia fluctuates over short periods of time; it may be absent in the morning and pronounced and disabling at night. Dystonia may also be paroxysmal, usually featuring abrupt onset of dystonic or choreoathetotic movements that may last seconds to hours. Such movements may involve the trunk or a single limb. Paroxysmal dystonia may be mistaken for a focal seizure. The movements are not associated with electroencephalographic abnormalities, but they often respond to anticonvulsants. Although there is no proof, it is possible to visualize these movements as resulting from abnormal paroxysmal discharges. Future understanding will come through the study of dystonia.

Blepharospasm

This well-recognized focal dystonia takes the form of an involuntary, bilateral eyelid closure. It results from spasmodic contraction of the orbicularis oculi muscles. It may occur alone (benign essential blepharospasm), but it is usually associated with dystonia of other craniocervical muscles. Blepharospasm often begins with increased blinking, but in time, the eyelids close forcefully, and the contractions become sustained and tonic. Eventually, patients have difficulty reading, watching television, and driving. Up to 15 percent become legally blind. Because light exacerbates blepharospasm, many patients wear sunglasses, even indoors.

Blepharospasm usually begins after age 50, and there is a 3:1 female preponderance. The initial symptoms include photophobia and blurred vision, misleading the patient to search for a primary ophthalmologic cause. Uncertainties as to the nature of the symptoms delay the diagnosis of blepharospasm by as long as 4 to 10 years in more than 50 percent of patients.

Blepharospasm is usually idiopathic, except that a variety of lesions in the basal ganglia and brainstem, including multiple sclerosis and encephalitis, can produce blepharospasm alone or in association with other dystonias. Blepharospasm and dystonia may occur during the course of levodopa treatment for Parkinson's disease or from withdrawal of dopamine antagonists. Approximately 30 percent of patients with essential blepharospasm have a relative with blepharospasm or spasmodic torticollis.

Botulinum toxin (Botox), 2.5 to 5.0 units injected into the orbicularis oculi, is the single best treatment, usually resulting in alleviation of symptoms for 2 to 6 months. Selective lysis of individual branches of the facial nerve is an alternative.

Dystonia Musculorum Deformans

Also known as *torsion dystonia* and *generalized dystonia,* dystonia musculorum deformans is a rare disorder than can be either sporadic or familial. It begins in childhood or adolescence and is variably progressive. It is not associated with cognitive, pyramidal, cerebellar, or sensory changes. In the absence of a family history, it is difficult to diagnose early on, but when fully developed, it is difficult to miss.

Stroke-Induced Dystonias

Two types have been described. *Action-induced rhythmic dystonia* begins as a sensorimotor stroke, which initially improves, but within a few months, the movement disorder begins, first in one of the limbs initially affected by the stroke and then spreading to involve the entire side. Clonazepam and 5-hydroxytryptophan are successful in suppressing the involuntary movement disorder.

The other comes from small deep (*lacunar*) infarction, which acutely precipitates a focal dystonia unaccompanied by weakness or sensory disturbances. Only a portion of the extremity may be affected. Haloperidol, 1 mg three times a day, has been effective.

Drug-Induced Dystonias

Levodopa-induced dyskinesias or dystonias are related to the severity of the underlying Parkinson's disease and to the amount and duration of therapy.

Dyskinesias are less likely to occur with dopamine agonists. Neuroleptic drugs may induce several movement disorders. Acute neuroleptic reactions are usually dystonic, occur in young people, and respond dramatically to anticholinergics. Chronic neuroleptic reactions include akathisias, dyskinesias, dystonias, and Parkinson's syndrome. Akathisia, not strictly a movement disorder, is a state characterized by a feeling of restlessness and a need to move. Parkinson's syndrome is due to blockade of striatal dopamine receptors and, unlike Parkinson's disease, responds better to anticholinergics than to levodopa.

Tardive dyskinesias develop after many months of continuous exposure to neurologic neuroleptics. Sometimes they develop after stopping neuroleptics. Although the temporal sequence of tardive dyskinesias is different from that of other dyskinesias, the similarity of the movements themselves suggests a common origin. Other drugs that occasionally and unexpectedly induce dyskinesias include the anticonvulsants: phenytoin, carbamazepine, and ethosuximide; oral contraceptives; anabolic steroids; and calcium channel blockers cinnarizine and flunarazine (not available in the United States). Acute dystonic reactions can also be caused by narcotic analgesics given during anesthesia. In some cases, the cause is never discovered.

WILSON'S DISEASE

Described by S. A. Kinnier Wilson (British neurologist, 1878–1937), Wilson's disease is a rare inherited disorder in which excessive copper is stored in the body, eventually reaching toxic levels. The excessive copper is associated with a deficiency in its carrier protein, ceruloplasmin. The gene for Wilson's disease is linked to the esterase-D locus on chromosome 13, and the ceruloplasmin gene is linked to the locus for transferrin on chromosome 3. The prevalence of Wilson's disease is probably about 1:50,000.

The normal human body contains about 80 mg of copper, depending on the balance between intestinal absorption, 1 to 5 mg per day, and biliary excretion. Copper is absorbed as a fixed percent of the amount ingested. Once copper reaches the liver, it is incorporated into an α-2 glycoprotein; ceruloplasmin. Ceruloplasmin consists of a single polypeptide chain, contains six copper atoms per molecule, and weighs 132,000 kD. Levels of ceruloplasmin are reduced in Wilson's disease as a result of the defective incorporation of copper into the glycoprotein rather than from a genetic deficiency of ceruloplasmin. Wilson's disease is not caused by a molecular defect in ceruloplasmin: ceruloplasmin levels can be normal in WD and may not be reduced in heterozygotes. The reduction in ceruloplasmin per se is not crucial to its pathogenesis. It is likely that the defect in the incorporation of copper into ceruloplasmin and the defect in the biliary excretion of copper are tied to an as-yet-unknown genetic defect.

Along with deposition in the liver, the most devastating consequence of the copper excess is its deposition in the brain. Copper deposition approximates the distribution of catecholamine neurons, accumulating in and damaging the substantia nigra, the caudate nucleus, putamen, and globus pallidus.

The failure in biliary excretion leads to excessive

accumulation of copper in the liver, resulting in cirrhosis and hepatic failure. This is the usual presentation of Wilson's disease in children. As copper spills out of the liver, it accumulates and damages other tissues. Copper deposition in the cornea produces the Kayser-Fleischer ring (B. Kayser, German physician, 1869–1954; B. Fleischer, German ophtalmologist, 1874–1965), the most important sign of Wilson's disease. The ring appears as a dull, yellow-brown, granular deposit on Descemet's membrane at the limbus of the cornea. It may be seen by direct inspection, but requires slit-lamp examination if the rings are not readily visible. They are present in 95 percent of all patients with Wilson's disease and in virtually all patients with Wilson's and neurologic disease. However, copper corneal rings are not specific for Wilson's disease and may occur in primary biliary cirrhosis and active hepatitis with cirrhosis. Furthermore, copper corneal rings are absent in a few well-documented cases of Wilson's disease. In the kidney, copper produces renal tubular damage; in the blood, it produces a hemolytic anemia; and in the bones and joints, it produces osteoporosis and arthropathy.

As a reflection of the damage to these areas, the brainstem, and the cerebellum, Wilson's disease may present with a number of different neurologic syndromes. It may present with dysarthria, pseudobulbar palsy, postural and kinetic tremor, and ataxia. These findings in a young person may, initially, suggest multiple sclerosis. It may present with bradykinesia, postural tremor, dystonia, and postural instability. Differential diagnoses include juvenile-onset Parkinson's disease or dystonia musculorum deformans. Wilson's disease may present with behavioral changes, psychiatric symptoms, intellectual deterioration, and choreoathetosis, suggesting Huntington's disease, or it may present with several different permutations and combinations of these symptoms.

Most patients with Wilson's disease present with symptoms of liver disease; therefore, the combination of hepatic failure and neurologic symptoms in a young person with a family history should suggest the diagnosis. Neurologic symptoms may be associated with hepatic failure of any cause. The neurologic symptoms associated with chronic hepatic insufficiency may simulate Wilson's disease, a condition known as *non-Wilsonian hepatocerebral dysfunction*. Such patients are usually older and have no family history of liver or CNS disease.

On the MRI scan, when neurologic symptoms are present, Wilson's disease shows a combination of increased signal, representing increased water content, and decreased signal, representing increased copper deposition, in the putamen and globus pallidus on high-field T_2-weighted images. There also may be ventricular dilation and cortical atrophy.

The diagnosis of Wilson's disease is made clinically by finding a combination of liver disease, evolving neurologic symptoms, and Kayser-Fleischer rings. Ceruloplasmin levels are usually but not invariably low. In normal adults, the serum ceruloplasmin level is 200 to 400 mg/L; in Wilson's disease, it is 0 to 200 mg/L. The serum copper level may be low. In normal adults, this ranges from 3 to 10 μmoll/L. In Wilson's disease, it ranges from 3 to 10 μmol/L. Urinary copper increases in Wilson's disease range from 100 to 1,000 μg per 24-hour specimen. Liver biopsy is the single most important test when Wilson's disease is suspected but not yet diagnosed. A combination of cirrhosis and increased copper deposition is virtually pathognomonic. A caveat is that not all laboratories can reliably assay tissue copper. When there is doubt about the diagnosis, then one of the few Wilson's disease experts should be consulted.

Although rare, the disease is treatable, and the extra effort in diagnosis should be made. As the fundamental problem in Wilson's disease is excessive accumulation of copper, the treatment consists of decreasing copper intake and increasing copper excretion. Penicillamine is the mainstay of treatment, resulting in increased copper excretion. Adverse effects of penicillamine range from the minor to life threatening and include aplastic anemia, immune complex nephritis, systemic lupus erythematosus, and myasthenia gravis.

TREMORS

Tremors are forms of involuntary movements that have a rhythmic and sinusoidal character.

Essential Tremor

By far the most frequent of the tremors is labeled essential (i.e., having no known cause). Essential tremor is often called *benign essential tremor*, but once developed, it is a lifelong malady, frequently resulting in emotional and functional disability. It is dominantly inherited with variable penetrance; approximately 30 to 50 percent of patients report familial occurrence.

Essential tremor may begin at any age and is slowly progressive. It is symmetric and of 7 to 12 Hz (slower and of higher amplitude than physiologic tremor) and may be postural or kinetic. It may involve the head, voice, and hands, but it usually spares the legs. It may be confined to the head, voice, or hands and, in some cases, is asymmetric. It usually is dramatically increased during specific activities, the best known being a writing tremor when it may be associated with dystonia.

Many patients do not seek medical advice, stoically

accepting their tremor as a family trait, part of growing old, or a case of "nerves." These features make epidemiologic studies difficult. Like other movement disorders, essential tremor is increased by stress, anxiety, and fatigue. Caffeine increases and alcohol decreases it.

Essential tremor is similar to *senile tremor* and differs only by the age of onset. It is similar to the postural and kinetic tremor of Parkinson's disease and spasmodic torticollis (see Ch. 75). *Hysterical tremor* may be difficult to distinguish from essential tremor, particularly because essential tremor is sensitive to emotional upset. Apart from the presence of suggestive psychiatric features, certain clues may indicate a functional tremor. The leading among them is that functional tremors usually cannot be sustained. They change in frequency and distribution during the examination or stop during voluntary activity of the opposite limb.

Although there are no pathologic changes in the brains of patients who die with essential tremor, it is thought, nonetheless, that essential tremor arises from a defective oscillator in the CNS. The neurons of the inferior olives, the dentate nucleus of the cerebellum, the red nucleus, the substantia nigra, and the ventral thalamus can generate tremors, and subtle defects in any or all may give rise to it. The similarity of essential tremor to the postural tremor seen in some cases of Parkinson's disease and spasmodic torticollis also suggest a central origin as does the fact that essential tremor may be abolished by CNS lesions: thalamotomy and pallidotomy. Alternatively, it could arise from oscillations around peripheral reflexes. This would explain the association of essential tremor with some peripheral neuropathies. What relationship exists between essential tremor and Parkinson's disease is unclear. Some patients in whom diagnostic features of Parkinson's disease later develop present with postural tremor, and initially, their condition may be diagnosed as essential tremor. Usually, within 2 to 5 years, other features of Parkinson's disease appear. A postural tremor, present for more than 5 years and unassociated with other features, is invariably essential tremor.

There is no cure for it, and treatment is symptomatic. Often, the treatment is worse than the tremor, and most patients take no medication. Propanolol, a central and peripheral β-adrenergic antagonist, is a mainstay of treatment. Clinical trials have demonstrated an approximately 50 percent reduction in amplitude in 50 percent of patients. There is little correlation between the dose and blood level of propranolol and the suppression of tremor. The drug is usually given as a long-acting preparation, 80 to 160 mg once a day. Occasionally, essential tremor may respond to peripheral β-adrenergic antagonists, raising the question as to whether it is solely a CNS disease. Adverse effects limit the usefulness of the β blockers. There effects include lethargy, fatigue, depression, and impotence. Primidone is another useful drug. Primidone is given as a bedtime dose of 50 to 250 mg. There is something specific about primidone that makes it more useful than other barbiturates for suppressing essential tremor. Benzodiazepines, with the exception of clonazepam, are rarely useful in essential tremor. The carbonic anhydrase inhibitors neptazane and acetazolamide are reported to be useful in essential tremor, but these findings must be confirmed. Levodopa, amantadine, and anticholinergics are rarely useful. If the tremor is disabling and refractory to medication, then stereotactic thalamotomy is the treatment of choice.

Drug-Related Tremor

Such tremor may be induced or aggravated by many drugs, including adrenocorticosteroids, β-adrenergic agonists, caffeine, calcium channel blockers, cardiac antiarrhythmics, lithium, nicotine, theophylline, thyroid hormone, tricyclic antidepressants, and valproic acid. Ethanol may both lessen and aggravate tremors.

ANNOTATED BIBLIOGRAPHY

Alvarez LA, Novak G. Valproic acid in the treatment of Sydenham chorea. Pediatr Neurol 1985;1:317–9.

Valproic acid therapy succeeded after diazepam and haloperidol failed.

Brewer GJ, Yuzbasiyan-Gurkan V. Wilson disease. Medicine (Baltimore) 1992;71:139–64.

Authoritative modern review.

Bruyn GW. Huntington's chorea. In Vinken PJ, Bruyn GW (eds). Handbook of Clinical Neurology, Disorders of the Basal Ganglia. Vol. 6. Elsevier, North Holland, 1968. pp. 289–378.

Full details.

Gowers WR. A Manual of Diseases of the Nervous System. P Philadelphia, Blakiston, 1888.

A neurologic classic, reprinted in 1981.

Gunne LM, Haggstrom JE, Johansson P et al. Neurobiochemical changes in tardive dyskinesia. Encephale 1988; 14:167–73.

The γ-aminobutyric acid thesis for dyskinesias.

Heye N, Jergas M, Hotzinger H et al. Sydenham chorea: clinical, EEG, MRI and SPECT findings in the early stage of the disease. J Neurol 1993;240:121–3.

Basal ganglia and substantia nigra lesions seen in an 18-year-old man with acute Sydenham's chorea.

Jankovic J, Schwartz K, Donovan DT. Botulinum toxin treatment of cranial cervical dystonia, spasmodic dysphonia, other focal dystonias and hemifacial spasm. J Neurol Neurosurg Psychiatry 1990;53:633–9.

More than 3,800 injections in greater than 450 patients with a variety of conditions with good results in most, lasting almost 3 months. Few complications encountered.

Jenkins IH, Bain PG, Colebatch JG et al. A positron emission tomography study of essential tremor: evidence for over-activity of cerebellar connections. Ann Neurol 1993;34: 82–90.

Those with essential tremor, compared with controls, showed bilaterally increased cerebellar blood flow at rest and during activation.

Kang UJ, Burke RE, Fahn S. Natural history and treatment of tardive dystonia. Mov Disord 1986;1:193–208.

Long review showing best results with tetrabenazine and reserpine.

Kase CS, Maulsby GO, deJuan E, Mohr JP. Hemichorea hemiballism and lacunar infarction in the basal ganglia. Neurology 1981;31:454.

Details of the syndromes.

Koller WC, Busenbark K, Gray C et al. Classification of essential tremor. Clin Neuropharmacol 1992;15:81–7.

Most patients have a tremor the frequency of which is less than 7.0 Hz, and the family history and response to alcohol are both positive. Less than one-half benefit from propranolol; more than 70 percent improve with primidone.

Lakie M, Arblaster LA, Roberts RC, Varma TR. Effect of stereotactic thalamic lesion on essential tremor. Lancet 1992;340:206–7.

Unilateral but not bilateral effects; site of essential termor still unknown.

Lou JS, Jankovic J. Essential tremor: clinical correlates in 350 patients. Neurology 1991;41:234–8.

Onset peaks occurred in the second and sixth. Tremor was most frequent in the hands and then the head, voice, tongue, leg, and trunk. Patients with low-frequency tremor are older.

Melamed E, Korn Lubetzki I, Reches A et al. Hemiballismus: detection of focal hemorrhage in subthalamic nucleus by CT scan. Ann Neurol 1978;4:582.

A convincing example.

Myers RH, Leavitt J, Farrer LA et al. Homozygote for Huntington disease. Am J Hum Genet 1989;45:615–8.

A rare instance of probable homozygote had the same age of onset as the heterozygote relatives and followed a similar course, suggesting the age of onset and severity of the disease is not a function of the density of genetic dosing.

National Institutes of Health. Clinical use of botulinum toxin. National Institutes of Health Consensus Development Conference Statement, November 12–14, 1990. Arch Neurol 1991;48:1294–8.

General advice.

Nausieda PA. Sydenham's chorea, chorea gravidarum and contraceptive-induced chorea, in Vinken PJ, Bruyn GW, Klawans HL (eds). Handbook of Clinical Neurology, revised series. Vol. 5. Elsevier, North Holland, 1985, pp. 359–65.

Thorough modern review.

Segawa Russo LS. Focal dystonia and lacunar infarction of the basal ganglia. Neurology 1983;40:61.

Delayed onset.

Sunohara N, Mukoyama M, Mano Y, Satoyoshi E. Action induced rhythmic dystonia: an autopsy case. Neurology 1984;34:321.

Subthalamic infarct initially beginning as sensorimotor stroke.

Thiébaut F. Sydenham's chorea. In Vinken PJ, Bruyn GW (eds). Handbook of Clinical Neurology. Vol. 6. Elsevier, North Holland, 1968, pp. 409–34.

Earlier version of the Nausieda (1985) chapter, rich with clinical and historic details.

Wertz DC, Fletcher JC, Mulvihill JJ. Medical geneticists confront ethical dilemmas: cross cultural comparisons among 18 nations. Am J Hum Genet 1990;46:1200–13.

Indecision on the use to be put to preclinical testing data.

78

Disorders of Sleep

C. M. Shapiro and J. A. Hicks

All clinicians deal with the sleep-related problems of their patients. For neurologists, this may be the primary disorder, as in the case of the presentation of excessive daytime sleepiness in the patient with narcolepsy (Greek, *narken,* dozing; *leptkos,* taking hold). It may be a facet of the disorder, for example, the nocturnal wanderings in the patient with dementia, or it may be a consequence of treatment, as in the case of sleep disruption in parkinsonian patients. There may be that the need to evaluate sleep as part of the diagnostic workup, for example, in patients with motor conversion disorders who show movements during sleep. In the specific sleep disorders that can be diagnosed with sleep laboratory evaluation, it may be that the specific neurologic disorder only manifests during sleep, for example, nocturnal epilepsy, and therefore, an inquiry about sleep-related events has paramount importance. For these reasons, it is necessary for the practicing neurologist to be familiar with the many facets of sleep and its disorders.

It is beyond the scope of this chapter to review the basic physiology of sleep (see the annotated bibliography for suggested sources). The focus of this chapter is to highlight a number of specific sleep disorders that may present to the neurologist and to discuss in some detail the sleep alterations that occur in the range of neurologic conditions.

The most recent classification of sleep disorders was the 1990 International Classification of Sleep Disorders produced by the American Sleep Disorders Association, which lists more than 80 specific sleep disorders. The general structure of the classification is provided in Table 78-1 with examples of specific disorders that may be of particular interest to neurologists indicated.

Within the section on sleep disorders associated with neurologic disorders, the following seven are specifically listed: cerebral degenerative disorders, dementia,

parkinsonism, fatal familial insomnia, sleep-related epilepsy, status epilepticus of sleep, and sleep-related headaches. This classification omits sleep disorders that are common in a number of other neurologic conditions such as multiple sclerosis and Gilles de la Tourette's syndrome. The authors have opted to provide information in some detail about some of these conditions but to omit others. The reader is referred to the 1992 work of Culebras for the items not discussed here.

BRIEF REVIEW OF SLEEP PHYSIOLOGY

Simply stated, sleep is an unconscious state in which the subject shows little responsiveness to the external world. There are two major sleep states that alternate through the night. *Rapid eye movement (REM) sleep* is associated with rapid eye movements and dream mentation. It usually occurs 90 to 100 minutes after sleep onset. This is followed by a further *non-REM* period of 1 to 1.5 hours followed by a further REM period. This cyclicity repeats four to five times during the night. Initially, REM episodes are short and become progressively longer through the night.

REM sleep consists of approximately 20 to 25 percent of a night's sleep but varies somewhat by age (e.g., in newborn infants it constitutes 50 percent of the total sleep time) (Fig. 78-1). Only in young children is it normal to have REM onset within a few minutes after sleep onset.

Non-REM sleep is divided into four sleep stages with stages 3 and 4 consisting of slow-wave sleep.

There is extensive evidence to suggest that *slow-wave sleep,* in particular, and non-REM sleep in general, provides a restorative function. The decline in total sleep time a night over adulthood is typically from an average of approximately 8 hours to perhaps 6. The decline in slow-wave sleep over this period is from 20

Table 78-1. International Classification of Sleep Disorders[a]

I. Dyssomnias
   A. Intrinsic sleep disorders
      Narcolepsy, periodic limb movement disorder, Restless legs syndrome
   B. Extrinsic sleep disorders
      Sleep-onset association disorder, stimulant-dependent sleep disorder, toxin-induced sleep disorder
   C. Circadian rhythm sleep disorders
      Delayed sleep phase syndrome
II. Parasomnias
   A. Arousal disorders
      Confusional arousals
   B. Sleep-wake transition disorders
      Rhythmic movement disorder
   C. Parasomnias usually associated with REM sleep
      REM sleep behavior disorder
   D. Other parasomnias
      Sleep bruxism, nocturnal paroxysmal dystonia
III. Sleep disorders associated with medical/psychiatric disorders
   A. Associated with mental disorders
      Panic disorder
   B. Associated with neurological disorders
      Cerebral degenerative disorders
   C. Associated with other medical disorders
      Fibrositis syndrome
IV. Proposed sleep disorders
   Terrifying hypnagogic hallucinations

[a] Listings of specific disorders are not exhaustive.

percent to approximately 5 percent of sleep time. It is this dramatic decline in the restorative aspect of sleep that occurs during middle age that probably leads to many complaints of poor sleep quality and the diminution of sleep continuity during the night in the later life.

The clinical significance of the decline in slow-wave sleep in adult life is becoming more appreciated. In the treatment of patients with complaints of sleep disruption, pharmacologic agents that lead to suppression of slow-wave sleep, such as benzodiazepines, should be avoided in favor of the newer generation of hypnotic drugs that do not suppress slow-wave sleep (e.g., cyclopyrrolones and imidazopyridines).

Sleep is far from an inactive state. During REM sleep, cerebral metabolism is elevated, and cerebral blood flow in excess of metabolic demand. During REM sleep, a number of homeostatically regulated systems are dysfunctional; included among them are an absence of thermoregulatory activity, both in heat and cold. There is a dramatic change in autonomic control of cardiac function; profound reduction in responsiveness to the partial pressures of oxygen and carbon dioxide; and the occurrence of vaginal lubrication in women and of penile erections in men. (The latter is used in a clinical test to assist in distinguishing psychogenic versus organically based impotence.) The clinical significance of this altered autonomic function may include the increase in cardiovascular and cerebrovascular events in the early hours of the day. The triggering of nocturnal asthma occurs in early REM periods, and the autonomic change in sleep may be a factor in kindling nocturnal panic.

SPECIFIC SLEEP DISORDERS

Excessive Daytime Sleepiness

A major category of disordered sleep is excessive daytime sleepiness. Its investigation is a common challenge for the neurologist. There are many causes, as is shown in Table 78-2, from the experience in Billiard's unit in Montpellier. A more comprehensive list of causes of hypersomnolence is given in the accompa-

---

DIFFERENTIAL DIAGNOSIS OF EXCESSIVE DAYTIME SOMNOLENCE

Sleep disorders
   Sleep apnea
   Narcolepsy
   Nocturnal myoclonus
   Circadian rhythm disorder
   Sleep restriction
   Klein-Levin syndrome
   Menstrual-associated syndrome
   Idiopathic hypersomnia
Medical
   Hypothyroidism
   Hypoglycemia
   Diabetes mellitus
   Adrenal insufficiency
   Myasthenia gravis
   Multiple sclerosis
   Epilepsy
   Diencephalic and mesencephalic lesions
   Head injury
   Encephalopathies
   Acute renal, liver, and respiratory failure
Physiologic
   Pregnancy (especially first trimester)
   Adolescence
Medication effects
   Stimulant withdrawal
   Sedative effects, including toxicity
   Alcohol or other drug abuse

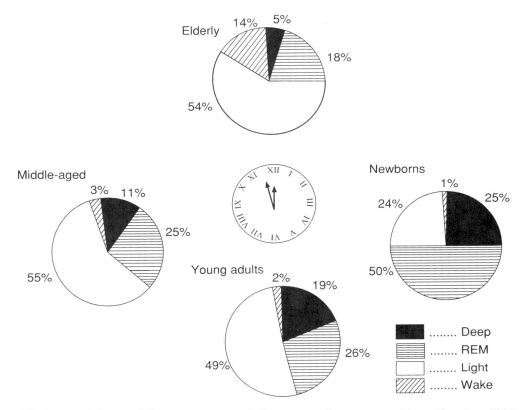

Figure 78-1. Breakdown of the components of sleep according to age. (From Shapiro, 1992, with permission.)

nying box. Daytime sleepiness has many practical implications, including an effect on motor vehicle accidents (Fig. 78-2).

Specific treatments exist for some patients, such as those with sleep apnea, who respond to continuous positive airway pressure. In others, such as those with hypersomnolence after head injury, it is extremely dif-ficult to achieve substantive clinical improvement, even with the use of stimulant medications.

Narcolepsy

Narcolepsy is a common disorder that is more frequent than multiple sclerosis but less so than parkinsonism (Fig. 78-3). It is reputed to be that condition

Table 78-2. Billiard's Series of ±957 Patients With Hypersomnolence

Condition	Percent
Sleep apnea	42.4
Narcolepsy	15.5
Atypical narcolepsy	2.0
Idiopathic hypersomnolence	2.6
With mental disorders	8.1
Recurrent hypersomnia	1.0
Periodic leg movements	3.3
Circadian disorder	2.9
Miscellaneous	4.3
Uncertain	8.8
No polysomnogram	8.3

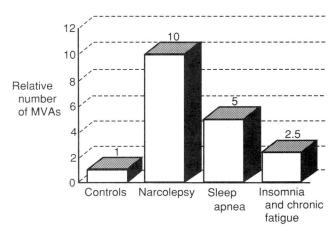

Figure 78-2. Effect of sleepiness on the number of motor vehicle accidents (MVAs). (From Shapiro, 1993a, with permission.)

Prevalence per 100,000 population of various neurologic diseases

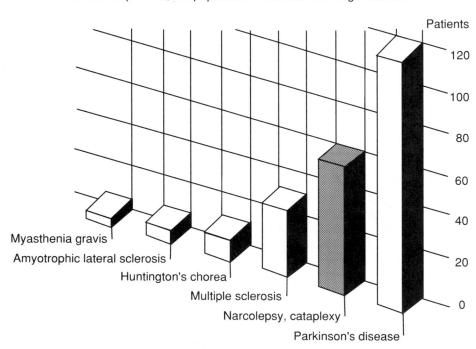

Figure 78-3. Prevalence per 100,000 population of various neurologic diseases.

in medicine in which there is the longest delay between the onset of symptoms and formal diagnosis, on average, between 9 and 10 years. This delay is all the more remarkable considering that the patient with narcolepsy has severe difficulties in coping with most aspects of daily living and it has a more profound impact on quality of life than almost any other neurologic condition.

It is a disorder described as classically having a tetrad of symptoms, namely, excessive daytime sleepiness; cataplexy (from the Greek for knock down). Narcolepsy-cataplexy is known as Gélineau's syndrome (J. B. E. Gélineau, French physician, 1859–1906). Also known as Gélineau's syndrome, it is a state of loss of muscle tone, which may be partial (e.g., the simple drooping of the head, dropping of a cup while drinking, or total muscle inhibition and a fall to the ground); sleep paralysis, and hallucinations in the hypnagogic (Greek: *hypnos*, sleep; *agogos*, leading; i.e., the state just before sleep) and hypnopompic states (Greek: *hypnos*, sleep; *pompe*, procession; i.e., state just after sleep). Each of these symptoms can occur on an independent time frame. The ease of diagnosis depends on the constellation of symptoms seen at any one time.

The onset is usually in the late teens and often may occur after psychological trauma. There is a clear linkage to human lymphocyte antigen (HLA) type,

SUGGESTED DIAGNOSTIC CRITERIA FOR NARCOLEPSY

History of excessive daytime somnolence.

Polysomnographic testing showing a mean sleep latency of less than 10 minutes on the Multiple Sleep Latency Test and the presence of at least two REM onset sleep periods out of five possible situations (overnight polysomnography plus the four nap periods of the test).

History of at least one of the following accessory symptoms is suggestive of the diagnosis: (1) cataplexy, (2) sleep paralysis, and (3) hypnagogic/hypnopompic hallucinations.

If other disorders of sleep are present (i.e., sleep apnea or circadian rhythm disturbance), they are treated before the diagnostic sleep studies.

Psychotropic medications are discontinued at least 2 weeks before the diagnostic sleep studies.

REM sleep deprivation, for example, because of discontinuation of the use of drugs that suppress REM sleep, has been excluded.

namely HLA-DR2 and -DQRwl on chromosome 6. These gene types are found in more than 90 percent of *Caucasian* white and Japanese patients with narcolepsy compared with a rate of 20 to 25 percent in the population at large. There is a wide discrepancy in figures regarding the epidemiology of narcolepsy, from 1:500,000 cases in Israel to 1:600 in Japan.

In almost all patients with narcolepsy, a multiple sleep latency test (see below) will reveal two episodes of daytime sleepiness in which there is a REM onset (i.e., an episode of REM sleep within 10 minutes of falling asleep). This pathognomonic feature of narcolepsy can be linked to all of the clinical manifestations of narcolepsy.

It is characteristic in patients with narcolepsy that the invariable naps that they have are of relatively short duration, 10 to 20 minutes, and almost always less than 1 hour, leaving the patient feeling fully refreshed, only to become sleepy again 2 to 3 hours later. This cycle is in contradistinction to the naps in patients with sleep apnea or patients with an affective disorder as a cause for their daytime sleepiness.

A standard protocol to evaluate the severity and frequency of symptoms in patients with narcolepsy is particularly useful (Table 78-3). During the course of treatment of this condition, the patient's subjective account of what has been and what has not been of benefit sometimes varies. In this circumstance, careful recording of the frequency and symptoms to establish whether different dosages and types of medications are beneficial is useful. In addition, a questionnaire is used to measure daytime sleepiness (Fig. 78-4), and monitoring the quality of nighttime sleep by nocturnal polysomnographic studies and assessment of alertness by means of the daytime Maintenance of Wakefulness Test described by Hanly and Shapiro (1993) provide objective information in this regard.

It is not often appreciated that it is common for patients with narcolepsy to have poor quality nighttime sleep. For them, the use of hypnotic medication is sometimes of great benefit. In rare, mild cases, the improvement in nighttime sleep quality may ameliorate the daytime features of narcolepsy so that no stimulant medication is required.

In the management of the patient with narcolepsy, it is incumbent on the physician to discuss sleep hygiene in some detail. This is often best done by directing the patient to written information on the subject; putting the patient in contact with self-help organizations and charities that deal with narcolepsy (e.g., Narcolepsy Network in the United States, Sleep-Wake Disorders Canada, and other societies in other countries), and intervening when appropriate in the workplace. A single letter to a teacher or employer that a student or worker has a disorder and that the availability of a

Table 78-3. Severity and Frequency of Symptoms of Narcolepsy

Excessive daytime somnolence
  Severe: Sleep attacks during activity (i.e., eating, driving, or conversing
  Moderate: Drowsiness and sleep during sedentary or "boring" situations (i.e. reading, watching television, or riding in a car)
  Mild: Somewhat drowsy, yawning at times with some impairment in concentration but able to stay awake and delay sleep until a more socially appropriate time
  Irritability: Often associated with excessive daytime somnolence; variability in severity and correlation with degree of sleepiness; diurnal variability
  Presence of "warning signals" before a sleep attack
Cataplexy
  Frequency and diurnal variability
  Severity: Total versus partial paralysis, body areas affected
  Ability to experience emotions without triggering a cataplectic attack, precipitating emotions and situations
Sleep paralysis
  Frequency
  Estimated duration of each episode
  Severity: Partial versus total paralysis; emotional distress associated with this symptom; variability in difficulty for the patient to end the attack
  May be associated with nocturnal sleep alone or also with daytime naps
  Sleep paralysis may occur on falling asleep, waking up, or both
Hypnagogic/hypnopompic hallucinations
  Severity: Degree of associated emotional distress content of hallucinations and type of sensory perception experienced (i.e. visual, auditory, tactile, olfactory, or gustatory)
  Estimated quality of nighttime sleep: Number of awakenings per night, estimate of sleep latency, number of minutes awake after each awakening
  Mood: Note the type and severity of mood disturbance if present (i.e., depressed mood, labile mood, elated mood)
  Automatic behavior: Type, frequency, consequences
  Cognitive complaints: Memory and concentration

place to sleep in the middle of the day is imperative to allow for better schooling and work performance often has a greater impact than regular visits to the physician and the prescription of stimulant drugs. The latter are mainstays of treatment, and Table 78-4 provides a summary of medications commonly used.

For the treatment of cataplexy, the most commonly used compounds are clomipramine 25 to 100 mg at night and fluoxetine 20 mg daily.

The diagnosis of narcolepsy may be a conversion reaction. We have recently seen such a patient. The diagnosis was made on the history, including cataplectic attacks; a sleep study, using the Multiple Sleep Latency Test (see below) showed one REM onset instead of the two REM onsets that are diagnostic for narcolepsy. HLA typing was negative, and subsequently, it

Epworth Sleepiness Scale

Situation	Chance of dozing
Sitting and reading	_____
Watching television	_____
Sitting, inactive in a public place (theater, meeting)	_____
Riding in a car for 1 hour without a break	_____
Lying down to rest in the afternoon when circumstances permit	_____
Sitting and talking to someone	_____
Sitting quietly after a lunch without alcohol	_____
Sitting in a car while stopped for a few minutes in traffic	_____
Total score	_____

Key: 0, would never doze; **1**, slight chance of dozing; **2**, moderate chance of dozing; **3**, high chance of dozing.

Figure 78-4. Epworth sleepiness scale. (Adapted from Johns, 1991, with permission.)

emerged that the patient had been engaged in a sexual relationship with the family physician that she was seeing about depression. The cataplectic attacks frequently occurred in the presence of her husband. The revelation of the relationship with her family physician to the sleep specialist lead to an abrupt resolution of daytime sleepiness and cataplexy. A repeat sleep study showed no shortening of either nocturnal or daytime REM onset.

Periodic Limb Movement Disorder

Periodic limb movement disorder is characterized by recurrent episodes of repetitive stereotyped limb movements during sleep. This most typically occurs

Table 78-4. Pharmacologic Treatment of Excessive Daytime Somnolence and Sleep Attacks in Narcolepsy

Drug (Class/Name)	Daily Dose (mg)	Plasma Elimination Half-Life (H)	Comments
Psychostimulant			
Methylphenidate hydrochloride	50–60	1–2	Clinical effect lasts for 3–6 h, usually associated with fewer side effects than dextroamphetamine. Should be taken 30–45 min before meals for proper absorption.
Methylphenidate extended release	20–40		Clinical effect lasts for about 8 h.
Dextroamphetamine sulfate	50–60	7–14	Clinical effect lasts for 3–6 h. Irritability and blood pressure changes may limit use.
Dextroamphetamine extended release	10–40		Clinical effect lasts for 10–12 h.
Pemoline	37.5–112	9–14	Structurally unrelated to amphetamine, once or twice daily dosing. Liver function needs to be monitored.
Anorexiant			
Mazindol	1–4	36	Structurally unrelated to amphetamine but with similar pharmacologic effects. Once or twice daily dosing with an 8–15 h duration of action. Should be taken 1 h before meals.
Selegiline hydrochloride	10–30		Two studies currently in press from different clinics showing the efficacy of this drug in narcolepsy. Has some effects on sleep architecture similar to those of methylphenidate.

(From Reinish and Shapiro, 1993, with permission.)

in the legs and consists of extension of the big toe and partial flexion of the ankle and knee. Each movement lasts between a 0.5 and 5 seconds and, depending on sleep stage, occurs with a periodicity of 20 to 40 seconds.

It is unusual before the age of 30 years, other than in pregnant women, but it occurs in one-third of those older than 50 and almost one-half of those older than 70. In one large series, it accounted for one-tenth of those patients presenting with hypersomnolence to a consortium of sleep clinics. The seemingly obvious connection of repeated disruptions during the night and arousals on the polysomnogram make the consequence of daytime drowsiness seem self-evident. However, careful studies concerning rate of limb movements and arousals on electroencephalography (EEG) have not shown a clear relationship with level of daytime sleepiness.

These periodic limb movements also occur in a number of medical disorders, including chronic myelopathies, peripheral neuropathies, end-stage renal disease, chronic lung disease, rheumatoid arthritis, and fibromyalgia. They also occur in narcolepsy, sleep apnea, and during the use of tricyclic or monoamine oxidase inhibitor antidepressants and are more frequent during the withdrawal of anticonvulsant and benzodiazepine medications.

Although there are no generally accepted measures indicating the severity of periodic limb movement disorder, a rule of thumb to describe its severity that has been applied is 5 to 25 movements/h of sleep would be considered mild; 25 to 50, moderate; and more than 50, severe.

Cases that are moderate to severe usually require treatment. An increasing dose of clonazepam to identify a dosage that is effective is one useful strategy in treatment. The authors have found that selegiline hydrochloride is useful in a proportion of patients. The elimination of caffeine and relaxation techniques can help some individuals. Many patients describe benefit from analgesics, particularly longer-acting medications and those containing codeine.

It has been speculated that the age-related decline in dopamine receptors relates to the occurrence of periodic limb movements in elderly people. Levodopa administration decreases the number of such movements. It has been suggested that there is a balance between protective factors and factors that stimulate the generation of periodic limb movements, for example, pain, spinal stenosis (particularly in the lumbosacral area), and proprioceptive feedback of limb position may all be factors in determining and initiating the movements. Other factors that have been considered to cause such movements, particularly in elderly people, include vascular insufficiency of the lower limbs and osteoarthritic changes.

Restless Legs Syndrome

Also known as Ekbom's syndrome, restless legs syndrome is characterized by an unpleasant sensation in the legs, usually occurring before sleep onset, and accompanied by an irresistible urge to move the legs. Many patients describe a need to put their feet into either warm or cold water to gain some relief or push their feet into the ground to try to create some tension in the leg muscles. The description of the sensation often comes across as formication (Latin, *formica*, ant), that is, a sensation as if small insects were crawling under the skin. Patients describe choosing to sit in an aisle seat when traveling long distances by air or rail or at the theatre so that they can get up and walk about. The problem may be exacerbated by being confined in a particular place for a long period (e.g., driving a motor car) or by strenuous exercise.

The condition occurs more frequently in pregnancy, end-stage renal failure, and Parkinson's disease. The pattern on polysomnography is typical and shows sustained tonic electromyographic (EMG) activity, which alternates from one leg to the other. The differential diagnosis includes peripheral neuropathy, akathisia (see Ch. 75), and chronic myopathy.

Treatment includes reduced use of caffeinated beverages. Benzodiazepines and high-dose selegiline hydrochloride may be beneficial.

Stimulant-Dependent Sleep Disorder

Stimulant-dependent sleep disorder is characterized by a reduction in sleepiness as a consequence of the use of central stimulants. There are a large number of prescribed and illicit compounds that cause alertness. They include amphetamines, caffeine and theophylline, and drugs used for their sympathomimetic effects, such as bronchodilators, antihypertensives, and decongestants (Table 78-5). During withdrawal of these compounds, excessive sleepiness may occur, which may lead to a relapse of overusage.

In many patients, chronic stimulants may be used to the point of abuse, and other psychiatric symptoms may be prominent. It is not always appreciated that the alerting effects of stimulants are highly individual and not simply dose dependent.

There are common features in the polysomnographic recordings of individuals who take similar medications. With stimulant drugs, REM latency is prolonged, and the total REM time is decreased. In some cases, in the treatment of narcolepsy with selegiline hydrochloride, there is a total absence of REM sleep. The authors have seen patients with drug-seeking behavior present an account of suffering from

Table 78-5. Drugs That Cause Insomnia With Sustained Use and/or Treatment

Central nervous system stimulants (sustained use)
    Sympathomimetics
        Ephedrine
        Pseudoephedrine
        Albuterol
    Theophyllines
    Amphetamines
    Cocaine
    Caffeine
        Chocolate, coffee, tea, cola
    Nicotine
Antidepressants (also cause drowsiness)
    Amitriptyline
    Clomipramine
    Imipramine
    Trimipramine
    Tranylcypromine
    Fluoxetine
    Trazodone
Cancer chemotherapeutic agents
    Aminoglutethimide
    Flutamide
Anticonvulsants
    Clonazepam
    Phenytoin
    Ethosuximide
Cardiovascular drugs (sustained use)
    Atenolol
    Propranolol
    Captopril
    Lisinopril
    Verapamil
Alcohol (sustained use and withdrawal)
Anti-inflammatories
    Diclofenac
    Ibuprofen
    Naproxen
Corticosteroids
Opiates (withdrawal)
Major tranquilizers
    Chlorpromazine
    Haloperidol
    Trifluoperazine
Thyroxine
Other
    Selegiline
    Levodopa
    Aspirin

narcolepsy. Paradoxically, the state of withdrawal leads to observations on the multiple sleep latency test, which mimics that seen in narcolepsy (i.e., short REM latencies as a consequence of the rebound in REM sleep that occurs after stimulant withdrawal). These may appear to confirm the diagnosis of narcolepsy and lead to unwarranted prescription of stimulant drugs.

Circadian Rhythm Disorders

Delayed Sleep Phase Syndrome

Delayed sleep phase syndrome occurs predominantly in adolescence and is a disorder in which the major part of sleep is delayed in relation to the desired clock time for sleep onset. Typically, patients with this condition fall asleep at approximately 4 A.M. and sleep continuously to midday with little difficulty in maintaining sleep once sleep onset occurs. The onset of sleep time is regular, and there is extreme difficulty in advancing (bringing forward) sleep onset time. Some evidence suggests that the pattern of circadian temperature rhythm is disrupted.

Occasionally, it is possible to reschedule sleep time by delaying such individuals' sleep time by encouraging them to go to bed 3 to 4 hours later each day on successive days until their sleep onset is at around midnight. They can usually maintain this midnight sleep onset but have a propensity to drift forward again to a sleep onset that is too late to allow for normal social functioning. In many such individuals, there are personality factors operative, and it is often difficult to disentangle the causative relationship between personality and clock time.

Some cases of circadian disruption have a clear organic basis. In one patient that the authors treated who had a free-running circadian rhythm in which there was a progressive daily 1 hour advance of sleep onset time, computed tomography scan showed a pineal tumor. This individual's inability to keep time on a regular basis had been present since childhood, leading to repeated canings at school and numerous failed work placements. When seen, this patient had a delusional disorder with grandiosity and persecutory features and had led a hermit's life, shunning social contact. Although he had an extremely high intelligence quotient, he had not succeeded in completing school because of the circadian rhythm disorder. This free-running rhythm was corrected with lithium.

Lithium, sodium valproate, and Carbamazepine can be beneficial in shifting circadian rhythms, both in patients with abnormal circadian rhythm problems and in patients with affective disorders.

Parasomnias

Parasomnias are sometimes colloquially referred to as those things that "bump in the night." Included among these are somnambulism (sleepwalking), enuresis (from the Greek for urination), pavor nocturnus (from the Latin for night terrors), and sleep seizures. Although these series of behaviors and actions are often harmless, they occasionally have the potential to cause morbidity and death. A somnambulator who walks through a plate glass window or performs homicidal acts clearly requires specific management.

The incidence of parasomnias is approximately 15 percent in children and 3 percent in adults. They may come to medical attention after some dramatic event, such as being arrested for driving while asleep. There are obvious forensic implications, and careful investigation and management are necessary.

The three most common precipitating factors in patients predisposed to parasomnias are alcohol ingestion, sleep deprivation, and psychosocial stress. The best course of action is usually the avoidance of these behaviors and ensuring that the sleep environment is safe. Low-dose benzodiazepines may help reduce the frequency of sleepwalking. Psychotherapy can be useful, but psychological problems are not paramount in most cases. A brief description of a few examples of parasomniac conditions are provided below.

Rhythmic Movement Disorder

Rhythmic movement disorder a group of stereotyped repetitive movements involving large muscles, often of the head and neck, which may occur before sleep onset and are sustained into light sleep. They may occur in any stage of sleep.

One common form of this condition is head banging, but it may include body rolling, arm swinging, or leg banging. This condition usually occurs in the early years of life and is unusual after the age of 5 or 6.

Rapid Eye Movement Sleep Behavior Disorder

REM sleep behavior disorder is a recently described condition that has been referred to as oneirism (Greek: *oneiros,* dream), that is, acting out of dreams, and REM motor parasomnia. It is characterized by loss of EMG atonia and the appearance of elaborate motor activity associated with dreams in patients. It occurs most commonly in older men who have a history of alcoholism or in the context of taking sedative-hypnotic drugs and during treatment with tricyclic antidepressants. The behavior may include physical violence in previously tranquil and sedate individuals. Instances have been described in which normal spouses are awakened to find that they are being strangled by their sleeping spouses. The time of onset is typically 1.5 hours after sleep onset.

In some cases, there has been an underlying diagnosis, such as subarachnoid hemorrhage, ischemic cerebral vascular disease, or multiple sclerosis. The polysomnographic features include persistent or augmented muscle tone in REM sleep.

The treatment of REM sleep behavior disorder is usually with the benzodiazepine clonazepam. A dose of 0.5 to 1 mg at bedtime is maximally beneficial after 1 week, with an improvement in vigorous problem behaviors and associated nightmares being reported by the bed partner and patient alike. It is suspected to be effective because of its serotonergic properties, and in practice, there seems to be little evidence of tolerance or abuse.

Although tricyclic antidepressants can be associated with the occurrence of REM sleep behavior disorder, desipramine has serotonergic properties and has been shown to be effective in the treatment of this condition. Other dopaminergic and serotonergic compounds (e.g., L-tryptophan, carbidopa/levodopa, and clonidine) may also be useful.

Nocturnal Paroxysmal Dystonia

Nocturnal paroxysmal dystonia is characterized by repeated dystonia or dyskinetic (ballistic or choreoathetoid) episodes that are stereotyped and occur in non-REM sleep. Two forms are described, one of short duration (less than 1 minute) and one of prolonged duration (up to 1 hour). The short version recurs repeatedly during the night, and the patient's eyes open with almost immediate dystonic posturing, for example, choreic and athetoid movements. There may be vocalizations in addition to other stereotyped movements. There is pronounced sleep disruption, and the sleep of the bed partner is often disturbed. Although there is no clear evidence that these disorders are related to frontal lobe seizures, carbamazepine in low doses has been described to be beneficial. These movement disorders occur typically in stage 2 sleep and may be related to changes in respiration, slowing in the electrocardiogram, and changes in electrical skin responses.

Sleep Disorders Associated With Mental Disorders

Almost every psychiatric condition has associated sleep disruption. It has become clear in recent years that sleep disruption can both trigger psychiatric illness and be the consequence of psychiatric illness. An impact on sleep patterns is well known from most psychotropic drugs and antidepressants, including monoamine oxidase inhibitors.

Alcohol-Related Sleep Disorders

Alcohol-related sleep disorders are common. It is not often appreciated that the return of normal sleep architecture in patients dependent on alcohol can take up to 2 years. The pattern of drinking may be determined in part by the suppression, in those who consume large amount of alcohol, of the normal secretion of growth hormone, which usually occurs during the first and second sleep cycles in association with slow-wave sleep. This suppression often leads the alcoholic person to experience a poor quality of sleep, which in turn, leads to repeated drinking in an attempt to obtain "deeper" sleep. In addition to this effect of alcohol, the withdrawal effects on sleep disruption are well known.

Panic Disorders

Panic disorders during sleep have been experienced by most patients with panic disorders. In a subgroup of patients, sleep panic is the predominant symptom, and in one-half, daytime panic attacks do not occur. The attacks occur in non-REM sleep, during the transition from stage 2 to δ sleep and during slow-wave sleep. They are preceded by autonomic activation; because they occur during non-REM sleep, they would seem to be triggered by autonomic nervous system variability rather than by psychogenic factors. However, some patients report having somatic sensations under other circumstances and maintain an anxiety about these sensations that is related to the belief that they are potentially harmful.

A number of studies have examined the sleep patterns of patients with panic with conflicting results. Some studies have found no differences between normal subjects and patients with panic disorder on any sleep variables; others have reported normal REM latency but a reduced total sleep time and lower sleep efficiency. Increased movement time has also been reported. Compared with control subjects, the panic disorder groups spend more time awake after sleep onset and have less slow-wave sleep.

The key issue is to inquire about panic if there are sudden nocturnal arousals. The mainstay of treatment is tricyclic antidepressants and benzodiazepines. Clonazepam and alprazolam, especially, have been shown to be effective. It is presumed, but not proved, that nocturnal panic is less amenable to psychological interventions.

Sleep in Neurologic Conditions

Parkinson's Disease and Sleep

Patients with Parkinson's disease are said to have "light and fragmented sleep." Until recently, most sleep studies of Parkinson's disease have not included healthy controls and, therefore, have not accounted for the changes in sleep accompanying natural aging. However, recent studies with age-matched controls have shown that patients with Parkinson's disease have more disturbed sleep maintenance because of nocturia, pain, stiffness, and problems of turning in bed. Altered dream experiences also occurred almost exclusively in such patients (these were frightening, intense dreams with some patients experiencing nocturnal visual hallucinations).

Excessive Daytime Sleepiness. This is a serious problem in patients with Parkinson's disease, with no relationship to any circadian factors. Among the multifactorial explanations are the degenerative processes, the aging processes, the dementing processes, and the dopaminergic and anticholinergic treatments.

Sleep Architecture. Thirty to 50 percent of patients with Parkinson's disease spend extended time awake at night. In general, studies have shown a reduction in stages 3 and 4 and REM sleep. A difference has been found in patterns of sleep, depression, and Parkinson's disease. Nondepressed patients have a decrease in REM latency, and depressed patients showed a further decrease in REM latency. The repetitive muscle contractions and periodic leg movements in patients with Parkinson's disease appear to inhibit the progression of deep slow-wave sleep, thus causing a light and fragmented sleep throughout the night.

Pain at Night. This has been reported in up to 75 percent of patients studied, who experience muscle cramps or tightness (typically in the neck, paraspinal, or calf muscles). Other forms of pain were experienced as a result of dystonia in the feet and neuritic or joint pain (mainly in the hips, knees, and ankles). Patients also attributed frequent awakening to their pain.

Respiration and Sleep. Disorganized respiration but no hypoventilation or sleep apnea has been seen in idiopathic Parkinson's disease or normal groups. The respiration is disorganized with frequent central and obstructive apneas in those with autonomic disturbance. More recent studies have described apneas in patients with Parkinson's disease without autonomic dysfunction.

Biologic Rhythms. The interrelationship between impaired circadian regulation and Parkinson's disease needs further research. It has been suggested that patients with Parkinson's disease function better in the morning. Overall symptoms have been shown to be less severe in those patients with no circadian variation in their Parkinson's disease symptoms. Sleep disorders were seen with equal frequency in the "morning better" and "morning worse" groups, which suggests that sleep does not have a direct effect on morning motor function.

Treatment of Nighttime Problems. Basic sleep hygiene is important, and medication adjustment should be considered to facilitate sleep. A relationship has been found between the improvement of light, fragmented, sleep in patients with Parkinson's disease and the decrease of muscle activity by means of dopaminergic drugs. Dopaminergic medications are known to have a biphasic action on sleep, that is, low doses are sedating, but high doses are arousing. Recommendations include the use of 100 mg of levodopa with 25 mg of carbidopa at bedtime with a second dose at 2 or 3 a.m. for those patients who awaken. (This would be recommended for the patient with insomnia but without nocturnal vocalizations.) The use of a sustained-release levodopa compound and decarboxylase inhibitor may improve nighttime akinesia, which is reflected by easier turning over in bed. Other medications used are tricyclic antidepressants and short-acting benzodiazepines, but dopaminergic medication should be used as first-line treatment.

Recently, clozapine has been studied and shown to improve sleep disturbances, such as nighttime vocalization and visual hallucinations. Because of its selective dopamine blocking of neurolimbic rather than nigrostriatal receptors, the problems of aggravation of parkinsonian symptoms with conventional neuroleptics are avoided. Occasionally, the "withdrawal" effects of medication lead to severe difficulties for the spouse or caregiver of the patient with Parkinson's disease during the night. Practical considerations, such as having a commode by the bedside, may lead to less sleep disruption for both patient and partner.

Huntington's Disease and Sleep

The EEG in Huntington's disease is generally flattened with suppression of α and the other regular rhythms, with poorly formed, low-voltage, irregular waves. The main findings are the absence of spindles, K-complexes, and responses to sounds; δ activity is intermittent and of low amplitude.

In mild disease, sleep recordings may be normal, but in moderate to severe disease, they show prolonged sleep onset latency, increased interspersed wakefulness, and reduced sleep efficiency, roughly correlating with the severity of the clinical disease. Slow-wave and REM sleep are reduced in moderate disease. An increase in sleep spindles in stage 2 is noticed, especially as the duration of disease increases, which suggests that an increased sleep spindle density during a nocturnal sleep EEG might disclose the development of Huntington's disease before the onset of clinical symptoms. However, no major differences have appeared overall in sleep recordings in patients with Huntington's disease and the control group. Global cerebral atrophy does not significantly correlate with sleep parameters, whereas atrophy of the caudate nuclei has been associated with decreased slow-wave sleep and time awake.

In summary, disturbed sleep occurs in Huntington's disease, especially late in the disease. Choreiform movements and the effects of medication may also contribute to disturbed sleep in some patients. Depres-

sion may alter sleep in Huntington's disease and is an important treatable cause of sleep disturbance. Nocturnal paroxysmal dystonia (see above) may antedate the onset of familial Huntington's disease by 15 to 20 years.

Sleep and Head Injury

There are a large number of patients who have sleep disorders, usually excessive daytime sleepiness, after head injuries. The polysomnographic features reported most frequently are a decrease in REM and slow-wave sleep and an increase in the number of awakenings from sleep, which result in a low sleep efficiency. It has been suggested that the duration of coma and the time elapsed since the occurrence of trauma play a critical role in determining sleep abnormalities. Sleep complaints are common in patients for a long time after the trauma, and the severity of excessive daytime somnolence correlated with the severity of the head injury. In one such study, most patients showed objective evidence of excessive daytime somnolence, but no patients had sleep onset REM sleep, as found in narcolepsy.

Comparisons of the sleep complaints of patients with recent traumatic head injuries with those of patients who sustained brain trauma 2 to 3 years before and of the relationship between sleep complaints and higher mental function show that disorders in waking and maintaining sleep are most common in patients with recent head injuries, whereas excessive daytime sleepiness was more common in those studied later on. In the discharged patients with sleep complaints, neurobehavioral impairments and a poorer occupational outcome were more common than in those discharged patients without sleep complaints. They suggest that early evaluation and treatment of sleep disturbances must be considered an integral part of the rehabilitation process. Several reports have now shown the narcoleptic syndrome is a recognized complication of head injury. However, it is now believed that the genetic HLA marker for narcolepsy, is still a prerequisite to developing true narcolepsy after head injury. Kleine-Levin syndrome (featuring periods of excess sleep, amnesia for the episodes, seen most often in boys) has also been related to head injury and precipitated by it. Lithium carbonate treatment has been reported to be useful in decreasing frequency of sleep attacks in this circumstance.

Sleep Patterns During Coma. Sleep patterns in recovery during post-traumatic coma have some prognostic significance. A more normal polysomnogram during coma indicates a good prognosis, and a relationship exists between cognitive recovery after head injury and normalization of a patient's sleep stages.

Treatment of Sleep Disturbances in Head-Injured Patients. Kowatch (1989) suggests the following points are useful.

1. Take a full sleep history, including 24-hour functioning and level of arousal.
2. Review the patient's medication, especially the timing of antiepileptic and stimulant medication (e.g., medication might not be given in the evening, only in the day).
3. Advise on basic sleep hygiene.
4. Refer all patients for a polysomnogram to rule out sleep apnea as a cause for excessive daytime somnolence.
5. Consider pharmacologic medical treatment (e.g., stimulants for attention deficits and hypnotics as appropriate).

Sleep and Stroke

The results of sleep studies in patients with stroke have not produced uniform results. The important role of brainstem structures in sleep regulation is generally accepted. Most patients with a locked-in syndrome show an absence of REM sleep and severe reduction or alteration of non-REM sleep, emphasizing the importance of pontine structures near the midline in the control of sleep states. An absence of REM sleep has been observed in pontine lesions, but in lower brainstem lesions, absent slow-wave sleep with sleep onset REM has been found.

There is also evidence that hemispheric lesions may also provoke changes in sleep behavior. In a small but homogeneous series of 19 patients with only cortical infarcts confined to the middle cerebral artery, disturbances in sleep have been seen compared with controls. A decrease in sleep efficiency has been found, with a higher amount of non-REM time and decreased REM sleep. Interhemispheric differences exist, with REM activity impaired to a high degree in right-sided hemispheric lesions and left hemispheric lesions showing only a slight decrease of REM activity.

Depression is a common sequela to stroke and its effects on the polysomnograph (e.g., shortened REM latency and decreased REM sleep overall) must be taken into account when sleep recordings are assessed from patients who have had a stroke.

Sleep and Headache

Headaches are known to occur during sleep, after sleep, and in relation to specific stages of sleep. The links between sleep and headache syndromes are complex. Migraine can occur in the middle of nocturnal sleep and after sleep. Nocturnal migraine seems to occur with REM sleep but has also been associated with excessive slow-wave sleep. It is a common observation that migraine symptoms improve after sleep. Some consider this to be unique within the field of pain research in which pain is almost always a noxious sensation that prevents sleep. In a prospective study of 310 consecutive patients with migraine, 50 percent of patients who slept showed complete recovery from their migraine, whereas only 31 percent of the patients who rested, but did not sleep, had a full recovery. Cluster headaches can occur during sleep, but there is no consensus in regard to a sleep stage association. Psychogenic headaches are not thought to be associated with a particular sleep state.

Sleep apnea and parasomnias are two important sleep disorders linked with headache. There is a strong association between sleepwalking and headache. Nocturnal enuresis and pavor nocturnus may also be linked to headache. Morning headaches are a common symptom of sleep apnea. Chronic recurring morning headaches should lead to inquiry about sleep apnea, and a polysomnographic recording may be indicated. The headache may be caused by the hypercarbia, vasodilation, or increased intracranial pressure that can occur with apneas. It is interesting to note that headaches, except perhaps the most severe, rarely disrupt sleep entirely. It is therefore important when a patient complains of long periods of sleep loss because of headache to consider anxiety and depression as a cause. Headache may also be associated with dreams, especially terror-like dreams, which may culminate in migraine. Because of the importance of the relationship between sleep and headache, as introduced above, sleep-related headache finds a place in the classification of sleep disorders.

Sleep in Gilles de la Tourette's Syndrome

Whereas 20 years ago it was commonly stated that most movement disorders subsided during sleep, current evident suggests that, in many movement disorders (e.g., Parkinson's disease, Huntington's chorea, primary or secondary torsion dystonia, and Gilles de la Tourette's syndrome), there is movement in most of these patients during sleep. These movements usually occur at times of lightening of sleep and in stage one sleep and rarely in the deeper phases of sleep. It is thought that there are changes in the generator systems or the "excitability of the final, motor pathway" at these points during sleep. Motor and vocal tics have been observed in all stages of sleep. In several questionnaire studies, the prevalence of sleep disorders in patients with Gilles de la Tourette's syndrome has been commonly reported. In some studies there appears to be an increased rate of sleep walking among affected patients. The associated sleep complaints are more frequent when there is accompanying attention deficit and a hyperactivity disorder. One may reasonably question the direction of causality, for example, is it the poor sleep that contributes to the attention deficit? The specific polysomnographic changes that have been observed include lower slow-wave sleep, increased awakenings, worse sleep efficiency, and reduced total sleep time. However, not all authors have found these sleep changes.

Sleep in Dementia

In dementia, the normal changes of sleep associated with aging are exacerbated. A degree of disruption parallels the severity of dementia. There is a greater decline in sleep efficiency; there are more arousals during the night. There is an increase in light stage 1 sleep and then a decrease compared with that in matched elderly people in slow-wave sleep. Sundowning, that is, the exacerbation of agitation and disruptive behavior in the evening or night, is commonly a feature that causes caregivers to be unable to continue in that role and is cited as the most common reason for hospitalization, together with nocturnal wandering and disrupted circadian rhythms, in demented patients.

The reason for disruptive nocturnal sleep may be the increasing disorganization of circadian rhythms and, in particular, core body temperature that has been found to be different in demented elderly patients compared with normal elderly people. There are several studies that suggest that nocturnal melatonin secretion is altered in dementia, and it has been suggested that changes in circadian rhythms in the elderly may be a causative factor in the increased incidence of psychiatric illness. In severely demented patients, a decline in REM sleep is seen. The increase in wakefulness in mild dementia compared with that in aged-matched controls is approximately 40 to 50 percent. Prinz's group has shown highly significant correlations between declining sleep quality and declining cognitive measures and functional status, which suggests that sleep-wake pattern disturbances parallel the decline in cognitive and functional ability as the Alzheimer's disease syndrome progresses. These changes in sleep-wake measures might serve as biologically based diagnostic markers for Alzheimer's disease.

Depression and hypnotic medication need to be taken into account when sleep problems in patients with Alzheimer's disease are assessed and treated. Benzodiazepines may exacerbate nocturnal confusion, and tricyclic antidepressants may worsen memory problems. Behavioral approaches and simple advice to caregivers may be more beneficial. This should include a reduction of daytime naps, an increase in exposure to ambient morning light, exercise during the day, and an attempt to keep regular hours.

Sleep in Multiple Sclerosis

One of the most common symptoms in multiple sclerosis is that of fatigue. The fatigue experienced interferes with activities of daily living and infringes on the perceived quality of life. The cause of fatigue in multiple sclerosis is poorly understood, and there is limited research in this area. In one study, almost 90 percent of the patients with multiple sclerosis described fatigue, but only 30 percent of the controls described themselves as suffering from fatigue. In many patients with multiple sclerosis, fatigue is considered the most troubling symptom.

Surprisingly, fatigue appears to be unrelated to the level of neurologic disability. In a survey of 656 patients with multiple sclerosis, almost four-fifths had fatigue, and more than two-fifths described sleepiness as a separate problem. In this latter group, sleep and naps appear to ameliorate the experience of fatigue. Sleep-related problems have also been reported, including difficulty in falling asleep, restless sleep, nonrestorative sleep, and early morning awakening. Among the causes for sleep disruption are anxiety, muscle spasms, and stiffness. The sleep disturbance in multiple sclerosis is often related to depression.

It has been suggested that the fatigue that does occur in this disease is related to the occurrence of disturbed sleep. One group showed that sleep difficulties were three times more likely than in a controlled group and the occurrence of sleep complaints was associated with high levels of depression. For a subgroup of patients with multiple sclerosis, the concurrence of sleep disturbance in depression may be attributed to the specific lesion present.

Epilepsy in Sleep

It is increasingly recognized that epileptiform activity may occur either exclusively during sleep or frequently during sleep, making sleep recordings in patients suspected of having epilepsy part of the standard evaluation.

At times, sleep disorders may present as epilepsy (these include nocturnal movements, narcolepsy, and parasomnias). Certain types of seizures are more likely to occur during sleep, for example, generalized tonic-clonic (grand mal) seizures, focal motor seizures, and complex partial seizures (see Ch. 79). For some patients, nocturnal seizures cause frequent awakenings, leading to daytime tiredness, which may be compounded by the use of sedating anticonvulsants. Of the patients presenting with recurrent sleep-related seizures, approximately 80 percent will continue to have seizures restricted to sleep. However, if there is only a single sleep-related seizure described, most will have seizures develop during the daytime. This rule of thumb applies to generalized tonic-clonic epilepsy but not to other forms of nocturnal seizures. Almost one-quarter of all patients with seizure disorders have either exclusively or predominantly sleep-related epilepsy. For some, there may be a predisposition to sleep-related seizures after irregularities of the sleep-wake cycle. There are clear diurnal variations in the peak time for seizures. Seizures during sleep affects approximately one-third of patients whose seizure type is of the tonic-clonic, partial simple, or partial complex variety. However, in the category of myoclonus and/or tonic-clonic generalized seizures, the figure is only 6 percent.

A single gene inheritance pattern has been described in which the seizure pattern is predominantly in the frontal lobes, with clusters of brief attacks occurring during sleep. A variety of diagnoses have been appended to these patients, including night terrors, nightmares, hysteria, and paroxysmal nocturnal dystonia, and the inheritance pattern not appreciated.

In general terms, non-REM sleep is an activator for sleep-related seizures, and REM sleep usually leads to a suppression in the frequency or the disappearance of seizure discharge. This applies to generalized tonic-clonic epilepsy during sleep, partial epilepsy, and benign focal epilepsy of childhood. It may be that the synchronous discharge of neurons during non-REM sleep provides a neural substrate for the propagation of seizure activity, but the underlying mechanism is still obscure. As noted above, closed-brain injuries are more likely to produce epilepsy restricted to sleep than open injuries.

In the 1962 classic paper by Janz, the link was made to frontotemporal contusions in closed-brain injuries, and the relationship of this to the forebrain substrate of sleep physiology was recognized. This is further supported by studies on epilepsy after brain surgery. It has been suggested that, for some patients, sleep-related epilepsy is a consequence of sleep state being too "deep." For other patients (particularly those with awakening epilepsy) sleep may be fragmented and incomplete. However, these generalizations are not easily supported by the research available. It is notable that sleep disruption may occur in patients who no longer have seizures and have had antiepileptic medication withdrawn for 4 to 5 months. In this situation, there is a temptation to attribute daytime sleepiness to continuing seizure activity, but this should be resisted.

The usual workup of patients with epilepsy is required. If sleep-related seizures are considered, polysomnography should be performed. This may elucidate other sleep disorders. In this circumstance, polysomnography with an EEG montage of 12 to 16 EEG channels is useful with the standard EEG speed changed to 30 mm/sec. (This is not the case for stan-dard polysomnography.) There is conflicting information in the literature as to whether sleep deprivation or drug-induced sleep is a better tool to detect seizure activity. The balance of evidence points to sleep deprivation, but in some patients, the sleep subsequent to sleep deprivation can be a useful time to detect epileptic activity. It is usually easier to use drug-induced sleep or natural sleep as a screening process in detecting EEG abnormalities, and the latter is probably currently underutilized.

There are many other interactions between neurologic disease and sleep and its disorders. For example, there is considerable evidence that snoring is an independent risk factor for stroke when factors such as arterial hypertension, coronary heart disease, age, obesity, smoking, and alcohol consumption are all taken into account. Although there is no single text to which the neurologist can be referred that covers these aspects, the one recent supplement (Culebras, 1992) on the neurology of sleep provides further information for the interested reader.

Sleep Disorders Associated With Other Medical Disorders

These conditions include sleep-related asthma, sleep-related gastroesophageal reflux, sleeping sickness, and chronic obstructive pulmonary disease. The authors chose to highlight the condition of fibrositis because this is a condition that may present to rheumatologists and neurologists as a condition of diffuse musculoskeletal pain, accompanied by chronic fatigue, unrefreshing sleep, and increased tenderness in specific localized anatomic regions. There is no evidence of contributing articular or nonarticular metabolic disease. This condition is known as fibromyositis, rheumatic pain modulation disorder, and fibromyalgia. There has been a rigorous debate as to the relationship of this condition with chronic fatigue syndrome, and the accompanying Table 78-6 emphasizes the similarities between these two conditions from all aspects of disease classification. The polysomnographic sleep shows characteristic α EEG activity during non-REM sleep. When this occurs during slow-wave sleep, the term α/δ activity is applied, and sleep architecture is often otherwise normal. Many patients with high α activity in their sleep recording describe a sense of being "partially awake while asleep." There are many patients presenting with chronic fatigue who are found to have other sleep disorders. In many patients with fibrositis, there are associated periodic limb movements during sleep, particularly in older subjects.

Proposed Sleep Disorders

In the state of evolution of this field, there are a number of descriptions of conditions that have not attained the status of being accepted by the scientific and medi-

Table 78-6. Similarities and Differences Between Chronic Fatigue Syndrome and Fibromyalgia

Features	Chronic Fatigue Syndrome	Fibromyalgia
Symptoms and signs		
Fatigue	+ + +(97%)	+ +(90%)
Pain	+	+ +
Sleep disturbance	+	+
α Pattern on EEG	+ ve	+ ve
Decreased slow-wave sleep	?	+
Depression	✔	✔
Tender points[a]	+	+ +
Other physical symptoms (e.g., paresthesias)	+/−	+/−
Epidemiology		
Preponderance among women	79%	87%
Age at presentation	25–40 yr	30–45 yr
Weather effects	?	?
Comorbid diagnosis (e.g., irritable bowel syndrome and premenstrual syndrome)	Common	Common
Evolution		
Sociocultural		
"Workaholism"	✔	✔
Masked depression	✔	✔
Western disease	✔	✔
Participation in self-help groups	+ +	?
Relapse triggered or precipitated by stress	✔	✔
No definitive investigations	True	True
Pathology delineated	No	No
Treatment response		
Cognitive therapy	Yes	Yes
Low-dose antidepressants	Improve sleep and muscular symptoms	Improve sleep and muscular symptoms
High-dose antidepressants	Improve comorbid mood disturbance	Improve comorbid mood disturbance
Improved sleep (e.g., with cyclopyrrolone)	Yes (anecdotal)	Yes
Exercise treatment	+/−	+/−
Light therapy	?	?

Symbols: +/−, may be present; ✔, present but no degrees; ?, uncertain.
[a] A normal tender point score is 3.5 ± 2.6. In patients with chronic fatigue syndrome, the score is 16.9 ± 14.1, and in patients with fibromyalgia, it is 33.0 ± 11.8.

cal community as constituting a clear-cut disorder. It is likely that some of these will fall by the wayside, but others will be more clearly defined. One such is menstrual-associated sleep disorder, which is currently described as a disorder of unknown cause, characterized by complaints of either insomnia or excessive sleepiness, that has a temporal relationship to the menses or menopause. The timing and relationship to the menstrual cycle is variable in such patients but occurs on a regular monthly basis. In some patients, there is characteristic pain in association with the change in sleep duration, and there may be some overlap with the condition described above. In many patients with narcolepsy, there are often complaints of menstrually related exacerbations of sleepiness, and this raises the possibility of a hormonal predisposition to increased sleepiness, particularly in a susceptible population. In someone with menstrually related fea-

tures of sleepiness, there are also changes in appetite and in libido, particularly an increase in both, which may be construed as atypical features of depression but are possibly indicative of Kleine-Levin syndrome, which was first described in adolescent men.

There are constellations of sleep alterations that have not achieved the status of "proposed sleep disorder" but seem to describe a distinct population of patients. The authors are particularly struck by those patients who complain of fatigue, tiredness, and sleepiness who have no other medical (including psychiatric disorder) and, on polysomnography, show a total absence of slow-wave (deep) sleep with no other specific sleep disorder. The authors anticipate "absence of slow-wave sleep" emerging as a disorder.

The impact of sleep disorders is profound. In one study, a quality-of-life comparison between patients with multiple sclerosis, paraplegia, end-stage renal disease, narcolepsy, and a number of other conditions concluded that, second only to paraplegia, narcolepsy was the most debilitating disorder. The point was noted in the section on narcolepsy that this is a condition that is both more common than is generally appreciated and very delayed in diagnosis. This speaks volumes to the absence of recognition of the impact of sleep disorders. The fact that patients with both excessive daytime sleepiness, whether it be as a consequence of sleep apnea, narcolepsy, or chronic insomnia, are severalfold more likely to have a motor vehicle accident and that such accidents are more likely to end in death (Fig. 78-3) raises the focus of sleep disorders in a societal context.

To think of sleep as only a litany of pathologic conditions is, of course, erroneous. There are many literary quotations that emphasize the restorative and positive qualities of sleep, for example,

> God bless the inventor of sleep,
> the cloak that covers all men's thoughts,
> the food that fuels all hunger . . .
> the balancing weight that levels the shepherd with
> the king and the simple with the wise.
> Miguel Cervantes (1547–1616),
> from *Don Quixote*

The many artistic depictions of people sleeping emphasizes these aspects of serenity and tranquility.

With the advent of nonbenzodiazepine hypnotics, notably the cyclopyrrolones and imidazopyridines, the treatment and management of insomnia has progressed. There is still much to learn in the field of treatment of patients with hypersomnolence and in ameliorating the sometimes very depressing consequences of sleep disruptions in patients with neurologic disease. There is relevance in treating sleep disruption. When a sleep problem occurs in conjunction with another medical disorder (e.g., end-stage renal failure or multiple sclerosis), the ability to cope with the primary illness is significantly compromised.

In the literary vein, Pope (1688–1744) wrote, "While pensive poets painful vigils keep, sleepless themselves to give their readers sleep." We keep sleepless ourselves to help our patients. The emergence of sleep disorders in medicine makes physicians and technicians keep late vigils to study the sleep of patients who have many types of sleep disorders. This chapter is but an introduction to these.

ANNOTATED BIBLIOGRAPHY

Aldrich MS. Cardinal manifestations of sleep disorders. In Kryger MR, Roth T, Dement WC (eds). Principles and Practice of Sleep Medicine. WB Saunders, 1989, p. 316.

Aldrich MS. Narcolepsy. N Engl J Med 1990;323;389–94.
Thorough review.

Aldrich MS. Insomnia in neurological diseases. Psychosom Res 1993;37(suppl 1):3–11.
Details in patients with Parkinson's disease.

Apps MCP, Sheaf PC, Ingram DA et al. Respiration and sleep in Parkinson's disease. J Neurol Neurosurg Psychiatry 1985;48:1240–5.

Ashton H. The effect of drugs on sleep. In Cooper R (ed). Sleep. Chapman and Hall Medical, London, 1994.
Antipsychotics and sleep.

Askercy JJM. Reversal of sleep disturbance in Parkinson's disease by antiparkinsonian therapy: a preliminary study. Neurology 1985;35:527–32.

Billiard M. Epilepsies and the sleep-wake cycle. In Sterman MB, Shouse MN, Passouant P (eds): Sleep and Epilepsy. New York, Academic Press, 1982, pp. 269–86.

Bliwise DL. Sleep in normal aging and dementia. Sleep 1993;16:40–81.
New data regarding changes in sleep in elderly people.

Broughton RJ, Shapiro CM. Parasomnias. In Shapiro CM (ed). Sleep Solutions. Vol. 8. Kommunicom Publications, St. Laurent, Quebec, 1993.
Description of many of the forms.

Carnazzo G, Patterno-Raddusa F, Travali S. Variations of melatonin secretion in elderly patients affected by cerebral deterioration. Arch Gerontol Geriatr 1991;suppl 2: 123–6.
Related to sleep disturbances.

Cohen M, Oksenberg A, Snir D et al. Temporally related changes of sleep complaints in traumatic brain injured patients. J Neurol Neurosurg Psychiatry 1992;55:313–5.
Excessive sleep in recent head injuries and complaints of daytime sleepiness in those seen later.

Craske MG, Krueger MT. Prevalence of nocturnal panic in a college population. J Anxiety Dis 1990;4:125–9.

Culebras A (ed). The neurology of sleep. Neurology 1992; 42(suppl 6):1–74.
Wide review of sleep disorders.

Dahl RE, Puig-Antich J. Sleep disturbances in child and adolescent psychiatric disorders. Pediatrician 1990;17:32–7.
Full review.

Devins GM, Edworthy SM, Paul LC et al. Restless sleep, illness intrusiveness, and depressive symptoms in three chronic illness conditions: rheumatoid arthritis, end-stage renal disease, and multiple sclerosis. J Psychosom Res 1993;37:163–70.

Dexter JD, Weitzman ED. The relationship of nocturnal headaches to sleep stage patterns. Neurology 1970;20: 513–8.
One of the first studies of nocturnal migraine and REM sleep.

Diagnostic classification of sleep and arousal disorders. Sleep 1979;2:1–137.

Douglas NJ, White NP, Weil JV et al. Hypoxic ventilatory response decreases during sleep in normal men. Am Rev Respir Dis 1982;125:286–9.

Drake ME Jr, Hietter SA, Bogner JE, Andrews JM. Cassette EEG sleep recordings in Gilles de la Tourette syndrome. Clin Electroencephalogr 1992;23:142–6.

Dube S, Jones DA, Bell J et al. Interface of panic and depression: clinical and sleep EEG correlates. Psychiatry Res 1986;19:119–33.

Sleep patterns the same for patients with sleep panic and normal individuals.

Dzvonik ML, Kripke DF, Klauber M, Ancoli-Israel S. Body position changes and periodic movements in sleep. Sleep 1986;9:484–91.

Feedback and other factors determining the concurrence of periodic movements in sleep.

Factor SA, McAlarney T, Sanches-Ramos JR, Weiner WJ. Sleep disorders. Movement Disorders 1990;5:280–5.

Comparison of sleep disorders in patients with Parkinson's disease.

Fish DR, Sawyers D, Allen PJ et al. The effect of sleep on the dyskinetic movements of Parkinson's disease, Gilles de la Tourette syndrome, Huntington's disease, and torsion dystonia. Arch Neurol 1991;48:210–4.

Visible even in sleep.

Flanigan M, Shapiro CM. MAOIs and sleep. In Kennedy S (ed). Clinical Advances in Monoamine Oxidase Inhibitor Therapies. Progress in Psychiatry, Series #43. American Psychiatric Press, Washington, DC, 1994, pp. 125–45.

Review of monoamine oxidase inhibtors.

Ford DE, Kamerow DB. Epidemiologic study of sleep disturbances and psychiatric disorders. An opportunity for prevention? JAMA 1989;15:1479–84.

Cause and results.

Freal JE, Kraft GH, Coryell KJ. Symptomatic fatigue in multiple sclerosis. Arch Phys Med Rehabil 1984;65:135.

Large cohort, fatigue common.

Gillin JC (ed). Psychiatric disorders (section XV). In Kryger MH, Roth T, Dement WC (eds). Principles and Practice of Sleep Medicine. 2nd Ed. WB Saunders, Philadelphia, 1994.

And changes in sleep. Descriptions of effects of alcohol are also included.

Goetz CG, Wilson RS, Tanner CM, Garson DC. Relationships between pain, depression and sleep alterations in Parkinson's disease. In Yahsand MD, Bergmann KJ (eds). Advances in Neurology. Vol. 45. Raven Press, New York, 1986, pp. 345–7.

Guilleminault C, Faull KF, Miles L et al. Posttraumatic excessive daytime sleepiness: a review of 20 patients. Neurobiology 1983;33:1584–8.

Sleep disorders are common, as is a type of narcolepsy.

Hanly PJ, Shapiro CM. Sleep Solutions: Excessive Daytime Sleepiness. Vol. 4. Kommunicom Publications, St. Laurent, Quebec, 1993, pp. 1–28.

Includes citation of the Maintainence of Wakefulness Test.

Jankovic J, Rohaidy H. Motor, behavioural and pharmacologic findings in Tourette's syndrome. Can J Neurol Sci 1987;14:541–6.

Movements also seen in sleep.

Janz D. The grand mal epilepsies and the sleeping-waking cycle. Epilepsia 1962;3:69–109.

Frontal lobe tumor and seizures cited.

Janz D. Epilepsy and the sleeping-waking cycle. In Vincken PJ, Bruyn GW (eds). Handbook of Clinical Neurology. Vol. 15. North Holland, Amsterdam, 1974, pp. 457–90.

Full review, including the correlations with brain lesions from work done in 1962.

Johns MW. A new method of measuring daytime sleepiness: the Epworth Sleepiness Scale. Sleep 1991;14:540.

Jones BE. Basic mechanisms of sleep-wake states. In Kryger MR, Roth T, Dement WC (eds). Principles and Practice of Sleep Medicine. WB Saunders, Philadelphia, 1989, pp. 121–40.

Review article.

Jouvet M, Delorme F. Locus coeruleus et sommeil paradoxal. CR Soc Seances Soc Biol Fil 1965;159:895–9.

In cats, locus ceruleus lesions produced the motor inhibition that was synonymous with REM sleep.

Korner E, Flooh E, Reinhart B et al. Sleep alterations in ischemic stroke. Eur Neurol 1986;25(suppl 2):104–10.

Sleep was markedly altered in 19 patients with middle cerebral artery territory infarction even when the lesions were confined to the cortical surface.

Kostic VS, Susic V, Prozedborski S, Stermic N. Sleep EEG in depressed and nondepressed patients with Parkinson's disease. Neuropsychiatry Clin Neurosci 1991;3:176–9.

Comparisons show non-depressed patients with Parkinson's disease have a decrease in REM latency while depressed patients have an even greater decrement.

Kowatch RA. Sleep and head injury. Psychiatr Med 1989; 7:37–41.

Prognostic factors for certain forms of sleep patterns.

Krupp LB, Alvarez LA, Larocca NG, Scheinberg LC. Fatigue in multiple sclerosis. Arch Neurol 1988;45:435–7.

High frequency of complaints in patients with multiple sclerosis compared with controls.

Lavie P, Peled R. Narcolepsy is a rare disease in Israel (letter). Sleep 1987;10:608.

Lees AJ, Blackburn NA, Campbell VL. The nighttime problems of Parkinson's disease. Clin Neuropharmacol 1988; 11:512–9.

Common problems with sleep in patients with Parkinson's disease.

Liesiene V, Adrien J, Benoit O. Effects of locus coerulus lesions on heart rate during sleep in the cat. Arch Ital Biol 1981;119:125–38.

Linazasoro G, Marti Masso JF, Suarez JA. Nocturnal akathisia in Parkinson's disease: treatment with clozapine. Mov Disord 1993;8:171–4.

Markand ON, Dyken ML. Sleep abnormalities in patients with brain stem lesions. Neurology 1976;26:769–76.

Most patients with the locked-in syndrome have absence of REM sleep and also a severe reduction or alteration of non-REM sleep.

Mellman TA, Uhde TW. Sleep panic attacks: new clinical findings and theoretical implications. Am J Psychiatry 1989;146:1204–7.

During non-REM sleep.

Montplaisir J, Godbout R, Poirier G, Bedard MA. Restless legs syndrome and periodic movements in sleep: physiopathology and treatment with L-dopa. Clin Neuropharmacol 1986;9:456–63.

Improved with levodopa administration.

Morrell MJ. Differential diagnosis of seizures. Neurol Clin 1993;11:737–54.

Review, including studies of disordered sleep in epilepsy.

Palomaki H, Partinen M, Erkinjuntti T, Kaste M. Snoring, sleep apnea syndrome and stroke. Neurology 1992; 42(suppl 6):75–82.

Pecknold JC, Lorenz L. Sleep studies and neurochemical correlates in panic disorder and agoraphobia. Prog Neuropsychopharmacol Biol Psychiatry 1990;14:753–8.

Pötzch R (ed). Sleep in Art. Editiones Roche, F. Hoffman-La Roche, Basel, Switzerland, 1993.

Prinz PN, Peskind E, Raskind M, Eisdorfer CC. Changes in the sleep and waking EEG in nondemented and demented elderly. J Am Geriatr Soc 1982 a;30:86–93.

Disturbances in sleep parallel the clincal disease and can be used to help make the diagnosis of dementia.

Prinz PN, Vitaliano P, Vitiello M et al. Mental functions changes in mild dementia of the Alzheimer's type. Neurobiol Aging 1982 b;3:361–370.

Reinish L, Sandor P, MacFarlane JG, Shapiro CM. Narcolepsy with selegiline. Sleep (in press).

Total absence of REM sleep in narcolepsy treated with selegiline.

Reinish LW, Shapiro CM. Narcolepsy-keeping your eyes open. Can J Diag 1993;10:61–79.

Sato S, Dreifuss FE, Penry JK. The effect of sleep on spike-wave discharges in absence seizures. Neurology 1973;23:1335–45.

Saunders J, Whitman R, Schaumann B. Sleep disturbance, fatigue, and depression in multiple sclerosis. Neurology 1991;41(suppl 1):320.

Scheffer IE, Bhatia KP, Andermann F, Andermann E. Autosomal dominant frontal epilepsy misdiagnosed as sleep disorder. Lancet 1994;343:515–7.

A new syndrome.

Shapiro CM (ed). ABC of Sleep Disorders. BMJ Publishing Group, London, 1993a.

Suitable for patients to read, too.

Shapiro CM. Sleep disorders. In Kendell RE, Zealy AK (eds). Companion to Psychiatric Studies. 5th Ed. Churchill Livingstone, Edinburgh, 1993b, pp. 543–552.

Includes description of sleep disorders in psychiatric states.

Shapiro CM. Dangers of sleep. In: Sleep Solutions. Vol. 3. Kommunicom Publications, St. Laurent, Quebec, 1992.

Shapiro CM. Health risks associated with autonomic nervous system malfunction. In Peter JH, Penzel T, Podszus T, von Wichert P (eds). Sleep and Health Risk. Springer-Verlag, Berlin, 1991, pp. 124–36.

Shapiro CM, Dement WC. Impact and epidemiology of sleep disorders. BMJ 1993;306:1604–7.

Shapiro CM, Driver H. Stress and sleep. NATO Colloquium: Plenum Press. Sommeil et ses implications militaires, In Roussel B, Jouvet M (eds). Proceedings of the 27th DRG Seminar. Laboratoire de Médecine Expérimentale, Université Claude Bernard, Lyon, France, 1988, pp. 133–146.

Shapiro CM, Moore AT, Mitchell D, Yodaiken ML. How well does man thermoregulate during sleep? Experientia 1974;30:1279–81.

Shapiro CM, Rosendorff C. Local hypothalamic blood flow during sleep. Electroencephalogr Clin Neurophysiol 1975;39:365–9.

Shouse MN. Epileptic seizure manifestations during sleep. In Kryger MH, Roth T, Dement WC (eds): Principles and Practice of Sleep Medicine. 2nd Ed. WB Saunders, Philadelphia, 1994, pp. 801–13.

Sishta SK, Troupe A, Marszalek KS, Kremer LM. Huntington's chorea: an electroencephalographic and psychometric study. Electroencephalogr Clin Neurophysiol 1974;36:387–93.

Early studies of sleep patterns.

Sloan EP, Shapiro CM. Sleep in panic disorder. Sleep Res 1994;22:237.

Stradling JR. Recreational drugs and sleep. BMJ 1993;306:573–5.

Alcohol and sleep patterns.

Tamura K, Karacan I, Williams RL, Meyer JS. Disturbances of the sleep-waking cycle in patients with vascular brain stem lesions. Clin Electroencephalogr 1983;14:35–46.

Taylor CB, Sheikh J, Agras WS et al. Self report of panic attacks: agreement with heart rate changes. Am J Psychiatry 1981;143:478–82.

Touitou Y, Reinberg A, Bogdan A et al. Age related changes in both circadian and seasonal rhythms of rectal temperature with special reference to senile dementia of Alzheimer type. Gerontology 1986;32:110–8.

Uhde TW, Roy-Byrne P, Gillin JC et al. The sleep of patients with panic disorder: a preliminary report. Psychiatr Res 1985;12:251–9.

Vaccarino K, Shapiro CM. Sleep in art. In Shapiro CM, Harkin A (eds). Sleep Solutions. Vol. 10. Kommunicom Publications, St. Laurent, Quebec, 1993.

Van Bemmel AL, Havermans RG, Van Diest R. Effects of trazodone on EEG sleep and clinical state in major depression. Psychopharmacol Bull 1988;24:164–7.

Antidepressants and sleep.

Van der Kechove, Jacquy J, Garce M, De Deyn PP. Sustained-released levodopa in parkinsonian patients with nocturnal disturbances. Acta Neurol Belg 1993;93:32–9.

Sustained-release levodopa compound with decarboxylase inhibitor improved nighttime akinesia.

Van Hilter JJ, Weggeman M, VanderVelde et al. Sleep, excessive daytime sleepiness and fatigue in Parkinson's disease. J Neural Transm 1993;5:235–44.

Studies with age-matched controls.

Vitiello MV, Poceta JS, Prinz PN. Sleep in Alzheimer's disease and other dementing disorders. Can J Psychol 1991;45:221–39.

Wand RR, Matazow GS, Shady GA et al. Tourette syndrome: associated symptoms and most disabling features. Neurosci Biobehav Rev 1993;17:271–5.

Wiegand M, Moller AA, Schreiber W et al. Brain morphology and sleep in patients with Huntington's disease. Eur Arch Psychiatry Clin Neurosci 1991b;240:148–52.

Correlates with caudate atrophy.

Wilkinson M, Williams K, Leyton M. Observation on the treatment of an acute attack of migraine. Res Clin Stud Headache 1978;6:141–6.

High incidence of headache improvement after sleep.

Will RG, Young JPR, Thomas DJ. Kleine-Levin syndrome: report of two cases with onset of symptoms precipitated by head trauma. Br J Psychiatry 1988;152:410–2.

Wong DF, Wagner HN, Dannals RF et al. Effects of age on dopamine and serotonin receptors measured by positron tomography in the living human brain. Science 1984;226:1393–6.

79

Epilepsies

P. Loiseau

Some Principles

The terms *epilepsy* and *epileptic seizures* cover different facts.

Epileptic seizures are *discrete clinical events* that reflect a temporary physiologic dysfunction of the brain, characterized by an excessive and hypersynchronous discharge of cortical neurons. Approximately 50 percent of epileptic seizures are acute symptomatic seizures caused by a direct or indirect cerebral insult, occurring during central nervous system (CNS) infection or after a head trauma or cerebrovascular disease or related to a metabolic derangement, such as hypoglycemia, hypocalcemia, or hypernatremia. In such cases, seizures can occur in a previously normal brain. They can also be isolated epileptic events (e.g., occasional seizures, without clinical, electroencephalographic [EEG] or neuroradiologic abnormality). These occasional seizures are epileptic events but do not constitute an epileptic disease. The main question for the clinician is, "What is the cause of the seizure?" Epilepsy is a chronic brain disorder of various causes that is characterized by recurrent seizures (World Health Organization definition, 1973). Epilepsy is also defined by the occurrence of at least two spontaneous seizures in a given patient. The main question for the clinician then is, "How can further seizures be prevented?"

Epileptic seizures are due to *cortical epileptic discharges.* The discharge may originate in various parts of the cortex, may spread more or less far and more or less quickly within the brain, and may be modified by subcortical centers. Hence, various and sometimes puzzling clinical manifestations. Of course, all paroxysmal events are not epileptic seizures; syncopal attacks, pseudoseizures, and transient ischemic attacks also occur. A good knowledge of the main clinical patterns of seizures is necessary to avoid diagnostic errors.

Various causes can provoke epileptic seizures or epilepsy. Some are genetic factors, and others are acquired pathologic conditions. Both being age dependent, the patient's age is a cornerstone for the diagnosis.

Treatment and prognosis depend on the background of seizures more than on the seizure type. Consequently, in clinical practice, the diagnosis of an epileptic syndrome is more important than a meticulous classification of the type of seizure. An epileptic syndrome is an epileptic disorder characterized by a cluster of symptoms and signs usually occurring together. It includes such items as type of seizure, cause, pathologic findings, precipitating factors, age of onset, severity, and chronicity. In contradistinction to a disease, a syndrome can have several causes; hence, it has not necessarily a common prognosis.

Both epileptic seizures and epilepsy are frequent. The global incidence rate of all epileptic events (i.e., recurrent spontaneous seizures plus acute symptomatic seizures plus isolated seizures is 71.3 per 100,000 persons per year). It is age dependent and higher in children and in elderly persons (i.e., more than 120 per 100,000) than in young adults. The estimated prevalence of active epilepsy (e.g., more than two seizures during the year preceding the point prevalence day) is 6.42 per 1,000.

EPILEPTIC SEIZURES

According to the International Classification (1981), there are two main categories of seizures: partial and generalized.

Partial or focal or local seizures are those in which, in general, the first clinical and EEG changes indicate an initial activation of a system of neurons limited to part of one cerebral hemisphere.

Generalized seizures are those in which the first clinical changes and bilateral EEG patterns indicate initial involvement of all or large parts of both hemispheres. In the past, they were said to be triggered by some subcortical pacemaker (centrencephalic seizures). Their cortical origin is now documented. Whereas in partial seizures, the spark comes from a constant focus and determines focal signs, in generalized seizures, either the cortical spread is extremely rapid and extended, resulting in a multisystem involvement (corticoreticular epilepsies), or the spark is multifocal, coming from one spot at one moment and from another spot at another moment, with a similarly fast generalization. Thus, by a strict definition, all seizures are focal, and the distinction between partial and generalized seizures is scientifically wrong but remains a useful clinical tool.

Partial Seizures

Many partial seizures include, simultaneously or successively, several clinical manifestations, for instance, visual symptoms, then turning of the head, then loss of consciousness, and finally generalized convulsions. Nevertheless, partial seizures are traditionally named according to their first symptom or sign because of its possible localizing significance (Jackson's signal symptom). This oversimplification is partly mended by the International Classification, which takes into account the successive manifestations occurring during a seizure.

There are thus three fundamental groups of partial seizures: first, *simple partial seizures,* during which consciousness is not impaired; second, *complex partial seizures,* during which consciousness is impaired; and third, *partial seizures secondarily generalized.* Either simple partial or complex seizures may evolve to generalized tonic-clonic convulsions. Consciousness refers to the degree of patient's awareness (i.e., the quality of the patient's contact with events during the attack and/or ability to carry out simple commands in response to external stimuli). As a matter of fact, a mild impairment of consciousness is very difficult to ascertain. Simple partial seizures may evolve into complex partial seizures or impairment of consciousness may be the first clinical sign.

Partial seizures are listed in the box. Any cortical function, hence any portion of the body, may be involved in focal seizure activity depending on the site of origin of the attack and the spread of the epileptic discharge. *Focal motor seizures* may remain strictly focal, with tonic and/or clonic contractions limited to some part of one side of the body or may produce a sequential involvement of body parts in a "Jacksonian march" (J. H. Jackson, British neurologist, 1835–1911), taken by many to represent the homuncular arrangement

---

PARTIAL SEIZURES

Simple partial seizures
    With motor signs
        Focal motor without march
        Focal motor with march (Jacksonian)
        Versive
        Postural
        Phonatory (vocalization or arrest of speech)
    With somatosensory or special-sensory symptoms
        Somatosensory
        Visual
        Auditory
        Olfactory
        Gustatory
        Vertiginous
    With autonomic symptoms or signs
    With psychic symptoms
        Dysphasic
        Dysmnesic (déjà vu)
        Cognitive (dreamy state, distortion of time)
        Affective (fear, anger)
        Illusions
        Structural hallucinations
Complex partial seizures
    Simple partial onset
        Followed by impairment of consciousness
        Followed by impairment of consciousness and automatisms
    With impairment of consciousness at onset
        Impairment only
        With automatisms
Partial seizures evolving to secondarily generalized seizures
    Simple partial seizures evolving to generalized seizures
    Complex partial seizures evolving to generalized seizures
    Simple evolving to complex evolving to generalized seizures

---

of the sensorimotor system in the rolandic cortex (see Chs. 22 and 25). Mainly in infants and young children, they may be followed by an hemiparesis lasting from 1 hour to 3 to 7 days and known as Todd's palsy (R. B. Todd, British physician, 1809–1860). Other focal motor attacks may be versive with head and/or eyes turning to one side. *Somatosensory seizures* are usually described as pins-and-needles or a feeling of numbness. They are often accompanied with motor signs. They may remain focal or extend through a march. *Visual, olfactory, and auditory seizures* vary in elaborateness, depending on whether the primary or association areas are involved, from flashing lights or crude auditory sensations to visual illusions (macropsia, and hallucinatory phenomena, including persons, scenes, or music. Autonomic manifestations are epigastric discomfort, vomiting, or borborygmi and, more rarely pallor, flushing, or sweating. Psychic symptoms are paroxysmal cognitive disturbances, such as dysphasia and aphasia, distortion of the time sense, sensation as if a present experience had been previously experienced (in French, déjà vu) or never previously experienced (jamais vu) or seemed familiar (déjà entendu) or unfamiliar (jamais entendu), and forced thinking. There may be affective symptoms, with fear being more frequent than pleasure. *Automatisms,* an important feature of complex partial seizures, are defined as coordinated, adapted or not, involuntary motor activity occurring during the state of clouding of consciousness either in the course of or after an epileptic seizure. The automatism may be simply a continuation of an ongoing activity (i.e., perseverative automatisms) or a new activity (i.e., de novo automatisms). There are oropharyngeal or gesturally crude or elaborate automatisms: chewing, swallowing, fumbling of the clothes, scratching, walking, or speech automatisms. Ictal and postictal automatisms are often difficult to distinguish. Automatisms are a common feature of different types of epilepsy: mainly temporal and frontal epilepsies but also absence seizures (for definition, see below). Postictal automatisms, usually associated with mental confusion, are also frequent after generalized tonic-clonic seizures.

The EEG pattern during simple partial seizures is a focal contralateral discharge of spikes or fast waves starting over the corresponding area of cortical representation. During a complex partial seizure, there is a less circumscribed discharge over the temporal or frontotemporal regions. Interictal EEG abnormalities are contralateral foci of spikes or slow waves. The ictal EEG is more reliable than the interictal recordings, but both may be misleading, especially when the epileptic focus is located in the mesial or inferior regions of the frontal or temporal lobes. EEG abnormalities may be present on standard recordings (Fig. 79-1) or appear only during drowsiness and slow sleep or from sphenoidal electrodes. In the present state of the art, brain mapping is informative in specialized laboratories but of little practical value in common practice. A normal EEG does not eliminate epilepsy (see also Ch. 11).

Generalized Seizures

A large number of epilepsies are characterized by generalized seizure type.

Absence Seizures and Atypical Absences

These are distinguished on the basis of the EEG pattern and clinical disorder. They consist in a sudden loss of consciousness, with interruption of ongoing activity, or less often with its continuation, a blank stare, and unresponsiveness. They usually are short, lasting from 2 to 60 seconds and generally occur many times a day. Many absence seizures present with other signs: clonic components, ranging from eyelid twitching to pronounced bilateral myoclonic jerks; tonic components, such as upward gaze deviation and backward pulling of the head; and atonic components, resulting in dropping of the head or in a fall and automatisms. In absence seizures, the ictal EEG shows a regular, symmetric discharge of 3-Hz spike-and-slow wave complexes, on a normal background activity. The interictal EEG also contains brief bursts of bilateral spike-waves. In atypical absences, the EEG is variable, with either irregular slow spike-waves or a fast low-voltage discharge on abnormal background activity.

Myoclonic Seizures

These are the only form of generalized seizures without loss of consciousness. They are sudden, brief, isolated, or rapidly repetitive jerks bilaterally affecting either the arms or the legs and then resulting in a fall. Ictal and interictal EEG patterns are bilateral polyspikes and waves.

Clonic, Tonic, and Atonic Seizures

Such seizures are observed mainly in infancy and childhood. Clonic seizures present with repetitive bilateral clonic jerks. Tonic seizures are a tonic contraction fixing the limbs in strained positions, either flexion or extension of the head, neck, trunk, and limbs. Atonic seizures result from a sudden decrease in muscle tone, leading to a head drop or a slumping to the ground. A loss of consciousness is difficult to ascertain in brief seizures in infants or young children. Ictal and interictal EEG are similar to those of atypical absences.

Tonic-Clonic Seizures

These, the so-called *grand mal* seizures, begin with a sudden loss of consciousness and a generalized tonic contraction of muscles. The patient falls to the ground. Breathing is arrested, and cyanosis occurs. The tongue may be bitten, and urine may be passed. Tongue bite is a hallmark of epileptic seizures, but urine loss is not specific, being more frequent indeed in syncopal attacks. Then the tonic contraction gives

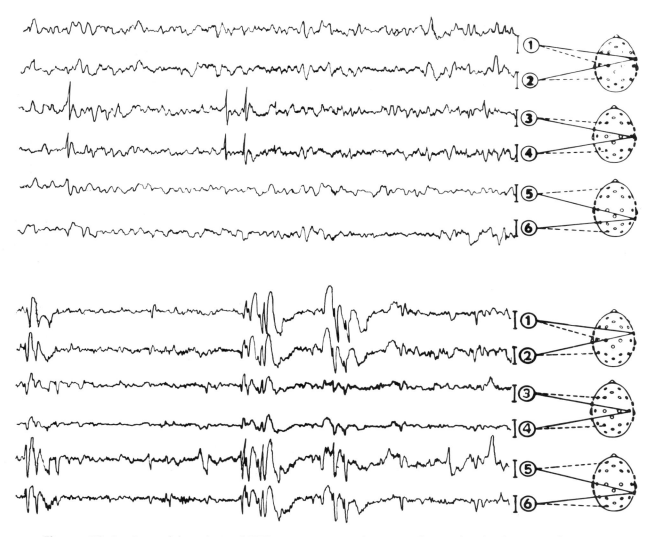

Figure 79-1. A careful analysis of EEG tracings is mandatory. Both samples display an epileptogenic focus, but in the upper part of the figure, spikes are located in the right rolandic area, and in the lower part, spikes and slow waves arise from the right temporal lobe.

GENERALIZED SEIZURES

Absence seizures; atypical absences
Myoclonic seizures
Clonic seizures
Tonic seizures
Tonic-clonic seizures
Atonic seizures

way to clonic jerks, with an increasing amplitude and a decreasing rate. After a last contraction, the muscles relax, and respiration starts again, with stertor and froth, often stained with blood, at the mouth. The patient remains unconscious for several minutes, progressively shifting from a comatose state to a confusional state and often to a deep sleep. A progressive return to normal consciousness is a useful diagnostic sign because, after a syncopal attack, the patient is immediately alert. The ictal EEG shows a repetitive fast activity, decreasing in frequency and increasing in amplitude during the tonic phase, interrupted by slow waves during the clonic phase, followed by a postictal depression of recordings in the high-voltage slow waves. The usual duration of a generalized tonic-clonic seizure is, not counting the postictal coma, 40 to 60 seconds. The interictal EEG depends on the epileptic syndrome (see below). A standard recording may be normal. Activation procedures are hyperpnea, intermittent light stimulation, and sleep deprivation (see also Ch. 11).

EPILEPTIC SYNDROMES

The diagnosis of a seizure type is necessary but is of limited value for treatment and prognosis. Epileptic syndromes are a more practical concept.

The present classification of epileptic syndromes (Table 79-1) is a description rather than a classification. It is not wholly satisfactory but has practical value. It is based on two major divisions: first, epilepsies with generalized seizures (generalized epilepsies) or with partial or focal seizures (localization-related epilepsies); and second, symptomatic, idiopathic, or cryptogenic epilepsies. The meaning of these terms is precise, and their comprehension is a prerequisite for using the classification. Symptomatic syndromes are considered the consequence of a known or strongly suspected disorder of the CNS. Idiopathic syndromes

have no underlying cause other than a possible hereditary predisposition. They are clear-cut syndromes, defined by age-related onset, clinical and EEG characteristics, and a presumed genetic cause. Cryptogenic epilepsies are defined on negative criteria. They are not related to a fixed or progressive cerebral injury, and they do not realize a characteristic electroclinical pattern of idiopathic epilepsy (see below).

The various epileptic syndromes are listed in Table 79-1. Some of them are frequent, whereas many others are rare conditions.

Focal Epileptic Syndromes

Two groups of focal epileptic syndromes are frequent (Table 79-1).

Idiopathic Localization-Related Epilepsies

These disorders are age-dependent syndromes, with an onset between 2 and 12 years of age. Their annual incidence rate in children 0 to 15 years of age is estimated to be 9 per 100,000, representing one-half of the cases of local epilepsies with an onset in this age range. They extend beyond the two main phenotypes:

Table 79-1. International Classification of Epilepsies, Epileptic Syndromes, and Related Seizures Disorders

1. Localization-related (focal, local, partial)
   1.1. Idiopathic
      Benign childhood epilepsy with centrotemporal spikes
      Childhood epilepsy with occipital paroxysms
      Primary reading epilepsy
   1.2. Symptomatic, defined by
      Seizure type and additional clinical features
      Anatomic localization
      Etiology
   1.3. Cryptogenic, defined by
      Seizure type
      Anatomic localization
         Lack of etiologic evidence
2. Generalized
   2.1. Idiopathic
      Benign neonatal familial convulsions
      Benign neonatal convulsions
      Benign myoclonic epilepsy in infancy
      Childhood absence epilepsy
      Juvenile absence epilepsy
      Juvenile myoclonic epilepsy
      Epilepsies with grand mal seizures on awakening
      Other generalized idiopathic epilepsies
      Epilepsies with seizures precipitated by specific modes of activation (e.g., photosensitive)
   2.2. Cryptogenic or symptomatic
      West's syndrome
      Lennox-Gastaut syndrome
      Epilepsy with myoclonic-astatic seizures
      Epilepsy with myoclonic absences

   2.3. Symptomatic
      2.3.1. Nonspecific etiology
         Early myoclonic encephalopathy
         Early infantile epileptic encephalopathy
         Other symptomatic generalized epilepsies
      2.3.2. Specific syndromes: metabolic or degenerative diseases in which seizures are a presenting or predominant feature
3. Epilepsies and syndromes undetermined whether focal or generalized
   3.1. With both generalized and focal seizures
      Neonatal seizures
      Severe myoclonic epilepsy in infancy
      Epilepsy with continuous spike-waves during slow wave sleep
      Acquired epileptic aphasia (Landau-Kleffner syndrome)
      Other
   3.2. Without unequivocal generalized or focal seizures: all cases with generalized tonic-clonic seizures in which clinical and electroencephalographic findings do not permit classification as clearly generalized or localization-related
4. Special syndromes
   4.1. Situation-related seizures
      Febrile convulsions
      Seizures occurring only when there is an acute metabolic or toxic event due to factors such as alcohol, drugs, eclampsia, or nonketotic hyperglycemia
   4.2. Isolated seizures

(From Commission on Classification and Terminology of the International League Against Epilepsy, 1989, with permission.)

benign childhood epilepsy with centrotemporal spikes, which is the most frequent, and the rarer childhood epilepsy with occipital paroxysms. Their main characteristics are as follows. They occur in normal children, without clinical or neuroimaging evidence of brain damage. The seizure patterns vary from case to case, with mostly focal sensorimotor signs. In three-quarters of patients, they occur during sleep. Characteristic interictal EEG abnormalities are mandatory for diagnosis. These are sharp waves, with characteristic morphology and variable location, on a normal background activity (see Fig. 11-13). Seizures always disappear during childhood or adolescence, with EEG normalization, hence the term of benign focal epilepsies of childhood. *Primary reading epilepsy* (Table 79-1) is a rare condition. Seizures are triggered by reading out aloud and occur only in this situation.

Symptomatic and Cryptogenic Focal Epilepsies

These disorders (Table 79-1) differ only by the presence or absence of an underlying cause. The more sophisticated the investigations are, the higher is the proportion of symptomatic versus cryptogenic focal epilepsies. Patients without a prior history and with a normal clinical examination may have an abnormal computed tomographic (CT) scan, and magnetic resonance imaging (MRI) may show an epileptogenic lesion in patients with a normal CT scan. Both symptomatic and cryptogenic focal epilepsies are defined by the type of seizures and their anatomic origin, documented by EEG and neuroimaging procedures. Syndromes related to localization are temporal lobe epilepsies, subdivided into lateral, temporal, and amygdalohippocampal (or mesiobasal limbic or rhinencephalic) epilepsies; frontal lobe epilepsies, with subdivisions, such as orbitofrontal, anterior frontopolar, supplementary motor, dorsolateral, opercular, and motor cortex epilepsies; and parietal and occipital lobe epilepsies. Many causative factors are age dependent, such as malformations, vascular injuries, perinatal anoxia, and rarely, brain tumors in childhood, brain tumors in middle-aged patients, and cerebrovascular disease in elderly patients. Others occur at all ages, for example, infections of the CNS and head trauma.

Generalized Epileptic Syndromes

Several forms exist in this group (Table 79-1).

Idiopathic Generalized Epilepsies

These are also age-related syndromes. The four main syndromes are as follows.

Childhood absence epilepsy, formerly known as petit mal, with an annual incidence rate estimated to be 6 per 100,000. It occurs in previously normal children,

with an onset between 2 and 10 years of age. It is characterized by many absence seizures per day and, on the EEG, 3 per second spike-wave bursts. A positive family history of epilepsy is found in 10 to 20 percent of children. Absence seizures tend to disappear spontaneously and, in 80 percent of cases, are controlled by specific antiepileptic drugs. A durable remission is not infrequent, but in 40 percent of patients, a mild generalized tonic-clonic epilepsy develops during adolescence or later in life.

The electroclinical pattern of *juvenile absence epilepsy* is the same as in childhood absence epilepsy, but its onset is after puberty, and an association with generalized tonic-clonic seizures is the rule, hence a prognostic significant distinction. Five to 10 percent of patients with epilepsy present with *juvenile myoclonic epilepsy.* Its mean age of onset is 12 to 14 years. Genetic predisposition is frequent. The diagnosis is easy, based on a cluster of clinical features: bilateral myoclonic jerks, mainly affecting the arms, specifically occurring on awakening, and triggered by sleep deprivation. Generalized tonic-clonic seizures are associated in 90 percent of patients. They also occur shortly after awakening. The EEG shows generalized spike-wave activity (see Fig. 11-5). Seventy percent of patients become seizure free with one-drug therapy, but treatment must be lifelong because relapses occur in more than 90 percent of cases after drug withdrawal, whatever the duration of the controlled period.

Epilepsy with grand mal on awakening is a syndrome close to juvenile myoclonic epilepsy. Indeed, a considerable overlap exists between these syndromes. Juvenile myoclonic epilepsy with an early onset may mimic absence epilepsy, absence seizures are present in 30 percent of cases of juvenile myoclonic epilepsy, and rare absence or myoclonic seizures may be noted in grand mal on awakening. The main syndromes probably represent different phenotypes of a common genetic disorder.

A similar remark may apply to *photosensitive epilepsies.* In some patients, all seizures are precipitated by a photic stimulation (television or other). In others, spontaneous seizures also occur, and paroxysmal responses to intermittent light stimulation during EEG are frequent in the various forms of idiopathic generalized epilepsies.

Cryptogenic or Symptomatic Generalized Epilepsies

Classifying them is less easy than describing cryptogenic and symptomatic (Table 79-1) generalized epilepsies. Most of them occur during infancy or childhood, with age-dependent electroclinical patterns.

West's syndrome has an onset between 2 and 8 months of age. It consists of a characteristic triad: infantile spasms (brief tonic seizures), arrest of psychomotor development, and typical EEG abnormalities, called hypsarrhythmia (Fig. 11-14). The spasms disappear within days with therapy with adrenocorticotropic hormone or oral steroids or spontaneously after some weeks or months. The mental prognosis is usually poor. It depends on the cause (see below) and on early therapy.

The *Lennox-Gastaut syndrome* has a later onset, between 1 and 8 years of age. It is also characterized by a triad: frequent seizures of different but suggestive forms, such as tonic and atonic seizures and atypical absences; a mental deterioration; and in the interictal EEG, long bursts of bilateral slow spike-wave complexes on an abnormal slow background activity.

A heterogeneous group of infants and children present with *myoclonic and/or myoclonoatonic or myoclonoastatic seizures,* possibly associated with mental impairment or neurologic signs and other types of partial or generalized seizures. The prognosis is variable and, in many cases, is unpredictable. Minor difficulties in classification arise because of patients moving from one syndrome to another during the evaluation of their epilepsy, for instance, presenting with West's syndrome and later with Lennox-Gastaut syndrome or partial epilepsy. Greater difficulties come from the fact that a given clinical pattern may have different causes. It may be cryptogenic or related to a fixed or progressive nonspecific or specific encephalopathy. For instance, West's syndrome may occur in previously normal infants or in brain-damaged patients or be related to tuberous sclerosis or an inborn error of metabolism. These patients could be classified under different headings.

Symptomatic Generalized Epilepsies

The situation is clearer in adolescents and adults. Most symptomatic generalized epilepsies (Table 79-1) are progressive myoclonic epilepsies, caused by specific rare diseases (e.g., Lafora's disease, mitochondrial encephalomyopathies, ceroid lipofuscinoses, or degenerative diseases, such as Unverricht-Lundborg disease).

Epilepsies and Syndromes Undetermined Whether Focal or Generalized

Finally, two groups of patients present with epileptic syndromes undetermined as to whether they are focal or generalized (Table 79-1). The first one covers clinically well-defined syndromes, with both focal and generalized seizures. The Landau-Kleffner syndrome presents as a progressive loss of language in previously normal children, accompanied by seizures of various clinical features. The second one is, in clinical practice, more important, because it covers all cases with tonic-clonic seizures apparently generalized from the onset or, rarely, occasionally secondarily generalized seizures in which neither clinical nor investigations allow a firm classification.

Special Syndromes

These disorders (Table 79-1) are not epilepsy, hence the terms of situation-related seizures and isolated seizures. Febrile convulsions are occasional epileptic seizures. Two to 5 percent of all children before the age of 5 years have seizures as a result of an individual susceptibility that is usually genetically determined. The incidence rate of epilepsy after febrile convulsions is only 2 to 5 percent. Isolated seizures are so-called spontaneous partial or generalized seizures, with a normal EEG and without cause.

DIAGNOSIS

Whenever possible, the clinician must answer two sets of questions: Is it a seizure and if so of what type? What is its cause?

Seizure Type

Ascertaining an epileptic disorder is like putting together a jigsaw puzzle. A correct arrangement of several pieces is necessary to guess the final pattern. The diagnosis of an epileptic seizure relies on history. If when alone the patient experiences a loss of consciousness, the history is likely to be poor. The diagnosis is more difficult after an isolated seizure than after repeated seizures. What the patients can tell and what the witnesses add must be carefully listened to. Personal and family history, clinical examination, EEG findings, and other investigations have to be put together and analyzed. The various presentations of epileptic seizures explain why numerous paroxysmal events may mimic epilepsy. In children, breath-holding attacks, night terrors, nightmares, tantrums, daydreams, abdominal pains, and reflex syncopal attacks can occur. In young people and adults, vasovagal syncopal attacks, migraine, narcolepsy-cataplexy, panic attacks and pseudoseizures, transient ischemic attacks, transient global amnesia, and cardiac syncopal attacks are possible. In practice, syncopal attacks are the major differentiating problem (see Ch. 34).

Cause

The extent of investigations depends on the epileptic syndrome suspected on a clinical basis, with three possible situations.

1. An idiopathic focal or generalized epilepsy is suspected. An EEG is mandatory to confirm the diagnosis. If it does, no other investigation has to be done. A CT scan is unnecessary when a typical

electroclinical pattern is present. When the EEG does not display a characteristic pattern, it must be done again, or a CT scan or MRI must be performed.

2. A symptomatic epilepsy is likely. An obvious cerebral insult is present. When an unequivocal correlation between its location and the type of seizures is present (e.g., an infantile palsy, a middle cerebral artery infarct, or a right craniocerebral wound and left-sided motor seizures), no other investigation is necessary. However, the insult has to be significant. Mild head trauma or a presumed perinatal anoxia are not serious epileptogenic factors. Pre-, peri-, or postnatal insults are considered to be a cause for epilepsy only when the patient also manifests either mental retardation or cerebral palsy. Post-traumatic epilepsy is a consequence of severe head trauma, with evidence of unconsciousness lasting more than 24 hours, a depressed skull fracture, an intracranial hematoma, or an open head injury. EEG and CT scan or MRI may be useful to confirm the clinical hypothesis.

3. A cryptogenic epilepsy is possible. There is no previous history, with a normal clinical examination and a normal or nonspecific EEG. In practice, 50 to 75 percent of epilepsies remain cryptogenic. Nevertheless, even after an isolated seizure, a CT scan or, better, MRI is mandatory. They can demonstrate a cerebral tumor, an arteriovenous malformation, a cavernous angioma, the scar of a forgotten or cryptic event, a cortical dysplasia, a temporal gliosis, or another lesion. The proportion of cryptogenic epilepsies dwindles with new and improved techniques and a timely re-evaluation of the etiologic diagnosis in uncontrolled patients is a wise attitude.

TREATMENT

Medical Treatment

Some preliminary remarks seem useful. First, epilepsy is not necessarily an unremitting disease. Some syndromes are of limited duration, whereas others are lifelong. Antiepileptic drugs control seizures but do not cure the basic disorder. The risk of relapse after their discontinuation depends on the natural history of the epileptic syndrome in the particular patient. So the duration of therapy should not exceed the period at risk for a given patient.

Second, antiepileptic drugs are used on a long-term basis. All of them have some toxicity; hence, a careful risk-benefit analysis is important to decide when to start an antiepileptic treatment and how high the dosage should be kept. Furthermore, poor compliance is common in patients receiving chronic therapies. Good communication between patient and physician is of prime importance. The diagnosis, necessity and methods of treatment, and a description of therapeutic effects and possible side effects of drugs should be clearly explained to patients. Routine follow-ups are most important.

Antiepileptic Drugs

Knowledge of the pharmacokinetic properties of antiepileptic drugs is especially important when attempting to achieve the most effective treatment with the fewest side effects. Common pharmacokinetic characteristics of the currently available drugs (in alphabetical order) are given in Table 79-2. Most antiepileptic

Table 79-2. Pharmacokinetic Properties of Antiepileptic Drugs

	CBZ	CZP	DZP	ESM	PB	PHT	PRM	VPA
Bioavailability	70–75	80–90	75–100	96–100	80–90	20–90	—	86–100
Time to peak levels (hours)	4–8	1–4	0.5–2	3–7	2–18	3–12 (DD)	2–6	1–8
% Protein bound	70–75	80–98	80–98	0	45–54 (A) 49–67 (C)	87–93	0–10	90 (DD)
Elimination half-life (hours)	5–6 (A) 8–19 (C)	19–60	20–90	60 (A) 30 (C)	50–160 (A) 37–73 (C)	8–60 (A) 12–22 (C) (DD)	9–22	8–17 (DD)
Steady state (days)	3	4–8	4–8	4–8	15–21	6–21 (DD)	3–4	2
P-450 system activity	Induced	No action	No action	No action	Induced	Induced	Induced	Inhibited
Recommended plasma level μg/ml	4–10	0.02–0.07	0.2–0.6	40–100	15–30	10–15	5–10	60–100
μmol/l	20–45	0.06–0.22	0.7–2.1	300–700	65–130	40–60	25–50	400–700
Toxicity above (μg/ml)	12	0.1	1	120	35–50	15–20	12	130–150
Usual adult doses (mg/kg/day)	10–15	0.05–0.15	0.2–0.3	15–20	2–3	4–8	15–20	10–15

Abbreviations: CBZ, carbamazepine; CZP, clonazepam; DZP, diazepam; ESM, ethosuximide; PB, phenobarbital; PHT, phenytoin; PRM, primidone; VPA, valproic acid; A, adults; C, children; DD, dose dependent.

drugs appear to be fully absorbed after oral administration. However, the rate and extent of absorption can be influenced by the biopharmaceutical formulation, the form of the preparation, the gastrointestinal contents, and coadministered drugs. Decreased protein binding may result from hypoalbuminemia or displacement by other drugs. In highly protein-bound drugs, an increase in their free fraction, which is the active part of the drug because it alone reaches the brain, may lead to toxic signs, without a change in the total blood concentration. The elimination half-life is theoretically important in regard to the number of daily doses. In practice, one or two daily doses are convenient for most patients. The relationship between clinical effect and serum level must be evaluated only during steady-state conditions.

The recommended plasma levels, the so-called therapeutic levels, are only a guideline to drug therapy because they are statistical figures but do not necessarily apply to the individual patient. With more than one drug, there is a risk for drug interactions in absorption, protein binding, excretion, and mainly metabolism. Antiepileptic or other drugs may either inhibit or accelerate the biotransformation of drugs in the liver (microsomial cytochrome P-450 system). The metabolism of most antiepileptic drugs is linear (i.e., concentration dependent). However, the metabolism of phenytoin is dose dependent and follows saturation (zero-order) kinetics. This means that, above a threshold, which is genetically determined (and, hence, different from one patient to another), a small dose increase will result in a nonproportional blood level increase. With phenytoin, dose escalation must be slow and cautious and phenytoin blood levels repeatedly checked.

Many side effects of antiepileptic drugs have been reported (Table 79-3). In the dose-related group are listed frequent but not life-threatening events. They are reported to occur in about 30 percent of patients. They may be considered as dose dependent because the higher the dose is, the more frequent or more pronounced are the side effects, according to individual thresholds. Some patients experience them with a dose or a level usually well tolerated by others. The opposite is sometimes true. Side effects may be partly avoided by a cautious drug escalation to reach the maintenance daily dose because, in most cases, a tolerance to these side effects develops. In the idiosyncratic reactions are listed rare but serious, sometimes fatal, adverse reactions, such as hypersensitivity reactions, Lyell's syndrome, bone marrow depression, and hepatitis. They can occur with any drug.

Table 79-3. Side Effects of Antiepileptic Drugs

	CBZ	CZP/DZP	ESM	PB	PHT	PRM	VPA
Dose related							
Sedation	+	+ + +	+	+ + +	+ +	+ + +	+
Subtle cognitive effects	+		+	+ + +	+ +	+ +	
Troubles of equilibrium	+ +	+ +	+	+	+ +	+ +	
Tremor							+ +
Behavior disorders	+	+	+	+ +			
Peripheral neuropathy							
Gastrointestinal	+		+ +		+	+	+ +
Weight gain		+					+ +
Gum hypetrophy					+ + +		
Coarse facies				+ +	+	+ +	
Folate deficiency				+	+	+	+
Metabolic bone disease				+	+	+	
Mild leukopenia	+		+	+	+		
Antidiuretic effect	+						
Idiosyncratic reactions							
Skin rash	+ +		+	+	+	+	
Hypersensitivity	+ +		+	+	+		
Systemic lupus erythematosus	+		+		+	+	
Megaloblastic anemia				+	+	+	
Bone marrow depression	+		+	+	+	+	+
Platelet dysfunction	+			+	+	+	+ +
Hepatitis	+			+	+	+	+ +
Acute psychosis	+	+	+ +				
Porphyria				+			

Symbols and Abbreviations: +, mild or unfrequent; + +, more serious or frequent; + + +, rather frequent; CBZ, carbomezepine; CZP, clonazepam; DZP, diazepam; ESM, ethosuximide; PB, phenobarbital; PHT, phenytoin; PRM, primidone; VPA, valproic acid.

Planning Therapy

Guidelines for therapy are summarized in Figure 79-2.

No rational policy determines the attitude to a first seizure. When it is precipitated by an acute illness or by sleep deprivation and when the ancillary investigation findings are normal, the risk of recurrence is lower than the risk of side effects of antiepileptic drugs. Conversely, when EEG epileptiform abnormalities are present, a risk of recurrence of about 80 percent justifies therapy.

About 75 to 80 percent of naive epileptic patients are controlled by adequate therapy. It is recommended to start with a relatively low dose of the chosen drug. The choice of the appropriate drug is dictated more by potential toxicity than by efficacy because there is no evidence of better efficacy among the major antiepileptic drugs. When the patient is seizure free, therapy is maintained during a time de-

pending on the epileptic syndrome: 2 or 3 years in partial epilepsies, at least 5 years in generalized epilepsies, and for life in juvenile myoclonic epilepsy and related conditions. Plasma level determinations are not necessary unless drug toxicity is suspected. Conversely, when seizures persist, plasma levels have to be checked, mainly for compliance assessment. The advantages of one-drug treatment are obvious. Furthermore, the administration of a second drug, even if sometimes necessary, does not control seizures in more than 15 percent of patients whose disease was uncontrolled with one drug.

Finally, a relatively small group of patients has uncontrolled epilepsy. For these drug-resistant, intractable seizures, the aim of the physician is to find an equilibrium between the risks caused by the seizures and the risks from too much therapy. Some patients' seizures are well controlled with persisting EEG abnormalities. Usually, the clinical condition is more impor-

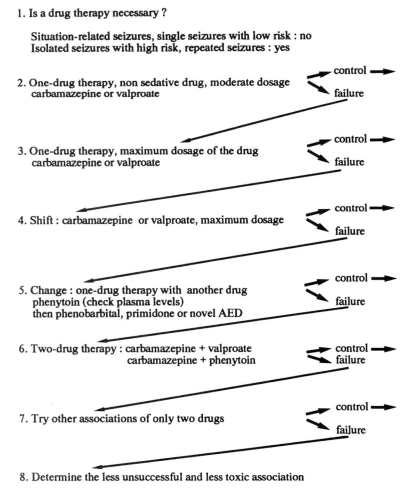

1. **Is a drug therapy necessary ?**

   Situation-related seizures, single seizures with low risk : no
   Isolated seizures with high risk, repeated seizures : yes

2. **One-drug therapy, non sedative drug, moderate dosage**
   carbamazepine or valproate — control → / failure

3. **One-drug therapy, maximum dosage of the drug**
   carbamazepine or valproate — control → / failure

4. **Shift : carbamazepine or valproate, maximum dosage** — control → / failure

5. **Change : one-drug therapy with another drug**
   phenytoin (check plasma levels)
   then phenobarbital, primidone or novel AED — control → / failure

6. **Two-drug therapy : carbamazepine + valproate**
   carbamazepine + phenytoin — control → / failure

7. **Try other associations of only two drugs** — control → / failure

8. **Determine the less unsuccessful and less toxic association**

Figure 79-2. Guidelines for therapy. AED, antiepileptic drug.

tant than is the EEG. However, frequent EEG epileptiform discharges are considered a source of neuropsychologic impairment, and therapy has to be increased.

Difficult problems arise with pregnancy or the risk of pregnancy. On the one hand, seizures during pregnancy may be harmful to the fetus. On the other hand, all antiepileptic drugs are mild teratogenic agents during the first 2 or 3 months of pregnancy, and the risk for malformations is twofold in treated epileptic mothers. The decision is an individual one. The drug should be stopped several weeks before pregnancy (whenever possible) because of the long-acting action of some drugs. When impossible, one-drug therapy is advised because the greater the number of antiepileptic drugs used, the greater is the risk for malformations. There is no teratogenic risk after the third month, and the only goal is the control of seizures. Pregnancy's influence on seizure frequency is unpredictable in a given woman and even can be different from one pregnancy to the following one. On the whole, epilepsy remains unchanged in 50 percent of the patients, improves in 25 percent, and worsens in 25 percent. Despite current opinion, breast feeding is possible in most cases. Many anticonvulsant drugs, such as carbamazepine, phenytoin, and phenobarbital, are metabolic inducers and may decrease the efficacy of birth control pills.

Surgical Treatment

When seizures persist after 2 years of aggressive medical therapy, the prognosis is poor, and a curative surgical treatment can be discussed. Such procedures mainly address partial epilepsies with a single epileptic focus in a cortical area, the excision of which will not lead to permanent interictal impairment.

The outcome of surgery for epilepsy must be assessed both in terms of effect on the seizures and in the changes in the patient's quality of life. In regard to seizures, 70 to 80 percent of temporal lobe epilepsies and 50 percent of extratemporal epilepsies can be cured by surgery. Surgery interferes also with the neurologic and psychological interictal state, which can be either improved or impaired. When both conditions are taken into account, more than 50 percent of patients with medically intractable epilepsy benefit from corticectomies. This overall benefit is greater when surgery is performed before the patient undergoes many years of recurrent seizures, wasting the quality of life of children or young adults.

Another group of patients with severe multifocal epilepsies who experience daily falls as a result of secondarily generalized seizures can benefit from palliative surgery, such as section of the corpus callosum that can suppress or reduce the generalization of seizures.

Treatment of Status Epilepticus

Status epilepticus is defined as a condition in which seizures repeat with a great frequency, more than three seizures per hour, or last more than 30 minutes (see also Ch. 83). There are as many types of status epilepticus as there are types of seizures. Generalized convulsive status epilepticus is an emergency because it can be fatal if untreated. Recurrent seizures should be treated with a benzodiazepine, such as diazepam, 0.25 to 0.5 mg/kg, up to 10 mgIV at no faster than 1 mg/min (risk of apnea). When seizures persist, the patient should be admitted to an intensive care unit, for repetition of intravenous diazepam, up to 100 to 120 mg/day; clonazepam, up to 6 to 12 mg/day; or intravenous infusion of phenytoin, with a loading dose of 16 mg/kg, no faster than 20 to 50 mg/min, with maintenance of airway, hydration, glucose, and electrolyte balance.

ANNOTATED BIBLIOGRAPHY

Commission on Classification and Terminology of the International League Against Epilepsy. Proposal for revised clinical and electroencephalographic classification of epileptic seizures. Epilepsia 1981;22:489–501.

The "Bible."

Commission on Classification and Terminology of the International League Against Epilepsy. Proposal for classification of epilepsies and epileptic syndromes. Epilepsia 1989;30:389–99.

Another "Bible."

Dasheiff RM. Epilepsy surgery: is it an effective treatment? Ann Neurol 1989;25:506–9.

A provocative review.

Delgado-Escueta AV, Treiman DM, Walsh GO. The treatable epilepsies. N Engl J Med 1983;308:1508–84.

An interesting review of the main types of epilepsy.

Gastaut H. Classification of status epilepticus. In Clifford Rose F (ed). Research Progress in Epilepsy. Pitman, UK, 1983, pp. 39–45.

An accurate description of the various forms of status epilepticus.

Mattson RH, Cramer JA, Collins JF et al. Comparison of carbamazepine, phenobarbital, phenytoin and primidone in partial and secondarily generalized tonic-clonic seizures. N Engl J Med 1985;313:145–51.

An astute multicenter clinical trial.

Rogawski MA, Porter RJ. Antiepileptic drugs: pharmacological mechanisms and clinical efficacy with consideration of promising developmental stage compounds. Pharmacol Rev 1990;42:224–86.

Extensive review of old and novel antiepileptic drugs.

Rougier A, Dartigues JF, Commenges D et al. A longitudinal assessment for seizure outcome and overall benefit from 10 cortectomies for epilepsy. J Neurol Neurosurg Psychiatry 1992;55:762–7.

Full assessment.

Scheuer ML, Pedley TA. The evaluation and treatment of seizures. N Engl J Med 1990;323:1468–74.

An interesting overview of modern trends in antiepileptic treatment.

Shorvon SD, Gram L, Meldrum BS et al. Epilepsy octet. Lancet 1990;336:93–6, 161–4, 231–4, 281–96, 350–4, 423–7, 486–91, 551–4.

A concise and commendable update on epilepsy.

80
Peripheral Nerve Disease

Dale J. Lange

There are many different types of peripheral nerves, each of which subserve different functions, such as light touch, temperature sensation, muscle innervation, and control of autonomic function. The manifestations of peripheral nervous system disease vary with the type of fibers affected. Based on the pattern of the nerves affected, the clinician can often determine the cause of the neuropathy (see Ch. 32).

ACQUIRED PERIPHERAL NEUROPATHY

Diabetic Neuropathy

The broad diversity of neurologic complications in diabetic patients is now generally accepted to consist of two distinct types: one in which the symptoms and signs are transient and another in which they progress steadily. The former category includes acute painful neuropathies, mononeuropathies, and radiculopathies and the latter, sensorimotor polyneuropathies with or without autonomic symptoms and signs. Although the actual cause of diabetic neuropathies is unknown, the origin of focal nerve involvement is considered to be vascular, whereas the progressive symmetric polyneuropathy more likely is due to a metabolic factor, a view not generally accepted.

Acute Painful Polyneuropathy

Acute painful polyneuropathy is characterized by acute continous pain of a disabling nature in a stocking distribution affecting the feet and legs or localized to the thighs as a femoral neuropathy (diabetic amyotrophy). Men are more often affected than women. The pain may last for several months and is often described as a burning sensation. However, recovery from severe pain is usually complete in less than 12 months, and the disorder does not necessarily progress to convential sensory polyneuropathy.

Mononeuropathies

It is generally believed but never shown by any comprehensive study that focal neuropathies are more frequent in diabetic patients than in the general population. They are usually localized to the common sites of entrapment or external compression and may reflect an increased liability to pressure palsies. This applies to the median nerve at the carpal tunnel, the ulnar at the elbow, and the peroneal at the fibular head. The electrophysiologic features are similar to those in nondiabetic patients with pressure palsies, except that abnormalities outside the clinically affected areas sometimes indicate that the palsies occur on top of a generalized neuropathy. Cranial nerve palsies are most often localized to the third and sixth nerves. They have an abrupt onset, are common in men, usually resolve completely within 3 to 6 months, and rarely relapse.

Diabetic Generalized Polyneuropathies

The most common type is a diffuse distal symmetric predominantly sensory neuropathy with or without autonomic manifestations. Distal motor involvement is usually relatively minor. The neuropathy develops slowly and is related to the duration of the diabetes, but not all patients are affflicted with it. Once present, it never remits or recovers. Whether there are any effective methods for changing its course is still a matter of debate. Most evidence suggests that small nerve fibers, myelinated and unmyelinated, are affected first in diabetic neuropathy. Thus, pain and temperature sensation transmitted through the smallest fibers my be affected before large-fiber modalities such as vibration, light touch, and position sense are involved. Small-fiber function can be investigated by determining the thresholds for warming and cooling or by the pinprick threshold technique with weighted needles.

MANIFESTATIONS OF PERIPHERAL NEUROPATHY AS A FUNCTION OF FIBER TYPE AFFECTED

Mononeuropathy/mononeuropathy
  multiplex
    Compression/trauma
    Polyarteritis
    HIV-1 infection
Sensory menifestations only
    Large-Fiber dysfunction
    Friedreich's ataxia
    Cisplatin
    Small-fiber dysfunction
        Amyloidosis
        Leprosy
        Diabetes
        Analphalipoproteinemia (Tangier)
        Fabry's disease
        AIDS neuropathy
    Unmyelinated
Autonomic only (unmyelinated)
    Heritary dysautonomia (Riley-Day syn-
        drome)
    Amyloidosis
    Pandysautonomic
Motor predominant
    Porphyria
    Chronic and acute inflammatory neu-
        ropathy
    Charcot-Marie-Tooth disease (types I
        and II)
    Lead neuropathy
Root only

The sensation of cooling and pinprick is conveyed by small myelinated fibers and that of warming, by unmyelinated fibers. The prevalence of diabetic autonomic neuropathy may be underestimated because patients may have nonspecific symptoms that remain undiagnosed or they may be asymptomatic. The development of symptoms appear to be relatively late, and the onset is often insidious. They progress slowly and are usually irreversible. It is essential to screen for autonomic involvement in diabetic patients because those with abnormal cardiovascular reflex function have an excess mortality risk of 56 percent when followed up to 5 years compared with 11 percent for the general diabetic population. Autonomic function tests include a determination of the heart rate at rest, during deep breathing, and during standing by measuring the R-R intervals (predominantly parasympathetic function); the change in mean arterial blood pressure from a supine to a standing position is used to test sympathetic function. Slowing in motor and sensory conduction is a common finding in diabetic patients, even among those without overt neuropathy. It is generally attributed to axonal degeneration with secondary demyelination.

Hypothyroid Neuropathy

Entrapment neuropathies are the most common neuropathy associated with hypothyroidism. The cause of these mononeuropathies is most likely the deposition of acid mucopolysaccaride protein complexes (mucoid). Less common is a diffuse sensorimotor neuropathy.

Patients usually complain of painful paresthesias in the hand and feet. Weakness is not common. Tendon reflexes are reduced or absent. When present, they may show the characteristic "delayed" response, and direct percussion of muscle produces transient mounding of the underlying skin (myoedema). Nerve conduction studies show mild slowing of motor nerve conduction with loss of sensory nerve-evoked response amplitude. However, morophologic studies show evidence of demyelination, axonal loss, and excessive glycogen within Schwann cells. The cerebrospinal fluid protein content is often markedly elevated (more than 100 mg/dl). Rarely, dysfunction of cranial nerves IX, X, and XII causes hoarseness and dysarthia, probably as a result of local myxedematous infiltration. Deafness has been reported in as many as 85 percent of hypothyroid patients. The peripheral neuropathy may occur before laboratory evidence of hypothyroidism is found.

Once identified, thyroid replacement causes clinical, electrophysiologic, and morphologic improvement.

Hyperthyroid Neuropathy

Hyperthyroidism can produce a syndrome consisting of diffuse weakness and fasciculations with preserved or hyperactive tendon reflexes, suggesting the presence of amyotrophic lateral sclerosis. It may also appear in association with Guillain-Barré syndrome. There are rare reports of chronic peripheral neuropathy occurring in association with hyperthyroidism with the use of electrophysiologic criteria, but none show pathologic changes, and the clinical relevance is doubtful.

Acromegalic Neuropathy

Entrapment neuropathy is also the most common manifestation of peripheral nerve disease in patients with acromegaly. Rarely, acromegalic patients complain of distal paresthesias, but in contradistinction to the findings in myxedematous patients, weakness may be severe, and peripheral nerves may be palpable. The enlarged nerves occur because of increased amounts of endoneurial and perineurial connective tissue, perhaps stimulated by the presence of increased levels of the mitogen, somatomedin C (insulinlike growth factor). Tendon reflexes are reduced.

Nerve conduction velocities are mildly slow with low evoked-response amplitudes. Morphologic changes suggest segmental demyelination.

Uremic Neuropathy

Peripheral neuropathy is only one of the clinical effects that chronic renal failure has on the neuromuscular system. Other manifestations, such as, "restless legs," cramps, and muscle twitching may also be due to dysfunction of the peripheral nervous system and may be one of the early manifestations of peripheral nerve disease. As many as 70 percent of patients with chronic renal failure have neuropathy, although most is subclinical. The neuropathy occurs most often in men (by severalfold) and correlates with the severity of the renal failure.

The neuropathy usually causes painful dysesthesias and a symmetric loss of sensation and weakness in distal muscles, in a stocking-glove distribution. Electrodiagnostic studies show a sensorimotor neuropathy with axonal features. Pathologic studies confirm the presence of axonopathy. Some investigators have shown sporadic segmental demyelination secondary to axonal loss.

Dialysis rarely reverses the neuropathy, but treatment usually stabilizes the progression of the neuropathy. Peritoneal dialysis is more effective than hemodialysis. Monitoring nerve conduction studies are used to measure the effectiveness of hemodialysis. However, successful renal transplantation often causes resolution of the neuropathy shortly after successful surgery.

Mononeuropathies, particularly carpal tunnel syndrome, are also common and often occur distal to an implanted arteriovenous fistula, suggesting distal ischemia as a possible mechanism. Distal ischemia from implanted bovine shunts may also cause a more severe ischemic neuropathy in the median, ulnar, and radial nerves, possibly from excessive arteriovenous shunting. Chronic hemodialysis (more than 10 years) causes excessive accumulation of β_2-microglobulin (generalized amyloidosis), which is another possible cause of carpal tunnel syndrome and peripheral uremic neuropathy. The cause of the neuropathy is uncertain, but accumulation of a toxic metabolite is the most likely explanation. However, its identity remains unknown.

Neuropathy Associated With Hepatic Disease

Peripheral neuropathy is rarely associated with primary diseases of the liver. A chronic demyelinating neuropathy may be associated with chronic liver disease, but it is usually subclinical. A painful sensory neuropathy occurs in patients with primary biliary cirrhosis and is probably caused by xanthoma formation in and around nerves. Electrodiagnostic study findings may be normal, or sensory-evoked response amplitudes may be low or absent. Nerve biopsies show loss of small-diameter nerve fibers. Sudanophilic-containing cells are often seen in the perineurium. Treatment is directed at pain control. Tricyclic antidepressants or anticonvulsants have been successful.

Infectious diseases that affect the liver may also be associated with peripheral neuropathies. Viral hepatitis, human immunodeficiency virus (HIV) infections, cytomegalovirus infection, and infectious mononucleosis may be associated with acute demyelinating neuropathy (Guillain-Barré syndrome), chronic demyelinating neuropathy, and mononeuropathy multiplex. Immunologically mediated diseases, such as polyarteritis and sarcoidosis, may also cause liver abnormalities and mononeuropathy multiplex.

Peripheral neuropathy is often seen in the presence of toxic liver disease and hepatic metabolic diseases such as acute intermittent pophyria, abetalipoproteinemia, and analphaproteinemia.

NEUROPATHIES ASSOCIATED WITH INFECTION

Human Immunodeficiency Virus Related Neuropathies

There are different neuropathies that afflict patients infected with the HIV virus, depending on the stage of the illness and the immunocompetence of the patient. Acute demyelinating neuropathy resembling Guillain-Barré syndrome occurs early in the course of infection, often when there are no signs of immunodeficiency, or at the time of seroconversion. Patients with Guillain-Barré syndrome associated with HIV infection differ from those with sporadic Guillain-Barré syndrome because of a greater incidence of generalized lymphadenopathy, more frequent involvement of cranial nerves, and a higher frequency of sexually transmitted disease.

Subacute demyelinating neuropathy, clinically indistinguishable from idiopathic non-HIV-associated chronic inflammatory demyelinating neuropathy is usually found in HIV-positive patients before the development of clinical acquired immunodeficiency syndrome (AIDS). The important difference between the two groups is the cerebrospinal fluid findings. Patients with HIV-associated demyelinating neuropathy have elevated levels of cerebrospinal fluid protein with lymphocytic pleocytosis. Patients with HIV-associated demyelinating neuropathy are treated identically to those without HIV infection. Steroids, plasmapheresis, and human immunoglobulin have been reported to be effective in these patients.

Patients with clinical manifestations of HIV infection who fulfill the criteria for AIDS rarely have demyelinating neuropathy. These patients often show a distal sensorimotor polyneuropathy with axonal features. The clinical syndrome is dominated by severe painful paresthesias that affect the feet first and most intensely. This painful neuropathy is often the most functionally disabling manifestation of AIDS. There is no treatment that reverses these symptoms, but relief is sometime achieved with drugs such as carbamazepine and amitriptyline.

Mononeuropathy multiplex occurs in HIV-infected patients at all stages of the disease. It may be found in association with hepatitis infection. When CD4 cells number less than 50, the likely cause of the mononeuroapthy is cytomegalovirus, and prompt treatment with gancicovir may be life saving. Cytomegalovirus infection is also associated with polyradiculopathy and Guillain-Barré syndrome in patients with HIV infection.

Lyme Disease

This disorder is being increasingly diagnosed in the United States and Europe. It is caused by a tick-borne spirochete infection, *Borrelia burgdorferi*, and may present as a multisystem infection. The most common clinical feature of neuroborreliosis is a painful sensory radiculitis, which may appear about 3 weeks after erythema migrans following a tick bite. The pain intensity varies from day to day and is often severe, jumping from one area to another and often associated with patchy areas of unpleasant dysesthesiae. Focal neurologic signs are common and may present as cranial nerve involvement (61 percent), limb paresis (12 percent), or both (16 percent). The facial nerve is most frequently affected, twice as often unilaterally as bilaterally. Abducens and oculomotor paresis may occasionally occur. Myeloradiculitis is a rare manifestation as is chronic progressive encephalomyelitis. Arthralgia is a common complaint among patients in the United States, but it is rare among Europeans (6 percent). The triad of painful radiculitis, predominantly cranial mononeuritis multiplex, and lymphocytic pleocytosis in the cerebrospinal fluid is known as Bannwarth's syndrome in Europe. Biopsies from peripheral nerves have shown signs of peri- and epineural vasculitis and axonal degeneration in agreement with electrophysiologic findings. The diagnosis of neuroborreliosis is based on the presence of inflammatory spinal fluid

changes and specific intrathecal *B. burgdorferi* antibody production. The prognosis is good after high doses of intravenous penicillin. Disabling sequelae are rare and occur mainly in patients with previous central nervous system involvement.

Herpes Zoster

Varicella virus infection of the dorsal root ganglion produces radicular pain that may precede or follow the appearance of the characteristic skin eruption. Herpes zoster infection may affect any level of the neuraxis, but it has the greatest predilection for thoracic dermatome levels and cranial nerves with sensory ganglia (V and VII). Ophthalmic herpes (cranial nerve V) occurs because of infection in the gasserian ganglion and characteristically involves the first division of the trigeminal nerve. Weakness of ocular muscles and ptosis may occur. Infection of the geniculate ganglion of the facial nerve (cranial nerve VII) causes a vesicular herpetic eruption in the external auditory meatus, vertigo, deafness, and facial weakness (Ramsey Hunt's syndrome).

The neuropathologic changes constitute a distinct syndrome characterized by a ganglionic lesion combined with degeneration of related sensory and motor nerve roots, severe neuritis, unilateral poliomyelitis, and localized leptomeningitis, findings that provide a reasonable explanation for the clinical symptoms and signs such as neuralgia and motor palsies.

Although primarily a sensory neuropathy, weakness from motor involvement may occur in 0.5 to 30 percent of infected patients, occurring more often in elderly patients and those afflicted with a malignancy and usually occurring in the same myotomal distribution as the dermatomal rash. Segmental zoster paresis caused by varicella viral infection parallels cutaneous pain and vesicular rash and affects predominantly middle-aged and elderly persons, equally often on the right as on the left side. Although thoracic segments are the preferred site for cutaneous zoster, they are relatively free of motor complications in contrast to herpes zoster, which is localized to the face and limbs. Electromyography reveal fibrillation potentials and positive sharp waves in affected muscles.

Zoster infections are also associated with the acute ascending paralysis of Guillain-Barré syndrome. Such patients often have a cellular pleocytosis in the cerebrospinal fluid. Because herpes infections often occur in patients with HIV infection and cerebrospinal fluid pleocytosis occurs in both conditions, the presence of herpes infection associated with weakness in a young person should alert the clinician to the presence of possible HIV infection.

Leprosy

The neuropathy associated with leprosy is caused by direct infiltration of small-diameter peripheral nerve fibers. It is the most common treatable neuropathy in the world. Leprosy is often seen in immigrants from India, Southeast Asia, and Central Africa, but small numbers of affected patients remain in parts of the southern United States.

Peripheral nerves are affected differently in tuberculoid and lepromatous forms. In tuberculoid leprosy, a small hypopigmented area with superficial sensory loss occurs, and the underlying subcutaneous sensory nerves may become visibly or palpably enlarged. Large nerve trunks, such as the ulnar, peroneal, facial, and posterior auricular, may be injured by inclusion in regions of granuloma formation and scarring. Endoneurial caseation necrosis may occur. The clinical picture is one of mononeuritis or mononeuritis multiplex.

In lepromatous leprosy, Hansen bacilli proliferate in large numbers within Schwann cells and macrophages in the endoneurium and perineurium of subcutaneous nerve twigs, particularly in cool areas of the body (pinnae of the ears, dorsum of the hands, forearms, and feet). Loss of cutaneous sensiblity is observed in affected patches; these may later coalesce to cover large parts of the body. Position sense may be preserved in affected areas, whereas pain and temperature sensibility is lost, a dissociation similar to that in syringomyelia. Tendon reflexes are preserved.

Acute mononeuritis multiplex may appear during chemotherapy of lepromatous leprosy in conjunction with erythema nodosum. This complication is treated with thalidomide.

Treatment with dapsone is designed to eradicate the bacterium and prevent secondary immune reactions, which may damage nerves. Because of the dense sensory loss, painless and inadvertent traumatic injuries, such as self-inflicted burns, may occur unless extreme caution is exercised to avoid trauma to the anesthetic areas.

Diptheria

Diphtheria and diphtheritic neuropathy are rare, occurring in approximately 20 percent of infected patients. The infecting organism is *Corynebacterium diphtheriae*. It usually infects the larynx or pharynx but may infect cutaneous wounds. The organisms release an exotoxin that causes myocarditis and, later, symmetric neuropathy. The neuropathy often begins with impaired visual accommodation and paresis of ocular and oropharyngeal muscles and is followed by quadriparesis. Nerve conduction velocities are very slow, reflecting the underlying demyelinating neuropathy.

Diphtheria and its neuropathy may be prevented by immunization and, if infection occurs, by antibiotic therapy. Recovery may be slow, and physiologic measures resolve after the clinical syndrome does.

Sarcoid Neuropathy

Some 4 percent of patients with sarcoidosis have involvement of the nervous system, most commonly single or multiple cranial nerve palsies that fluctuate in intensity. Of the cranial nerves, the seventh is most commonly affected, and as in diabetes mellitus, the facial nerve syndrome in sarcoidosis is indistinguishable from idiopathic Bell's palsy. In some instances, cranial neuropathies in patients with sarcoid neuropathy result from basilar meningitis. A distinguishing feature of the mononeuropathy associated with sarcoid is the appearance of large areas of sensory loss on the trunk.

In patients with sarcoidosis, symmetric polyneuropathy occasionally develops months to years after the diagnosis is established. The neuropathy may become apparent before the diagnosis is made, and the associated clinical syndromes may include Guillain-Barré syndrome, lumbosacral plexopathy, mononeuritis multiplex, and pure sensory neuropathy. However, almost all patients have cranial nerve involvement. Nerve biopsy shows a mixture of wallerian degeneration and segmental demyelination with sarcoid granulomas in the endoneurium and epineurium. Sarcoid neuropathy generally responds to steroid therapy.

POLYNEUROPATHY ASSOCIATED WITH DIETARY DEFICIENCIES

Thiamine Deficiency

The existence of peripheral neuropathy in alcoholic persons is well known, but its cause is still debated. There is no unequivocal evidence to support the concept that alcohol is toxic to peripheral nerves. A widely held belief is that the neuropathy associated with alcoholism is due to nutritional deficiency, particularly of vitamin B_1 (thiamine).

Thiamine deficiency may cause two different clinical syndromes. The first is called "wet beriberi", in which congestive heart failure is the predominant syndrome. The second is called "dry beriberi," in which peripheral neuropathy is the predominant symptom. The signs and symptoms of this neuropathy closely resemble that found in alcoholic persons.

Patients with thiamine deficiency have severe burning dysesthesias in the feet more than the hands; weakness and wasting of distal more than proximal muscles; trophic changes (shiny skin and hair loss); and sensory loss, worse in distal portions of the legs. Electromyography and nerve conduction studies reveal the presence of a diffuse sensorimotor peripheral neuropathy, which is axonal in nature. Axonal degeneration is also the principal finding seen on nerve biopsies.

Treatment of both beriberi and alcoholic neuropathy should be initiated with parenteral B-complex vitamins followed by oral thiamine. Recovery is slow; there may be residual muscular weakness and atrophy.

Niacin (Nicotinic Acid) Deficiency

This causes pellagra, characterized by hyperkeratotic skin lesions. Peripheral neuropathy is usually present in patients deficient in niacin, but the neuropathy does not improve with niacin supplements; only when thiamine and pyridoxine are added to the diet do the symptoms improve.

Vitamin B$_{12}$ Deficiency

This causes the classical clinical syndrome of subacute combined degeneration of the spinal cord (see also Ch. 71). Separation of the peripheral neuropathic symptoms from spinal cord involvement is difficult. The painful paresthesias accompanying vitamin B$_{12}$ deficiency are probably the result of the spinal cord involvement.

Vitamin B$_6$ (Pyridoxine) Deficiency

This produces a peripheral neuropathy, and the most common cause of vitamin B$_6$ deficiency is ingestion of the antituberculous drug, isoniazid. This drug increases the excretion of pyridoxine. The resulting neuropathy affects sensory more than motor fibers and is caused by axonal loss. Treatment consists of administering excessive amounts of pyridoxine to compensate for the added excretion. The neuropathy can be prevented by prophylactic vitamin B$_6$ administration. Isoniazid also can occasionally elicit a vasculitic mononeuropathy multiplex.

Vitamin E Deficiency

This contributes to neuropathy in fat malabsorption syndromes such as in chronic cholestasis. The clinical syndrome that results from vitamin E deficiency resembles spinocerebellar degeneration with ataxia and severe sensory loss of joint position and vibration with hyporeflexia. Peripheral motor nerve conduction study results are normal, but sensory-evoked responses are of low amplitude or absent. Somatosensory-evoked responses show a delay in central conduction. Electromyographic results are usually normal. Vitamin E deficiency occurs in most fat malabsorption disorders, abetalipoproteinemia, congenital biliary atriesia, pancreatic dysfunction, or surgical removal of large portions of the small intestine.

NEUROPATHY PRODUCED BY METALS

Arsenic

Damage to peripheral nerves may follow chronic exposure to small amounts of arsenic or ingestion or parenteral administration of a large amount of the metal. Chronic exposure may occur in industries where arsenic is released as a by-product, such as the copper smelting industry. Because of the prevalence of such by-products in the industrial community, arsenic neuropathy is the most common of all heavy metal-induced neuropathies. Gastrointestinal symptoms, vomiting, and diarrhea occur when a toxic quantity of arsenic is ingested, but these symptoms may be absent if the arsenic is given parenterally or taken in small amounts over long periods. In acute arsenic poisoning, the onset of polyneuropathy is delayed 4 to 8 weeks; once symptoms develop, they reach maximum intensity within a few days. The evolution of polyneuropathy is much slower in patients with chronic arsenic poisoning. Sensory symptoms are prominent in the early stages. Pain and paresthesias in the legs may be present for several days or weeks before the onset of weakness. The weakness progresses to complete flaccid paralysis of the legs and sometimes the arms. Cutaneous sensation is impaired in a stocking-glove distribution, with vibration and position sensation being affected most. Tendon reflexes are lost. Pigmentation and hyperkeratosis of the skin and changes in the nails ("Mees' lines") are frequently present. Arsenic is present in the urine in the acute stages of poisoning and in the hair and nails in the late stages. Nerve conduction velocities may be normal or mildly diminished; the amplitude of sensory-evoked responses may be reduced. Pathologic examination of nerves shows axonal degeneration. A chelating agent is used to treat arsenic polyneuropathy. The effectiveness of chelation therapy can be monitored by measuring arsenic excretion rates in 24-hour samples.

Lead

Most toxic neuropathies cause a symmetric weakness and loss of sensation in distal more than proximal regions, with the feet worse than the legs. In contrast to most other toxic neuropathies, lead poisoning causes focal weakness of the extensor muscles of the fingers and wrist. Lead neuropathy occurs almost exclusively in adults. Infants poisoned with lead usually develop encephalopathy. Lead may enter the body through the lungs, skin, or gut. Occupational lead poisoning is encountered in battery workers, painters, and pottery glazers. Accidental lead poisoning follows ingestion of lead in food or beverages or among children who ingest lead paint. Lead poisoning may cause abdominal distress (lead colic). By its effect on renal tubules, lead poisoning often causes urate retention and gout. Weakness usually begins in distinct muscles innervated by the radial nerve, sparing the brachioradialis; it is often bilateral. Later, the weakness may extend to other muscles in the arms and, occasionally, to the legs. Sensory symptoms and signs are usually absent. Rarely, upper motor neuron signs may occur with the lower motor neuron disorder and mimic amyotrophic lateral sclerosis. Laboratory findings include anemia with basophilic stippling of the red cells, increased serum uric acid, and slight elevation of cerebrospinal fluid protein content. Nerve conduction velocities are usually normal, raising the possibility that a disorder may be an anterior horn cell disorder rather than a neuropathy. Urinary lead excretion is elevated, particularly after administration of a chelating agent. Urinary porphobilinogen excretion is also elevated, but the β-aminolevulinic acid level is normal. The primary therapy is prevention of further exposure to lead. When exposure ceases, recovery is gradual over several months.

Mercury

Mercury is used in the electrical and chemical industries. There are two forms of mercury, elemental and organic. The organic form of mercury (methyl and ethyl mercury) is the most toxic to the central nervous system, although distal paresthesias are prominent symptoms (presumably due to dorsal root ganglion degeneration). Ventral roots are spared.

Inorganic mercury may be absorbed through the gastrointestinal tract, and elemental mercury may be absorbed directly through the skin or lungs (it is volatile at room temperature). Elemental mercury exposure primarily causes weakness and wasting more than sensory symptoms. Because of the prominent motor manifestations, confusion with amyotrophic lateral sclerosis can occur. Treatment with vitamin E or selenium may be beneficial.

Thallium

This element is used as a rodenticide and in other industrial processes. As with lead, children exposed to thallium are more likely to have encephalopathy, whereas adults have neuropathy. In contrast to lead poisoning, however, thallium neuropathy is primarily sensory and autonomic. Severe disturbing dysesthesias appear acutely, and the course is complicated in many patients by tachycardia and hypertension. Quadriplegia, dysphagia, and dysarthria may occur in severe cases. Most patients have partial or total alopecia after the onset of the neuropathic symptoms. The diagnosis is by history of thallium exposure. The typical syndrome of acute dysesthesias, autonomic dysfunction, and subsequent alopecia and the identifica-

tion of thallium in the urine are of diagnostic value. Nerve conduction velocities are usually normal. Nerve biopsy or autopsy shows axonal degeneration. Thallium excretion can be accelerated by potassium administration, but potassium therapy may transiently worsen the pain and autonomic signs. Complete recovery usually occurs after exposure to thallium ends.

Gold

Gold neuropathy occurs only as a side effect when patients are receiving it as a treatment for rheumatoid arthritis. Clinically, it is characterized by a progressive sensorimotor neuropathy that can rapidly evolve to tetraplegia over days. Clinical muscle twitching is frequent, and electromyographic findings show myokymia.

NEUROPATHY PRODUCED BY ALIPHATIC CHEMICALS

Solvents

Carbon disulfide, hexane, and methyl-N-butyl ketone are industrial solvents. Carbon disulfide toxicity was once frequent in rayon workers but is now rare. Hexane and methyl-N-butyl ketone are inhaled for pleasure by some adolescents and cause subacute or chronic symmetric neuropathy, frequently with prominent weakness of proximal and distal limb muscles. Symptoms may worsen for several weeks after exposure is discontinued, but recovery eventually occurs. Nerve biopsy shows focal dilations of axons that are filled with neurofilaments. Paranodal retraction of myelin caused by these "axonal balloons" is believed responsible for the considerable slowing of nerve conduction velocities.

Other Chemicals

Tri-ortho-cresyl phosphate ("ginger jake"), an adulterant used in illegal liquor (moonshine) and as a cooking oil contaminant, has been responsible for epidemics of neuropathy. Symmetric distal, primarily motor, polyneuropathy is seen, which progresses over 2 to 3 weeks, causing confusion with amyotrophic lateral sclerosis. Furthermore, in the later stages, upper motor neuron findings appear. However, electrophysiologic studies show axonal loss in both motor and sensory nerves. Nerve biopsy shows distal axonal fragmentation. As the neuropathy clears, evidence of previously unrecognized irreversible damage to corticospinal tracts may become apparent, and late spasticity is common.

Acrylamide monomer is used to prepare polyacrylamide. It is used in chemical laboratories and to treat liquid sewage. Exposure produces a distal sensorimotor neuropathy that may be associated with trophic skin changes and a mild organic dementia. Nerve biopsy shows axonal degeneration with accumulations of neurofilaments in affected axons.

INJURIES TO PERIPHERAL NERVES

The anatomic basis and the clinical syndromes of the many sites of trauma as a cause of peripheral neuropathy have been detailed in Chapter 34. What follows emphasizes the various sites and causes to roots, plexuses, and individual nerves.

Median Nerve

A supracondylar bony spur with a ligament spanning between the spur and the lateral epicondyle can compress the median nerve, causing dysfunction in all median innervated muscles (ligament of Struthers syndrome). Compression of the nerve in the pronator muscle can cause aching of the forearm, particularly during pronation and supination movements (pronator syndrome). Denervation on needle electromyography can be seen in median innervated forearm muscles distal to the pronator teres. However, these muscles may often be normal. The existence of this syndrome has been questioned because of the frequent finding of median nerve compression in cadavers that had no symptoms of pronator teres syndrome. Also in the forearm, the anterior interosseous nerve may be injured by trauma or by compression of the pronator teres or flexor digitorum superficialis. A variant of brachial plexitis may also appear as an isolated anterior interosseous nerve lesion.

After giving off the anterior interosseous nerve, the median nerve continues in the forearm to pass under the transverse carpal ligament along with the long flexor tendons, lying between the tendons of the flexor carpi radialis and flexor digitorum superficialis. In the wrist, entrapment of the median nerve beneath the transverse carpal ligament site is the basis of carpal tunnel syndrome, the most common entrapment neuropathy. Median nerve entrapment at the wrist is usually caused by hypertrophy of the flexor retinaculum. Although this may occur without cause, it is often associated with particular occupations that require repeated wrist flexion and extension, such as jack hammer operators, secretaries and keyboard operators, carpenters, and housewives. It affects women more than men, and although symptoms usually occur in the dominant hand first, disease is found bilaterally in up to 40 percent of patients. Other causes of median nerve entrapment include tenosynovitis associated with rheumatoid arthritis, hypothyroidism, acromegaly, multiple myeloma, amyloidosis, pregnancy, ganglia, and tophi from gout. Carpal tunnel syndrome may be the presenting sign of generalized neuropathies, such as diabetes, and may occur because of an inherited tendency to develop pressure palsies (tomaculous neuropathy). The diagnosis is best established through electromyography and nerve conduction studies. Specialized conduction studies enabling isolation of conduction through the carpal tunnel increase the diagnostic sensitivity as do conduction studies of the dual innervated digit 4. Differential diagnosis is rarely difficult, but cervical radiculopathy (C6 and C7 levels), and the neurogenic thoracic outlet syndrome should be considered. For carpal tunnel syndrome, treatment should be directed to the cause, whether it is medical (hypothyroid, acromegaly, myeloma, and so forth) or surgical (ligamentous hypertrophy). Although conservative therapy is available (wrist splinting and steroid injection), surgical treatment is so refined and recuperation is so short that few patients with established disease should not have surgery. The most common reason for failed response to surgery is probably a wrong preoperative diagnosis.

Ulnar Nerve

The ulnar nerve is most often entrapped in the region of the elbow; however, entrapment at the wrist may also occur and cause some diagnostic confusion. Compression at the elbow is the second most common cause of nerve compression. The nerve may be injured by chronic stretch and trauma around a cubitus valgus deformity or previous trauma to the lateral epicondyle. It may also be compressed in the aponeurosis between the two heads of the flexor carpi ulnaris (cubital tunnel syndrome). Because surgical treatment is different for both of the sites of compression, it is important to differentiate between the two sites of compression preoperatively with electrodiagnostic studies. The nerve passes through the wrist through Guyon's canal where compression distal to Guyon's canal causes a pure motor syndrome of wasting of hand intrinsic muscles, sparing the hypothenar muscles and sensation. Ulnar nerve compression may occur at the wrist in bicyclists and those with amyloidosis; the neuropathy causes wasting and weakness of small hand muscles that may be confused with amyotrophic lateral sclerosis, thoracic outlet syndrome, cervical radiculopathy, syringomyelia, and lower trunk brachial plexopaties.

Radial Nerve

Trauma is a common cause of radial neuropathy, especially in conjunction with fractures of the distal third of the humerus. Spontaneous recovery is the rule (up to 95 percent). Some systemic diseases have a predilection for the radial nerve (wrist drop), including lead intoxication, polyarteritis nodosa, diabetes mellitus, and leprosy.

The most common sites of compressive radial neuropathy are at the humeral head, proximal or at the spiral groove (Saturday night palsy), or after pressure from a crutch at this site. Compression of the radial nerve in the arm may be caused by tourniquets, and in the forearm, the superficial sensory nerves can be compressed by tight watchbands or handcuffs. The purely sensory syndrome of pain and paresthesias from dysfunction of the radial sensory nerve is called cheiralgia paresthetica. Entrapment of the posterior interosseous branch of the radial nerve in the vicinity of the elbow can produce chronic pain and tenderness, which is difficult to differentiate from tennis elbow (lateral epicondylitis), but in the former condition, the hallmark finding is pain over the posterior interosseous nerve, not over the lateral epicondyle.

Musculocutaneous Nerve

Injury to the muculocutaneous nerve is uncommon, but excessive stretching during surgery and after heavy exercise has been reported.

Axillary Nerve

Axillary nerve injury often occurs during shoulder trauma or dislocation and fractures of the neck of the humerus.

Suprascapular Nerve

Suprascapular nerve injury causes weakness of shoulder abduction (supraspinatus) and external rotation (infraspinatus). The injury most often occurs from falls during downward traction of the shoulder. Entrapment can occur in the suprascapular notch, and selective weakness of the infraspinatus can occur from suprascapular injury at the spinoglenoid notch or from ganglion cysts.

Long Thoracis Nerve

The long thoracic nerve is subject to trauma during tennis, knapsack carrying, direct trauma, stretch injury during surgery, or even maintenance of a particular position during sleep. It may also occur as an isolated manifestation of brachial plexitis (see below). Scapular winging also occurs as a result of trapezius weakness from a spinal accessory nerve neuropathy. This neuropathy usually causes drooping of the shoulders and scapular winging. However, the scapular winging associated with trapezius weakness is accentuated by abduction, not forward flexion.

Brachial Plexopathy

The most common cause of brachial plexopathy is trauma, either direct because of its superfical location, or from stretch or traction injuries. Postoperative brachial plexopathy is common because of the susceptibility of the brachial plexus to stretch injuries during operative positioning. Such injuries complicate 5 to 15 percent of postoperative periods in patients undergoing open heart surgery. The specific cause is usually not identifiable. It is also a risk in patients undergoing surgery for thoracic outlet syndrome (see below).

Thoracic Outlet Syndrome

Compressive lesions of the brachial plexus are rare, but one that is frequently cited is thoracic outlet syndrome. The incidence of true neurogenic thoracic outlet syndrome has been estimated to be 1 per 1,000,000. Many patients lack the classic physical and electrophysiologic findings of thoracic outlet syndrome. Such patients may be considered to have disputed thoracic outlet syndrome. In these patients, the pathologic condition is less well defined, and physiologic study results are usually normal. Surgical intervention should be reserved for patients with objective evidence, establishing the presence of true neurogenic thoracic outlet syndrome. The characteristic electrophysiologic findings consist of low motor-evoked responses in the APB with normal sensory-evoked response amplitude; low amplitude ulnar sensory-evoked response with lesser affected motor response from the ADM; and fibrillations and positive sharp waves with neurogenic motor units in the ADM and APB. This syndrome is called true neurogenic thoracic outlet syndrome. The treatment for true neurogenic thoracic outlet syndrome is surgical removal of the rib and compressive fibrous band.

Radiation-induced Plexopathy

Irradiation for carcinoma may cause damage to nervous tissue and more often so after the introduction of high-voltage therapy. Radiogenic lesions of the brachial plexus may be encountered after treatment for breast cancer or lymphoma. The initial symptoms are usually severe pain followed by paresthesias and sensory loss. They may occur after a latent period of 12 to 20 months, although in milder cases, several years may elapse before the symptoms appear. Motor deficits reach a peak many months later. Long latent intervals of up to 20 years have been reported. The nerve damage may affect a single peripheral nerve initially and then progress slowly to involve more nerves. Clinically, tendinous reflexes disappear before muscle weakness and atrophy become obvious, and fasciculation and myokymia are often prominent features. Electromyographic and conduction studies reveal changes consistent with axonal damage and myokymic discharges are frequent and believed to be helpful in differentiating plexopathy from radiation-induced neuropathy from plexopathy caused by infiltration of the malignancy.

Brachial Plexitis

An autoimmune reaction or an infectious agent has been suggested as the cause of this syndrome, but the etiologic agent is obscure in most instances. Some cases have been described in small epidemics among military personnel and, occasionally, after intravenous heroin administration.

The typical electromyographic findings, including motor and sensory nerve studies, are consistent with a predominantly axonal type of involvement, although demyelination may play a role in rare instances. The diversity of affection of different nerves and even within the same nerve can be accounted for by assuming involvement of the terminal nerve twigs or patchy damage of discrete bundles of fibers within the cords or trunks of the brachial plexus or its branches. Recovery depends on the degree of the initial involvement. It is considered good in about two-thirds, fair in one-fifth, and poor in approximately one-sixth. Clinical recovery may take 2 months to 3 years.

MONONEUROPATHIES OF THE LOWER LIMB

Lateral Femoral Cutaneous Nerve

The lateral femoral cutaneous nerve originates from the second and third lumbar nerves and supplies sensation to the anterolateral and lateral portions of the thigh. It passes into the thigh under the lateral edge of the inguinal ligament, just distal to the anterior iliac spine. The most common site of entrapment is at the lateral edge of the inguinal ligament. There is usually no etiology but it occurs most often in pregnancy or obese patients. Wearing tight belts may also predispose to compression of this nerve. Compression of this nerve by pelvic tumors or hematomas is rare. The numbness that results from compression may be particularly painful, explaining the name of the resulting clinical syndrome meralgia paresthetica (see Ch. 32).

Obturator Nerve

The origin of the obturator nerve is from the second, third, and fourth lumbar nerves, the same roots that compose the femoral nerve. It winds around the pelvic cavity and exits through the obturator foramen to supply the thigh adductors (adductor longus, brevis, and adductor magnus). It supplies sensation to a small area of skin on the medial portion of the proximal thigh. Injuries are rare. It may be injured during labor, hip dislocation, or during hip replacement. Pelvic malignancies may also invade the nerve.

Ilioinguinal, Iliohypogastric, and Genitofemoral Nerves

These nerves supply the skin to the inguinal region, part of the genitalia, and upper and medial thigh. They arise from the upper lumbar plexus containing fibers from T12, L1, and L2. The ilioinguinal nerve innervates the inguinal region and base of the scrotum or labia. The genitofemoral nerve is often injured during appendectomy or from adhesions. Its injury produces pain in the inguinal ring with sensory impairment in the femoral triangle. Hip flexion relieves compression of both nerves. Injury to the iliohypogastric nerve usually occurs during surgery in the lower quadrant and produces minimal sensory deficit in the suprapubic region.

Femoral Nerve

The femoral nerve originates from the lumbar plexus (lumbar roots 2, 3, and 4) within the psoas muscle. The psoas muscle is innervated by direct branches of the plexus just proximal to the origin of the femoral nerve, from the L2 and L3 roots. In the abdomen it gives a branch to the iliacus before emerging from the pelvis beneath the inguinal ligament, lateral to the femoral artery. It then divides into the anterior division, supplying sensation to the anterior thigh and innervating the sartorius muscles, and posterior division, which supplies motor innervation to the quadriceps muscle (vastus medialis, vastus lateralis, rectus femoris, and vastus intermedius). It continues as the saphenous nerve, which supplies sensory innervation to the medial side of the leg to the medial malleolus.

The femoral nerve may be damaged by direct trauma, intrapelvic tumors, aneurysms, abscess, and fractures. Procedures requiring protracted and extreme hip abduction have been associated with femoral neuropathy. Femoral nerve injury within the pelvis produces weakness of hip flexion because of involvement of the iliacus muscle. Prominent hip flexion weakness implicates iliopsoas involvement and plexus injury. Diabetes is often associated with proximal leg weakness and pain resembling femoral neuropathy, often bilateral. However, careful clinical and electrodiagnostic studies suggest more extensive involvement more compatible with a plexus involvement.

The prominent clinical deficit seen in femoral nerve injuries is weakness of knee extension and loss of the quadriceps reflex.

Sciatic Nerve

The sciatic nerve originates from fibers from the lower portions of the lumbosacral plexus fibers containing the L4, L5, and S1 and S2 nerve roots. It is formed by two physically separable trunks (the medial, which becomes the tibial nerve, and the lateral, which becomes the peroneal). The two trunks separate just proximal to the popliteal fossa. All hamstring muscles (semitendinosis, semimembranosus, biceps, [long head], adductor magnus, and biceps [short head]) are supplied by the medial trunk of the sciatic nerve except for the short head of the biceps. The sensory innervation of the sciatic nerve is along the posterior thigh, the posterior and lateral aspects of the leg, and the sole of the foot. In lesions of the sciatic nerve, the Achilles reflex is lost. Most injuries are caused by fracture-dislocations of the hip and complications of hip replacement procedures. Vasculitis, injection of toxic substances into the lower gluteal region, tumors, cysts, and trauma from stabbing or gunshots may injure the sciatic nerve. Weakness of gluteal muscles suggests a more proximal plexus localization.

Superior and Inferior Gluteal Nerves

The gluteal nerves branch from the plexus just proximal to the sciatic nerve. The superior gluteal nerve contains fibers from L4, L5, and S1 and innervates the gluteus medius. The inferior contains fibers from L5, S1, and S2 and innervates the gluteus maximus. The gluteal nerves may be damaged by misplaced injections but they are most helpful in differentiating plexus from sciatic nerve lesions.

Posterior Cutaneous Nerve of the Thigh and the Pudendal Nerve

These nerves arise from the lower plexus containing S1, S2, and S3 roots (posterior cutaneous nerve) and S2, S3, and S4 (pudendal) roots. The posterior cutaneous nerve supplies the skin of the lower buttock and posterior thigh. Lesions are rare but have occurred from injections and prolonged cycling. The pudendal nerve supplies the external anal sphincter, perineum muscles, erectile tissue of the penis, and external urethral sphincter. It also supplies the skin of the penis and labia majora. It can be damaged by injections, cycling, and as a result of complications from hip surgery.

Common Peroneal Nerve

Just above the popliteal fossa the sciatic nerve separates into the peroneal and tibial division. Just distal to the bifurcation, the common peroneal nerve gives off the branch to the short head of the biceps, a useful anatomic fact when attempting to separate peroneal neuropathies at the fibular head from sciatic neuropathy and L5 radiculopathy. It descends in the popliteal fossa and winds around the fibular head, where it divides into the superficial and deep branches. The superficial innervates the peroneal longus and brevis and continues as the superficial peroneal (sensory) nerve, supplying skin of the distal lateral leg and dorum of the foot. The deep peroneal nerve supplies the dorsiflexors, the tibialis anterior, and extensor hallicus longus, and terminates in a sensory branch that supplies the skin between the first and second toes.

The common peroneal nerve is vulnerable to compression at the fibular head. This occurs during protracted periods of knee crossing, prolonged bed rest during coma or during immobility of other reasons, and from wearing plaster casts and leg braces; there may be no obvious cause. Patients with hereditary tendency to pressure palsies may be especially vulnerable. It may also be compressed by ganglia, cysts, tumors, or lipomas.

Tibial Nerve

The other division of the sciatic nerve is the tibial nerve. It passes through the popliteal fossa into the leg deep to the gastrocnemius muscle. It gives off branches to the calf muscles that plantar flex the foot, such as the gastrocnemius and soleus muscles. The sural nerve is formed by branches from the tibial and peroneal nerves and supplies the lateral aspect of the foot.

The tibial nerve enters the foot by winding around the medial malleolus. In the foot the nerve separates into the medial and lateral plantar nerves. Compression of the tibial nerve at the ankle (tarsal tunnel syndrome) produces pain and paresthesias in the distribution of one or both branches. Interdigital nerves may be compressed between adjacent metatarsal heads, stretched by crossing ligaments, or compressed by small tumors (Morton's neuroma). Focal pain is the most common symptom and the third metatarsal space is the most frequently involved.

LUMBOSACRAL PLEXOPATHY

The lumbosacral plexus is formed by the ventral nerve roots from L1 through S3. The many different causes of lumbosacral plexus disease include tumor infiltration, compression by tumors and other masses, hemorrhage, aneurysms, radiation, and complications of pregnancy. The clinical syndromes are defined by muscle weakness implying plexus involvement beyond the distribution of single peripheral nerves or roots. The weakness is typically unilateral and is exacerbated by flexion of the hip in sciatic lesions and extension of the hip in femoral lesions.

Lumbar Plexitis

Lumbar plexitis is a clinical diagnosis; it is a diagnosis of exclusion. Lumbar plexitis is similar to brachial plexitis (see above). It begins with severe back and leg pain and is followed by weakness, sensory loss, and reflex changes. Immunosuppressive medication may be helpful.

Electrodiagnostic findings help certify plexus involvement from any of the various causes, and may demonstrate abnormalities when the plexus involvement is not evident by clinical findings. One feature separating plexus and nerve disease is the presence of sensory nerve action potential, which is missing in lumbosacral plexus lesions.

DRUG-INDUCED NEUROPATHIES

There are many medications currently in use that may cause peripheral neuropathy as a side effect. Sometimes the neuropathy may be the limiting factor of treatment. For example, patients with HIV infection receiving dideoxycytosine (ddC) may be unable to continue treatment because of disabling symptoms from the neuropathy. Vinca alkaloids such as vincristine and vinblastine cause a peripheral neuropathy that may limit their use in needed cancer therapy. Cisplatin is another antineoplastic treatment use of which is complicated by peripheral nerve impairment (primarily sensory neuropathy with ataxia).

Other medications that are complicated by neuropathy, usually of the sensorimotor type and axonal in nature, include phenytoin, disulfiram, gold, dapsone (motor neuropathy), and thalidomide. Isoniazid causes a sensorimotor peripheral neuropathy, often with prominent muscle cramps. It antagonizes the effects of B6 and is prevented by simultaneous administration of B6. However, large doses of B6 will cause a sensory neuropathy with prominent ataxia.

IMMUNOLOGICALLY-MEDIATED PERIPHERAL NEUROPATHIES

Although the particular event stimulating the immune response is not certain, some neuropathies are caused by an immune attack directed against some component of peripheral nerve. Therapies that modulate the immune system are frequently effective.

Guillain-Barré Syndrome

First described by Landry (J. B. O. Landry, French physician, 1826–1865) in 1859 as an acute ascending paralysis, the syndrome was more completely described by Georges Guillain, J. A. Barré, and A. Strohl in 1916, who noted changes in tendon reflexes and cerebrospinal fluid content (see below). This syndrome is now known as the Guillain-Barré syndrome, although many still refer to it as Landry's ascending paralysis. How Strohl's name came to be omitted is uncertain.

The cause of Guillain-Barré syndrome is uncertain. Many of the clinical and neuropathologic features (see below) are reproduced in the animal model of experimental allergic neuritis induced by immunizing animals with P2 protein and galactocerebroside protein from peripheral nerve. The ganglioside GM1 is suspected to be the target of immunologic attack in some forms of Guillain-Barré syndrome as well as some

forms of pure motor neuropathy. Thirty percent of patients with the axonal form of the disease have immunoglobulin G (IgG) forms of antibodies to GM1; of these, 50 percent have evidence of *Campylobacter jejunii* infection, which has shown cross reactivity. One form of acute paralysis found in China is associated with *Campylobacter* infection in more than 90 percent of affected children. However, direct correlation with anti-GM1 titers and disease activity has not been observed.

Guillian-Barré syndrome occurs at an incidence of 2 per 100,000 population. It affects all age groups but the average age of onset is 40 years. There is a slight male preponderance. Although no proof has emerged of a seasonal variation, some studies have shown clustering in autumn and winter. More than 50 percent of patients report a previous respiratory or gastrointestinal infection. Antecedent infections frequently associated with Guillian-Barré syndrome include cytomegalovirus, Epstein-Barr virus, *Campylobacter jejunii*, *Mycoplasma pneumoniae*, measles, varicella, and possibly influenza. *Campylobacter* infection may predispose individuals to a particularly severe Guillain-Barré syndrome. Coexisting diseases include HIV, hepatitis, and Hodgkin's disease. A syndrome indistinguisable from Guillain-Barré syndrome occurs after use of rabies vaccine prepared from desiccated spinal cord and nerve roots from rabbits.

The most prominent clinical manifestation of Guillain-Barré syndrome is weakness. Areflexia is an early finding. Usually preceded by paresthesias in the hands or feet, the weakness often progresses day by day. It begins in the legs, with patients experiencing difficulty in weight-bearing and hip flexion and extension (e.g., in climbing stairs and getting up from chairs); such symptoms are quickly followed by hand and arm weakness. Impaired breathing occurs in 50 percent of patients; 25 percent require mechanical ventilation. Cranial nerve involvement is frequent, usually manifesting as bifacial weakness, a clinical feature rare in other neuropathies. Ophthalmoparesis occurs in 10 percent of patients, some of whom have pupillary abnormalities.

Pure sensory and pure autonomic forms occur but are uncommon. Sensory involvement is minimal although painful paresthesias may be prominent sequelae. Besides respiratory failure, autonomic insufficiency is the most common cause of death. This is manifested as blood pressure lability, postural hypotension, supraventricular tachycardia, and bradycardia.

Laboratory abnormalities show the characteristic albuminocytologic dissociation in the cerebrospinal fluid by the first week, usually well established within 7 to 14 days after initial onset. By dissociation is meant an elevation of protein (often over 200 mg/dl) with no accompanying increase in cell counts. Pleocytosis is unusual enough that its presence should cause consideration of another diagnosis, or Guillain-Barré syndrome with coexisting Lyme disease or HIV infection.

Electrophysiologic findings of peripheral nerves and muscles are often normal, reflecting the proximal nature of the disease (polyradiculoneuropathy). The most common finding is conduction block in proximal nerve segments. F responses may be absent or prolonged. Distal motor latencies are often prolonged, particularly in the median nerve. Biopsy of the sural nerve shows few abnormalities. Teased fiber studies often show segmental demyelination.

The course of the illness is variable, with weakness progressing at a variable pace over hours to days, but is often rapid, resulting in respiratory arrest within days of onset. Progression stops in 50 percent of patients within 2 weeks, and in 90 percent in 4 weeks. Progression continuing longer than 6 weeks should prompt reassessment of the diagnosis.

Plasmapheresis shortens the time of recovery if given within 2 weeks of symptom onset. Intravenous immunoglobulin may also be effective, but relapses may be a common complication. Apart from these attempts to shorten the course, the most important is treatment directed against complications. Subcutaneous injection of heparin and the wearing of elastic stockings should provide prophylaxis against thromboembolism. Patients with autonomic instability require electrocardiograph monitoring, and some require pacemaker placement to prevent the consequences of associated arrhythmias. Physical therapy, at least passive range of motion exercise, should be employed early in the course of the illness.

Despite maximal treatment, 5 percent of patients with Guillain-Barré syndrome die in the acute phase of the illness. Poor prognostic signs include advanced age, initially rapid evolution, ventilator dependence, and severe loss of motor evoked response amplitudes from peripheral nerve stimulation. Among the survivors, 60 percent make full functional recovery, the remainder showing some residual deficit. Ten percent are left with a severe deficit. Recurrence of Guillain-Barré syndrome occurs in 3 to 5 percent of patients.

Miller Fisher Syndrome

Miller Fisher syndrome, one of the variants of Guillain-Barré syndrome, consists of acute onset of ophthalmoparesis, ataxia, and generalized loss of reflexes. Clinical overlap with other features of Guillain-Barré syndrome may occur. The spinal fluid shows albuminocytologic dissociation (i.e., protein is increased without pleocytosis). Electrodiagnostic studies show axonal changes with low evoked response amplitudes and normal motor and sensory nerve conduction velocities. Sensory nerve evoked responses may be absent.

The clinical features occasionally make differential diagnosis between Miller Fisher syndrome and brainstem encephalitis difficult. Brainstem encephalitis is characterized by an abnormal MRI evaluation of the brainstem and by abnormal evoked potentials.

Miller Fisher syndrome seems to be associated with antibodies to GQ1b. Plasmapheresis and immunoglobulin have been reported to be effective in uncontrolled trials.

Chronic Inflammatory Demyelinating Neuropathy

Separated from Guillain-Barré syndrome primarily by the time course, chronic inflammatory demyelinating neuropathy (CIDP) is a diffuse sensorimotor polyneuropathy that is thought to be immunologically mediated. It, too, occurs in all age groups with a slight predominance in men. A previous infection is found to have occurred in 30 percent of patients.

The syndrome is defined using clinical and electrophysiologic criteria. It is a progressive symmetric polyneuropathy, typically evolving over longer than 8 weeks, affecting both motor and sensory nerves of the limbs, but rarely involving cranial nerves (ophthalmoparesis, facial weakness, or bulbar nerve signs). The characteristic symptoms are weakness, sensory loss, and paresthesias. An irregular tremor is frequently seen. Proximal and distal limb weakness is usually evident and hypo- or areflexia is necessary, although there are rare reports of concomitant CNS involvement. The course is progressive in approximately two-thirds of CIDP patients; in one-third of patients the course is stepwise or relapsing.

The CSF protein level is elevated without significant pleocytosis (usually less than $5/mm^3$ and not more than $50/mm^3$). On electrophysiologic testing, motor and sensory conduction velocity are lower than 80 percent of the lower limit of normal with temporal dispersion and conduction block. Sural nerve biopsy results show both axonal and demyelinating changes. Rarely hypertrophic (onion bulb) formations are observed. Teased fiber preparations show segmental demyelination. Inflammatory cell infiltrates are sometimes found in the endoneurium.

Immunosuppression is usually effective. Response occurs to steroids (1 to 1.5 mg/kg/day). Anecdotal reports have indicated success using intravenous immunoglobulin (2 gm/kg over 1 week) but the clinical improvement rarely lasts more than 8 weeks. Plasmapheresis may also be effective.

Paraproteinemic Neuropathy

Ten percent of patients with peripheral neuropathy have a circulating monoclonal protein (M-protein). M-proteins are the result of a proliferation of a single clone of plasma cells that secrete an antibody in blood, urine, or both. They consist of a single heavy chain, from either immunoglobulin M (IgM), IgG, IgA, or IgD, and a single light chain κ or λ.

The M-protein may be directed against specific antigens, often having activity against specific idiotypes. Patients with M-proteins often have low total γ globulin levels, elevated α_2-globulins, and a low albumin level. A sensitive test for an M-protein is immunofixation electrophoresis, allowing separation by light chain subtypes. Monoclonal light chains (Bence Jones proteins) can be seen in urine, particularly in multiple myeloma, light chain amyloidosis and γ-heavy-chain disease.

In some patients with peripheral neuropathy, often those with pure motor neuropathies, M-proteins are found to have activity against ganglioside antibodies (GM1).

The medical condition most commonly associated with an M-protein is multiple myeloma. Many other patients with M-proteins are eventually found to have lymphoma, amyloidosis, Waldenstrom's macroglobulinemia, osteosclerotic myeloma, or γ-heavy-chain disease. In myeloma patients, peripheral neuropathy occurs in less than 5 percent of cases; it is usually axonal in nature, involving both sensory and motor fibers. Other patients have amyloid neuropathy. Patients with osteosclerotic myeloma have a distinctive demyelinating sensorimotor neuropathy that sometimes occurs in association with organomegaly, endocrinopathy, and skin disease (POEMS). Radiation therapy of the bone lesions and chemotherapy is often effective.

M-proteins are found in some patients with cryoglobulins. The neuropathy in cryoglobulinemia is usually a sensorimotor stocking and glove type of neuropathy with axonal features. Most, however, have no underlying disease (monoclonal gammopathy of undetermined significance).

Monoclonal Gammopathy of Uncertain Significance

Although by definition patients with monoclonal gammopathy of uncertain significance (MGUS) have no other identifiable disease at the time of diagnosis, almost 20 percent are eventually diagnosed as having a plasma cell dyscrasia. The clinical syndrome associated with IgM-associated neuropathies is characterized by sensory loss, sometimes severe enough to lead to ataxia. Nerve thickening is sometimes observed. CSF protein levels may be elevated and nerve biopsy results show axonal and demyelinating features; immunostaining of the nerve often shows the M-protein.

Of patients with IgM MGUS without an underlying disorder, 50 percent show activity against myelin-associated glycoprotein (MAG). Patients with anti-MAG neuropathy have slowing of sensory and motor conduction velocity to less than 30 m/s in the arms and 20 m/s in the legs, compatible with a demyelinating neuropathy.

Patients with MGUS but with no evidence of anti-MAG activity also show demyelinating features during nerve conduction studies. Most IgM, MAG-nonreactive patients have chronic axonal neuropathies, and serum rarely reacts with peripheral nerve obtained during biopsy in such patients. In some, the M-protein may react with other nerve antigens. Many will respond to immunosuppressive therapy.

Patients with IgG and IgA M-proteins are rare, but when encountered, they usually have a predominately axonal sensorimotor peripheral neuropathy.

Multifocal Conduction Block Neuropathy

Patients with multifocal motor neuropathy with conduction block (MMNCB) appear as if they have motor neuron disease (amyotrophic lateral sclerosis [ALS]; see Ch. 63). The recognition of this group of patients owes much to the intensive study of patients diagnosed clinically as having ALS and whose electrophysiologic studies revealed conduction block. Like those with ALS, this group of patients develops weakness and wasting of muscles, usually in the arms, with fasciculations; reflexes are often absent in affected nerve territories, but in other territories they are normal or brisk; the clinical course if often protracted.

Antibodies to GM1 are seen in 30 percent of patients. Electrodiagnostic studies show multifocal conduction block, often in proximal nerve segments.

Treatment with intravenous immunoglobulin has been reported to be effective.

VASCULITIC NEUROPATHIES

The characteristic pathologic finding in vasculitis is inflammatory cell infiltration of the blood vessel wall with necrosis. Infarction of the tissues supplied by the affected arteries is usually the cause of the clinical syndromes. Therefore, the clinical manifestations of this pathologic process in the peripheral nervous system is multiple mononeuropathies, often misnamed as "mononeuritis multiplex."

The vasculitides may be divided into systemic forms that also affect peripheral nerve and the nonsystemic vasculitides that affect peripheral nerve exclusively (see also Ch. 38).

Systemic Vasculopathies

Polyarteritis Nodosa

Polyarteritis nodosa is the classic example of systemic vasculitis with prominent peripheral nervous system manifestations. The vasculitis affects small and medium-sized arteries. Renal disease and skin lesions typically accompany the neurologic manifestations. The neuropathy usually occurs as multiple mononeuropathies but cranial neuropathy and brachial plexopathy have also been reported.

Hepatitis B is found in 10 to 50 percent of patients with polyarteritis nodosa. The basis of this relationship is unclear but may be due to the hepatitis B virus forming immune complexes that are deposited within the blood vessel wall, promoting complement deposition with inflammatory cell infiltration and necrosis. Biopsy of the affected nerve shows necrotizing vasculitis.

Treatment with steroids is usually effective. Other immunosuppressive agents and plasmapheresis may also be effective.

Churg-Strauss Syndrome (Allergic Angiitis and Granulomatosis)

The characteristic features of the Churg-Strauss syndrome is asthma, eosinophilia, and peripheral neuropathy, typically of the multiple mononeuropathies type. The pathologic findings are usually identical to those found in polyarteritis nodosa; eosinophil infiltrates are not common. Immunosuppressant medication has been effective.

Connective Tissue Disease

Rheumatoid vasculitis is the second most common cause of vasculitic neuropathy. The manifestations of peripheral nervous system involvement is varied. Most common is a chronic symmetric sensorimotor neuropathy but multiple mononeuropathies, including entrapment neuropathy, also occur. Cranial neuropathy may occur. Elevated sedimentation rate and elevated titers of rheumatoid factor are common. Pathologic findings resemble polyarteritis nodosa with necrotizing vasculitis involving epineural arterioles.

Patients with peripheral nervous system disease in association with systemic lupus erythematosus (SLE) often have distal, symmetric sensorimotor neuropathy. Less often Guillain-Barré syndrome, chronic inflammatory demyelinating peripheral neuropathy, and multiple mononeuropathies occur. Necrotizing vasculitis is not common, but lymphocytic infiltrates around blood vessels are common.

Wegener Granulomatosis

Multiple mononeuropathy and cranial neuropathy are common. Systemic peripheral neuropathy may also occur. Diagnosis is suspected from associated respiratory and renal involvement. Serum autoantibodies to neurotrophil cytoplasmic antigens (ANCA) are common and may mark disease activity.

Sarcoid Neuropathy

For discussion of sarcoid neuropathy, see above.

Nonsystemic Vasculitic Neuropathy

In some patients, vasculitis affects the peripheral nervous system exclusively. Peripheral nerves, plexus, roots, and cranial nerves may be affected. Rarely, such patients have a symmetric, distal sensorimotor peripheral neuropathy. Biopsy of the involved nerve shows inflammatory cell infiltration of the vessel wall in the epineurium or perineurium. However, muscle biopsy shows increased sensitivity in detecting arteritis.

INHERITED NEUROPATHIES

Charcot-Marie-Tooth Disease

Named after the French neurologist J. M. Charcot (1825–1893) and P. Marie (1853–1940) and the British physician H. H. Tooth (1856–1925), Charcot-Marie-Tooth disease (CMT) is a diverse group of inherited neuropathies. The term *hereditary motor and sensory neuropathy* (HMSN) and its subtypes (see below) have been preferred in the past, but recent advances in molecular biology suggest that the basis for future classification may change. There are different modes of inheritance in the forms of CMT including autosomal-dominant and -recessive with variable penetrance. Many instances of familial occurrence may be missed if family members with subclinical involvement are not tested.

In this group of disorders, patients present at any age. Motor and sensory function are usually affected, although the most common presenting sign is peroneal muscular atrophy and foot drop.

Charcot-Marie-Tooth Disease Type I

This is the most common form of CMT, affecting 1 in 2,500 individuals. Inheritance is usually autosomal-dominant. Chromosome studies have proven linkage to the Duffy blood group locus on chromosome 1 (CMT b) and to chromosome 17p11.2-12 (CMT Ia). The molecular basis form the majority of CMT IA patients is DNA duplication in chromosome 17p11.2-12. The duplication can also arise spontaneously. It is possible that peripheral myelin protein 22 gene (PMP-22) maps to this region. Human myelin protein zero gene (Po) has been mapped to the first chromosome making point mutations in this gene attractive candidates for CMT IB. Autosomal-dominant forms of CMT I that map neither to chromosome 1 or 17 are designated CMT IC.

The first clinical manifestation is often pes cavus (from the Latin meaning hollow foot, so named because of the exaggerated depth of the arch of the sole).

Distal foot and leg weakness is usually evident within the first decade of life. Distal wasting of the legs causes them to resemble inverted champagne bottles. Hand weakness and wasting occurs later in the illness. Postural tremor is common. Paresthesias are unusual but loss of all sensory modalities in distal segments of the limbs is common. Loss of ankle reflexes occurs early and most show areflexia later in the disease. Clinically detectable hypertrophic nerves are found in 30 percent of patients.

The electrophysiologic hallmark of CMT I is marked slowing of conduction velocity (30 to 40 m/s in the arms, 20 to 30 m/s in the legs). Distal latencies are prolonged but conduction block is not found. Sensory responses are typically absent in CMT I. Sural nerve biopsy shows hypertrophic onion-bulb changes and reduced density of myelinated fibers.

Charcot-Marie-Tooth Disease Type II

CMT II is less common than type I. For some patients with CMT II the gene locus has been mapped to the short arm of chromosome 1 but this finding has not occurred with all cases, indicating the presence of genetic heterogeneity.

The syndrome begins later in life, usually in the second or third decade but sometimes it first appears in old age. Pes cavus and scoliosis is present but less often than in CMT I. The clinical presentation is usually because of bilateral foot drop but a distal sensorimotor glove and stocking-type distribution evolves. Ankle reflexes are absent. Nerve thickening and enlargement do not occur. Progression is slow, sometimes producing little change over many years.

Motor nerve conduction velocities are normal or borderline slow with low-amplitude evoked responses. Sensory nerve evoked responses are low or absent. The CSF protein level is normal. Nerve biopsy shows axonal loss with no evidence of demyelination but rarely, small hypertrophic onion bulbs are seen.

Dejerine-Sottas Disease

Dejerine-Sottas disease (HMSN III) was described by J. Dejerine (French neurologist, 1849–1917) and J. Sottas (French neurologist, 1866–1943). Inheritance for this distinctive syndrome is often thought to be autosomal-recessive. However, this clinical syndrome has been reported to be associated with a point mutation in Po and P22 genes. There is evidence to suggest that this disorder is actually a heterozygote. Therefore, this disorder may not be distinct from CMT I and assignation of HMSN III seems inappropriate.

The peripheral neuropathy closely resembles CMT I but features enlarged and palpable peripheral nerves. Ataxia may be prominent.

Motor nerve conduction velocity is far slower than in CMT I, often less than 12 m/s. Spinal fluid protein is often increased. Nerve biopsy results may show marked hypertrophy with onion bulbs or hypomyelination, which portends a poor prognosis.

Charcot-Marie-Tooth Disease Type IV

CMT 4 (HMSN IV) is an autosomal-recessive sensorimotor peripheral neuropathy. Some families, but not all, have been mapped to chromosome 8q. Families with axonal change and others with demyelinating change have been reported.

Hereditary Susceptibility to Pressure Palsies

Peripheral nerves may be compressed at specific anatomic sites prone to compression. Examples include the median nerve in the carpal tunnel and the peroneal nerve at the fibular head. In some patients whose disorder is often inherited as an autosomal-dominant trait, symptomatic nerve compression occurs even during only slight compression and does so recurrently. Recurrent brachial plexopathy may also occur. Nerve biopsies often show tomaculous (sausage-shaped) swellings. The molecular basis of this disorder has been assigned to a deletion in chromosome 17p11.2-12, in contrast to the duplication in CMT 1A.

Hereditary Sensory and Autonomic Neuropathies

There are several types of inherited neuropathies affecting small-diameter and nonmyelinated peripheral nerve fibers. Inheritance may be dominant or recessive. Foot ulcers and anhydrosis are common.

Inherited Neuropathies With Identified Metabolic Defects

Adrenoleukodystrophy

Adrenoleukodystrophy is an X-linked inherited defect of very long chain fatty acids (VLCFAs). The diagnostic abnormality is abnormally elevated levels of VLCFAs. The clinical syndrome is usually localizable to the spinal cord with peripheral nerve involvement (adrenomyeloneuropathy).

Fabry Disease

Fabry disease is an X-linked peripheral neuropathy affecting small fibers. The disease, described by J. Fabry (German dermatologist, 1860–1930), begins in childhood or early adult life with burning pain and paresthesiae. A maculopapular rash is present in a bathing suit distribution. Stroke, hypertension, renal disease, and corneal opacification are common. The diagnosis is revealed by low levels of blood leukocyte lysosomal alpha galactosidase.

Porphyric Neuropathy

Porphyric neuropathy is part of an autosomal-dominant disorder. Peripheral neuropathy often develops in acute intermittent and variegate porphyria and less often in hereditary coproporphyria and δ-aminolevulinic acid dehydrase. The clinical features of all four disorders are similar with attacks of muscle weakness, often precipitated by drugs, particularly barbiturates. The distribution of weakness may be symmetric and proximal, affecting arms more than legs, or asymmetric. A generalized quadriparesis may be present. Tendon reflexes are reduced or absent. Sensory loss is minimal. Cranial nerves are often affected, particularly bulbar dysfunction. Autonomic dysfunction is also common.

Refsum's Disease

Refsum's disease is an autosomal-recessive disorder caused by deficiency of phytanic acid. It is sometimes referred to as hereditary motor and sensory neuropathy, type 4. Clinical manifestations include retinitis pigmentosa, cerebellar ataxia, and chronic polyneuropathy with increased blood serum phytanic acid. Cardiomyopathy, pupillary abnormalities, cataracts, deafness, ichthyosis, anosmia, and night blindness and also associated with the disorder. Nerve biopsy shows hypertropic changes, although they are usually not clinically palpable. CSF protein is often increased.

Metachromatic Leukodystrophy

Metachromatic leukodystrophy (MLD) (sulfatide lipidosis) is an autosomal-recessive disease caused by deficiency of arylsulfatase causing accumulation of sulfatide throughout the peripheral and central nervous systems. Clinically, hypotonia, loss of reflexes, and demyelinating changes are seen on sensory and motor nerve conduction studies. Cerebral involvement is common. MLD is characterized by demyelination in peripheral and central nervous systems. It is associated with arylsufatase deficiency.

Tangier Disease

Tangier disease, a rare autosomal-recessive disease described in families from Tangier Island, Virginia, is characterized by a deficiency of high-density lipoprotein, low cholesterol, low phospholipids, and high triglycerides. Enlarged yellow (cholesterol-laden) tonsils are a constant finding. Sensory loss is primarily small fiber with loss of pain and temperature sensation. The loss of sensation occurs over all aspects of the body, particularly the trunk. Weakness also affects proximal muscles, especially in the arms. Tendon reflexes are often preserved.

Abetalipoproteinemia

Abetalipoproteinemia (Bassen-Kornzweig disease) features sensorimotor peripheral neuropathy coexisting with ataxia, retinitis pigmentosa, fat malabsorption, and acanthocytes in peripheral blood. The disease is due to an autosomal-recessive disorder associated with a defect in absorption of fat-soluble vitamins. Vitamin E therapy may halt progression and produce improvement.

Amyloid Neuropathy

Amyloidosis is caused by deposits of proteins that characteristically produce apple-green birefringence after being stained with congo-red dye and viewed in a polarizing light. The proteins vary in composition but all assume the configuration of a β-pleated sheet. In types I, II, and IV familial amyloidosis, the deposited proteins are the result of single amino acid substitutions into transthyretin (pre-albumin). In type III, the deposited abnormal protein results from an amino acid substitution in apolipoprotein A1. In primary amyloidosis, immunoglobulin light chains usually derived from plasma cell tumors accumulate in tissues.

In familial amyloidosis, numbness and loss of pain and temperature in a stocking glove distribution is typical. Trophic ulcers and severe pain is common. Loss of reflexes and distal weakness occurs later in the illness. Autonomic neuropathy is common and manifested as orthostatic hypotension, impotence, impaired intestinal motility, and pupillary abnormalities. Type II familial amyloidosis often presents with carpal tunnel syndrome due to amyloid deposition. Transthyretin amyloidosis may improve after after liver transplant.

Peripheral neuropathy occurs in one-third of patients with primary amyloidosis. Associated paraproteinemia and free light chains in the urine (Bence-Jones proteins) are frequent. The paraproteinemia may be benign or associated with an underlying lymphoproliferative disorder. Hypernephroma may also occur. Initial symptoms are usually sensory with loss of pain and temperature sensation. Autonomic symptoms are common. Muscle weakness and reflex loss are not prominent. Electrophysiologic findings reveal an axonal neuropathy.

Inherited Neuropathies Without Identified Metabolic Defect

Giant Axonal Neuropathy

Giant axonal neuropathy features a sensorimotor neuropathy typically beginning in childhood, often accompanied by ataxia resembling spinocerebellar degeneration. Most affected children have abnormally curly hair. Electrodiagnostic findings are axonal in nature.

Chédiak-Higashi Syndrome

Chédiak-Higashi syndrome is a rare autosomal-dominant disorder characterized by mental retardation and peripheral neuropathy.

Familial Multiple Symmetric Lipomatosis

Familial multiple symmetric lipomatosis is an autosomal-recessive syndrome characterized by the development of large symmetric lipoma on the back neck, shoulders, and upper limb. Electrodiagnostic studies show an axonal neuropathy.

CRITICAL ILLNESS POLYNEUROPATHY

Severe sensorimotor peripheral neuropathy complicates the clinical course of many patients who are critically ill, with sepsis and multiple organ failure. Although this disorder may be suspected from the clinical state, it is usually suspected when patients have difficulty being weaned from ventilators. Electrodiagnostic studies show a severe sensorimotor axonal neuropathy, but some pathologic studies have shown little axonal loss and extensive type 1 and 2 fiber atrophy. Such muscular atrophy might occur because of pharmacologic denervation or treatment with other medications capable of interfering with neuromuscular transmission. Recovery of neuronal function may occur if the underlying cause of the multiple organ failure is successfully treated. The cause of this condition is unknown, but a dietary deficiency is not considered a candidate. Many patients with respirator dependence with critically ill neuropathy have received neuromuscular blocking agents, which some authors believe may be involved in causing this neuruopathy. Mononeuritis or mononeuritis multiplex occurs in 2 percent of patients with bacterial endocarditis because of septic emboli to peripheral nerves. Some patients with bacterial endocarditis may experience a severe axonal neuropathy, thought to be similar to the axonopathy seen in patients with critically ill polyneuropathy.

BIBLIOGRAPHY

Adams CR, Ziegler DK, Lin JT. Mercury intoxication simulating amyotrophic lateral sclerosis. JAMA 1983;250: 642–63.

Albers JW, Allen AA, Bastron JA, Daube JR. Limb myokymia. Muscle Nerve 1981;4:494–504.

Albers JW, Kelly JJ. Acquired inflammatory demyelinating polyneuropathies: clinical and electrodiagnostic features. Muscle Nerve 1989;12:435–51.

Asbury AK. Renal failure, hepatic disorders, respiratory insufficiency, and critical illness. In Dyck PJ, Thomas PK, Griffin JW et al. (eds). Peripheral Neuropathy. WB Saunders, Philadelphia, 1993, pp. 1251–65.

Behar R, Wiley C, McCutchan JA. Cytomegalovirus polyradiculopathy in AIDS. Neurology 1987;37:557–61.

Bird TD, Ott J, Giblett ER. Evidence for linkage of Charcot Marie Tooth neuropathy to the Duffy locus on chromosome 1. Am J Hum Genet 1982;34:388–94.

Bolton CF. Peripheral neuropathies associated with chronic renal failure. Can J Neurol Sci 1980;7:89–96.

Bolton CF, Gilbert JJ, Hahn AF, Sibbald WJ. Polyneuropathy in critically ill patients. J Neurol Neurosurg Psychiatry 1984;47:1223–31.

Bolton CF, Laverty DA, Brown JD et al. Critically ill polyneuropathy: electrophysiological studies and differentiation from Guillain Barré syndrome. J Neurol Neurosurg Psychiatry 1986;49:563–73.

Bolton CF, Young GB. The Neurological Complications of Renal Disease. Butterworths, Boston, 1990.

Brown WF, Feasby TE, Hahn AF. Electrophysiological changed in the acute "axonal" form of Guillain-Barré syndrome. Muscle Nerve 1993;16:200–5.

Buchthal F, Behse F. Electromyography and nerve biopsy in men exposed to lead. Br J Ind Med 1979;36:135–47.

Burgdorfer W, Barbour AG, Hayes SF et al. Lyme disease—a tick-borne spirochetosis? Science 1982;216: 1317–19.

Castro LHM, Ropper AH. Human immune globulin infusion in Guillain-Barré syndrome: worsening during and after treatment. Neurology 1993;43:1034–6.

Chance PF, Matsunami N, Lensch MW et al. Analysis of the DNA duplication 17p11.2 in Charcot Marie Tooth neuropathy type 1 pedigrees: additional evidence for a third autosomal CMT1 locus. Neurology 1992;42: 2037–41.

Chaudhry V, Corse AM, Cornblath DR, et al. Multifocal motor neuropathy: response to immune globulin. Ann Neurol 1993;33:237–42.

Chiba A, Kusunoki S, Obata H et al. Serum anti-GQ1b IgG antibody is associated with ophthalmoplegia in Miller Fisher syndrome and Guillain Barré syndrome: clinical and immunohistochemical studies. Neurology 1993;43: 1911–17.

Clarke DJ, Ewing J, Campbell JW. Diabetic autonomic neuropathy. Diabetologia 1979;ZS17:195–212.

Cornblath DR, McArthur JC, Kennedy PGE et al. Inflammatory demyelinating peripheral neuropathies associated wtih human T-cell lymphotropic virus type III infection. Ann Neurol 1987;21:32–40.

Costa PMP, Teixeira A, Saraia MJM, Costa PP. Immunoassay for transthyretin variants associated with amyloid neuropathy. Scand J Immunol 1993;38:177–82.

Dawson DM. Entrapment neuropathies of the upper extremities. N Eng J Med 1993;329;2013–8.

Modern overview.

Dutch Guillain-Barré study group: treatment of Guillain-Barré syndrome with high-dose immune globulin combined with methylprednisoolone: a pilot study. Ann Neurol 1994;35:749–52.

Dyck PJ, Prineas J, Pollard J. Chronic inflammatory demyelinating neuropathy. In Dyck PJ, Thomas PK, Griffin JW et al (eds). Peripheral neuropathy. 3rd Ed. WB Saunders, Philadelphia, 1993, pp. 1488–1524.

Fisher M. Syndrome of ophthalmoplegia, ataxia, and areflexia. N Engl J Med 1956;255:57–65.

Fross RD, Daube J. Neuropathy in Miller-Fisher syndrome: clinical and electrophysiological findings. Neurology 1987;37:1493–8.

Gilliatt RW. Thoracic outlet compression syndrome. BMJ 1976;1:1274–6.

First clinical and electrophysiologic description of true neurogenic thoracic outlet syndrome.

Glass JD, Cornblath DR. Chronic inflammatory demyelinating polyneuropathy and paraproteinemic neuropathies. Current Opinion in Neurology 1994;7:393–7.

Gorson KC, Ropper AH. Acute respiratory failure neuropathy: a variant of critical illness polyneuropathy. Crit Care Med 1993;21:267–71.

Griffin JW, Ho TW-H. The Guillain-Barré syndrome at 75: the campylobacter connection. Ann Neurol 1993;34: 125–7.

Hansen K, Lebech A-M. The clinical and epidemiological profile of Lyme neuroborreliosis in Denmark 1985–1990.

A prospective study of 187 patients with B. burgdorferi-*specific intrathecal antibody production.*

Hanson MR, Breuer AC, Fulan AJ et al. Mechanism and frequency of brachial plexus injury in open heart surgery: a prospective analysis. Ann Thorac Surg 1983;36: 675–82.

Details frequency and severity of brachial plexopathy after cardiac surgery.

Harding AE, Thomas PK. Clinical features of hereditary motor and sensory neuropathy types I and II. Brain 1980;103:259–80.

Holmgren G, Ericzon BG, Groth CG et al. Clinical improvement and amyloid regression after liver transplantation in hereditary transthyretic amyloidosis. Lancet 1993;341: 1113–16.

Hughes RAC, Rees JH. Guillain-Barré syndrome. Curr Opin Neurol 1994;7:386–92.

Inoue A, Tsukada M, Koh CS, Yangisawa N. Chronic relapsing demyelinating polyneuropathy associated with hepatitis B infection. Neurology 1987;37:1663.

Irani DN, Cornblath DR, Chaudry V et al. Relapse in Guillain-Barré syndrome after treatment with human immune globulin. Neurology 1993;43:872–5.

Jamal GA, Kerr DJ, McLellaan AR et al. Generalized peripheral nerve dysfunction in acromegaly: a study by conventional and novel neurophysiological techniques. J Neurol Neurosurg Psychiatry 1987;50:886–94.

Johnson RK, Spinner M, Shrewsbury MM. Median nerve entrapment syndrome in the proximal forearm. J Hand Surg 1979;4:48.

Khaleeli AA, Levy RD, Edwards RHT et al. The neuromuscular features of acromegaly: a clinical and pathological study. J Neurol Neurosurg Psychiatry 1984;47:1009–15.

Lange DJ, Trojaborg W, Uncini A et al. Multifocal motor neuropathy with conduction block: is it a distinct clinical entity? Neurology 1992;42:497–505.

Lange DJ, Trojaborg W, McDonald TD. Persistent and transient conduction block in motor neuron disease. Muscle Nerve 1993;16:896–903.

Lange DJ, Britton CB, Younger DS, Hays AP. The neuromuscular manifestations of human immunodeficiency virus infections. Arch Neurol 1988;1084–8.

Logigian EL, Kaplan RF, Steere AC. Chronic neurologic manifestations of Lyme disease. N Engl J Med 1990;323: 1438–44.

Logigian EL, Steere AC. Clinical and electrophysiologic findings in chronic neuropathy of Lyme disease. Neurology 1992;42:303–11.

Matthews WB. Sarcoid neuropathy. In Dyck PJ, Thomas PK, Griffin JW et al. (eds). Peripheral neuropathy. WB Saunders, Philadelphia, 1993, pp. 1418–23.

McDonald WI. Diphtheritic neuropathy. In Dyck PJ, Thomas PK, Griffin JW et al. (eds). Peripheral Neuropathy. WB Saunders, Philadelphia, 1993, pp. 1412–7.

McKhann GM, Griffin JW, Cornblath DC et al. Plasmapheresis and Guillain-Barré syndrome: analysis of prognostic factors and the effect of plasmapheresis. Ann Neurol 1988;23:347–53.

McKann GM, Cornblath DR, Griffin JW et al. Acute motor axonal neuropathy: a frequent cause of acute flaccid paralysis in China. Ann Neurol 1993;33:333–42.

Mendell JR. Chronic inflammatory demyelinating polyradiculoneuropathy. Ann Rev Med 1993;44:211–19.

Miller RG, Storey JR, Greco CM. Ganciclovir in the treatment of progressive AIDS-related polyradiculopathy. Neurology 1990;40:560–74.

Nemni R, Bottacchi E, Fazio R et al. Polyneuropathy in hypothyroidism: clinical, electrophysiological and morphological findings in four cases. J Neurol Neurosurg Psychiatry 1987;50:1454.

Nielsen VK. Toxic neuropathies. In Brown WF, Bolton CF (eds). Clinical Electromyography. Butterworth-Heinemann, Boston, 1993, pp. 601–21.

Pollard JD. Neuropathy in diseases of the thyroid and pituitary glands. In Dyck PJ, Thomas PK, Griffin JW et al. (eds). Peripheral Neuropathy. WB Saunders, Philadelphia, 1993, pp. 1266–74.

Rao SN, Katiuar BC, Nair KRP, Misra S. Neuromuscular status in hypothyroidism. Acta Neurol Scand. 1980;61: 167.

Roberts M, Willison H, Vincent A, Newsom-Davis J. Serum factor in Miller-Fisher variant of Guillain-Barré syndrome and neurotransmitter release. Lancet 1994;343: 454–55.

Ropper AH. The Guillain-Barré syndrome. N Engl J Med 1992;326:1130–6.

Sabin TD, Swift TR, Jacobson RR. Leprosy. In Dyck PJ, Thomas PK, Griffin JW et al. (eds). Peripheral Neuropathy. WB Saunders, Philadelphia, 1993, pp. 1354–79.

Said G, Lacroix C, Chemoulli P et al. Cytomegalovirus neuropathy in acquired immunodeficiency syndrome: a clinical and pathological study. Ann Neurol 1991;29:139–95.

Solders G, Nennesmo I, Persson A. Diphtheritic neuropathy, an analysis based on muscle and nerve biopsy and repeated neurophysiological and autonomic function tests. J Neurol Neurosurg Psychiatry 1989;52:876–80.

Stewart JD. Focal Peripheral Neuropathies. Elsevier, New York, 1987.

Thomas PK. Diabetic neuropathy; models, mechanisms and mayhem. Can J Neurol Sci 1992;19:1–7.

Thornton CA, Latif AS, Emmanuel JC. Guillain Barre syndrome associated with human immunodeficiency virus infection in Zimbabwe. Neurology 1991;41:812–5.

Tsukada N, Koh CS, Inoue A, Yanagisawa N. Demyelinating neuropathy associated with hepatitis B virus infection: detection of immune complexes composed of hepatitis B virus antigen. Neurol Sci 1987;77:203.

Vallat JM, Hugon J, Lubeau M et al. Tick bite meningoradiculoneuritis: clinical, electrophysiologic, and histologic findings in 10 cases. Neurology 1987;37:749–53.

Van der Meche FGA, Schmitz PIM. Dutch Guillain-Barré Study Group: a randomized trial comparing intravenous immune globulin and plasma exchange in Guillain-Barré syndrome. N Engl J Med 1992;326:1123–9.

Wilborurn AJ. Thoracic outlet syndrome surgery causing severe brachial plexopathy. Muscle Nerve 1988;11: 66–74.

Review of neurologic complications of surgery for thoracic outlet syndrome and a review of the two types of thoracic outlet syndromes (true and disputed). Clinical and electrophysiologic features of eight patients with surgical complications are discussed.

Windebank AJ. Metal neuropathy. In Dyck PJ, Thomas PK, Griffin JW et al. (eds). Peripheral Neuropathy. WB Saunders, Philadelphia, 1993, pp. 12549–1570.

Wokke JH, Jennekens FG, vandeOord CJ et al. Histological investigations of muscle atrophy and end plates in two critically ill patients with generalized weakness. J Neurol Sci 1988;88:95–106.

Wulff CH, Hansen K, Strange P, Trojaborg W. Multiple mononeuritis and radiculitis with erythema, pain, elevated CSF protein and pleocytosis (Bannwarth's syndrome). J Neurol Neurosurg Psychiatry 1983;46: 485–90.

Yuki N, Taki T, Inagaki F et al. A bacterium lipopolysaccharide that elicits Guillain-Barré syndrome has a GM1 ganglioside-like structure. J Exp Med 1993;33:563–7.

Zochodne DW, Bolton CF, Wells GA et al. Polyneuropathy associated with critical illness: a complication of sepsis and multiple organ failure. Brain 1987;110:819–42.

Zuniga G, Ropper AH, Frank J. Sarcoid peripheral neuropathy. Neurology 1991;41:1558–61.

81

Myasthenia Gravis and Disorders of Neuromuscular Transmission

Dale J. Lange

The great common feature of disorders of neuromuscular transmission is the enormous variation that occurs from time to time in strength. By the astute use of history, examination, and diagnostic tests, the clinician can arrive at a proper diagnosis. Accurate diagnosis is essential because treatment exists for many disorders of neuromuscular transmission and the treatment is specific for each type of disorder.

Myasthenia gravis occurs in 5 per 100,000 people. Except for the congenital form, onset before the teenage years is rare. There is a bimodal age distribution with a peak frequency occurring in the 20 to 30-year-old age range, and there is another peak at 50 to 70 years. Women outnumber men 2:1 in the younger patient population; men and women have an equal disease prevalence in the older age group.

MYASTHENIA GRAVIS

Pathophysiology

Myasthenia gravis is an immunologically mediated disease in which autoantibodies directed against the acetylcholine receptor (AChR) cause impaired receptor function, inefficient neuromuscular transmission, and weakness. This process was first suggested in 1973 when Patrick and Lindstrom showed that a syndrome indistinguishable from myasthenia gravis could be produced in rabbits after immunization with AChRs from the electric eel. The critical role of immunoglobulins (Igs) was demonstrated by the observation that the clinical syndrome was produced in mice after injection with myasthenic serum containing IgG. Morphologic studies show that affected neuromuscular junctions have smaller than normal nerve terminals, widening of the primary synaptic cleft, and simplification of the postsynaptic membrane.

AChR antibodies are thought to be essential for the development of the disease. Elevated titers of antibodies to the AChR are found in 80 to 90 percent of myasthenic patients. Plasmapheresis is an effective means of treatment in many patients. Infants born of myasthenic mothers have myasthenia gravis until the maternal antibody is cleared (see below). There is a general correlation with the disease activity and level of antibody titer. However, some observations suggest that other factors are involved. First, antibodies are not found in 10 to 20 percent of patients; such seronegative myasthenic patients respond to immunosuppressive therapy in a manner no different from that of those with antibodies. Second, in an individual patient, the disease course may be completely independent of the antibody titer. Third, plasmapheresis may be ineffective. It is possible that the antibody assayed in the diagnostic test is not the one that is responsible for disease. Recent evidence suggests that the antibody that blocks the AChR binding region correlates best with disease activity.

The mechanism by which antibodies induce disease is uncertain. Three possibilities include blocking the main site necessary for muscle activation, immunomodulation, and enhanced destruction of AChRs.

The stimulus for AChR antibody generation is uncertain; however, the thymus gland seems to be an important factor. The thymus is the most important organ responsible for developing T lymphocytes, which disseminates T cells to the rest of the body. However, most patients with myasthenia gravis have persistently active thymus glands. Pathologic findings in patients with generalized myasthenia show profuse activity in the thymus, with lymphoid follicles present. There is considerable evidence to suggest that the thy-

935

mus is the site where the body is first sensitized to the AChR.

Myasthenia Gravis and the Thymus Gland

The suggestion that the thymus gland might play some role in the pathogenesis of myasthenia gravis first came from an observation by Blalock et al. in 1939 when the removal of a thymoma caused a dramatic improvement in a patient's myasthenic symptoms. The thymus gland is the primary source of T cells and generally becomes atrophic by the age of 12. However, 70 percent of myasthenic patients show hyperplastic and enlarged thymus glands, which suggests continued immunologic activity. The typical histopathologic abnormalities consist of hyperplasia of the lymphoid follicles. The cells in the hyperplastic follicles are B cells, plasma cells, and helper T cells.

The exact connection between myasthenia and the thymus is uncertain. Myoid cells in the thymus may result from a mechanism of sensitization of the immune system to the AChR protein. In 10 percent of myasthenic patients, a thymic tumor is present. Fasciculations and continuous muscle fiber activity have been reported in patients with thymomas and may be the presenting signs. Metastases from thymomas are rare, but local invasion of the pleura and pericardium can be life threatening. Patients may have thymomas without myasthenia.

Autoimmune Disorders

Coexisting autoimmune diseases are common in myasthenia. Thyrotoxicosis occurs in about 5 percent of patients with myasthenia. Other autoimmune diseases also occur in myasthenic patients and their families, including polymyositis, lupus, Gougerot-Sjögren syndrome, pernicious anemia, and rheumatoid arthritis. The coexistence of polymyositis and myasthenia gravis makes specific diagnosis difficult because small inflammatory infiltrates, known as lymphorrhages, may occur in patients with otherwise typical myasthenia.

Neonatal Myasthenia Gravis

Neonatal myasthenia gravis is a special form of myasthenia that is completely due only from the presence of maternal AChR antibodies that have crossed the placenta during pregnancy. This form of the disease therefore only occurs in children born to myasthenic mothers. The level of the infant's antibody titer is similar to the mother's and determines the degree of weakness, which is often proportionate to the magnitude of the titer.

The pregnancy is characterized by small amounts of prenatal movement and floppiness at birth. The child is unable to suck or feed. Respiratory distress may occur. The weakness usually lasts 2 weeks (the half-life of maternal antibody is 2 to 3 weeks and is usually completely absent from the infant's blood in 5 months) but may last up to 12 weeks, the time required for the infant to develop its own IgG response to infection. There is no increased risk for developing myasthenia gravis in later life.

Clinical Features

The two most important features of the weakness associated with myasthenia gravis are the distribution and the fluctuation in severity of the weakness. The predominance of impairment of ocular motility and the swallowing and speech disorders help to distinguish myasthenia gravis from other diseases. The diagnosis may be difficult in the early stages of the disease when the symptoms are frequently worse than the findings on clinical examination.

Several features help distinguish myasthenia from other disorders. Ocular pareses occur that cannot be explained by paresis of one oculomotor nerve (e.g., ptosis and exotropia), but the pupil is normal. Usually, the weakness is more marked in the evenings than in the mornings.

Weakness in eyelid and ocular muscles occurs in more than 90 percent of patients at some point of their disease. The typical complaints are loss of vision (because of eyelid drooping below the pupil) and double vision that varies in severity. Although the weakness may be asymmetric and even unilateral, the details of the clinical history usually indicate a bilateral syndrome. Red glass testing for diplopia (see Ch. 26) is a very sensitive way to detect subtle weakness of ocular muscles. Despite the occasional occurrence of ocular weakness simulating brainstem lesions, such as internuclear ophthalmoplegia, it is the fluctuation in severity that stamps the process as myasthenia gravis.

The muscles of facial expression, speech, and swallowing are also commonly affected. Approximately 60 percent of all myasthenic patients have difficulty smiling (so-called *myasthenic snarl* in which the upper lip elevates transversely in an apparent snarl while the patient is attempting to smile), difficulty chewing (hanging jaw sign in which the patient supports the drooped jaw with the hand), nasal speech, and difficulty swallowing. The fluctuation in strength is often shown by the inability to finish a meal because of inability to chew the food. Rarely, patients may present solely with weakness of neck flexors, resulting in *floppy head syndrome*. In some, the first problem is noted at the movies when it becomes necessary to support the head in mild elevation using the hands.

Limb weakness occurs in 40 percent of patients. The distribution is most often in proximal muscle groups and is manifested as difficulty rising from chairs or lifting the arms over the head. However, the author has seen two patients in whom the only limb muscle affected was the triceps. Some patients have shown weakness resembling a radial nerve palsy with wrist drop. Muscles with marked weakness may show significant atrophy. The pattern of involvement in the limbs is rarely distinctive enough to make a diagnosis of myasthenia. Reflexes are usually preserved. The exhaustion of muscular strength can sometimes be elicited by having the patient perform sustained elevation of the eyelids or arms for 1 minute, when worsening weakness can be observed (see Ch. 26). The diagnosis usually is made from the more typical pattern of involvement in the ocular and bulbar musculature.

The onset of the disease is usually insidious and over 4 to 6 months, but considerable variation has been documented. Rapid evolution of weakness over days with respiratory failure shortly after the onset of symptoms has been reported. More often, the disease slowly progresses to involve all muscles of the body. In perhaps 15 percent of patients, the weakness remains limited to the eyes (*ocular myasthenia*), but this variant is considered to exist only when ocular signs (ptosis and ophthalmoparesis) are the sole manifestations and have been present for 2 years or more. Rarely, after the beginning with myasthenia, the syndrome resolves spontaneously.

Rapid changes in muscle strength can occur from external influences. Many medications and altered physiologic states may cause worsening of myasthenia because of their effects on neuromuscular transmission. Included in this group are quinine sulfate, aminoglycoside antibiotics, curarelike agents, calcium channel blockers, hypocalcemia, hypokalemia, hypo- and hyperthyroidism, and pregnancy. Some pharmacologic agents, such as D-penicillamine and benzodiazepines, can produce the disease in an otherwise asymptomatic person. Coincident infections are a particularly common cause of myasthenic exacerbations. If respiratory failure occurs, *myasthenic crisis* exists.

The ranking of severity is conveniently accomplished using a modified Osserman scale:

Class 1. Ocular only
Class 2. Mild generalized symptoms sparing oculopharyngeal muscles
Class 3. Moderate, generalized weakness with mild to moderate oropharyngeal symptoms
Class 4. Severe disability, including oropharyngeal and respiratory muscles
Class 5. Myasthenic crisis

The diagnosis is often difficult to establish if limb weakness in the predominant complaint. However, the characteristic exhaustion of strength in muscles that are seemingly uninvolved may be demonstrated by having the patient perform sustained muscular effort, such as raising of the eyelids for 1 minute and watching for worsening ptosis or ophthalmoparesis. Reversal of these signs with edrophonium (see below) confirms the diagnosis.

Clinical and Laboratory Diagnosis

Edrophonium Test

To establish the presence of a disorder of neuromuscular transmission, the edrophonium test remains one of the most useful tests. In the presence of obvious weakness, such as ptosis, diplopia, or nasal speech, one mg IV of edrophonium is injected as a test dose. If no response is obtained in 1 minute, a dose of 5 mg is injected. If no response is observed within 2 minutes, the remaining 4 mg is injected. The effect is a normalization of the weakness pattern, which appears within 30 to 60 seconds after injection, and all effects are gone within 5 minutes.

Side effects include nausea, lightheadedness, bradycardia (necessitating the injection of 0.4 mg of atropine IV). A control injection of saline is useful, especially if the objective measure is limb strength. The effects are often negative in ocular myasthenia.

Injection of 1.5 mg IM of neostigmine may also be used for the same purpose, with a maximal effect being apparent 30 minutes after injection.

Regardless of the route of administration, there are few false-positive tests. Patients with amyotrophic lateral sclerosis (ALS) and Lambert-Eaton syndrome have been reported rarely to have a positive test result.

Antiacetylcholine Receptor and Antistriated Muscle Antibodies

Serum antibodies are found in 80 to 90 percent of patients with myasthenia gravis. There are few, if any, other diseases that yield strongly positive results (i.e., false positive). A few patients with ALS (see Ch. 63) have been found to have borderline or mildly increased titers. Patients with Lambert-Eaton syndrome (see below) may show increased titers, but this may represent coexisting diseases.

In general, antibody titers among myasthenic patients are lower in those with ocular disease and higher in those with thymomas. Elevated titers of antistriated muscle antibodies are present in all patients with thymomas and in about one-third of patients with myasthenia but no thymomas.

The magnitude of the titer generally correlates with disease severity. Most patients show a decrease in antibody titer as the disease improves, but some show no correlation, supporting the hypothesis that the antibody measured in the clinical assay may not be responsible for the disease process.

Muscle Biopsy

In contrast to the distinctive histologic appearance of some other forms of muscle disease (see Ch. 82), routine staining of muscle biopsy specimens for light microscopy generally shows no major abnormalities. Rarely, small inflammatory cell infiltrates (lymphorrhages) are seen.

Electrophysiologic Studies

Nerve conduction velocity and evoked-response amplitude (see Ch. 12) are normal. However, while performing studies, the examiner may note variation in the evoked-response amplitude during repeated stimuli. The results of needle electromyography (see Ch. 12) are usually normal, but in the presence of severe weakness and atrophy, spontaneous activity in the form of positive sharp waves and fibrillation potentials may be seen. During voluntary activation, motor unit form is normal. But in severely weakened muscles, motor unit duration may be short, and variation in amplitude of the motor unit potential may be observed on repeated firing of the motor unit.

Weakness from myasthenia gravis occurs because transmission between nerve and muscle fibers within motor units is blocked. The more muscle-nerve interactions are blocked, the greater the weakness is. The likelihood of blocked transmission increases during exercise. The electrophysiologic correlate of exercise is to deliver repetitive supramaximal electrical stimuli to a muscle at 2 to 3 Hz (more than 5 Hz facilitates neuromuscular transmission). The classic electromyographic response seen in myasthenic patients is a progressive decrement of the compound muscle action potential amplitude from 1 to 4 or 5, which then slowly increases. Immediately after a brief (15-second) period of maximal exercise, the decrement is usually abolished, and the initial compound muscle action potential is larger (postexercise facilitation). This is a short-lived phenomenon, lasting between 15 and 40 seconds. Thereafter, the decrement may get worse for 2 to 4 minutes after 1 minute of sustained muscle contraction (postactivation exhaustion) (see Ch. 12).

Repetitive stimulation study results are more often positive in muscles that are weak. As many as 99 percent of weak muscles show excessive decrement. In clinically normal muscles, stimulation of proximal muscles systems (accessory/trapezius or axillary/deltoid) is often abnormal when distal systems are normal.

Single-fiber electromyography (SFEMG) (see Ch. 12) is a technique that uses a needle electrode with a special recording electrode with a small recording area that allows recording from single muscle fibers. The needle is positioned within a motor unit such that at least two time-locked fibers belonging to the same motor unit are firing repeatedly. The machine triggers on one spike, and the variability in firing between the two time-locked potentials is measured and referred to as jitter. Jitter is a measure of the efficiency of neuromuscular transmission. If fewer receptors are available to react with the acetylcholine released from the presynaptic terminus because of antibody-induced receptor dysfunction, the efficiency of neuromuscular transmission decreases, and the time it takes for enough receptors to be activated to produce a propagated action potential increases. Although muscle fiber contraction occurs and weakness is not present, the inefficient manner of muscle fiber activation is documented in the recording of increased jitter measurements. Therefore, abnormal jitter values can be recorded in clinically strong muscles, making this a sensitive tool for diagnosis. When weakness is found, blocking is usually observed during the SFEMG examination. In addition, when clinically weak muscles show normal jitter measurements, the diagnosis cannot be myasthenia gravis.

The sensitivity of SFEMG has been established in several studies. As many as 95 percent of patients with mild myasthenia show abnormalities if proximal muscles (frontalis or orbicularis oculi) are studied with SFEMG. Patients with suspected myasthenia should have the extensor digitorum communis studied first because normal values are most secure for this muscle and patient tolerance is best. If this examination is normal and the clinical suspicion is high, the examination should then be carried out in the frontalis or orbicularis oculi.

Improvement in disease status is usually accompanied by improvement in decrement and SFEMG abnormalities. However, the correlation is not sensitive enough to use as a predictor of disease activity.

Differential Diagnosis and Diagnostic Evaluation

The clinical presentation of patients with myasthenia gravis is often so distinctive that the diagnosis is obvious. Despite an easy diagnosis, concomitant diseases need to be sought. Patients should be screened for other autoimmune diseases (see above), such as thyroiditis, lupus, rheumatoid arthritis, and pernicious anemia. The possible existence of a thymoma should be pursued with a chest computed tomographic scan, which is preferable to the magnetic resonance imaging scan. With EMG, repetitive stimulation studies should be obtained on all patients during evaluation to serve as a baseline for future reference. After the diagnosis of myasthenia is established, pulmonary function tests should also be obtained early in the diagnostic evaluation to serve also as a reference point.

Patients with prominent swallowing and speech

problems may be difficult to distinguish from the bulbar form of amyotrophic lateral sclerosis (see Ch. 63). To confuse matters further, patients with bulbar ALS may also show mild decrement during repetitive stimulation studies, anti-AChR titers may be borderline elevated, and an edrophonium test result may be interpreted as mildly positive. However, if tongue movement is monitored closely, there is no doubt that edrophonium does nothing to improve strength in ALS. In myasthenia, tongue bulk is usually normal without fasciculations, whereas in ALS, it is wasted with fasciculations. Finally, there is never significant variation in strength in patients with ALS.

There are other disorders that may be difficult to distinguish from myasthenia gravis. Progressive external ophthalmoplegia (PEO) may be especially difficult to separate from ocular myasthenia. However, patients with PEO report little fluctuation in weakness, and ophthalmoparesis is rarely accompanied by disturbed vision (such as blurriness or double vision). SFEMG studies of facial muscles may be abnormal in both groups of patients, but proximal arm muscles in patients with PEO usually show myogenic change on quantitative EMG, even in clinically normal muscle. Myogenic change may also be seen in myasthenia gravis, but this occurs only in weak muscles. Patients with PEO often show ragged red fibers revealing the nature of the myopathy (mitochondrial) (see Ch. 82).

Prognosis

The course is usually progressive. In those in whom generalized disease develops, 77 percent do so within the first year of symptoms. The maximum severity of the disease occurs within the first year in 60 percent of patients. Left untreated, one-third die of respiratory failure.

Treatment

Anticholinesterase Medications

The therapeutic benefit of anticholinesterase medication has been known since the 1930s. The presumed mechanism of action is to inhibit cholinesterase to allow increased time for effective interaction between the acetylcholine released from the presynaptic terminal and the AChR on the postsynaptic membrane.

Three forms of the medication are in use. Edrophonium is too short acting to be useful for anything other than a diagnostic test. Neostigmine bromide may be given intramuscularly, and its duration of action is a little longer than edrophonium. The doses range from 7.5 to 45 mg every 2 to 6 hours. The most commonly used anticholinesterase medication is pyridostigmine because it is available in oral (capsule) form and has the longest half-life and the fewest anticholinergic side effects. The dose generally ranges from 30 to 90 mg every 4 to 6 hours; however, there is really no maximum dose. Enough drug should be given to the patient to alleviate the symptoms without causing significant side effects.

There are drawbacks to the use of anticholinesterase agents. First, chronic use of anticholinergic agents may damage the neuromuscular junction. Second, large doses predispose the patient to the development of cholinergic crisis (see below). Symptoms may develop from overstimulation of the muscarinic cholinergic system, such as nausea, vomiting, diarrhea, increased salivation, and increased weakness. Fasciculations may also occur. Differentiating between the weakness induced by too little medication or too much is sometimes difficult. When such symptoms occur, it is advisable to admit the patient to an intensive care setting and withdraw the anticholinesterase medication while using other modes of therapy (see below) for the myasthenia.

Steroids

Because the disease is presumed to be mediated through an autoantibody, the use of steroids is a logical choice. They are usually used in a setting of generalized myasthenia, although success has been reported in ocular disease. The largest consideration in the decision to start steroid use is the exposure of the patient to potential side effects. These include weight gain and moon facies, important manifestations, especially in younger patients. Steroid-induced hypertension, diabetes, ulcers, and osteoporosis are particularly important in older patients. Therefore, close monitoring and reduction of dosage to the lowest possible level is required.

Although daily use of prednisone, 60 mg/day, is often the starting dose, higher doses can be used in settings where close monitoring is available. Clinical worsening may occur within the first week of treatment, which suggests that inpatient observation during institution of steroid therapy is advisable. As the clinical condition stabilizes and improves, the dose is slowly reduced. Alternate-day therapy may produce fewer side effects.

Immunosuppression

Immunosuppressant agents are used to treat generalized myasthenia gravis in patients who are not candidates for steroid therapy or have not received sufficient benefit from other modes of therapy, or immunosuppressive agents are added to an existing regimen to enhance the clinical response.

There are several different drugs available, but three of the more commonly used drugs are azathioprine, cyclophosphamide, and cyclosporine. The dose of azathioprine is 2.5 mg/kg/day (150 to 250 total daily dose). Clinically evident side effects are often minimal, and patients are free of the disfiguring side effects seen with steroid use. Unfortunately, it may take up to 6 months to see a clinical effect. Success has also been reported with cyclophosphamide. The time between the onset of therapy and the observation of clinical response may be shorter when cyclosporine is used.

The side effects of all immunosuppressant agents involve bone marrow suppression. Accordingly, blood counts need to be measured routinely. In addition to the bone marrow suppression, patients receiving cyclophosphamide risk the development of hemorrhagic cystitis. The development of lymphoma associated with long-term use of azathioprine rarely occurs but must be considered in the decision to initiate therapy.

Plasmapheresis

Shortly after the autoimmune basis for myasthenia was reported, plasmapheresis was shown to be effective in reversing the weakness associated with myasthenia. It consists of having one blood volume undergo pheresis and may result in striking clinical improvement. Unfortunately, the improvement is temporary, lasting at most 4 to 6 weeks. This treatment is used only as a temporizing measure while other treatments are initiated (e.g., during myasthenic crisis to product a more rapid improvement in muscle strength or as a means to improve strength preoperatively in preparation for thymectomy).

Thymectomy

There are two indications for thymectomy in patients with myasthenia gravis. One is the presence of a thymoma. Patients with thymomas are more likely to have more severe weakness that is difficult to control with immunosuppressant medications. Furthermore, although the tumor rarely metastasizes outside of the thoracic cavity, its ability to spread locally can induce life-threatening complications. It is important to remove the surrounding thymic tissue in addition to the tumor to maximize the clinical response to surgery. The second indication is for generalized myasthenia gravis. Removal of the thymus gland is the only therapy that offers a complete cure.

There is much discussion about the technique used to perform the thymectomy. One method is a suprasternal method, which removes all visible thymus from an incision well above the anatomic placement of the gland. A modification of this technique described by Cooper et al. in 1988 uses a special retractor to maximize visualization of the thymus. Although these techniques afford the patient the benefit of a small postoperative scar, the lack of complete removal of the gland, especially in the case of tumors, makes reoperation by

a transsternal method a possibility. The author has found the hyperactive thymus in myasthenic patients to be so extensive, sometimes tracking well into the neck or deep into the thoracic cavity, that it is only by direct visualization of the gland by a transsternal approach that can complete removal be achieved.

Although some centers restrict thymectomy to younger patients, the author recommends it for all patients with definite generalized myasthenia whose general medical health is good enough to tolerate surgery and whose life expectancy is long enough to benefit from the expectation that the opportunity to see a change in clinical condition may take as long as 1 year after thymectomy. About 80 percent of patients without thymomas will become asymptomatic with medication or go into complete remission (asymptomatic without medication) within 5 years of thymectomy.

Myasthenic Crisis

Myasthenic crisis is defined as the need for assisted ventilation because of myasthenia-induced weakness of the muscles of respiration. Once mechanical ventilation is initiated, anticholinergic medications are stopped to decrease the problems induced by secretions from cholinergic stimulation. Most instances of myasthenic crises are caused by concurrent infections or unstable metabolic conditions. Plasmapheresis is initiated while investigation for the underlying cause is pursued. When the underlying cause is identified and treated appropriately, the weakness usually improves gradually with previously effective therapy.

LAMBERT-EATON SYNDROME

Usually found in patients with oat cell carcinoma of the lung, patients with Lambert-Eaton syndrome have a disorder of neuromuscular transmission in which the release of vesicles containing acetylcholine in the presynaptic axonal terminal is impaired. Presynaptic destruction in the vicinity of the voltage-sensitive calcium channels is seen on electron microscopic examination. In fact, many patients show increased titers of antibodies directed against these channels.

The defect in acetylcholine release is maximal during low rates of activation. As the axon is stimulated with increasing frequency, more acetylcholine is released, and successful neuromuscular transmission occurs at individual neuromuscular junction, causing improvement in strength. Patients complain of weakness of the legs and arms, causing difficulty getting up from chairs, climbing stairs, and combing or washing the hair. Dryness of the mouth with associated hoarseness occurs in more than 50 percent of patients because of autonomic involvement. Unlike myasthenia gravis, cranial nerve dysfunction (ptosis, diplopia, and swallowing problems) is rare. The clinical examination confirms the proximal weakness, and reflexes are hypoactive or absent.

The presence of Lambert-Eaton syndrome may be suspected from the physical examination on finding improving muscle strength with effort or enhanced reflexes after activation of the muscle being tested (reflex facilitation). In this circumstance, a reflex originally absent may become normal if tested immediately after maximal contraction of that muscle for 10 seconds. This effect is lost within 15 seconds of the exercise.

The presence of Lambert-Eaton syndrome is defined by the electrophysiologic finding of incrementing amplitude of the compound muscle action potential in response to rapid repetitive stimulation (20, 40, or 50 Hz) or immediately after exercise. There are other disorders that show an incrementing response after exercise, most commonly myasthenia gravis. However, these two diseases may coexist, and precise separation is impossible.

Lambert-Eaton syndrome is often associated with systemic malignancies; the most frequent tumor seen is small cell carcinoma (oat cell) of the lung. However, it has been described in association with breast, prostate, stomach, and rectal cancer and lymphoma. The clinical signs may predate discovery of the cancer. In almost one-half of the patients with Lambert-Eaton syndrome, no cancer is found, but other autoimmune diseases are often present. The presumed mechanism in all types of Lambert-Eaton syndrome is an autoimmune destruction of the voltage-gated calcium channel by antibodies directed against this channel. These antibodies are detectable in the serum of most patients with this disease and are helpful in establishing the diagnosis.

BOTULISM

Botulism occurs from the ingestion of botulinus toxin produced by spores from the bacterium *Clostridium botulinum*. It is one of the most toxic substances known, being able to kill humans in microgram amounts. It is a rare syndrome in the United States; however, this toxin is now being used in a very diluted form to control involuntary movements (focal dystonia) (see Chs. 22 and 77). The toxin impairs the release of acetylcholine at all cholinergic synapses (muscarinic and nicotinic); therefore, autonomic effects are common. Although never reported, clinicians must be aware of the severe weakness that may accompany systemic botulism. Weakness may cause respiratory suppression, swallowing difficulty or paralysis, absent gag reflex promoting aspiration, and pupillary paralysis. Differ-

entiating the acute patient with botulism from one with a brainstem stroke may be difficult.

Treatment consists of supportive care, mechanical ventilation, and antitoxin.

ANNOTATED BIBLIOGRAPHY

Bever CT, Aquino-AV, Penn AS et al. Prognosis of ocular myasthenia. Ann Neurol 1983;14:516.

Established that patients whose symptoms remain localized to the eyes for 2 years or less have virtually no risk of generalization.

Blalock A, Mason MF, Mogan HJ, Riven SS. Myasthenia gravis and tumors of the thymus region. Ann Surg 1939; 110:544–59.

First report of improvement in myasthenia gravis in response to thymectomy.

Cherington M. Electrophysiologic methods as an aid in diagnosis of botulism: a review. Muscle Nerve 1982;5(Suppl 9):S28–29.

Cooper JD, Al-Jilaihawa AN, Pearson FG et al. An improved technique to facilitate transcervical thymectomy for myasthenia gravis. Ann Thorac Surg 1988;45:242–7.

Donaldson DH, Ansher M, Horan S et al. The relationship of age to outcome in myasthenia gravis. Neurology 1990; 40:786–90.

Excellent review of results from one center using their own approach to treatment.

Drachman DB, Adams RN, Josifek LF et al. Functional activities of autoantibodies to acetylcholine receptors and the clinical severity of myasthenia gravis. N Engl J Med 1982;307:769.

An attempt to correlate disease severity with different modes of action of antibody.

Drachman DB. Medical progress: myasthenia gravis. N Engl J Med 1994;330:1797–810.

Extensive review article.

Eaton LM, Lambert EJ. Electromyography and electric stimulation of nerves and diseases of motor unit: observations on myasthenic syndrome associated with malignant tumors. JAMA 1957;163:1117.

The original description of the myasthenic syndrome.

Engle AG. Myasthenia gravis and myasthenic syndromes. Ann Neurol 1984;16:519–34.

Excellent review of the myasthenia gravis and myasthenic syndromes.

Engel AG, Lambert EJ, Santa T. Study of long term anticholinesterase therapy: effects on neuromuscular transmission and motor end plate fine structure. Neurology 1973; 23:1273–81.

These investigators conclusively showed that that use of anticholinesterase agents has the potential to cause damage to the neuromuscular junction without impicating a disease process.

Engel AG, Santa T. Histometric analysis of the ultrastructure of the neuromuscular junction in myasthenia gravis and in the myasthenic syndrome. Ann N Y Acad Sci 1971;183:46–63.

The first study to show conclusively the intrasynaptic abnormalities in myasthenic patients by electron microscopy. This study showed striking changes in the postsynaptic membrane, consisting of simplification, that exist in myasthenic muscles.

Fisher RC, Schwartzmann RJ. Oral corticosteroid in the treatment of ocular myasthenia gravis. Ann N Y Acad Sci 1976;274:652–4.

These investigators show that oral steroid therapy is effective in ocular myasthenia. The issue is whether the treatment is worth the induced side effects.

Garcia-Merino A, Cabello A, Mora JS, Liano J. Continuous muscle fiber activity, peripheral neuropathy, and thymoma. Ann Neurol 1991;29:215–18.

This report emphasizes that myasthenia gravis is not the only neurologic syndrome encountered in patients with thymomas. Rarely, a syndrome of continuous muscle fiber activity and fasciculations may be found.

Gilchrist JM, AAEM Study Group. Single fiber EMG reference values: a collaborative effort. Muscle Nerve 1992; 15:151–61.

A multicenter study of SFEMG findings (jitter and fiber density) in normal subjects in a various muscles.

Jaretzki A III, Penn AS, Younger DS et al. Maximal thymectomy for myasthenia gravis: results. J Thorac Surg 1988;45:242–7.

Krendel DA, Sanders DB, Massey JM. Single fiber electromyography in chronic progressive external ophthalmoplegia. Muscle Nerve 1987;10:299–302.

This report summarizes the electrophysiologic findings that may cause confusion when the physician is trying to differentiate progressive external ophthalmoplegia from ocular myasthenia.

Lennon VA, Lambert EJ, Whittingham S, Fairbanks V. Autoimmunity in the Lambert Eaton myasthenic syndrome. Muscle Nerve 1982;5:224–6.

Lindstrom JM, Seybold ME, Lemon VA et al. Antibody to acetylcholine receptor in myasthenia gravis: prevalence, clinical correlates and diagnostic value. Neurology 1976; 26:1054–9.

A large study that attempts to correlate antibody titer with severity of disease.

McEvoy KM, Windebank AJ, Daube Jr, Low PA. 3,4 Diaminopyridine in the treatment of Lambert-Eaton syndrome. N Engl J Med 1989;321:1567–71.

Nath A, Kerman R, Novak IS, Wolinsky JS. Immune studies in human immunodeficiency virus infection with myasthenia gravis: a case report. Neurology 1990;40:581–3.

A patient with clinically typical myasthenia gravis is described that improved after human immunodeficiency virus infection caused a loss of CD4 cells with a corresponding reduction in anti-AChR antibodies.

Oh SJ, Eslami N, Nishirira T et al. Electrophysiological testing in myasthenia gravis. Ann Neurol 1982;12:348–54.

This study nicely demonstrates that the yield of repetitive nerve stimulation increases as the muscle group being tested weakens.

O'Neill JH, Murray NMF, Newsome-Davis J. The Lambert Eaton myasthenic syndrome: review of 50 cases. Brain 1988;111:577–96.

Ozdemir C, Young RR. Electrical testing in myasthenia gravis. Ann Neurol 1971;183:287–302.

This was the first study to show that testing proximal muscle systems increases the diagnostic yield of repetitive stimulation.

Pacher AR. Anti-acetylcholine receptor antibodies block bungarotoxin binding to native human acetylcholine receptor on the surface of TE671 cells. Neurology 1989; 39:1057–61.

Reports that disease severity is best correlated with the amount of blocking activity for the AChR in the neuromuscular junction.

Patrick J, Lindstrom J. Autoimmune response to acetylcholine receptor. Science 1973;180:871–2.

The first report of an experimental autoimmune model of myasthenia gravis.

Roberts A, Perera S, Lang B et al. Paraneoplastic myasthenic syndrome IgG inhibits Ca flux in a small cell carcinoma line. Nature 1985;2:737–9.

Solivan B, Lange DJ, Penn AS et al. Seronegative myasthenia gravis. Neurology 1998;38:514–7.

A clinical, electrophysiologic, and immunologic review of patients with myasthenia but no detectable antibodies.

Toyka KV, Drachman DB, Pestronk A, Kao I. Myasthenia gravis: passive transfer from man to mouse. Science 1975;190:397–9.

The first documentation of passive transfer of disease with Igs.

Walker MB. Treatment of myasthenia gravis with physostigmine. Lancet 1934;1:1200.

Original observation of improvement of weakness after receiving anticholinesterase.

Witte AS, Cornblath DR, Parry GJ et al. Azathioprine in the treatment of myasthenia gravis. Ann Neurol 1984;15: 602.

Younger DS, Jaretzki AJ III, Penn AS et al. Maximum thymectomy for myasthenia gravis. Ann N Y Acad Sci 1983;505:832–5.

Provides data to support surgical methods to visualize the thymus and obtain maximum removal.

82
Disorders of Muscle

Dale J. Lange and Salvatore DiMauro

Diseases of muscle are characterized according to age of onset, mechanism (acquired or inherited), tempo of illness (acute or chronic), and areas affected (proximal, distal, or selective as in fascioscapulohumeral and oculopharyngeal dystrophy). The classification used in this chapter relies on the point of view of the clinician when the patient is first seen and before physiologic, morphologic, or biochemical information becomes available. It is, therefore, based largely on the distribution of weakness.

MYOPATHIES PRESENTING WITH PREDOMINANTLY PROXIMAL WEAKNESS

Genetically Transmitted Diseases

Duchenne's Muscular Dystrophy

This disorder, named for the French neurologist G. B. A. Duchenne de Boulogne (1806–1875) is described in some detail because it is perhaps the best known of all diseases of muscle. It occurs in 20 of every 100,000 male births and is transmitted as an X-linked recessive disease: thus it is passed to boys from clinically unaffected mothers. One-third of patients have negative family histories, which suggests that spontaneous mutations are not infrequent. The affected gene of the X chromosome codes for a protein in the muscle cell membrane called dystrophin (see Ch. 4). This very large protein seems to be important in the maintenance of the structural integrity of the muscle membrane. Its absence may cause the membrane to be more porous and leaky. This inferred porosity could explain the greatly elevated levels of creatine kinase (CK) that are so characteristic of patients with Duchenne's dystrophy.

Clinical Features. All motor milestones of infancy and early childhood are usually normal in children with Duchenne's dystrophy. The first manifestations of the disease occur at 3 or 4 years of age when clumsiness is noted. The child also "feels heavy" when lifted, tends to toe-walk, and needs to use the arms to "climb up the legs" when getting up from the floor (Gowers' sign, named after W. R. Gowers, British neurologist, 1845–1915). By the time the boy is 4 or 5 years old, he has difficulty climbing stairs and keeping up with his peers.

On examination, there is exaggerated lumbar lordosis and waddling gait. Parents tell of slowness when climbing stairs. The tendency to walk on the toes is due to contractures in heel cords, which occur early in the disease (before age 5). Ankle reflexes may be blunted because of this, whereas other reflexes are usually preserved. Enlargement of the calf (pseudohypertrophy) is characteristic of Duchenne's dystrophy and occurs because of excessive fatty replacement of calf muscles.

The disease is relentlessly progressive, affecting most skeletal muscles of the body. Interestingly, hip adductors are usually spared. Cardiac and respiratory muscles are also affected, and cardiopathy or respiratory failure are common causes of death. Usually, children stop climbing stairs by age 10 and are confined to a wheelchair by age 12. Death usually occurs before age 20, but a few live beyond the age of 30.

Laboratory Findings. A dramatic increase of serum CK level (several thousand units) is found in all patients with Duchenne's dystrophy, even in early infancy before the disease is clinically evident. In fact, CK levels may be increased in the amniotic fluid of the fetus. CK levels fall later in the disease as the muscles atrophy. Other laboratory results (blood counts and chemistries) are normal.

The electrocardiogram (ECG) is abnormal in as many as 80 percent of patients. There may be conduction abnormalities and rhythm disturbances (often tachyarrhythmias).

Identification of the X-linked muscular dystrophies (Duchenne's and Becker's types) is facilitated by DNA analysis and immunologic studies of dystrophin. The amount of dystrophin appears to be inversely proportional to the severity of the clinical syndrome. Most patients with Duchenne's dystrophy have no detectable dystrophin by immunoblotting and by immunohistochemistry.

Nerve Conduction Studies and Electromyography. Motor and sensory nerve conduction studies are normal; electromyography (EMG) usually shows no spontaneous activity, but mild to moderate amounts of positive sharp waves and fibrillation potentials may occur early in the disease. Motor unit potentials are of short duration and low amplitude. Linked or satellite potentials are common, and recruitment in weak muscles is usually full if maximal effort is achieved.

The morphologic findings seen in patients with Duchenne's dystrophy are usually held as the paradigm for myogenic disease. There is excessive variation in muscle fiber diameter, hypertrophied muscle fibers, central nuclei, excessive amounts of interstitial fibrosis, and necrotic and regenerating muscle fibers.

Treatment. There is no effective treatment that will reverse the disease process of Duchenne's dystrophy. Chronic administration of prednisone (0.75 mg/kg/day) has been shown in controlled trials to slow the decline of muscle strength and increase muscle mass, especially in boys between 5 and 15 years of age. Myoblast transfer studies have shown no positive results to date.

Becker's Muscular Dystrophy

The ability to walk after age 12 essentially excludes the diagnosis of Duchenne's dystrophy. However, some boys manifest the proximal weakness pattern typical of Duchenne's dystrophy later in life. The symptoms may not start until age 8 or 9. This too is an X-linked disorder and was first described by Becker in 1962. The genetic errors affect the same gene as in Duchenne's dystrophy, but it is often the size of the essential membrane protein, dystrophin, that is altered (decreased or increased), although the amount of dystrophin is considerably more than that seen in patients with Duchenne's dystrophy.

Clinical Features. Clinically, children with Becker's dystrophy are similar to boys with Duchenne's dystrophy, except for the age difference. After they achieve all motor milestones at expected ages, weakness begins in the legs and is manifested as difficulty in climbing stairs or getting up from chairs

and very slow running and walking. On examination, proximal weakness is best manifested by the Gowers' maneuver (see above). Reflexes and sensation are preserved. Calf hypertrophy is present. The patient may not require a wheelchair until 30 years of age, and death usually occurs by age 50.

Laboratory Findings. The Serum CK level is dramatically increased (as much as 25 times normal). All other hematologic measurements are normal. ECG abnormalities are found in fewer than 40 percent of patients, but isolated cardiomyopathy has been reported in a few cases.

Nerve conduction studies are normal. EMG may show spontaneous activity (fibrillations and positive sharp waves), and motor units are myogenic in form (low amplitude and short duration). During maximal voluntary activation, recruitment is full in weak muscles.

Muscle biopsy findings are similar to those in patients with Duchenne's dystrophy, except for greater amounts of dystrophin by immunoblotting and immunohistochemical analysis.

Emery-Dreifuss Muscular Dystrophy

Emery-Dreifuss dystrophy is another X-linked recessive disorder with proximal muscle weakness as one of the cardinal manifestations. Most severely affected are the biceps and periscapular muscles with selective sparing of the deltoids. However, a more distinctive feature of the disorder is the presence of contractures at the elbow and neck. A potentially life-threatening feature of Emery-Dreifuss dystrophy is the presence of cardiac conduction defect.

The CK levels are moderately increased in patients with Emery-Dreifuss muscular dystrophy. Motor nerve conduction studies are normal, but EMG shows motor units of short duration and low amplitude. Recruitment patterns in weak muscles are normal.

Muscle biopsy shows myogenic change with type I fiber predominance and type I atrophy.

Limb-Girdle Muscular Dystrophy

This term is used to describe proximal muscle weakness of uncertain cause in patients with laboratory study findings (CK, EMG, and muscle biopsy) that suggest a myogenic disorder. In some instances, more sophisticated studies have revealed an underlying metabolic cause (e.g., acid maltase deficiency, see below).

Metabolic Myopathies
Acid Maltase Deficiency

Deficiency of the glycogenolytic enzyme acid maltase (α-1,4-glucosidase) causes two distinctive syndromes. The enzyme is found in lysosomes and catalyzes the breakdown of glycogen to glucose. In infants, glycogen accumulates in skeletal muscle, heart, and nervous system (Pompe's disease), causing a multisystem disorder that results in death, usually before 1 year of age. In children or adults, the deficiency causes progressive proximal muscle weakness. In both forms, the disease is inherited as an autosomal recessive trait. The gene that codes for acid maltase has been mapped to the long arm of chromosome 17 (see Ch. 4). The reason for the different clinical syndromes is uncertain at present.

In the adult form, proximal muscle weakness begins in the third or fourth decade in otherwise health people. It occurs with equal frequency in men and women. Of note is that there is striking focality in patients with acid maltase deficiency superimposed on the proximal weakness. For example, the iliopsoas may be strong, yet the quadriceps may be severely affected. Respiratory weakness may be out of proportion to limb weakness and may result in death. Reflexes and sensory examination are normal.

The serum CK concentration is elevated in all patients, sometimes substantially so. The ischemic exercise test result is normal. Nerve conduction studies (sensory and motor) are normal. EMG shows profuse spontaneous activity, usually in the form of complex repetitive discharges and even true myotonic discharges. Quantitative EMG studies may show long-duration motor units with reduced recruitment, suggestive of neurogenic disease.

Muscle biopsy shows periodic acid-Schiff-positive vacuoles. Electron microscopy shows intralysosomal glycogen but also clusters of glycogen granules free in the cytoplasm (these are most commonly found in affected muscles).

There is no known treatment for acid maltase deficiency. The prognosis of the adult form of the illness is very slow (progression in the childhood form, known as Pompe's disease, is rapid).

Sporadic Diseases

Polymyositis

Accurate studies of the incidence and prevalence of polymyositis are few, but one estimate of prevalence is 8 per 100,000. Part of the problem is definition. Polymyositis is a syndrome with multiple causes that share one common pathologic feature, mononuclear cell infiltration of skeletal muscle. This may be due to direct infection (influenza viral myositis), may be part of a more diffuse disease process (such as Gougerot-Sjögren's disease, lupus, or sarcoidosis), or may present as an idiopathic disorder the cause of which is uncertain. There is general agreement that idiopathic polymyositis is an autoimmune disease. Because circulating antibodies against muscle components have not been convincingly demonstrated in polymyositis, attention has been directed to alterations in cellular immunity. Lymphocytes from patients with polymyositis produce a lymphotoxin when cultured in the presence of autologous muscle and are cytotoxic to chick and human fetal muscle cultures, making sensitized cytotoxic T lymphocytes possible causes of the disease. The initial event that causes sensitization of the lymphocytes is unknown, but it may involve a persistent viral infection. Nonetheless, a virus has never been cultured from affected muscles despite numerous reports of viruslike particles in electron microscopic studies.

In contrast to myasthenia gravis, there is no good animal model of experimental myositis. However, injection of mitochondrial and microsomal fractions from muscle preparations in rats have induced myositis with increased levels of serum CK, and the disease could be passively transferred with lymphocytes.

Clinical Features. Patients with polymyositis have proximal muscle weakness of either acute or chronic onset. There is no characteristic clinical feature, but several findings argue against the diagnosis. These include rash (making the diagnosis of dermatomyositis more likely, as described below), clinical or laboratory evidence of dysfunction of the central or peripheral nervous system, use of drugs or alcohol, evidence of metabolic myopathy, endocrine dysfunction, clinical or laboratory evidence of specific bacterial or viral infections (such as human immunodeficiency virus [HIV] infection, trichinosis, or influenza), or morphologic evidence of granulomatous disease, such as sarcoidosis.

The diagnosis of polymyositis may be considered definite, probable, or possible, depending on whether all of four typical features (weakness, inflammatory cell infiltrates in muscle biopsies, increased serum CK levels, and myogenic changes on EMG) are present, or only three or two. Accordingly, the diagnosis of polymyositis is one of exclusion.

Although the distribution of weakness is usually proximal, involving arms and legs, patients with this disease may also have distal muscle involvement, problems in swallowing, and facial weakness. Myalgia may be present but is variable in occurrence. The presence of dysphagia is useful in differentiating this disease from dystrophies when present. Respiratory muscles are rarely affected. Deep tendon reflexes are usually preserved, and muscle wasting is not apparent until late in the course of the disease. In fewer than 50 percent of patients, systemic symptoms, including fever, arthralgia, and Raynaud's phenomenon, are present.

Laboratory Findings. Serum enzymes, particularly CK, are increased in more than one-half of the pa-

DIFFERENTIAL DIAGNOSIS OF POLYMYOSITIS

Etiology unknown: Idiopathic polymyositis

Collagen vascular disease: Systemic lupus erythematosus, rheumatoid arthritis, periarteritis nodosa, systemic sclerosis, giant cell arteritis, Gougerot-Sjögren syndrome

Infections: Toxoplasmosis, trichinosis, schistosomiasis, cysticercosis, Chagas' disease, legionnaires' disease, candidiasis, influenza virus, rubella, hepatitis B, Behçet's disease, Kawasaki's disease, *Mycoplasma,* coxsackievirus, echovirus, acquired immunodeficiency syndrome

Immunization

Drugs: Systemic ethanol, penicillamine, clofibrate, steroids, emetine, chloroquine, kaliuretics, aminocaproic acid, rifampin, ipecac, intramuscular meperidine, pentazocine

Systemic diseases: Carcinoma, thymoma, sarcoid, amyloid, psoriasis, hyperglobulinemia (plasma cell dyscrasias), celiac disease, papular mucinosis, graft versus host disease after transplant, alcoholism

Endocrine disease: Hyperthyroidism, hypothyroidism, hyperadrenocorticism, hyperparathyroidism, Hashimoto's thyroiditis

Metabolic disease: Therapeutic starvation, anorexia nervosa, hypocalcemia, osteomalacia, chronic renal disease, chronic K^+ depletion, carnitine deficiency, acid maltase deficiency, phosphorylase deficiency, phosphofructokinase deficiency

(Adapted from Rowland, 1989, with permission.)

---

tients. There is some relationship between activity of disease and serum enzyme levels, but the correlation is not tight. Spontaneous clinical improvement may be accompanied by a decrease or normalization in serum enzyme levels, but corticosteroids alone also lower serum enzyme concentrations, independent of any clinical effect and should not be used as a criterion of therapeutic success.

Additional laboratory tests are necessary to exclude other disease processes. These include thyroid profile, antinuclear antibody, latex fixation, erythrocyte sedimentation rate, HIV antibodies, and quantitative immunoglobulins.

Nerve conduction study results are normal. EMG often shows moderate or profuse amounts of spontaneous activity in the form of positive sharp waves and fibrillation potentials. Complex repetitive discharges are common. Motor unit potentials are of short duration and low amplitude. The changes are most prominent in symptomatic muscles, with proximal muscles being most affected. In fact, sometimes, the only muscles to show prominent spontaneous activity in mildly symptomatic patients are paraspinal muscles.

Muscle biopsy is the basis for the diagnosis. Characteristic features include perivascular and interstitial inflammatory cell infiltration with evidence of degeneration and regeneration. However, the inflammatory process is patchy and may not always be seen in the portion of muscle sampled. To increase the likelihood of finding characteristic pathologic features, the muscle chosen for biopsy should be moderately affected, and physiologic study results on the contralateral muscle should be abnormal. Sometimes, more than one site should be sampled. At the very least, a neurogenic disorder or a storage myopathy (particularly glycogen storage disease and carnitine deficiency) should be excluded.

Treatment. Because of the presumed autoimmune basis, treatment options consist of various means of immunomodulation. Anecdotal reports of dramatic reversal of symptoms in response to prednisone, methotrexate, cyclophosphamide, cyclosporine, and other agents have made double-blind controlled trials difficult to perform. Instead, most studies compare different treatments. Unfortunately, there is no uniformly accepted therapeutic regimen. A regimen followed by many neurologists consists of prednisone beginning at doses of 60 to 100 mg/day. Higher doses are advocated by some investigators. A clinical response may occur within days, but a period of 3 months is recommended before reconsidering the use of this agent. In the presence of a clinical response, prednisone is gradually tapered with close clinical monitoring. Some patients require chronic steroid administration. The lowest effective dose should be established with intermittent attempts at further reduction. Monitoring of steroid-induced side effects is essential. Administering this dose of steroids in an alternate-day regimen may further reduce the risk of side effects.

If a patient does not respond to corticosteroids, alternative immunosuppressive agents should be tried. These include azathioprine (50 to 150 mg/day), methotrexate (40 mg/day), and cyclosporine (serum levels of 500 mg/dl). A full understanding of the side effects of each agent is essential. Plasmapheresis has produced temporary improvement in some patients. There is no clinical experience with human gamma-globulin at this time.

Dermatomyositis

This is a better defined syndrome than polymyositis because a characteristic skin rash occurs together with the presence of proximal weakness. Dermatomyositis occurs more frequently in children; in adults, it is often associated with an underlying malignancy. The autoimmune basis of this disease is supported by the presence of antigen-antibody complexes in the walls of blood vessels, especially in children. Other organs may be involved in childhood dermatomyositis, particularly the gastrointestinal tract.

Clinical Features. The skin lesion is the most prominent clinical finding in patients with dermatomyositis. It consists of an erythematous rash with lilac hue and edema affecting the eyelids and malar area, upper portion of chest, knuckles, periungal area, and less commonly, elbows and knees. The rash may be so subtle that it is overlooked. Calcifications in the interstitial and subcutaneous tissue (calcinosis) are common and may be seen on routine radiographs. Small granules of calcium may exude through the skin as a white pasty discharge. The weakness is proximal and symmetric, and progression may be rapid. Ocular muscles are spared, but swallowing and respiratory muscle weakness may occur. Reflexes are normal. Myalgia is a frequent but inconsistent symptom. The course may be relapsing.

In adults, particularly in men older than age 40, there is an increased frequency of malignancy, making a thorough search for occult cancer necessary once the diagnosis is established.

Laboratory Findings. Serum CK levels may be increased during the acute phase of the illness but are often normal. Nerve conduction studies are normal. EMG shows abnormal amounts of spontaneous activity in the form of positive sharp waves, fibrillation potentials, and complex repetitive discharges, particularly in proximal muscles. Motor units are of short duration and low amplitude. Recruitment in weak muscles is full with low amplitude.

Muscle biopsy shows abnormal fiber size variation, necrosis and regeneration, and a characteristic distribution of atrophic fibers at the periphery of the muscle fascicles. Inflammatory cell infiltrates are seen in 75 percent of patients.

Treatment. In adult patients, therapy is similar to that of polymyositis, with daily or alternate-day high-dose corticosteroid therapy (60 to 100 mg/day of prednisone) for 2 or 3 months followed by a slow taper. In children, a common mode of treatment is prednisone 1 mg/kg/day with appropriate reduction as clinical recovery occurs. Other immunosuppressive drugs (azathioprine and methotrexate) may be tried in patients with steroid-resistant disease. Preliminary studies have shown that immunoglobulin administration (2 g/kg IV over 5 days) is an effective treatment for patients with dermatomyositis.

Inclusion Body Myositis

This is a pathologic diagnosis based on the finding of characteristic inclusions in skeletal muscle. There is no distinctive clinical or EMG pattern. There are, however, suggestive features: It usually occurs in patients older than age 50, more frequently in men (3:1); it affects proximal leg muscles most (iliopsoas, quadriceps). Quadriceps reflexes are also reduced early in the disease, and a concomitant peripheral neuropathy is common. Serum CK levels are usually normal or mildly elevated. Treatment with steroids has little or no effect on the progression of disease.

Systemic Illness

There are many systemic illnesses that present with proximal muscle weakness and may therefore be confused with polymyositis (see box, above). Many endocrine disorders and collagen-vascular diseases produce proximal muscle weakness, which may be the sole manifestation of sarcoidosis. Acute viral syndromes may be associated with myalgia, weakness, and myoglobinuria.

Myopathy may be caused by many toxins. For example, most cholesterol-lowering agents have the potential to cause myopathy. Painful proximal weakness is the most common symptom. The serum CK level may be elevated, and acute necrosis may be observed on muscle biopsy. Patients may have myoglobinuria. EMG shows profuse spontaneous activity.

Zidovudine, a treatment for HIV infection, may also cause proximal muscle weakness, elevated CK level, and inflammation on muscle biopsy. Differentiation between this and HIV-associated inflammatory myopathy is difficult and probably the best way to differentiate the two is withdrawal of the drug and monitor for clinical response.

Inherited Metabolic Disease

Carnitine Deficiency

Carnitine is an essential cofactor involved in the transport of long chain fatty acids across the mitochondrial membrane. Myopathic carnitine deficiency is an autosomal recessive disorder that usually begins in childhood with symptoms of mild proximal weakness. Slow progression and spread to the neck, palate, and face may occur.

Laboratory studies may show electrocardiographic abnormalities. The serum CK level is usually mildly elevated. Nerve conduction studies are normal. EMG shows short-duration and low-amplitude motor units. Serum carnitine concentrations are normal, contrasting with low carnitine concentrations in muscle. Muscle biopsy shows lipid storage myopathy with vacuoles that stain positive with Sudan black or oil red O.

Treatment with carnitine has produced variable results; some patients respond to corticosteroids.

Debrancher Deficiency (Type III Glycogenosis)

Deficiency of debrancher enzyme is an inherited autosomal recessive disease, usually found in children and characterized by liver dysfunction, stunted growth, and fasting hypoglycemia with ketonuria. In adults, debrancher deficiency is associated with slowly progressive weakness, which usually affects distal muscles. This distribution of weakness and the frequent finding on EMG of abundant fibrillation potentials makes the diagnosis of amyotrophic lateral sclerosis (ALS) a consideration. Muscle biopsy, however, shows a severe vacuolar myopathy with periodic acid-Schiff-positive material within the vacuoles.

MYOPATHIES PRESENTING WITH SELECTIVE MUSCLE INVOLVEMENT

Fascioscapulohumeral Disease

Fascioscapulohumeral dystrophy is inherited as an autosomal dominant trait. The gene responsible for the clinical syndrome has been localized to chromosome 4 (see Ch. 4). However, neither the gene nor the gene product has been identified.

Clinical Features

The diagnosis of fascioscapulohumeral dystrophy is suggested by the peculiar distribution of weakness. The onset is between ages 6 and 30, but initial symptoms may go unnoticed. Many patients report lifelong inability to whistle or draw fluid through a straw. Some patients are told they sleep with the whites of the eyes visible. At the other extreme, facial weakness may be a prominent clinical problem.

Limb weakness is of variable severity and is symmetric. The neck is characteristically elongated. The deltoid is spared, but periscapular muscles (infraspinatus, supraspinatus, and other periscapular muscles) are weak, causing the characteristic appearance of scapular winging. Selective wasting in the biceps and triceps produces a "Popeye" appearance because of the relatively large forearm muscles and deltoid contrasting with wasted biceps and triceps. There is variation in the distribution of weakness, and the legs are sometimes involved (so-called *scapuloperoneal dystrophy*). However, small foot muscles, such as the extensor digitorum brevis are hypertrophied. Many patients have

congenital absence of muscles or parts of muscles, especially the pectoralis.

The illness is usually slowly progressive. Examination of family members is important to establish the nature of transmission.

Laboratory Findings

Serum CK levels are often normal. Nerve conduction studies are normal. EMG shows little or no spontaneous activity, but motor units are of short duration and low amplitude with full recruitment in weak muscles. It is important to examine the most affected muscles, such as facial and periscapular muscles.

Muscle biopsy findings are varied. It is important to choose a symptomatic muscle or at least one that shows electrophysiologic abnormalities on the opposite side. Pathologic changes include increased fiber size variability and interstitial fibrosis. Few patients have inflammatory cell infiltrates, others show nemaline bodies, and still others show neurogenic changes (group atrophy). One family had abnormal lipid storage and mitochondrial proliferation.

Treatment

There is no specific treatment for fascioscapulohumeral dystrophy. Physical and occupational therapy and strengthening exercises are useful to help patients live and function independently. Genetic counseling is also important.

Oculopharyngeal Dystrophy

Oculopharyngeal dystrophy is a rare autosomal dominant disorder, in which the molecular defect has not been established. It is a disorder of later life, usually beginning in the fifth decade. It is particularly common in patients of French Canadian descent in whom the disease has been traced back to a common ancestor who landed in Quebec in the 1600s.

Ptosis is usually the first clinical finding, followed by difficulty swallowing and facial weakness. Limb weakness is variably present. The CK levels are often normal and are rarely significantly elevated. Nerve conduction studies are usually normal, but axonal neuropathy has been described. EMG of proximal muscles shows motor units of short duration and low amplitude, especially in periscapular muscles. Muscle biopsy shows myogenic changes with intranuclear filamentous inclusions, which are characteristic of this disease. Differentiation from ALS (bulbar palsy, see Ch. 63) and myasthenia gravis (see Ch. 81) may be difficult. There is no treatment available.

Distal Myopathy

First described in Sweden, there are now four different forms of this disease. Welander's myopathy occurs primarily in older people (mean age, 47 years; male-to-female ratio, 1.5:1). It is an autosomal dominant disorder found most often in patients of Scandinavian origin. Distal extensor muscles are most affected, and vasomotor instability (coldness of hands and feet) is present in more than 90 percent of patients. Despite the neurogenic distribution of weakness, EMG and muscle biopsy indicate a myogenic process.

A second form is Finnish tibial dystrophy, an autosomal dominant disorder beginning after age 35 with selective involvement of the anterior tibial muscle and, in advanced stages, the long toe extensors. The serum CK level is mildly increased and muscle biopsy confirms the dystrophic process. Electron microscopy shows occasional vacuoles with tubulofilamentous inclusions.

Distal myopathy can occur in younger patients, and two types are primarily in Japanese patients. In one form, there is weakness of the gastrocnemius muscles, and the CK level is dramatically increased. Patellar and ankle jerks may be absent. The onset is in the early 20s, and the mode of transmission is autosomal recessive. Morphologic analysis shows dystrophic changes. Another form affects mainly muscles in the anterior compartment of the leg. The CK levels are modestly increased, and transmission is autosomal recessive. Morphologic analysis reveals rimmed vacuoles.

Other disorders to consider in patients with suspected distal myopathy include myotonic dystrophy, inclusion body myositis, motor neuropathy (e.g., lead toxicity or porphyria), neuronal form of the Charcot-Marie-Tooth disease, centronuclear myopathy, debrancher deficiency myopathy, and lipid storage myopathy.

Progressive External Ophthalmoparesis

Selective weakness of ocular movement is sometimes caused by myogenic disease. It may be familial or sporadic. It begins in childhood or early adulthood with ptosis followed by limitation of ocular movements. Double vision does not occur. Examination shows paralysis of ocular movements and ptosis that does not vary in severity.

Progressive external ophthalmoparesis (PEO) may also be part of a more generalized disorder, which is termed Kearns-Sayre syndrome. In these patients, PEO occurs in association with two other obligatory features: onset before age 20 and pigmentary retinopathy, plus one of the following: heart block, cerebellar syndrome, or cerebrospinal fluid protein level greater than 100 mg/dl. Using this definition, Kearns-Sayre syndrome is never familial. Laboratory abnormalities include raised blood and spinal fluid lactate and pyruvate levels. Ragged red fibers are characteristically found on muscle biopsy. Ragged red fibers contain increased numbers of lipid droplets and subsarcolemmal accumulations of mitochondria, best seen on the Gomori's trichrome or succinate dehydrogenase stains.

Recent evidence has shown that mitochondrial DNA deletions (a single deletion in each patient) are found in virtually all patients with Kearns-Sayre syndrome. Mitochondrial deletions are also found in about one-half of patients with non-Kearns-Sayre syndrome sporadic PEO.

Two other forms of PEO with ragged red fibers, both hereditary, are due to mutations in mitochondrial DNA. Patients with maternally inherited PEO usually have a point mutation at nucleotide 3243, in the transfer RNA Leu (UUR) gene. Autosomal dominant PEO (often associated with proximal limb and respiratory weakness) is seen in patients with multiple deletions of mitochondrial DNA, that is, each patient has more than one deletion in the mitochondrial genome.

Quadriceps Myopathy

Patients with selective involvement of the quadriceps present a difficult diagnostic challenge. Muscle biopsy often shows nonspecific myogenic changes. Recent advances have shown that some patients have defects of dystrophin similar to those seen in patients with Becker's muscular dystrophy.

Inflammatory Myopathies

Polymyositis (see above) may rarely affect distal and pharyngeal muscles. Isolated weakness of the neck extensors (floppy head syndrome) may be caused by polymyositis or sclerodermatomyositis. Inclusion body myositis has a preference for distal muscles and forearm flexors.

Metabolic Myopathies

Metabolic diseases rarely present with focal weakness. Case reports of acid maltase deficiency with prominent respiratory involvement have been reported. Patients with carnitine deficiency may have prominent neck weakness.

MYOPATHIES ASSOCIATED WITH PREMATURE FATIGUE AND CRAMPS

Inherited Disease

McArdle's Disease (Myophosphorylase Deficiency)

McArdle's disease is a rare autosomal recessive disorder caused by a defect in glycogen metabolism (myophosphorylase deficiency), making muscle unable to use glycogen as a source of energy for short-term exercise. This disorder is also known as type V glycogenosis.

Clinical Features. The characteristic clinical feature of McArdle's disease is painful cramps after intense exercise, a symptom often disregarded because of the lack of atrophy or weakness. Some patients show dark, "Coca-Cola"-colored urine after exercise (myoglobinuria). The pain may be so severe that muscle activity ceases. However, if exercise is resumed at low effort, a "second wind" phenomenon occurs, and the person can continue exercise without discomfort.

Molecular analysis has shown 10 different mutations in the myophosphorylase gene. Because one of these is common in Anglo-Saxon individuals, detection of the mutation in genomic DNA from leukocytes may provide diagnostic information in affected patients without the need of a muscle biopsy.

Examination in the asymptomatic state is usually normal. However, when patients are asked to exercise anaerobically, painful cramps develop, which are not accompanied by electrical discharge of motor units, thus making the phenomenon a true contracture. Proximal weakness often develops late in life and may dominate the clinical picture in some patients.

Laboratory Features. The serum CK level is variably increased in most patients. Analysis of the venous blood lactate after a standardized period of exercise under ischemic conditions provides unequivocal proof of a glycolytic defect (although not specifically of McArdle's disease). The forearm ischemic lactate test is performed as follows: A catheter is placed in a superficial vein, and a resting blood sample for venous lactate is withdrawn and placed on ice. The patient is asked to grip a dynamometer repetitively at 60 strokes/minute, which is sufficient to produce a work load of 5 to 6 kpm for 1 minute. Clinical analysis for contracture is made, and observations are noted. Venous blood for lactate analysis is withdrawn at 1, 3, 5, 10, and 20 minutes after exercise, with the tubes kept on ice. Peak lactate occurs at 3 minutes and should be at least three times the baseline value. In patients with McArdle's disease, there is no rise in venous lactate concentration; small rises of lactate (less than three times baseline) are more difficult to interpret but may suggest a defect in terminal glycolysis.

Nerve conduction studies are normal. EMG shows no spontaneous activity, and motor unit form is normal, except for occasional triplets and doublets. The EMG silent contracture is the hallmark EMG finding.

Muscle biopsy shows subsarcolemmal deposits of glycogen. Histochemical staining for phosphorylase is absent. Specific biochemical analysis of myophosophorylase confirms the enzyme defect.

Treatment. No effective treatment exists for this disease. However, high protein diets has been attempted with some reported benefits.

Phosphofructokinase Deficiency

Phosphofructokinase (PFK) deficiency is another disorder of glycogen metabolism. Deficiency of PFK prevents the conversion of fructose-6-phosphate to fructose-1,6-diphosphate, an essential glycolytic step. PFK deficiency is also known as glycogenosis type VII (or Tarui's disease). It is a genetic disorder transmitted as an autosomal recessive trait, and in some countries, it is prevalent among Ashkenazi Jewish individuals.

Clinical Features. Patients with PFK deficiency complain of muscle pain and cramps after intense exercise. Fixed weakness is rare, but it has been reported in both infants and adults.

Laboratory Findings. Because PFK in erythrocytes shares a common subunit with PFK in muscle, patients with muscle PFK deficiency show a mild hemolytic anemia with increased bilirubin and reticulocyte count. Serum CK levels are often elevated. Myoglobinuria can occur. Nerve conduction studies are normal, but EMG often shows short-duration, low-amplitude motor unit potentials. Ischemic exercise testing does not show a rise in venous lactate level.

Muscle biopsy shows accumulation of periodic acid-Schiff-positive material. PFK deficiency can be demonstrated directly through the lack of histochemically identified PFK or lack of measurable PFK biochemically. Recently, several molecular defects in the PFK gene have been documented in Ashkenazi patients.

Treatment. There is no specific treatment for PFK deficiency. Management of symptoms is achieved through awareness of exercise limitations.

Defects of Terminal Glycolysis

Intolerance to intense exercise, cramps, and myoglobulinuria also characterize the clinical presentations of three rare defects of terminal glycolysis involving the following enzymes: phosphoglycerate kinase, phosphoglycerate mutase, and lactate dehydrogenase. Phosphoglycerate kinase deficiency (glycogenosis type IX) is transmitted as an X-linked trait, whereas phosphoglycerate mutase (glycogenosis type X) and lactate dehydrogenase deficiencies (glycogenosis type XI) are causes of a blunted (but not absent) increase in venous lactate level.

Carnitine Palmityl Transferase Deficiency

Carnitine palmityltransferase (CPT) occurs in two forms: one (CPT I) bound on the inner surface of the outer mitochondrial membrane and the other (CPT

II) on the inside of the inner mitochondrial membrane. By catalyzing the conversion of long-chain acetyl coenzyme A to acylcarnitine and back to acetyl coenzyme A, CPT, together with carnitine, facilitates transport of fatty acids into the mitochondrial matrix where they are oxidized. CPT II deficiency, which causes recurrent myoglobinuria, is transmitted as an autosomal recessive trait. The gene encoding CPT II is located on chromosome 7, and several mutations have been identified (see Ch. 4).

Fatty acids are a critical energy source for muscle during fasting and prolonged exercise, and it is during these conditions that manifestations of this disease are most likely to occur. They consist of muscle pain and stiffness accompanied by myoglobinuria. CPT deficiency appears to be the most common metabolic cause of recurrent myoglobinuria in adults.

The serum CK level at rest is usually normal, and ischemic exercise causes a normal rise in venous lactate level. EMG and nerve conduction study results are normal. Muscle biopsy findings may be normal, or it may show a variable degree of lipid storage.

Myoadenylate Deaminase Deficiency

Myoadenylate deaminase deficiency is transmitted as an autosomal recessive trait and is found in about 2 percent of all muscle biopsy specimens examined histochemically. The wide variety of clinical syndromes associated with myoadenylate deaminase deficiency has raised doubts about the pathogenic significance of the enzyme defect. Two main clinical subgroups exist. Two-thirds of patients complain of cramps or pain after exercise, usually mild and almost never incapacitating. Myoglobinuria has been reported in very few patients, and fixed weakness is rare. A second group of patients have clinically well-defined but diverse neurologic diseases, including ALS, spinal muscular atrophy, dermatomyositis, and periodic paralysis. In these patients, the association of myoadenylate deaminase deficiency with specific neuromuscular disease is likely to be purely coincidental. Therefore, the significance of this defect is uncertain at best.

DISORDERS OF MUSCLE WITH MYOTONIA

Myotonia refers to delayed relaxation after muscle contraction elicited by voluntary effort, mechanical stimulation, or electrical excitation. The EMG correlate of clinical myotonia is high-frequency motor unit discharges the amplitude and frequency of which wax and wane. Many observers liken the sound produced by these discharges to that of a "dive bomber." These discharges are resistant to peripheral nerve block or curare, which suggests that the discharges originate in the muscle itself.

There are several clinical syndromes in which myotonia is the only or the prominent clinical manifestation. Recent advances have localized the defect to the sodium or chloride channel within the muscle membrane.

Myotonic Dystrophy

Myotonic dystrophy is a clinical syndrome characterized by distal limb weakness and wasting, myotonia, cataracts, heart conduction defects, multiple endocrine abnormalities associated with infertility, premature frontal balding, and often, mild mental retardation. It is transmitted as an autosomal dominant trait, occurring in 5.5 per 100,000 population. The disease is transmitted by a mutation in the myotonin protein kinase gene on chromosome 19 (see Ch. 4). The mutation is characterized by a repeating sequence of three base pairs (CTG). The longer the CTG repeat sequence is, the more severe the clinical syndrome is. The clinical severity of myotonic dystrophy increases in succeeding generations (the phenomenon known as "anticipation"), and this is correlated with lengthening of the repeat sequence.

The mutation that causes myotonic dystrophy is thought to affect a membrane-bound protein kinase that is essential for proper functioning of the sodium channel. The impaired enzyme function prevents efficient closure of the channel after activation, causing impaired relaxation.

Clinical Features

Weakness is usually the first symptom noticed by patients with myotonic dystrophy. The age of onset varies within the same family, but most patients become symptomatic by the end of the second or beginning of the third decade. Patients with myotonic dystrophy rarely complain of symptoms caused by myotonia (muscle cramps and difficulty relaxing muscles). Later in the disease, many patients complain of diffuse muscle stiffness and vague muscle pain.

Examination shows a characteristic elongated facies with frontal balding, ptosis, and wasting of the temporalis and sternocleidomastoid muscles. The wasting of neck muscles causes a "swan-neck" appearance. Neck flexors are weak. Distal muscles in the arms and legs are weak and wasted in contradistinction to other myogenic disorders. Myotonia is easily demonstrated by voluntary contraction (e.g., during sustained upgaze with rapid downgaze, the eyelids are slow to follow; after vigorous contraction of the hand, there is a marked slowness of relaxation) or by direct percussion of a muscle (including the tongue). Sometimes, exposure of the muscle to cold temperatures enhances the myotonic response.

Weakness of the pharyngeal muscles causes a nasal

voice with difficulty swallowing. Associated involvement of smooth muscle may also impair esophageal and intestinal motility and cause uterine dystocia. Cardiac involvement consists mainly of conduction disturbances, usually requiring pacemaker placement.

The disease is progressive, although the rate of progression varies.

Myotonic dystrophy may affect infants. The disease is limited to children born of mothers with myotonic dystrophy. The severity of the maternal disease is not correlated with that of the infant. Affected infants have severe hypotonia, bilateral facial weakness, difficulty sucking, weak cry, respiratory distress, and multiple contractures (one cause of arthrogryposis multiplex congenita). An important negative feature is the absence of clinical and often electrical myotonia. Therefore, evidence of clinical or electrical myotonia in the affected mother is an important diagnostic clue. If death caused by respiratory failure does not occur in the neonatal period, there is usually some improvement of motor function. However, facial diplegia persists, and affected children have lack of expression and a characteristic "tented" upper lip or "fish mouth." Mental retardation is common. The exclusively maternal transmission has been attributed to the combined effect of the mutant gene and an intrauterine maternal factor, the nature of which, however, remains obscure. Genetic imprinting has also been considered.

Laboratory Findings

The serum CK level may be mildly elevated. Genetic screening shows the GTC repeat sequence on chromosome 19 (see Ch. 4). ECG may show bradycardia with a prolonged PR interval. Nerve conduction velocities are usually normal, although the evoked-response amplitudes may be low. Needle EMG shows profuse amounts of myotonic discharges with characteristic waxing and waning of amplitude and frequency. Motor unit potentials are often difficult to isolate from the myotonic discharges but, when visualized, show short duration and low amplitude.

The muscle biopsy is not distinctive and may show only hypertrophy of type II fibers in subclinical cases. Later in the course of the disease, there are increased numbers of internal nuclei, ring fibers, sarcoplasmic masses, and accumulation of fat and connective tissue.

Treatment

There is no treatment for the progressive weakness associated with myotonic dystrophy. Physical and occupational therapy is required to assist walking and maintain independent living as long as possible. Attention should be directed to the non-neurologic features of myotonic dystrophy. For example, periodic cardiac assessment, cataract assessment, and endocri-

nologic screens are necessary. Excessive fatigue and daytime sleepiness may be due to ventilatory disorders, and appropriate consultation with the sleep disorders laboratory and ventilatory monitoring may be necessary.

Myotonia can sometimes be controlled through medications, such as phenytoin or carbamazepine. Recently, the use of mexiletine has been reported to be particularly effective and well tolerated. Other therapeutic options, quinine and procainamide, carry risks of aggravating cardiac conduction defects.

Myotonia Congenita

Myotonia congenita is inherited as an autosomal dominant (Thomsen's) or recessive (Becker's) disorder the primary manifestation of which is myotonia. Therefore, unlike myotonic dystrophy, in myotonia congenita, myotonia is the disabling symptom. This disease is due to malfunction of the chloride channel, and has been linked to a gene on chromosome 7 (see Ch. 4). The characteristic history involves a prominent "warm-up" phenomenon in which the patient is very stiff at the onset of activity but loosens up as exercises continues. Most muscles are affected, including the hands, face, tongue, and pharynx. Myotonia is easily elicited by strong hand grasp or direct percussion of the muscle and is shown by difficulty opening the eyes after forced closure. The muscles are usually large with a peculiar firmness. The habitus of these patients is often described as "herculean." In the dominant form, there is no progression, and weakness does not occur. In the recessive form, a slowly progressive weakness may be observed. Treatment consists of anticonvulsant agents or specific sodium channel blockers, such as mexiletine.

Paramytonia Congenita

Paramyotonia begins in late childhood, and the cardinal feature is muscle stiffness triggered by cold. It is an autosomal dominant disorder with a high degree of penetrance. Repeated muscle contractions may lead to weakness, particularly in the face, hand, tongue, and pharynx. Rarely, repeated muscle contractions in cold muscles lead to flaccid paralysis. Some patients have episodes of generalized paralysis. In some patients, weakness develops in response to potassium infusion much like that in patients with hyperkalemic periodic paralysis. Examination usually shows a very muscular habitus with normal strength. Percussion myotonia is usually present but may require cooling for demonstration. Delayed opening after eye closure is invariably present.

Diagnostic studies show normal sensory and motor conduction studies. Needle EMG shows diffuse myotonic discharges. Motor unit form is normal. Repetitive stimulation may show a decrement in motor evoked-response amplitude, especially after cooling.

The cause of myotonia congenita has been linked to the occurrence of single amino acid substitutions in the voltage-gated sodium channel caused by mutations in a gene on chromosome 17 (see Ch. 4). The treatment of choice is the sodium channel blocking agent, mexiletine.

Hyperkalemic Periodic Paralysis

Hyperkalemic periodic paralysis is an autosomal dominant disorder that usually begins in childhood and occurs equally in men and women. It is manifested as attacks of weakness after exercise, either generalized or limited to the exercised muscle. In some patients, weakness may be prevented by continuing exercise, causing some patients to pace all night to ensure proper strength in the morning for important events.

Hyperkalemic periodic paralysis was the first neuromuscular disease shown to be due to genetically determined defects in an ion channel. Several mutations that cause amino acid substitutions in the voltage-gated sodium channel of the muscle cell membrane have been documented in patients with this disorder. These mutations affect the gene encoding the sodium channel on chromosome 17 (see Ch. 4).

Examination between attacks shows no evidence of weakness. Some families show no clinical or EMG evidence of myotonia in between attacks, but most show some type of myotonia (clinical or electrical). The presence of myotonia differentiates familial hyperkalemic periodic paralysis from hypokalemic periodic paralysis.

The serum potassium level is normal between attacks but is often high during an attack. Rarely, the serum potassium content may be low during the attack of weakness. ECG may show signs of hyperkalemia during the attack (tall, slender T waves). The serum CK concentration may be elevated between attacks. Nerve conduction study results are normal, but during repeated stimulation (repetitive stimuli), the motor-evoked response may lose amplitude (decrement). EMG shows myotonic discharges.

Muscle biopsy may show mild myopathic changes and empty vacuoles.

The diagnosis is confirmed if weakness is observed during an oral loading dose of potassium chloride (0.05 to 0.5 g/kg). Unfortunately, false-negative results are common.

Treatment is directed toward avoiding known precipitants of attacks, such as exercise, cold, hunger, and emotional stress. Most attacks are brief and require no treatment. If severe and prolonged, measures to lower the serum potassium level are needed. Administration of glucose (100 g PO) and insulin (10 units

subcutaneously) is effective. Some investigators have found chronic use of acetazolamide effective in preventing attacks of hyperkalemic periodic paralysis. The interictal myotonia may respond to membrane-stabilizing agents, such as phenytoin or carbamazepine. Recent experience with mexiletine has been favorable. The weakness may be permanent and progressive, resulting in a limb-girdle clinical syndrome.

Schwartz-Jampel Syndrome

Schwartz-Jampel syndrome is a rare autosomal recessive disorder that begins in childhood. The clinical examination reveals three characteristic features: percussion myotonia with muscle stiffness, especially in facial muscles resulting in an abnormal facial appearance ("frozen smile"); skeletal abnormalities (spondyloepiphysial dysplasia and short stature); and joint contractures. Grip myotonia is also present.

EMG shows continuous muscle fiber activity that is resistant to ischemia and curare, which suggests the generator is within the muscle fiber itself. Abnormal sodium channel opening has been proposed, and this is supported by the observation that procainamide, which blocks sodium channels in nerves, abolishes the spontaneous activity and the afterdischarges.

DISORDERS CHARACTERIZED BY ACUTE MUSCLE WEAKNESS

Hypokalemic Periodic Paralysis

Acute and episodic generalized weakness associated with hypokalemia is usually inherited as an autosomal dominant disorder, occurring in men more than women (3:1). The symptoms are often more severe in men. The disease usually becomes clinically apparent by the age of 30. The history is characteristic. Patients tell of awakening with generalized weakness or paralysis after carbohydrate-rich meals (such as pasta or pizza) or after excessive exercise the night before. The attacks occur most often in the morning but may be triggered by rest after strenuous exercise. Cold exposure, stress, and alcohol may also trigger an episode.

Examination during the episode of weakness shows greatest involvement of proximal muscles, and reflexes are absent. Respiratory muscles and cranial nerve-innervated muscles are spared. Accordingly, there is little danger of respiratory insufficiency. The duration of the attack is usually less than 24 hours but may last up to 72 hours. The frequency of attacks varies between individuals but usually decreases with age.

Between attacks, examination is usually normal, but proximal fixed weakness may evolve after repeated episodes. Induction of weakness with hypokalemia is possible and, when observed, is diagnostic. Administration of 100 g of glucose usually reduces the serum potassium level to a significant degree, which induces weakness in the patient. If this is unsuccessful, an insulin challenge is necessary. In this test, the patient is given 1.5 to 2 g/kg of glucose orally with 20 units of insulin subcutaneously. Maximum lowering of the potassium level occurs within 2 to 3 hours with weakness occurring several hours later. The ECG and serum potassium level should be monitored closely.

Laboratory findings are significant only for a mild elevation of the serum CK concentration. Potassium levels between attacks are often normal, but during the attack, levels between 2 to 3 mEq/L are common. ECG changes of hypokalemia are common (bradycardia, U waves, flattened T waves, and lengthening of the PR and QT intervals).

Muscle biopsy specimens are usually normal, but if affected muscles are sampled during an attack, vacuoles are often seen, which may disappear as the symptoms resolve. With subsequent episodes, the vacuoles persist between attacks. The vacuoles result from the proliferation of T tubules and dilation of the sarcoplasmic reticulum.

Treatment consists of administration of 5 to 10 g PO of potassium chloride, which is repeated in 2 hours if there is no improvement. Attacks can be prevented by avoiding high carbohydrate meals and excessive amounts of physical activity. Acetazolamide (125 to 150 mg/day), which promotes metabolic acidosis and opposes movement of potassium into cells, is often effective as a prophylactic agent.

Acute Myopathy Associated With Corticosteroids and Neuromuscular Blocking Agents

This is a syndrome usually seen in asthmatic patients in the intensive care unit on a ventilator requiring neuromuscular blocking agents (usually vecuronium or pancuronium). The weakness may be severe and results in flaccid quadriplegia. The weakness is discovered only after the neuromuscular blocking agent is tapered. The serum CK level is elevated. EMG is usually myogenic. Muscle biopsy shows loss of adenosine triphosphatase staining in a patchy distribution. Recovery is common, although it may take months. The cause of this disorder is uncertain, but it has been suggested that the functional denervation may enhance myosin degradation.

DISORDERS CHARACTERIZED BY MUSCLE HYPERACTIVITY

Isaacs' Syndrome

In this syndrome, first described in 1961, patients complain of muscle stiffness, cramps, and twitching. Myalgia may be a prominent complaint, and excessive perspiration is common. The onset is usually in early adulthood. Examination shows muscle hypertrophy and twitching. Reflexes may be absent. Although there is obvious difficulty in muscle relaxation, percussion myotonia is usually not evident.

The syndrome is defined by the characteristic response to pharmacologic agents. The muscle activity is blocked by curare but not by peripheral nerve block, sleep, general anesthesia, or spinal anesthesia. Activity increases during hyperventilation or ischemia.

Nerve conduction studies may reveal evidence of sensorimotor neuropathy. Afterdischarges follow the electrically evoked compound muscle action potential or even direct percussion of the peripheral nerve. These afterdischarges are responsible for the difficulty in relaxation. Needle EMG shows continuous muscle fiber activity, neuromyotonic discharges, myokymia, and myotonic discharges. Pathologic studies have found evidence of a sensorimotor neuropathy of variable severity.

Isaacs' syndrome may be an autoimmune disease, in which immunoglobulins increase the amount of neurotransmitter released from nerve terminals. Treatment usually consists of anticonvulsant medication, either phenytoin or carbamazepine, although one patient improved after plasmapheresis.

Stiff-Man Syndrome

Patients with stiff-man syndrome show a gradual progression of muscle stiffness, first affecting trunk and neck muscles. Episodic spasms are superimposed on generalized stiffness. They may be precipitated by sudden stimuli and may involve laryngeal and respiratory muscles. The absence of trismus differentiates this from tetanus.

Laboratory studies show normal nerve conduction studies. EMG shows only protracted, involuntary firing of normal motor units. The abnormal activity is abolished by sleep, general anesthesia, and intravenous diazepam, which suggests that the abnormal generator is in the central nervous system. Antibodies against glutamic acid decarboxylase are found in these patients. This enzyme synthesizes γ-aminobutyric acid, an inhibitory neurotransmitter.

Treatment with high-dose diazepam is sometimes beneficial.

MORPHOLOGICALLY DEFINED CONGENITAL MYOPATHIES

This is a group of hereditary myopathies, which share several features as follows: distinct, but not absolutely specific, structural abnormalities in the muscle biopsy; presence of weakness at birth or onset soon thereafter, although presentation may occasionally be in adult life; in most cases, a benign and nonprogressive course, with proximal or diffuse weakness; frequent association with skeletal anomalies, such as pes cavus and dislocated hip; and normal or only slightly elevated serum enzyme levels.

At least eight disorders have been described. *Central core disease,* transmitted as an autosomal dominant trait, shows central or paracentral areas (cores) on biopsy, which usually extend along the entire length of the muscle fibers and show decreased stains with reactions for oxidative enzymes and phosphorylase. The lesions are generally limited to type I fibers. Most patients show a marked type I fiber predominance. Some of the cores are composed of closely packed but normally striated myofibrils ("structured cores"); others show disorganized myofibrils ("unstructured" cores).

As suggested by the name, *multicore (minicore) disease* features multiple small cores on biopsy, ultrastructurally similar to unstructured central cores but which do not extend along the entire length of the fiber. This is a disease of children.

Nemaline (rod) myopathy is usually transmitted as an autosomal dominant trait, with females more frequently affected than males. Although the onset is in infancy, with hypotonia, weak cry, feeding difficulties, and delayed motor development, the diagnosis may not be made until adulthood in some cases. The myopathy is accompanied by a dysmorphic appearance with slender habitus, high-arched palate, kyphoscoliosis, pigeon chest, and pes cavus. The muscle biopsy features multiple "rod" structures in muscle fibers, which are not seen in hematoxylin and eosin-stained preparations but are revealed by the Gomori's trichrome stain or the phosphotungstic acid hematoxylin stain. Rods tend to be more abundant in type I fibers, and there is usually type I fiber predominance. Ultrastructurally, nemaline bodies are similar to Z-discs, from which they appear to originate.

Myotubular (centronuclear) myopathy is a rare disorder usually transmitted as an autosomal dominant trait, although X-linked recessive cases have been described. The disease usually affects children with ophthalmoplegia and facial diplegia. Weakness is usually evident at birth, but the onset may be later in childhood or even in the second or third decade. The clinical course also varies in different patients, from a benign, virtually static myopathy to severe generalized weakness with respiratory failure. Muscle biopsy characteristically shows rows of central nuclei, predominantly in type I fibers, surrounded by an area of cytoplasm devoid of myofibrils and containing variably increased oxidative enzymes, phosphorylase and glycogen. These abnormal fibers resemble immature muscle fibers (myotubes), which suggests that the disorder may be due to an arrest of normal muscle development.

Several other types of histopathologically distinctive myopathies have also been described in rare cases, most of them sharing childhood onset and a static course. They include *sarcotubular myopathy,* a congenital nonprogressive myopathy with abnormal accumulations of sarcotubular vesicles mostly in type II fibers; *fingerprint body myopathy* the morphologic abnormalities of which are not visible by light microscopy, but they appear ultrastructurally as concentric lamellae reminiscent of fingerprints; *reducing body myopathy,* featuring multiple inclusion bodies within the fibers, staining with sulfhydryl group reagents; and *fiber type disproportion* in which histochemical stains of muscle biopsy specimens show a marked predominance of type I fibers, uniformly smaller than type II, although in normal children, the two types of fibers have comparable size. Although most patients begin in childhood with weakness, the disorder becomes static and may actually improve.

ANNOTATED BIBLIOGRAPHY

Baumann N, Serratrice G (eds). Mitochondries et maladies du système nerveuse. Rev Neurol (Paris) 1991;147: 413–548. (Special issue on mitochondrial myopathies.)

Thorough update, 13 papers in English and 9 in French.

Becker PE. Two new families of benign sex-linked recessive muscular dystrophy. Rev Can Biol 1962;21:551–66.

The original description.

Bonilla E, Samitt CE, Miranda AF et al. Duchenne muscular dystrophy; deficiency of dystrophin at the muscle cell surface. Cell 1988;54:447–52.

Polyclonal antibody studies to localize dystrophin.

Bradley WG. Adynamia episodica hereditaria. Brain 1969; 92:345–78.

Review article.

Dalakas MC, Illa I, Dambrosia JM et al. A controlled trial of high-dose intravenous immune globulin infusions as treatment for dermatomyositis. N Eng J Med 1993;329: 1993–2000.

Studied 15 patients with significant benefits.

DiMauro S, Trevisan C, Hays A. Disorders of lipid metabolism in muscle. Muscle Nerve 1980;3:369–88.

Review article.

Drachman DA. Ophthalmoplegia-plus; a classification of the disorders associated with progressive external ophthalmoplegia. In Vinken PJ, Bruyn GW (eds). Handbook of Clinical Neurology. Vol. 22. Elsevier-North Holland, New York, 1975, pp. 203–16.

Review article.

East C, Alivizatos PA, Grundy SM et al. Rhabdomyolysis in

patients receiving levostatin after cardiac transplantation. N Eng J Med 1988;318:47–8.

Case reports.

Griggs RC, Engel WK, Resnick JS. Acetazolamide treatment of hypokalemic periodic paralysis. Ann Intern Med 1970; 73:39–48.

Useful in some cases.

Hays AP, Hallett M, Delfs J et al. Muscle phosphofructokinase deficiency: abnormal polysaccharide in a case of late onset myopathy. Neurology 1981;31:1077–86.

A patient with proximal weakness and metabolic myopathy with PFK deficiency.

Hirano M, Ott BR, Raps EC et al. Acute quadriplegic myopathy: a complication of treatment with steroids, nondepolarizing blocking agents, or both. Neurology 1992;42: 2082–7.

Case reports.

Hoffman EP, Fischbeck K, Brown KH et al. Characterization of dystrophin in muscle biopsy specimens from patients with Duchenne's or Becker's muscular dystrophy. N Eng J Med 1988;318:1363–8.

Correlations of clinical phenotype and dystrophin deficiency.

Holt IJ, Harding AE, Morgan-Hughes JA. Deletions of mitochondrial DNA in patients with mitochondrial myopathies. Nature 1988;331:717–9.

Genetic studies.

Isaacs H. A syndrome of continues muscle fiber activity. J Neurol Neurosurg Psychiatry 1961;24:319–25.

The original article.

Karpati G, Ajdukovic D, Arnold D et al. Myoblast transfer in Duchenne dystrophy. Ann Neurol 1993;34:8–17.

Not much benefit from myoblast transfer.

Layzer RB. Stiff-man syndrome—an autoimmune disease. N Engl J Med 1988;318:1060–1.

Review article.

Layzer RB, Lovelace RE, Rowland LP. Hyperkalemic periodic paralysis. Arch Neurol 1967;16:455–72.

Review article.

Leger JM (ed). Rev Neurol (Paris) 1991;147:413–548. (Special issue on mitochondrial myopathies.)

Thorough update, 13 papers in English and 9 in French.

Lehman-Horn F, Iaizzo PA, Franke C et al. Schwartz-Jampel syndrome 2. Na+ channel defect causes myotonia. Muscle Nerve 1990;13:528–35.

Case report.

Lehmann-Horn F, Rudel R, Dengler R et al. Membrane defects in paramyotonia congenita with and without myotonia in a warm environment. Muscle Nerve 1981; 4:396–406.

Biopsy findings from three patients.

Lotz BP, Engel AG, Nishino H et al. Inclusion body myositis. Observations in 40 patients. Brain 1989;122:727–47.

Large series and update on concepts.

McEvoy KM, Windebank AJ, Daube JR, Low PA. 3,4 Diaminopyridine in the treatment of Lambert-Eaton myasthenic syndrome. N Engl J Med 1989;321:1567–70.

Effective in double-blind design.

Medori R, Brooke MH, Waterson RH. Genetic abnormalities in Duchenne and Becker dystrophies: clinical correlations. Neurology 1989;86:59–70.

The first demonstration that clinical deficit may correlate with the degree of dystrophin content.

Mendell JR, Moxley RT, Griggs RC et al. Randomized, double-blind six-month trial of prednisone in Duchenne's muscular dystrophy. N Engl J Med 1989;320:1592–7.

Benefits in both prednisone treatment groups.

Moersch FP, Woltman WH. Progressive fluctuating muscular rigidity and spasm (stiff-man syndrome): report of a case and some observations on 13 other cases. Proc Mayo Clin 1956;31:421–7.

The original case report.

Munsat TL. A standardized forearm ischemic exercise test. Neurology 1970;20:1171–8.

Original description of the 1-minute forearm ischemic lactate test.

Olafson RA, Mulder DW, Howard FM. Stiff man syndrome: a review of the literature, report of three additional cases and discussion of pathophysiology and therapy. Proc Mayo Clin 1964;39:131.

Update.

Pascuzzi RM, Gratiane R, Azzarelli B, Kincaid JC. Schwartz-Jampel syndrome with dominant inheritance. Muscle Nerve 1990;13:1152–63.

Genetics.

Ptacek LJ, Johnson KJ, Griggs RC. Genetics and physiology of myotonic muscle disorders. N Engl J Med 1993;38: 482–9.

Review article.

Riggs JE. The periodic paralyses. Neurol Clin North Am 1988;6:485–98.

Review article.

Rowland LP. Progressive external ophthalmoplegia. In Vinken PJ, Bruyn GW (eds). Handbook of Clinical Neurology. Vol. 22. Elsevier-North Holland, New York, 1975, pp. 177–202.

Textbook chapter.

Rowland LP. Clinical concepts of Duchenne muscular dystrophy: the impact of molecular genetics. Brain 1988; 111:479–95.

A comprehensive review of how advances in molecular genetics have influenced concepts of how inherited myopathies occur.

Rowland LP. Polymyositis. In Rowland LP (ed). Merritt's Textbook of Neurology. 8th Ed. Lea & Febiger, Philadelphia, 1989, p. 77.

Textbook chapter.

Shillito P, Lang J, Newsom-Davis J et al. Evidence for an autoantibody mediated mechanism in acquired neuromyotonia. J Neurol Neurosurg Psychiatry 1992;55:1214(abstract).

Simpson DM, Citak KA, Godfrey E et al. Myopathies associated with human immunodeficiency virus and zidovudine. Can their effects be distinguished? Neurology 1993;43:971–6.

Myopathy is due to HIV but not easy to distinguish on clinical grounds.

Sinha S, Newsom Davis J, Mills K et al. Autoimmune etiology for acquired neuromyotonia (Isaacs' syndrome). Lancet 1991;338:75–7.

Case report.

Solimena M, Foli F, Denis-Donini S et al. Autoantibodies to glutamic acid decarboxylase in patient with stiff-man syndrome, epilepsy, and type I diabetes mellitus. N Engl J Med 1988;318:1012–20.

γ-Aminobutyric acid pathway involved.

Spaans F, Theunissen P, Reekers AD et al. Schwartz-Jampel syndrome: 1. Clinical, electromyographic and histologic studies. Muscle Nerve 1990;13:516–27.

Case reviews.

Tarui S, Okuno G, Ikua Y et al. Phosphofructokinase deficiency in skeletal muscle. A new type of glycogenosis. Biochem Biophys Res Commun 1965;19:517–23.

Original report.

Thompson PD. Stiff muscles. J Neurol Neurosurg Psychiatry 1993;56:121–4.

Review article.

Tome FM, Fardeau M. Nuclear inclusions in oculopharyngeal dystrophy. Acta Neuropathol (Berl) 1980;49:85–7.

Tubular filaments in biopsies of three cases.

Victor M, Hayes R, Adams RD. Oculopharyngeal muscular dystrophy: a familial disease of late life characterized by dysphagia and progressive ptosis of the eyelids. N Engl J Med 1962;267:1267–72.

Original case reports.

Wada Y, Itoh Y, Furukawa T et al. "Quadriceps myopathy": a clinical variant form of Becker muscular dystrophy. J Neurol 1990;237:310–12.

Case reports.

Zeviani M, Moraes CT, DiMauro S et al. Deletions of mitchondrial DNA in Kearns-Sayre syndrome. Neurology 1988;38:1339–46.

Genetic studies.

Section V
Emergencies

83

Emergencies in Neurology

J. C. Gautier and J. P. Mohr

DIAGNOSIS OF NONTRAUMATIC COMA

Nontraumatic or medical coma (hereafter termed *"coma"*) is common and often is potentially lethal or liable to leave disabling sequelae. It obviously calls for prompt and correct diagnostic procedures that allow immediate and adequate treatment.

In practice, it may be difficult to exclude traumatic coma or the late consequences of previous trauma (e.g., subdural hematoma). However, by history taking, systematic examination of the head and neck, and imaging this question is usually solved.

The priority in a comatose patient is to ensure that the airway is free, breathing is acceptable (in terms of oxygenation), and the hemodynamic state is stable (see Severe Head Injury below and also Ch. 6).

Clinical History

History taking is not always possible, especially in large urban communities where social isolation is common, coma from drugs is frequent, and nobody is willing to act as a witness. When available, the history can be invaluable. Among the main points are the following.

1. Physical and mental health before the present coma.
2. Sudden onset of coma, suggesting an intracerebral catastrophe.
3. Progressive onset, suggesting metabolic disturbances or self-poisoning.
4. Was the patient harboring a cerebral tumor, depressed with suicidal ideas, or found among empty bottles?
5. Was the patient a known diabetic treated with insulin or even oral hypoglycemic agents? In the last case, blood would be immediately withdrawn for glucose dosage (the results will come later), and a bolus of 25 to 50 g of dextrose should be injected intravenously. Lasting hypoglycemia causes irreversible brain lesions, and it is now admitted that such a quantity of glucose cannot be really harmful, were cerebral ischemia present (see Ch. 5). Recent hypoglycemic coma dramatically disappears during or just after the injection.

6. If there is a suspicion of alcoholism, a bolus of thiamine is injected after dextrose to prevent Wernicke's encephalopathy (see Chs. 67 and 71). It should be remembered that alcohol can precipitate hypoglycemia and that alcohol can be taken with sedatives in suicide. Until proved otherwise, it is a safe rule to admit that alcohol is responsible for coma only when the blood level exceeds 2 g/L.

Examination

While the history is taken, the general examination is ongoing. The skin, nails, and mucous membranes can suggest anemia, cyanosis, jaundice, or carbon monoxide poisoning (cherry-red skin). The following rather long list of points to be examined can in fact be checked out in a few moments, leaving time for assessment of the neurologic condition.

Skin

Hyperpigmentation evokes Addison's disease, the facies can be myxedematous in hypothyroidism, or a sallow complexion suggests hypopituitarism. Bullous skin lesions are frequent in barbiturate poisoning. Petechiae can be due to meningococcemia or acute bacterial endocarditis. Diaphoresis suggests hypoglycemia or shock. Kaposi's sarcoma, oral candidiasis, and anogenital herpes all make acquired immunodeficiency syndrome possible and hence a variety of brain lesions (see Ch. 49). As mentioned elsewhere in this chapter, examination of the head and neck for evidence of trauma is part of the examination in all cases of coma.

Breath

The odor can reflect alcohol intake (vodka is scentless), acetone (diabetes mellitus), cholemia (the musty tang of fetor hepaticus), or uremia (uriniferous odor). Apart from alcohol, these time-honored changes in breath odor are now of secondary interest in Western-style medicine, but it should be kept in mind that, currently, in many regions of the world, physicians have to examine cases of coma in medically underequipped settings so that these traditional signs may still help.

Temperature

This is rectally recorded. Save for rare cases (diencephalic lesions, heat stroke), fever indicates infection, either "neurologic" (meningitis, abscess, or encephalitis) or systemic (septicemia or urinary tract or lung infections). Hypothermia may indicate hypopituitarism or myxedema. Often, it results from alcohol or barbiturate intoxication or from exposure to cold after a cerebrovascular accident.

Cardiovascular Examination

Cardiovascular examination may reveal valvular disease, cardiac failure, or atrial fibrillation, which all support the likelihood of cerebral embolic infarction. However, atrial fibrillation is frequent in elderly people and can be a chance finding (see Ch. 35). In a comatose patient, at some time in the examination, an electrocardiogram (ECG) should be recorded for the possible evidence of a recent and silent myocardial infarction.

Hypotension

Hypotension may be due to diabetes mellitus, Addison's disease, shock, or intake of drugs. *Hypertension* is a feature of hypertensive encephalopathy, generally with convulsions in a previously normotensive young patient (see Ch. 35).

Respiratory Rate

Respiratory rate is recorded. The specifics of respiration are considered below with the neurologic assessment.

Fundoscopy

Fundoscopy rarely shows a subhyaloid hemorrhage, diagnostic of subarachnoid hemorrhage (see Chs. 26 and 37). No mydriatics should be used in comatose patients. The absence of papilledema by no means rules out raised intracranial pressure.

Neurologic Examination

The pathophysiology of coma, considered in Chapter 17, makes it clear that the three essential points are (1) the evaluation of the depth of the coma, (2) the evaluation of brainstem functioning, and (3) the assessment of the presence or absence of lateralizing signs. In coma with fever, assessment for meningism would come first.

Depth of Coma

The level of consciousness must be assessed serially with the Glasgow Coma Scale (see Ch. 6). To test eye opening, the patient's name is called with increased loudness; the first name is more effective than the surname. Short interrogations are also effective and should be alternated with short commands, such as, "Bill, how are you?," "Look," "Do you have a pain in your head?," or "Open your eyes!" Some patients will open their eyes only when called within the second that follows a strong painful stimulation. Note that "opening the eyes" does not mean staring. An incomplete opening or even a lifting of an eyebrow is a token of a responsive nervous system.

Painful stimuli go from light pricking to pinching to strong pressure on the supraorbital nerve at the superior orbital ridge or on the posterior edge of the jaw to pressure on the nail beds with an interposed pen.

Best Motor Responses. Before testing the response to ordered movements, clinicians note the patient's posture. A comfortable-looking patient with the appearance of natural sleep is almost always in a light coma. Similarly, yawning and sneezing indicate light coma. Spontaneous swallowing movements mean that the medullary and lower pontine circuitry is functioning. Myoclonus is prominent in uremia and anoxic encephalopathy. Muscle twitching and fasciculations are frequent in brain infarction and hemorrhage and also in hyponatremia and hypoglycemia. Focal motor epilepsy of course is a lateralizing sign (see below). It can be continuous or permanent. Some forms require careful observation because they involve only the eyelids, the eyeballs, the corner of the mouth, or one or two fingers.

Movements of the face and all four limbs are assessed on command and in reaction to pain. Pain can elicit a variety of responses, from adapted (chasing the offending stimulus) to decerebrate or decorticate responses (see Ch. 22). Therefore movements in reaction to pain are not always a simple and straightforward indication of the depth of coma. Because reflex responses may sometimes mimic voluntary movements, it is a safe rule to consider abduction movements of the limbs or parts of the limbs as tokens of light coma. Until disproved, flexion, extension, and adduction are to be regarded as reflexes and thus indicative of deep coma. (It is worth noting in passing that the stimulus required to elicit responses need not be severely painful. The light movement of a tip of paper along the external auditory meatus or nostril, mimicking the march of an insect, may suffice for arousal and should be attempted before more punitive measures such as firmly pinching the patient or other cruder maneuvers, which could leave signs of contusions in those patients with hemorrhagic disorders.)

In the initial emergency setting, it is not possible to record the amazing variety of movements that can occur in coma and that have utmost neurologic interest. Such signs should be studied when therapy has been instituted. For these, the reader is referred to the masterful article by C. Miller Fisher (1969) and Plum and Posner's book (1980).

Verbal Responses. However minimal a mumble or a grunt may be, it indicates a light coma. The voice of loved ones (e.g., mother or companion) can be a better stimulus than the examiner's voice.

Brainstem Functions

Respiration. Various respiratory changes are possible. The cyclic Cheyne-Stokes pattern, the classic poor prognosis of which should be revised, is commonly encountered. Less often, it is possible to observe central neurogenic hyperventilation, apneustic breathing, ataxic breathing, and gasping respiration, with the latter heralding death after a short delay (see Ch. 17). Rapid, regular breathing with fever may indicate pulmonary infection.

Pupillary Reactivity. The examination of the pupils provides vital information on the site and severity of the nervous lesions, but pupillary reactions do not directly correlate with the depth of coma.

The size and reactivity to light (bright and focused) are recorded. No mydriatics should be instilled. Clinicians are encouraged to have a magnifying glass that allows them to see responses to light in pinpoint miosis.

Equal pupils of intermediate or small size that react to light indicate the absence of structural lesions of the brainstem and, consequently, suggest the coma is of metabolic or toxic origin.

Midbrain lesions cause midposition pupils with loss of the light reflex. Pontine lesions cause pinpoint miosis with retained response to light. Fixed dilation of both pupils is a sign of diencephalic herniation or diffuse anoxia.

Unilateral pupillary dilation that is unresponsive to light and caused by compression of the parasympa-

thetic fibers of the oculomotor nerve is a major sign of tentorial herniation (see Chs. 17, 25, and 27).

An oculosympathetic syndrome (Bernard-Horner syndrome) with miosis can occur with lesions of the central part of the sympathetic, from the hypothalamus to the brainstem, but also with lesions of the extra-axial sympathetic (e.g., in dissections of the internal carotid artery) (see Ch. 35).

Eye Position and Movements. With few exceptions, patients in coma lie with their eyes closed. Blinking in response to bright light or to an auditory stimulus such as loud hand clapping indicates light coma. When lifted, the lids close briskly in light coma and slowly and incompletely in deep coma.

Before passive head movement, the eyeballs may be immobile. A symmetric divergence of the globes has no predictable pathologic significance and may represent the eye position that is normal for the patient during sleep. Fixed eyeballs in the presence of reactive pupils and deep coma with normal respiration are diagnostic of barbiturate or other hypnotic intoxication. Downward and inward deviation of one or both eyes and roving movements are seen in light coma, with ocular bobbing in low pons or cerebellar lesions and in hydrocephalus (see Ch. 28).

The oculovestibular reflex movements of the eyeballs can be tested either by moving the head (oculocephalic reflexes, the so-called doll's eyes) or by caloric vestibular stimulation (oculovestibular reflexes, see Chs. 17 and 29). Oculocephalic (doll's eyes) reflexes are tested by rotating the head from side to side. The eyes should normally move conjugately in the horizontal plane in the direction opposite to the head's rotation. In pontine lesions, this response is lost, and the eyes remain in the midposition. (The authors have often found the results of this maneuver difficult to interpret and advise caloric testing.)

In caloric testing, 20 to 100 ml of cold water is instilled successively into each ear canal through a rubber tube or nozzle. (When the water is ice cold, its low temperature is beyond doubt, but a temperature cold enough to be refreshing when drunk is usually sufficient for this test.) The normal response is a conjugate deviation of the eyes toward the irrigated ear ("cold attracts," see Ch. 29). Nystagmus away from the stimulated side, also a part of the normal response (see Ch. 29), is impaired or absent in coma. A tonic (i.e., nonnystagmoid) conjugate deviation indicates a normal functioning in the pons; the absence of a nystagmus indicates the cerebrum is not functioning well enough to mediate the expected nystagmoid response to the cold water-induced deviation. A dysconjugate or absent response means a brainstem lesion or drug overdose, in which irrigation of one ear may also cause vertical nystagmus because of the profound depression of the horizontal gaze circuitry by many drugs.

Corneal Reflex. The corneal response persists until the coma is deep, and its abolition is a sign of a poor prognosis. An absent corneal response should raise the possibility of corneal lenses and, in the presence of light coma, is suggestive of drug overdose.

Lateralizing Signs

During the Glasgow coma scale scoring and examination of brainstem functions, evidence of a focal lesion at the origin of the coma may have been gathered. Additional tests are asymmetry of facial grimacing in response to pain (facial paralysis, see above and Ch. 29); greater flaccidity of the hemiplegic side, which when lifted and released falls more like a dead weight on the bed; and of course, signs of tentorial herniation (see above) that point to an ipsilateral supratentorial mass. Hemisensory deficit is suggestive of a contralateral focal lesion, but it can be difficult to demonstrate in deep coma so that painful stimuli on the midline are recommended to show asymmetry of the motor response, that is, firm rolling of the examiner's knuckles on the sternum.

Meningism. Neck stiffness and Kernig's and Brudzinski's signs (see Ch. 39) are an essential part of the examination because subarachnoid hemorrhage, meningitis, and meningoencephalitis are possible causes of coma. In subarachnoid hemorrhage, lumbar puncture is no longer considered mandatory when magnetic resonance imaging (MRI) or current-generation computed tomography (CT) are available (see Ch. 37). In meningitis, associating meningism with fever, a full examination of the cerebrospinal fluid (CSF) is mandatory, with cell count, determination of total protein and sugar, Gram stain, culture, and viral antibody titers (see Ch. 9).

When there is concern about raised intracranial pressure, an immediate imaging study can rule out a cerebral mass or obstructive hydrocephalus. However, prudence would dictate that, if the opening pressure is markedly elevated, only the minimum amount of fluid necessary should be removed, and then treatment of intracranial hypertension should be instituted with mannitol.

Investigations

These include a full blood count, erythrocyte sedimentation rate, urea and glucose level, estimation of the alkaline reserve, electrolyte concentrations, liver function tests, and tests of coagulation. If indicated by clinical findings, other assessments include toxicologic and alcohol levels and determination of the arterial gases.

In most Western-style countries, some form of imaging is readily available. Where it can be accomplished without delay, CT is invaluable to rule out antecedent or current silent structural pathologic conditions. MRI is likely to be as good or better, but problems may arise from a nontotal immobility of the patient and difficulties in the insertion of the patient into the machine with all the life-support devices.

Differential Diagnoses

It is customary to cite clinical states that could resemble coma.

Persistent Vegetative State

The persistent vegetative state (see Ch. 17) follows coma and, when present, should not raise difficulties in diagnosis.

Akinetic Mutism

In akinetic mutism, the patient cannot move, but there is clinical and electroencephalographic (EEG) evidence of apparent alertness.

Locked-In Syndrome

In the locked-in syndrome, which is caused by bilateral ventral infarction of the pons, the patient lies immobile, generally with eyes closed. However, because the neural circuitry of the oculomotor nerve is spared, the eyes can be opened and moved in the vertical plane. Such patients are conscious and can communicate with the examiner through a code based on assent/dissent expressed by blinks or vertical eyes movements (e.g., one for "yes" and two for "no"). The EEG confirms the responsiveness to external stimuli. It is sound practice to begin the examination of cases suspected of coma by asking the patient to open the eyes and blink to rule out a locked-in syndrome. This avoid distress from possible remarks on the severity or poor prognosis that the patient can understand. More generally, physicians, technicians, and nurses should refrain from such comments at the bedside, however deep a coma appears. Many regrettable instances of patients emerging from coma and understanding inappropriate comments are known.

Pseudocoma

Psychogenic states can superficially mimic coma. First, there are disorders in coma that cannot be duplicated voluntarily (e.g., a slow gradual closure of an eyelid after it has been lifted or roving eye movements). Second, irrigation of the ears (see above) and EEG findings are normal in psychogenic coma.

SEVERE HEAD INJURY

Blunt trauma, in the management of which neurologic knowledge plays a key role, is the most common neurologic emergency in general practice in Western countries; most cases are due to road accidents, falls, sports, or assaults. Missiles and sharp blows cause open, often depressed, fractures with destruction of brain tissue and driven-in scalp and bone fragments. They require immediate neurosurgery.

By severe head injury is meant cases of coma scoring 8 or less with no eye opening to command or pain on the Glasgow Coma Scale (see Ch. 6). This simple and practical scale, which is useful for triage and based only on the level of consciousness, has an important reservation, namely, that patients with lesser degrees of decreased alertness, and presumably less severe or no brain lesions, may have significant lesions of the skull, that is, linear fractures involving air or venous sinuses, depressed fractures, or small penetrating wounds (see Ch. 6).

Assessment and Management of Severe Head Injury

The primary effect of severe acceleration-deceleration of the head, that is, diffuse axonal injury and its consequences, are described in Chapter 6. Among these are cerebral edema and bleeding. Both cause raised intracranial pressure, which carries risks of cerebral herniation and compromises cerebral perfusion pressure (see below). The various forms of bleeding are intra- or extracerebral hematomas, among which extradural and acute subdural hematomas are priority emergencies.

In addition, the autoregulation of the cerebral circulation (see Ch. 5) is lost in severe head injury so that the supply of oxygen and glucose are no longer locally regulated according to the requirements of brain tissue. The brain must passively sustain whatever energy supply is provided by respiration and circulation. Breathing and circulation are commonly compromised in severe head injury because of associated multiple injuries (occluded airway; chest trauma; pneumo- or hemothorax; hypovolemic or hemorrhagic shock with hypotension; or collapse from chest, abdomen, pelvic, or limb injuries) and also because the cerebral trauma per se causes respiratory disorders and bradycardia. A fall in the mean blood pressure to values below 60 to 80 mmHg for more than a few minutes, in the presence of raised intracranial pressure, may cause ischemic cerebral damage.

In severe head injury, it must be remembered that neurologic deterioration can be due not only to the primary brain injury but also to hypoxia or hypoperfusion. Therefore, prevention of anoxia and collapse is the basic priority for both life and brain-saving emergency procedures, as described below.

Infection is immediately a risk when there is a cerebral wound, depressed fracture tear, fracture with leakage of CSF, or fracture sinuses (see above and Ch. 6). Neurosurgical repair and antibiotic therapy are mandatory.

Because multiple injuries besides head trauma are present more often than not in severe head injury and must be considered present until proved otherwise, their assessment is vital. Bleeding to death is, along with severe head injury, the leading cause of death within hours of hospitalization. However, in the following neurologic guidelines, multiple injuries will only be mentioned.

On the Scene of the Accident

The primary survey and resuscitation go hand in hand, in an orderly fashion, which is well summarized by the mnemonic ABCD for airway, breathing, circulation, and disorders of the nervous system.

If obstructed, the airway must be freed. In any case, dentures are removed. Orotracheal intubation is generally recommended with 100 percent oxygen. It is most important, during these maneuvers, and before, during the extraction of the patient from the vehicle, to assume that the cervical spine is fractured, and the neck is not moved from its original position, if at all possible. A rigid collar should be applied to protect the neck and spine. Breathing is assessed by looking and auscultating both sides of the chest. The respiratory rate is noted. A tension pneumothorax must be immediately treated by chest tube.

Assessment of circulatory status involves control of major external hemorrhages and monitoring of pulse and blood pressure. Central and intravenous lines are inserted to measure central venous pressure and give, where needed, colloid solutions or blood.

Disorders of the brain and cord are assessed roughly by talking to the patient and asking for elementary movements: put the tongue out, squeeze the hand, and wriggle the toes. In severe head injury, no response is obtained. Pupils are evaluated and their state noted. Evaluation of the depth of coma is then carried out with the Glasgow Coma Scale.

Blood is taken for a complete blood count, urea and electrolyte concentrations, grouping and cross match, and the tension of blood gases, and it is sent for alcohol and drug screening.

In tetraplegic patients and in cold climates, the risk of poikilothermia must be prevented by thermal blankets.

The patient is carried supine on a firm stretcher by four people to prevent movements of the spine and transferred whenever possible to a hospital with an accident center.

In the Emergency Room

The priority is still security of the airway and a stable circulation. These points must be achieved before considering further neurologic investigations.

At the scene of the accident or at admission, it is, of course, most important, whenever feasible, to gather as many data as possible on the circumstances of the accident and the medical history of the patient.

The clinical neurologic assessment is limited to essential points. The evolution of coma is judged according to the Glasgow Coma Scale. The state of the pupils is compared with that noted on the spot of the accident and is regularly watched; this prohibits the use of any mydriatics. The pupils must be examined with a bright, focused light. Bilaterally unresponsive pupils indicate a brainstem lesion. Unilateral unresponsive mydriasis is suggestive of temporal herniation (see Chs. 17, 25, and 27). Unilateral loss of response can be due to a lesion of the optic nerve; in this case, the pupil contracts on illumination of the other eye. Funduscopy, when possible, rarely shows papilledema, which by no means excludes raised intracranial pressure, and also rarely, a subhyaloid hemorrhage, which is indicative of subarachnoid hemorrhage (see Ch. 26).

Next is the search for focal or lateralizing signs. Some asymmetric grimacing in response to pain, indicative of a facial palsy, can often be elicited by symmetric pressure on the upper orbital ridges, mastoid processes, or on the posterior edges of the mandibles. Pressure is then applied on the nail beds of the thumb and big toe, which, when accompanied by asymmetric withdrawal, can indicate lateralized lesions in addition to those primarily responsible of coma (see Ch. 17).

The next neurologic step is to get images of the skull, cervical spine, and brain, in that order. Radiographs of the spine can detect linear, compound, or depressed fractures, sometimes with a fluid level in the sphenoid sinus, or air in the ventricles or brain. Linear fractures mean an increased possibility of intracranial hematoma. Lateral radiographs of the cervical spine should be taken with the patient's arms pulled toward the feet to show all seven cervical vertebrae, and possibly the small telltale flake of bone from the seventh vertebra that is diagnostic of extension fracture of the cervical spine (see Ch. 6). For a complete radiographic assessment of the cervical spine, an anteroposterior view and a view of the odontoid process are necessary but are often performed later.

Whenever possible, severe head injury is subjected to CT scan. MRI is more sensitive for brain lesions, but it is not widely available in emergency settings, takes more time, and has yet not been proved to be superior to CT in the diagnosis of early lesions. CT is excellent to pick up blood, either extracerebral (extradural and acute subdural hematomas or intracerebral, see Ch. 6). CT can still detect smaller quantities of blood within contusions and lacerations, although artifacts caused by bone are commonly prominent due to the frequent location of the lesions on the orbital aspect of the frontal lobe and on the temporal pole. CT, in addition, is useful for the diagnosis of raised intracranial pressure by showing a midline shift greater than 10-mm, dilation of the contralateral ventricle or the absence of the normal images of the third ventricle and cisterns around the high brainstem.

Monitoring the Evolution

In some patients, the neurologic status is severely impaired from the onset or deteriorates rapidly with a unilateral mydriasis. In such cases, there is usually evidence of a linear fracture that involves the groove of the middle meningeal artery, and CT shows the epidural hematoma or, more rarely, an acute subdural hematoma. Surgical evacuation of the hematoma can be life saving if it is performed immediately. When imaging facilities are lacking, clinical evidence alone would indicate immediate burr holes, with the first being adjacent to the fracture (if plain radiographs have been performed), or in the absence of a fracture or normal radiographs, in the temporal region, 2.5 cm above the zygoma and 2.5 cm behind the zygomaticofrontal ridge. The authors can cite several instances in which the patient's life was spared by such dramatic interventions done on clinical grounds alone.

In most patients there is no indication for surgical intervention. Such patients are usually intubated and artificially ventilated. Monitoring involves the main following points.

Oxygenation. Arterial oxygen saturation is continuously monitored by pulse oximetry. The oxygen saturation should be kept as close to 100 percent as possible and the partial arterial carbon dioxide pressure in the range 3.5 to 4.5 kPa. Full blood counts should be frequently available. The risk of a missed chest or abdominal hemorrhage decreases rapidly but should be borne in mind.

Circulation. Pulse, blood pressure, and ECG are continuously monitored. As already stated, even brief falls in cerebral perfusion pressure can be disastrous to the brain. Common causes of such falls are hypovolemia and sedative drugs such as barbiturates. Transcranial Doppler, in expert hands, can provide useful information on middle cerebral artery flow velocity, which thus indicates possible vasospasm (when flow velocity increases) and or decreasing cerebral perfusion pressure (when flow velocity decreases and resistance to flow increases, as reflected by a peak velocity profile) (see Ch. 17).

Insonation of the carotid and vertebral arteries in the neck is also useful to detect any previous lesion in aged patients and, in all, to diagnose arterial dissection, a possible consequence of trauma to the head and neck.

Raised Intracranial Pressure. The intracranial pressure should be below 20 mmHg. Figures up to 30 mmHg are acceptable if the blood pressure is sufficient to maintain adequate cerebral perfusion pressure. Monitoring intracranial pressure is somewhat controversial because it is invasive with risks, admittedly very small, of infection, hemorrhage, and epilepsy. Continuous monitoring of jugular venous saturation is useful because values below 55 percent signify increased oxygen extraction that can occur when blood flow is reduced. Below 45 percent, there is ischemia. As stated before, CT can be helpful in the diagnosis of raised intracranial pressure.

Elevation of intracranial pressure can be due to simple causes, which should be first looked for, such as airway obstruction merely from inordinate flexion or rotation of the head; insufficient relaxation of the patient with resulting efforts against the ventilator; or epileptic fits, which can be difficult to diagnose in patients treated with muscle relaxants. They should be suspected when bilateral pupillary dilation occurs with a rise in blood pressure and a larger rise in intracranial pressure. EEG monitoring would help the diagnosis.

When simple causes of raised intracranial pressure have been excluded and high pressure persists, the best, when possible, would be to diagnose the cause of this pressure increase. An overload of water with hyponatremia should be corrected. Delayed intracerebral hemorrhage or swelling (see Ch. 6) should be shown by CT. When there are reasons to think that vasodilation is a significant factor, hyperventilation, which causes vasoconstriction, can have a good, albeit temporary, effect. This supposes, however, that the brain vessels have still some reactivity. When hyperventilation is effective, the risk is to provoke ischemia. Close monitoring of jugular venous saturation, see above, is then indicated.

When it is deemed that raised intracranial pressure results from brain swelling, intravenous mannitol is generally used. Steroids have no acute benefits. Mannitol, 20 percent solution with the lowest effective dose, is given usually as 0.5 g/kg of body weight, later adjusting the doses according to the effects. Furosemide given concomitantly, and an albumin infusion after mannitol, could improve the results. Mannitol should not be given when the serum osmolality is greater than 320 mmol/kg because it then carries a

strong risk of causing renal failure and, in addition, would be ineffective.

Epileptic Seizures. These are usually treated with phenytoin and, if necessary, with clonazepam or diazepam. For precaution, see Chapter 79 and Status Epilepticus below.

Infection. Temperature is recorded and clinical examinations methodically include a search for signs of infection. Infection is not rare in this setting, and nosocomial infections are kept in mind. Antibiotics are given in cases of proved meningitis, basal fractures, and compound vault fractures. Prophylactic antibiotic therapy is controversial.

Neuroprotective Drugs. Experimental evidence shows, as would be expected, that delayed ischemic injury is a process that takes some time to achieve its end. This can be compared with the fine analysis of the death of neurons in infarction (see Ch. 5); similarly, hopes have arisen that it could be possible to halt or to minimize delayed ischemic injury with appropriate drugs given early after the injury. Trials have been organized to test calcium ion channels, N-methyl-D-aspartate-type glutamate receptor blocking agents, or antioxidants. Firm conclusions have not yet been reached.

STATUS EPILEPTICUS IN ADULTS

Clinically, epilepsy is essentially a paroxysmal event, with more or less frequent seizures (fits) that last a matter of minutes. In some cases, however, the epileptic discharges can become protracted and cause status epilepticus, that is, seizures lasting more than 30 minutes, or repeated seizures between which the patient does not regain consciousness.

There are as many kinds of status epilepticus as there are varieties of epilepsy, namely generalized convulsive (tonic-clonic), partial convulsive (epilepsia partialis continuans), and nonconvulsive partial or generalized (absences) (see Ch. 79).

Generalized Convulsive Status Epilepticus

Generalized convulsive status epilepticus is an emergency because the mortality rate is about 10 percent, and when it continues more than 2 hours, it may cause sequelae as a result of neuronal degenerative changes in the hippocampus (particularly, the endfolium and CA1 zone) (see Ch. 25) and cortex. Moreover, the longer the seizures are, the more difficult it is to control them. In most cases, the seizures can be stopped, but a few are resistant to therapy, either primarily or because they have a strong tendency to recur after they have been stopped. Such cases, fortunately rare, raise difficult problems.

CHIEF CAUSES OF GENERALIZED CONVULSIVE STATUS EPILEPTICUS

Prior epilepsy
  Poor compliance with therapy
  Reduction or discontinuation of therapy
  Alcohol, barbiturate withdrawal
No prior epilepsy
  Head trauma
  Meningoencephalitis
  Cerebrovascular disease, including arteritis
  Tumor, abcess, often frontal
  Metabolic disorders (e.g., hypoglycemia, hyponatremia, renal failure, hepatic encephalopathy, and anoxic encephalopathy)
  Drug overdose (e.g., cocaine, tricyclic antidepressants, theophylline, isoniazid, phenothiazines)
  Alcohol, barbiturates, and benzodiazepine withdrawal

Generalized convulsive status epilepticus can occur in a known epileptic patient (it is rare in idiopathic grand mal) or as the first manifestation of epilepsy, either generalized or partial, usually in the wake of a partial fit. The accompanying box lists the main causes. The differential diagnosis includes pseudostatus epilepticus (i.e., psychogenic or hysteric seizures). This differentiation is important because, when not controlled by therapy, generalized convulsive status epilepticus can lead to death, with a rising temperature and circulatory collapse.

Emergency Treatment

The plan for emergency treatment can vary slightly, but its main points are usually accepted as follows.

At the Scene. Immediately, remove dentures and contact lenses. Place the patient in a lateral semiprone position. Secure the airway. Give an intravenous benzodiazepine, usually diazepam (some prefer lorazepam). First, 10 mg is injected smoothly but not as a sudden bolus. If the seizures continue, a further 10 mg intravenously is given slowly over 30 seconds. Diazepam must not be injected intramuscularly or subcutaneously, added to an intravenous infusion, or given with phenobarbital unless mechanical ventilation is at hand. Benzodiazepines can depress respiration, but apnea is uncommon. Diazepam can be used rectally where there is no venous access. As soon as possible, give oxygen by mask, at high flow rates (i.e., 10 L/min). Transfer the patient to the hospital.

In the Emergency Department. If seizures continue, additional intravenous diazepam can be used (20 mg injected slowly). Take blood for anticonvulsant, glucose, urea, electrolyte, calcium, and magnesium levels; blood count; arterial gases; and screen for alcohol, and drug abuse.

Phenytoin (some neurologists start therapy with phenytoin) is given intravenously, 15 to 18 mg/kg in 0.9 percent saline at 50 mg/min or 20 to 30 mg/min in elderly patients. Because phenytoin can cause hypotension and cardiac arrhythmia, the infusion has to be made under ECG monitoring, watching for widening of the Q-T interval, which, when seen, should prompt cessation of treatment. Given its high pH, phenytoin must not be given intramuscularly or subcutaneously, by central line, or added to dextrose infusions or any other drug.

If the patient is thought to be hypoglycemic or the blood glucose level is low, 25 ml of 50 percent glucose is given intravenously.

If the patient is an alcoholic, 100 mg of thiamine is given intramuscularly.

Long-lasting convulsions can cause acidosis from a rise in lactic acid and respiratory disorders. However, bicarbonate, in general, should not be given because it could lower the convulsive threshold, and the acidosis usually quickly regresses when convulsions are controlled.

As soon as possible, an EEG and a CT scan should be done. In patients known to harbor tumors, arteritis, or brain parasites, a high dose of dexamethasone is given intravenously.

Resistant Status. Such patients should be transferred to an intensive care unit. There, several therapeutic schemes can be considered.

1. *Clomethiazole.* An infusion of 40 to 100 ml of an 0.8 percent solution is given over 10 minutes. This is particularly advised when alcoholic withdrawal is the cause of status. Respiration should be monitored. If the convulsive status stops, reduce the infusion rate to 0.5 to 1 ml/min.
2. *Paraldehyde.* This drug is usually given as a continuous infusion of 15 to 30 ml every 3 hours of a solution of 15 ml in 500 ml of 5 percent dextrose. The solution should be made fresh every 3 hours.
3. *Phenobarbital.* It is highly effective but can cause sedation, respiratory depression, and hypotension. Careful respiratory monitoring is mandatory. Phenobarbital 15 mg/kg should be injected no faster than 100 mg/min, provided that the

patient has not already received phenobarbital or primidone.

4. Lidocaine. Given as 100 mg by slow intravenous injection, it has a potent but short-lived action. If effective, 5 to 10 mg of lidocaine is given in 250 ml of 5 percent dextrose, at a rate of 1 to 2 mg/min. ECG should be monitored for widening of the QRS.

5. *Pentobarbital or thiopental.* These are general anesthetics and short-lived (mostly pentobarbital) barbiturates. They must be given only in an intensive care unit setting, in an intubated, mechanically ventilated patient. Monitoring of the ECG and blood pressure is mandatory.

Whatever the therapy, the patient should never be left until the seizures have been controlled. Oral therapy should be instituted without delay. For the first few days after status epilepticus, carbamazepine liquid can be given by a nasogastric tube. Sodium valproate can be given intravenously. Oral phenytoin is a frequent choice in a previously untreated patient. The dose is established from the concentrations found after intravenous infusion. A loading oral dose may be necessary.

Partial Convulsive Status Epilepticus

This less dangerous state is controlled by phenytoin intravenously (for doses and monitoring, see above). After a few hours, if necessary, one-half of the initial dose could be infused. Clinically, nystagmus is the first sign of overdosage. When a focal lesion is identified, high-dose dexamethasone given intravenously may be used.

Nonconvulsive Status Epilepticus

Nonconvulsive status epilepticus usually presents with decreased alertness or stupor. Facial or distal myoclonia or stereotyped movements suggest the diagnosis, which is established by EEG.

Intravenous benzodiazepines (see above) are generally effective in petit mal status. In temporal absences or pseudoabsences (see Chs. 25, temporal lobe, and 79), phenytoin given intravenously (see above for doses and monitoring, or carbamazepine orally are usually effective.

STROKE

Stroke is one of the most common emergencies in all its clinical variants. The emergency is self-evident for severe attacks with disorders of consciousness but still true for mild deficits because, before (and even after) detailed investigations, the wise neurologist always formulates a cautious prognosis in the early course of a stroke. In transient ischemic attacks, it is urgent to know their cause to take immediately preventive measures against a possibly impending infarction.

The subject of stroke is addressed in Chapters 5, 35, 36, and 37; the authors only intend here to give guidelines for the workup of the first examination of a recent case by a neurologist. As in all emergencies, the history, even when negative, is invaluable, but the clinician must be prepared to get none.

Is It a Stroke?

The essential mark of cerebrovascular accidents, whatever their cause, is the *sudden* onset of a *focal* deficit. The exceptions are so few as to have almost no practical importance. An occasional postepileptic paralysis or rare bleeding within a tumor (really a cerebrovascular accident) are nevertheless kept in mind. There are also pseudo–transient ischemic attacks, such as brief episodes of sensory or jerking deficit, loss of consciousness, and arrest of speech that imply the possibility of a tumor.

Even when a patient is in coma and no details on the onset are available, it is usually possible to diagnose a hemiplegia (facial paralysis, head and eyes turned toward the involved hemisphere, greater flaccidity of limbs on the paralyzed side, and on that same side, a Babinski's sign) (see Ch. 17). Experience shows that family doctors rarely miss the diagnosis of stroke.

Because the diagnosis of stroke is a very general one, several additional diagnostic steps are to be taken without delay.

Ischemia or Hemorrhage?

The clinical examination cannot settle this question safely, although it is a basic one because anticoagulation is at stake. Severe headache with focal signs suggests lobar hemorrhage, but this only occurs as a distinct syndrome rarely and even then can only be a suggestion of the cause.

Some constellations of signs strongly suggest lesions within an arterial territory, hence ischemia, whereas strokes without this arterial pattern suggest hemorrhages. However, when it comes to the decision of whether to attempt to intervene in an acute ischemic stroke with anticoagulation, these, too, are only bedside guesses. Even with Wallenberg's syndrome, the archetype of ischemic syndromes, few neurologists would dispense with a CT or MRI scan that ensure the diagnosis of ischemia versus hemorrhage. This applies even to transient ischemic attacks, except amaurosis fugax (in that case, CT or MRI are performed to check the brain). When CT and MRI are not available, a spinal tap is the last resort. If it is done well and it shows bloody CSF, hemorrhage has occurred; if the CSF is clear, it should mean ischemia, but there are false negatives because small brain hemorrhages may not stain the CSF with blood. Furthermore, in syndromes that suggest large infarcts, lumbar puncture is not without risks (herniation); it should be done with caution, tapping only a few milliliters of CSF.

Subtypes of Ischemic Strokes

Before CT or MRI, the clinical examination, directed toward essential points, can generate data highly important for treatment.

1. Is the patient already receiving anticoagulants, and if so, why? (A stroke in an anticoagulated patient is presumed to be hemorrhagic until proved otherwise, and the prothrombin time should be measured immediately.)
2. Early stupor or coma, early vomiting, bilateral Babinski's signs (indicative of temporal herniation) (see Chs. 17 and 25) and severe hypertension suggest hemorrhage.
3. Antecedent transient ischemic attacks, particularly amaurosis fugax, and coronary or peripheral arteriopathy suggest an ischemic accident.
4. Aphasia, neglect, and apraxia can be detected with simple bedside tests in an alert patient (see Chs. 18 and 19) and suggest retrorolandic surface infarcts. Pure Wernicke's aphasia and pure hemianopia point to occlusion of surface arteries and hence to embolism (usually of cardiac origin).
5. Hemiparesis involving equally the face, arm, and leg in an alert patient makes a lacunar infarct likely, whereas fractional arm weakness (i.e., shoulder different from hand) suggests high convexity and often a border-zone infarction. Dense sensory deficit that goes to the midline and involves the ear and genitalia is highly suggestive of a thalamic lesion; however, infarction and hemorrhage are both possible, with the latter less frequent and usually accompanied by ocular signs (skew deviation) (see Ch. 28).
6. Pain in the neck, side of the face, teeth, or jaw or an oculosympathetic syndrome strongly suggest an internal carotid dissection, which can also cause paralysis of cranial nerves IX to XII (see Ch. 35).
7. Where one radial pulse is weak and the blood pressure is low on that side, a subclavian steal (see Ch. 35) is likely, but it is unlikely to be the cause of the stroke. Leg phlebitis and the conditions that foster it (surgery, puerperium, and oral contraceptives) and a Valsalva-like activity at the stroke onset all make the diagnosis of paradoxic embolism a possibility.
8. Auscultation of the neck and eyeball is routine (see Ch. 35), as are cardiac auscultation and ECG.

Carotid or Vertebrobasilar?

This is an often difficult question in completed strokes and also in transient ischemic attacks. The best markers of vertebrobasilar disease are disorders of ocular movements: diplopia and gaze paralyses. Aphasia, apraxia, and amaurosis fugax are carotid markers. However, even here, scores of cases remain in which the wise clinician is only guessing.

In many cases, a sure diagnosis comes with imaging. Some 2 to 3 hours, sometimes more, are necessary for lucencies to appear on CT and high signals to appear on T_2-weighted MRI scans (see Ch. 10). CT often does not show small lesions in the posterior fossa because of an insufficient resolution and frequent artifacts from bone. MRI is to be preferred whenever possible.

Quest for the Cause

Cardiac embolism and artery-to-artery embolism (ATAE) are the first and second most frequent causes of ischemic arterial strokes. Rare causes are not considered here, with the exception of a significantly raised hematocrit that requires phlebotomy.

The chief cause of cardiac embolism is valvular or nonvalvular atrial fibrillation, followed by myocardial infarction, cardiomyopathies, and a host of rare cardiac conditions. Transcardiac ("paradoxic") emboli are an expanding subtype of cardiac disease (see Ch. 35). The chief cause of ATAE is atherosclerosis of the internal carotid artery (ICA), vertebral artery, or aortic arch. Other sources from other sites in the cerebral arterial tree (e.g., the basilar artery) are possible but probably rare and less well known.

There are currently no satisfactory clinical neurologic criteria to separate infarctions caused by cardiac embolism from those due to ATAE. In both cases, the onset is sudden. Emboli of arterial origin are probably smaller, on average, than those that come from the heart, but this point applies mainly to statistical analyses because examples exist of small cardiac emboli and large strokes from ATAE. The basic criteria for the diagnosis of ATAE is the presence of an arterial source and the absence of a cardiac source. When both conditions coexist, a variety of cryptogenic stroke is realized.

Detection of a cardiac source of embolism presents various degrees of difficulty. Evidence of atrial fibrillation, myocardial infarction, or cardiac failure can be obvious on the first examination. Such findings do not relieve the duty to search for a source of ATAE (see below) because, again, both conditions can coexist. When there is no clinical suggestion of cardiac disease, 24-hour Holter monitoring is very likely to be negative and should be considered a last-resort investigation.

Transthoracic or, better, transesophageal echocardiography (TEE), or still better, TEE with contrast can show valvular abnormalities, intracardiac thrombus, or patent foramen ovale.

Sources of ATAE can be suspected by auscultation and demonstrated by noninvasive methods such as duplex ultrasonography and magnetic resonance angiography. Duplex studies have a sensitivity and a specificity in the range of 80 percent. They can miss the rare instances of stenoses so severe that flow is reduced to a trickle, and the findings in all cases are highly dependent on the operator's skill. There are a few false-positive and negative results. Magnetic resonance angiography has a sensitivity in the 90 percent range and a specificity in the 75 percent range, but in current stages of development, it tends to overestimate the degree of stenoses and is still less precise in this respect than x-ray angiography. The latter, however, tends to be now reserved for particular cases (e.g., those with a stenosis of borderline degree, for which surgery is considered). TEE also allows imaging of parts of the aortic arch, which thus begins to enter into the field of reliable and noninvasive procedures.

Despite the full use of this impressive armamentarium and all the investigations that take place later on, some 30 to 40 percent of patients leave good neurologic departments with no cause found for the infarct, with the diagnosis in such cases being the unsatisfactory term cryptogenic infarction.

Immediate Therapeutic Measures

Animal studies and anecdotal observations in humans show beyond doubt that clinical deficits do not necessarily mean tissue necrosis (see Ch. 5) and that, for a few hours, in some cases, much could be done to head off infarction, particularly by restoring the blood supply. This possibility implies that patients with strokes should be brought to (well-equipped) hospitals as quickly as those with myocardial infarction. In many countries, to the authors' knowledge, this notion has not stirred public opinion, which still considers strokes with fatalism as inherent to old age. In this domain of neurology, efforts to inform the public and health agencies are urgently needed.

During the few early hours of a proved ischemic stroke, there are several ideal therapeutic goals, namely, to restore the patency of the occluded artery, minimize neuronal damage, oppose secondary thromboembolism, and oppose the development of cerebral edema. For the theoretical bases of such therapies, see Chapters 5 and 35.

Deoccluding the Artery

Thrombolytic therapy is, in principle, the same as is used for myocardial infarction. For brain arteries, much of the limited experience comes from tissue plasminogen activator, but urokinase and streptokinase have also been used. Several ongoing trials compare the benefits and dangers (symptomatic intracerebral hemorrhages) of thrombolysis and try to separate deocclusions caused by thrombolysis from those that occur spontaneously fairly frequently in cerebral embolism. Whatever the ultimate results, acute thrombolysis is currently reserved to a few university hospitals (i.e., a very small minority of patients), and it is too soon to know its future.

Some 20 years ago, a few emergency *surgical* deocclusions of the ICA and even of the middle cerebral artery were performed, some with encouraging results. Currently, few examples of this practice and no ongoing surgical study have come to the authors' attention.

Neuronal Rescue

Calcium entry into the neurons is a major concomitant of ischemia (see Ch. 5). Among agents that block calcium entry, oral nimodipine (30 mg every 6 hours, within 12 hours of the onset of a stroke) is beneficial. Those treated within 12 to 24 hours have shown no improvement, and those treated after 24 hours have been shown to have a slightly worse outcome. Plans for trials of other neuroprotective agents are in the offing, but either have not yet begun or are not yet completed.

Preventing Thromboembolism

Heparin, available for more than one-half century and in widespread use, has never been subjected to well-designed trials. Its use thus remains controversial. An ongoing trial is comparing a form of synthetic heparin with placebo. The less disputed indication of heparin is as part of a plan to prevent recurrence of cardioembolic stroke, provided some conditions are met; that is, the infarct should not be hemorrhagic on CT and it should not be too large because large infarcts would be more often spontaneously hemorrhagic and tend to produce herniations with hemorrhagic brainstem lesions (Duret's hemorrhages) (see Ch. 25). With such precautions, the authors use heparin in small or moderate-sized infarcts by intravenous infusion, maintaining a partial thromboplastin time 1.4 to 2.5 times the control value. Heparin perhaps also opposes the extension of secondary thrombi and certainly has the major advantage of reducing the risk of leg phlebitis and pulmonary embolism. CT monitoring of the brain lesions, of course is necessary in anticoagulated patients.

Cerebral Edema

Cerebral edema is part of all infarcts, large or small (see Ch. 5), but in large infarcts, the volume of edema is large and threatens life through herniations. Drugs to prevent this complication such as steroids and hyperosmolar agents are of unproved value. This is one of the main pitfalls of acute therapy of large infarcts.

A particular case arises with cerebellar infarcts that affect the territory of the posterior inferior cerebellar artery, which because of edema, can cause acute hypertension in the posterior fossa and rapidly cause death from compression of the brainstem and herniations. Such patients require the closest supervision and an emergency surgical removal of the infarcted tissue can be lifesaving. The peak risk for this type of compression occurs between the third and fourth day after the onset of the stroke, which provides ample time for close monitoring. Unhappily, no distinctive syndrome heralds fatal compression; so surgical plans, if made, are based on a large infarct seen on CT scan and repeat CT scans that show enlarging ventricles.

Hypertension

The authors caution against lowering blood pressure more than 20 to 30 mmHg within the first 3 days after the onset (see Ch. 35).

Hemorrhage

Emergency treatment of nontraumatic intracerebral hemorrhages has three main goals. The first is to prove the hemorrhage, evaluate its location, size, and to diagnose intraventricular bleeding and herniations; these are achieved by CT.

The second goal is to look for a possible vascular malformation, (berry) aneurysm, or arteriovenous malformation. Sometimes, CT with contrast yields a positive diagnosis, but when negative, angiography is considered immediately when the history, clinical examination, and CT suggest an aneurysm (see Ch. 37). When this early angiogram is positive, the aneurysm is operated on as soon as the state of the patient permits. When this early angiogram is negative, for fear that the hematoma has precluded contrast to enter the aneurysm, angiography is repeated, some weeks or some months later. In the authors' experience, the yield of repeat angiograms for the diagnosis of the cause of hemorrhage is very low. When early investigations have shown an arteriovenous malformation, surgery is usually delayed until the resorption of blood allows good operative conditions.

The third goal is immediate treatment. Small to middle-sized hemorrhages require no more than rest under observation in a hospital and cautious hypotensive therapy when needed. For large supratentorial hemorrhages, direct removal and endoscopic evacuation of blood have not yet been widely accepted because of the attendant unavoidable injury to healthy brain from the surgery. Medical therapy aims to prevent rebleeding (which is uncommon except from an

aneurysm and arteriovenous malformation), to minimize edema (see Infarction, above), to lower blood pressure when necessary (see Infarction, above), and, where abnormal, rapidly to restore the prothrombin time with intravenous vitamin K (intravenous injections should be undertaken very slowly to avoid the rare hypotensive response) in those who are overanticoagulated.

Nursing and early rehabilitation are of the utmost importance. Prevention of recurrences, including advice on long-term anticoagulation, carotid surgery, and reduction of risk factors for atherosclerosis, are an essential part of the neurologist's tasks but do not belong in the setting of emergency procedures (see Ch. 35).

DELIRIUM

Delirium (Latin: *delirare;* to get off the groove) is the term currently used in acute confusional states to indicate a global psychological dysfunction with impaired consciousness and attention. *Acute organic reaction* or *acute brain syndrome* are other synonyms that the reader might still meet occasionally, but their imprecision makes them inadvisable.

Delirium is a common condition, with a frequency rising steeply with age. It is particularly frequent in elderly inpatients admitted for surgery and for medical reasons. Therefore, the opinion of a neurologist might be sought in various settings.

Some definitions of delirium state include the point that it is a transient disorder. This is somewhat equivocal. Fortunately, it is true that most cases recover in a matter of days or weeks, but the mortality rate is still high, reaching 25 percent in elderly inpatients. Delirium requires urgent diagnosis and treatment.

Pathogenesis of Delirium

Pathologic examination of brains has not shown lesions specific for delirium. Clinical evidence suggests a functional disorder (i.e., one that acts at the cellular or molecular level). Claims of impaired cerebral oxidative metabolism and of specific failure in acetylcholine transmission await confirmation.

Causes of Delirium

The causes of delirium are many; some are primary nervous diseases, but others, more common, are systemic illnesses. A nonexhaustive list is presented in the accompanying box.

Stroke

Stroke is an uncommon cause of delirium, but infarction in the territory of the right middle cerebral or posterior cerebral arteries can cause acute delirium.

MAIN CAUSES OF DELIRIUM

Diseases of the nervous system
    Head trauma
    Subdural hematoma, subarachnoid hemorrhage, hypertensive encephalopathy, stroke[a]
    Raised intracranial pressure
    Encephalitis, meningitis
    Epilepsy, ictal, postictal
Systemic causes
    Infections, particularly lungs and urinary tract
    Trauma (e.g., fractures, surgery,[a] cataract operations[a])
    Myocardial infarction,[a] cardiac failure
    Metabolic (e.g., hypo- or hyperglycemia, hepatic, renal failure, porphyria, hyponatremia, hypercalcemia)
    Drugs, overdosage or withdrawal (e.g., anticholinergics, hypnotics, antidepressants, anxiolytics, cimetidine, and polypharmacy)
    Drug abuse (e.g., ethanol, drug withdrawal,[a] and Wernicke's encephalopathy)
    Miscellaneous (e.g., systemic lupus erythematosus, pellagra, deficiency in vitamin B_{12} or folate, hypothyroidism, hypopituitarism)

[a] Indicates comment in text.

In the authors' experience, delirium is not a transient ischemic attack.

Trauma

Trauma and consequent surgery is a frequent cause of delirium, particularly in elderly patients. A cataract operation is a classic cause of delirium in which long sensory deprivation followed by sudden return of normal stimulations probably plays a pathogenic role. In myocardial infarction, emotional stress and admission into an intensive care unit (see above) can play a role, together with possible withdrawal of alcohol and habitual drugs, as well as cardiac failure.

Drugs

Drugs, either overdosage or withdrawal, may account for delirium on admission in surgical wards; the polypharmacy that results in noncompliance or mixing up doses and drugs is a common cause of delirium. A careful check of the pills and tablets that pile up on the bed table is necessary, as is ascertaining which drugs are actually taken and at which dosages.

In delirious patients recently taken from home (see above), it is good practice to inquire tactfully about their drinking habits. Many decent elderly people drink more alcohol than believed at first sight, for instance, one, two, or more alcoholic drinks before and/or after dinner. Sudden withdrawal can be the cause of a mild delirium. Giving a small, rapidly declining quantity of alcohol at the usual hours for a few days can do good.

Diagnosis

Delirium is caused by a concomitant systemic or nervous disease so that the diagnosis implies, first, the recognition of delirium, and second, the identification of the underlying disease.

The onset is rapid, in a matter of hours or days, and characteristically, the course fluctuates, often with unexpected lucid intervals by day and worsening by night.

The clinical picture is complex because all psychological functions are, as it were, depressed. Because they are probably fundamental and account for the patient's appearance, disorders of consciousness are of prime importance. For practical, clinical purposes, the word "consciousness" means alertness and awareness (see Ch. 17). Alertness is that normal psychological state of awake people who are watchful of external events and synthesize their mental flow into adapted behavior. Awareness is a related normal state in which correct inferences are drawn from current experiences and the self is distinguished from the nonself (i.e., the external world).

In delirium, awareness is decreased so that present external events (e.g., visual stimuli) cannot be sorted out from internal experiences (e.g., visual hallucinations), and past experiences (i.e., memories) cannot be clearly sorted out from present experiences. With this chaotic mental flow, the patient looks perplexed and anxious. This also is the cause of the major symptom of disorientation in time and, in the more severe cases, in place as well.

Alertness can be altered in two opposite ways. First, it can be lowered, with patients being immobile with no mimicry and unconcerned by what is going on around them. Movements are rare, and language is reduced to short, laconic responses that come through long delays after simple questions. Mutism and stupor are possible. This state of reduced activity is chiefly a feature of metabolic encephalopathies. On the other hand, alertness can be increased, with agitation resulting from hallucinations, usually visual, that drive the patient to grab at or struggle with imaginary threats (e.g., animals) or fearfully crouch in a corner of the room. Such overactivity is characteristic of delirium tremens caused by withdrawal from alcohol, barbiturates, or other sedatives. During an episode of delirium, hypo- and hyperactivity can alternate.

Impaired attention is a core disorder. During examination, the patient's attention wanders, easy distractibility breaks up history taking, and focused attention is obtained for brief periods of time or is totally wanting. Bedside tests such as serial sevens or digit span usually fail. Often simple tasks such as giving the months of the year or the days of the week in reverse also fail.

As can be expected in such patients, memory is severely disturbed. Immediate and short-term recall are mediocre at best, and long-term memory is poor but relatively spared. During delirium, there is anterograde amnesia so the episode will be covered by lacunar amnesia. The time of the first clear memory is a clinical hallmark of recovery.

Abnormal perceptions, mostly in the visual modality, are almost always present. Some are misperceptions (illusions) in which an external stimulus (e.g., a shadow on the ceiling or a crack in the wall painting) are misinterpreted as threatening persons or animals. Such illusions are typical of delirium tremens. Others are hallucinations, namely perceptions without external stimuli.

The sleep-wake cycle is always disrupted, with drowsiness during day and poor sleep with nightmares at night. In severe cases, insomnia can be total. The return of sleep to normal is a major predictor of a good prognosis.

Differential Diagnosis

It is usually not difficult to separate delirium from dementia. *Alzheimer's disease* has an insidious, progressive onset. Memory, language, and praxic disorders predominate in a normally alert patient. However, the frequent case is delirium in a slightly demented patient. The cerebral decline fosters delirium, for instance, when patients are uprooted from their usual surroundings to be admitted in a hospital or nursing home. *Multi-infarct dementia,* a rare condition in the authors' experience, has a history of successive strokes, increased deep reflexes, upgoing toes, and several infarcts on CT.

In *schizophrenia,* the onset is insidious, and alertness and memory are usually in the normal range. Attention is normal, albeit parasitized by auditory, not visual, hallucinations, which are highly suggestive of the diagnosis.

Some transient *acute psychotic states* often follow emotional stress and can mimic delirium. Some correspond to the clinical onset of schizophrenia; most have a good prognosis with the reservation of possible recurrences.

Particular clinical forms of *affective disorders* prima facie can resemble delirium. In acute endogenous depression, the severely apathetic patient is immobile, immersed in sorrow, silent, or uttering laconic responses. There may be an appearance of obtundation or stupor. Insomnia (early morning waking) is present. Beyond this clinical picture, there is self-depreciation, culpability (guilt), and a conviction of incurability (hopelessness). Suicidal thoughts are frequent. In some cases, instead of hypoactivity, there is anxious agitation. Endogenous depression and delirium both require urgent and specific treatment and must be distinguished without delay.

In *mania,* the patient is usually agitated and garrulous with a flight of ideas, that is, incessantly changing ideas that chase out each other. The patient skips from one subject to another. There are grandiose projects and delusions of grandeur. Some patients abound in jokes, puns, and spoonerisms. However, others are irritable and deny examination. When available, a history of bipolar illness, of course, is essential.

More frequent than these classic diagnoses is the common problem of aged people who have just been taken away from home to live with a relative or to be admitted in a hospital, especially in intensive care units with their strange environment and the usual deprivation of sleep. Such people are often mildly disoriented for time and, sometimes, for place. Consciousness is normal. This is not delirium, and the prognosis is generally relatively good. If such patients were submitted to formal testing, it is likely that a fair number would have incipient dementia.

Investigations

A clinical neurologic and general examination is the first step. History taking is of course difficult at best, and interviews with kin and relations can be vital. Investigations to be undertaken include the usually routine full blood count, erythrocyte sedimentation rate, electrolytes, glucose, calcium, creatinine, and blood urea nitrogen assessments, urine or blood drug screen, and electrocardiogram. Other studies that may be helpful are spinal fluid examination, blood gases, serum folate, and vitamin B_{12} measurements, assessment of blood transketolase activity, and urine porphyrins measurement.

Management

The patient is placed in a well-lit, still room devoid of potentially dangerous implements. The frequent presence of quiet, sympathetic, close relatives should be encouraged. Of essence is an experienced nursing staff.

Most agitated patients are given haloperidol. Contraindications are withdrawal delirium, intoxication with anticholinergics, and hepatic failure. In mild to moderate cases, haloperidol can be given orally at a dose of 5 to 10 mg three times a day and gradually increased when necessary. Intramuscularly, haloperidol acts in about 30 minutes with usual doses from 2 to 10 mg. Sedation is maintained with 5 mg every 1 to 8 hours, according to the patient's clinical status. Intravenous haloperidol is not available in all countries. When it is not, intravenous droperidol can be used in extreme emergencies; 5 to 15 mg is repeated every 4 to 6 hours. As a general rule, these drugs are given at half doses to elderly and debilitated patients.

Benzodiazepines are used in delirium caused by withdrawal of alcohol or benzodiazepines and in hepatic failure. Diazepam is given in divided doses up to 30 mg/day and then gradually reduced over 7 to 10 days. Benzodiazepines are contraindicated in respiratory failure and myasthenia. Withdrawal syndromes can cause convulsions that require anticonvulsants.

The utmost attention is paid to nutrition and fluid and electrolytes balance. Acute dehydration is common and must be corrected without delay. An intravenous line is placed as soon as sedation permits. Whenever possible, the patient is presented with abundant liquid nutrients as soups, fruit juices, and the like. Diuresis is noted, and a distended bladder is regularly sought. Prevention of pressure sores and contractures is achieved by adequate nursing and physiotherapy.

In the meantime, the treatment of the condition underlying delirium must be vigorously pursued. For this aspect of the management of delirium, the collaboration of internists, of course, may be necessary.

MALIGNANT NEUROLEPTIC SYNDROME

The malignant neuroleptic syndrome is rare, occurring in about 1 percent of treated patients. It is potentially rapidly lethal and hence is an emergency.

Phenothiazines, especially depot forms of fluphenazine and haloperidol, are the drugs most often held responsible, but all neuroleptics can cause the syndrome, including the substituted benzamides and metoclopramide, an antiemetic related to chlorpromazine. Drugs not expected to alter brain dopamine have also been implicated such as clozapine, lithium, and carbamazepine. Causal drugs have usually been given in the therapeutic, not toxic, doses.

Malignant neuroleptic syndrome often arises at the start of treatment, while dosage is being increased, or when a second drug is introduced. Abrupt cessation of treatment with anticholinergic drugs (given against the neuroleptic-induced extrapyramidal syndrome or in parkinsonism), previous dehydration, and malnutrition can also foster malignant neuroleptic syndrome. Young male patients, usually schizophrenic, and alcoholic patients treated for delirium tremens are considered at special risk for malignant neuroleptic syndrome.

Pathogenesis

The pathogenesis of the syndrome is still obscure. An increased sensitivity to caffeine of the sarcoplasmic reticulum of muscle fibers has been reported, which thus shows an analogy to anesthesia-induced malignant hyperthermia (see below). However, it is currently considered unlikely that the two syndromes are related. Sustained muscular contraction caused by a disorder of calcium transfer across the membrane of striate muscle cells is accepted as the source of hyperthermia in malignant neuroleptic syndrome, but its cause is unknown. Blockade of pre- and postsynaptic D_2 receptors can also cause a central disorder of heat regulation.

Diagnosis

The syndrome typically develops clinically in 24 to 72 hours. Among the warning signs are tachycardia, hypersalivation, sweating, and labile blood pressure, which denote autonomic dysfunction.

The full-blown clinical picture includes three major disorders: hyperthermia, muscular rigidity, and myoglobinuria. The patient's temperature rises to 40°C or more. There is muscle rigidity. Catatonia and mutism can progress to stupor and coma. Dehydration is prominent with oliguria and myoglobinuria.

Laboratory studies show that the creatinine phosphokinase level is increased, due to muscle breakdown, and increases are also found in the hematocrit and serum protein concentrations as a result of dehydration. Leukocytosis is frequent.

The differential diagnosis is from malignant hyperthermia, an autosomal dominant disease with variable penetrance, in which hyperthermia, muscle rigidity, and myoglobinuria immediately succeed anesthesia with volatile agents, especially halothane, or medication with succinylcholine. Malignant hyperthermia is associated with central core disease and possibly with other neuromuscular conditions (see Chs. 4 and 33), lethal catatonia, and the side effects of monoamine oxidase inhibitors with other drugs and foods.

In the malignant neuroleptic syndrome, the risks of hypoventilation and aspiration pneumonia (because of decreased chest compliance), acute renal failure, and cardiovascular collapse imply transfer to an intensive care unit.

Management

The first step of treatment is withdrawal of neuroleptics. Cooling; rehydration; and prevention of renal failure, respiratory complications, and collapse are mandatory (see below, Heat Stroke). Bromocriptine, a dopamine agonist, is given orally or by nasogastric tube at a dose of 5 mg three times a day. Dantrolene sodium, a muscle relaxant, is given intravenously at doses of 50 mg every 12 hours, with watching for signs of hepatotoxicity. Such a regimen has considerably improved the outcome of malignant neuroleptic syndrome. Obviously, the best treatment is prevention. In neuroleptic-treated patients with fever of unknown cause, neuroleptics should be immediately withdrawn.

HEAT STROKE

Heat stroke, is a medical emergency with still a high mortality rate. It can occur in two main settings. First, it may occur in high ambient temperatures (e.g., during extreme heat waves, especially when there is high humidity that impedes sweating, one of the most potent ways for the body to lose heat). The patients most affected are those who are elderly with cardiac ailments or those who take anticholinergic drugs (e.g., antiparkinsonism medication or phenothiazines). Uncommonly, heat stroke may affect those who have special difficulties in evacuating heat such as patients with ectodermal dysplasias, severe ichthyosis, extensive scleroderma, or congenital absence of sweat glands. Second, heat stroke may occur when there is high internal caloric production. Because such states usually result from strenuous and protracted physical activity, the patients are mostly young people: marathon runners, cyclists, or soldiers on long marches. Youngsters who take 3,4-dimethylenedioxymetamphetamine ("ecstasy") for dancing ("dance of death") can die from disorders that are heat stroke or close to it.

Exposure to the sun is not a prerequisite for heat stroke.

Diagnosis

Clinically, heat stroke may be heralded by muscular cramps, abdominal pains, confusion, and irritability, but in some cases, the onset can be rapid or sudden. The patient sinks into coma, and seizures, even focal deficits, are possible. The skin is hot and dry, although profuse sweating can be encountered. The rectal temperature is between 40 and 43°C. When the temperature is more than 42°C, the prognosis is particularly severe.

Polypnea and tachycardia are present, with a strikingly low diastolic pressure. Muscular rigidity from rhabdomyolysis can be prominent, with oliguria and a brownish urine, a major increase in the serum creatinine phosphokinase level, and the attendant risk of renal failure. A syndrome of disseminated intravascular coagulation has been reported, featuring purpura, hemorrhages at puncture points, and epistaxis; this is a poor prognostic sign. Hemoconcentration is evident, and serum calcium and magnesium levels are low. The serum potassium level is normal or low.

Management

Immediately cooling is mandatory. Clothes are removed, and the patient is placed in a cool atmosphere, covered with ice or, better for some, permanently aspersed with cold water. Transfer to an intensive care unit whenever possible is mandatory.

Cooling can be further achieved by transfusion of fresh-frozen plasma. Forced diuresis with mannitol can enhance myoglobin clearance and prevent anuria, which could require dialysis. Diazepines are given against seizures. When there is disseminated intravascular coagulation, heparin intravenously 1.5 mg/kg is also given.

Intravenous dantrolene 2 to 4 mg/kg has been recommended. It may cause the rigidity to subside quickly with a concomitant fall of temperature. It is however far from being always effective. Survivors often have neurologic sequelae, among which cerebellar ataxia is prominent, because Purkinje cells are particularly vulnerable to heat.

ACUTE RESPIRATORY FAILURE

Acute respiratory failure caused by neuromuscular dysfunction, the topic considered here, is really an acute mechanical ventilatory failure. There are many causes, from disorders of the brainstem area that operates the respiratory cycles to paralysis of the nerves that innervate the respiratory muscles to malfunction of the neuromuscular junction to diseases of the respiratory muscles. So defined, acute respiratory failure is distinct from acute respiratory failure caused by lung disease. Actually, acute mechanical ventilatory failure is all too often compounded by lung lesions because of the risk of aspiration pneumonia and nosocomial infection in ventilated patients.

Either form of failure is obviously an emergency. The onset can be insidious because an increase in the partial arterial carbon dioxide pressure, the traditional hallmark of acute mechanical ventilatory failure, is a late event and means impending respiratory arrest. Therefore, the clinician's aim is to detect earlier symptoms and signs to take emergency preventive steps.

Diagnosis

Fundamentally, it rests on the diagnosis of weakness of the muscles that enlarge the rib cage rhythmically.

The chief respiratory muscle is the diaphragm (see Ch. 22). When the diaphragm contracts, its dome flattens, pushing down the abdominal contents and thus causing the abdominal wall to bulge. When the diaphragm is paralyzed, and the accessory respiratory muscles (intercostals, pectorals, scalenes, and sterno-cleidomastoids) maintain the expansion of the rib cage, the inert diaphragm is aspirated into the thorax together with the abdominal viscera. After that movement, the abdominal wall moves upward. This upward movement is the major sign of paralysis of the diaphragm. It is more obvious in the supine patient than in the standing patient because, in the former, gravity assists the ascending movement of the abdominal viscera. The supine position further reduces the capacity of the rib cage and, consequently, the volume of inhaled air.

The diaphragm is almost the only muscle that works during sleep, so its paralysis is particularly likely to cause hypoventilation at night. Patients with neuromuscular disease may complain of waking headache because of a high carbon dioxide partial pressure, which indicates ventilatory assistance at night.

Paralyzed intercostal muscles are passively drawn in during inspiration, but this movement can be seen only in slim patients and only when the diaphragm functions enough to lower intrapleural pressure during inspiration. The diaphragm and intercostals are muscles that fatigue easily.

The diaphragm is innervated by the phrenic nerve (see Ch. 22), and it is a safe clinical rule to look for its paralysis when the deltoid or biceps (C5-C6) are paralyzed.

In impending acute mechanical ventilatory failure, there may be headache, dyspnea with rapid and shallow respiration, and tachycardia, but these also can be late signs. As vital capacity decreases, there is, in succession, weak cough with poor clearing of secretions and the attendant risk of aspiration pneumonia, dysfunction of the sigh mechanism, hypoventilation, and lately, as already stressed, hypercapnia. In some cases, there is papilledema. Clinical signs of fatigue, flapping tremor (see Ch. 22), diaphoresis, tachycardia, drowsiness, growing anxiety, and insomnia herald the necessity of prompt intubation with mechanical ventilation.

Management

Frequent evaluation of ventilatory capacity is mandatory. The ability to count rapidly from 1 to 25 on one breath roughly means a ventilatory capacity above 2 L; counting to 10 means a ventilatory capacity of 1 L. Measuring ventilatory capacity by forced exhalation is a cause of atelectasis and can be replaced by measurements of inspiratory ventilatory capacity or inspiratory force. Currently, bedside electronic devices can monitor respiratory rate, tidal volume, and ventilatory capacity in spontaneously breathing patients.

All patients should be regularly monitored by pulse oximetry to detect early falls in partial oxygen pressure.

The decision to start artificial ventilation depends primarily on the clinical assessment. The level of the ventilatory capacity that dictates mandatory ventilatory support depends on the predicted normal value for the patient's age and weight. Usually, however, artificial ventilation is used in an adult when ventilatory capacity falls below 1 L. Elective intubation is far better than intubation in a hurry, which carries risks of aspiration pneumonia. Patients for whom intubation is a possibility should be told so well in advance, and the major advantages of ventilatory support should be explained. Whenever possible, intubation should be performed by a skilled physician in an intensive care unit.

The indications and timing of tracheostomy are debatable. Many wait until the end of the second week of mechanical ventilation to ascertain whether clearing secretions, and the patient's comfort, indicate a tracheostomy. By waiting 2 weeks, many patients are spared tracheostomy.

During mechanical ventilation, in the intensive care unit, the main points of management are to ensure a permanent appropriate ventilation, to maintain nutrition, and to prevent nosocomial infections. Prevention of deep vein occlusion with heparin and passive mobilization of limbs; prevention of bed sores, contractures, and nerve compressions by physiotherapy; adequate bedding and frequent changes in position; and psychological support are other important tasks of the intensive care unit team.

Withdrawal of ventilatory assistance, of course, varies with the causal disease, possible complications, and general health status. Weaning is progressive, with particularly, a longer maintenance of light support at night. A number of patients grow anxious when they are separated from their machines, and this implies extra psychological support is needed.

Causes of Acute Mechanical Ventilatory Failure

Brainstem and Cord

The most common disorder in practice is respiratory depression caused by ethanol (see Ch. 67), sedatives (barbiturates or benzodiazepines), and opioids (see Ch. 68) for patients in coma (see Ch. 17). Several central nervous diseases (e.g., tumors, hemorrhage, and motor neuron disease) can raise difficult problems when the time comes to decide whether mechanical ventilation is used.

Poliomyelitis is still frequent in some parts of Eastern Europe and in the Middle and Far East. The diagnosis should be considered wherever there is a flaccid

---

CAUSES OF ACUTE MECHANICAL VENTILATORY FAILURE: BRAINSTEM AND CORD DISORDERS

Alcohol, sedatives, opioids
Metabolic encephalopathies
Infarction, hemorrhage
Motor neuron disease
Tumors, intrinsic, extrinsic
Encephalitides, myelitides
Poliomyelitis

CAUSES OF ACUTE MECHANICAL VENTILATORY FAILURE: NEUROMUSCULAR JUNCTION DISORDERS

Myasthenia gravis
Anticholinesterase overdose
Eaton-Lambert syndrome
Hypermagnesemia
Antibiotic-induced paralysis
Botulism
Spider, scorpion, snake, fish, crab or other shellfish bites
Tick paralysis

---

paralysis, often asymmetric, without sensory deficit, with a pleocytosis in the CSF (see Ch. 48).

Peripheral Nerves

Peripheral neuropathies usually have a progressive, ascending course, with numbness, sensory deficit, and dulled or absent deep reflexes, although rare cases are purely motor and rapidly evolving. The major disease in this group is the Guillain-Barré syndrome (see Chs. 32 and 80). Therapy rests on plasma exchanges and intravenous immunoglobulins. In principle, the diagnosis of Guillain-Barré syndrome should be accepted only after the other neuropathies listed in the box are excluded (see Chs. 72 and 80).

CAUSES OF ACUTE MECHANICAL VENTILATORY FAILURE: PERIPHERAL NEUROPATHIES

Guillain-Barré syndrome, demyelinating, axonal forms
Chronic idiopathic demyelinating polyradiculoneuropathy
Critical illness polyneuropathy
Toxins (e.g., thallium, arsenic, lead, organophosphates, lithium)
Hereditary tyrosinemia
Drugs (e.g., vincristine)
Lymphoma
Systemic lupus erythematosus
Acute porphyria
Diphtheria
Buckthorn neuropathy in Mexico

Neuromuscular Junction

Myasthenia gravis and anticholinesterase overdosage, or cholinergic block depolarization, are the most common causes of acute mechanical ventilatory failure in western countries, but in other parts of the world, insects, crab, fish, and shellfish can be the culprits.

Rarely, acute mechanical ventilatory failure is the first presenting sign of myasthenia gravis (see Ch. 81). Usually, acute mechanical ventilatory failure appears in a treated patient, either with a causal circumstance (contraindicated drugs, surgery, infection, or pregnancy) or without obvious cause. The vital point is to distinguish a myasthenic crisis from a cholinergic crisis.

Cholinergic crises are due to the permanent depolarization of the motor end-plate by anticholinesterase drugs, either as a result of overdosage or a well-tolerated dose until some other drug has been introduced, particularly when there is rapid improvement after plasma exchange. Depolarization cholinergic block causes hypersalivation, small pupils, colic, diarrhea, and muscle fasciculations. Moreover, it causes excessive bronchial secretions that obviously can aggravate the consequences of the acute mechanical ventilatory failure because of paralysis of the respiratory muscles.

Intravenous injection of edrophonium that worsens rather than improves the disorders is proposed as a diagnostic test. Actually, the results are not always clear-cut; when in doubt, it is advisable to resort to mechanical ventilation, which allows anticholinesterase drugs to be stopped and resumed progressively later, under close supervision.

For the Eaton-Lambert syndrome, see Chapter 81.

Several varieties of *Clostridium botulinum*, the agent in botulism, produce about 10 varieties of toxins. Type A predominates in the Western parts of the United

States; type B predominates in the Eastern states. Type E predominates in Europe, along the shores of seas and lakes. The toxin blocks cholinergic transmission, particularly in postganglionic parasympathetic synapses and in motor end-plates. Contamination through wounds is rare. Usually, the clinical onset follows (by 12 to 36 hours) the ingestion of tainted food, more commonly home-preserved vegetables. There is early vomiting and colic. Autonomic disorders are prominent: dry mouth, poorly reactive mydriasis, and constipation. Extrinsic ocular and swallowing paralyses are frequent. Besides mechanical ventilation, the treatment rests on antitoxin.

Hypermagnesemia can result from taking magnesium-rich antacids or laxatives. Magnesium can interfere with the release of acetylcholine and cause acute mechanical ventilatory failure. Aminoglycoside and polymyxin antibiotics can cause similar disorders.

For the effects of toxins from spiders, snakes, scorpions, fish, and so forth, see Chapter 72. Female tick bites in North America can cause acute mechanical ventilatory failure, probably because the animal's saliva contains a toxin that blocks the neuromuscular junction. Reportedly, removal of the tick is curative. It can be difficult to locate, however.

Muscles

The main muscle disorders that can cause acute mechanical ventilatory failure are listed in the accompanying box. Acute mechanical ventilatory failure that occurs within a few hours in the setting of flaccid paralysis, with normal deep reflexes and no sensory deficit, suggests first hypokalemia (see Chs. 69 and 82). Severe hypophosphatemia, a rare cause of acute mechanical ventilatory failure, can be precipitated by glucose infusions in alcoholic people (see Ch. 67).

Acute rhabdomyolysis can cause muscle weakness and, consequently, acute mechanical ventilatory failure. The creatinine phosphokinase level is very high. Biopsy shows massive muscle fiber necrosis. The prognosis depends primarily on myoglobinuria and renal failure. The possible causes are many: alcohol, viruses, a variety of drugs, heat stroke (see above), malignant neuroleptic syndrome, and malignant hyperthermia (see above).

Polymyositis can rarely present as acute mechanical ventilatory failure, and acute mechanical ventilatory failure is a relatively frequent cause of death (see Chs. 33 and 82). Lung lesions can aggravate acute mechanical ventilatory failure.

In dystrophies, acute mechanical ventilatory failure is a late event. Intercurrent lung infections can precipitate acute mechanical ventilatory failure in patients whose vital capacity has been slowly reduced. Acid maltase deficiency is characterized by marked wasting of paraspinal muscles, in addition to proximal upper limb weakness, and periodic acid-Schiff-positive (glycogen-containing) lymphocytes.

ACUTE COMPRESSION OF THE SPINAL CORD

In acute compression of the cord, the chief factors of prognosis are the severity of primary injury and the elapsed time before decompression, which thus makes acute cord compression an emergency. By "acute" is meant not only those cases that arise from trauma but also those for whom the cause of cord compression develops over hours to days (e.g., abscess, hemorrhage, and malignancies). With few exceptions, nontraumatic diseases that cause acute compression actually induce a prior subacute compression, so that, for a short period beforehand, an opportunity exists to make the diagnosis with better chances of prompt treatment and a good prognosis.

Syndromes

In acute compression, the predominant symptom is pain somewhere along the spine. The importance of back pain means that any occurrence of localized spinal pain (inasmuch as pain is exacerbated by gentle pressure or tapping with the reflex hammer) should prompt a neurologic examination in which the first concern is to determine whether incipient cord compression is the explanation.

The principles of the clinical diagnosis of cord compression are considered in Chapters 22 and 31 but are here summarized briefly. There are two components. First, there is the syndrome at a certain level, which features radicular pain, abolished tendon reflexes, and in chronic cases, wasting of muscles supplied by the affected segment(s). In many cases, the focal spinal pain could also be viewed as a part of the "level" syndrome, taking in account the shift of levels between cord and spine (see Chs. 31 and 32). Second, there is a syndrome below the affected level, with

---

CAUSES OF ACUTE MECHANICAL VENTILATORY FAILURE: MAIN MUSCLE DISORDERS

Hypokalemia
Acute rhabdomyolysis
Acid maltase deficiency
Polymyositis
Hypophosphatemia
Dystrophies

weakness, which can amount to para- or tetraplegia; exaggerated tendon reflexes; Babinski's signs; and sensory deficit for pain and temperature, position of limbs, and perception of the vibrations of a tuning fork. For the various significances of the components of both syndromes, see Chapter 31.

In the acute cord compression syndrome, the presence or absence of sensory deficit dissociations, such as sacral sparing (spinothalamic tract) or sparing of position and vibration perception (posterior columns), can be useful prognostic indicators (see Ch. 31).

In settings that require it (e.g., in acute cord compression caused by trauma), the detailed neurologic examination is performed after the vital functions have been controlled (see "ABCD" in the section Severe Head Injury earlier in this chapter).

Special Effects

Compression of the high thoracic and cervical cord disrupts autonomic functions because the sympathetic control is lost due to spinal shock (see Ch. 31). This has several consequences that should not mislead the clinician. One is peripheral vasodilation, hence mild hypotension and bradycardia, which do not by themselves indicate volume loading or vasopressors. There may also be hypovolemic shock (e.g., in traumatic acute cord compression with multiple injuries), and such expected signs as pallor and tachycardia may be lacking. Severe hypotension in a patient with acute cord compression who is receiving fluids is presumed not to be due to spinal shock and thus has another cause.

The bladder and rectum are paralyzed. Catheterization of the bladder and prevention of gastric dilation (it may not be known well enough that gastric rupture can be a frequent cause of early death) by a nasogastric tube are mandatory.

Another point is that, in such patients, signs of peritoneal irritation are lacking, even with massive abdominal hemorrhage or severe infection.

Radiologic Assessment

Acute cord compression should lead to a radiologic assessment as soon as possible. *Plain radiographs* are the first step with anteroposterior, lateral, and oblique views and views of special sites when indicated (e.g., for the atlanto-occipital or atlantoaxial joints. For the cervical spine, lateral views must, whenever possible, show the lowest vertebrae (see Chs. 6 and 31). Flexion-extension views may show the abnormally excessive movements that are consistent with fractures or dislocations, but such maneuvers should be reserved for experienced practitioners.

CT scan has been a significant advance, showing fractures, particularly of pedicles, in many patients whose plain films had been considered normal. It can show bony fragments in the spinal canal or root foramen. CT myelography is now possible.

MRI has the advantage of showing, with a high sensibility, damage to discs, ligaments, and prevertebral tissues.

Whatever the cause of acute spinal cord compression, the immediate goals are, first, to relieve compression and, second, to stabilize the spine in good alignment. This, of course, means surgery, and the patient should be transferred without delay to a neurosurgical unit, ideally to an acute spinal cord injuries unit such as those currently organized throughout Western Europe, the United States, and Japan. Transfer obviously requires that temporary immobilization of the spine has been achieved. For some clinicians, in addition, some causes of acute cord compression call for immediate medical therapy (methylprednisolone in cases caused by trauma, see below) or neuroprotective drugs such as N-methyl-D-aspartate receptors blockers, which are given to suppress or minimize the catabolic chain of pathologic events set up by the primary insult to the cord (see Severe Head Injury, above).

Causes

Trauma

In general practice, the cervical spine is involved in 50 percent of cases, and most patients are young because the main causes are traffic and sports accidents. Falls happen in the young and in the aged (stairs or tripping on mats, see Ch. 6). According to the forces at play, various fractures at various levels can occur. It should be realized that compression of the cord can have taken place even with normal plain radiographs in the neutral position. The spine may nevertheless be unstable, as shown by radiographs in flexion and extension and CT or MRI (see above).

On the scene of the accident, there can be evidence of cord damage or severe head injury (see above), in which case, fracture of the cervical spine is presumed until proved otherwise. Patients must be extracted from vehicles with the least possible movement of the neck. From the site of the accident to the hospital, the spine should be immobilized by traction or a Philadelphia-style collar. In the United States, it is now usual to inject a loading dose of 30 mg/kg of methylprednisolone over 15 minutes, followed by 5.4 mg/kg/h for the next 23 hours.

Only the most general principles of surgery can be considered here. Compression and misalignment must be corrected. Surgical interventions are often indicated in thoracolumbar or lumbar fractures because many of these fractures are compounded and traction alone is unlikely to relieve the contractures of large muscular masses. Surgery may also be necessary because of the risks of high instability in some atlanto-occipital or atlantoaxial dislocations.

Eventually, bone, particularly cancellous bone, heals well if well immobilized, whereas the healing of ligaments is at best slow. This is obviously significant for the indications of spine-stabilizing surgery.

Tumors

Metastases are the common cause of cord compression, usually by invasion of the epidural space from deposits in the vertebral body or pedicles. Most of them involve the thoracic spine, and the primary tumors are lung, breast, prostate, digestive tract, or kidney cancers and myeloma or lymphoma. Acute cord compression can occur when a vertebral body collapses or a tumor enlarges very rapidly, but commonly, the compression is subacute with the patient complaining for weeks of focal spinal pain and leg weakness.

Plain radiographs or, better, CT or MRI are the decisive diagnostic steps. The characteristic features are loss of vertebral height, irregular low-density lesions within the vertebral bone, and preservation of the intervertebral disc. When no primary tumor is found, it might be necessary to resort to vertebral biopsy. Between T5 and L5, a percutaneous vertebral body biopsy can be carried out under biplanar image intensifier control, or at almost any level, a CT-guided needle biopsy may provide tumor tissue adjacent to the vertebra.

Infections

Tuberculosis of the spine is now rare in Western-style countries but still frequent in developing countries (see Ch. 46). Brucellosis (see Ch. 47) or vertebral osteomyelitis from *Staphylococcus aureus*, streptococci or *Escherichia coli* can generate extradural abscesses that can compress the cord. Besides signs of cord dysfunction, focal spinal pain is the major symptom. Tuberculosis and brucellosis usually cause subacute compressions. MRI or CT myelography are the key investigations in neurosurgical emergencies. Extradural abscesses are neurosurgical emergencies.

Hemorrhages

Epidural hematomas are more frequent than subdural hematomas. They can occur without detectable reason. Some occur in anticoagulated patients, sometimes after a lumbar puncture. MRI or CT are the investigations of choice. Immediate evacuation is realized through a laminectomy.

Inflammatory Diseases

Rheumatoid disease commonly affects the cervical spine but usually spares its lower part. The brunt of the lesions bear on the atlanto-occipital and atlantoax-ial joints. The most frequent consequence is anterior subluxation of C1 on C2. A few cases have been reported of acute cord compression with the patient collapsing suddenly because of odontoid luxation. Most cord compressions are subacute but are always liable to a sudden aggravation. MRI or CT myelography should be done with the patient extending and flexing the neck.

Degenerative Diseases

Acute disc protrusions occur mainly in the lower lumbar spine. Consequently, they can cause an acute compression of the cauda equina, which is a neurosurgical emergency. Acute cervical disc protrusions can occur. In aged people, there is often a degree of disc protrusion associated with spondylosis. In such patients, hyperextension of the neck can cause an acute cord compression (see Ch. 6).

ANNOTATED BIBLIOGRAPHY

Diagnosis of Nontraumatic Coma

Bates D. Management of medical coma. J Neurol Neurosurg Psychiatry 1993;56:589–98.

Good recent review.

Fisher CM. The neurological examination of the comatose patient. Acta Neurol Scand 1969;45 (suppl 36):1–56.

Outstanding article. Should be read by all those who are fond of neurology.

Plum F, Posner JB. The Diagnosis of Stupor and Coma. 3rd Ed. FA Davis, Philadelphia, 1980.

The classic monograph.

Severe Head Injury

Miller JD. Head injury. J Neurol Neurosurg Psychiatry 1993;56:440–7.

Good, detailed, recent review.

Skinner D, Driscoll P, Earlam R (eds). A B C of Major Trauma. British Med Journal, London, 1991.

Clear and precise guidelines. With articles on initial assessment and management.

Trunkey D. Initial treatment of patients with extensive trauma. N Engl J Med 1991;324:1259–63.

Multiple injuries. A surgeon's point of view.

White RJ, Likavec MJ. The initial diagnosis and management of head injury. N Engl J Med 1992;327:1507–14.

Good update.

Status Epilepticus in Adults

Bauer J, Elger CE. Management of status epilepticus in adults. CNS Drugs 1994;1:26–44.

Thorough review with many references.

Brodie MJ. Status epilepticus in adults. Lancet 1990;336:
551–2.

Concise, precise review.

Editorial. Pseudostatus epilepticus. Lancet 1989;2:485.

Diagnosis of psychogenic or pseudoseizures.

Meldrum BS. Anatomy, physiology, and pathology of epilepsy. Lancet 1990;336:231–4.

Highly commendable update.

Nouailhat F. État de mal épileptique, In Goulon M (ed). Les Urgences. Edisem, St. Hyacinthe, Quebec, Maloine SA, Paris, 1990.

Comprehensive and practical review of kinds of status epilepticus.

O'Brien MD. Management of major status. BMJ 1990;301:
918.

Hyperconcise review.

Shorvon S. Tonic-clonic status epilepticus. J Neurol Neurosurg Psychiatry 1993;56:125–34.

Full review.

Stroke

Borges LF. Management of non traumatic brain hemorrhage, in Ropper AH (ed). Neurological and Neurosurgical Intensive Care. 3rd Ed. Raven Press, New York, 1993, pp. 279–90.

Balanced review.

Caronna JJ. Carotid artery disease: a comparison of DUS, MRA, and x-ray angiography. Neurol Alert 1994;12:
57–64.

Conventional angiography better than Doppler ultrasound and magnetic resonance angiography to evaluate the degree of carotid stenoses.

Gautier JC, Loron P, Juillard JB. Traitement des accidents vasculaires cérébraux, in Goulon M (ed). Les Urgences. Edisem, St. Hyacinthe, Quebec, Maloine SA, Paris, 1990.

Guidelines for emergencies.

Humphrey P. Stroke and transient ischaemic attacks. J Neurol Neurosurg Psychiatry 1994;57:534–43.

Review and personal views.

Marshall RS, Mohr JP. Current management of ischaemic stroke. J Neurol Neurosurg Psychiatry 1993;56:6–16.

Recent update with recommendations on management.

Delirium

Awada A, Poncet M, Signoret JL. Troubles du comportement soudains avec agitation chez un homme de 68 ans. Rev Neurol (Paris) 1984;140:446–51.

Infarct in the right middle cerebral artery territory. Early French references.

Critchley EMR. Delirium as a General Medical Condition in Neurological Emergencies. WB Saunders, London, 1988.

Good diagnostic discussion.

Medina JL, Rubino FA, Ross E. Agitated delirium caused by infarctions of the hippocampal formation and fusiform and lingual gyri: a case report. Neurology 1974;24:
1181–3.

Infarcts in the posterior cerebral artery territory.

Mesulam MM, Waxman SG, Geschwind N, Sabin TD. Acute confusional states with right middle cerebral artery infarctions. J Neurol Neurosurg Psychiatry 1976;39:84–9.

Seminal case in English.

Taylor D, Lewis S. Delirium in Neurological Emergencies. BMJ Publishing Group, London, 1994.

Recent review.

Malignant Neuroleptic Syndrome

Adnet P. Le syndrome malin des neuroleptiques, in Viars P (ed). Anesthésie, Réanimation, Urgences, Tl. Université Paris VI, Médecins du Monde. Imprimerie Nationale, Paris, 1994.

Good overview.

Araki M, Takagi A, Higuchi I, Sugita H. Neuroleptic malignant syndrome: caffeine contracture of single muscle fibers and muscle pathology. Neurology 1988;38:
297–301.

Caffeine-induced contracture of skinned muscle fibers in six of eight cases of meuroleptic malignant syndrome.

Editorial. Neuroleptic malignant syndrome. Lancet 1984;1:
545–6.

Clear account.

Kellam AMP. The neuroleptic malignant syndrome, so-called. A survey of the world's literature. The (frequently) neuroleptic (potentially) malignant syndrome. 1987;150:
752–9.

Historic review.

Kellam AMP. The (frequently) neuroleptic (potentially) malignant syndrome. Br J Psychiatry 1990;157:169–73.

Good review of diagnostic problems.

Rohan-Chabot P de. Reconnaitre et traiter une hyperthermie maligne, in Goulon M (ed). Les Urgences. Edisem, St. Hyacinthe, Quebec, Maloine SA, Paris, 1990.

Overview of the various malignant hyperthermias.

Wedel DJ. Malignant hyperthermia and neuromuscular disease. Neuromusc Disord 1992;2:157–64.

Thorough review of malignant hyperthermia with certainly, possibly, and not related neuromuscular conditions.

Heat Stroke

Adnet P. Coup de chaleur, in Viars P (ed). Anesthésie, Réanimation, Urgences. Université Paris VI, Médecins du Monde. Imprimerie Nationale, Paris, 1994.

Concise pathophysiology and therapeutic guidelines.

Henry JA. Ecstasy and the dance of death. BMJ 1992;305: 5–6.

Dancing to heat stroke.

Henry JA, Jeffreys KJ, Dawlings S. Toxicity and death from 3,4-dimethylenedioxymetamphetamine ("ecstasy"). Lancet 1992;340:384–7.

Seven cases with fulminant hyperthermia.

Rohan-Chabot P de. Reconnaitre et traiter une hyperthermie maligne, in Goulon M (ed). Les Urgences. 2nd Ed. Edisem St. Hyacynthe, Quebec, Maloine SA, Paris 1992.

Clear survey of pathogenesis. Clinical features and treatment.

Screaton GR, Cairns HS, Sarner M et al. Hyperpyrexia and rhabdomyolysis after MDMA ("ecstasy") abuse. Lancet 1992;339:677–8.

Three more cases.

Acute Respiratory Failure

Goulon M. Crise myasthénique, in Goulon M (ed). Les Urgences. Edisem, St. Hyacinthe, Quebec, Maloine SA, Paris, 1990, pp. 543–52.

Clear and concise account with good advice.

Hughes RAC, Bihari D. Acute neuromuscular respiratory paralysis. J Neurol Neurosurg Psychiatry 1993;56: 334–43.

Detailed, recent review with a personal experience flavor.

Ropper AH. Neurological and Neurosurgical Intensive Care. 3rd Ed. Raven Press, New York, 1993.

Most facets of neurologic intensive care, with a particularly wide experience on Guillain-Barré syndrome.

Acute Compression of the Spinal Cord

Editorial. Steroids after spinal cord injury. Lancet 1990;336: 279–80.

Review of the pathophysiological primary events in spinal cord injury and of the results of the first and second trials of methylprednisolone in the United States.

Grundy D, Russel J, Swain A (eds). ABC of Spinal Cord Injury. 3rd Ed. British Medical Journal Publishing, London, 1990.

Guidelines for early and late managemrnt.

Johnston RA. The management of acute spinal cord compression. J Neurol Neurosurg Psychiatry 1993;56: 1046–54.

Recent and comprehensive review with experience.

Ogilvy CS, Heros RC. Spinal cord compression. In Ropper AH (ed). Neurological and Neurosurgical Intensive Care. 3rd Ed. Raven Press, New York, 1993.

Detailed review of cervical trauma.

Young W. Medical treatments of acute spinal cord injury (Editorial). J Neurol Neurosurg Psychiatry 1992;55: 635–9.

Review of results with methylprednisolone and comments on then-promising new treatments.

Index

Page numbers followed by f *indicate figures; those followed by* t *indicate tables.*